Advances in Intelligent Systems and Computing

Volume 1018

AF800662

The series "Advances in Intelligent Systems and Computing" contains publications on theory, applications, and design methods of Intelligent Systems and Intelligent Computing. Virtually all disciplines such as engineering, natural sciences, computer and information science, ICT, economics, business, e-commerce, environment, healthcare, life science are covered. The list of topics spans all the areas of modern intelligent systems and computing such as: computational intelligence, soft computing including neural networks, fuzzy systems, evolutionary computing and the fusion of these paradigms, social intelligence, ambient intelligence, computational neuroscience, artificial life, virtual worlds and society, cognitive science and systems, Perception and Vision, DNA and immune based systems, self-organizing and adaptive systems, e-Learning and teaching, human-centered and human-centric computing, recommender systems, intelligent control, robotics and mechatronics including human-machine teaming, knowledge-based paradigms, learning paradigms, machine ethics, intelligent data analysis, knowledge management, intelligent agents, intelligent decision making and support, intelligent network security, trust management, interactive entertainment, Web intelligence and multimedia.

The publications within "Advances in Intelligent Systems and Computing" are primarily proceedings of important conferences, symposia and congresses. They cover significant recent developments in the field, both of a foundational and applicable character. An important characteristic feature of the series is the short publication time and world-wide distribution. This permits a rapid and broad dissemination of research results.

**** Indexing: The books of this series are submitted to ISI Proceedings, EI-Compendex, DBLP, SCOPUS, Google Scholar and Springerlink ****

More information about this series at http://www.springer.com/series/11156

Tareq Ahram · Redha Taiar ·
Serge Colson · Arnaud Choplin
Editors

Human Interaction and Emerging Technologies

Proceedings of the 1st International Conference on Human Interaction and Emerging Technologies (IHIET 2019), August 22–24, 2019, Nice, France

Springer

Editors
Tareq Ahram
Institute for Advanced
Systems Engineering
University of Central Florida
Orlando, FL, USA

Redha Taiar
Université de Reims
Champagne Ardenne, GRESPI
Reims, France

Serge Colson
Laboratoire Motricité Humaine,
Expertise, Sport, Santé
Université Côte d'Azur
Nice Cedex 3, France

Arnaud Choplin
IFMK Niçois
Université Côte d'Azur
Nice Cedex 3, France

ISSN 2194-5357 ISSN 2194-5365 (electronic)
Advances in Intelligent Systems and Computing
ISBN 978-3-030-25628-9 ISBN 978-3-030-25629-6 (eBook)
https://doi.org/10.1007/978-3-030-25629-6

This Springer imprint is published by the registered company Springer Nature Switzerland AG
The registered company address is: Gewerbestrasse 11, 6330 Cham, Switzerland

Preface

This book, entitled *Human Interaction and Emerging Technologies*, aims to provide a global forum for presenting and discussing novel human interaction, emerging technologies and engineering approaches, tools, methodologies, techniques, and solutions for integrating people, concepts, trends, and applications in all areas of human interaction endeavor. Such applications include, but are not limited to, health care and medicine, transportation, optimization and urban planning for infrastructure development, manufacturing, social development, a new generation of service systems, as well as safety, risk assessment, and cybersecurity in both civilian and military contexts. Indeed, rapid progress in developments in cognitive computing, modeling, and simulation, as well as smart sensor technology, will have a profound effect on the principles of human interaction and emerging technologies at both the individual and societal levels in the near future. This interdisciplinary book will also expand the boundaries of the current state of the art by investigating the pervasive complexity that underlies the most profound problems contemporary society is facing today. Emerging technologies included in this book cover a variety of technologies such as educational technology, information technology, nanotechnology, biotechnology, cognitive science, robotics, and artificial intelligence.

The book, which gathers selected papers presented at the 1st International Conference on Human Interaction and Emerging Technologies (IHIET 2019), to be held on August 22–24, 2019, at Université Côte d'Azur, Nice, France, and the 3rd International WAVEX Conference: Physical and Cognitive Research, to be held on August 29–31, 2019, at CHU-Université de Reims Champagne-Ardenne, France, focuses on advancing the theory and applications for human interaction requirements as part of an overall system development life cycle, by adopting a human-centered design approach that utilizes and expands on the current knowledge of user-centered design and systems engineering supported by cognitive software and engineering, data analytics, simulation and modeling, and next-generation visualizations. This book also presents many innovative studies with a particular emphasis on the development of technology throughout the lifecycle development process, including the consideration of user experience in the design of human interfaces for virtual, augmented, and mixed reality applications.

Reflecting on the above-outlined perspective, the papers contained in this volume are organized into nine sections, including:

Section 1: Human-centered Design
Section 2: Computation and Intelligent Design
Section 3: Augmented, Virtual and Mixed Reality Simulation
Section 4: Wearable Technologies, Social and Affective Computing
Section 5: Human–computer Interaction
Section 6: Medicine, Biomechanics, Sports and Healthcare
Section 7: WAVEX: Physical and Cognitive Research
Section 8: Human-Technology and Future of Work
Section 9: Emerging Technologies and Business Applications

We would like to extend our sincere thanks to the IFMK Niçois and Université Côte d'Azur for their kind support. Our appreciation also goes to the members of the Scientific Program Advisory Board who have reviewed the accepted papers that are presented in this volume.

We hope that this book, which presents the current state of the art in human interaction and emerging technologies, will be a valuable source of both theoretical and applied knowledge enabling the human-centered design and applications of a variety of products, services, and systems for their safe, effective, and pleasurable use by people around the world.

August 2019

Tareq Ahram
Redha Taiar
Serge Colson
Arnaud Choplin

Contents

Human-Centered Design

Social Robots: Development and Evaluation of a Human-Centered Application Scenario

Kaspar Kaufmann(✉), Eleni Ziakas, Marco Catanzariti, Giancarlo Stoppa, Roger Burkhard, Hartmut Schulze, and Alexandra Tanner

School of Applied Psychology, University of Applied Sciences and Arts Northwestern Switzerland, Riggenbachstrasse 16, 4600 Olten, Switzerland
kaspar.kaufmann, eleni.ziakas, marco.catanzariti, giancarlo.stoppa, roger.burkhard, hartmut.schulze, alexandra.tanner@fhnw.ch

Abstract. This study aimed to develop and evaluate an application scenario for the use of a social robot, following a human-centered design approach. The social robot, which assisted the reception desk staff of a hotel by answering simple, repetitive and time-consuming questions (e.g. parking information, directions), was perceived predominantly positive by employees and guests of the hotel. However, the results suggested that to effectively reduce the employees' workload and to provide a reliable source of information for the guest, the robot had to work on a high level of autonomy and technological stability. Additionally, the use of a social robot may estrange guests and employees alike, as they prefer human interaction or are fearful of job loss, respectively. An early inclusion of the employees in the design process has shown to reduce fears and increase acceptance towards the social robot and its integration into the workforce.

Keywords: Human-centered design · Social robot · NAO · Hotel · Human-robot interaction

1 Introduction

Social robots are being introduced in various fields such as healthcare, education and public spaces as artificial companions and helpers [1]. Social robots can express and perceive emotions and conduct sophisticated dialogues with human interaction partners [2]. While research interest has increased in recent years [3] and several studies investigated the use of social robots in hotels [4–6], the focus has been limited mainly to technical aspects. Further studies in the real-world context of hotels are widely seen as a prerequisite in order to gain in-depth knowledge about the productive use of a robot in a hotel [4]. Various works show that a user-centered design of human-robotics interaction covering user needs in the service area remain a challenge [5–8]. This refers to the development of suitable application contexts and use cases, and to the technical restrictions that render applications difficult to implement beyond entertainment functionalities [7, 8]. In a case study in Switzerland, several social robot deployments

T. Ahram et al. (Eds.): IHIET 2019, AISC 1018, pp. 3–9, 2020.
https://doi.org/10.1007/978-3-030-25629-6_1

were investigated; the study showed that the robots are valuable in attracting attention, but do not generate any meaningful benefit or reduce the effort for the staff in terms of support [7]. Another example of limited deployment is the Henn na robot hotel in Japan, which gained a lot of media attention after it recently had to cut more than half of their robot workforce and replace them by returning to traditional human-provided services [9]. The robots in the Henn na hotel could neither reduce the workload for their human counterparts nor reduce costs. Another recent study with 393 respondents in five different hotels warned of possible resistance by employees when introducing a robot into the workforce [10].

On this basis, a case study was conducted in a Swiss hotel which aimed to answer three research questions applying a human-centered design (HCD) [11] approach:

- Which area of the hotel offers a high potential for the use of a social robot?
- Which application scenario with a social robot offers an added value for employees and guests in the hotel?
- Can early involvement of staff in the human-centered design process reduce concerns about social robots from an employee perspective?

2 Methodology

2.1 Context of Use Analysis

In the initial context of use analysis five semi-structured interviews [12] were conducted with management and entry-level employees. The focus was laid on identifying use cases of social robot employment, and chances and risks regarding the use in the hotel. The employees were asked about their attitude towards robots and their willingness to work with a robot. In the interviews the reception was identified as a suitable location for the application of a social robot. Subsequently, four observations [12] were carried out by using a standardized observation sheet. Particular attention was paid to employee work processes, which could potentially be standardized and carried out by a social robot to support the staff.

2.2 Specification of User Requirements and Development of Application Scenario

With the help of the data obtained in the context of use analysis, nine user requirements were specified bottom-up. An application scenario was developed, in which a social robot would support the employees by answering simple and repetitive questions (e.g. directions, parking information) asked by guests of the hotel. In addition, the robot would be able to perform a number of entertainment tasks (e.g. telling jokes). The programming of the robot NAO (version 6) by SoftBank Robotics was a continuous process that took place iteratively over several phases of the human-centered design process. Speech, movement, gestures and visual expressions were developed with the software Choreographe provided by SoftBank Robotics.

2.3 Evaluation of Application Scenario

The developed application scenario and the programmed robot were first evaluated with employees (n = 6) in a workshop, where they had the opportunity to be acquainted with the robot and the scenario, and give feedback. Second, the application scenario was evaluated along six days in the hotel under natural conditions. In order to facilitate the interaction a poster with guiding questions was placed behind the robot. The robot was positioned next to the reception approximately at guest eye level. Throughout the evaluation, two members of the study team were present to help with technical problems and answer staff or guest questions. The guests interacting with the robot were observed and subsequently interviewed [12]. The observation was carried out with a standardized observation sheet and focused on the interaction quality. In the interview, the guests were asked how they experienced the interaction. Additionally, two self-designed questionnaire items on the usage potential of the robot were asked.

During the evaluation, a semi-standardized interview [12] was conducted with the reception employees in a weekly interval. The receptionists were asked about how they perceived the guests' interactions and how they felt about having the robot as a team member.

2.4 Process Evaluation with Employees

In a final process evaluation, a group interview [12] was conducted with three employees of the reception, in which fears and expectations raised at the beginning of the study and possible changes were addressed. Furthermore, the use of a social robot in the hotel context and the employees' involvement in the entire HCD process was reflected. Finally, the receptionists were asked about the robots usage potential at the reception.

3 Results

The context of use analysis showed that the reception is particularly suitable for the use of a social robot in a hotel. The robot can relieve the reception staff by answering repetitive, simple yet time-consuming questions. The reception is also ideal to leave a lasting impression on the guests through the presence of a robot, the application of which is still novel in the hotel industry. The use of a social robot was not only seen as a potential relief for the employees and a possible added economic value, but also as a possibility to entertain and delight the guests. Other areas of the hotel (e.g. restaurant, room cleaning) were excluded from the study because of technical limitations of the robot or lack of interaction possibilities. The interviewees saw risks and uncertainty of jeopardizing the existing highly positive guest-reception relationship, which could lead to guest abandonment; such a relationship should be preserved when introducing the robot. Furthermore, no additional work should be generated for the employees and the data privacy may not be compromised at any time. The most prominent fear in management interviews was the employees' acceptance of the robot. The reception staff emphasized that they see little added value in the use of a social robot and that the risks listed above outweigh the potential added value. Fear of job loss was also mentioned in isolated cases.

In the development of the resulting application scenario, the emphasis was placed on ensuring that the natural course of interaction between guests and employees remained intact. The employees therefore should direct the guests to the robot if it can answer the questions. An overview about the setting can be seen in Fig. 1.

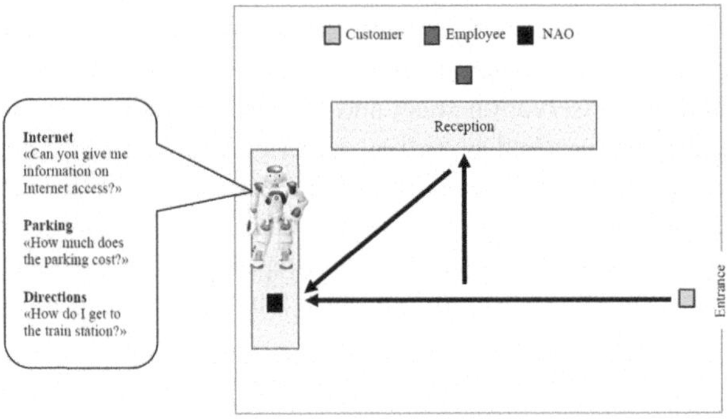

Fig. 1. Layout of reception area with positions of involved actors and guest paths.

In the evaluation of the application scenario and the robot, the employees responded positively. The reluctance and the skepticism towards the use of the robot could be visibly reduced by role-playing and interacting with the robot without restrictions.

During the evaluation of the application scenario in the hotel, a total of 37 people who interacted with the robot were interviewed. These interviews were conducted with 20 men (54%) and 17 women (46%). Of the sample, 27 persons (73%) were on their own and 10 (27%) in a group of two or more. When asked whether they would use the robot again in its current state, seven people (19%) responded "No", six (16%) "More likely No", 10 (27%) "More likely Yes", and 14 (38%) "Yes". When asked if they would use a future improved version of the robot, five people (13%) responded "No," with several people saying that they generally prefer contact with people. One (3%) responded "More likely No," one (3%) "Maybe," seven (19%) "More likely Yes," and 23 (38%) "Yes".

The guests felt predominantly positive about the interaction, with occasional negative statements such as "I'm just talking to a robot to see how ridiculous and stupid this is". When asked what they wished for future interactions, aspects of further conversational flexibility, autonomy, and functionality were most frequently mentioned (24 mentions). For example, the guests desired more leeway in the questions that the robot could be asked, as well as the answers it could give. Furthermore, according to various guest statements, the robot should be able to take on more tasks, in both the reception and other areas of the hotel, however specific activities were rarely mentioned. Almost the same number of requests for improvement were made about the individual language (14 mentions) and speech recognition (13 mentions). According to many guests, it would be advantageous if the robot could speak more languages than just German, the language used in this study. The guests also demanded more proactivity by the robot (6 mentions) when approaching it (e.g. the robot recognizing the guest and greeting the person by name).

From the weekly interviews and the group interview with the reception staff, it can be concluded that the majority of them observed enjoyment and satisfaction among the guests when interacting with the robot. The question of whether the receptionists could imagine the robot as a member of the team at this time did not lead to a conclusive result. On the one hand, the robot was attributed to a certain entertainment value for the receptionists themselves as well as the guests. On the other hand, they only saw limited added value in the answering of routine questions, since difficulties in speech recognition and thus interaction difficulties arose multiple times. Regarding their attitude towards the robot, the reception staff noted that their initially prevailing fears were gradually diminished by active participation in the process and finally completely dissolved. In the beginning, the receptionists were overwhelmed by the idea of a robot in their workplace. This, however, changed when they got to know it during the scenario evaluation. Especially the robots' appearance, which was positively perceived as cute or adorable, was mentioned in this context. In conclusion, all receptionists were of the opinion that they would accept the robot as a team member despite its technical deficiencies, which they regretted, because it did not offer them enough added value in their daily business on top of the other.

4 Discussion and Conclusion

As mentioned in the introduction, previous studies have shown that a challenge is to find an economic benefit of social service robots in a hotel that goes beyond the pure entertainment factor [4]. In this study, the reception area proved to be a suitable area for future use of social robots in hotel operations, since repetitive work processes could be taken over by social robots. This would free employees from monotonous tasks and save time for guests if long waiting times occur at the reception [13]. While employees and guests acknowledged the positive potential of the social robot in this study, it could not be proven that economically relevant effects such as shortened waiting times actually occurred by letting the robot answer recurring guest questions.

Apart from the potential economic benefit, this study also showed by interviewing both employees and guests that the entertainment factor can be a significant reason for the introduction of a robot in the reception area, because compared to other information providers its attractive nature enables a positive interaction [13]. The entertainment factor for guests and employees may also have been so prominent because the robot stood in an exposed position near the reception desk. This was the first point of contact, thereby leaving a lasting impression, which is decisive for a positive customer experience [14]. However, in order to be able to exploit the aforementioned usage potential, the technical restrictions have to be solved.

Robots can nevertheless make us feel uncomfortable, especially if a robot is introduced without involving the human factor [8, 9]. The use of social robots can alienate guests and employees alike, as they prefer human interaction and are afraid of losing their jobs. The results have shown that the early involvement of employees in the design process leads to a reduction of fears and increases acceptance of the social robot and its use. This was achieved by applying the HCD approach. The continuous involvement of the employees led to a more realistic classification of the robot and its capabilities. A further factor for the increased acceptance is the robot's appearance, especially its face, which was assessed positively as cute or sweet. The positive evaluation of the robot as cute is related to theories that say that humans tend to recognize human traits in robots [15]. Whether the appearance of a robot and its way of interacting has an influence on the acceptance by employees must be investigated in more detail in further studies.

This case study shows the value of applying human-centered design in the field of social robots and that the hotel's employees constitute the necessary link between guests and the robot for its successful application in working environments. Only by empowering the employees in the process of the robot's implementation in the hotel can their fears concerning job security be reduced, which, eventually, increases their willingness to support the guest-robot interaction in the hotel, in spite of its technical restrictions. Finally, the acceptance of a robot by employees and guests can be a prerequisite for a successful human-robot interaction that can compensate for its current technical limitations.

References

1. Broadbent, E.: Interaction with robots: the truths we reveal about ourselves. Annu. Rev. Psychol. **68**, 627–652 (2003)
2. Fong, T., Nourbakhsh, I., Dautenhahn, K.: A survey of socially interactive robots. Robot. Auton. Syst. **42**, 143–166 (2003)
3. Bensch, S., Jevtić, A., Jevtić, A., Hellström, T.: On interaction quality in human-robot interaction. In: 9th International Conference on Agents and Artificial Intelligence, pp. 182–189. Scitepress, Setúbal (2007)
4. Zalama, E., García-Bermejo, J.G., Marcos, S., Domínguez, S., Feliz, R., Pinillos, R., López, J.: Sacarino, a service robot in a hotel environment. In: Armada, M.A., Sanfeliu, A., Ferre, M. (eds.) ROBOT 2013. AISC, vol. 253, pp. 3–14. Springer, Cham (2014)
5. Pinillos, R., Marcos, S., Feliz, R., Zalama, E., Gómez-García-Bermejo, J.: Long-term assessment of a service robot in a hotel environment. Robot. Auton. Syst. **79**, 40–57 (2016)
6. Tussyadiah, I.P., Park, S.: Consumer evaluation of hotel service robots. In: Stangl, B., Pesonen, J. (eds.) Information and Communication Technologies in Tourism 2018, pp. 308–320, Cham (2018)
7. Tanner, A., Schulze, H., Burkhard, R.: Soziale Roboter - Erfolgsfaktoren für die Umsetzung ihrer Potenziale. Ergebnisse einer Fallstudie in der Schweiz. In: 65. Frühjahrskongress der Gesellschaft für Arbeitswissenschaft (GfA) (2019)
8. Willis, M.: Human centered robotics: designing valuable experiences for social robots. Proceedings of HRI2018 Workshop (Social Robots in the Wild). ACM, New York (2018)

9. The Wall Street Journal. https://www.wsj.com/articles/robot-hotel-loses-love-for-robots-11547484628
10. Ivanov, S.H., Webster, C., Berezina, K.: Adoption of Robots and Service Automation by Tourism and Hospitality Companies: Revista Turismo & Desenvolvimento **27**(28), 1501–1517 (2017)
11. ISO 9241-210 Ergonomics of human-system interaction – Part 210: human-centred design for interactive systems (2010)
12. Flick, U.: An introduction to qualitative research. Sage, Los Angeles (2009)
13. Pan, Y., Okada, H., Uchiyama, T.: Listening to vs overhearing robots in a hotel public space. In: 8th ACM/IEEE International Conference on Human-Robot, Interaction, pp. 205–206. IEEE Press, Tokyo (2013)
14. Bruhn, M.: Servicequalität: Konzepte und Instrumente für eine perfekte Dienstleistung. Deutscher Taschenbuchverlag, München (2013)
15. Mori, M., MacDorman, K.F., Kageki, N.: The Uncanny Valley. IEEE Robotics & Automation Magazine 19, 98–100 (2012)

Addressing Accountability in Highly Autonomous Virtual Assistants

Fernando Galdon[1(✉)] and Stephen Jia Wang[2]

[1] Department of Global Innovation Design, School of Design, Royal College of Art, London, UK
fernando.galdon@network.rca.ac.uk
[2] Department of Innovation Design Engineering, School of Design, Royal College of Art, London, UK

Abstract. Building from a survey specifically developed to address the rising concerns of highly autonomous virtual assistants; this paper presents a multi-level taxonomy of accountability levels specifically adapted to virtual assistants in the context of Human-Human-Interaction (HHI). Based on research findings, the authors recommend the integration of the variable of accountability as capital in the development of future applications around highly automated systems. This element inserts a sense of balance in terms of integrity between users and developers enhancing trust in the interactive process. Ongoing work is being dedicated to further understand to which extent different contexts affect accountability in virtual assistants.

Keywords: Human factors · Human-systems integration · Systems engineering · Trust · Virtual assistant · Highly automated systems · Autonomy · Automation · Accountability

1 Introduction

With the rise of highly autonomous systems concerns in the field of human factors are focusing on designing appropriate tools to address this new class of technology [1]. Recent investigations, such as MIT's research paper on who should kill a self-driving car, are pointing to ethical decision making in the context of highly autonomous systems (HAS) [2]. Furthermore, due to its persuasive capabilities, concerns are also rising in the area of virtual assistants (VA) with the introduction of Duplex and Alexa by Google and Amazon. In this context, Amazon has recently filed a patent to transform its systems into a doctor diagnosing and providing treatment in the process [3]. Further innovations are transforming the VA into legal or financial advisers, set up romantic dates and provide jobs. They will engage with us, and by combining and inferring preliminary knowledge and in situ interaction they will have the potential and capability to change our preliminary decisions and take actions on our behalf on highly sensitive areas such as health and wellbeing, identity, social interactions or economically related activities. However, one fundamental question remains, if something goes wrong, who should be accountable for the action?

As we are moving into a machine-human paradigm questions of accountability remain unsolved. This fact positions highly autonomous systems at the centre and

T. Ahram et al. (Eds.): IHIET 2019, AISC 1018, pp. 10–14, 2020.
https://doi.org/10.1007/978-3-030-25629-6_2

re- search must try to address the implications of trust from their perspective [4]. Traditionally, accountability in complex autonomous virtual assistants has been out of research due to the automated nature of the interactions. They were based on one-off query focused on non-dangerous outcomes such as playing songs. Nowadays, as systems become more autonomous and unsupervised, the potential outcomes of these interventions are probing capital for the successful development and implementation of these systems in society. Humans, therefore, must be considered as a key component in even a fully automated system [5], and implement a human-centred approach to tackle this challenge [6].

Recent research in the area of robustness in HAS shows 0% adversarial accuracy when evaluating a deep network against stronger adversaries [7, 8]. In order to address this problem they are using interval bound propagation [9, 10, 11] to great success. However, as the researcher acknowledge "no amount of testing can formally guarantee that a system will behave as we want. In large-scale models, enumerating all possible outputs for a given set of inputs…is intractable due to the astronomical number of choices for the input perturbation" [12].

In the context of unsupervised HAS constantly evolving we must change our approach. Instead of talking about transparency we have to start talking about trust and accountability as an a priori and a posteriori elements to address. Although I agree that preventive strategies must be seen as the preferred area of intervention, systems of accountability must be put in place to address errors and failures in the system.

In this paper the authors minds the warning and propose a human-centred approach aimed at ensuring that these highly automated interactions remain focused on the user's interests and protection.

2 Method

Research into the area of automation present levels as a tool to address trust in automated systems. In this context gradient-base models of approximation has been embodied through the concept of scales or Level of trust (LoT). This approach of different levels of automation has been persistent in the automation literature since its introduction by Sheridan and Verplanck [13]. Kaber [14] emphasises that levels of automation (LoA) is a fundamental design characteristic that determines the ability of operators to provide effective oversight and interaction with system autonomy. According to Endsley [15], although they represent a simplification of reality, they provide a tool. This method has proven successful in providing a solid foundation to understand HAI at a deeper level. This is highly relevant when confronting an invisible entity making decisions while working in the background.

Levels aim to improve transparency by simplifying interactions. In this context, transparency refers to the extent to which the actions of the automation are understandable and predictable [15]. According to research in the area, automated systems which clarify their reasoning are more likely to be trusted [16, 17, 18].

In this context, a multi-level taxonomy of levels of accountability specifically designed to address the increasing autonomy of highly automated virtual assistants was designed by the authors. It integrated a gradient spectrum of levels ranging from the system to the user. It was structures in four distinctive levels; the platform hosting all the interactions (Level 1), the developer/designer designing the actions/skills algorithms (Level 2), due to its unsupervised and evolutive nature I decided to include the algorithm performing the action (Level 3), and finally, the user (Level 4) (Table 1).

Table 1. Proposed levels of accountability.

Levels	Subject	Explanation
Level 1	Platform	*The company who owns the platform*
Level 2	Developer	*The designer who designed the action*
Level 3	Algorithm	*The algorithm performing the action*
Level 4	User	*The user performing the action*

3 Discussion

Due to the highly contextual nature of virtual assistants, a co-design workshop with students from the Royal College of Art underpinned four highly sensitives areas where highly automated VAs may impact significantly users; health and wellbeing, identity, economically related activities and social interactions.

From the areas aforementioned and based on demos, patents and prototypes, eight case studies were built to address different outcomes. Two cases addressed each sensitive area ranging from low to high impact. Then, a survey was designed to establish whether the proposed levels of accountability in highly automated virtual assistants were sufficient to address all the cases.

To test the scale, the main technique consisted on integrating an *other* tab in each case. This space allowed the participant to propose a new level or area missing, questioning the existing scale in the process. Participants engaged with the *other* tab though the survey at different points.

50 participant, 21 men, 27 women and 2 who didn't want to identify themselves, from 14 different countries with an age range between 18–67 years old from different professions have undertaken the survey (Table 2).

Table 2. Survey results.

	Unhappy service medicine	Unhappy service newspaper	Ends in violence addiction	Ends in violence raped	Wrong prediction sexuality	Wrong prediction jailed	Loses money	Loses job	Total
Level 1 Platform	20%	26%	12%	6%	14%	22%	18%	8%	15.75%
Level 2 Designer	18%	**28%**	18%	14%	22%	24%	32%	8%	20.50%
Level 3 Algorithm	16%	20%	8%	6%	**38%**	**30%**	16%	8%	17.75%
Level 4 User	**38%**	24%	**56%**	**38%**	24%	22%	**34%**	**74%**	38.75%
Other	8%	2%	6%	36%	2%	2%	0%	2%	7.25%

In average, 38, 75% of participants found that the user is the main element accountable for unexpected consequences. This result was highly unexpected as in all cases the VA was initiating and doing actions on behalf of the user. The designer/developer is placed second with 20.50% of participants pointing them as accountable. Third position is for the algorithm with 17.75%. Finally, the platform would be the least accountable level with 15.75% of the participants. Other elements (third-parties) add the other 7.25%.

4 Conclusion

The survey aimed to understand whether or not contexts and actions affected the level of accountability. In the main area of levels of accountability, contexts and actions play a role in determining which level of accountability is needed. In addition, they did play a role in determining the spectrum. These elements demanded the integration of a third-party level in the scale. However, at the same time, a generic granular scale of 5 levels covering from platform to user and integrating third-parties is capable of addressing different contexts and actions in highly automated virtual assistants.

Finally, if we combine Level 1 (platform), 2 (designer), and 3 (algorithm) 54% of participants place accountability in the system's side. Therefore, inserting the accountability variable in the design process is capital for the correct integration of Highly Automated Systems in society, as this element inserts a sense of balance in terms of integrity between users and developers enhancing trust in the interactive process (Table 3).

Table 3. Final levels of accountability.

Levels	Subject	Explanation
Level 1	Platform	*The company who owns the platform*
Level 2	Developer	*The designer who designed the action*
Level 3	Algorithm	*The algorithm performing the action*
Level 4	Third party	*A third party affecting the service*
Level 5	User	*The user performing the action*

References

1. Hancock, P.A.: Imposing limits on autonomous systems. Ergonomics **60**(2), 284–291 (2017)
2. Awad, E., Dsouza, S., Kim, R., Schulz, J., Henrich, J., Shariff, A., Bonnefon, J.F., Rahwan, I.: The moral machine experiment. Nature (2018). https://doi.org/10.1038/s41586-018-0637-6
3. Jin, H., Wang, S.: Voice-based determination of physical and emotional characteristics of user (2018). http://patft.uspto.gov/netacgi/nph-Parser?Sect1=PTO2&Sect2=HITOFF&u=%2Fnetahtml%2FPTO%2Fsearch-adv.htm&r=1&p=1&f=G&l=50&d=PTXT&S1=10,096,319&OS=10,096,319&RS=10,096,319

4. Ortega, B.P.A., Maini, V.: Building safe artificial intelligence: specification, robustness, and assurance specification: de ne the purpose of the system. Medium. Retrieved from https://medium.com/@deepmindsafetyresearch/building-safe-artificial-intelligence-52f5f75058f (2018)
5. Wang, S.J.: Fields interaction design (FID): the answer to ubiquitous computing supported environments in the post-information age. Homa & Sekey Books (2013)
6. Wang, S.J., Moriarty, P.: Big Data for Urban Sustainability. Springer (2018)
7. Athalye, A., Carlini, N., Wagner, D.: Obfuscated gradients give a false sense of security: circumventing defenses to adversarial examples. Proceedings of the 35th International Conference on Machine Learning. Stockholm, Sweden, PMLR 80 (2018)
8. Uesato, J., O'Donoghue, B., van den Oord, A., Kohli, P.: Adversarial risk and the dangers of evaluating against weak attacks. Proceedings of the 35th International Conference on Machine Learning. Stockholm, Sweden, PMLR 80 (2018)
9. Ehlers, R.: Formal verification of piece-wise linear feed-forward neural networks. BT - Automated Technology for Verification and Analysis - 15th International Symposium, ATVA 2017, Pune, India, October 3–6, 2017, Proceedings (2017)
10. Katz, G., Barrett, C.W., Dill, D.L., Julian, K., Kochenderfer, M.J.: Reluplex: an efficient SMT solver for verifying deep neural networks. BT - Computer Aided Verification - 29th International Conference, CAV 2017, Heidelberg, Germany, July 24–28, 2017, Proceedings, Part I (2017)
11. Mirman, M., Gehr, T., Vechev, M.: Differentiable abstract interpretation for provably robust neural networks. Proceedings of the 35th International Conference on Machine Learning, in PMLR 80, pp. 3578–3586 (2018)
12. Kohli, P., Gowal, S., Dvijotham, K., Uesato, J.: Towards robust and verified AI: specification testing, robust training, and formal verification. Deepmind. Medium 28 March 2019. https://deepmind.com/blog/robust-and-verified-ai/ (2019). Accessed 29 Mar 2019
13. Sheridan, T.B., Verplank, W.L.: Human and computer control of Undersea teleoperators: Fort Belvoir, VA: Defense Technical Information Center (1978). https://doi.org/10.21236/ADA057655
14. Kaber, D.B.: Issues in human-automation interaction modeling: presumptive aspects of frameworks of types and levels of automation. J. Cogn. Eng. Decis. Making **12**(1), 7–24 (2018). https://doi.org/10.1177/1555343417737203
15. Endsley, M.R.: From here to autonomy: lessons learned from human–automation research. Hum. Factors: The J. Hum. Factors Ergon. Soc. **59**, 5–27 (2017). https://doi.org/10.1177/0018720816681350
16. Simpson, A., Brander, G.N., Portsdown, D.R.A.: Seaworthy trust: confidence in automated data fusion. In: Taylor, R.M., Reising, J. (eds.) The Human-Electronic Crew: Can We Trust the Team, pp, 77–81. Hampshire, UK: Defence Research Academy. Retrieved from http://www.dtic.mil/dtic/tr/fulltext/u2/a308589.pdf (1995)
17. Hoff, K.A., Bashir, M.: Trust in automation: integrating empirical evidence on factors that influence trust. Hum. Factors: The J. Hum. Factors Ergon. Soc. **57**, 407–434 (2015)
18. Galdon, F., Wang, S.J.: Designing trust in highly automated virtual assistants: a taxonomy of levels of autonomy. International Conference on Industry 4.0 and Artificial Intelligence Technologies. Cambridge, UK. ISBN: 978-1-912532-07-0 (2019)

From Aggregation to Navigation: Large Image Collections Seeking and Exploration

Ole Goethe(✉)

Kristiania University, Oslo, Norway
ole.goethe@kristiania.no

Abstract. In this paper, we evaluate managing huge sets of visual content as we know handling large image collections has always been a challenge for technologists. With the rise of various social media platforms that aggregate a vast amount visual data it causes new implications not only for the computer scientists but also for curators, designers, social scientists, statisticians and end users: how to navigate the data efficiently, access to new levels of exploration and visualize the content without too many details being lost. With more and more such platforms, the bigger this challenge is going to get. In 22 semi structured surveys in Oslo (Norway), we find that a set of factors intermix to inform perceptions about large image collections - including how often they look-over large image collections.

Keywords: Human factors · Aggregation · Design · Exploration · Navigation · Performance · Visualization

1 Introduction

Exploring large image sets can lead to valuable insight despite that research shows that an average human can perceive only 20 to 50 unsorted images at a time, and can easily lose the track if the number exceeds [1]. Through the previous work that has been done regarding content-based image retrieval, the exploratory image browsing is still in its infancy stage in terms of research. In order to support millions of images and more, given the high dimensionality of the image space, the challenge is in creating a cohesive grid that preserves the relations among all images.

2 Related Work

To address these needs, some research systems focus on supporting various browsing capabilities to enable navigating through images [2]. For example, browsing specific clusters of images [3], browsing hierarchies that are automatically built according to visual and semantic similarities [4–6], or browsing along conceptual dimensions according to hierarchical faceted metadata [7], or use techniques like self-organizing image maps to generate visually sorted arrangements of search results. The short-coming of these approaches is also evident. Though these approaches provided an overview, their interface was all based on not regularly positioned images and

T. Ahram et al. (Eds.): IHIET 2019, AISC 1018, pp. 15–20, 2020.
https://doi.org/10.1007/978-3-030-25629-6_3

overlapping images [8]. In most of the previous works we studied, we infer that just a few images of the entire image sets were displayed and the users were unable to determine the relationships with other images.

While text-based directed search can be effective for image search, studies have shown that image search is often more exploratory in nature than text search, and that browsing is an essential strategy when looking for images [9–11].

Unlike text search, the content of an image can be grasped at a glance, and a large number of images can be presented to a user at once. In image search, often the user does not have an exact target in mind [12]. Furthermore, images often lack textual cues and might have many different meanings embedded in a single image [13], making them difficult to support with only text-based search.

Finally, much of work done on image retrieval focuses on the back end of the search in image indexing and content-based image retrieval [14]. However, in our study, we tend to focus on an image browsing user interface, the user experience side and reviews the two different systems that support image browsing. We then took the feedback of the survey participants to determine their perceptions regarding our chosen platforms that they used for their image browsing.

3 Study

We performed a survey with students in Oslo with the goal of capturing initial perceptions of exploring and navigating large image collections.

Motivation. To create a basis for discussion, we designed a photo sharing application called Picturemarks with a zoom/pan based 2d image map that can aggregate and navigate a plethora of images and compared it to a well-known animated GIF platform named Giphy that use a more conventional scroll-based navigation to browse and search (Fig. 2) images. These two representations were chosen to evaluate a small set of features, including navigation, exploration, and source (Table 1). For the context of this study, we define source as the search-word in which the image collection was discovered. Each image collection was presented to participants in a browser on a desktop computer.

Table 1. When interpreting frequencies, the participants were asked to comment on the use of the Picturemarks application

#	Website	Type	Found on (source)	Perceptions (code frequency)
A	Picturemarks	2d-mage map	picturemarks.com	Easier analysis of images (2), More chances of exploration (4), A faster way to get an overview (5), Higher visibility of all your images (5), All of the above (1), Other (5)
B	Giphy	Scroll-based	giphy.com	

Participants. We recruited 22 participants (11 females), aged 20–39, from our local university community. The participants came from different academic programs including film and media, technology, marketing and innovation, and design and communication.

For each participant, we collected their age, gender, how often they look at large image collections ("never" (1) to "often" (7)), and the extent to which a 2d-image map based versus a scroll-based navigation has any advantages with an option to add custom rationale (see Fig. 1).

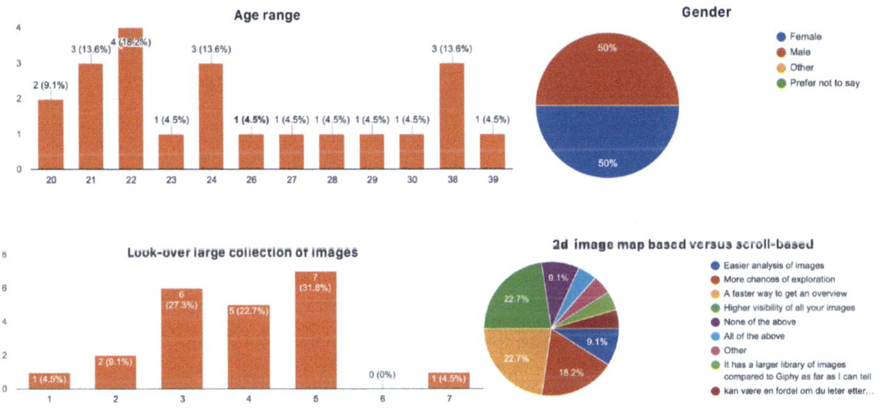

Fig. 1. Demographics and engagement with large image collections of the students we surveyed. Our participants represented educational backgrounds and young adults in the creative field

Procedure. We followed a semi-structured hallway testing process that varied depending on participant situation. Below, we give an overview of the survey structure, as well as the number of participants that were asked each question.

1. Introduction and consent

2. Sources are revealed: The sources of the photo sharing platforms were revealed in an email (Table 1). The researcher provided a brief background of the exemplified keywords (e.g. "Disney", "Barack Obama", "Beyonce", "Ronaldo"). After the sources where revealed, participants were not asked which one they choose, as well as their rationale.

3. Large image sets presentation. Participants were given as much time as needed to consider them before responding to the following prompt: "How often do you look through a large collection of images?". The framing of this prompt is critical and can guide participants in a number of directions.

4 Analysis

The goal of our study is to compare the usefulness of the 2d-image map-based navigation for supporting large image collection information seeking and exploration during users' every day browsing interactions.

Easy to Get Lost in the Large Image Collection? In our motivation, we presented two photo sharing applications (A and B) - both of which were identical in the content. Perceptions of large image collections between the two applications were diverse, with some participants gained a better overview (coded 6 times) or liked the interface (4), found it to be engaging (5) representations of data and others believing them to be confusing (7) or cluttered (7).

"There is too much. I don't understand it. I get distracted by it. It's hard to structure the information in my mind." - P6, 30 years old, male

"I'm not sure how I'm supposed to navigate. There is simply too much information." - P3, 26 years old, female

"Too much information. Would much rather scroll through, than see everything at once." - P18, 28 years old, female

"The format seems messy. Unlike similar platforms it's harder to tell exactly where I am, what I'm looking for or if I've already seen an image before." – P8, 21 years old, male

However, the notion gaining a better way to get an overview manifested itself in perceptions of these websites. When participants commented about how the exploration of a large collection of images influence your decision, we found at 16 instances in which said yes:

"It's easier to get an overview." - P1, 38 years old, female

"Easier interface and you can see more pictures." - P4, 38 years old, male

"Good overview, but a lot of images to process." - P7, 27 years old, female

"I think I would use this because I will be able to see almost all of the pics that have been made" - P12, 20 years old, female

"I can skim through a lot of information in a short amount of time." – P9, 22 years female

"I like the layout, and I can see a lot of gifs at the same time. But It could be too much, when I found the zoom in feature it got a lot easier, it was refreshing that all the pics were shown despite their popularity." – P15, 21 years old, male

These perceptions held for large image collections with any indications of more visibility, overview and exploration.

"Slightly messy / disturbing and cluttered. You could see more pictures at the same time, but they were too small, but fun to place the cursor over the pictures. One could also choose to tap one image and continue." – P10, 22 years old, female

"A fun way of showing thoughts and emotions." – P11, 24 years old, male

"Due to large collection that can be displayed without navigating to other pages too much, this platform it's kinda great." – P19, 20 years old, male

While trends with larger image collections may more accurately be centered searching a particular image, our participants' focus on their navigation design implications for more effective support of exploratory image browsing (and perhaps more broadly).

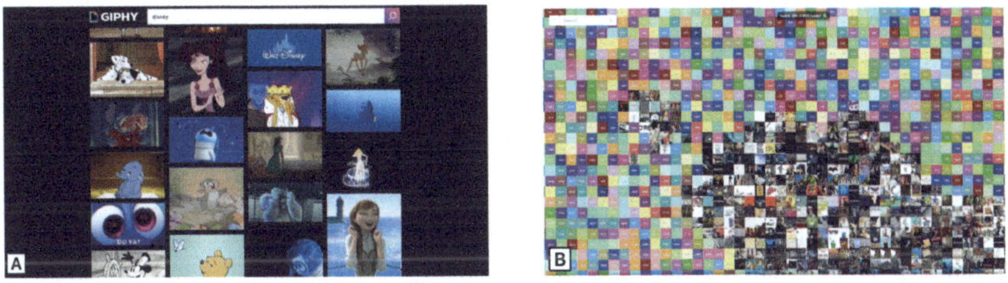

Fig. 2. The websites shown to participants. The image collection was presented in a browser on a desktop computer

Large Image Collections: Clarity and Exploration. To navigate large image sets have been a growing challenge for human perception aligning with previous analyses of searching for particular images in very large, untagged image collections [15], and our surveys were no exception.

As the codes in Table 1 reveal, participants who had positive feelings about the 2d-image map-based website (second image in Fig. 2) found it to be explorative (4), furthering the overview (5), and give a higher visibility of the image sets (5), or all of the above (1). However, participants that had other types of perceptions of the 2d-image map were more diverse in their rationales, saying that "it can be god if you are looking for a specific picture" (1), easier form of analysis (2) or one participant assumed the platform had a larger library of images (1). Those participants that were more critical said none of the above (2), or other (1).

5 Discussion

Our survey aimed to determine the perceptions on browsing large image collections using two different key sources; Picturemarks and Giphy, both of which are based on an image exploration interface. More often than not, studies of this nature often leave us with more questions than answers.

People that were using Picturemarks, found it a useful tool to have quick image overview and more chances of exploration. Other people tended to value the easy user interface. One participant even suggested that the platform could evoke thoughts and emotions.

On other hand, we also ended up with some negative perceptions as well. As we know the average human perceptions have limitations when presented huge sets of images, which reflected our expectations that some participants articulated clutter and confusion. This could be attributed to the small previews which distracts those users who lose direction when presented with a huge amount of visual information.

Broader Engagement. This paper aims to improve and support interaction design practice for people that are seeking for simple and easy to use interface for exploring large image collections based on their specific objectives. We believe that our research will help redefine the design of the future image retrieval, exploration and navigation platforms that primarily focuses user interface, access to large image sets and quick analysis for enhanced user engagement.

References

1. Barthel, K., Hezel, N.: Graph navigation for exploring very large image collections. In: Proceedings of the 12th International Joint Conference on Computer Vision, Imaging and Computer Graphics Theory and Applications, pp. 411–416 (2017)
2. Heesch, D.: A survey of browsing models for content-based image retrieval. Multimedia Tools and Appl. Arch. **40**(2), 261–284, November (2008)
3. Pečenovic, Z., Do, M.N., Vetterli, M., Pu, P.: Integrated browsing and searching of large image collections, pp. 279–289. In Advances in Visual Information Systems. Springer, Berlin Heidelberg (2000)
4. Jing, Y., et al.: Google image swirl: a large-scale content-based image visualization system. Proceedings of WWW, pp. 539–540 (2012)
5. Strong, G., Hoque, E., Gong, M., Hoeber, O.: Organizing and browsing image search results based on conceptual and visual similarities. In: ISVC, pp. 481–490 (2010)
6. Wang, J., Jia, L., Hua, X.-S.: Interactive browsing via diversified visual summarization for image search results. Multimedia Syst. **17**(5), 379–391 (2011)
7. Yee, K.P., Swearingen, K., Li, K., Hearst, M.: Faceted metadata for image search and browsing. In: Proc CHI 2003, pp. 401–408. ACM Press (2003)
8. Barthel, K., Hezel, N.: Graph navigation for exploring very large image collections. International Conference on Computer Vision Theory and Applications (2017)
9. André, P., Cutrell, E., Tan, D.S., Smith, G.: Designing novel image search interfaces by understanding unique characteristics and usage. INTERACT '09, pp. 340–353 (2009)
10. Chew, B., Rode, J.A., Sellen, A.: Understanding the everyday use of images on the web. In: Proc. NordiCHI'10, pp. 102–111. ACM Press (2010)
11. Markkula, M., Sormunen, E.: End-user searching challenges indexing practices in the digital newspaper photo archive. Inf. Retrieval **1**(4), 259–285 (2000)
12. Chung, E., Yoon, J.: Image needs in the context of image use: an exploratory study. J. Inf. Sci. (2011)
13. Shatford-Layne, S.: Some issues in the indexing of images. J. Am. Soc. Inf. Sci. **45**(8), 583–588 (1994)
14. Datta, R., Li, J., Wang, J.Z.: Content-based image retrieval: approaches and trends of the new age. In: Proc. of SIGMM, pp. 253–262. ACM Press (2005)
15. Barthel, K., et al.: ImageMap - visually browsing millions of images. Multimedia Modeling; 21st International Conference (2010)

Levels of Driving Automation from a User's Perspective: How Are the Levels Represented in the User's Mental Model?

Hendrik Homans(✉), Jonas Radlmayr, and Klaus Bengler

Chair of Ergonomics, Technical University of Munich, Boltzmannstraße 15, 85747 Munich, Garching, Germany
{hendrik.homans, jonas.radlmayr, bengler}@tum.de

Abstract. In this explorative study, we focused on the number of levels of driving automation as part of the mental model, using a newly created online questionnaire and analyzing results using Principal Component Analysis. The online questionnaire consisted of 20 automated driving functions that were described in short sentences. The 247 participants subjectively rated the degree of automation of the 20 functions on a 7-point rating scale. Using Principal Component Analysis, the ratings were summarized into groups represented by the components based on correlative relationships. The results yielded three components, which can be interpreted as three levels of driving automation. These three levels differ from the well-established taxonomies, showing that users do not differentiate between five or six levels of driving automation.

Keywords: Mental models · Levels of automation · Vehicle automation · Human-automation interaction · Analysis and evaluation · Autonomous driving

1 Introduction

Automated driving has recently become a big topic in society, research and development. From a human factors point of view, a lot of research is done on topics such as driver attention [1] or take-over performance [2]. All these studies and publications refer to comparable taxonomies of automation from different organizations like SAE [3], NHTSA [4] or the German Federal Highway Research Institute BASt [5]. This work takes a critical view of these levels of driving automation and their perception with the general driver. To describe and distinguish the capabilities of automated driving functions, several organizations created levels of driving automation that follow a similar classification of automation in vehicles. The most common taxonomies refer to either 5 or 6 levels of driving automation and range from "Driver Only" or "No Automation" to "Driverless" or "Full Automation." The higher the degree of automation, the greater the part of the driving task that is taken over by the technical system [6]. Mental models reflect the individual understanding of a user interacting with a system: which parts the system consists of, how the system works, and why it works [7]. If mental models are wrong or incomplete, wrong actions may consequently be chosen, which may result in unsafe or inefficient use and operation [6]. Based on a

T. Ahram et al. (Eds.): IHIET 2019, AISC 1018, pp. 21–27, 2020.
https://doi.org/10.1007/978-3-030-25629-6_4

mental model of automated systems, users can derive the fundamental allocation of control and responsibility between humans and machines [6]. This helps the user to derive the functional and responsibility limits of the automated systems. The driver needs to be aware of these limits to enable a safe interaction with the system [8]. There are various methods to measure or assess mental models, such as questionnaires, interviews, behavioral observations and card sorting. If the mental models of the users are unknown, there is the probability of a mismatch to the real world, which can be associated with different risks. This effect is well known from human computer interaction and was discussed by [9]. Original Equipment Manufacturers (OEMs) communicate their system dissimilarly, e.g. comparable systems are called "Autopilot" [10] or "Traffic Jam Assist" [11]. In comparison to other domains that establish automation (aviation, process control), there is no dedicated process of teaching and training, which could lead to an inconsistent model between the developer, organization and user. Based on the literature and the well-established taxonomies, this work addresses the following research questions: How are the levels of automation represented from the user's perspective?

2 Method

The users rated 20 automated driving functions subjectively on a scale regarding the degree of automation in an online questionnaire. With the Principal Component Analysis (PCA), these driving functions can be divided into groups based on correlative relationships. The method can be used to reduce a larger set of measured variables or items to a smaller group of underlying dimensions [12], called components or factors. With the PCA, the rated driving functions can be summarized into groups represented by the components. Therefore, it is suitable for this research question: in which and how many groups can the functions be summarized based on their degree of automation? At the end of the survey period, 280 complete datasets were gathered. Four records were excluded due to missing preconditions. In addition, 29 records were excluded from the analysis due to unrealistically quick completion. This was based on system-generated values from *Soscisurvey*. The final sample consisted of n = 247 participants. The sample consisted of n = 135 male and n = 108 female participants, with 4 participants not providing their gender. The mean age was m = 32.71 years (range: 19–74 years, *SD* = 10.72). All participants had a valid driver's license and German as their native language. The theoretical knowledge of automated driving functions, in general, is balanced: 41% stated they had "moderate" knowledge; 23% had "low" and 23% had "high" knowledge. Practical experience was less present in the sample compared to theoretical knowledge: 42% only had "low" experience with automated driving functions; 23% had "none" and 21% "moderate" practical experience. Almost 14% in total had "high" or "very high" experience. The 20 driving functions were described in short sentences. Every driving function was described by name and a brief description focused on functionality and constraints, for example:

Cruise Control: The driver sets a speed that is kept by the car. The driver must steer and, if necessary, adjust the speed and brake.

Robot Taxi: Allows for autonomous driving from start to finish - without restrictions: a driver is not necessary.

The names of the 20 driving functions in the order they were presented in the questionnaire were: 1. Robot Taxi ($M = 6.87$, $SD = 0.57$), 2. Night Vision ($M = 1.81$, $SD = 1.15$), 3. Cruise Control ($M = 5.28$, $SD = 1.12$), 4. Collision Protection ($M = 4.18$, $SD = 1.28$), 5. Chauffeur ($M = 5.28$, $SD = 1.09$), 6. Evasive Assistant ($M = 4.32$, $SD = 1.22$), 7. Extended Chauffeur ($M = 5.89$, $SD = 0.97$), 8. Lane Departure Warning ($M = 1.94$, $SD = 1.01$), 9. Emergency Stop Assist ($M = 4.67$, $SD = 1.52$), 10. Traffic Jam Assistant ($M = 4.51$, $SD = 1.20$), 11. Lane Keeping Assist ($M = 3.67$, $SD = 1.23$), 12. Collision Warning ($M = 1.96$, $SD = 1.00$), 13. Traffic Jam Pilot ($M = 5.62$, $SD = 1.22$), 14. Autobahn/Highway Pilot ($M = 6.18$, $SD = 0.96$), 15. Shift Support ($M = 1.50$, $SD = 0.91$), 16. Park Steering Assist ($M = 3.54$, $SD = 1.21$), 17. Adaptive Cruise Control (3.56, $SD = 1.22$), 18. Remote Parking, ($M = 5.43$, $SD = 1.39$) 19. Adaptive Cruise Control with Steering Assistance ($M = 4.57$, $SD = 1.20$), 20. Parking Garage Pilot ($M = 6.49$, $SD = 1.00$). The 20 driving functions in the questionnaire were rated on a 7-point rating scale. All 20 functions cover all driving situations of automated driving and the full range from manual driving to autonomous driving and contained already implemented and future functions. This was ensured by experts researching this topic.

For the statistical calculation it was important that the items in an online questionnaire cover the whole spectrum of the rating scale [13]: "no automation" and "full automation." In an expert discussion, it was ensured that the complete range of driving functions was evenly represented within the 20 functions. The scale was presented as an optical numeric rating scale with 7 levels (unipolar). The number of scale points is chosen based on the literature and the results of the pre-tests. [14] concluded that a 7-point scale corresponds to people's natural judgement, which is why it is preferable to all other scales. The driving functions in the questionnaire were not grouped according to the levels of driving automation or functional areas but are randomly arranged as far as possible. The two pre-tests were conducted with a total of 41 participants to uncover possible weaknesses in the formulation, sequence, length and design of the questionnaire and the items. The online questionnaire was implemented on the platform www.soscisurvey.de and the survey period lasted six weeks. The questionnaire was mainly distributed via social networks and email. In addition to the online questionnaire, 11 questionnaires were completed in printed form.

As a precondition for participation, a valid driver's license and German as their native language was required on the first website to avoid possible language barriers. Both preconditions were verified in the demographic data. The participants could take part in a raffle for online shopping vouchers: 2 × 50 Euro and 4 × 25 Euro. Anonymity was ensured by all participants via the system *Soscisurvey*.

Statistical evaluations were performed in SPSS 21 (IBM). The descriptive evaluation shows that the lowest mean of level of automation are the functions "Shift Support", "Night Vision" and "Lane Departure Warning". The highest ratings of the degree of automation are the functions "Robot Taxi", "Parking Garage Pilot" and "Highway Pilot". The largest standard deviation exists in the function "Emergency Stop Assist".

With 0.86, the Kaiser–Meyer–Olkin measure of sampling adequacy (MSA) is "meritorious" [15]. Bartlett's test of sphericity was significant ($\chi^2(190) = 2403$, $p < .001$). Mean communalities over 20 functions are $M = 0.62$ (Range: 0.31–0.74). The lowest communalities can be found for "Robot Taxi" with $h^2 = 0.31$ and "Cruise Control" with $h^2 = 0.36$. There should be at least three variables per factor for the factor extraction [13]. Factor loadings <0.3 can be neglected [13]. A principal component analysis was performed with 20 variables using a varimax rotation. The varimax rotation was chosen to simplify the interpretation of the components. The extraction was based on substantive considerations and interpretations of the factor loadings as well as on the Scree-Test according to [16] and the Kaiser-Guttman criterion [17]. The rotated solution shows a relatively unique structure in which all major components have high factor loadings. There are no high transverse loads, which is why many functions only load on one main component, which simplifies a clear assignment of the functions to one group. Exceptions are the following functions:

- The "Adaptive Cruise Control" function heavily loads on components 1 (.546) and 2 (.542)
- The "Lane Keeping Assist" function loads on components 1 (.369), 2 (.470) and 3 (.467)
- The "Robot Taxi" loads negatively only on component 1 but with −.516. It can also be seen in the correlation matrix that this function does not correlate positively higher with any other function than with r = .19 (Motorway Pilot). In addition, this function has the lowest commonality of $h^2 = 0.31$, so suitability for the PCA should be considered critical.
- The "Chauffeur" was taken out of the statistical calculation because two functions were named very similarly: "Chauffeur" and "Extended Chauffeur". Analysis with both functions within one PCA showed one component with only these two functions. A PCA with only one of the "Chauffeur"-functions showed more perspicuous results. Further analysis was conducted leaving out each one of the "Chauffeur"-functions: both PCAs showed a very similar result with similar statistical values for both "Chauffeur"-functions.

The analysis shows a 3-component solution. Based on the online questionnaire and the principal component analysis, a mental model of levels of driving automation could be established. It was possible to extract a clear 3-component solution based on the used driving functions. The components contain the following driving functions with their factor loadings in brackets.

Component 1 (Eigenvalue: 6.625): None to low automation: Lane Departure Warning System (.821), Shift Support (.821), Night Vision (.788), Collision Warning (.767), Cruise Control (.565), Adaptive Cruise Control (.546).

Component 2 (Eigenvalue: 3.22): Medium automation: Evasive Assistant (.807), Extended Chauffeur (.604), Collision Protection (.569), Emergency Stop Assist (.561), Lane Keeping Assist (.479).

Component 3 (Eigenvalue 1.169): High to very high automation: Remote Parking (.799), Parking Garage Pilot (.793), Traffic Jam Pilot (.672), Autobahn/Highway Pilot (.663), Adaptive Cruise Control with Steering Assistance (.660), Park Steering Assist (.535), Traffic Jam Assistant (.507).

3 Discussion and Limitations

The results on the mental models of automation levels are not in line with the taxonomies that are used by OEMs and the community of experts. This suggests that automated driving functions are not sophistically distinguished between 5 or 6 levels from a current user's point of view. The China Industry Innovation Alliance for Intelligent and Connected Vehicles [18] also utilizes a taxonomy with three groups of automated and connected driving, supporting the need for a new understanding and critical view of the established taxonomies. If users are to understand and interact with automated driving functions in a safe and acceptable way, their mental model should match the functions they interact with in the future. If the results are compared to the existing taxonomies, from a user's point of view, the differences between functions are considered in less detail (Table 1).

Table 1. Comparison between taxonomies and the results of our study

	Level 0	Level 1	Level 2	Level 3	Level 4	Level 5
NHTSA [4]	No automation	Function-specific automation	Combined function automation	Limited-self-driving automation	Full self-driving automation	
SAE [3]	No automation	Assisted	Partial automation	Conditional automation	High automation	Full automation
Mental model	None to low automation		Medium automation		High to very high automation	

It is understandable that technical experts rely on another understanding and view in comparison to non-expert users (see [9]). For example, in research and functional development, technical possibilities and limits need to be identified, which may require detailed technical and functional taxonomies. However, especially in complex and safety-critical systems, development and design should be user-centered. The different understanding and mental models between experts and users present a problem when users get in touch with the products made by these experts without focusing on the user's mental models. Here, the HMI of automated driving functions and the advertisement of such functions plays a predominant role to avoid wrong expectations, misuse and frustration. A stronger orientation in the development and introduction of automated systems, especially considering existing mental models, will increase acceptance and system trust.

The automated driving functions were only described textually. The correct understanding of the functions cannot be guaranteed. One option would be to let the participants experience the functions themselves in simulators or real vehicles (see for example [8]). The names of the functions could, regardless of their function, provide hints to the classification; such as the words "Assistant" and "Pilot." For example, all driving functions that include the word "Help" or "Warning" are summarized in the first component. Also, the functions with the addition "Pilot" can be found in one component. However, it would be conceivable that these functions would be assessed differently by the participants if they had a different (or no) name. On the one hand, it is unclear whether the 3-level model is also demonstrably present in the population. On the other hand, the study was conducted in Germany in German, which is the reason why the results are based on German terms. It would be reasonable to replicate this study in other language and cultural areas. In addition, mental models differ between different people: there is not only one mental model. They change and vary depending on expertise and experience. It would be conceivable to collect and compare the mental models of non-experts and experts with a sufficiently large sample and to quantify distances within and between groups.

References

1. Radlmayr, J., Brüch, K., Schmidt, K., Solbeck, C., Wehner, T.: Peripheral monitoring of traffic in conditionally automated driving. Proc. Hum. Factors Ergon. Soc. Annu. Meet. **62**, 1828–1832 (2018)
2. Gold, C., Körber, M., Lechner, D., Bengler, K.: Taking over control from highly automated vehicles in complex traffic situations: the role of traffic density. Hum. Factors **58**, 642–652 (2016)
3. Society of Automotive Engineers: Taxonomy and Definitions for Terms Related to Driving Automation Systems for On-Road Motor Vehicles. (SAE Standard J3016_201609). PA: SAE International, Warrensdale (2016)
4. National Highway Traffic Safety Administration: Preliminary Statement of Policy Concerning Automated Vehicles. http://www.nhtsa.gov/staticfiles/rulemaking/pdf/
5. Gasser, T.M. (ed.): Rechtsfolgen zunehmender Fahrzeugautomatisierung; Gemeinsamer Schlussbericht der Projektgruppe; Bericht zum Forschungsprojekt F (Legal consequences of increasing vehicle automation; joint final report of the project group; Report on the research project F). Wirtschaftsverl. NW Verl. für neue Wiss, Bremerhaven (2012)
6. Flemisch, F., Heesen, M., Hesse, T., Kelsch, J., Schieben, A., Beller, J.: Towards a dynamic balance between humans and automation: authority, ability, responsibility and control in shared and cooperative control situations. Cogn. Technol. Work **14**, 3–18 (2012)
7. Rouse, W.B., Morris, N.M.: On looking into the black box: prospects and limits in the search for mental models. Psychol. Bull. **100**, 349–363 (1986)
8. Beggiato, M., Krems, J.F.: The evolution of mental model, trust and acceptance of adaptive cruise control in relation to initial information. Transp. Res. Part F: Traffic Psychol. Behav. **18**, 47–57 (2013)
9. Norman, D.: The design of everyday things. Basic Books, New York, NY (2013)
10. Tesla, I.: Autopilot: Full Self-Driving Hardware. https://www.tesla.com/autopilot
11. Volkswagen AG: Traffic Jam Assist. http://www.volkswagen.co.uk/technology/proximity-sensing/traffic-jam-assist
12. Field, A.: Discovering Statistics Using IBM SPSS Statistics and Sex and Drugs and Rock 'n' Roll. Sage, Los Angeles, London, New Delhi, Singapore, Washington DC (2013)
13. Bühner, M.: Einführung in die Test- und Fragebogenkonstruktion (Introduction to Test Design and Questionnaire Design). Pearson Studium, München (2006)
14. Krosnick, J.A.: Response strategies for coping with the cognitive demands of attitude measures in surveys. Appl. Cognit. Psychol. **5**, 213–236 (1991)
15. Kaiser, H.F.: An index of factorial simplicity. Psychometrika **39**, 31–36 (1974)

16. Cattell, R.B.: The scree test for the number of factors. Multivar. Behav. Res. **1**, 245–276 (1966)
17. Kaiser, H.F.: The application of electronic computers to factor analysis. Educ. Psychol. Measur. **20**, 141–151 (1960)
18. Li, K.: The Base Platform of ICV System and Its Industrialization Approach. SIP-adus Workshop; Cross-Ministerial Strategic Innovation Promotion Program, Council for Science, Government of Japan. Tokyo, Japan (2018)

What Do You Do? An Analysis of Non-driving Related Activities During a 60 Minutes Conditionally Automated Highway Drive

Tobias Hecht(✉), Anna Feldhütter, Kathrin Draeger, and Klaus Bengler

Chair of Ergonomics, Technical University of Munich, Boltzmannstr. 15, 85748 Garching, Germany
{t.hecht,anna.feldhuetter,ga73bet,bengler}@tum.de

Abstract. Conditionally automated driving (CAD) allows the driver to deal with non-driving related activities (NDRA) whenever the automation is active. We have analyzed video data from a one hour driving simulator study with free naturalistic NDRA. Most time was spent watching videos on a pre-installed tablet, looking at the surrounding traffic and landscape, listening to music and using the phone for multiple activities. The latter was undertaken by 75% of the participants, followed by reading books and magazines (60%) and browsing the tablet (50%). There was a wide variety of observed activities and also a high variance in both total time spent on such activities and their mean duration. Participants engaged in NDRA about 2 min after switching on the automation. Older participants spent significantly more time looking at the surrounding traffic and less time using their phone or playing video games.

Keywords: Non-driving related activities · Automated driving · HMI design

1 Introduction

With the ongoing automatization in the automotive industry, new human factors questions arise. Level 2 systems, such as Tesla Autopilot and Mercedes Drive Pilot, are already on the market. Unlike these partially automated systems, Level 3 or conditional driving automation allows the driver to disengage from the driving task with no supervision of the vehicle needed [1]. This allows the driver to deal with non-driving related activities (NDRA) whenever the automation is active. However, the driver has to maintain readiness to react to requests to intervene (RtI) within a given time budget to fully take back control. So far, many studies have focused on the take-over process, HMI design and driver state aspects such as fatigue [2, 3]. NDRA have mainly been researched using standardized tasks (e.g. n-back task, SURT) to assess their impact on the take-over performance [4]. When looking at real-life NDRA that people are likely to engage in during automated driving, research has mainly focused on surveys: Similarly to today's manual driving, people want to talk to other passengers, listen to music or drink, eat, write messages look at the surroundings [5]. Thus, another approach is to investigate bus and train rides. For short trips like metro or suburban

T. Ahram et al. (Eds.): IHIET 2019, AISC 1018, pp. 28–34, 2020.
https://doi.org/10.1007/978-3-030-25629-6_5

train rides, listening to music, talking, looking at the surroundings, doing nothing and phone use are popular activities [5]. For long distance train and bus rides, Russel et al. [6] observed people mainly looking at the surroundings, listening to music or talking to other passengers. Reading, writing, sleeping and the use of electronic devices are popular for train rides. In an online survey amongst users of the long distance high-speed train Thalys [7], the most popular activities were reading, relaxing, sleeping and using electronic devices such as tablet, laptop or phone. On business trips, working is more important with sleeping and reading less so [7, 8]. Another approach is the performance of driving simulator studies with free and real-life NDRA. The authors are only aware of one study by Large et al. [9] that adopted this approach. In a week-long driving simulator study with two identical 30 min drives per day and five participants, they found users mainly engaging in media use (magazines, books), laptop, tablet and smartphone. The researchers also highlight large individual differences.

Therefore, the aim of the current analysis is to enhance knowledge about actual activities to allow researchers and developers to design optimum future car interior including seat and seating position, to assess the likelihood of motion sickness and to design the HMI and the automated driving functions according to user needs. This is why we have analyzed video data from a driving simulator experiment originally dealing with the development of fatigue in CAD [3]. In the study, two activity conditions were chosen: the natural load (with real-life NDRA) and the underload condition (with no NDRA allowed). For this paper, video data of the natural load condition during a steady and uninterrupted one-hour drive was coded and analyzed to describe activities and their share of the driving time. Also the average activity duration is reported to enhance the findings of Metz et al. [10] for automated driving. Furthermore, different behaviors in relation to the participants' age are researched.

2 Method

The experiment was conducted in a high-fidelity, fix-based driving simulator comprising of a full-vehicle BMW series 6 mock-up. Seven projectors created a > 180° field of view and allowed the use of side and rear mirrors. All participants underwent a test drive to get used to the simulator and the automation including engagement and disengagement of the conditionally automated driving function. Next, they completed an uninterrupted 60 min drive with conditional automation at a constant speed of 120 km/h on a three-lane highway. After 60 min of CAD, a broken-down vehicle suddenly appeared in the ego-vehicle lane, prompting a RtI. Participants in the natural load scenario were instructed to bring personal items they would want to use. Additionally, there was a tablet installed in the simulator offering videos, audio books, games, music and radio. Magazines, Wi-Fi and reading lights were also provided to ensure a large range of possible NDRA. Participants were told in advance that they would experience a 75 min drive to ensure they were not expecting an RtI after 60 min. A camera was used to film the drivers during the experimental drive. Also, the remote eye-tracking system Smart Eye with three cameras was implemented. More details on study design, apparatus and procedure can be found in Feldhütter et al. [3].

A total of 42 drivers in two age groups (young: 23–38 years; old: 60–77 years) participated in the experiments, 22 in the natural load group. For technical reasons, two participants in the latter group were excluded. Six of the remaining 20 participants were female (30%). On average, the young drivers were 24.91 years old (*SD* = 1.14), old drivers 66.22 years (*SD* = 4.76). Twelve participants had taken part in a driving simulator study before. It was possible to undertake two activities at the same time, which was coded as two ongoing activities (e.g. watching video and phone use). When watching a video, the preceding process of selecting the video was included in the activity. For the use of the tablet, the activities video, games, music, audiobook and browsing were coded. However, for phone and laptop use, no further sub-activities except for phone calls and listening to music via phone could be differentiated. Activities were considered to have been interrupted after an interruption time of approximately 15 to 20 s. The last activity which was interrupted by the RtI was not included, unless it had been ongoing for more than ten minutes. This was to achieve realistic average times. "Other" activities include scratching one's head, changing volume and drinking. The eye-tracking system was used to determine the amount of time participants spent looking at the surrounding traffic and landscape through the windshield.

3 Results

75% of the passengers used their phone during the drive, 60% read and 50% used the tablet for browsing the content. The least popular activities were sleeping, phoning and listening to music via a private phone. Table 1 displays the amount of time spent on each NDRA during the drive subdivided by age group. Qualitatively, it is apparent that there are large differences between age groups for almost all activities: old participants spent more time watching videos, looking at the surroundings, listening to music (tablet) and reading, and less on phone and laptop use, music (phone) and playing games. However, due to the small sample size and the high variance in activities, differences are only significant for time spent looking at the surroundings through the windshield ($t(10.083) = -2.673$, $p = .023$, $d = 1.297$). Old participants spent almost 20 min on this activity, young drivers only about eight.

As can be seen in Fig. 1 the participants spent most of the 60 min drive watching videos on the pre-installed tablet and on looking at the surrounding traffic and landscape. The average duration of watching videos was 17:36 min (*SD* = 19:10 min), approximately as long as listening to music on the phone (*M* = 18:23, *SD* = 17:33) or playing games on the tablet (*M* = 16:47, *SD* = 14:18). The third most time was spent using the phone, which has a short average duration of 2:27 min (*SD* = 3:46). More than three hours were spent listening to music/radio on the tablet (*M* = 24:17, *SD* = 25:08).

Using a personal laptop was the activity with the highest average duration (*M* = 55:20, *SD* = 5:06): two out of three drivers used it for the whole drive. Reading (books, magazines or newspapers) totaled 2:39 h and was a rather short-duration activity (*M* = 5:18, *SD* = 6:34). Two participants listened to music on their phone for a total of 1:32 h. Less time was spent on playing games, listening to audio books,

Table 1. Participation by number of participants (rank) and average time spent per activity in minutes (n = 20)

Activity	Participants	Time young (n = 11)		Time old (n = 9)	
	(Rank)	*M*	*SD*	*M*	*SD*
Videos (tablet)	9 (4)	13:49	23:33	16:21	18:54
Surroundings	20 (-)	08:15	04:55	19:55	12:19
Phone usage	15 (1)	14:47	16:46	05:57	08:48
Music (tablet)	7 (5)	05:27	12:33	14:55	25:41
Laptop usage	3 (6)	15:05	25:57	00:00	–
Reading	12 (2)	06:06	11:11	10:12	13:48
Music (phone)	2 (7)	08:21	18:36	00:00	–
Games (tablet)	3 (6)	07:04	15:43	00:41	02:04
Audio books	7 (5)	01:27	04:11	02:39	04:23
Tablet browsing	10 (3)	00:49	01:27	01:33	01:51
Sleeping	1 (8)	00:00	–	01:40	04:59
Phone calls	1 (8)	00:00	–	00:27	01:21
Others	20 (-)	01:12	01:35	05:26	06:54

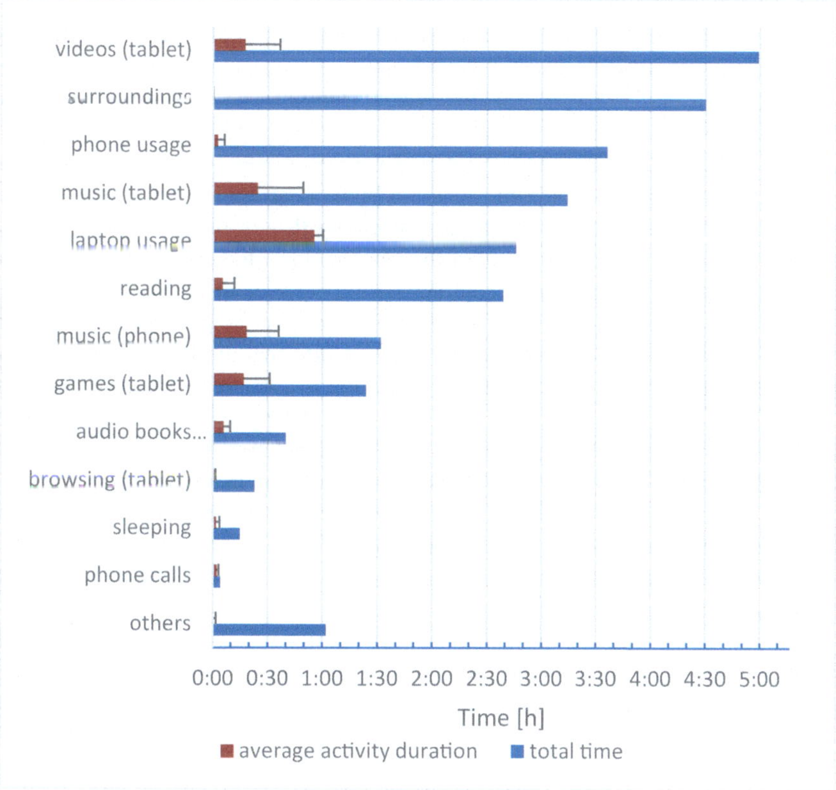

Fig. 1. Average activity duration and total time spent on activities when driving automated (n = 20), error bars represent standard deviation

sleeping and phone calls. Short moments of sleep occurred very rarely and only one participant used his time for (two) phone calls. Tablet browsing without a subsequent activity amounted to 23 min in total (*M* = 0:37, *SD* = 0:48).

We also analyzed the time before participants took up an activity after the automated driving function was activated. Therefore, only activities differing from those that can be conducted while driving manually have been considered. This means that drinking, turning on the radio, changing volume, etc. have not been counted as first NDRA. One participant had to be excluded because there was no such activity. The remaining 19 passengers engaged in an activity after a mean time of 2:06 min (*SD* = 5:13 min), ranging from five seconds to 22:30 min.

4 Discussion and Conclusion

Analyzing the video data of this 60 min steady and uninterrupted conditionally automated highway drive reveals high differences between individuals in respect of the activities they undertake and the average activity durations. The high variance confirms findings by Large et al. [9] and Metz et al. [10] and indicates different motivations and influencing factors for the starting of activities. Nonetheless, phone use could be identified as the activity most people participated in and also the total time spent on this activity indicates that phone use is very popular. This is probably due to the short time needed to interact with the phone and the high variety of possible activities. However, even more time was spent looking at the surroundings and especially watching videos, which almost half of the drivers did. However, it should be noted that watching videos can easily be combined with control glances or even longer periods of observing traffic or landscape. Activities performed on internal devices similar to the tablet used in this experiment (videos, games, radio/music/audio books) can be helpful when communicating the automation system's intentions, prompting RtIs or blocking the activity and to force the driver to take-over control of the vehicle [11]. However, with other devices such as phone, books or magazines, communication between driver and the automation system becomes more difficult. HMI designers either have the problem of interrupting the driver's NDRA when communicating relevant information, most likely with negative effects for the driver [12], or, if the HMI design is less noticeable, running the risk that the driver will miss information and that trust in the system, as well as mode and situation awareness will be decreased [13]. The challenge is to design the HMI according to user needs, with NDRA being one of the main needs identified for automated driving [14]. Especially for activities like laptop usage, there is a need for long uninterrupted periods. A good HMI thus supports the driver in the choice of activities by providing the required information to plan the drive and the activities accordingly.

Nevertheless, the findings of this study were obtained in a static driving simulator. The participants experienced no dynamics and there was no risk of injury. Also, the purpose for the choice of NDRA in this study was unclear. For future studies, experiments under actual driving conditions and more specific set-ups are recommended. However, we have been able to provide more detailed insights into possible NDRA during automated driving, allowing researchers and developers to use this as input for further studies. Furthermore, we have expanded the findings of Large et al. [9] as well as those of surveys and observations on NDRA in automated driving.

Acknowledgements. This report is based on parts of the research project carried out at the request of the Federal Ministry of Transport and Digital Infrastructure, represented by the Federal Highway Research Institute, under research project No. 82.0628/2015. The author is solely responsible for the content.

References

1. SAE International: Taxonomy and Definitions for Terms Related to Driving Automation Systems for On-Road Motor Vehicles(SAE J3016) (2018)
2. Naujoks, F., Forster, Y., Wiedemann, K., Neukum, A.: A human-machine interface for cooperative highly automated driving. In: Stanton, N.A., Landry, S., Di Bucchianico, G. (eds.) Advances in Human Aspects of Transportation: Proceedings of the AHFE 2016 International Conference on Human Factors in Transportation. Springer International Publishing, Cham (2017)
3. Feldhütter, A., Hecht, T., Kalb, L., Bengler, K.: Effect of prolonged periods of conditionally automated driving on the development of fatigue. With and without non-driving-related activities. Cognition, Technology & Work (2018). https://doi.org/10.1007/s10111-018-0524-9
4. Radlmayr, J., Fischer, F.M., Bengler, K.: The influence of non-driving related tasks on driver availability in the context of conditionally automated driving. In: Bagnara, S., Tartaglia, R., Albolino, S., Alexander, T., Fujita, Y. (eds.) Proceedings of the 20th Congress of the International Ergonomics Association (IEA 2018). Springer International Publishing, Cham (2019)
5. Pfleging, B., Rang, M., Broy, N.: Investigating user needs for non-driving-related activities during automated driving. In: Alt, F. (ed.) MUM 2016. 15th International Conference on Mobile and Ubiquitous Multimedia: Proceedings: Dec 12 - Dec 15, 2016, Rovaniemi, Finland. The 15th International Conference, Rovaniemi, Finland, pp. 91 99. The Association for Computing Machinery, Inc, New York (2016). https://doi.org/10.1145/3012709.3012735
6. Russell, M., Price, R., Signal, L., Stanley, J., Gerring, Z., Cumming, J.: What do passengers do during travel time? Structured observations on buses and trains. JPT (2011). https://doi.org/10.5038/2375-0901.14.3.7
7. Thalys: Umfrage im Auftrag von Thalys: Wie reisen Europäer? Studie unter europäischen Reisenden zeigt länderspezifische Unterschiede und Gemeinsamkeiten im Reiseverhalten, Köln (2013)
8. Susilo, Y.O., Lyons, G., Jain, J., Atkins, S.: Rail passengers' time use and utility assessment. Transp. Res. Rec. (2013). https://doi.org/10.3141/2323-12
9. Large, D., Burnett, G., Morris, A., Muthumani, A., Matthias, R.: Design implications of drivers' engagement with secondary activities during highly-automated driving – a longitudinal simulator study. In: Road Safety and Simulation International Conference (RSS2017), The Hague, Netherlands, 17–19 October 2017 (2017)
10. Metz, B., Landau, A., Just, M.: Frequency of secondary tasks in driving – results from naturalistic driving data. Saf. Sci. (2014). https://doi.org/10.1016/j.ssci.2014.04.002

11. Wandtner, B., Schömig, N., Schmidt, G.: Effects of non-driving related task modalities on takeover performance in highly automated driving. Hum. Factors (2018). https://doi.org/10.1177/0018720818768199
12. Naujoks, F., Wiedemann, K., Schoemig, N.: The importance of interruption management for usefulness and acceptance of automated driving. In: Proceedings of the 9th International Conference on Automotive User Interfaces and Interactive Vehicular Applications, Oldenburg, Germany (2017). https://doi.org/10.1145/3122986.3123000
13. Miglani, A., Diels, C., Terken, J.: Compatibility between trust and non-driving related tasks in UI design for highly and fully automated driving. In: Green, P. (ed.) Adjunct Proceedings of the 8th International Conference on Automotive User Interfaces and Interactive Vehicular Applications. The 8th International Conference, pp. 75–80. Ann Arbor, MI, USA. ACM, New York, NY (2016). https://doi.org/10.1145/3004323.3004331
14. König, M., Neumayr, L.: Users' resistance towards radical innovations. The case of the self-driving car. Transp. Res. Part F: Traffic Psychol. Behav. (2017). https://doi.org/10.1016/j.trf.2016.10.013

Virtual Workshops on the Road: Co-designing with Drivers, Within Context in Real-Time

Daniel de la Flor Aceituno[1(✉)], Joseph Giacomin[1], Alessio Malizia[2], and Lee Skrypchuk[3]

[1] Human Centred Design Institute, Brunel University, UB8 3PH London, UK
{daniel.delafloraceituno, Joseph.Giacomin}@brunel.ac.uk
[2] School of Creative Arts, University of Hertfordshire, AL10 9AB Hertfordshire, UK
a.malizia@herts.ac.uk
[3] Human Machine Interface Research, Jaguar Land Rover, CV3 4LF Coventry, UK
lskrypch@jaguarlandrover.com

Abstract. An investigation was performed of the characteristics of real-time, virtually present, contextual inquiry between automobile drivers and automotive designers. 28 participants were remotely interviewed while they were in one of two contexts: either sitting in a bare isolated meeting room or when operating a driving simulator. Open questions of the type involved in concept design were used as the basis of the real time interview. The interview transcripts were analysed by means of discourse analysis, thematic analysis and evaluations of degree of creativity. The results revealed that the real time automotive interview context provided richer information in terms of the quantity of the words expressed, the variety of the words expressed, and in terms of the judged degree of creativity of the statements.

Keywords: Human centred design · Co-design, design · Contextual inquiry · Interviewing · Discourse analysis · Thematic analysis · Creativity · Driving · Automobile · Simulator

1 Introduction

The automotive industry is currently facing an era of rapid evolution driven by the development of sophisticated electronics and algorithms, which are affecting user behaviour, and gradually changing customer experience [1]. In order to explore the implications of this evolution, automotive designers currently apply methodologies such as online surveys, telephone interviews and more recently, trend analysis [2, 3]. These tend to focus on drivers' opinions, not necessarily capturing how they actually experience the automobiles. In addition, the methods rely on human long-term memory which is affected by a large list of cognitive processes [4]. These processes include the "location updating effect" [5], which refers to a decline in memory when people move from one place to another, and the "fading affect bias" [6], which involves affect

T. Ahram et al. (Eds.): IHIET 2019, AISC 1018, pp. 35–41, 2020.
https://doi.org/10.1007/978-3-030-25629-6_6

associated with negative memories fading faster than affect associated with positive memories. These processes lead to inaccuracies and biases [4].

Aiming to improve the situation, researchers have recently shifted their interest towards Human-Centred Design, which can be considered as a form of structured empathy [7]. In turn, there is an increasing tendency to collaborate with customers [8]. Part of this community focus is on contextual inquiry [9], which in the automotive context refers to collaborating with drivers while they are inside the automobile. This reduces several cognitive biases including the "location updating effect" [5].

Most recently, researchers started exploring the possibility of connecting designers with users in real-time while they are driving [10, 11]. Those researchers advocate for the use of the co-design approach in order to provide carmakers with both ethnographic data and creative ideas generated through contextual inquiry [9]. This paper describes a research study which was performed to investigate the possibilities of real-time collaborative dialogue between drivers and designers, and to evaluate the benefits of within context interaction on the quantity and creative qualities of the information which can be gathered.

2 Method

2.1 Real-Time Collaboration Taxonomy

Participants were interviewed in one of two study contexts. The contexts were when sitting in a bare and isolated meeting room or when using a driving simulator. The interviews were transcribed, and the information was subsequently analysed to explore its usefulness.

Literature in innovation frequently uses the term 'useful' interchangeably with the term 'creative' [12]. Further, literature advocates that the collection of greater amounts of information correlates with the collection of more creative ideas [13]. Therefore, the information collected in this study was considered to be more 'useful' and 'richer' when it involved a greater number of words, a greater variety of words, a greater number of themes, or when it was assessed as more creative by an independent panel of experts. The research hypotheses of the current study were the following:

- Within context interviews provide richer information in terms of word quantity and variety.
- Within context interviews provide richer information in terms of number of themes.
- Within context interviews provide richer information in terms of creativity.

2.2 Stimulus Materials

The Bare and Isolated Meeting Room. To simulate the typical context in which most interviews and focus groups are held in current practice, a small and bare room (no decoration or items of equipment other than table and seat) of the university was chosen for the activity. The room provided no obvious visual or acoustic texture or distractions.

The Driving Simulator. The simulator was composed of three elements: a BMW MINI body shell, a computer under the bonnet which processed the within-vehicle systems (i.e. steering wheel, gearbox, pedals, etc.) and a computer installed outside the vehicle which hosted the "XPI DS2 Full Car Simulator" [14] simulation and monitoring software.

The Interview. The interview questions were based on the verbal version of the Torrance Test of Creative Thinking [12] and the structure of the interview was designed to prompt a creative dialogue based on the principles of effective interviewing [15]. The subject selected for the creative conversation was the In-Vehicle Navigation System (IVNS) due to it being one of the main sources of distraction inside cars and, hence, a target for possible future improvements [16].

2.3 Participant Recruitment

The sample size adopted for the study was 28 participants. Fourteen were interviewed through a telephone while sitting in the bare and isolated meeting room, while fourteen were interviewed through a telephone while steering the driving simulator (each participant was interviewed only once to reduce learning effects). Each group of 14 participants consisted of equal numbers of men and women. The participants had an average age of 26 (SD = 3) with a range of 21 to 36 years old and an average of 6 years of experience driving (SD = 4) with a range of 1 to 18 years holding the driving license.

2.4 Measurement Instruments

Discourse Analysis. The objective metrics adopted for the study were the total number of words spoken, the word variety (number of unique words occurring in the transcripts) and the word frequency (number of times that a given word occurred in the transcripts) [17]. The automated tool used to conduct the analysis was "Word Smith Tools 7.0" [18].

Thematic Analysis. The method selected for the thematic analysis was the General Inductive Approach, due to its clarity and effectiveness in exploring repeating topics [19]. The approach leads to the creation of summary themes or categories from the raw data. The aim of the thematic analysis was the selection and categorisation of ideas which could help to improve the IVNS. Four independent coders were selected from different professional backgrounds, age groups and genders to obtain a range of perspectives. The procedure followed an approach outlined by Thomas [19]. The metric used to measure inter-coder consistency was the percentage of agreement in assigning ideas to categories [20].

Creativity Analysis. The Consensual Assessment Technique [12] was used to estimate the degree of creativity of the interview contents. The technique relies on the judgement of a panel of experts for the evaluation of creative achievement. Six professionals were selected for the expert panel. The main criteria used to select the professionals was that of having a PhD or significant industrial experience in psychology, design or engineering, and a minimum of 3 years of working experience in their respective sector [21].

3 Results

3.1 Discourse Analysis

Participants who answered the interview questions from the driving simulator provided longer answers in terms of the number of words than those who were interviewed from the bare isolated meeting room ($F = 9.830$, $p = 0.004$). Regarding the variety of vocabulary used, the within context interview of the driving simulator provided more varied vocabulary than the interview from the bare isolated meeting room ($F = 7.618$, $p = 0.010$). The interviews which took place while the respondents were driving the simulator did not however last longer[1] than the interviews that took place while the participants were located in the bare isolated meeting room ($F = 0.171$, $p = 0.683$). Table 1 presents the summary values.

Table 1. Mean and standard deviation (SD) values of the number of words, variety of words, and interview time durations determined across the complete set of participants.

		Word quantity	Word variety	Seconds	Minutes
Isolated room	*Mean*	586	200	575	9'35"
	SD	205	43	129	2'9"
Driving simulator	*Mean*	880	249	552	9'12"
	SD	285	52	164	2'44"

In terms of word frequency, the ten nouns which were used most frequently in both contexts were: *car, navigation, GPS, time, maps, places, example, Google, road* and *way*.

3.2 Thematic Analysis

The coders extracted 40 improvement ideas from the raw data of the transcribed interviews, which were subsequently clustered into three main themes with an inter-coder agreement of 0.9. The three main themes were:

Navigation Instructions. The suggestions which were made in relation to improving how the instructions were given (n = 14) ranged from visual issues, such as the use of real pictures of the street, to verbal issues such as the anticipation or the wording used when providing instructions to the driver.

Connectivity & Software Updates. The proposals made to improve the connectivity of the device to the network (n = 10) included the ability to download maps in order to facilitate operation in zones of degraded GPS coverage, and the inclusion of an on-board AI such as *Siri* or *Alexa*.

[1] Time length refers to the number of seconds between the instant in which the interviewer started asking the first question and the moment in which the respondent stopped answering the last question.

Customised Experience. The ideas in relation to the customising of the user experience (n = 16) ranged from passenger monitoring, to suggesting alternative destinations, to tracking nearby friends and notifying the driver about their presence.

Table 2 below presents the number of independent improvement ideas extracted from the transcripts of the interviews performed in each of the two study contexts.

Table 2. Number of improvement ideas extracted by the coders in each context.

	Isolated room	Driving simulator	Both contexts	Total
Navigation instructions	2	5	7	14
Connectivity & software updates	1	2	7	10
Customised experience	3	9	4	16

3.3 Creativity Analysis

Each of the six professional experts was first asked to articulate his or her own personal definition of creativity, and to define criteria for measuring it across a set of statements. The declared self-selected criteria of creativity included the concepts of positive thinking, elaboration, surprise, originality, abstractness and novelty.

Each professional expert was next provided an individually randomised list of the 28 statements which had been provided by the participants in response to the question: *"If you were to write a newspaper headline to summarise your experience with navigation system what would it be?"*. The core creative question provided an opportunity for the interviewees to furnish high level conceptual accounts of their experience, leveraging any relevant metaphors which were being used to make sense of the situation.

Each professional expert was asked to organise the 28 statements from the first (most creative) to the last (least creative) using his or her own self-selected criteria. The method of analytic hierarchy process [22] was then used to assign a numerical value to the rank order position of each statement, and to calculate the average score (from 0 to 100) of the statement across the complete ensemble of expert opinions.

A statistically significant difference was found between the creativity scores of the statements made in the bare isolated meeting room with respect to those expressed in the driving context ($F = 7.188$; $p = 0.013$). The statements made while driving were scored as more creative ($M = 59.4$; $SD = 15.5$) than those expressed in the meeting room ($M = 44.2$; $SD = 14.6$). To illustrate the nature of the differences, Table 3 below provides the five statements which were judged to be the most creative, the five which were judged to be the least creative, along with the context in which each statement was made.

Table 3. The five most creative statements, the five least creative statements and the context in which the statement was provided.

Answer provided by the respondents	Mean score	Isolated room	Driving simulator
A great power takes a great responsibility	86.3	X	
Lifesaver	82.7		X
My salvation	77.4		X
Your friendly virtual co-pilot	73.8		X
SAT NAV saves the day!	71.4		X
Useless navigation	36.9	X	
My hard experience with the GPS	36.3	X	
Useful but the voice is annoying	30.4	X	
Not a very intuitive system	25.0	X	
Travel guide to getting you from A to B	29.2		X

4 Discussion

The results of the all three analysis confirmed the hypotheses that the within context interview provided richer information in terms of word quantity, word variety, and creativity. However, the results of all three analysis performed in the current study rejected the hypothesis that the within context interview provided richer information in terms of the number of themes covered.

The driving simulator context was found to produce an increased number of words and an increased variety of words, on average, with respect to the bare isolated meeting room. The greater number and variety appeared to be attributable to the interviewees providing greater detail in their explanations. Significant differences were not noted in the number of themes which were expressed, but the level of detail and the degree of creativity was greater in the case of the interviews which were performed within the driving context.

Acknowledgements. This research was funded and supported by Jaguar Land Rover.

References

1. Smith, T., Vardhan, H., Cherniavsky, L.: Humanising Autonomy: Where are We Going. USTWO, London (2017)
2. Seat: Annual Report. Retrieved from https://www.seat.com/company/annual-report/management.html (2017)
3. Audi: Annual Report. Retrieved from https://www.audi.com/en/company/investor-relations/reports-and-key-figures/annual-reports.html (2017)
4. Benson, B.: Cognitive bias cheat sheet. Better Humans (2016)
5. Radvansky, G.A., Krawietz, S.A., Tamplin, A.K.: Walking through doorways causes forgetting: further explorations. Q. J. Exp. Psychol. 1632–1645 (2011)

6. Walker, W.R., Skowronski, J.J.: The fading affect bias: but what the hell is it for? Appl. Cogn. Psychol. **23**(8), 1122–1136 (2009)
7. Giacomin, J.: What is human centred design? Des. J. **17**(4), 606–623 (2014)
8. Ramm, S., Giacomin, J., Malizia, A., Anyasodo, B.: Using participatory design workshops to identify what feels natural about using a car's secondary controls. ATA – Ing. dell'Autoveicolo **68**, 46–52 (2015)
9. Gkatzidou, V., Giacomin, J., Skrypchuk, L.: Automotive habitat laboratory: a facility for automotive co-design. Proceedings of the 7th International Conference on Applied Human Factors and Ergonomics. Orlando, Florida, USA (2016)
10. Martelaro, N., Ju, W.: WoZ way: enabling real-time remote interaction prototyping & observation in on-road. CSCW '17 Proceedings of the 2017 ACM Conference on Computer Supported Cooperative Work and Social Computing, pp. 169–182. ACM, Portland, Oregon, USA (2017)
11. Giuliano, L., Germak, C., Giacomin, J.: Effect of driving context on design dialogue. International Conference on Applied Human Factors and Ergonomics: Advances in Ergonomics in Design. Orlando, Florida, USA, 134–144 (2017)
12. Said-Metwaly, S., Noortgate, W.V., Kyndt, E.: Approaches to measuring creativity: a systematic literature review. Creativity: Theor. Res. Appl. **4**(2), 238–275 (2017)
13. Pedersen, T.: Recipe for creativity: crank out ideas and step away. PsychCentral (2019)
14. The Driving Simulator Company. http://www.xpisimulation.com/products/full-car-simulator
15. Strachan, D.: Making Questions Work: A Guide to What and How to Ask for Facilitators, Consultants, Managers, Coaches, and Educators. Wiley (2007)
16. Lee, B., Lee, Y.J.N., Park, S., Kim, H., Lee, S.J., Kim, J.: Driver's distraction and understandability (EOU) change due to the level of abstractness and modality of GPS navigation information during driving. Procedia Comput. Sci. **39**, 115–122 (2014)
17. Baker, P.: Using Corpora in Discourse Analysis. Continuum International Publishing Group, London (2006)
18. Word Smith Tools. https://www.lexically.net/wordsmith/
19. Thomas, D.R.: A general inductive approach for analyzing qualitative evaluation data. Am. J. Eval. **27**(2), 237–246 (2006)
20. Lombard, M., Snyder-Duch, J., Bracken, C.C.: Content analysis in mass communication: assessment and reporting of intercoder reliability. Hum. Commun. Res. **28**(4), 587–604 (2006)
21. Origgi, G.: Reputation: What It Is and Why It Matters. Princeton University Press, Oxfordshire, UK (2018)
22. Saaty, T.L.: Decision making with the analytic hierarchy process. Int. J. Serv. Sci. **1**(1), 83, 98 (2008)

From Apology to Compensation: A Multi-level Taxonomy of Trust Reparation for Highly Automated Virtual Assistants

Fernando Galdon[1(✉)] and Stephen Jia Wang[2]

[1] Department of Global Innovation Design, School of Design, Royal College of Art, London, UK
fernando.galdon@network.rca.ac.uk
[2] Department of Innovation Design Engineering, School of Design, Royal College of Art, London, UK

Abstract. This paper presents a multi-level taxonomy of reparation levels specifically adapted to virtual assistants in the context of Human-Human-Interaction (HHI) with a specific focus on maintaining trust in the system. This taxonomy ranges from current models of apology to the newly integrated compensation area via a range of case studies specifically developed to address the rising concerns of unsupervised interactions in the context of Virtual Assistants (VA). Based on preliminary research, the author recommends the integration of reparation strategies as a fundamental variable in the ongoing development of VAs, as this element inserts a sense of balance in terms of vulnerability between users and developers to enhance trust in the interactive process. Present and future work is being dedicated to further understand how different contexts may affect integrity in highly automated virtual assistants.

Keywords: Human factors · Human-systems integration · Systems engineering · Trust · Virtual assistant · Highly automated systems · Autonomy · Automation · Reparation strategies

1 Introduction

Recent developments of machine learning and deep learning are leading the rise of a new type of technology; highly automated systems (HAS). In this context, experts in the field of human factors [1] and data related human factors [2, 3] are calling for the development of tools and strategies to address the implications of autonomy in this type of systems. In this area, Virtual Assistants (VA) such as Google's Duplex are raising concerns due to an extraordinary level of autonomy, fluency and interactivity never seen before.

Literature in the area of automation are calling for the development of reparation strategies [4–6]. These strategies are becoming capital not only to address engagement but to maintain trust in these systems. According to research in the area, VAs need to generate less than 30% of errors, otherwise, the user would stop using them [7–9]. As these systems become more autonomous, ubiquitous and unsupervised, the

T. Ahram et al. (Eds.): IHIET 2019, AISC 1018, pp. 42–46, 2020.
https://doi.org/10.1007/978-3-030-25629-6_7

development of reparation techniques becomes fundamental for the adequate development and integration of these systems in society.

Traditionally, these papers focus on different types of reparations such as apologies or denials and the timing to deliver them. Bansal and Zahedi [10] investigated how trust may be rebuilt after it is violated by negative events in data privacy, including the efficacy of the three most used response types—apology, denial and no response. After conducting controlled experiments their results showed that apology emerged as a universally effective response, although its reparative power was far less effective in unauthorised sharing than in hacking. Denial emerged as a complex response and as a very negative approach. Finally, they also reported that is critical to investigate the typology of violation events.

Their research was groundbreaking, however, it was based on current models of automated VAs which are equipped with the capacity of responding to queries. However, with the emergence of highly autonomous systems such as *Duplex* (capable of getting the initiative of the interaction and establishing and maintaining conversations) and recent patents by Amazon to transform the VA into a medical adviser, it seems that reparation strategies around apology become limited in scope. In this paper the authors mind this evolution and propose a human centred approach aimed at ensuring that these highly automated interactions remain focused on the user's interests and protection. In this scenario, the authors have structured a scale and integrated a gradation of compensation levels to test whether they could account for the type of interactions [3] emerging from highly automated virtual assistants.

2 Method

Research into the area of automation present levels as a tool to address trust in automated systems. In this context gradient-base models of approximation have been embodied through the concept of scales or Level of trust (LoT). This approach of different levels of automation has been persistent in the automation literature since its introduction by Sheridan and Verplanck [11]. Levels of automation (LoA) is acknowledged by Kaber as a fundamental design characteristic that determines the ability of operators to provide effective oversight and interaction with system autonomy [12]. According to Endsley, although Levels present a simplification of reality, they provide a system by which different stakeholders understand the full scope of the system at hand [13]. This method has proven successful in providing a solid foundation to understand automated systems at a deeper level. This is highly relevant when confronting an invisible entity making decisions while working in the background.

Levels aim to improve transparency by simplifying interactions. In this context, transparency refers to the extent to which the actions of the automation are understandable and predictable [13]. According to research in the area, automated systems which clarify their reasoning are more likely to be trusted [14–16].

In this context, a multi-level taxonomy of levels of reparation specifically designed to address the increasing autonomy of highly automated virtual assistants was designed by the lead author. It integrates a gradient spectrum ranging from no apology to high compensation. It is structured in seven distinctive levels organised in three main areas:

no apology (Level 1), a triple gradient around apology (Level 2, 3 and 4), and a triple gradient around compensation (Level 5, 6 and 7) (Table 1).

Table 1. Levels of reparation.

Levels	Subject	Explanation
Level 1	No apology	*The company who owns the platform*
Level 2	Basic apology	*The designer who designed the action*
Level 3	Generic apology	*The algorithm performing the action*
Level 4	Public apology	*The user performing the action*
Level 5	Low compensation	*Between 0$ and 100000$*
Level 6	Medium compensation	*Between 100000$ and 1 Million $*
Level 7	High compensation	*+ 1 Million $*

3 Discussion

Although the responsibility to design the scale remains in the designer, Kaber calls for empirical studies to address Level of Automation (LoA) [10]. Due to the highly contextual nature of VAs, a co-design workshop with students from the Royal College of Art underpinned. On one hand, four highly sensitives areas where high-level automated VAs may impact users significantly; health and wellbeing, identity, economically related activities and social interactions. On the other hand, four major unintended consequences; unhappy services, wrong predictions, unintended loses related to the service and an action unexpectedly ending violently.

From the areas aforementioned and based on demos, patents and prototypes, eight case studies were built to address different contexts and unintended consequences. Two cases addressed each sensitive area ranging from low to high impact. Then, a survey was designed to establish whether the proposed levels of reparation in highly automated virtual assistants were sufficient to address all the spectrum.

To test the scale, the main technique consisted on integrating *an other* tab in each case. This space allowed the participant to propose a new level or area missing, questioning the existing scale in the process. Participants engaged with the other tab though the survey at different points.

50 participant, 21 men, 27 women and 2 who didn't want to identify themselves, from 14 different countries with an age range between 18–67 years old from different professions have undertaken the survey (Table 2).

In average, 48,75% of participants found that no reparation is the best option when the system generate an unintended consequence in highly sensitive areas. Thus, placing the responsibility in the user. This result was unexpected as the initiative of the action was placed in the system. 23.25% of participants would accept some sort of apology. Finally, 23.00% in average would demand some sort of compensation to repair trust in

Table 2. Survey results.

	Unhappy service medicine	Unhappy service Newspaper	Ends in violence addiction	Ends in violence raped	Wrong prediction sexuality	Wrong prediction jailed	Loses money	Loses job	Total
Level 1 No reparation	36%	48%	56%	64%	46%	56%	40%	44%	48.75%
Level 2 Basic apology	10%	8%	10%	6%	10%	4%	4%	6%	7.25%
Level 3 pers. Personal apology	22%	12%	2%	0%	24%	2%	2%	6%	8.75%
Level 4 Public apology	6%	20%	6%	4%	4%	4%	6%	8%	7.25%
Level 5 low compensation	6%	2%	4%	4%	2%	0%	10%	4%	4.00%
Level 6 medium compensation	6%	0%	10%	2%	10%	8%	14%	18%	8.50%
Level 7 full compensation	4%	6%	10%	12%	2%	20%	20%	10%	10.50%
Other	10%	4%	2%	8%	2%	6%	4%	4%	5.00%

the system. If we combine reparation strategies (apology and compensation) a total of 46.25% of participants would request them to keep using the system. Other elements such as third-parties were not present in the other tab. Responses in this area demanded combinations of apologies and compensation to repair trust in the system. None of the participants demanded a new level.

4 Conclusion

The survey aimed to understand whether or not contexts and actions affected the level of reparation. They partially determine the level of reparation, however, they did not play a role in determining the spectrum. A generic granular scale of 7 levels covering from no reparation to high compensation would be capable of addressing different contexts and actions in highly automated virtual assistants.

From the survey conducted, contexts (highly sensitive areas) and actions (unintended consequences) play a role in determining user engagement. The 50/50 split presented by this research presents an empirical need for approaching the design of these system equally from a preventive *a priori* strategies to reparative *a posteriori* strategies. Therefore, inserting the reparation variable in the design process is as important as preventing strategies for the correct integration of Highly Automated Virtual Assistants in society.

Based on the results, the author recommends the integration of reparation strategies as a fundamental variable in the ongoing development of virtual assistants, as this element inserts a sense of balance in terms of vulnerability between users and developers enhancing trust in the interactive process.

References

1. Hancock, P.A.: Imposing limits on autonomous systems. Ergonomics **60**(2), 284–291 (2017). https://doi.org/10.1080/00140139.2016.1190035
2. Wang, S.J., Moriarty, P.: Big Data for Urban Sustainability. Springer (2018)
3. Wang, S.J.: Fields Interaction Design (FID): The Answer to Ubiquitous Computing-Supported Environments in the Post-Information Age. Homa & Sekey Books, Paramus (2013)
4. Bottom, W.P., Gibson, K., Daniels, S.E., Murnighan, J.K.: When talk is not cheap: substantive penance and expressions of intent in rebuilding cooperation. Organ. Sci. **13**(5), 497–513 (2002)
5. Kim, P.H., Ferrin, D.L., Cooper, C.D., Dirks, K.T.: Removing the shadow of suspicion: the effects of apology versus denial for repairing competence-versus integrity-based trust violations. J. Appl. Psychol. **89**(1), 104 (2004)
6. Kohn, S.C., Quinn, D., Pak, R., de Visser, E.J., Shaw, T.H.: Trust repair strategies with self-driving vehicles: an exploratory study. Proc. Hum. Factors Ergon. Soc. Annu. Meet. **62**(1), 1108–1112 (2018). https://doi.org/10.1177/1541931218621254
7. Parasuraman, R., Sheridan, T.B., Wickens, C.D.: A model for types and levels of human interaction with automation. IEEE Trans. Syst. Man Cybern. A Syst. Hum. **30,** 286–297 (2000)
8. Wickens, C.D., Dixon, S.R.: The benefits of imperfect diagnostic automation: a synthesis of the literature. Theor. Issues Ergon. Sci. **8**, 201–212 (2007)
9. Wang, L., Jamieson, G.A., Hollands, J.G.: Trust and reliance on an automated combat identification system. Hum. Factors **51**, 281–291 (2009)
10. Bansal, G., Zahedi, F.M.: Trust violation and repair: The information privacy perspective. Decis. Support. Syst. **71**(2015), 62–77 (2015)
11. Sheridan, T.B., Verplank, W.L.: Human and Computer Control of Undersea Teleoperators. Defense Technical Information Center, Fort Belvoir, VA (1978). https://doi.org/10.21236/ADA057655
12. Kaber, D.B.: Issues in human-automation interaction modeling: presumptive aspects of frameworks of types and levels of automation. J. Cogn. Eng. Decis. Mak. **12**(1), 7–24 (2018). https://doi.org/10.1177/1555343417737203
13. Endsley, M.R.: From here to autonomy: lessons learned from human–automation research. Hum. Factors: J. Hum. Factors Ergon. Soc. **59**, 5–27 (2017). https://doi.org/10.1177/0018720816681350
14. Simpson, A., Brander, G.N., Portsdown, D.R.A.: Seaworthy trust: confidence in automated data fusion. In: Taylor, R.M. Reising, J. (eds.) The Human-Electronic Crew: can we Trust the Team, pp. 77–81. Defence Research Academy, Hampshire, UK (1995). http://www.dtic.mil/dtic/tr/fulltext/u2/a308589.pdf
15. Hoff, K.A., Bashir, M.: Trust in automation: integrating empirical evidence on factors that influence trust. Hum. Factors: J. Hum. Factors Ergon. Soc. **57**, 407–434 (2015)
16. Galdon, F., Wang, S.J. (2019). Designing trust in highly automated virtual assistants: a taxonomy of levels of autonomy. In: International Conference on Industry 4.0 and Artificial Intelligence Technologies. Cambridge, UK. ISBN: 978-1-912532-07-0

Ethics in Designing Intelligent Systems

Pertti Saariluoma[1(✉)] and Jaana Leikas[2]

[1] University of Jyväskylä,
Box 35, Mattilanniemi 3, 40014 Jyväskylä, Finland
ps@jyu.fi

[2] VTT Technical Research Centre of Finland Ltd.,
Visiokatu 4, 33101 Tampere, Finland

Abstract. The idea of Hume's guillotine contains the argument that one cannot derive values from facts. As intelligent systems operate with facts, Hume's famous dilemma seems to contradict the very idea of being able to create ethical intelligent systems. In a closer look, ethics is a system of rules guiding actions. Actions always have factual or cognitive aspects, as well as evaluative or emotional aspects. Therefore, Hume's juxtaposition of facts and norms is not well-founded. Instead of separating the facts and norms it should rather ask what kinds of facts are associated to what kinds of norms. Consequently, Hume's guillotine sets no limits in processing ethical information, as one can combine facts and values while constructing information processes. However, intelligent machines cannot process ethical information independently of the human mind, as one cannot discuss 'relevance' in any formal language. Intelligent systems can be given descriptions of ethical situations and related norms, but machines cannot initiate ethical rules themselves.

Keywords: Ethics · Hume's guillotine · Appraisal · Designing intelligent systems · The problem of relevance

1 Introduction

Human research is receiving an increasingly important position in technology desing discourses. Intelligent machines are replacing people in tasks which have traditionally been carried out by humans [1]. Therefore, it is expected that intelligent machines act and think like people, or at least, be able to reach the same or a higher level of performance when carrying out the tasks. To reach this goal, it is necessary to keep in mind that practical human actions have ethical dimensions. A relevant question is how machines can follow the ethical aspects of human actions.

The increasing performance capabilities of intelligent machines justify why the ethical and juridical problems associated to intelligent systems deserve serious attention [2]. An uncontrolled transition to AI society may have numerous risks. An overuse or misuse of AI in the society may cause e.g., misaligned incentives, greed and malicious intent, unequal distributions of costs and benefits, social disintegration, violation of human rights, or disruption of the job market and redundancy [3]. In addition, the underuse of AI technologies may cause risks, such as heavy-handed or misconceived regulations, under-investment or public backlash, and thus, a lack of trust in public

T. Ahram et al. (Eds.): IHIET 2019, AISC 1018, pp. 47–52, 2020.
https://doi.org/10.1007/978-3-030-25629-6_8

authority and resistance to change. This is why the ethics of intelligent technologies has become a vital issue [1, 4].

The basic model of intelligent technologies is the Turing machine, as it can carry out actions typical to people [5]. Turing argued that computers could think like people [6]. Though he did not explicitly focus on the problems of ethical thinking, it makes sense to ponder on whether intelligent systems could be able to reflect ethical issues the way human beings do. If they cannot think ethically, it is impossible to imagine machines with the human capability to think.

From the human point of view, ethics concerns the content and quality of human actions [7]. Ethics provides concepts, questions, norms and discourses about how some actions should be carried out with regard to ethical thinking. Two important challenges arise here: (1) Can facts-processing machines process values? and (2) Can machines know what is ethically relevant?

The difference between facts and values has been central in ethics. If we know facts, can we derive values from facts? Can the knowledge of 'is' lead to the knowledge of 'ought-to'? It is well-known that smoking causes cancer and other illnesses, but does this fact really mean that one should not smoke? The problem of the relations between facts and values is called Hume's guillotine. Hume was the first to argue that one cannot derive 'ought from 'is', that is, values cannot be derived from facts. Facts and values are just two different types of information, which cannot be linked to each other. Similarly, to Hume, G.E. Moore argued that it is a naturalist fallacy to think that natural laws and ethical principles represent the same kind of knowledge [8]. Further, one can ask if machines can also discriminate relevant values from irrelevant data.

Intelligent machines should solve these fundamental problems. Computers and intelligent systems may operate on factual information having truth-values, but does it mean that they are able to process ethical information? What does it actually mean to have ethical information processing systems?

2 Ethics and Emotions

Factual information can be true or false. It has a binary truth-value. However, ethical information is different. It is more or less moral or justified. Factual information is about how things are, whereas values express how things should be. Facts can be compared with their references in order to define their truth-value. However, one cannot determine the ethical value of information in this manner. Thus, it is essential to study the grounds of ethical information.

The key concept in ethics is action. Ethics is a system of principles, which are guiding human actions. Actions are products of human mind, A major division in understanding ethics is to separate cognitive information processing from dynamic ones or from emotions [9].

Cognitive processes such as perception, attention, memory language and thinking processes are mainly factual information, which describe what people do, and what the situation is like. Emotions are an independent information processing system, and despite many integrating connections, emotions are neutrally and functionally different from cognitions [10]. Cognitive information processes construct factual contents in mental representations, while emotions are decisive in evaluating the value of things to people [10, 11]. For example, cognitive processes tell a person that there is a bear nearby, but emotions tell that the situation is dangerous. Thus, cognitive and emotional systems have different roles in processing facts and values.

Thanks to their evaluative functions, emotions form the fundament of ethical information processes. They tell that some situations and actions are unpleasant, and some others are pleasant. They tell what kinds of situations are worth aspiring for and what situations should be avoided. Cognitions tell what the actions and situations are like.

From a modern psychological point of view, it seems, thus, that emotional valence, i.e., positivity or negativity of emotions, is crucial in evaluating the pleasantness and unpleasantness of situations. Consequently, emotional experiences pave the way to the preliminary grounds to ethics, the idea of which has been noticed in intuitionist, emotionalist and utilitarian schools of ethics [6, 7]. In addition to emotional experience, it is essential to consider the integration of cognition and emotions in human action control. This key process is called appraisal [12].

3 Appraisal, Experience and Discourse in Ethics

The fact that ethical evaluation of the actions begins with the emotional experiences associated to these actions and their outcomes does not mean that ethical analysis should result in emotional analysis. Emotions are to some degree like observations: they are experiences. In appraisal, human mind unifies emotional experience with a cognitive analysis of situations.

Human actions are controlled by mental representations. Mental representations are the "programs" in mind, which tell the human body what to do. The cognitive system makes it possible for the person to act rationally, to register what is happening, what has happened, what can happen and how it would be possible to make things happen. Emotions define the value of those issues.

Cognition and emotions are intimately linked in human action control. One cannot really understand human actions unless one has encoded and represented actions and the related contexts both cognitively and emotionally. Emotions without cognition are empty and cognitions without emotions do not have value.

Appraisal is a core process in human mentality. Primary appraisal is a subconscious process [13, 14]. Emotions are integrated to cognitions before people are conscious of them. However, appraisal also operates on a conscious level. An example of secondary appraisal is feeling good with another person for a lifetime.

Appraisal provides people with representations unifying cognitive and emotional aspects of the situation they operate. It provides the basics for an ethical experience of any situation. The human mind gradually unifies individual experiences into ethical stands of the individual. Cognitive analysis of situations is integrated with emotional evaluations and thus people can consider a specific situation as negative and some other situations as positive in an ethical sense. Finally, the ethical conceptions of individuals are unified into social conceptions.

Ethics can be seen to originate from the positive and negative experiences of individuals. The pursuit to moral good means the pursuit to positive experiences and feelings. Appraisal associates an individual's positive and negative experiences to a cognitive analysis of moral situations [12]. Normal human generalisation mechanisms enable people to have moral representations. The social analysis of individuals' moral representations and the communication between people creates moral discourse [14].

Moral discourses are dynamical. People recognise tacit pieces of moral knowledge, arguments, hidden agendas and other presuppositions in prevailing social situations. Old ideas are critically revised, and what used to be important will become past [14]. Present and future shall revise old norms. For example, many traditional moral norms have changed within a hundred years. The traditional ways of experience have been replaced by new ones, and what has been unpleasant or disgusting in past may become a new norm in the future.

Social discourse is the mechanisms which construct ethical norms. Owing to the industrial revolution, people have moved from the countryside to cities, and along with this change many earlier ethical norms have altered. Technology has had many functions in this process. Technologies enable people to communicate, but they also change the existing forms of life. For example, people have learnt new ways to make their living by means of new technologies in new ways. Since technologies have strong influence on how people live, it is obvious that new technologies create new ethical experiences, as well. These experiences in turn activate new social discourses. At the same time, new possibilities and new threats are created. The rise of emerging technologies, especially the increased performance capacities of technical artefacts makes it necessary to consider ethics from a new angle and to develop special codes of ethics for emerging new technologies.

Hume's guillotine has one special presupposition. It juxtaposes reason and emotion, that is, cognition and emotion. Respectively, Hume could have argued that facts and values are different and separated issues in ethics. However, in human actions, facts and values are always unified. One cannot have actions without associated values and facts. Emotions provide the value and cognitions with the contents of ethical analysis. Thus, values are not derivative from facts, but a factual analysis of a situation has its emotional aspects. For this reason, ethics has two aspects: factual or cognitive, and emotional or evaluative. Individual thinking unifies the experiences of individuals with ethical experiences with cognitive and emotional dimensions. Ethical discourse creates social norms on the basis of these experiences.

Finally, we argue that Hume's basic question, the Hume's guillotine, is misplaced. Instead of arguing that facts cannot be used in creating values, he should have asked what kinds of facts are associated with what kinds of values. If we proceed with this way of thinking a bit further, and connect it with the present discussion of artificial intelligence, it can be argued that there is no real obstacle to process ethical information by means of machines. Consequently, it can be said that Hume's guillotine is not an obstacle for ethical information processing in machines. However, this does not yet indicate that intelligent systems could process ethical information in he way humans do. This problem is further studied in the following chapter.

4 The Limitations of Intelligent Systems

Research has been increasingly carried out on the possibility of designing ethical systems, which refer to ethical algorithms for e.g., robots and autonomous systems. The ground question here is the ability of intelligent machines to process ethical information in the same way that humans do.

Intelligent machines have some necessary properties. First, they have a set of internal memory states, e.g., tape in a Turing machine, with different combinations of ones and zeros. Second, they have a set of functions, which can manipulate in an orderly manner the memory states. Thus, they have the capacity to manipulate symbols and in this way generate new memory states. They can also modify themselves by the following rules, and thus they have a capacity to learn. However, the formal theory of intelligence has a crucial weakness. It cannot really speak about ethics.

Intelligent machines are designed relying on mathematics and formal theory-languages. They are studied syntactically rather than semantically. The problem is in the power of expression of formal languages. Formal languages are not able to express what is relevant. A good example of the limits of theory languages is the proof that no natural number can express the ratio of the side and diagonal of a square. To solve the problem, it was necessary to find a new theory language – the real number. However, all too seldom, it has been understood that not only natural numbers are limited in their power of expression, but mathematics by itself has its limits in its poser of expressions.

There is no formal way to define why some functions have a relevant form, and why some elements in a set are relevant while the others are irrelevant. This means that issues, which presuppose discussions of what is relevant and what is not are beyond formal theory languages [14]. However, relevance is a key concept of any ethical theory.

There is no mathematical conceptualisation which could express what is right and what is wrong. There are no mathematical arguments which convey why something is justified. For this reason, it is impossible to have formal automata such as Turing machines, which could create ethics independent of human research notions and philosophical concepts. Consequently, the construction of machines with the capacity to process information ethically requires theory languages outside the scope of formal machines or automata.

5 Ethics of Technology Supported Actions

Human life can be seen as a web of actions. People set goals for themselves and pursuit towards their goals. Ethics provides a set of norms that explain the quality of actions, that is, how the actions should be carried out. There is no logical obstacle to unify ethical and emotional evaluations with factual and cognitive analysis of the situation in machines. It is possible, however, to provide intelligent machines with descriptions of factual situations and unify these with ethical norms [15].

However, formal machines are still unable to know what is relevant and what is irrelevant. They can process information states, but one cannot rely on ones and zeros when discussing the issues of right or wrong, good or bad or allowed and forbidden.

Thus, intelligent machines cannot create information independently, without information provided by humans, to construct ethical information processing systems. People always have to provide the information for ethical information processing. People can provide information indirectly by programming suitable learning functions and creating information contents to the systems.

Machines are created to support human actions. However, they cannot know what is relevant and thus they cannot have independent ethics. But machines can help people in ethics in many ways. For example, they can provide information about the consequences of some ethical principles, although they cannot be aware that those principles are ethical.

Programming, which processes ethical information, is the normal use of intelligent machines. Ada Lovelace argued long ago that computers cannot originate anything. They cannot create new ethical rules, because they do not know that the rules are new or that they are ethical [16]. Intelligent machines can generate new rules of ethics, but they cannot know whether these are relevant without people deciding it. Thus, it is possible to have ethical information processing in intelligent machines, but not without human beings to conduct the processes.

References

1. Saariluoma, P.: Four challenges in structuring human-autonomous systems interaction design processes. In: Williams, A.P., Sharre, P. (eds.) Autonomous Systems. NCI, The Hague (2015)
2. Lin, P., Jenkins, R., Abney, K.: Robot Ethics 2.0. Oxford University Press, Oxford (2017)
3. Floridi, L., Cowls, J., Beltrametti, M., Chatila, R., Chazerand, P., Dignum, V., Luetge, C., Madelin, R., Pagallo, U., Rossi, F.: AI4People—an ethical framework for a good AI society. Minds Mach. **28**, 689–707 (2018)
4. Tegemark, M.: Life 3.0. Penguin Books, Harmondsworth (2018)
5. Turing, A.: On computable numbers, with an application to the Entscheidungsproblem. Proc. Lond. Math. Soc. **42**, 230–65 (1936–1937)
6. Turing, A.: Computing Machinery and Intelligence. Mind LIX, 433–60 (1950)
7. Piper, A.: Einfuerung in die Ethik. A. Franke, Tuebingen (2007)
8. Moore, G.E.: Principia ethica. Cambridge University Press, Cambridge (1993)
9. Saariluoma, P., Cañas, J., Leikas, J.: Designing for Life. PalgraveMacmillan, London (2016)
10. Rolls, E.T.: Precis of the brain and emotion. Behav. Brain Sci. **23**, 177–191 (2000)
11. Frijda, N.: The Emotions. Cambridge University Press, Cambridge (1986)
12. Arnold, M.: Emotions and Personality. Columbia University Press, New York (1960)
13. Oatley, K., Keltner, D., Jenkins, J.: Understanding Emotions. Basil Blackwell, Oxford (2007)
14. Habermas, J.: Diskursethik. Surkamp, Frankfurth am Main (2009)
15. Leikas, J., Koivisto, R., Gotcheva, N.: Ethical framework for designing autonomous systems. J. Open Innov.: Technol., Mark., Complex. Special Issue on Technology Driven Innovation, Research Management and Policy Making, **5**, 18 (2019)
16. Saariluoma, P.: Foundational Analysis. Routledge, London (1997)

Implementing Workplace Technologies: A Motivation-Oriented Approach

Yvonne Schmid(✉) and Julia Auburger

University of Regensburg, Universitätsstr. 31, 93053 Regensburg, Germany
{Yvonne.Schmid, Julial.Auburger}@UR.de

Abstract. The accelerating evolution of workplace technologies and employees' changing demands pose an increasing challenge for management to implement technologies and improve the motivation potential of jobs. In this paper, we examine technological opportunities in workplace design based on the Job Characteristics Model. For a holistic understanding, we chose a qualitative approach with interviews and case studies. Our results show various effects of technology application based on employees' perception. Especially the characteristics skill variety and autonomy can be affected by technology selection and workplace design.

Keywords: Workplace technologies · Motivation · Strategic workplace design · Job characteristics model · Virtual and augmented realities · ICT · Mobile devices · Digital workplace · Qualitative research · Case study approach · Qualitative content analysis

1 Introduction

Today's working world is changing fast and continually placing new and complex demands on companies and their employees. These requirements can be met faster and more effectively with the support of new technologies [1]. For example, sophisticated information and communication technologies (ICT), mobile devices, and artificial intelligence (AI) lead to new business models and opportunities for success as a company. However, the use of new technologies offers additional—though still underrated—potential: the possibility to increase employee motivation. According to an Eventboard survey among 1,000 professionals, 38% claim to be motivated by innovative gadgets [2]. This topic is particularly important for younger people in the workforce: The Future Workforce Study 2016 shows that "[n]early half of American Millennials (42%) say they'd likely quit a job if workplace tech didn't meet their standards" [3]. Thus, procuring technologies and designing modern, technologically advanced workplaces should be integrated into the companies' strategies [4–6]. To implement workplace technologies effectively and strategically so as to foster employee motivation, it is necessary to understand the individual needs and motivators. To investigate the potential of new technologies for employee motivation, we use the Job Characteristics model as theoretical basis, as it offers the possibility to connect well-researched theory with new technologies as a new aspect of future work.

T. Ahram et al. (Eds.): IHIET 2019, AISC 1018, pp. 53–58, 2020.
https://doi.org/10.1007/978-3-030-25629-6_9

2 Technologies Influencing Job Characteristics

According to the Job Characteristics Model, specific core job dimensions influence the motivation potential of a job. These core dimensions are skill variety, task identity, task significance, autonomy, and feedback. They influence employee motivation and other personal and work outcomes via three critical psychological states. *Skill variety*, *task identity*, and *task significance* influence the experienced meaningfulness of the work. *Autonomy* influences the experienced responsibility for the outcome of the work, and *feedback* influences the knowledge of the actual results of the work activities [7].

We chose a holistic approach to investigate how modern workplace technologies influence job characteristics and, in turn, employee motivation. We derived the theoretical frameworks and implications from an extensive literature review. Our empirical data stems from fourteen qualitative, semi-structured interviews with professionals and managers, whose expertise lies in implementing information and communication technologies like mobile devices, social platforms as well as augmented and virtual reality applications. To obtain results applicable to different sectors and companies, we acquired a heterogonous pool of experts. We coded the results and inductively assigned them to the factors using a qualitative content analysis [8]. Additionally, we created two case studies on the implementation of such technologies using a triangular approach on diverse data.[1]

In the following section, the results of our study are presented based on the five job characteristics. The findings are clustered according to their influence on the critical psychological states.

2.1 Skill Variety, Task Identity, and Task Significance

Skill Variety. "The degree to which a job requires a variety of different activities in carrying out the work, which involve the use of a number of different skills and talents of the person" [7].

Throughout the last decades, motivational approaches to job design have mainly focused on enrichment practices to enhance skill variety [9]. Yet, it is not only the tasks that define the competencies needed. The implementation of new devices and technologies in the workplace also demands new processes and the skills to handle them [4, 10]. Various research projects examined the question of which skills will be needed in the future [11]. One skill prominently mentioned with regards to new technologies is digital fluency: the ability to choose the appropriate tool depending on the situation and utilize it according to one's needs [12]. Applying these skills can lead to a more diverse and motivating job profile [13]. When interviewed, a sales manager highlighted the potential of mobile devices during clients' appointments. The seamless access to data enables in-depth negotiations without back-office assistants needing to research product specifications and availability.

[1] Part of this data collection was conducted by Elisabeth Sauer and Helen Holland in the context of their respective master thesis at the Department of Innovation and Technology Management at the University of Regensburg.

Yet, too many and too carelessly implemented innovations may lead to overload and a loss of control [14–16]. Advanced data processing and human-centric user interfaces may have the opposite effect. Augmented and virtual reality (AR/VR) applications, voice-activated systems, and virtual personal assistants provide necessary information in a context sensitive manner as well as suggestions for how to solve the problems at hand based on visual and other sensorics information. These simplifications–sometimes even viewed as a return to scientific management or referred to as 'Neo-Taylorism'–cause a loss in skill variety [17–19]. During an interview, a senior manager specializing in research on new technologies and labor markets described the trend of digital technologies substituting human tasks. She estimated that currently about 90% of the implementations follow such a cost-saving paradigm and only 10% pursue the goal of creating value-adding processes through human-machine collaboration.

Task Identity. "The degree to which the job requires completion of a 'whole' and identifiable piece of work; that is, doing a job from beginning to end with a visible outcome" [7].

Technology can have a twofold influence on Task Identity. First, ICT provide transparency. It becomes easier for employees to track the product (or "piece of work") and identify their own contribution. Second, technology can change the processes and tasks altogether. Interviewees describe the application of AR/VR as a seamless experience, enabling them to work on a greater range within the processes while additional information is provided automatically [17]. The previous example with the sales manager highlights this aspect. Data access enabled him to provide all services to his client without having to integrate other colleagues into the process.

Task Significance. "The degree to which the job has a substantial impact on the lives or work of other people, whether in the immediate organization or in the external environment" [7].

Again, technologies do not necessarily change the impact a person has directly. Yet, modern ICT creates visibility and transparency. This changes how the significance for others can be perceived by a person.

2.2 Autonomy

"The degree to which the job provides substantial freedom, independence, and discretion to the individual in scheduling the work and in determining the procedures to be used in carrying it out" [7].

The use of mobile devices and ICT applications enables tele-working, hoteling, and other location independent workplace concepts. Having the choice of where to work—and in some cases even when to work—provides autonomy to employees [20]. Moreover, the access to information enables staff to work independently of their offices and colleagues [21, 22]. Yet, this improved access to information may also lead to decreasing autonomy. Management does not necessarily have to delegate decisions when the possible alternatives can be accessed anytime and anywhere. An international corporation provided us with a case highlighting this aspect. After the company introduced a new digital travel-booking system that provides all time and paperless access to bookings and approval procedures for sales and procurement staff, adoption rates remained below expectations. Investigations provided an explanation: team assistants and administrative personnel were still using the outdated processes to prevent their manager from handling the bookings alone for fear of being substituted.

These opportunities for automatized processes are widespread: One VR designer explained throughout the interview that the glasses provide information on process relevant tasks and next steps for the user. Particularly in shop floor use-cases, this leads to practically remote-controlled employees.

2.3 Feedback

"The degree to which carrying out the work activities required by the job results in the individual obtaining direct and clear information about the effectiveness of his or her performance" [7].

While ICT can enhance information flow and, therefore, feedback from the job and from others, the content of feedback still comes from management and colleagues [17]. Gamification elements in particular enhance the social exchange and instant feedback through competitive situations, awards, or team achievements [23]. An IT company provided a vivid case on how to facilitate feedback with ICT: The employees were asked to give general feedback once a week through a mobile app. They clicked on a smiley or a frowney[2] and had the option of adding a comment with max. 140 characters anonymously. These comments could be rated by others. The highest ranked comments were addressed by management towards staff every Friday.

Again, this information transparency can have its downsides: mobile devices and wearables can be used as monitoring/tracking devices [21]. Being always on causes a perceived lack of control, inter-role conflicts as well as physical effects like stress [24]. A manager described his experiences during an interview: "I feel permanently stressed [...] having the systems and the smartphone available [...] you keep looking at it all the time—it is awful!" [25].

3 Conclusion

While some effects of technologies on the job characteristics seemed obvious initially, interviewees provided us different and sometimes contradicting perceptions. Our interviews showed that new technologies influence all five job dimensions are, but skill variety and autonomy to be the most conspicuous and challenging characteristics. Our results suggest that these dimensions should be addressed when companies introduce new technologies in workplaces. Also, we found another explanatory approach for different perceptions besides the various individual needs:

Modern technologies offer great potential for new processes and interactions. Implementing a new tool has various consequences for other organizational features. How these innovations are perceived depends on aspects such as company culture,

[2] A frowny is a sad-faced emoticon. In this context, it is used to express negative emotions (in contrast to a smiley).

leadership style, individual skills, etc. The perception of technologies determines whether employees sense opportunities or threats in these innovations [15]. Other factors the interview results provided refer to the characteristics of the technologies themselves. The VR/AR experts in particular highlighted the increasing efficiency through an intuitive and hands-free handling of the technology. Users claimed they have fun at work with these gadgets as they can be handled intuitively [17]. Our results also highlight the benefits of new technologies in existing processes. The seamless access to information anytime and anywhere was praised by sales managers and service technicians. Those categories can be associated with factors identified by the Technology Acceptance Model and its successors: 'Perceived Ease of Use' and 'Perceived Usefulness' [26].

Implementing new structures in a holistic manner is more important than ever before. Implications for companies can already be derived from these first qualitative results. For managers in particular, the awareness of company culture and the needs of their employees determines strategic decisions on workplace design and technologies. In addition, our contribution plants the seeds for a fruitful future research area as these results can be further strengthened through quantitative studies with employees to validate the qualitative findings. The technologies themselves can make a big difference, but the way they are implemented can make an even bigger one.

Acknowledgments. We wish to thank various people for their contribution to this project; Elisabeth Sauer, Helen Holland, and Marija Durkovic, for their valuable support on collecting and interpreting data for this project. Special thanks should be given to Prof. Dr. Michael Dowling and Prof. Dr. Roland Helm, our research project supervisors for their professional guidance and valuable support and to Suzanne Weinberger for her useful and constructive recommendations on this project.

References

1. Brynjolfsson, E., McAfee, A.: The Second Machine Age: Work, Progress, and Prosperity in a Time of Brilliant Technologies. Norton & Company, New York (2016)
2. Eventboard.io: You Can't Buy Workplace Happiness. But Tech Helps Teem, 9 Feb 2019. http://pages.teem.com/rs/379-VML-039/images/Workplace-Happiness-Infographic-600px.jpg
3. Dell Technologies, Intel: Future Workforce Study (2016)
4. Chan, J.K., Beckman, S.L., Lawrence, P.G.: Workplace design: a new managerial imperative. Calif. Manage. Rev. **49**(2), 6–22 (2007)
5. Kampschroer, K., Heerwagen, J.H.: The strategic workplace: development and evaluation. Build Res. Inf. **33**(4), 326–337 (2005)
6. Vischer, J.C.: The Concept of Workplace Performance and its Value to Managers. Calif. Manag. Rev. **49**(2), 62–79 (2007)
7. Hackman, R.J., Oldham, G.R.: Motivation through the design of work: test of a theory. Organ. Behav. Hum. Perform. **16**(2), 250–279 (1976)
8. Mayring, P.: Qualitative Inhaltsanalyse. Grundlagen und Techniken. Beltz, Weinheim (2010)

9. Oldham, G.R., Hackman, J.R.: Not what it was and not what it will be: the future of job design research. J. Organ. Behav. **31**(2–3), 463–479 (2010)
10. Colbert, A., Yee, N., George, G.: The digital workforce and the workplace of the future. Acad. Manag. J. **59**(3), 731–739 (2016)
11. Bughin, J., Hazan, E., Lund, S., Dahlström, P., Wiesinger, A., Subramaniam, A.: Skillshift. Automation and the future of the workforce (May 2018)
12. Wang, R., Wiesemes, R., Gibbons, C.: Developing digital fluency through ubiquitous mobile devices: findings from a small-scale study. Comput. Educ. **58**(1), 570–578 (2012)
13. Morgeson, F.P., Campion, M.A.: Work Design, pp. 423–452. Wiley, Hoboken, New Jersey (2003)
14. Demerouti, E., Bakker, A.B.: The job demands–resources model. Challenges for future research. J. Ind. Psychol. **37**(2) (2011)
15. Bala, H., Venkatesh, V.: Changes in employees job characteristics during an enterprise system implementation: a latent growth modeling perspective. MIS Quart. **37**(4), 1113–1140 (2013)
16. Boxall, P., Macky, K.: Research and theory on high-performance work systems: progressing the high-involvement stream. Hum. Resour. Manag. J. **19**(1), 3–23 (2009)
17. Sauer, E.S.: Auswirkungen neuer Technologien am Arbeitsplatz auf die Motivation von Mitarbeitern am Beispiel von Augmented and Virtual Reality, Regensburg (2019)
18. Hannola, L., Richter, A., Richter, S., Stocker, A.: Empowering production workers with digitally facilitated knowledge processes – a conceptual framework. Int. J. Prod. Res. **56**(14), 4729–4743 (2018)
19. Niepce, W., Molleman, E.: Work design issues in lean production from a sociotechnical systems perspective: neo-taylorism or the next step in sociotechnical design? Hum. Relat. **51**(3), 259–287 (1998)
20. Nicklin, J.M., Cerasoli, C.P., Dydyn, K.L.: Telecommuting: What? Why? When? and How? pp. 41–70. Springer, Singapore (2016)
21. Martin, L.: Do Innovative work practices and use of information and communication technologies motivate employees? Ind. Relat. **56**(2), 263–292 (2017)
22. Karanika-Murray, M., Michaelides, G.: Workplace design. JOEPP **2**(3), 224–243 (2015)
23. Liu, M., Huang, Y., Zhang, D.: Gamification's impact on manufacturing: enhancing job motivation, satisfaction and operational performance with smartphone-based gamified job design. Hum. Factor Ergon Man **28**(1), 38–51 (2018)
24. Bader, V., Kaiser, S.: Autonomy and control? how heterogeneous sociomaterial assemblages explain paradoxical rationalities in the digital workplace. Manag. Rev. **28**(3), 338–358 (2017)
25. Interview in Holland, H.J.: Auswirkungen des steigenden Einsatzes von mobilen Technologien am Arbeitsplatz auf die Mitarbeitermotivation, Regensburg (2019)
26. Davis, F.D., Bagozzi, R.P., Warshaw, P.R.: User acceptance of computer technology: a comparison of two theoretical models. Manag. Sci. **35**(8), 982–1003 (1989)

'3DPix' - Design Thinking for Desktop Personal 3D-Printers–A Project Oriented Training Method

Zuk N. Turbovich(✉) and Iko Avital

Department of Mechanical Engineering,
SCE–Shamoon College of Engineering, Beer-Sheva, Israel
{zuktu, ikoav}@sce.ac.il

Abstract. This paper introduces '3DPix' a new Project Oriented training method that integrates and interacts between personal 3D printer and design thinking processes, when using grafting method as a creative platform for innovative product design. The integration of personal 3D orienting praxis with Insertix model enrich ideation processes with varied alternatives. Through detailed prototype designer can examine well function and form in his output along creative process. 3DPix offers hundreds by hundreds of "jumping together" stimulus that helps ideates from human-center design and advance technology gap by embracing personal and cultural perspectives as well.

Keywords: 3D training · Creative modeling · Design thinking

1 Introduction

In recent years desktop personal 3D printers (P3DP) have become accessible and affordable for the general public. Even though there is no standard that defines what type of 3D printers can be considered as desktop P3DPs, and in particular that are suitable for personal environment, there is a wide range of relatively inexpensive desktop P3DPs which can be found for sale over the Internet. According to "Wohlers" report the definition for desktop 3DP is: "An additive manufacturing (AM) systems that sell for less than $5,000" [1]. Under this independent definition, approximately 530 K of this type of 3DPs have been sold globally during 2017. An impressive data in comparison to 2007, where only 66 desktop 3DPs were sold.

The possibility that anyone who wishes, consumers and designers, can own a desktop P3DP is already here, and it brings with it many new opportunities. Out of the perspective of the product designers (PD), the proximity to the mean of the manufacturing, which is also the mean that produces prototypes along the Development Process, is significantly shortening the period of today processes and enables to dedicate time for the empowerment of the 'What', and the 'How' pre-design strategy. Moreover, the ability to produce alternatives, and "changes of product designs without cost penalty in manufacturing" [2] can lead to a flexible thinking, and innovative designs.

T. Ahram et al. (Eds.): IHIET 2019, AISC 1018, pp. 59–65, 2020.
https://doi.org/10.1007/978-3-030-25629-6_10

Out of the perspectives of all parties, the value of mass-customization (MC), i.e. that the same large number of customers can be reached as in mass markets of the industrial economy, and simultaneously treated individually as in the customized market of pre-industrial economies [3], can be applied much more cheap and easily. Therefore, it requires from the PD's to flex their creative thinking skills, and consider how to get unique advantages, and benefits in product design, according to the available options in the desktop P3DP market. Since the idea of MC was presented, many researchers and industries investigated and developed models and processes that enable MC in products under certain conditions, e.g. the automotive industry [4], Nike ID program [5], and the very interesting jewelry studio "Nervous System" (https://n-e-r-v-o-u-s.com/), which offers few open-architecture customized jewelry through a unique cybernetic dynamic platform, and by using 3DPs. "Nervous System" demonstrates how can cybernetic platform hand-with-hand with 3DPs can produce benefits both for the customer and designers. From the business perspective, there is an ability to produce "custom products at relatively low prices, and with low inventory risk" [6], and from the customer perspective, there is an option to buy a customized product at relatively low price, and to undergo a unique buying experience with significant control over the final design and the price. The value chain that links between designers and consumers becomes much shorter, and in general, the connection between designers and consumers becomes a direct one, with one well known intermediate, the Internet.

2 3DPix: Behind the Method

One of the powerful motors for innovation lies on Design Education that encourages synergy between two main processes: one, creative thinking that produces many conceptual alternatives, and the second is the design flexibility of technological knowledge accumulated in the design process. Out of this perspective, our Project Oriented (PO) training method integrates two theoretical branches:

1. Design methodology for PD in the context of desktop P3DPs [7] – The branch that directs how to strategically engage with the desktop P3DPs market.
2. 'Insertix' – A creative thinking generator of design alternative [8]. 'Insertix' is a method the links together Design and Graftage to a Consilience method. Graftage is a process of making a graft in horticulture, the technique in which the separate parts of some plants are caused to grow together as one plant: hook, punch, slice, wrap, bunch, and mix techniques. Graftage is used to produce such novelty plants in basic technique, when a plant is selected for its roots, the other plant is selected for its stems, leaves, flowers, or fruits and is contains the desired genes to be supplicated in future production.

The general structure of 3DPix training method was constructed out of combination of conservative and up-to-date perceptions. The brief of the course/workshop (C/W) is supposed to be formulated from the integration and interaction of these two branches.

2.1 Brief and Re-brief

Every development process begins with identifying potential solutions that result in an official, or an unofficial freeform design-brief. Since our training method focuses on desktop P3DPs, the tutor, and the students/designers (S/D) must be aware to the implications of the project theme. The theme can be both specific/generic, and Wide/narrow (Table 1), and it must be determined based on 2 considerations.

Table 1. Examples for project themes.

	Project theme	
	Generic	*Specific*
Wide	Generic-wide Examples: "babies", "Light", or any philosophical statement"	Specific-wide Examples: "Toys for babies", "lighting fixtures for hotel lobby", or any product for defined end-user/environment
Narrow	Generic-narrow Examples: "Keep my baby busy", "Lighting fixtures", or any generic theme	Specific-narrow Examples: "Completing forms toy for babies", "Desk lamp", or any specific product for a defined environment

The first 3DPix re-brief consideration relates to the type of the product in context of the desktop P3DPs market, based on the taxonomy matrix that classifies types of products in the desktop P3DPs market [9]. A revised pedagogical version of the taxonomy matrix (Table 2) presents the available options, which should be determined as part of the formulation of the design-brief. For instance, if the theme of the of the C/W is lighting fixtures, so the tutor must be aware that this subject relates to the section of products that depend on complementary parts/components, e.g. lighting bulb socket, cable and switch, etc., and these complementary components must be accessible for the S/D, as well as for potential consumers.

The second consideration relates to the field of study of the students/field of creation of the designers. In case the theme of the C/W belongs to the section of products that depend on complementary components, then the tutor must make sure that these components are accessible to the students/designers, as well as to the potential consumers.

Table 2. Examples for project themes.

		Product dependency on complementary parts/components	
		Independent	Dependent
Architecture of the product	Open	*Modifiable* *Fully 3D-Printable Product*	*Modifiable* *Partially 3D-Printable Product*
	Close	*Inalterable* *Fully 3D-Printable Product*	*Inalterable* *Partially 3D-Printable Product*

Once the theme of the project task has been determined, the story of the brief is required to be completed by the S/D. This 'What' abstractive question (regardless to the specificness of the theme) is recommended to be answered by following the "Insertix Matrix" (Fig. 1). It is important that the ideas for the project will be creative and authentic, and therefore the awareness of the combination of these factors should assist the S/D to come up with ideas as such.

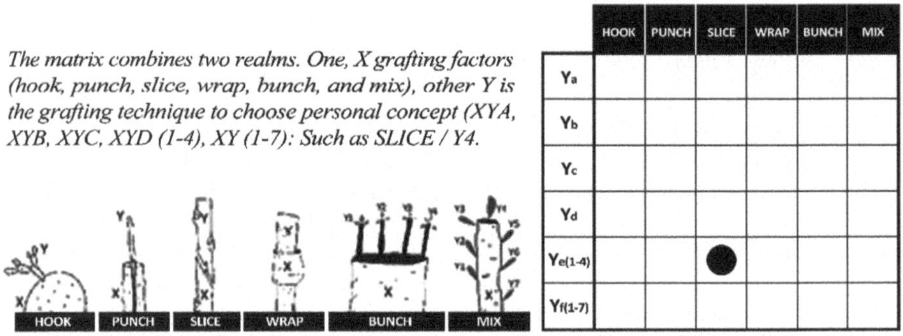

Fig. 1. "Insertix matrix".

2.2 The Development Process

Once the formulation of the brief has been completed, the development process begins. The structural core of the development process of our PBL training method is inspired by a few sources of product design methodologies that define the required phases in the product designing process, and that specify the actions to be taken, from the task to the solution, e.g. French, Pahl & Beitz, VDI 2221 [10], and Baxter's methodology [11]. In context of this paper, there is a suggested design methodology that refers specifically to products intended to be manufactured by desktop P3DP [7], and that is based on examination of few methodologies, inter alia the mentioned above methodologies. The general structure of the suggested methodology (Fig. 2) has an expansion that relates to the characterization of the product, based on the taxonomy matrix the classifies type of products in the desktop P3DPs market (Table 2) as mentioned in context earlier.

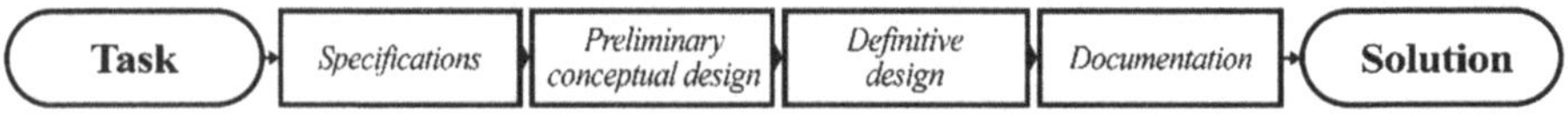

Fig. 2. The general structure of the development process.

The Specification Phase. At this stage, it is important to determine whether the architecture of the product is modifiable or inalterable. This decision affects the design dramatically and should be taken attentionally. If for instance the theme of the project is lighting fixtures, and if the S/D finds benefits in designing an open architecture product, so there must be an awareness that there are certain features in the product that must remain inalterable, otherwise the ability to integrate complementary parts can be affected. There are also cases of fully 3D printable products e.g. rehabilitation devices, which are highly recommended to be modifiable, and most likely that these devices have certain functional features that must remain inalterable so the device will function. This way or another, the S/D must be aware to the following factors and considerations:

1. The effect of the modifications on the functionality.
2. Complementary components integration considerations.
3. How the modifications can be applied, i.e. if it is a matter of scaling only, then every slicing software can apply it easily. If it is a matter of personalizing the product by adding text, then a very few file-sharing websites enable to do online modification as such. If the design is intended to be highly modifiable, same as "Nervous-System" customizable jewelries, then a creative way of how the potential consumer can bring his/her inputs, must be found in principle, or in practical.

More data that needs to be collected at the specification phase regards to the method of operation of the 3DP, the specifications of the 3DP (build volume, X/Y tolerance, Z-layer thickness, and the available materials. Additionally, the specifications should include conventional design considerations, e.g. end user requirements, environmental effects, safety considerations, etc.

The 3DPix Method Process. It is highly important that once the design process begins, participants will get immediate access to a desktop P3DP. We highly recommend starting the design process with hand sketching, as conventionally done, but in parallel to explore the ideas with 3D printed models. Notice that the proximity to the mean of the manufacturing is a key factor, and it is highly important that the S/D feel the advantage of it during the design process. The required time for answering the 'What' question as part of the design-brief, as well as formulating the specifications document cannot be shortened, but the design process can be shortened without quality compromises, and it is must be reflected.

Documentation: Using Wisdom of the Crowd. As part of the evaluation process, next step is to combine conventional academic evaluation methods with evaluation by file-sharing websites users. We recommend that right after the development process ends, the S/D will upload the files to a file-sharing selected website, and get genuine feedback (like, make, share and free comments) from websites users. Therefore, the documentation phase is highly important, since the required documents (not including the files) are mostly marketing oriented. The quality of the pictures, images, and instructions for assembly if necessary, should intrigue users to watch and evaluate the design.

3 The Structure of the Method and Summary

The principle structure of the PBL training method (Fig. 3), based on the theoretical knowledge that was presented, shows the principle creative fluency of the C/W. This principle structure should be adjusted to the amount of time that can be devoted for the training, according to the suggested percentage of time column.

It is a matter of short time until 3D printing will become an inseparable factor from human society, same as the computer, the Internet, the smartphone and the tablet. For the industry and professional product designers & engineers, 3D printing has become already an inseparable part of the design and manufacturing processes, and we strongly believe that our PBL training method will advance the 3D printing market in context of personal use, which is currently the weakest sub-market.

	Tutor	Students/ Designers	% of time	Comments
Pre-training preparations	- Determine the theme of the project - Get the complementary components (in case of partially 3D-printable products)/ instruct the students/ designers where to get/ buy these components. - Schedule setting.	- Get the complementary components (if instructed - in case of partially 3D-printable product).	-	-
Formulation of a design-brief	- Introducing the 'Insertix' method. - Assistance in completing the design-brief.	- Formulate a design-brief.	7.5%	Tutor: Encourage the students/ designers to come-up with authentic ideas by using the 'Insertix' method.
The specification phase	- Introducing the 3D printer, the method of operation and the available materials. - Introducing the taxonomy matrix that classifies types of products in the desktop P3DP market. - Assistance in completing the specifications, and in making a decision regarding the product architecture.	- Take a decision regarding the product architecture (modifiable/ inalterable). - Formulate a specification document.	7.5%	Tutor: make sure that the decision regarding the product architecture does not cause excessive complexity, which will make difficulties in producing a final product at the end of the training.
The development process	- Encourage the students/ designers to engage with the the 3D printer as soon, and as much as possible. - Assistance in the design process.	- Preliminary conceptual design. - Definitive design.	35% 35%	Strive to generate designs that do not require support material.
The Documentation phase	- Assistance in the graphic designing of the marketing page, and the assembly instructions (if necessary). - Writing recommendations for a successful printing.	- Generate high quality renderings of the product. - Generate .stl files. - Prepare marketing page, assembly instructions (if necessary), and write recommendations for a successful printing.	15%	Tutor: show examples of good pages.
Evaluation	- Assistance in uploading the files and the pages to a selected file-sharing website. - Create an evaluation index.	- Upload the files and the pages to the file-sharing website, as instructed by the tutor.	-	We recommend uploading to 'My-mini-factory', or to 'Thingiverse'.

Fig. 3. The principle structure of the training method.

References

1. Wohlers Associates: Wohlers Report 2018. Wohlers Associates Inc., Fort Collins (2018)
2. Weller, C., Kleer, R., Piller, F.T.: Economic implications of 3D printing: market structure models in light of additive manufacturing revisited. Int J. Prod. Ergonomics. **164**, 43–56 (2015)
3. Davis, S.M.: Future Perfect. Addison Wesley, Boston (1987)
4. Alford, D., Sackett, P., Nedler, G.: Mass customization – an automotive perspective. Int J. Prod. Economies. **65**(1), 99–110 (2000)
5. Ramaswamy, V.: CO-creating value through customers' experience: the Nike case. Strat. Leadersh. **36**(5), 9–14 (2008)
6. Berman, B.: 3-D printing: the new industrial revolution. Bus. Horiz. **55**(2), 155–162 (2012)
7. Turbovich, Z.N.: Design Methodology for Product Designer in the Context of Personal 3D-Printing. IIT-Guwahati, North Guwahati (2018)
8. Avital, I., Monga, C.: Insertix: Grafting 'XY' factor in engineering and design creativity. In: Consilience and Innovation, Japan (2014)

9. Turbovich, Z.N., Das, A.K., Avital, I., Mazor, G.: Personal 3D-printing: a remapping of the relationship between product designers, product and users. In: NordDesign2016, pp. 12–21. Design Society, Trondheim (2016)
10. Roozenburg, N., Ekeles, J.: Product Design: Fundamentals and Methods. Wiley, Chichester (1995)
11. Baxter, M.: Product Design: Practical Methods for Systematic Development of New Product. CRC Press, Boca Raton (1995)

Concepts for Improving Employee Qualifications for Resource-Efficient Chipping Production

Leif Goldhahn(✉), Christina Pietschmann, Robert Eckardt, and Sebastian Roch

Faculty Engineering Sciences, InnArbeit – Centre of Innovative Process Planning and Ergonomics, University of Applied Sciences Mittweida, Technikumplatz 17, 09648 Mittweida, Germany
{Goldhahn,Pietschm,Eckardt,Roch}@hs-mittweida.de

Abstract. In the field of parts production of highly stressed components, qualification concepts are absolutely necessary. Process planners, foremen, workers and other actors ought to be sensitized to and purposefully trained in the topic of resource-oriented production. According to the current state and depending on the respective work task, employees should develop and improve their skills and knowledge through motivation, methodological guidance, computer-aided models of selected equipment and manufacturing processes. Within the ESF junior research project "MoQuaRT - models and qualification concepts for resource-efficient parts production" a qualification concept was exemplary developed. In addition to the fundamental possibilities for saving resources, the concept focuses on the topics of energy, material and time resource savings. Among other things, an energetic comparison of different production variants, based on models for the energy demand forecast, is embedded. Thus, this topic makes a significant contribution to saving resources in chipping production.

Keywords: Qualification concepts · Chipping production · Resource-oriented production · Manufacturing process · Knowledge management · Organizational learning

1 Introduction

Current economic developments, new technologies and resource depletion contribute to the increasing awareness of resource savings. Legal restrictions as well as the necessity to reduce process-related energy costs urge the companies to rethink their production [1–3]. Varieties of processes, especially in the field of chipping production, are currently not questioned regarding resources. In the field of aircraft components, for example, components with an extremely high cutting volume of up to 97% are machined. These cause a high loss of material and lengthy production times [4]. For materials with difficult cutting characteristics, the technological conditions for machinability must be established in order to limit tool wear and enhance cutting performance. A conscious selection and a skillful use of tools by choosing more

T. Ahram et al. (Eds.): IHIET 2019, AISC 1018, pp. 66–72, 2020.
https://doi.org/10.1007/978-3-030-25629-6_11

efficient cutting parameters can also reduce the energy demand of the chipping process up to 24% [3, 5]. Rapid product changes together with more complex and flexible work and production systems require new, flexible concepts and strategies in order to advancement and qualification of the employees. Therefore, the employees' lifelong learning is more important than ever [6, 7].

Based on these circumstances, a qualification concept was developed and is depicted in this article. The concept not only discusses the basic possibilities for conserving resources but also, more thoroughly, the issue of energetic, materialistic and temporal savings.

2 Background

2.1 Transfer of Knowledge

Didactics describes the art and science of teaching and learning [8]. With the help of different learning concepts, knowledge is meant to be transferred goal-driven to certain groups of people. Here, the learning environment describes the spatial, temporal and instrumental characteristics of the learning process [9]. The learning process can be supported by different kinds of media, such as the incorporation of videos or interactive elements [10]. There are "active" and "passive" methods to introduce the learner to (new) knowledge. If the learner is directly integrated in the process of knowledge transfer, an active method. A passive method is mentioned, when the knowledge is brought to the learner [11].

2.2 Actual Learning Environment

The *Training Plant 4.0* (see Fig. 1) represents the actual (physically existing) learning environment for the compiled qualification concept. It is composed of a 3-axis-CNC-milling machine, a 2-axis-CNC lathe, a collaborative robot, an automatic high bay warehouse and an automatic belt conveyor system with a by-pass function.

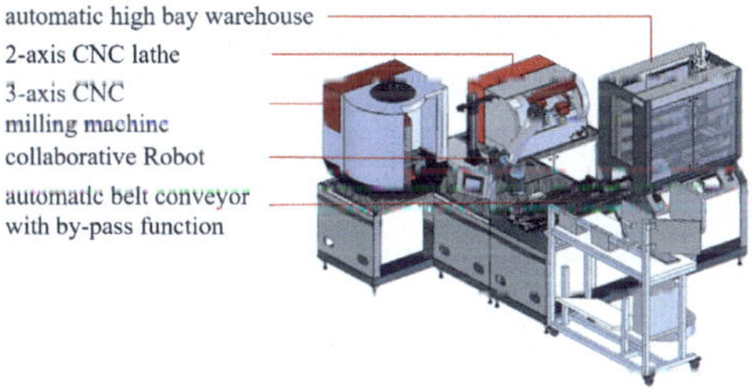

Fig. 1. CAD model of the Training Plant 4.0

2.3 Digital Learning Environment - Learning Platform

A digital learning environment or learning platform enables the knowledge transmission via intranet, internet or mobile applications. The necessary materials for the communication of knowledge are digitally provided. This online learning method is also called e-learning. The greatest advantage of e-learning is that the learner can autonomously decide on his learning rate and learning needs [12]. E-learning scenarios can vary in the amount of online work. The intensity of the online part and the amount of virtualization determine how the attendance and self-study periods are distributed and characterized [13].

2.4 Blended-Learning-Concept

The Blended-Learning-Arrangement is the most used learning approach to support the attendance period. The close correlation between attendance and self-study period is not only an option. It is also a precondition of the next attendance period. The Blended-Learning-Concept serves as the basis for the established qualification concept. The first part of the knowledge transfer takes place during an attendance period. There, the basic approach and learning objectives as well as first foci will be discussed. In the subsequent self-study periods, knowledge should be replicated, deepened and consolidated (online). Virtualization, interactive animations, self-tests and self-study materials support this. The knowledge conveyed online will subsequently be taken up in the next attendance period. Where appropriate, the knowledge will be deepened and further consolidated by means of practical applications [13, 14].

3 Pilot Qualification Concept

3.1 Goal of the Qualification Concept

The skills development of current and future planners is the goal of the qualification concept. By means of a procedure developed based on the *Blended- Learning-Concept*, cognitive abilities, skills and knowledge are conveyed. These contribute to the skills development. This procedure primarily supports a sensitization and motivation of sustainable thinking in the field of chipping production, depending on the already existing skills of the planner.

3.2 Focus of the Qualification Concept

Resource-oriented process planning and the subsequent realization in producing the sample part *Koordinatensystem* (see Fig. 2) make up the focus of the qualification concept [15]. The participants are provided with the task and the reference part. On this basis, the participants are asked to create a work schedule and the NC-program for a sample solution. They have to set up the machinery, record important test parameters and evaluate them. This process takes part under the guidance of an instructor. Thereafter, the participants independently work on an alternative solution. The alternative solution has to be implemented and evaluated now. Very important is the comparison of the alternative solution with the sample solution. The process planning and implementation has to be realized with the aids from the Training Plant 4.0 (see Fig. 1).

3.3 Realization of the Qualification Concept

The developed qualification concept with the sample part is exemplary implemented in a digital learning environment. The digital learning environment is created with the markup language HTML. The structure follows the phases of the Blended-Learning-Concept (compare 2.4). It provides this learning approach with digital documents, media such as videos or pictures as well as exercises (see Fig. 2).

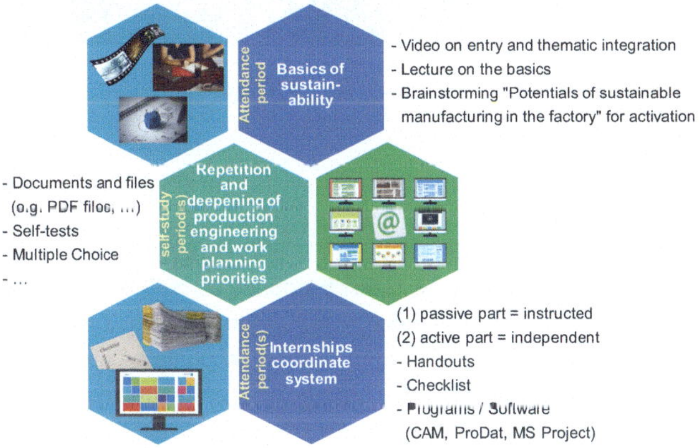

Fig. 2. Developed blended learning-concept

Attendance and self-study periods are changing iteratively. During the attendance period, digital media such as the already compiled video and a lecture with a PowerPoint presentation are initially used to sensitize the participants. The attendance period focuses on the issue-specific establishment of basic knowledge for the resource-oriented planning and production. In the following self-study period, a targeted repetition and deepening of the newly acquired knowledge are used to activate the participants. This can be done, for example, with the help of multiple-choice tests. The homepage of the digital learning environment is displayed in Fig. 3. It is the starting point for all actions and shows an overview of the topics.

The topics *Qualification Concept* and *Basics* support the attendance period. The goals and motivations for this concept as well as a first sensitization for the topic of resource efficiency are outlined in a video and can be looked up. The documents used for the lecture of the introductory attendance period are also retrievable. The topic *Repetition and Deepening* is planned for the work during a self-study period. The participants can acquire relevant knowledge individually and with thematic focus. The participants may determine their learning content and speed for themselves. Process planning and manufacturing engineering represent the main focus. The implementation of the deepened and consolidated basics takes place in the *Practical Training* topic.

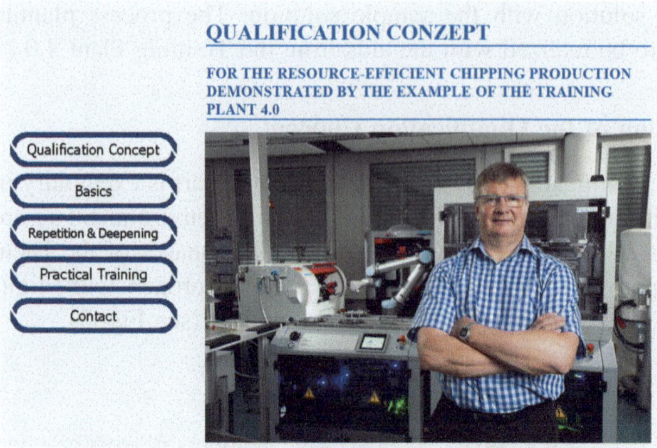

Fig. 3. Homepage in an HTML-based environment

It initially describes the concept and basic construction of the task. These topics and contents are specified more closely in Table 1.

The practical training concerning the sample part is divided into two subphases, an active and a passive part. In the passive part guidance as well as the sample solution is provided for every part of the task. All necessary documents are available in the passive and active part. With this Practical Training, the participants create a resource-oriented production strategy. In parallel, they obtain a significant reduction of material requirements.

Table 1. Topics learning environment

Topic	Content	Attendance period	Self-study period
Qualification concept	• Definition Qualification Concept • Overview goals and concept • Link to the stages and foci **Basics, Repetition and Deepening** as well as **Practical Training**	**X**	**X** additionally available online
Basics	• Short film as Introduction • Definition and link to further information on **Sustainability, Resources** and **Sustainable Action** • Link to the ESF project MoQuaRT	**X**	**X** additionally available online

(*continued*)

Table 1. (*continued*)

Topic	Content	Attendance period	Self-study period
Repetition and deepening	• Overview and link to further information on the foci of **Process Planning and Manufacturing Engineering**		**X**
Practical training	• Explanation of **Task** and **Approach** concerning the sample part • Guidance for "passive" part • Task for "active" part • Instruction and application of a tool to predict energy demands of the production variant • Comparison of variants	**X** active part is worked out with the participants corporately	**X** active part additionally available online; instruction and hints for passive part additionally available online
Contact	• Contact details		**X**

4 Summary

The pilot qualification concept discusses in its sample solution the issue of a high cutting volume. The sample solution also represents the first production strategy. The participants gain knowledge about the resource-oriented tasks in process planning. This mainly relates to the planning of raw material measurement and raw material types, production processes, the selection of machinery and tools or the specification of cutting parameters. Furthermore, the skills to compare technological variants concerning material and energy demands are developed. These skills rely on energetic machine models. The practical training shows the participants that the necessary amount of chipping energy can vary evidently. This is in part depending on machining task, production variant and the used machinery including integrated components. Additionally, the tool selection and the specification of cutting strategy and cutting parameters can result in an evident reduction of the demand of cutting energy. With the help of the qualification concept, a systematic, resource-oriented, creative and analytic working method will be promoted.

Acknowledgments. The authors thank the European Social Fund (ESF) and the Federal State of Saxony for supporting the junior research group MoQuaRT as well as the project executing organisation Sächsische Aufbaubank – Förderbank.

References

1. Goldhahn, L., et al.: Ressourceneffiziente technologische Planung. ZWF Zeitschrift für Wirtschaftlichen Fabrikbetrieb **112**(5), 332–336 (2017)
2. Hesselbach, J.: Energie- und klimaeffiziente Produktion: Grundlagen, Leitlinien und Praxisbeispiele, 1st edn. Vieweg+Teubner (GWV), Wiesbaden (2012)
3. Neugebauer, R., Götze, U., Drossel, W.-G. (eds.): Energieorientierte Bilanzierung und Bewertung in der Produktionstechnik - Methoden und Anwendungsbeispiele: 2. Methodenworkshop der Querschnittsarbeitsgruppe 1. In: "Energetisch-Wirtschaftliche Bilan-zierung" des Spitzentechnologieclusters eniPROD. Verl. Wiss. Scripten, Auerbach (2013)
4. Goldhahn, L., Eckardt, R.: Sustainable process planning of manufacturing variants for high-precision parts. CIRP **46**, 344–347 (2016)
5. Goldhahn, L., Pietschmann, C., Eckardt, R.: Process for the machine specific analysis and modeling of the technology based energetical demand forecasts. CIRP **77**, 405–408 (2018)
6. Bauer, W., Schlund, S. (eds.): Wandel der Arbeit in indirekten Bereichen - Planung und Engineering. In: Digitalisierung industrieller Arbeit. Die Vision Industrie 4.0 und ihre sozialen Herausforderungen. Nomos edition sigma, Baden-Baden (2015)
7. Hirsch-Kreinsen, H. (ed.): Digitalisierung industrieller Arbeit. In: Digitalisierung industrieller Arbeit Die Vision Industrie 4.0 und ihre sozialen Herausforderungen. Nomos edition sigma, Baden-Baden (2015)
8. Universität Münster. www.uni-muenster.de/griesha/fsu/mtd/begriffe.html
9. Reinmann, G., Mandl, H.: Unterrichten und Lernumgebungen gestalten. In: Krapp, A., Weidenmann, B. (eds.) Anwendung Psychologie. Pädagogische Psychologie. Ein Lehrbuch, 5th edn. Beltz PVU, Weinheim (2006)
10. Martin-Luther-Universität Halle-Wittenberg. wiki.llz.uni-halle.de/Virtualisierungsgrad
11. Quilling, E., Nicolini, H.J.: Erfolgreiche Seminargestaltung: Strategien und Methoden in der Erwachsenenbildung (2., erweiterte Auflage). VS Verlag für Sozialwissenschaften / GWV Fachverlage GmbH Wiesbaden, Wiesbaden (2009)
12. Onpulson. www.onpulson.de/lexikon/e-learning/
13. Bremer, C.: www.bremer.cx/material/Bremer_Szenarien.pdf
14. Rohs, M. (ed.): Handbuch Informelles Lernen. Springer Reference Sozialwissenschaften. Springer VS, Wiesbaden (2016)
15. Goldhahn, L., et. al.: Mitarbeiterorientiertes Qualifizierungskonzept für die ressourcenorientierte spanende Fertigung. GfA 65, C.7.5, pp. 1–6 (2019)

Selecting AAC Tools and Strategies for Interactions with Teachers and Students at Special Needs School for Children with Intellectual Disabilities

Tetsuya Hirotomi(✉)

Institute of Science and Engineering, Academic Assembly,
Shimane University, 1060 Nishikawatsu-cho, Matsue, Shimane 690-8504, Japan
hirotomi@cis.shimane-u.ac.jp

Abstract. Successful communication between children with complex communication needs and their partners often relies on selecting appropriate augmentative and alternative communication (AAC) tools and strategies to fit their opportunity. Mobile apps are powerful AAC tools for presenting visual aids with synthesized voice. However, special needs school teachers sometimes do not use these apps actively even they recognize the usefulness. The purpose of this study is to examine the teacher's selection process of AAC tools and strategies at special needs schools for children with intellectual disabilities. We had developed STalk2 mobile app and unstructured focus group interviews were conducted at the end of 8–11 months of STalk2 trial use. The results suggest that teachers select AAC tools and strategies for interaction with their students based on characteristics of communication tools and strategies, environments, and/or knowledge and experience on the use of communication tools and strategies.

Keywords: Augmentative and alternative communication · Special needs school for children with intellectual disabilities · Complex communication needs · Selection of AAC tools and strategies

1 Introduction

If children with pervasive developmental and/or intellectual disabilities have complex communication needs caused by the limitation in the use of speech, a set of augmentative and alternative communication (AAC) tools and strategies are used with their communication partners to solve everyday communication challenges [1, 12]. Printed cards of pictorial symbols and photographs are popular tools [3, 4]. Mobile apps are more powerful tools because they can present these visual aids with synthesized voice. These tools are used along with vocalizations, facial expressions, and gestures in order to express and/or understand messages more intelligibly and specifically.

Communicative competence of children who requires AAC consists of intrinsic factors related to them and extrinsic factors related to the environment [10]. Communication partners, a part of the environment, play an important role to facilitate or impede the realization of communicative competence [2].

T. Ahram et al. (Eds.): IHIET 2019, AISC 1018, pp. 73–77, 2020.
https://doi.org/10.1007/978-3-030-25629-6_12

We focused on communication partner's process to select AAC tools and strategies because school teachers sometimes do not use AAC apps actively even they recognize the usefulness [6]. The purpose of this study is to examine the teacher's selection process at special needs schools for children with intellectual disabilities.

2 STalk2 Mobile App

We had developed STalk2 mobile app running on Android OS [7]. We adopted "reduction" and "self-monitoring" persuasive technology principles [5, 11] for increasing opportunities to present visual aids with verbal messages to children with complex communication needs.

Figure 1 shows an overview of the app. The users can compose a message as a set of visual aids, i.e., images with captions, allocated into five columns for answering the following questions: when (time), where (place), who (subject), how (feeling, language, method, tool, transportation, or material), and what (action).

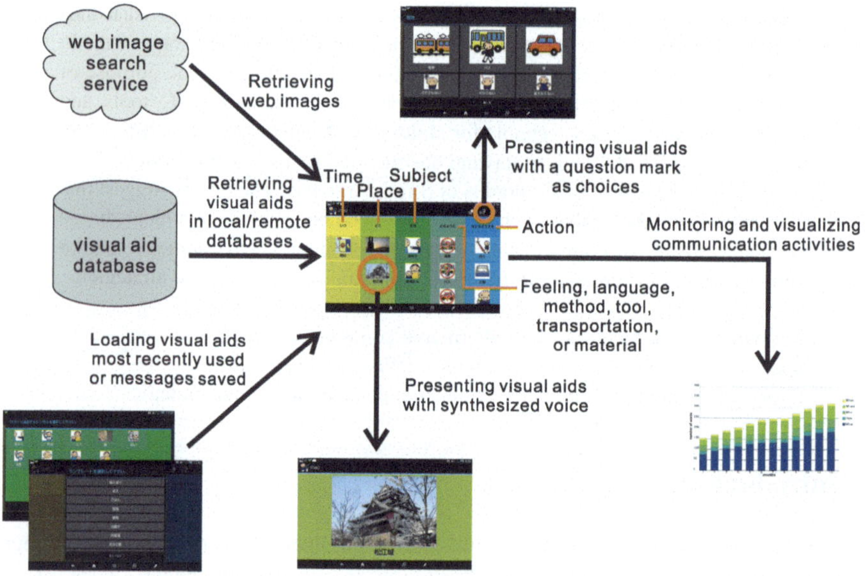

Fig. 1. Overview of STalk2 mobile app

To compose a message, the users can retrieve web images and visual aids in local/remote databases by speech recognition or typing keywords. They can also load visual aids most recently used or messages saved. They can place a question mark or slash symbol over any visual aid. By touching one of the visual aids in the message, STalk2 presents its enlarged image, caption, and synthesized voice of the caption. They can also open a dialog designed for choosing among several visual aids with a question mark. STalk2 has a special function to visualize data by monitoring and analyzing user activities.

3 Method

Unstructured focus group interviews were conducted to gather the usage of AAC tools and strategies at the end of 8–11 months of STalk2 trial use. The interviewees were five school teachers of special needs schools. They had in charge of students with complex communication needs ages 8, 11 and 12. The interview for each class lasted approximately one hour. Interviews were digitally recorded and transcribed verbatim. We performed grounded theory analysis of the interview transcripts and examined the selection process of AAC tools and strategies for interactions with teachers and students.

4 Results and Discussion

In grounded theory [9], collection of codes that describe similar contents are grouped together to form higher level concepts. Concepts can then be grouped to form categories (and subcategories). After that, relationships between categories and concepts are identified.

Our study outcomes include identification of AAC tools and strategies used in interaction with teachers and students as well as their selection process. First, STalk2 app, printed cards, real objects, hand-written schedule, and speech were identified as AAC tools and strategies used. Consequently, Fig. 2 was derived as the process for selecting one or a few of them. In this figure, ≪ ≫, < >, and " " denote categories, subcategories, and concepts, respectively. Rectangles and arrows indicate inclusion and interaction between them.

Teachers conduct ≪selection and the use of AAC tools and strategies≫ for interaction with a student. ≪Factors affecting teacher's judgement≫ are <characteristics of communication tools and strategies>, <environments>, and/or "knowledge and experience on the use of communication tools and strategies." <Characteristics of communication tools and strategies> are comprised of "expected vocabularies," "physical portability," "efforts to prepare visual aids for communication (e.g., taking photographs in advance)," and "estimated time to be spent in composing and presenting messages." <Environments> are comprised of characteristics of "student" with whom teachers try to communicate, "activity" that AAC tools and strategies are applied, and "context" including supports from other teachers and behaviors and attitudes of other students in a classroom, as well as AAC tools and strategies are used to interact with "individual or group." As a result of the communication, "knowledge and experience on the use of communication tools and strategies" will be updated for future selections.

In our former study, STalk2's simple steps for creating, searching, editing, and presenting visual aids reduced the burden of communication partners and increased the frequency of presenting visual aids with verbal messages [7]. In other words, that study examines the effects of the improvements on time and efforts in <characteristics of communication tools and strategies>.

In Fujino and Noh's survey, 61% of special needs school teachers responded that computers were necessary for their communication with students, but only 34% of

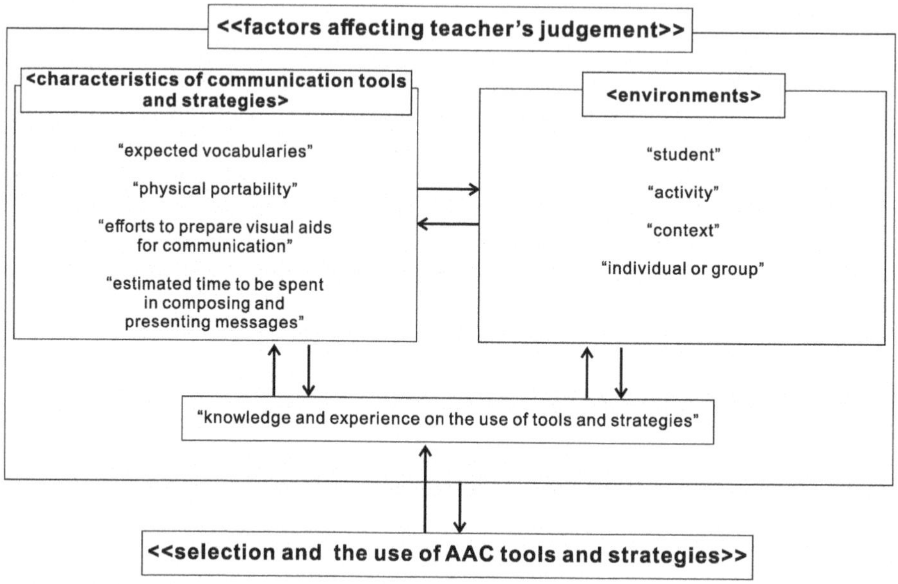

Fig. 2. Teacher's process for selecting AAC tools and strategies to interact with a student of special needs school for intellectual disabilities

them used [6]. They also reported that the usage rate in high school was higher than that in elementary school. These facts can be explained by "knowledge and experience on the use of tools and strategies" and different <environments>. That is why, communication partner instruction can be an effective intervention component for individuals with complex communication needs as Kent-Walsh et al. reported [8].

The development of AAC apps are usually focusing on how to improve <characteristics of communication tools and strategies> and how to support a variety <environments>. The results suggest that more attention should be directed toward accommodating with the diversity of teacher's knowledge and experience on AAC apps.

5 Conclusion

In this study, we have examined the teacher's selection process of AAC tools and strategies at special needs schools for children with intellectual disabilities. The results of grounded theory analysis on transcripts of focus groups suggest that teachers select AAC tools and strategies for interaction with their students based on characteristics of communication tools and strategies, environments, and/or knowledge and experience on the use of communication tools and strategies. Our future work will be the development of adaptive AAC apps to improve behaviors of teachers with a variety of knowledge and experience.

Acknowledgments. This work was supported by JSPS KAKENHI Grant Number JP16K01553. We thank Shunsuke Kyo for providing insight and expertise to conduct this research, and Honoka Hyodo for assistance with data collection and analysis.

References

1. Beukelman, D.R., Mirenda, P.: Augmentative and Alternative Communication: Management of Severe Communication Disorders, 2nd edn. Paul H. Brookes Publishing Co, Baltimore (1998)
2. Blackstone, S.W., Williams, M.B., Wilkins, D.P.: Key principles underlying research and practice in AAC. Augmentative and Altern. Commun. **23**, 191–203 (2007)
3. Bondy, A.S., Frost, L.A.: The picture exchange communication system. Focus Autism Other Dev. Disabil. **9**, 1–19 (1994)
4. Charlop-Christy, M., Carpenter, M., Le, L., LeBlanc, L., Kellet, K.: Using the picture exchange communication system (PECS) with children with autism: assessment of pecs acquisition, speech. Soc.-Communicative Behav. **35**(3), 213–231 (2002)
5. Fogg, B.J.: Persuasive Technology: Using Computers to Change What We Think and Do Morgan Kaufmann Publishers Inc., San Francisco (2003)
6. Fujino, H., Noh, H.: Usage of augmentative and alternative communication (AAC) systems in special schools for children with intellectual disabilities: current status. Jpn. J. Special Educ. **48**(3), 181–190 (2010) (in Japanese)
7. Hirotomi, T.: An AAC system designed for improving behaviors and attitudes in communication between children with CCN and their peers. In: Antona, M., Stephanidis, C. (eds.) UAHCI 2018. LNCS, vol. 10907, pp. 530–541. Springer, Cham (2018)
8. Kent-Walsh, J., Murza, K.A., Malani, M.D., Binger, C.: Effects of communication partner instruction on the communication of individuals using AAC: a meta-analysis. Augmentative Altern. Commun. **31**(4), 271–284 (2015)
9. Lazar, J., Feng, J.H., Hochheiser, H.: Research Methods in Human-Computer Interaction. Wiley, Chichester (2010)
10. Light, J., McNaughton, D.: Communicative competence for individuals who require augmentative and alternative communication: a new definition for a new era of communication? Augmentative Altern. Commun. **30**(1), 1–18 (2014)
11. Oinas-Kukkonen, H., Harjumaa, M.: A systematic framework for designing and evaluating persuasive systems. In: Proceedings of Persuasive 2008, pp. 164–176 (2008)
12. Therrien, M.C.S., Light, J., Pope, L.: Systematic review of the effects of interventions to promote peer interactions for children who use aided AAC. Augmentative Altern. Commun. **32**, 81–93 (2016)

Judgment Analysis for Real-Time Decision Support Using the Cognitive Shadow Policy-Capturing System

Daniel Lafond[1(✉)], Katherine Labonté[2], Aren Hunter[3], Heather F. Neyedli[4], and Sébastien Tremblay[2]

[1] Thales Research and Technology, Quebec City, QC, Canada
daniel.lafond@ca.thalesgroup.com
[2] School of Psychology, Université Laval, Quebec City, QC, Canada
[3] Defence Research and Development Canada - Atlantic, Halifax, NS, Canada
[4] School of Health and Human Performance, Dalhousie University, Halifax, NS, Canada

Abstract. The present work introduces a prototype intelligent cognitive assistant that continuously learns the decision pattern of the user online, instantly recognizes deviations from that pattern as potential errors and then alerts the user accordingly. We investigated the potential of this prototype system using a human-in-the-loop experiment designed to assess impacts on decision making performance, workload and trust in the decision support capability. Study participants interacted with a naval air-defence testbed to classify radar contacts as friendly, uncertain or hostile based on track parameters displayed on screen. The between-group experimental design included a control condition and two decision support conditions (with system reliability provided either offline or online). Results showed that both decision support conditions significantly improved task accuracy compared to the control condition. The advisory system was successful at improving human performance without burdening the user with excessive additional workload, even when providing reliability information in real time.

Keywords: Judgment analysis · Policy capturing · Decision support · Trust · Machine learning · Classification · Cognitive engineering · Dynamic decision making · Workload · Cognitive modeling · Human-in-the-loop experiment

1 Introduction

Policy capturing is a judgment analysis method relying on statistical or machine learning techniques to understand and predict human decisions [1]. This methodology allows inferring a decision model based on a list of observed decisions (a target behavior or judgment) and a set of predictors (features or variables) associated to each decision. For example, policy capturing has been used to infer clinical decisions based on patient attributes and symptoms [2–5] and has been applied in various other domains such as education [6, 7], finance [8, 9], judicial decision making [10],

T. Ahram et al. (Eds.): IHIET 2019, AISC 1018, pp. 78–83, 2020.
https://doi.org/10.1007/978-3-030-25629-6_13

personnel selection/training [11] and environmental risk management [12]. Policy capturing constitutes an alternative to classic approaches requiring the verbal elicitation of human knowledge to manually generate complex if-then rule sets (expert systems). Indeed, a known limitation of verbal protocol analysis is that human experts may not be fully able to verbally express their knowledge, partly in the case of implicit/procedural knowledge. Linear regression models (logistic regression when the output is a category) have dominated this approach and were found in a recent meta-analysis to provide decision models that are on average 10% more accurate than individual experts [13]. While the strength of linear models is their robustness to noise, more flexible machine learning models were found to be superior in a task domain involving non-linearly separable categories [14]. Another important finding in [14] was that no single model appears to be always best across decision makers and across tasks. This result is attributable to the well-known "no free lunch" theorem stating that given the full range of possible classification problems, the distinct bias of different inference models will necessarily be favorable for some problems and unfavorable for others [15]. The performance benefit of policy capturing is called the "judgmental bootstrapping" effect, which can be observed when modeling groups of experts or individuals [2, 14]. This effect speaks to the notion that models tend to capture the regularities in a decision pattern without replicating a minority of idiosyncratic decisions (likely errors due to fatigue, stress, distraction, mental overload, and so on).

1.1 Policy-Capturing System

Thales has developed a prototype policy capturing tool called the Cognitive Shadow to automatically learn an operator's decision pattern and provide advisory warnings in real-time when a mismatch is detected between a given decision by the user and the inferred decision policy. Advisory warnings present the current and expected decision in a notification window, and optionally present a reliability estimate of the system's prediction. The decision model is built by the cognitive assistant through interactions with an expert. The system adopts a multi-model approach to compare several linear and non-linear models to dynamically select the one with the best predictive accuracy. Four learning algorithms were used herein: logistic regression, decision trees, k-nearest neighbors and support vector classifier. The Cognitive Shadow is implemented as a web service with a representational state transfer application programming interface (REST API) and a relational (PostgreSQL) database. Python scripts are used to train the four machine learning algorithms available in Scikit-Learn. The system allows configuring new tasks using the web interface and deploying this capability either on premise or in the cloud to enable interactions with different computerized task environments.

By running multiple models in parallel and evaluating automatically their predictive accuracy, this policy capturing system can dynamically select the most effective model at a given time and for a given context, at the group or individual level. In the present study, individual-level models were retrained in real-time once every three decisions. Predictive accuracy was estimated using a ten-fold cross-validation procedure. Just like a human, a model may not always be right. If an expert accepts warnings when the model is correct and correctly rejects warnings when the model is wrong, then the human-machine team will have a higher accuracy than each team component.

The system's display of reliability in a warning may help the user appropriately make that final choice. While supervised learning applications typically focus on modeling the ground truth using very large datasets, the Cognitive Shadow is geared towards learning to predict human behavior or decisions (no ground truth needed, but can be used if available), by relying on relatively small datasets (i.e., online frugal learning). One way to support frugal learning is to represent the problem space at a higher and more parsimonious abstraction level based on domain expert knowledge (i.e., making continuous variables categorical if possible).

1.2 Research Objective

While policy capturing has been successfully applied for decades through post-hoc analysis, it has yet to be automated and applied in real-time for error prevention in safety-critical tasks. The present work introduced the Cognitive Shadow into a dynamic decision making environment in a first-ever test of an online policy capturing system. Accordingly, the main objective of this study was to experimentally test the Cognitive Shadow prototype to measure its impact on human performance, trust and workload. Additionally, this research aimed to determine how model reliability information should be presented along with the advisory warnings to improve performance and trust without increasing workload. Reliability information may help the user rely on the system more appropriately, which may consequently improve overall task performance [16].

2 Method

2.1 Simulated Task Environment

The dynamic decision making testbed used in the following experiment is the Simulated Combat Control System (S-CCS; see [14]). S-CCS is a low-fidelity simulation of a naval air-defence task, designed for experimental control, behavior analysis and accessibility to non-experts. As the tactical coordinator in the operations room of a frigate, the operator is required to monitor the operational environment, detect significant changes, classify potential threats, determine the temporal immediacy of a threat, and coordinate responses to threats (i.e., engage hostile aircraft).

Figure 1 shows the user interface of S-CCS. It includes a main geospatial display that is representative of typical radar systems, including a black screen, a central point corresponding to the ownship and four concentric circles specifying different hit probability regions. Aircraft appear as dots with a green squared contour, moving on at various speeds, proportional to the length of the line indicating the track's current heading. A ship hit is recorded when a hostile aircraft reaches the ownship.

During each scenario, participants were required to classify radar contacts, assess the temporal immediacy of threats and engage hostile aircraft. Classifying aircraft threat level required considering five parameters: (1) origin (hostile territory or not), (2) altitude (low, high), (3) Identify friend or foe signal (IFF; friendly, neutral, or enemy), (4) weapon systems detected (yes/no), and (5) military electronic emissions detected (yes/no). Aircraft could be associated to one of three levels of threat depending

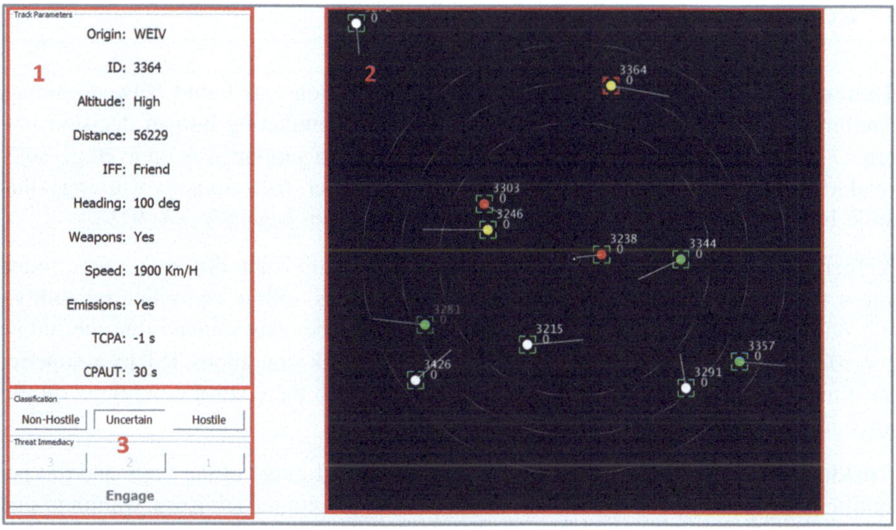

Fig. 1. Simulated Combat Control System interface. (1) Parameter list. (2) Radar screen. (3) Action buttons.

on the number of threatening cues (0–1 = non-hostile, 2–3 = uncertain, 4–5 = hostile). Assessing threat immediacy involved calculating the temporal proximity of the aircraft (1 = under 15 s, 2 = between 15 and 30 s, 3 = over 30 s).

Participants. Fifty-six university students took part in the experiment. Five participants were removed from the analysis due to a human and/or model accuracy below 75%. Participants were randomly assigned to either the control (n = 18), offline reliability (n = 17), or online reliability (n = 16) condition.

Apparatus. Participants interacted with the S-CCS testbed on a standard personal computer with a flat-screen monitor, a keyboard and a mouse. The NASA-TLX questionnaire [17] was used to measure subjective workload. The 12-item questionnaire on trust in the automated decision support system [18] allowed us to capture subjective impressions of users about their confidence in the advisory support received.

Procedure. Participants took part in a single, 60-min experimental session. The experiments started with a task tutorial, followed by nine static practice trials (screenshots with no time pressure and experimenter verification/guidance). Two dynamic practice scenarios then followed, lasting 3 min each. The test session comprised three experimental blocks lasting 5 min each. After each block S-CCS displayed the amount of ship hits, of correctly neutralized threats, and of non-hostile aircraft erroneously engaged. The Cognitive Shadow was used here to specifically learn from the user's threat classification judgments. An advisory warning appeared at the center of the screen when a divergence from the inferred decision pattern was detected.

3 Results

Human Versus Model Accuracy. A significant relation was found between human classification accuracy and the system's accuracy at predicting human decision patterns, r (31) = .774, p < .001. Human accuracy with no support was on average 86%. Final model accuracy was also 86% on average. However, with advisory warnings (that could be rejected or accepted) the joint cognitive system accuracy was 91%.

Performance (Threat Evaluation Accuracy). A significant difference was found across the three decision support conditions (control vs. offline vs. online reliability), $F(2, 48) = 3.20$, $p = .0498$. Unilateral pairwise post-hoc tests showed that the offline ($p = .0225$) and online ($p = .0272$) reliability feedback conditions led to a superior performance (on average 5% better) when compared to the control condition, yet did not significantly differ between each other.

Workload. Subjective workload was overall at the mid-range of the scale and did not significantly differ across conditions, either with or without advisory warnings and across reliability presentation modes.

Trust. Trust in the advisory system was overall at the mid-range of the scale and was not significantly impacted by the reliability presentation mode.

4 Discussion

This paper has reported the first "proof-of-concept" experimental test of an online policy capturing system for decision support in a dynamic decision making environment. The Cognitive Shadow prototype was successful at improving human performance without significantly burdening the operator with additional workload, even when providing reliability information in real time. Trust in the system was moderate and could be improved by explaining to the operator how the Cognitive Shadow operates and by using a more prolonged training and experimental session (allowing model accuracy to further improve over time). The strong relation observed between human and model accuracy speaks to the notion that modeling human decisions requires a reliable decision making pattern (i.e., from an expert) to be accurately inferred by the system. One appealing prospect of this work is the potential to leverage artificial intelligence to increase safety and human effectiveness while keeping the human decision maker fully in charge and accountable. This approach also offers a unique potential for training applications by helping novices using real-time feedback from advisory models derived from experts. Ongoing work includes adding new algorithms and testing this new policy-capturing system on experts using a high-fidelity simulator. Future work will also further investigate how artificial and human intelligence may work as team players in a synergistic and complementary manner.

Acknowledgments. We are thankful to Wheejae Kim for assistance in data collection and to Frédéric Morin, Philippe Michaud-Côté, Sébastien Carrier, Jean-Sébastien Thivierge, Jonathan Ouellet, Jonathan Richard, Jean-Baptiste Bebaah, Michel Mercier, Marlène Gauthier and Nicolas

Déry for software development and testing. This work was supported by an R&D partnership grant awarded to Sébastien Tremblay and to Heather Neyedli from the National Sciences and Engineering Research Council of Canada (NSERC) with Defence R&D Canada – Atlantic and Thales Research and Technology Canada.

References

1. Cooksey, R.W.: Judgment Analysis: Theory, Methods, and Applications. Academic Press, San Diego (1996)
2. Meehl, P.E.: Clinical Versus Statistical Prediction: A Theoretical Analysis and a Review of the Evidence. University of Minnesota Press, Minneapolis (1954)
3. Hammond, K.R.: Probabilistic functioning and the clinical method. Psychol. Rev. **62**, 255–262 (1955)
4. Hoffman, P.J.: The paramorphic representation of clinical judgment. Psychol. Bull. **57**, 116–131 (1960)
5. Wigton, R.S.: Social judgment theory and medical judgment. Think. Reason **2**, 175–190 (1996)
6. Dawes, R.M.: A case study of graduate admissions: application of three principles of human decision making. Am. Psychol. **26**, 180–188 (1971)
7. Heald, J.E.: Social judgment theory: applications to educational decision making. Educ. Adm. Q. **27**, 343–357 (1991)
8. Ebert, R.J., Kruse, T.E.: Bootstrapping the security analyst. J. Appl. Psychol. **63**, 110–119 (1978)
9. Waller, W.S.: Brunswikian research in accounting and auditing. In: Human Judgment: The SJT view, pp. 247–272. North-Holland, Amsterdam (1988)
10. Dhami, M.K.: Psychological models of professional decision making. Psychol. Sci. **14**, 175–180 (2003)
11. Carretta, T.R.: U.S. Air Force pilot selection and training methods. Aviat. Space Environ. Med. **71**, 950–956 (2000)
12. Cropp, N., Banks, A., Elghali, L.: Expert decision making in a complex engineering environment: a comparison of the lens model, explanatory coherence, and matching heuristics. J. Cogn. Eng. Decis. Mak. **5**, 255–276 (2011)
13. Karelaia, N., Hogarth, R.M.: Determinants of linear judgment: a meta-analysis of lens model studies. Psychol. Bull. **134**, 404–426 (2008)
14. Lafond, D., Vallières, B.R., Vachon, F., Tremblay, S.: Judgment analysis in a dynamic multi-task environment: capturing non-linear policies using decision trees. J. Cogn. Eng. Decis. Mak. **11**, 122–135 (2017)
15. Wolpert, D.H.: The lack of a priori distinctions between learning algorithms. Neural Comput. **8**, 1341–1390 (1996)
16. Lee, J., See, K.: Trust in automation: designing for appropriate reliance. H. Factors **46**, 50–80 (2004)
17. Hart, S.G., Staveland, L.E.: Development of NASA-TLX (Task Load Index): results of empirical and theoretical research. In: Human Mental Workload, pp. 139–183. North Holland Press, Amsterdam (1988)
18. Jian, J.-Y., Bisantz, A.M., Drury, C.G.: Foundations for an empirically determined scale of trust in automated systems. Int. J. Cognit. Ergon. **4**, 53–71 (2000)

Impact of Disruptive Technologies on the Human Attitude

Vaclav Jirovsky[(✉)] and Vaclav Jirovsky Jr.

Faculty of Transportation Sciences,
Czech Technical University in Prague, 110 00 Prague, Czech Republic
{jirovsky,xl.jirovsky}@fd.cvut.cz

Abstract. The article deals with current problems of IT deployment in different segments of human activities. In the introduction the similarity of Industrial Revolution in 18 century and IT revolution today are compared. Following chapter deals with the impact of broad deployment of IT on human mental and decision process. Following chapter discuss changes in capability of human to memorize information and to judge based on information memorized and impact of IT on these abilities. The filtering model of human information processing introduce simple novelty approach using two separated filters – the knowledge filter and emotional filter. The conclusion emphasizes the thread of changes in people way of information processing, especially impact on people attitude and simple perception management.

Keywords: Disruptive technology · Human attitude · Big data · Knowledge filter · Knowledge database · Impact of IT deployment · Primary and secondary memory

1 Introduction

The disruptive technologies bring some new approach for access to information stored somewhere every day. The disruptive technology generates or allow to generate incredible amount of data hour by hour, filling the data to the internet often without any meaningful usage. Such a way, the internet, starting from the scratch in past, becomes a busy place. There is over 500 million tweets sent every day, over 5 billion Google searches, nearly two billion are expected to purchase something online in 2019 [6]. From the time when first website was published on August 6, 1991 by British physicist Tim Berners-Lee, the number of web sites had increased to nearly 2 billion, where the Google is world's most visited web site[1]. While internet traffic and speed had increased every day, cumulative speed of internet traffic is about 60 TB/s, only 48,2% comes from humans remaining 51,8% of all Internet traffic comes from bots or belongs to internet overheads [7]. Over 90,000 websites are hacked every day.

[1] Followed by Youtube, Facebook and Chinese search engine Baidu.

T. Ahram et al. (Eds.): IHIET 2019, AISC 1018, pp. 84–89, 2020.
https://doi.org/10.1007/978-3-030-25629-6_14

The internet servers keep over 15 ZBytes of data[2], some of them usable and trusted, some of them not. Because of such high data penetration, humans do not care for the knowledge, their own retained information, just relying on the search engine to find out the response to their requests. Incredible storage capacity of the internet doubles every three years while world computing capacity doubles every 18 month. All these numbers give an impression of incredible power of the internet and IT technology, giving to journalist open space for talking and writing about artificial intelligence. Even we should expect artificial intelligence in many ways, the artificial intelligence itself is still far from outperforming human cognitive capacity, humanlike intelligence.

Martin Hilbert, a professor of communications at the Davis University of California said: “We’re going from an information age to a knowledge age” [2]. This idea is very popular, but misleading – we are going to age of comfortable amnesia. This article is going to show some elementary models of interactions in the process how society and technology interact, how new disruptive technology beats traditional human way of thinking and decision making with devastating impact on the human. The conclusion described below are based on the data model of processing information rather than on physiological processes in the human brain.

2 Historical Analogy

In 18th century Britain was the world’s leading commercial nation, controlling a global trading empire with activities from North America to Indian subcontinent. The development of trade and the rise of business were leading factors of the Industrial Revolution raising in the middle of 18th century, lately broaden all around the world [3]. It makes a major turning point in history; almost every aspect of daily life was influenced in some way. The transition to new manufacturing processes from hand production methods to machines and the development of mechanized factory system relieve humans from heavy manual work transferring them to the machines. Although the workers destroyed new machines in the belief that they were overtaking their jobs, necessity of using at least some mental power to work with the machines led to the rise of educated workers class using their skills to control machines. At the end, the people enjoy their power, their intellectual superiority in thinking and making decision while machines relieve them off the heavy manual work[3]. Nevertheless, the human remains only the “system element” who has an ability to think, with right to make a decision, to be creative and to behave indeterministically.

Similarly, we can describe the situation in the information age, when we are in the middle of IT revolution. Broad deployment of the information technology in all segments of human doings, starting from accounting to the art, human activity is replaced by cold machine calculation. The transfer, likewise during the Industrial Revolution, is done from people to the machines, under conviction that machines will do it better with no errors and faster. Similarly, as manual work in the Industrial Revolution, had been

[2] One ZByte is 10^{21} bytes of data.

[3] This situation also leads to the rise of materialism and consumerism.

transferred from human to the machine, thinking and decision making is now reassigned from human to the machines. The human is losing the privilege of thinking and making decision.

The situation has many consequences starting from impression of freedom on one side to the total apathy on the other side. The decision made by algorithms are predictable, the world is going to be changed from indeterministic process to algorithmized deterministic process. The human became only the part of the implemented algorithm, being forced to behave algorithmically according to commands or requests of the machine. Continual loss of memorized information and the knowledge is observable.

Another problem, related to the automatic decision making, remains in the amount of information available for construction of the decision. Usually, the data available for decision never form a full set. Although general data space is enormous, the data available for the decision making and the data which would be evaluated as a truthful base are usually insufficient for algorithmic decision. The human substitutes this data insufficiency by intuition, having on the mind the necessity of the decision even not all facts are known. The machine not having such a quality as the intuition is, replaces intuition by very complex computation, usually based on the multi-criteria statistic methods. The fact, which is being often omitted, is that stochastic process undergoing statistical evaluation has to be stationary and ergodic. If not, the statistical processing could fail.

Another case could be the completeness of the set of possible states. Again, the set is already incomplete, so decision making could only estimate on the remainder of the set and generate remainder of the information by mathematical processing of the data already available. This approach brings further errors to the process of machine decision making[4]. People, using their intuition, are able make a decision even faster and more accurate than machine, if this is the case.

There is many articles and discussion about artificial intelligence and using the artificial intelligence in the decision making process. But what we have to accept today, there is no artificial intelligence build into any machine. The most of it are very sophisticated self-learning algorithms – we still have to go a very long way to achieve common quality of "the intelligence", to implement basic abilities of human as deep association, intuition or subliminal perception. And, as a matter of fact, we cannot expect introduction of such an attributes as morality or ethics.

3 Primary and Secondary Memory

The human memory is usually described as the ability of the brain by which information is encoded, stored, and retrieved when needed. The scientist had created very sophisticated apparatus of different descriptive vocabulary for a different portions of memory or their function. For us, to show the impact of disruptive technologies on the

[4] In this chapter we are dealing with high level decision making, not with an elementary decision where full set of data is known, as is e.g. temperature control etc.

human behavior we are going to extremely simplify the memory description just dividing it into two parts – primary memory and secondary memory. As mentioned above, our judgement is based rather on information processing point of view then on physiological model on human brain.

The primary memory is the functionality of the memory to store and use the information which we have already learned. Primary memory is the functionality used on its own, without any supporting elements. As an example, we have learned how to count numbers in elementary school. When we need to sum two numbers, we just use our primary memory associating these two numbers with information already learned and we get immediate results. In the case when numbers are too large, we recall the mechanism in our primary memory, how to add two numbers using elementary information about adding small numbers and we get a result.

Another situation is in the case of secondary memory. The secondary memory is the part of the memory where we store the information about places, where the requested answer could be found. As an example we know, in our secondary memory, that information about solving partial differential equation could be found in mathematical library. So, it's more associative memory which associate particular "questions" with "places". By influence of disruptive technologies this secondary memory gets shortened to the name of internet search engine.

With growing influence of the technology, the human, naturally lazy animal, is shorting the amount of the information stored in the primary memory, relying on technology support. Again, why to remember how to add numbers if I do have calculators? The knowledge of adding is moved to the skill of handling the calculator. So, the primary memory is still keeping some information, but this information is kept without the relation to other information[5]. The knowledge is going to be replaced by skills.

4 Knowledge Filter Model

The amount of information coming to senses of the human is growing day by day. The scientists had published many theories and estimations of human information channel capacity from tens of bits/s [4] to several tens of Mbit/s [5], even higher. Also the discussion on the brain functionality leads scientist to surprising conclusion, that biological organisms must violate the second law of thermodynamics by keeping their long term average entropy low[6]. In our study we try another view of human processing of the information, which is generated by general environment and provided via technology, attacking human cognitive system, see Fig. 1.

The huge amount of information attacking human cognitive system is filtered by knowledge filter using current knowledge and when evaluated creates new records in

[5] Students using calculators losing their sense of the dimension and even the numbers in result of calculation are corresponding to correct result, the dimension is far away, even several orders of magnitude.

[6] In another words, it means to push "surprises" of the organism as low as possible. To make AI working means to design a mechanism that can avoid being surprised as often as possible.

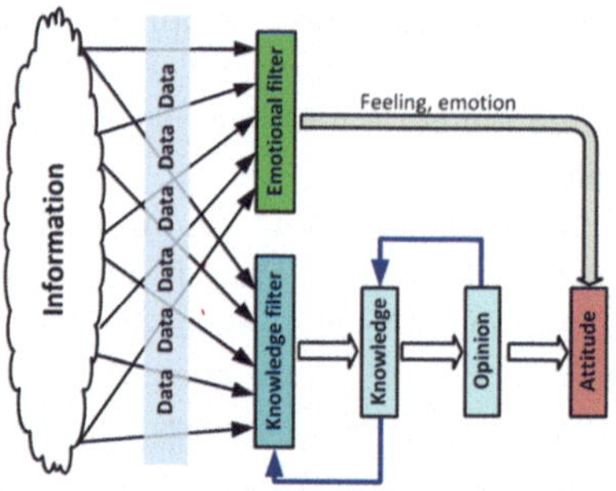

Fig. 1. Filter model of information processing.

human "knowledge database". We assume that "knowledge" is according to Plato "justified true belief"[7], where justification is done in knowledge filter based on truthfulness and believeness of incoming information. The result of justification depends on the amount of information in the "knowledge database", related to the evaluated information, and on the confidence in the source of the information. The new knowledge updates the knowledge filter with new setup, if necessary, which will be used when evaluating new incoming information.

The knowledge, stored in "knowledge database" is periodically evaluated to form non conclusive judgment or viewpoint – the opinion, supported by gained knowledge. When new knowledge become available, the mechanism transforming knowledge into opinion is taking place and new opinion is formed, old opinion is modified or remains unchanged. Based on the result of evaluation of the knowledge, the new "knowledge record" in "knowledge database" will be kept, deleted or marked as "less important". The opinion mechanism would be responsible for taking care of "garbage collecting" which saves the "storage space" wiping useless information out of the knowledge database. Last but not least, based on formed opinion, the human attitude is developed and presented to outer world as a mental and emotional entity that inheres in, or characterizes a person.

The critical situation in this model happens, when the amount of the information coming from outer world overwhelms the processing capacity of knowledge filter. The filter becomes saturated and release fully its functionality to more simple method of filtering – emotional filter. The decision rule of emotional filter is simple – either I like it or I dislike it. The decision is based only on the emotional value of the information not on its factual value and without involving further elements of filter chain – knowledge and opinion. The result of emotional decision forms immediately the human attitude without any reasoning, without ability to discuss the issue, to be able to defend the attitude by some reasoning based on opinion or knowledge. The example of such situation, when knowledge filter is saturated, is the emotional sundering of society during the time of political election. The society is undergoing high pressure from

[7] Even there are some examples of incompleteness of the definition as Gettier problem etc. for our purposes the definition is quite satisfactory.

advertisement, the discussion on social networks, internet blogs and other kind of information sources which leads to giving up the analytical thinking and making decision based on functionality of emotional filter. After all, the society losing the speed of development, becoming the confirmation society dependent on the information presented on the open media.

5 Conclusions

We have shown elementary model of human behavior under stress of information flow. Also we have pointed out the possible influence of broad deployment of the IT technologies into decision making process and shortening the primary and secondary memory, where secondary memory gets shorten to one word only, the name of internet browser. All of these finding are warning signs of the impact of new disruptive technologies deployment, meaningless big data collection and losing the mental abilities of the society.

References

1. Stevens, J.: Internet stats & facts for 2019. 17 December 2018. https://hostingfacts.com/internet-facts-stats/. Accessed 22 Jan 2019
2. Paloheimo, L.: To "know" is for Gods (and possibly for A.I.). To "learn" is Human. Panda. 20 April 2017. https://panda training.com/blog/2017/4/20/to know is for gods-and-possibly-ai-to-learn-is-human. Accessed 22 Jan 2019
3. Horn, J., Rosenband, L., Smith, M.: Reconceptualizing the Industrial Revolution. MIT Press, Cambridge, MA and London (2010)
4. Fitts, P.M.: The information capacity of the human motor system in controlling the amplitude of movement. J. Exp. Psychol. **47**, 381–391 (1954)
5. Koch, K., et al.: How much the eye tells the brain. Curr. Biol. **16**, 1428–1434 (2006)
6. Pappas, S.: How big is the internet, really? 18 March 2016. https://www.livescience.com/54094-how-big-is-the-internet.html
7. Lucas, R.E.J.: Lectures on Economic Growth, pp. 109–110. Cambridge, Harvard University Press (2002)

Transnational Communities and Vernacular Expressions in Abu Dhabi's Industrial Spaces

Mohamed El Amrousi, Mohamed Elhakeem(✉), and Evan K. Paleologos

Abu Dhabi University, Abu Dhabi, United Arab Emirates
mohamed.elhakeem@adu.ac.ae

Abstract. Today, identity and social status are increasingly being manifested by housing typologies. The massive construction industry that has mushroomed in the Gulf region and parts of Asia is being supported by a large population of workers requiring accommodation. In the Industrial City, on the mainland of Abu Dhabi (ICAD) labor housing conglomerated on a large scale with a capacity of 40,000 workers, with other camps on a smaller scale existing on the islands of Yas and Al-Reem. One of the challenges is the design and sustainability of such building stocks. This article studies the design of vernacular architecture in the industrial areas of Abu Dhabi as representations of urban enclaves, continuity and discontinuity from tradition. It also highlights the importance of safety guidelines in spaces where multi-cultural communities co-exist.

Keywords: Abu Dhabi · Industrial urbanism · Industrial architecture · Shared space · Safety guidelines

1 Introduction

The urban footprint and construction industry in Abu Dhabi has increased significantly in the last five decades as major construction projects emerge on mainland and the recently developed islands of Al-Saadiyat, Al-Reem and Yas Island. The Industrial City of Abu Dhabi (ICAD) re-contextualizes and re-interprets workers' residences much needed to support the construction industry. ICAD Residential City is a labor accommodation complex located in Mussafah, Abu Dhabi, and the first of its kind and scale, to be constructed as a residential city for workers, covering an area of 1.0 million square meters. The workers city that can accommodate up to 40,000 people has been hailed for the sanitized conditions it offers to multi-national workers. The city is well organized and has a predominantly unified modern design within its walled enclosure (Fig. 1). However, because of its large scale, the style of buildings and geometry of its spaces it poses questions of shared spaces of integration with the surrounding urban context, and the kind of activities that can offered for the personal development of migrant workers. Industrial housing and labor camps rely on pragmatic engineering solutions, such as modularity, pre-fabrication, and materiality, which play an important role in facilitating construction. On the other hand, they have been criticized for neglecting socio-cultural aspects and the potential for human development. A revisiting of the design perception of such housing typologies is needed in order to evaluate

T. Ahram et al. (Eds.): IHIET 2019, AISC 1018, pp. 90–97, 2020.
https://doi.org/10.1007/978-3-030-25629-6_15

designs that would support social interaction: spaces of belonging, shared spaces, and a form of advocacy planning that supports entrepreneurial projects and businesses. The shortage and inequity in the distribution of shared space in the walled urban enclaves of labor camps are symptomatic of a design that had been predominantly governed by pragmatism and the need to offer low cost housing. The concrete/brick wall around the workers city creates a gated community of a different kind, one that gathers transnational workers. While walls and gated communities are common in Gulf State cities as they reflect cultural values of privacy, here a walled enclosure hinders urban connectivity to surrounding landscapes and it isolates possible transformations of public space within and outside the walled city. Eliminating or changing the materials of such boundaries can integrate this type of communities into the public realm, as exemplified by the Workers Village in Al-Reem Island (Fig. 2). This paper studies the multi-layered land-use in vernacular architecture in the industrial areas of Abu Dhabi as representations of human interaction, experimental trans-disciplinary design, which includes continuity and discontinuity from tradition. This paper also highlights the importance of safety guidelines in spaces where multi-cultural communities co-exist.

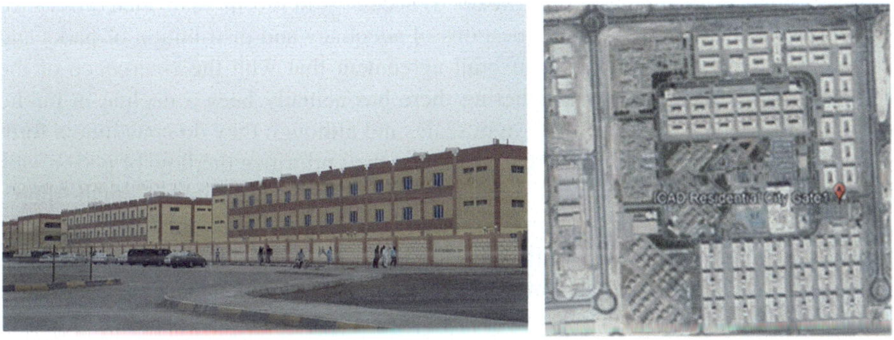

Fig. 1. ICAD residential city in Mussafah.

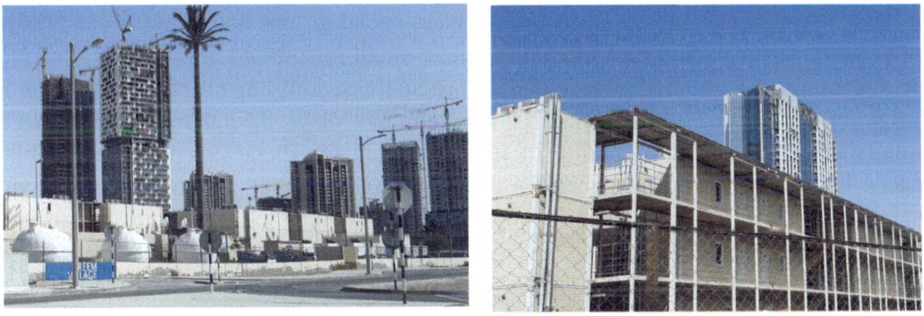

Fig. 2. Workers village in Al-Reem Island- Abu Dhabi.

2 Identity and Shared Space in the Modern City

Abu Dhabi is best understood as a simultaneously modern and traditional city, its contemporary styled high-rise buildings and emerging cultural centers, such as the Louvre Abu Dhabi, showcasing the state's policy to represent itself as contemporary, yet adhering to cultural norms and retaining its traditional community values. The space under the Louvre's dome is a good example of the multi-culturalism of the city and the diversity of its expatriate communities. On the other hand, Abu Dhabi is also a city that is protective of its local culture and family values, as reflected in its socially sanitized spaces. Sanitization of public spaces is not only emerging in Abu Dhabi but it has become a global phenomenon visible, among others, in Singapore, Hong Kong, and Seoul. It has become part of a new world order in which global cities are re-negotiating the concept of urban-mixing social stratification by designing modern cities where public space is associated with museums, cultural clusters, theme parks, and gated beaches, safe environments that are accessible to certain social groups. While public spaces are important for the wellbeing of a city and the health of its society here design of the built environment plays a role to direct physical movement and accessibility through walls, freeways and (ticketed) accesses. In recent years the concern for public space has extended beyond questions of adequacy and distribution of parks and open spaces, but rather there is an overall agreement that with the emergence of the mall as a major space of social gathering there has actually been a decline in public realm [1]. Malls have become massive in scale, and although they do constitute a form of public space they are not accessible to all, and they prioritize the flow of pedestrians through a physical space that is subject to surveillance. In contrast small shops, especially in industrial areas of a city represent spaces of gathering that are accessible to all, particularly if provided with sidewalks, shade, and public transport (Fig. 3). Architected urban landscape regulates the walkability of a city and can create features of the built environment that foster pedestrian accessibility and preserve property values [2]. Accessibility to open/shared space needs to be addressed in relation to identification forms, domesticity, and landscape in order to improve the integration of transnational worker communities in the broader context of the socio-cultural factors of the expatriate communities in the United Arab Emirates (UAE). Creating public spaces and pedestrian routes, which lower middle class social groups and workers can access is essential, as for example in Mussafah where small businesses are emerging having the ability to create shared spaces and to provide essential amenities. In this regard, designing appropriate spaces for labor communities plays a vital role in creating a sustainable city, and a community of living in need for social amenities and public spaces [3]. A decrease in spaces for social interaction that people can walk and socialize promotes car-based communities, with concomitant gas emissions, heat-island effects, deterioration of the air over a city, and health effects from a sedentary lifestyle [4]. Open space revitalization aims not only to improve the ecological function of a city, but to improve also its social function in the public realm. This includes a revival of the traditional coffee houses, and facilities that offer recreational opportunities for the public, beyond the sanitized space of museums and malls.

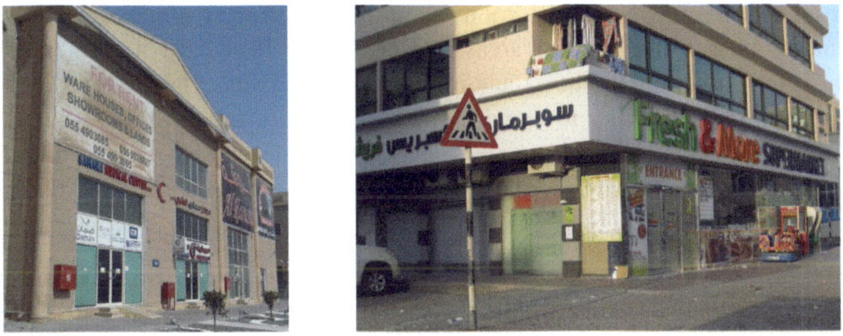

Fig. 3. Labor housing on the upper floor and small businesses on the ground floor-Mussafah.

3 Design Guidelines and Safety Regulations for Labor Housing

In the modern Arab city transnational laborers share similar physical living conditions in spite of coming from different socio-cultural backgrounds. Adopting an inclusive design strategy, rather than one based on pragmatic engineering solutions can improve shared spaces, and foster socio-cultural interaction and a self-sustaining community, through offering entrepreneurial-based development opportunities. In recent years regulations have been put in place to improve the physical conditions of transnational workers, however designing industrial workers' housing is no easy task. This problem has existed since the beginning of the first industrial revolution in the 19th century with, among others, Garnier's theories on the Cite Industrialle attempting to resolve the maladies of overcrowded metropoles through zoning that would isolate migrant workers in the urban fabric. Garnier's city was divided into four main functions: Work, housing, health and leisure, with his tenant being the separation of urban spacing by function [5]. Aldo Rossi refers to this kind of design as an architecture that fosters segregation, an "Analogue Architecture" that manifests bi-lateral plan-form, a central axis, and which is marked by geometric plans (circular or a square elements), usually associated with prisons, hospitals and asylums [6]. Peter Behrens attempted to improve the architecture associated with industrial plants, keeping in mind a clear separation between Art and Engineering. His design for the Allgemeine Elektricitäts-Gesellschaft AEG in Germany was characterized by a composite effort of rational and pseudo-aesthetic attempts, manifested in straight linear compositions, which aimed to improve the street facades of industrial plants without venturing into the excessive curvilinear compositions of Art Nouveau Architecture. Behrens' designs of the facades incorporated modern engineering construction forms, yet were governed by order, organization, and formal Constructivist Ideals [7]. These same cultural norms still dominate the design of industrial housing, as manifested by the Workers village in Yas Island (Fig. 4), even though guidelines were issued by the Ministry of Human Resources and Emiratization in Abu Dhabi (MoHRE), which aimed to improve design and living conditions of workers. These standards are related to the area occupied by each person in worker residences, which should not be less than 3 sq. m, and also that the maximum number of people allowed per bedroom should range from 8–10 persons. Additional requirements include the kitchen areas that are required to have a drainage system, there should exist ventilation holes and/or chimneys, and gas cylinders must be located outside the building in order to avoid the risks of fires or other hazards [8].

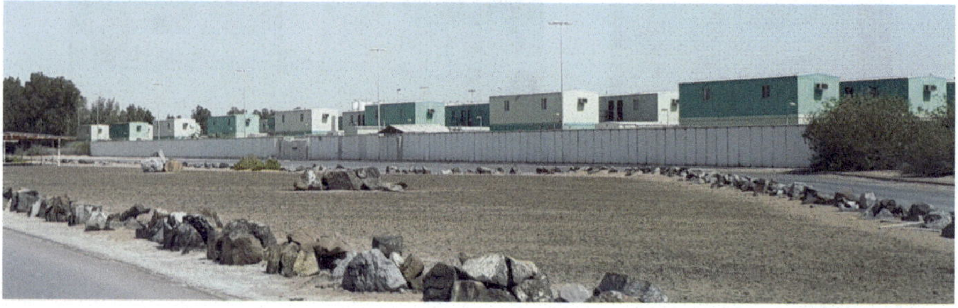

Fig. 4. Workers village in Yas Island- Abu Dhabi.

Several values and equations have been proposed to estimate the water demand for firefighting. A range of 0.032 – 0.075 m^3/s is proposed for a single fire action and if simultaneous fire occurs an amount of 0.125 – 0.5 m^3/s must be added [9]. Typical fire duration is 3 h at minimum, and for simultaneous fires it increases to 4 to 7 h. Classification of fire demand based on the type of residential status of the plot area is proposed [10] in the range of 0.032 – 0.126 m^3/s for a single family residential areas, in the range of 0.095 – 0.189 m^3/s for multi-family residential areas and in the range 0.158 – 0.315 m^3/s for commercial buildings. The following equation was also proposed to estimate the flow rate required for fire demand [11]:

$$Q = 1020\sqrt{p}(1 - 0.01\sqrt{p}) \tag{1}$$

where Q is the flow rate of fire in gpm, p is the population in thousands. This flow rate must be guaranteed for duration of at least 4 h for 1000 population, and 5 h for 1,500, 6 h for 2,000, 7 h for 3,000, 8 h for 4,000, 9 h for 5,000, and 10 h for 6,000 or more.

In addition, [12] provided the following equation for the flow rate required for fire demand:

$$Q = 18F\sqrt{A} \tag{2}$$

where Q is the flow rate of fire in gpm, A is the effective area includes all stories in the building except the basement in ft square, and F is a constant that depends on building construction material: 1.5 for wood frame, 1.0 for ordinary joisted masonry, 0.8 for noncombustible masonry, and 0.6 for fire resistant construction. Special rules are used to find the area for multistory, fire-resistant structures, buildings with various fire loading, and buildings with sprinkler systems. Q should not be less than 0.032 m^3/s (500 gpm), or more than 0.379 m^3/s (6,000 gpm).

The second requirement after estimating the water demand is to satisfy the pressure ranges for fire fighting systems. The pressure required for a domestic water system depends on various factors such as building height, the maximum instantaneous flow rate, and the friction losses. Pressure zoning is arranged wherever possible to limit the maximum static pressure at any point to 60 m head (6.0 bars) unless otherwise higher pressure is needed in the network for elevated areas or varying ground elevations. The pipeline test pressure shall be 1.5 times the design. Water distribution system shall be sized to ensure that the minimum residual pressures at the customer connection boundary shall be generally not less than 12.5 m head (1.25 bar) at all times for standard length connections or sufficient to meet the supply to the roof tank for low-rise buildings. The following four methods were proposed to achieve the firefighting pressure [11]: (1) The maintenance of sufficient pressure on the network at all times for direct hydrants service for hose streams; (2) The use of emergency fire pumps to boost the pressure in the distribution system during fires; (3) The use of mobile pumping engines which takes suction from the hydrants; and (4) The use of a separate high pressure distribution system for fire protection only.

The first method is more ordinarily economical for large communities, but is usually the best method for villas not provided with full time fire departments and mobile pumps. The second method is applicable to villas requiring higher pressures for firefighting than the desirable for normal consumption, and in which there are no mobile pumps. It is more economical but less reliable than the first method. The third method is preferable for all communities large enough to maintain modern and well-trained fire departments. The fourth method is in use only in portions of some of large cities. Separate high pressure systems are usually supplementary to the main distribution system and thus give added fire protection in high value districts. All public fire hydrants shall be installed at street intersections where possible. Public hydrant spacing shall be measured along vehicle access routes. In areas zoned for single-family residential use, public hydrants shall be spaced no more than 200 m apart. If dead-end streets, or driveways, singly or in combination, are over 110 m long, additional public hydrants shall be installed so that the public hydrant spacing is not over 200 m [9].

For the fire system, the Abu Dhabi water municipality requires any building to have at least two of the following three fire systems [13]:

1. Dry riser is a technique used to fight the fire action in which they design pipes along all floors of the building but in a dry status (pipes are empty with no water), and once the firemen come to the site, they use the water inside their cars and pump it through the inlet cabinet and then it fills the pipes along all the floors.
2. Wet Riser is another technique in which the pipes for the fire fighting through all floors are getting their water demand from the main tank under the building by a certain pump that allows the water to reach all the floors in the building at sufficient flow rate and pressure head.

3. Sprinkler system is the fire fighting system used for firefighting. It uses the same water resource and method of the wet riser, but it is provided with sensors that monitor the heat of the area around the building and once it reaches a certain limit, it automatically opens the sprinklers to pump the water and help in shutting off the fire. This system does not give sufficient amount of water therefore it has to be combined with one of the above described systems to meet the water municipality regulations.

4 Conclusion

Much has changed in terms of architecture and urban landscape in Abu Dhabi in the past decade. Gentrification of the downtown area and a notable growth in open spaces and cultural institutions have improved the quality of life in the city and have been felt by the expatriate community. However, in order to foster sustainable urban growth it is essential to design by keeping in mind the equity of open space and the public realm, in order to create a city environment that ensures better quality of city life. Collaboration between Municipalities, urban planners, and policy makers is necessary in creating solutions that would improve accessibility to public space. Industrial housing and labor villages have taken on more permanent forms in some cases representing part of the building stock of the city. They and can be designed to represent alternative forms of housing, as in the case of the workers village in Al-Reem Island that represents a positive example of shared space that connects between diaspora, memory and identity in a rapidly urbanizing Arab city. These labor villages/cities can play their parts as a key element in the modern city, and to manifest cultural sensitivity towards a new world order that is more interconnected, and where homogenization, interaction and social exchange become part of the living city.

References

1. Banerjee, T.: Public space, beyond invented streets and reinvented places. APA J. Win-ter 2001, **67**(1) (2001)
2. Schindler, S.: Architectural exclusion: discrimination and segregation through physical design of the built environment, 124 Yale L. J. 1934 (2015)
3. Cakmak, C.: Dubai: re-designing labor worker communities (2014)
4. Wikantiyoso, R., Suhartono, T.: The role of CSR in the revitalization of urban open space for better sustainable urban development. IRSPSD International **6**(4), 5–20 (2018)
5. Wiebenson, D.: Utopian aspects of Tony Garnier's Cité Industrielle. J. Soc. Architectural Historians **19**(1), 16–24 (1960)
6. https://cameronmcewan.wordpress.com/tag/aldo-rossi/
7. Anderson, S.: Modern architecture and industry: Peter Behrens and the cultural policy of historical determinism. J. Ideas and Criticism in Architect. **11**, MIT Press (1977, reprint 1981)
8. (https://government.ae/en/information-and-services/jobs/labour-accommodation)
9. Linsley, R.K., Franzini, J.B.: Water Resources Engineering. McGraw-Hill, NY (1979)

10. Mays, L.R.: Hydraulic Design Handbook. McGraw-Hill, NY (1999)
11. Davis, C.V., Sorensen, K.E.: Handbook of Applied Hydraulics. McGraw-Hill, NY (1969)
12. Lindeburg, M.R.: Civil Engineering Reference Manual, 9th edn. Professional Publications, CA (2003)
13. Fire Code. Retrieved 6 14, 2014, from Code Publishing. http://www.codepublishing.com/wa/edmonds/html/Edmonds19/Edmonds1925.html

Space Architecture: The Rise of a New Discipline in Architecture and Design Curricula

Paolo Caratelli(✉)

Department of Architecture and Design, College of Engineering, Abu Dhabi University, 59911, Abu Dhabi, United Arab Emirates
paolo.caratelli@adu.ac.ae

Abstract. The amazing endeavors of space missions on 1960s and 70s pushed the human knowledge and technology beyond the physical threshold of our planet, seemingly opening to infinite possibilities. With the ingress of private developers in space business, the exploration of outer space seems resurged to a new vitality in public opinion. Usually paired with aerospace engineering and advanced sciences, the new space business is asking today also for new competencies and expertise. In this view, disciplines associated with study programs in architecture and design seem particularly appropriated, offering the requested multidisciplinary education to shape high talented skills in a highly regulated environment. Space Architecture has the full potential to become a discipline of study within the usual curriculum in 'terrestrial' architecture, filling a gap in between the engineering approach of system design for space vehicles and habitats, and the interdisciplinary complexity associated to human oriented design. This paper explores the potentialities of Space Architecture as discipline, and definition of the field of study in which architects' education can offer a fundamental contribution towards a better integration between human crew and a sounding reliable spacecraft.

Keywords: Human-machine integration · Extreme environments · Space habitats · Space architecture · Moon-Mars missions

1 Introduction

In recent years, a new interest towards space exploration and connected sciences has been revitalized by initiatives fueled by private and governmental agencies, after the extraordinary development of these fields during the 'space race' leaded by United States and Soviet Russia, which ended with the Moon landing on July 20th, 1969.

Since then, space exploration has influenced dramatically culture and sciences at global level, unleashing an extraordinary power of imagination. Not only space sciences, but also arts, music, literature, fashion, movies, design and education were energized by this power, inspiring people that nothing is deemed impossible to human creativity and determination [1]. The term *Space Age* became synonymous of an unavoidable step in human civilization towards other worlds, from seafaring to spacefaring, and popular culture delved between science fiction and popular myths.

T. Ahram et al. (Eds.): IHIET 2019, AISC 1018, pp. 98–104, 2020.
https://doi.org/10.1007/978-3-030-25629-6_16

Ulysses and Christopher Columbus clothed with astronaut suit, settlers on board of space-wagons, and glowing cities floating on black seas of space vacuum became popular images of a coming future. Politics and fluctuating economy, shocking accidents and increasing environmental concerns obfuscated for a while this alluring image of limitless evolution in outer space.

After a period of quiescence, following the conclusion of Apollo program and the huge economic effort spent on ISS Alpha and Shuttle program, human spaceflight seems resurged to a renovated vitality, especially due to the ingress in the civilian space business of private commercial companies such as Elon Musk's SpaceX [2], Bigelow Aerospace [3], and Richard Branson's Virgin Galactic, which is planning to start a pioneering 'space tourism' enterprise. Most of the latest improvements in the aerospace sector belong to the last decade, and several of them drafted by private commercial companies. Between these, large part of research and development is currently concentrated on habitats, both as permanent habitats on planetary surfaces, orbiting stations, and deep space habitats. The huge amount of technical and scientific knowledge and experience accrued with the early generation of crewed orbiting stations such as Skylab (1973–1979), Salyut (1971–1982), Mir (1986–2001), International Space Station (ISS Alpha, completed 2015), and the Shuttle Transport System (1981–2011), are forming the backbone on which governmental space agencies, and the abovementioned group of private companies, are looking towards future steps. Plans for a Moon permanent habitat foresaw on 2020's, and human exploration of Mars surface within 2030's are still under development on the boards of major space agencies and aerospace contractors R&D's offices. Furthermore, the joining of emergent countries in the then restricted 'Space Club', preannounces a rapid escalation of technological, industrial, and economic efforts towards these expected goals.

The early fundamental contribution to the knowledge of outer space and planetary physics given by automatic exploration provided by unmanned probes, paved the way for a direct exploration of outer space by human beings. Issues related to the time spent in isolation, distances, and hazards never affronted before are now concentrating all the efforts, besides the outnumbered technical and logistic aspects that such a mission will face. The psychophysical needing of the crew, and definition of their habitation facility, is going well beyond a list of components between many others in a highly sophisticated engineered system. Other than technical, also physiological, psychological, medical, and operational issues need to be duly analyzed, assessed, and verified, before to plan any prolonged crewed mission out of Earth's orbit [4]. If the early stage of space exploration was primarily concentrated on drafting, assessing and testing in real conditions of an accrual of system technologies, materials, and procedures never tested before, now it is the time for further development and implementation of these systems, especially in terms of time spent in the most extreme of known environments. During the early stage of human spaceflights, the efforts of space scientists, aerospace engineers, and contractors focused mainly in accumulating data and experience in order to design and build an efficient and fully reliable vehicle first, leaving the habitation needing of the crew, intended as beyond the pure sustainment of biological life and operational activity, as secondary importance. Conceptually, the first generation of manned spacecraft were conceived as ballistic capsules in which the limited cramped space left by the huge amount of hardware was occupied by a living being for the needed operational time. Further observations and psychometric tests elaborated during this first period of spaceflights, revealed the fundamental importance of habitable environment in terms of operational efficiency and fully accomplishment of the assigned tasks, especially in prevision of prolonged missions [4]. Therefore, the psychological and physiological comfort of the crew associated with the quality of habitable environment, its design, features and ergonomics, represented since then as a major task and challenge for aerospace engineers and designers, becoming an ineludible requirement for future manned missions beyond earth's orbit. Nevertheless, limitations given by cost-cutting, technology readily available, political and economic obstacles due government subsides, and eradicated mindsets still belonging to the early period of spaceflights, still considered the human crew as a component in a list of many others, deemed to be extremely flexible and adaptable to all conditions and situations, keeping its operational efficiency unaltered.

Researches in this field concur on the idea that future generations of space vehicles designed to go beyond Low Earth Orbit (LEO) will need a different methodological approach to their design and implementation, placing the human psychophysical comfort as the core of the system first, hence shaping the hardware around this vital inner space then, obviously within the unavoidable limitations in terms of mass, loads, and available technology. In fact, current researches in the field of habitable spaces in low and microgravity are looking in this direction, creatively suggesting the starting points in developing new materials, procedures and technologies such as inflatable structures, bio-regenerative life support systems, and 3D printed habitats using in situ resources [5]. Therefore, opportunities for research sharing and multidisciplinary collaboration at academic, governmental, and industrial level are extremely promising. In this scenario, the role of aerospace engineers, architects, industrial designers, physicists, psychologists, and physiologists become even more tight than in the past, opening a variety of possible spin-offs and expertise available also for terrestrial 'ordinary' applications, such as sustainable design applied to the built environment, energy systems, aircraft interiors, medical design, interior design, and industrial manufacturing.

2 Space Architecture as Discipline

The subject of habitable spaces in manned spacecraft, in terms of dimensions, life support systems and safety requirements, has necessarily informed the entire development of space vehicles from the beginning, with ballistic capsules Mercury, Gemini and Vostok, and spacecraft like Apollo, Voskhod, and Soyuz. Since the mid-70's with Skylab, Salyut and Mir orbiting stations, until the recent ISS Alpha and Chinese Tiangong 1, the internal habitable space occupied by crew for prolonged missions became an autonomous subject for study and further development, within the traditional aerospace system engineering. Initially considered as an empty space left in the hardware, instead of a habitable space with operational and intrinsic characteristics, the design and formal definition as an ultra-specialized habitat for human permanence in the most extreme environment, attracted interests and expertise of architects, industrial designers, physiologists, psychologists, botanists, and environmental engineers, beyond to physicists and aerospace engineers as traditionally involved. Architectural design of space habitats is not totally new, but has been constantly emerging since 1967, with the involvement of architect Maynard Dalton and designer Raymond Loewy during Apollo-Saturn and Skylab's projects [6]. The architects' contribution revealed to be particularly important during the Skylab Space Station project, still the largest orbiting station ever built in a single module[1], with the presence of industrial designer Raymond Loewy leading the habitat's design team since the initial concept stage. Under his supervision, eight habitability studies were conducted in strict collaboration with final users, the astronauts, to achieve the optimal habitat's configuration. His fundamental role in this achievement is expressed in a letter sent to Loewy on 1974 by Dr. George Mueller, NASA's deputy administrator for manned spaceflights: "I do not believe, that it would have been possible for the Skylab crews to have lived in relative comfort, excellent spirits, and outstanding efficiency had it not been for your creative design, based on a deep understanding of human needs, of the interior environment of Skylab and the human engineering of the equipment and furnishings which the astronauts used" [7].

Despite these initial outstanding achievements, however the contribution and role of architects in design configuration of space habitats seemed largely underestimated, often relegating their expertise to a later stage of development, just filling the gap between the machinery and the needs of whom will operate it. Has been only recently that Space Architecture received a defined mission statement as an autonomous discipline and specialization, stated during the World Space Congress in Houston in 2002 by members of the Technical Aerospace Architecture Subcommittee of the American Institute of Aeronautics and Astronautics (AIAA) as follows: "*Space Architecture is the theory and practice of designing and building inhabited environments in outer space, responding to the deep human drive to explore and occupy new places. Designing for space requires specialized knowledge of orbital mechanics, propulsion, weightlessness, hard vacuum, psychology of hermetic environments and other topics. Space Architecture has complementary relationships with diverse fields such as aerospace engineering, terrestrial architecture, transportation design, medicine, human factors, space science, law, and art*" (ŚATC 2002). As per this definition, Space Architecture would be regarded as an autonomous discipline which comprises the design, planning and implementation of living and working environments in space and planetary bodies such as Moon and Mars, including also Earth analogs such as Antarctic, airborne, desert, high altitude, underground, undersea, and closed ecological systems [8].

Available literature on the subject is quite extensive, even if large part of it presented as NASA papers and reports not necessarily in a systemized manner. However, specialized literature is growing since the interest on this particular subject is constantly rising, defining Space Architecture as an advanced field of studies such as Architecture in extreme environments, which embraces several disciplines at technical and scientific

[1] The Skylab Space Station was realized converting the third stage of a Saturn V rocket into a two-storey living and working space, with an overall internal volume of 320 m^3 and permanent habitable volume of 270.2 m^3. By comparison, the Mir station had an internal volume of 380 m^3 split into 7 modules, and ISS in its final configuration has an internal volume of 935 m^3 divided into 11 modules [7].

level. With renovated interests towards lunar missions, and efforts addressed towards a supposed manned mission on Mars within 2030's, the potentials for advanced studies on the specific subject of human habitats in low and microgravity, besides terrestrial extreme environments such as arid, cold, high, and water, could represent by itself a discipline to be included in architecture and design curricula. In this regard, the rigorous analysis of the engineer and creative synthesis of the architect could be integrated, joining the best for both types of education, surpassing a still diffused mindset that these two approaches are difficult to integrate if not mutually excluding. The plans for a new generation of space vehicles and habitats, necessary for extended length of crewed missions towards Moon and Mars, coupled with habitability issues related to long permanence in conditions of low and microgravity associated to unavoidable psycho-physical comfort, functionality of habitable spaces, and protection against multiple hazards of extended spaceflight, are requesting the contribution of other expertise other than engineering in shaping the habitats' requirements, which it would be part of architect's competency and education.

Since the beginning of their study program, architects are educated to approach problems differently by their engineering colleagues, privileging a heuristic approach open to multiple solutions which in cascade could generate other alternative options along the process. Engineering privileges the linear process, in which the problem is decomposed in multiple subsystems that once proved reliable singularly are then aggregated into one system, who would be reliable itself due transitivity. If different subsystems fail to work once integrated, the linear process restart from the beginning for the failing subsystems, and it is repeated until all of them are properly integrated. Architecture design instead is assimilated to a cyclical process, in which each element is integrated in the whole from the beginning, with different levels of definition at each turn of the cycle, roughly at the early stage and increasingly detailed at the later, iterating a sequence of conception, representation and evaluation until a satisfactory solution is achieved [8]. The difference between *systems engineering* and *systems architecting* basically resides in the way final product is conceived from the early stage: as an aggregation of multiple subsystems analytically responsive to technical requirements and integrated in a final design for the former; an envisioned integrated design solution from the beginning which is analyzed and decomposed to achieve that initial vision for the latter [6]. The contribution that architects could bring to the aerospace sector, traditionally undisputed competence of aerospace engineering, is the focus on human factors and integration of habitability issues with the hardware, in terms of physical and psychological comfort and ergonomics, features which are part of architects' expertise. Such competence would be unavoidable once it will be necessary to figure out habitats and vehicles occupied by a human crew for an undefined period of time, confined in a relative isolation at distances never reached before, immersed in the most hostile and lethal environment ever known by human beings.

3 Conclusions

Opportunities to study and specialize in Space Architecture are still rare, and only a handful of universities are currently offering study programs dedicated to this specialist discipline at master or undergraduate level [8]. However, a growing interest towards STEM disciplines by academic institutions and governmental education bodies worldwide, joined with a rising popularity of space sciences between students' communities and funding research sponsorships by industry and governments, could stimulate also other universities with architecture and design programs to integrate their curricula with subjects related to habitats' design in extreme environments, including low and microgravity. The preliminary knowledge required to student candidates is quite vast and comparable to what an architecture student should have at its fifth year of study or at master's program. As per the NASA document 'Curriculum for Aerospace Architecture', drafted by Dr. Donna P. Duerk, Professor of Architecture at California Polytechnic State University, the students interested in Space Architecture should demonstrate knowledge and ability in architectural history and theory, basic design skills, structural engineering, basic psychology and sociology, basics of biology, physics and chemistry, critical thinking, mathematics, computer literacy, basic human physiology, literature, and principles of sustainability [9]. Architecture per se is a multidisciplinary specialty, and the ideal candidate for this kind of advanced study should have received preliminarily an architectural education, which is making a program in Space Architecture particularly suitable as master's level specialization. Moreover, the multidisciplinary aspect traditionally associated with this type of studies, would represent by itself the optimal way for an academic institution to strengthen internal and external collaboration between different colleges and departments, with other academic institutions, and with industry and research institutions, in terms of expertise and funding. Technical and procedural spin-offs from advanced systems developed for habitats in reduced gravity and extreme environments, are currently used in 'ordinary' built environment in order to enhance its sustainability, or in habitable systems to improve their performance and reliability, receiving particular attention both from private and governmental stakeholders in terms of research funding and investments. The recent involvement of well-known international architectural firms in design competitions for lunar and Martian habitats, such as Foster + Partners, BIG and SOM, and a growing number of specialized publications and articles addressed to this specific subject, reveals a rising interest in this field from design community at large.

References

1. McCurdy, H.E.: Space and the American Imagination. Johns Hopkins University Press, Baltimore (2011)
2. Seedhouse, E.: SpaceX: Making Commercial Spaceflight a Reality. Springer-Praxis, Heidelberg (2013)
3. Seedhouse, E.: Bigelow Aerospace: Colonizing Space One Module at a Time. Springer-Praxis, Heidelberg (2015)

4. Connors, M., Harrison, A., Akins, F.: Living Aloft: Human Requirements for Extended Spaceflight. NASA SP-483, Ames Research Center (1985)
5. Leach, N. (ed.): Space architecture: the New Frontier for design research. Architectural Design No. 232. Wiley, London (2014)
6. Howe, A.S., Sherwood, B.: Out of This World: The New Field of Space Architecture. AIAA, Reston (2009)
7. Häuplik-Meusberger, S.: Architecture for Astronauts: An Activity Based Approach. Springer, Wien (2011)
8. Häuplik-Meusberger, S., Bannova, O.: Space Architecture Education for Engineers and Architects. Springer, Heidelberg (2016)
9. Duerk, D.P.: Curriculum for aerospace architecture with emphasis on lunar base and habitat studies. NASA/CR-2004-212820, Ames Research Center (2004)

Application of Fuzzy Evaluation Methods on Campus Security Awareness

Shu Wang, Qiang Qu, and Xue-bo Chen(✉)

School of Electronic and Information Engineering,
University of Science and Technology Liaoning,
Anshan 114051, Liaoning, People's Republic of China
xuebochen@126.com

Abstract. Traditional safety evaluation methods, most of which rely on the experience of experts and managers to draw conclusions, lack of scientific. In this paper, the fuzzy comprehensive evaluation method is used to establish a campus security valuation index system. Firstly, the analytic hierarchy process is used to calculate the single factor evaluation decision matrix, and calculate the weight of each factor in different levels. Secondly, using fuzzy evaluation method, membership function, fuzzy operator and linguistic variables for security evaluation. Finally, we conclude that the school's students, front-line teachers, and managers have a higher overall security awareness according to the evaluation of the maximum membership degree principle. Therefore, it is recommended that schools further strengthen students' security awareness through security education lectures and other training lessons.

Keywords: Campus security · Fuzzy comprehensive evaluation method · Security awareness

1 Introduction

With the rapid development of higher education, the number of college students is increasing, and the campus security issues are becoming more and more prominent [1]. Campus security issues have become a major concern for governments, schools and the security community. College campus is the basic place for college teachers and students to study, work and live. The security of campus is related to the normal development of teaching, research, study and life. At present, universities do not have a uniform set of standards to check the school's security status, and the indicators used for inspections cover a narrow range of issues, involving one or several aspects of the school. Therefore, the establishment of a scientific, reasonable and systematic campus safety evaluation system has become one of the important topics in college research. Various scholars have achieved some research results in improving campus safety evaluation. Such as Xin Qu [2] from the existing security risks of colleges and universities, in-depth analysis of the countermeasures to solve campus security problems. Wuyu Xu [3] analyzed the hidden dangers and causes of the safety of most college campuses, and proposed solutions. Analytic hierarchy process, or AHP for short, is a decision-making method that decomposes the elements always related to decision-

T. Ahram et al. (Eds.): IHIET 2019, AISC 1018, pp. 105–109, 2020.
https://doi.org/10.1007/978-3-030-25629-6_17

making into levels of objectives, criteria and schemes, etc., on which qualitative and quantitative analysis can be carried out. AHP is to break down complex problems into no. The same various elements, according to the affiliation between the elements and mutual shadow Ringing hierarchical clustering to form a hierarchical, ordered hierarchical structure. The importance of the factor is based on the expert's judgment on reality. Represents the importance order weight of each level factor. Based on the characteristics of the research object, using the analytic hierarchy process.

2 Paper Preparation

2.1 Evaluation Factor Sets

$$U = \{U_1, U_2, \ldots, U_n\}$$

There are n evaluation indexes, indicating that the object to be evaluated will be judged and described [4].

2.2 The Establishment of Evaluation Result Sets

$$V = \{V_1, V_2, \ldots V_n\}$$

The indicators are divided into five levels, which are none, very low, low, high, and very high, and scores are assigned.

2.3 Determining the Weight of Indexes Using AHP Method

AHP combines qualitative and quantitative analysis and could solve complicated multi-factor problems. Therefore, this paper adopts the analytic hierarchy process to construct the enterprise security situation system.

(1) Structural hierarchy model.
The evaluation index system of petrochemical plants security situation can be divided into three layers: target layer, criterion layer and scheme layer.
(2) Build judgment matrix of pairing comparison.
The method of AHP is used to seek the weights of various factors. Evaluation indexes in the same factor set are pairwise compared by panel of experts for their importance to the upper criterion or target based on the 1–9 scale in order to establish the judgement matrix of the factor set [4].
(3) The weight calculation procedure is as follows:
1. The sum of each column of the judgement matrix is calculated H_{ij}.
2. Each column of the judgment matrix can be normalized W_{ij}.
3. The average of each row of the judgment matrix is calculated W_i. W_i is the weight of each index.

2.4 Single Factor Evaluation, Fuzzy Relation Matrix R

Judging by a single factor and determining the membership degree of the evaluation object to the element, it is called the single factor fuzzy evaluation. It is necessary to establish a fuzzy relation matrix R for single factor evaluation.

2.5 Comprehensive Fuzzy Evaluation

The weight set A and fuzzy relation matrix R are obtained by analytic hierarchy process, a comprehensive risk evaluation model is established. The calculation formula is B = A*R.

3 Empirical Analysis

3.1 Model Establishment of Fuzzy Comprehensive Evaluation

Nine evaluation indexes were selected from the three aspects of students, school environment and school management. There are three first-grade evaluation indicators and nine second-grade evaluation indicators included in this study [5, 6]. This can be seen in Table 1.

Table 1. Campus safety evaluation index system.

Code	Factor subset	Code	Factor
C_1	Campus safety assessment student	C_{11}	Anti-theft awareness
		C_{12}	Safety awareness level
		C_{13}	Emotional and academic pressure
C_2	School environment	C_{21}	Campus health security
		C_{22}	Campus road traffic
		C_{23}	Campus security measures
C_3	School management	C_{31}	Emergency drill
		C_{32}	Lecture training exercise on campus safety issues
		C_{33}	Security staff processing

3.2 Weight Calculation

The weight result is shown in Table 2.

3.3 Single Factor Evaluation Matrix

Making a comprehensive assessment by using five-level division method, that is none, very low, low, high, and very high, the worst in five grades [7]. Additionally, Five experts to evaluate. Statistical evaluation results as shown in Table 3.

Table 2. The weight result form.

Code	Weight	Code	Weight
C_1	0.333	C_{11}	0.120
		C_{12}	0.631
		C_{13}	0.248
C_2	0.333	C_{21}	0.682
		C_{22}	0.182
		C_{23}	0.135
C_3	0.333	C_{31}	0.634
		C_{32}	0.260
		C_{33}	0.106

Table 3. Evaluation form.

Evaluation indicator number	Very high	High	Low	Very low	None
C_{11}	3	1	0	1	0
C_{12}	3	2	0	0	0
C_{13}	2	2	1	0	0
C_{21}	2	2	1	0	0
C_{22}	2	2	1	0	0
C_{23}	0	0	3	2	0
C_{31}	1	3	1	0	0
C_{32}	2	2	1	0	0
C_{33}	2	2	1	0	0

3.4 Fuzzy Comprehensive Evaluation

(1) First order fuzzy comprehensive evaluation
First-Grade indicator fuzzy comprehensive evaluation of the petrochemical campus security situation as follow:

$$B1 = A1 * R1 = (0.550 \quad 0.376 \quad 0.050 \quad 0.024 \quad 0)$$

$$B2 = (0.346 \quad 0.346 \quad 0.254 \quad 0.054 \quad 0)$$

$$B3 = (0.273 \quad 0.527 \quad 0.200 \quad 0 \quad 0)$$

(2) Second order fuzzy comprehensive evaluation

$$B = A * R = (0.389 \quad 0.415 \quad 0.164 \quad 0.026 \quad 0)$$

It can be seen from the evaluation results that the largest relative membership degree is 0.415, campus security awareness is high.

4 Conclusion

This paper uses AHP and fuzzy mathematics comprehensive evaluation method. A scientific, reasonable and operational university campus safety evaluation Model are established, which can objectively evaluate the security level of college campuses, The model is highly adaptable. The example proves that the model is in the campus safety evaluation is effective. The improvement of school campus safety management provides a scientific basis and method law. But the model is only some of the discussions in the campus safety evaluation. There are many methods and theories that deserve further study. According to the maximum membership degree [8], College students, administrators, and front-line teachers have a higher awareness of campus security.

Acknowledgments. This research reported herein was supported by the NSFC of China under Grants No.71571091 and 71771112.

References

1. Fan, T., Li, Z.: College campus security based on interpretative structural model method problem exploration. J. Educ. Explor. **10**, 64–65 (2014). (in Chinese)
2. Qu, X.: Analysis of university campus security problems and countermeasures. Jiamusi Univ. J. Sci. **28**(2), 130–131 (2010). (in Chinese)
3. Xu, W.: Reflections and countermeasures on campus safety in colleges and universities. J. Mudanjiang Jiao J. Educ. Coll. **117**(5), 66–67 (2009). (in Chinese)
4. Yang, W., Xia, X., Pan, B., Gu, C., Yue, J.: The fuzzy comprehensive evaluation of water and sand inrush risk during underground mining. J. Intell. Fuzzy Syst. **30**, 2289–2295 (2016)
5. Zhang, S.Y., Wu, M.: A fuzzy analytic hierarchy process based model for assessing material suppliers. Logistics Sci.-Tceh. **6**(2), 89–90 (2007)
6. Zhou, Z., Zhang, X., Dong, W.: Fuzzy comprehensive evaluation for safety guarantee system of reclaimed water quality. Procedia Environ. Sci. **18**, 227–235 (2013)
7. Bao, J., Zhang, J., Li, F., Liu, C., Shi, S.: Social benefits of the mine occupational health and safety management systems of mines in China and Sweden based on a fuzzy analytic hierarchy process: a comparative study. J. Intell. Fuzzy Syst. **31**, 3113–3120 (2016)
8. Chen, D., Tian, H.: Behavior based safety for accidents prevention and positive study in China construction project. Procedia Eng. **43**, 528–534 (2012)

Diurnal Temperature Variation in an Idealized Room for Different Wall Materials Using a Thermal Load Model in the Philippine Setting

Neil Martin Manaoat[1(✉)], Johnrob Bantang[2], and Luis Maria Bo-ot[3]

[1] National Graduate School of Engineering, University of the Philippines, 1101 Diliman, Quezon City, Philippines
ngmanaoat@up.edu.ph
[2] National Institute of Physics, University of the Philippines, 1101 Diliman, Quezon City, Philippines
jbantang@nip.upd.edu.ph
[3] College of Architecture, University of the Philippines, 1101 Diliman, Quezon City, Philippines
ltboot@up.edu.ph

Abstract. A simple thermal model is used to simulate the heat load received by an idealized room incorporating climatological factors and daily weather patterns in the Philippine setting. The model provides diurnal temperature variation of the idealized room with varying wall materials situated in Quezon City during the cool-dry and hot-dry seasons in the country. The model was used to calculate the heat load to keep the temperature of the room less than 25 °C. Rooms with walls made of bamboo and oak were demonstrated to perform better than those which are made of concrete, bricks and sandstone. The room with oak walls were shown to provide up to 3 × savings in terms of computed daily energy consumption during the hot-dry season. This study can help us provide design and structural considerations in relation to energy utilization and possibly conservation.

Keywords: Thermodynamics · Air conditioning · Temperature · Regulations · Simulation · Energy conservation

1 Introduction

One of the challenges of building simulations is choosing the right model. According to Saltelli et al. [1], models can be *diagnostic* or *prognostic,* and *law-driven* or *data-driven.* In summary, diagnostic models are used to identify the cause of some phenomenon while prognostic models predict the behavior of a system given a set of laws. A law-driven model works forward by simulating output data using a detailed physical model while data-driven works backward by inputting data to statistical models to output detailed physical models. The kind of model that building energy simulations commonly use can be classified as a *prognostic law-driven* model because of the set of laws used to predict the behavior of the system in study [2].

T. Ahram et al. (Eds.): IHIET 2019, AISC 1018, pp. 110–116, 2020.
https://doi.org/10.1007/978-3-030-25629-6_18

There are comprehensive multi zonal models like Mendonca et al.'s where simultaneous heat and mass transfer model was created using SPARK but doesn't include radiation [3]. A multi zonal model divides the room in study in smaller units and were then solved numerically. Some studies like Lu et al's opted to analytical approach instead of the more commonly used numerical approach [4]. This paper intends to apply a prognostic law-driven model that uses recorded publicly available local weather data and simulated solar radiation to simulate the temperature variation of a room with varying wall materials. The model used in this paper is single zonal computation. The model is detailed enough to include terrestrial and atmospheric radiation, and air temperature but does not include mass transfer between the walls.

In the Philippine setting, daily conditions (with average year-round temperature around 27 °C but can even reach a high around 40 °C) are deemed uncomfortable [5]. Therefore, air conditioning has been profusely used locally. This paper focuses on minimizing energy consumption without compromising thermal comfort. While thermal comfort is composed of several factors like clothing and humidity, only the room air temperature was initially considered.

2 Atmospheric Variables

A weather generator was created to output hourly shortwave and longwave radiation, air temperature, dew point, humidity, and cloud cover for a chosen day. Except for the radiation outputs, all variables are downloaded from www.wunderground.com.

Humidity, and Air and Dew Point Temperatures. The hourly values for humidity, and air and dew point temperatures were acquired by averaging hourly records based on the month and day from 1997 to 2016. This is an approximation and should not be used for applications relying on forecast or accuracy. The generator simply provides plausible and acceptable values of variables needed for the simulation.

Cloud Cover. Cloud cover is needed to calculate the atmospheric longwave radiation which contributes to the overall longwave radiation received by the outside walls of the room [6]. The downloaded dataset included description of the cloud cover. However, cloud cover is commonly measured in terms of *okta*. Okta is a measuring system ranging from integers 1 to 8. Each number refers to an eight of the sky covered. Table 1 shows the conversion from the terms in the dataset to the okta system.

Radiation. Datasets which includes solar radiation values are very rare (if not available at all) for the case of the Philippines. This is why solar radiation is simulated using different algorithms and formulas. To provide a detailed simulation on solar radiation, the sun path was calculated first. To calculate these angles, a simple algorithm provided by the website www.pveducation.org was used. The absolute intensity of solar radiation varies throughout the day due to sun path and the air mass. Given the airmass, the direct normal irradiance can be calculated [7].

Table 1. The corresponding conversion to okta values of the six available cloud cover terms in the dataset. (Note: this conversion is subjected to author's prerogative)

Description	Okta value
Haze	1
Heavy Haze	2
Scattered clouds	3
Partly cloudy	4
Mostly cloudy	6
Overcast	8

3 Thermodynamics of the System

The model included all modes of heat transfer namely (1) conduction, (2) convection, and (3) radiation. In the case of the room, heat transfer through conduction occurs in the walls because of the temperature difference of its outside and inside surfaces. The model assumes the homogeneity of the wall materials. The ceiling and the floor are assumed to be adiabatic. Convection happens due to the air, and radiation happens through the absorption of shortwave and longwave radiation. There is a convenient way to allow the calculation of both convection and radiation in a single formula but would introduce the concept of *sol-air temperature.* Sol-air temperature T_{sa} is a fictitious temperature that can account solar radiation and longwave exchanges from the environment in addition to convection when substituted to Newton's Law of Convection [8]. All radiation calculations were based from Kehrer et al's study [9]. Another assumption is that the heat transfer is one dimensional.

3.1 Thermal Load Model

The heat transfer equation of the whole room is equated to the sum of all heat transfer processes it received given by the set of equations

$$C\frac{dT_{w,out}}{dT} = A(h_c + h_r)(T_{sa} - T_{w,out}) + \frac{T_{w,in} - T_{w,out}}{R} \tag{1}$$

$$C\frac{dT_{w,in}}{dT} = h_c A(T_{rm} - T_{w,in}) + \frac{T_{w,out} - T_{w,in}}{R} \tag{2}$$

$$C_{air}\frac{dT_{rm}}{dT} = \sum_{wall}^{6walls} h_c A_{wall}(T_{wall} - T_{rm}) + q_{input} \tag{3}$$

where C is thermal capacitance of the wall, A is area of the wall, $T_{\mathrm{w,out}}$ is the temperature of outside wall, $T_{\mathrm{w,in}}$ is temperature of inside wall, C_{air} is thermal capacitance of air, q_{input} is power input and R is thermal resistance.

In Eqs. 2 and 3, the heat transfer received by the outer wall through radiation and convection was included as a single term using a sol-air formula. The terms with R is the heat transfer due to conduction. The cooling load refers to the rate of energy needed to cool a structure to a certain temperature.

This set of equations was calculated numerically with a time step of 24 × 3600/1000 or 86.4 s using the forward Euler method of solving differential equations. For the room model, it is assumed to be situated at Quezon City, Philippines and has outer dimensions of 6 × 3 × 3 (length × width × height) m^3. The length by height surfaces of the room (longer walls) were facing the east and west directly. The walls have a thickness of 0.2000 m. The thermal properties of the wall (Table 2) depend on what material is it made of. All materials included are assumed to be painted white at the outside. There are no doors and fenestrations in the room since the focus of the study is to compare the materials with each other. There is no present literature on the thermal properties of local lumbers like coconuts, bamboo, acacia, narra and other popular lumbers used in the Philippines. The closest that was found was a study done by Shah et al. [10] on the thermal conductivity of engineered bamboo composites. Oak was chosen even though it's not particularly used in the country to know how hardwood compares to the other materials.

Table 2. Thermal properties of the specified wall materials

Material	Specific heat c ($J/kg{\cdot}K$)	Thermal conductivity k (W/m·K)	Density ρ (kg/m^3)
Concrete	880	1.13	2320
Brick	1000	1.2	2165
Sandstone	801	1.23	1867
Processed bamboo	1759	0.26	714
Oak	2000	0.17	750

4 Results and Discussion

The temperature variations of each room with different wall materials were compared in a 7-day simulation for each season. The two seasons are the cool-dry (December–February) and hot-dry (March–May) seasons. For each simulation, two temperature variations with that same material is calculated. The first one is the temperature variation when the room has no other external power input. The second is when external power is applied to maintain the temperature of 25 °C. As we can see in Fig. 1, there is a phase difference with the outside and inside temperature. The attenuation is due to the decrement factor of the wall. The time lag and the decrement factor are dependent on the following: thermal capacitance, thermal conductivity, thickness, convective heat transfer coefficient on both side of the wall and the angular frequency [11].

Time lag is helpful when occupants need heat during the night like in deserts where night temperatures can reach up to negative Celsius. The dispersal of heat through the night absorbed during the day can be used as a passive source of heating. However, in the Philippines, like most tropical countries, day and night temperatures can still be

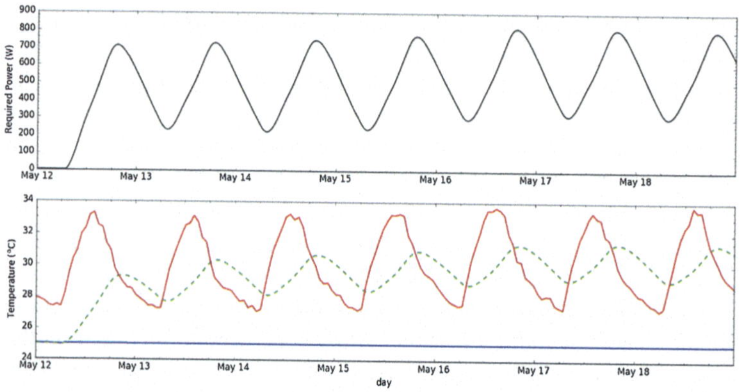

Fig. 1. Output of the model for the concrete walls during the hot-dry season. (above) variation of power required to maintain the temperature to 25 °C. (below) The red plot is the outside air temperature. The dotted green line is the temperature variation for free-floating conditions (qinput = 0) while the solid blue line is when air conditioning is turned on.

deemed uncomfortably hot. A high time lag might be detrimental specifically for residential buildings since the occupancy generally peaks during the night when people rest and sleep after a day's work. Figure 2 shows the summary of the cooling energy for 7 days during the cool-dry and hot-dry seasons. We can see that the hot-dry season cooling load is much higher than in the cool-dry season. The two lumbers, oak and bamboo, also performed better than the other three.

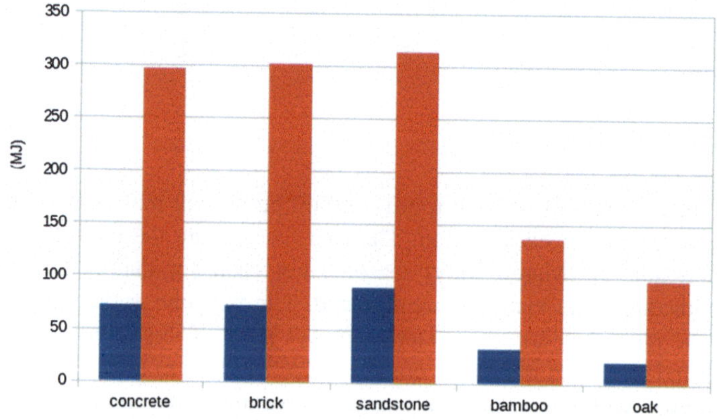

Fig. 2. Calculated total cooling energy for each room with different wall materials during the 7-day exposure to the cool-dry and hot-dry seasons.

By total cooling energy alone, it seems like there is not much of a difference between concrete, brick, and sandstone walls. However, if we are going to compare the temperature variations of the three in Fig. 2, the sandstone room becomes colder than concrete and brick from about 12 midnight to about 12 noon. If the expected occupancy is at this span of time, the sandstone room is the better choice than concrete and brick. It is important to note that the power requirements calculated here belongs to an empty room. No other heat sources like furniture surfaces or appliances are given so the calculated cooling load is lower than in real life.

5 Conclusions and Recommendations

Using a simple model that uses local climatological factors and daily weather patterns in the Philippine setting, the temperature variation and thermal load requirements of the idealized rooms were compared. It was shown that oak, or lumber in general, performs better in Philippine conditions. Oak walls provided up to $3\times$ savings in terms of total daily energy consumption compared to the commonly used concrete. This is true when the room needs to be cooled throughout the day.

However, if the purpose of a building is to avoid the usage of air conditioning as much as possible, occupancy should be considered. It should be noted when the occupants need to be the most comfortable. For example, if the occupancy of a certain building is during the day, it would be good to have a high decrement factor to decrease the effect of the outside temperature to the indoor temperature. However, for buildings that has occupancy during the night, it would be good to have wall materials that respond to outside environment as fast as possible since you want to maximize the colder temperature of the night.

References

1. Saltelli, A., Ratto, M., Andres, T., Campolongo, F., Cariboni, J., Gatelli, D., et al. Global sensitivity analysis: the primer. Wiley, Chichester, West Sussex PO19 8SQ, England (2008). ISBN: 978-0-470-05997-5
2. Coakley, D., Raftery, P., Keane, M.: A review of methods to match building energy simulation models to measured data. Renew. Sustain. Energy Rev. **37**, 123–141 (2014). https://doi.org/10.1016/j.rser.2014.05.007 URL https://escholarship.org/uc/item/88z3g017
3. Mendonca, K.C., Inard, C., Wurtz, E., Winkelmann, F.C., Allard, F.: A zonal model for predicting simultaneous heat and moisture transfer in buildings. In: Proceedings of Indoor Air (2002)
4. Lu, X., Lu, T., Viljanen, M.: A new analytical method to simulate heat transfer process in buildings. Appl. Therm. Eng. **26**(16), 1901–1909 (2006)
5. Cui, W., Cao, G., Park, J., Ouyang, Q., Zhu, Y.: Influence of indoor air temperature on human thermal comfort, motivation and performance. Build. Environ., 114–122. ISSN 0360-1323 (2013). https://doi.org/10.1016/j.buildenv.2013.06.012
6. Lauster, M., Remmen, P., Fuchs, M., Teichmann, J., Streblow, R., Muller, D.: Modelling long-wave radiation heat exchange for thermal network building simulations at urban scale using Modelica (2014)
7. Kasten, F., Young, A.: Revised optical air mass tables and approximation formula. Appl. Opt., **28**(22), 4735–4738 (1989). https://doi.org/10.1364/ao.28.004735, http://ao.osa.org/abstract.cfm?URI=ao-28-22-4735

8. Stephenson, D.: Thermal radiation and its effect on the heating and cooling of buildings. In: Technical Report June, National Research Council of Canada – Division of Building Research, Ottawa (1961)
9. Kehrer, M., Schmidt, T.: Radiation effects on exterior surfaces. In: Proceedings of the 8th Symposium on Building Physics in the Nordic Countries, pp. 207–212 (2008)
10. Shah, D., Bock, M., Mulligan, H., Ramage, M.: Thermal conductivity of engineered bamboo composites. J. Mater. Sci. **51**, 2991–3002 (2015)
11. Luo, C., Moghtaderi, B., Sugo, H.: Time lags and decrement factors under air-conditioned and free-floating conditions for multi-layer materials. Building Simulation, pp. 95–100 (2007)

User Experience of a Social Media Based Knowledge Sharing System in Industry Work

Susanna Aromaa[1(✉)], Maria Tsourma[2], Stylianos Zikos[2], Eija Kaasinen[1], Mariia Kreposna[3], Anastasios Drosou[2], and Dimitrios Tzovaras[2]

[1] VTT Technical Research Centre of Finland Ltd., Tampere, Finland
{susanna.aromaa,eija.kaasinen}@vtt.fi
[2] Information Technologies Institute Centre for Research and Technology Hellas, Thessaloniki, Greece
{mtsourma,szikos,drosou,dimitrios.tzovaras}@iti.gr
[3] FINN-POWER Oy, Seinäjoki, Finland
mariia.kreposna@primapower.com

Abstract. With increasing automation, the work in manufacturing industry is getting knowledge intensive: workers need to solve complex problems to keep systems running. The knowledge needed in these situations often cannot be found in ready-made manuals but it is tacit knowledge possessed by co-workers. This paper presents a user study of a knowledge sharing platform. The platform integrates production information and social media features, thus connecting discussions to specific machine states or error situations. The platform was evaluated with factory workers in a workshop. The results show that integration of production information and social media features such as messaging is valuable, as it proactively provides practical solutions to the problem at hand. The results also show that the use of social media features in industrial environment requires changes in organizational policies, processes and culture. The findings of this study can be considered when developing social media applications for industrial use.

Keywords: Knowledge sharing · Social media · User evaluation · Production · Gamification · Industry work

1 Introduction

Industry 4.0 factories require smart and skilled operators because work in manufacturing industry is getting knowledge intensive. Recovering from an alarm situation requires knowledge but access to the knowledge can be challenging as situations are different and most of them are not documented in the official manuals for end-users. The operators recover from alarms by learning by doing or by contacting their colleagues. In these cases, the shared knowledge remains known by few. Therefore, there is a need to share the knowledge more widely to make good practices visible and accessible for all.

T. Ahram et al. (Eds.): IHIET 2019, AISC 1018, pp. 117–123, 2020.
https://doi.org/10.1007/978-3-030-25629-6_19

A promising approach to support knowledge sharing is social media technologies. Social media can be defined as a combination of various forms of media content that are publicly available in a platform and that are created by end-users in a participatory and collaborative fashion [1]. Currently, the use of social media technologies and social messenger systems in the work context has grown as organizations have begun to realize that social media might aid organizational knowledge sharing [2, 3]. Aromaa et al. [4] report user studies of an augmented reality (AR) based, knowledge-sharing system in industrial maintenance. In their study, the social media features for adding and sharing one's own comments, notes and pictures embedded with AR on physical objects was seen very useful.

The use of social media to support knowledge sharing in work environments has still challenges to overcome. Mere installation of social media platforms is not enough: success in adoption and effectiveness in full exploitation will be dependent on reconfiguration and redesign of the whole socio-technical and managerial system [5]. According to Kassner et al. [6], "no manufacturing-specific approach for integrating social media into the shop floor workspace currently exists".

Key challenge in knowledge sharing is how to motivate the employees to participate. Swacha [7] has proposed gamification as an effective way to increase motivation to share knowledge. Gamification is commonly defined as the use of gaming elements to improve user experience and user engagement in non-game services and applications [8]. It is widely used in the domains of marketing, health and education. However, in factory floor environments, it is a new concept [9].

This paper describes the design and user study of a knowledge sharing platform targeted to factory floor workers. The platform integrates social media features to the production information. This facilitates connecting discussions e.g. to certain machine alarms, as the relevant discussions can be shown to the user when an alarm occurs. Messages can be complemented with photos and videos to visualize proposed solutions. In addition, gamification features aim to motivate workers to share knowledge.

2 Social Media Platform

The Social Media Platform (SoMeP) is a web-based application, which aims to increase interaction, communication and socialization among workers through the use of various social media technologies such as discussion forums, instant messaging, news feeds, and gamification. The main novelty of SoMeP is that it integrates social media features with production information. By using SoMeP, workers are able to share multimedia content, exchange opinions with their colleagues, as well as find and provide solutions to problems. SoMeP is able to receive alarms from machines of the production line and visualize them in real-time, as shown in Fig. 1. When a user faces an alarm situation, s/he can find information about the alarm codes on the production view available in SoMeP. By selecting a specific alarm in the view, the system makes a query to the knowledge base for relevant discussions in the forum based on the alarm ID and machine ID, and presents the list of relevant discussions found. The list can be filtered by creation time and popularity. The user is able to add a new post related to the specific alarm ID and to attach a file in a discussion. In addition, user feedback mechanisms such as text replies to posts and 'Like' buttons are implemented in SoMeP.

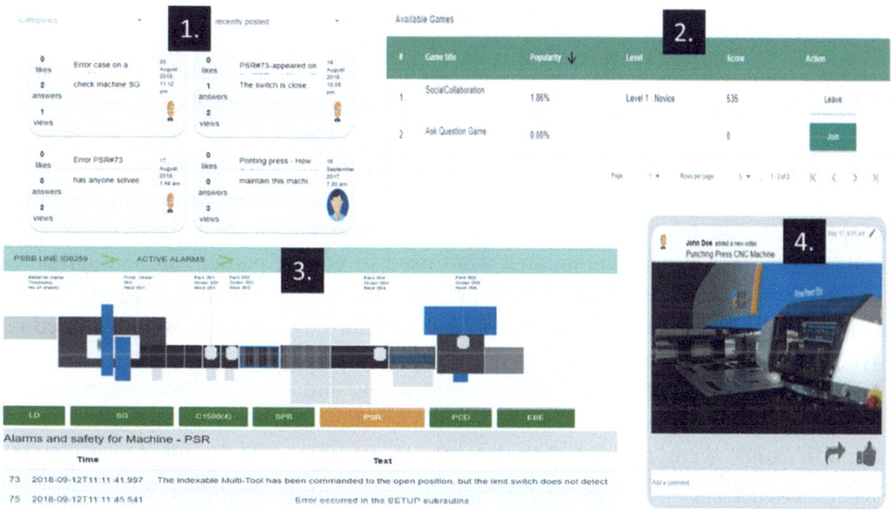

Fig. 1. SoMeP screenshots: (1) discussions in the forum, (2) user participation in games, (3) production status monitoring and machine error alarms and (4) news feed.

A gamification module is integrated into the SoMeP, aiming at increasing workers' motivation and participation in knowledge sharing. It implements a rating system, through which users can earn points and awards when sharing their knowledge and when others assess the shared knowledge valuable. Moreover, predefined levels can be unlocked based on the collected points, indicating user engagement. Awards in the form of badges can be earned when a user has performed certain number of actions. Actions, rules and awards are defined in games that are created by the administrator, targeting to motivate users to participate in discussions and share good solutions to work-related problems. A personal profile dashboard informs the user about the collected points per game, current level and earned awards (Fig. 1).

SoMeP is intended to be deployed inside the local network of the factory and can be accessed via PC as well as mobile devices such as tablets located at the shop floor. The platform supports two types of users, administrators and regular users. All users are able to login to the system, view current active alarms, search for already stored solutions, provide feedback, and upload new information on how a specific alarm can be resolved. In alarm situations, the system displays the alarm code and the "official" guidance related to it. If the user cannot resolve the alarm with the guidance, s/he can open the SoMeP discussion related to the alarm. If the discussion does not help, either s/he can request support via instant messaging or e-mail. Administrators can additionally perform content moderation operations and set up games.

3 Methods

Nine male participants took part to the evaluation. Their age range was 24–56 years (average 46 years). They were all working in a company that manufactures highly automated metal sheet processing machines. Their professions were automation designer, technical specialist, electrician, technician, two engineers, quality expert, manager and head of design. Four of them were active messenger users and five did have some experience of messenger systems (e.g., WhatsApp, Facebook messenger).

A focus group approach was used as a data collection method. The SoMeP usability, pros/cons and development ideas were discussed in two groups. In addition, a project specific evaluation framework [10] was used when creating questionnaires and discussion topics. The questionnaires were used to collect participant demographics, UX (with smiley faces on 5 point Likert scale), the system usability scale (SUS) [11] and knowledge sharing questions (5 point Likert scale). Discussions were recorded via a voice recorder. Data was analyzed qualitatively.

First, the participants signed the consent forms and filled in demographic information. The SoMeP was introduced briefly to the whole group with a live demo. Then, the participants were divided into two focus groups with 5 and 4 participants, respectively. Three facilitators were collecting data: one in the first group and two in the second group. Within both groups, participants were encouraged to try out different features of the SoMeP running on a PC such as discussion forums, instant messaging, news feed, production alarm views, and the games. After trying each feature, participants gave comments and facilitators asked questions related to the pros and cons as well as further development ideas. Each participant filled in an evaluation questionnaire at the end of the focus group.

4 Results

4.1 User Experience, Usability and User Acceptance

The overall user experience of the SoMeP was good: most of the participants felt using the system as a positive experience. In addition, the usability of the system was rated to be on a good level: the SUS score was 75. It can be perceived that the participants would like to use the system frequently. They agreed that the system was easy to use and they would not need guidance from an expert. They thought that the system was not complex, nor did it have too many inconsistencies. Most of them agreed that the system would be easy to learn to use and felt quite confident while using it.

Regarding user acceptance, the participants agreed that integrating discussions with production system information was beneficial. In addition, they agreed that the system could increase knowledge sharing within the factory. Most of the participants thought that seeing how many had liked the comments was good when evaluating the usefulness of the comments. However, 3 participants neither agreed nor disagreed with it. The ability to add videos to the discussions was referred as beneficial.

The participants gave contradictory comments regarding the gamification features. They mentioned that gamification could motivate workers to share knowledge but on the other hand, one participant said that gathering points does not belong to the work. In the knowledge sharing platform, the gamification scores are seen only by the worker him/herself. Still the participants wondered if other people could see their personal scores. The participants were concerned that managers may think that workers are only playing and not doing their work. They also thought that there might be cultural differences on accepting games, and gamification might not work in less developed countries due to workers' skill level and workplace hierarchy.

4.2 Comments and Development Ideas

The participants suggested some usability improvements during the discussions. For example, more text could be visible of the messages before opening them, the text and icons could be larger throughout the platform, and several alarms should be shown simultaneously.

The participants claimed that the production view was the best feature in the system. They commented that it is useful because it was possible to search messages based on the alarm code. However, they noticed that for a successful search, the users should write alarm codes in similar formats. The participants thought that the filtering and sorting of messages could be improved to manage all the messages better. Adding videos to the messages was seen useful: with them novice workers can concretely see how to perform an assembly task. However, the participants wondered how the overall content moderation would be organized.

In addition, the SoMeP could be useful in knowledge sharing between different groups (e.g., worker-worker, worker-maintenance, worker-management, company-customer). The participants pointed that the knowledge sharing community would probably influence the knowledge sharing activity and the content. This is because sharing within a familiar, limited group, is easier.

The cultural differences were discussed too. In some less developed countries, it is hard to imagine workers sharing knowledge via the system. In addition, cultural differences exist between companies for example in the form of different policies for knowledge sharing. The participants also raised a concern that some people do not want to share their expertise to others, e.g. because they may fear losing their power as acknowledged experts.

The participants commented that SoMeP could be useful if a company has lot of rented workforce. They suggested that by using this platform new people could ask questions easily even if they do not know who to ask. In addition, it would help company's workers learn to know new workers if their profiles (name and photo) are accessible through the platform.

5 Conclusions

It can be concluded that most of the participants liked SoMeP and found it useful and easy to use. Particularly, integration of production information and messages was seen valuable. The participants thought that SoMeP would increase knowledge sharing but they were questioning whether gamification is the right way to motivate workers to participate. The use of social media features in industrial environments requires changes in organizational policies, processes and cultures. It is important to define the community who shares the knowledge and who else can access the shared knowledge. Content moderation is needed to make sure that false information is not shared. As a future work, we plan to exploit the feedback received from the workers in order to improve the usability of the platform, re-design the interface and enrich it with additional features. In addition, the acceptance of gamification use in a production environment needs to be evaluated thoroughly. In general, social media technologies should be studied in a long-term use to understand better the needs for content supervision and company policies.

Acknowledgments. This project has received funding from the European Union's Horizon 2020 research and innovation programme under grant agreement No. 723277 (project Factory2Fit). This paper reflects only the authors' view and the Commission is not responsible for any use that may be made of the information it contains. The authors are grateful to all researchers, concepts' developers and company representatives who have contributed to and supported the work presented in this publication.

References

1. Kaplan, A.M., Haenlein, M.: Users of the world, unite! The challenges and opportunities of social media. Bus. Horiz. **53**(1), 59–68 (2010)
2. Leonardi, P.M.: Ambient awareness and knowledge acquisition: using social media to learn 'who knows what' and 'who knows whom'. MIS Q. **39**(4), 747–762 (2015)
3. Jarrahi, M.H., Sawyer, S.: Social technologies, informal knowledge practices, and the enterprise. J. Org. Comp. Elect. Com. **23**(1–2), 110–137 (2013)
4. Aromaa, S., Väätänen, A., Hakkarainen, M., Kaasinen, E.: User experience and user acceptance of an augmented reality based knowledge-sharing solution in industrial maintenance work. In: 8th International Conference on Applied Human Factors and Ergonomics, pp. 145–156. Springer, Cham (2018)
5. Denyer, D., Parry, E., Flowers, P.: "Social", "open" and "participative"? Exploring personal experiences and organisational effects of enterprise 2.0 use. Long Range Plann. **44**(5–6), 375–396 (2011)
6. Kassner, L., Hirmer, P., Wieland, M., Steimle, F., Königsberger, J., Mitschang, B.: The social factory: connecting people, machines and data in manufacturing for context-aware exception escalation. In: 50th Hawaii International Conference on System Sciences, pp. 1673–1682 (2017)
7. Swacha, J.: Gamification in knowledge management: motivating for knowledge sharing. Polish J. Manag. Stud. **12**(2), 150–160 (2015)
8. Deterding, S., Sicart, M., Nacke, L., O'Hara, K., Dixon, D.: Gamification: using game design elements in non-gaming contexts. In: CHI'11 Extended Abstracts on Human Factors in Computing Systems, pp. 2425–2428. ACM (2011)
9. Korn, O., Funk, M., Schmidt, A.: Design approaches for the gamification of production environments: a study focusing on acceptance. In: 8th ACM International Conference on Pervasive Technologies Related to Assistive Environments, p. 6. ACM (2015)

10. Kaasinen, E., Liinasuo, M., Schmalfuß, F., Koskinen, H., Aromaa, S., Heikkilä, P., Honka, A., Mach, S., Malm, T.: A worker-centric design and evaluation framework for operator 4.0 solutions that support work well-being. In: Human Work Interaction Design. Designing Engaging Automation. HWID 2018. IFIP Advances in Information and Communication Technology, 544, pp. 263–282. Springer, Cham (2018)
11. Brooke, J.: SUS-A quick and dirty usability scale. In: Usability Evaluation in Industry, pp. 189–194. Taylor & Francis, London (1996)

User Interface Design for Remote Small Airport Operation

Satoru Inoue[1(✉)], Kazuhiko Yamazaki[2], and Taro Kanno[3]

[1] Electronic Navigation Research Institute, National Institute of Maritime, Port and Aviation Technology, 7-42-23, Jindaiji-Higashi-Machi, Chofu, Tokyo 182-0012, Japan
s-inoue@enri.go.jp
[2] Department of Creative Innovation, Musashino Art University, 1-4, Ichigayata-Machi, Shinjuku-Ku, Tokyo 162-0843, Japan
designkaz@gmail.com
[3] Department of Systems Innovation, School of Engineering, The University of Tokyo, 7-3-1, Hongo, Bunkyo-Ku, Tokyo 113-8656, Japan
kanno@sys.t.u-tokyo.ac.jp

Abstract. Remote aerodrome operation is a new type of airport tower operation. To introduce this type of a new technology for the tower operation, we considered user interface design is also an important element to perform as effective systems. In this research, we discuss about the practical design process for developing user interfaces based on Human Centered Design (HCD) approach for applying the remote airport traffic control operation. We discuss about how we introduced human centered approach to specialized and complicated work process. After that, we show an result of analysis. We also examined to create a prototype interface design concept for the future systems derived from the result of task analysis.

Keywords: Human Centered Design · Design process · Remote aerodrome operation systems

1 Introduction

Small class airports have a few numbers of aircraft operating in a day. However, operators control condition and provide services for keeping safety at the tower of airport. In such a small airport, an operator carries out providing information that is necessary for the aircraft flying from the control tower in the airport through radio communication systems. However, in recent years, with the development of Information and network technology, a remote type of aerodrome operation is considered one of attractive solution in the world. This type of system is called a "remote tower". The operator works their operational work with cameras and surveillance sensors remotely which are installed at the airport. And, the information data is sent to the operation room at a distance from the airport through the network, reproducing the environment as well as the real airport. The operator operates with images on the display sent from other located actual airport environment. However, it has sufficient

T. Ahram et al. (Eds.): IHIET 2019, AISC 1018, pp. 124–129, 2020.
https://doi.org/10.1007/978-3-030-25629-6_20

support functions for carrying out operation in the system. Thus, they can operate in remote environments. In air traffic service, it is important to optimize the user interface for the operator as well as the design of system functions in order to achieve a higher level of safety and reliability. Therefore, in this research, we discuss the design method of the user interface for this remote system and introduce the approach.

2 Design Process

In order to achieve sufficient performance as a system, it is important to consider user's potential and to perform user's full ability [1]. From a human factors perspective, we believe designing high usability interface optimized for the user's work is a key element to get user's maximum capability.

In this study, in order to design an optimized specific user interface for remote small airport operation, we tried to design interfaces based on the idea of Human Centered Design (HCD) approach. In this research, we report a practical design process for developing system user interfaces for remote aerodrome flight information services of Japan along with HCD approach.

2.1 Survey of Target Operations (Remote Aerodrome Flight Information Services: AFIS)

The purpose of survey is to understand and find out problems through observing a real work flow how an operator use the interface of the systems as first step of HCD process [2]. We observed real operators' work at the actual small airport. When changing from conventional control tower operation to remote control systems, the major difference is the out of the tower window view. The view of the out of the window changes to an image on the panorama displays which provided from fixed cameras of the airport through network. Usually, in small-scale airport operations, the operator checks the state of the airport surface and the area around the airport from the tower and provides information to the aircraft. It is expected to develop a system with enhanced visual monitoring information in order to control a safer and more air traffic efficiently by carrying out the tower operation at the airport as a remote operation. As shown in Fig. 1, the remote tower system has fixed cameras and panoramic views to provide out of the window view as well as the real control tower at the airport. Furthermore, based on the surveillance sensor information, the position data of the aircraft around or in the airport is combined with the panoramic view on the display as operational support information shown as augmented reality (AR). These functions can improve efficiency of controllers' work as well as improving safety. The AR information is linked to the video and the location information from the surveillance sensor, so that unique information associated with the aircraft can be displayed as an aircraft information label. The display of the task support information by the AR can contribute to reduce workload of the operator. The operator can understand the position of the aircraft intuitively. Because, the position of the aircraft is displayed as composite image information as a label even though it is in case of low visibility condition such as night-time or bad weather. In addition, the Pan-Tilt-Zoom (PTZ) camera is equipped for zooming up a specific area instead of binocular. PTZ cameras have the ability to zoom up on a specific location and link with the information of the position sensor for tracking a specific target. With these functions, the operator can monitor the aircraft from the operation center located far from the airport and can provide information and control operations to aircraft.

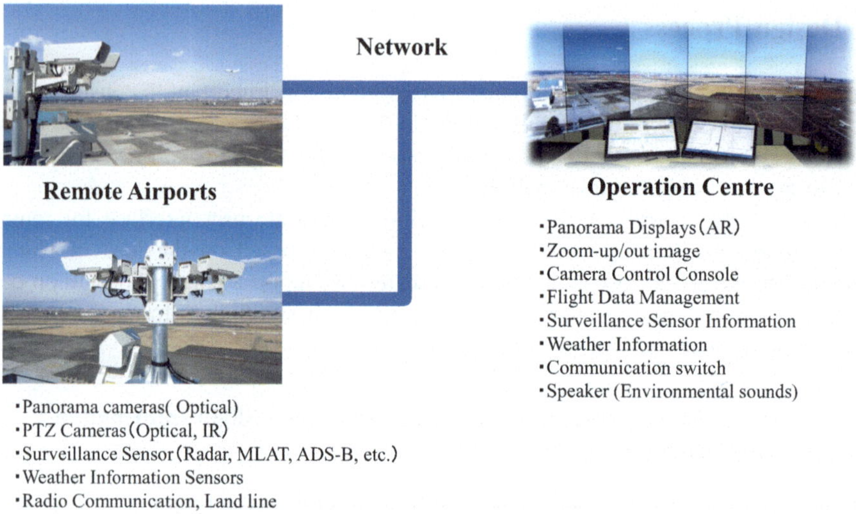

Fig. 1. Systems concept of remote tower

3 Create an Interface Design Idea

Based on the results of analysis, we created prototype ideas of user interface design. We also tried to develop "easy-to-use" design for remote AFIS operators. As an example of a concept design, a current system does not provide information of camera direction. Therefore, the operator cannot know the PTZ camera direction intuitively from the analysis. That's because current systems don't show the camera's direct position intuitively. To solve this problem, we created an indicator function on the concept interface that shows the map of PTZ camera direction. The operator can intuitively know the direction of the camera using this map interface.

3.1 Consider Space Design and Layout Design

In this research, our concept design is consisted of panoramic displays provided out of the window view and system console interfaces to provide information for remote AFIS operation. The panoramic display consists of several LCD displays that provide out of the window view of the airport which connected from the camera system in the real airport as well as the airport control tower window view. The benefits of a panoramic view give you an overview of the airport. We also proposed an interface function of the PTZ camera from the viewpoint of controllability. The operator knows the state of the zooming-up of the camera with the "level-gauge" on the display screen.

As next step, we tried to integrate the weather information onto the panoramic view. We also take into account the physical layout of the desktop console displays. In this study, we analyzed the frequency of interface usage. Frequency of usage is defined as not only the number of times an interface is physical touch, but also includes monitoring actions. We recognized the work can be divided into two types: "monitoring or checking" and "operating" from the analysis. Therefore, we proposed the system interface concept which has two touch panel displays as the desktop consoles. One display mainly shows information that is automatically updated. The other display has an input console or manual switch button for AFIS operation. Second, in order to operate the access control panel easily, it should be set closer to the operator. We've tried some prototype ideas to consider physical positioning.

3.2 Simple Prototype

We developed the initial simple prototype model. We designed some ideas of prototype interface based on the analysis for remote AFIS concept. At first, we considered layout of the display with touch panel consoles and the physical layout arrangement of desktop consoles. We tested prototype ideas such as function layout of buttons, key, signs on the console interfaces. The initial layout and display design ideas are shown in Fig. 2. The prototype design consisted of a panoramic display and two control console touch displays. Weather information is displayed on the right of the bottom of Fig. 2. The control console interface is divided into two displays. The display of left side shows a radar information, airport map and daily operational information. The second display of right hand side also has a flight information console where operator needs to enter or update information about takeoffs and landings. In addition, this display also has a camera control interface.

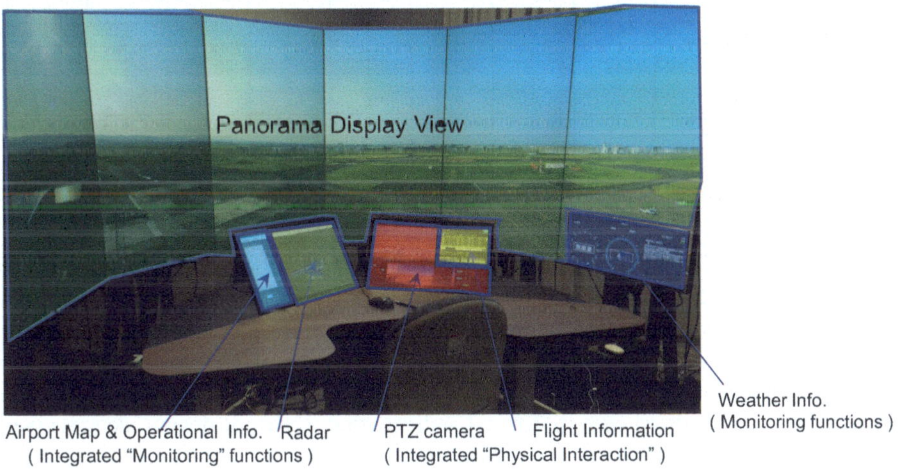

Fig. 2. Concept user interface design idea of remote AFIS

4 User Test and Evaluation

User testing is one of the important steps in the HCD process,. User testing is a valuable chance to catch user feedback in order to achieve a user-oriented design. In this research, we made user scenarios based on the persona method [3]. Test users can use all functions designed for specific AFIS operation in this user scenario. They can also check the usefulness of the proposed system with the scenario from the usability perspective. The test scenario has 17 tasks and 50 actions in about 15 min. As a first step, we tested three types of design ideas. The purpose of the three layouts is to evaluate the console design such as layout, process of use, action of function, window size, buttons, keys, etc. such as interactivity and ease of use. Three test users who were genuine AFIS operators in Japan participated in the test.

Table 1 shows the results of user tests of three design proposals. The scores in Table 1 indicate that the test user selected a score of 1 to 7. "1" means that the user has a negative impression or usability for the proposed function. "4" means "average" or "no change" compared to current remote AFIS systems. "7" means that the user gave a positive or positive impression of using the proposed function or design.

Table 1. The result of user test of user interface design ideas

Design Ideas		1			2			3		
Test User		A	B	C	A	B	C	A	B	C
Task	1	5	4	4	7	4	4	7	4	4
	2	7	4	4	7	4	4	3	1	2
	3	7	4	4	7	4	4	3	3	2
	4	5	5	5	5	5	4	5	5	5
	5	7	4	5	7	4	5	3	2	3
	6	4	4	4	4	4	4	4	4	4
	7	3	3	4	7	2	4	3	3	3
	8	7	4	5	7	4	5	7	4	5
	9	5	5	5	5	5	5	5	5	5
	10	7	7	7	7	5	7	7	4	7
	11	7	4	5	6	4	6	6	4	7
	12	5	4	4	5	4	4	5	4	4
	13	7	4	5	7	4	5	7	3	5
	14	5	5	5	5	5	4	7	5	5
	15	7	4	1	7	4	4	3	1	2
	16	7	4	1	7	4	4	7	4	4
	17	4	4	4	1	4	4	1	2	2

We created design ideas with three concepts of working manners. The feature of the first idea is that the operation can be specified in a simple process. The second is a design that displays all the information. Although this idea displays a lot of information in the screen space due to the large amount of information displayed, it was expected to be easy to operate. The third is an idea to enlarge individual views and show them exclusively. The results shown in Table 1 indicate that the Third design idea received negative evaluations in this test. As a third idea, we proposed the idea of setting some function keys and buttons to keep large information space for easy-to-watch observation and monitoring in a hidden hierarchical panel. In this case, once they have to open the panel manually to use some specific function. This means that users need to waste time for using the function and increase steps in the process to use. Therefore, an operator with expert knowledge can understand that displaying a large amount of information is not a problem, and can selectively acquire necessary information. We can recognize and confirm that operators prefer to use simple step functions. As results of the display layout test, we understood the pros and cons of each design. Moreover, from the test user's interview, our proposed layout design could provide more useful space in front of the operator. The test user gave a positive rating that this free space could be used as a flight information sheet while their working. However, on the other hand, they also pointed out some drawbacks of the idea of our layout design ideas. For example, an adverse situation occurs when the operator has to simultaneously control the left panel while looking at the right side of the screen. The results of our user tests show that our ideas still have some drawbacks to be improved. At the same time, we also confirmed the usefulness of our user-oriented consideration.

5 Summary

We discuss about practical design process for creating user interface of a small remote aerodrome operation based on HCD. As a practical process, we showed how we could apply ideas of design process along with HCD approach such as "survey and analysis, design prototyping and user test". For the future work, we will improve our practical design to brush up ideas from usability perspective. User-oriented and higher usability products contribute to reduce human errors and increase safety of operation system.

References

1. Norman, D.: The Design of Everyday Things. Basic Books, New York (1988) ISBN 978-0-465-06710-7
2. ISO 9241-210: Ergonomics of human-system interaction - part 210: human-centred design for interactive systems. ISO, Geneva (2010)
3. Goodwin, K.: Making personas work (without breaking the bank). London (2011). http://www.slideshare.net/KimGoodwin/making-personas-work-breaking thux london 2011

Motion Capturing for the Evaluation of Ergonomically Designed Guitars

Stijn Verwulgen[1(✉)], Sofia Scataglini[1], Thomas Peeters[1], Emilie Van Campenhout[2], Stijn Verheyen[2], and Steven Truijen[2]

[1] Department of Product Development, Faculty of Design Science, University of Antwerp, Antwerp, Belgium
{Stijn.Verwulgen, Sofia.Scataglini, Thomas.Peeters}@uantwerpen.be

[2] Department MOVANT, Faculty of Health and Health Science, University of Antwerp, Antwerp, Belgium
Steven.Truijen@uantwerpen.be

Abstract. Many musicians such as guitarists have to practice in very unnatural positions for several hours while making repetitive movements. Specific for guitar players, problems can occur in the long term, at the wrists, shoulders, neck, and low back. Based on user feedback, questionnaires and observations, two types of ergonomic adaptations have been proposed and implemented by (semi) professional instrument builders, while maintaining the original sound quality. The aim of this study is to assess the differences in body kinematics (neck, shoulder, right and left wrist) playing three different kinds of guitars (classical guitar and two adapted guitars) in order to monitor the ergonomic effect on two different players preventing injuries and a decrease of performance. The 3D human movements of two professional guitar players (more than 40 years of experience), one female (age: 53y, body height: 1.64 m) and one male (age: 60y, body height: 1.77 m), were measured using a Vicon motion capturing system while playing the same piece two times on three different guitars (one normal and the two ergonomic adapted guitars).

Results indicate that guitars need to be ergonomically adapted for each player, considering gender and anthropometry. Future studies should address ergonomic adaptation using inertial system together with Vicon and video recording.

Keywords: Ergonomically designed guitar · Mocap · Prevention

1 Introduction

Guitarists represent a popular group of musicians [1]. The movements that guitar players perform are often unnatural and they present an example of highly skilled and sophisticated task performance. It is almost certain that all guitarists will experience an episode of problems that will affect the upper extremity, back and neck during their career [2, 3]. The 1-year prevalence of pain varied from 26% to 93%, examined in symphonic orchestras and pianists. The prevalence of pain where the playing capacity was also affected, ranged from 41% to 73% [4, 5]. The prevalence varied from 57% to

T. Ahram et al. (Eds.): IHIET 2019, AISC 1018, pp. 130–135, 2020.
https://doi.org/10.1007/978-3-030-25629-6_21

68% for all musculoskeletal complaints, and from 9% to 68% for playing-related complaints [6]. Due to the different definitions of 'musculoskeletal complaints' and 'pain', the ranges were rather large. These complaints can have physical, psychological and social consequences so they will also have an impact on the Quality of Life (QoL) [7]. It is known that in case of injury, 40.7% did never consult any health care and because of this, 59.3% evolved to chronic complaints [8].

The reasons for these musculoskeletal problems among guitarists are not fully comprehended. Physical demands such as unnatural postures while playing, repetitive arm and finger movements and a certain required force while playing have been proposed as a cause [9]. A good posture is when all segments align perfectly to each other and when there is a certain symmetry between left and right. While playing the guitar, maintaining this is rather difficult due to the design of the instrument. For a classical guitar, the instrument has to be hold against the body with the right (dominant) arm. Depending on the size of the guitar, the arm exerts a certain pressure on the side of the guitar which could impact the blood flow to the muscles [9]. Often the guitarist puts the left leg on a footstool to prevent the guitar from slipping away and to rotate the neck of the guitar upwards for a more comfortable wrist position [10, 11]. This is not a healthy position for the left wrist because the playing still happens with a flexed wrist. This can be avoided by flexing the elbow, so the wrist remains neutral but then the problem moves on to another segment. The compromise for this problem is holding the neck of the guitar at 45°, as is the recommended classical guitar position. When playing, the guitarist has to flex and rotate the neck in order to see the frets. This position is very unnatural and can tend to complaints [9]. Next, the movements of the fingers and the grip force is a subject to attend to. The grip force can vary depending on what music piece is played. In fact, it is known that when playing a fret, there must be a counterforce on the back of the neck, otherwise the neck of the guitar will sway. It is also needed as an orientation for the fingers on which fret they are playing. It is highly understood that the movements of the fingers while playing are widespread. Always extending the fingers and maintaining the necessary force on the fret, is very demanding. Due to the shape of the guitar, all the above factors that can cause complaints are difficult to avoid [9].

Only a minority of guitar players had ever received some training in ergonomics when practicing [10]. The prevention of musculoskeletal disorders includes knowledge of intrinsic (flexibility, strength, stature of the musician) and extrinsic (posture while playing an instrument) factors, while taking the playing environment into account (duration of breaks, hours of practice). It is known that a warm-up, education and taking micro-breaks can help in decreasing the unease [11]. Investigating the unnatural positions and being able to decrease them would be an enormous help in preventing these problems [12].

Most of the research is done in a population of string players or pianists. In string players, it is examined that ergonomic adaptations can substantially help in the prevention and reduction of complaints [11]. However, not many studies are specific for guitar players. One study concluded that some ergonomic changes can reduce the need for external low technology tools while remaining the character of the instrument [13]. Nonetheless, it states that not all problems regarding playing the guitar can be eliminated, only with ergonomic adaptations [13]. Another study showed that strength training and stability exercises of the hand could play a substantial part in preventing complaints [14].

It is obvious that guitar players are at risk for medical problems. In order to acknowledge an understanding of the injury mechanism, a biomechanical analysis of the playing is needed. The aim of this study is to assess the differences in body kinematics (neck, shoulder, right and left wrist) playing three different guitars (classical guitar and two adapted guitars) in order to monitor the ergonomic effect on two different players eventually preventing injuries and with a increase of performance.

2 Methods

This study was approved by the ethical committee of UA/UZA (18/49/579). Recruitment of musicians was done by contacting conservatoria and music schools.

The including criteria were semi-professional guitarists who could speak Dutch.

From twenty-four subjects contacted only by mail or phone only two (right handed, >43 years of experience) corresponding to our inclusion criteria (Table 1).

Table 1. Main anthropometric data of the individuals that participated in the study

Subject	Gender	Height (cm)	Body mass (kg)	BMI (kg/m^2)
1	Female	164	54	20.1
2	Male	177	73	23.3

The two players played on three different guitars, one classical instrument and two instruments with ergonomic adaptations such as the torsion of the neck of the guitar turn up (ergo guitar 1) or down (ergo guitar 2, Fig. 1) or a small body guitar (ergo guitar 1).

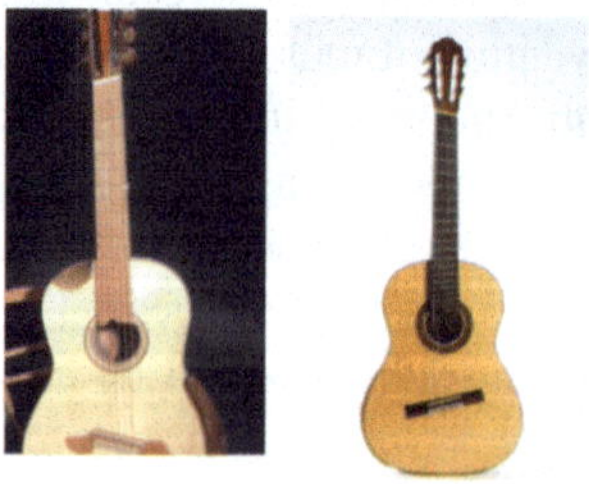

Fig. 1. Ergonomic guitars

Three trials were performed on each different instrument. The different guitars were handed in a random order to the guitar player and they were given five minutes of playing to get used to the new instrument. The musicians were instructed to play the same piece out of "Suite Espagnola", namely "Canarios" by Gaspar Ganz for one minute in each separate trial. Whenever there was a mistake that made them stop playing, they could start over that specific trial. The three different instruments were all tuned to the same level prior to the trials.

Body kinematics and kinetics of the upper body of two players were collected by a Vicon camera system in the M^2OCEAN laboratory (UZA, Antwerp).

Musicians were asked to fill a comfort questionnaire attributing a score from 0 to 10 (most comfortable playing sensation) investigating comfort perception at upper body such as back, neck, shoulder, wrist during the play.

2.1 Motion Capturing

A motion capture protocol was designed specifically for this study. The subjects wore well-fitted and tight garments to minimize the restrictions. A total 36 markers were placed (26 on the body of the subject, four on a headband and two plates of three markers that were placed on each upper arm) to collect the data of the head, cervical spine, thorax and left and right upper extremity.

The dynamic trials were processed by extracting the marker tracks, spline interpolation of gaps and low pass filtering to reduce noise and smooth data.

Kinematic variables and angles between anatomical segments were computed in Vicon ProCalc and then were exported directly to Excel. Data selection was done by visually searching for usable frames in the graph and extrapolating the right angles in an Excel file. Then, the minimum, maximum and mean score were calculated. Of the three trials recorded from each subject only trial 2 and 3 were used for the results due to the 'learn effect' that was noticed in trial 1.

3 Results and Discussion

For the Z-axis, the classical guitar produced the smallest range of motion in subject one in all angles. Also, in the shoulder for X-axis, Y-axis and Z-axis the classical guitar provided the smallest range of motion. For movements in the other planes and other body parts the ergonomic guitars and classical guitar vary in producing the best result. In subject two, different results were found. For the shoulder and right wrist, the ergonomic guitars gave the best range of motion in X-axis, Y-axis and Z-axis. For the left wrist the classical guitar provided the smallest range of motion for all three axes. In the neck ergo guitar 1 gave the smallest range of motion for the X-axis and the Y-axis while the classical guitar gave the best results in the Z-axis.

Comfort scores were attributed by the two players during the trials and are presented in Table 2.

Both subjects preferred a different guitar when looking at comfort. This could be explained by the inter-subject differences. Also playing style and personal preference have to be taken into account. This brings us to another limitation of the study; the sample size should have been much larger. In this study, both subjects were two completely opposite scenarios. One was male and one was female. They both had lot of playing experience, but they did have different demographics. Also, subject one had

Table 2. Comfort Scores

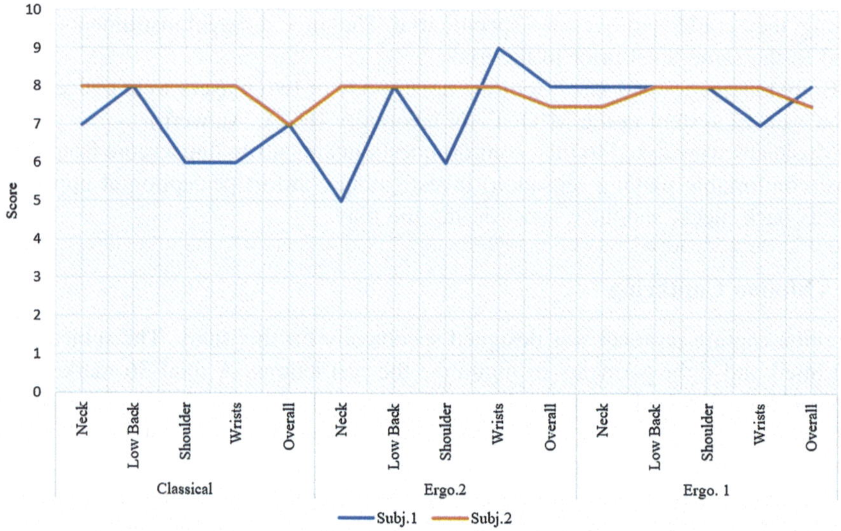

already played more often on the ergonomic guitars then the other one, which made subject one more comfortable with the adaptations than subject two.

4 Conclusion

In this study, differences in the mobility of guitar players between a classical and two ergonomic guitars were analyzed. Three-dimensional neck, shoulder and wrist angles were captured in a motion lab for two subjects while playing the same piece of "Suite Espagnola". The results show no consistent difference in range of motion between the three guitars. The study indicates that the guitar should be redesigned considering the anthropometry of the guitar player, where the size of the body of the guitarist plays an important factor. The adaptations of the ergonomic guitars can help guitar players in playing music pieces in a more comfortable way. Only the neck rotation of the ergonomic guitars scores lower in comfort and range of motion. In future research a larger sample size with differences in gender, height, body weight and playing experience is recommended to give a more complete overview of the influence of the ergonomic adaptations. Future perspective will be addressed to study ergonomic adaptation using inertial system (IMU) together with Vicon and video recording. Using these additions, the advantages of the ergonomic guitar against a classical guitar in the prevention of musculoskeletal problems in guitar players can be shown.

References

1. Guitars Are Getting More Popular. So Why Do We Think They're Dying? Rolling Stone Magazine. https://www.rollingstone.com/music/music-news/guitars-are-getting-more-popular-so-why-do-we-think-theyre-dying-630446/. Accessed May 2019
2. Heijink, H., Meulenbroek, R.G.: On the complexity of classical guitar playing: functional adaptations to task constraints. J. Mot. Behav. **34**(4), 339–351 (2002)
3. Fjellman-Wiklund, A., Chesky, K.: Musculoskeletal and general health problems of acoustic guitar, electric guitar, electric bass, and banjo players. Med. Probl. Perform. Artist. **21**(4), 169–176 (2006)
4. Silva, A.G., La, F.M., Afreixo, V.: Pain prevalence in instrumental musicians: a systematic review. Med. Probl. Perform Art. **30**(1), 8–19 (2015)
5. Baadjou, V.A., Roussel, N.A., Verbunt, J.A., Smeets, R.J., de Bie, R.A.: Systematic review: risk factors for musculoskeletal disorders in musicians. Occupational medicine, Oxford, England (2016)
6. Kok, L.M., Huisstede, B.M., Voorn, V.M., Schoones, J.W., Nelissen, R.G.: The occurrence of musculoskeletal complaints among professional musicians: a systematic review. Int. Arch. Occup. Environ. Health **89**(3), 373–396 (2016)
7. Zaza, C., Charles, C., Muszynski, A.: The meaning of playing-related musculoskeletal disorders to classical musicians. Soc. Sci. Med. 1998 **47**(12), 2013–2023 (1982)
8. Sánchez-Padilla, M., Bayo-Tallón, V., Esquirol-Caussa, J., Guerrero-Forteza, E., López-Iglesias, I., Salas-Gómez, D.: Incidencia de lesiones en profesionales de la guitarra clásica. Fisioterapia **35**(6), 243–251 (2013)
9. Genani, G.: Biomechanics of Playing electric guitar (2013)
10. Valenzuela-Gómez, S.A., Rey-Galindo, J.A., Aceves-González, C.: Evaluation of posture, self-efficacy, comfort and discomfort in Guitarists while using auxiliary implements for instrument positioning. In: Goossens, R. (eds.) Advances in Social & Occupational Ergonomics. AHFE 2017. Advances in Intelligent Systems and Computing, vol. 605. Springer, Cham (2018)
11. Prado León, L.R., Rey Galindo, J.A., Zambrano Prado, P.L.: Human factors in musicians: design proposals. Procedia Manufacturing, vol. 3, 6th International Conference on Applied Human Factors and Ergonomics. AHFE, 6124–6132 (2015)
12. Spahn, C., Hildebrandt, H., Seidenglanz, K.: Effectiveness of a prophylactic course to prevent playing-related health problems of music students. MPPA **16**, 24–31 (2001)
13. Marmaras, N., Zarboutis, N.: Ergonomic redesign of the electric guitar. Appl. Ergon. **28**(1), 59–67 (1997)
14. Butler, K.: Preventing injuries in Guitarists ergonomics, strengthening and surgery. Acoustic Magazine (2011)

User Test: How Many Users Are Needed to Find the Psychophysiological Pain Points in a Journey Map?

Charles Lamontagne[1(✉)], Sylvain Sénécal[1], Marc Fredette[1], Shang Lin Chen[1], Romain Pourchon[2], Yohan Gaumont[2], David De Grandpré[2], and Pierre-Majorique Léger[1]

[1] HEC Montréal, 3000 Chemin de La Côte-Sainte-Catherine, Montréal, Qc H3T 2A7, Canada
{charles.lamontagne,sylvain.senecal,marc.fredette, shang-lin.chen,pierre-majorique.leger}@hec.ca

[2] Deloitte Digital, La Tour Deloitte, 1190, Avenue Des Canadiens-de-Montréal, Bureau 500, Montréal, Qc H3B 0M7, Canada
{rpourchon,ygaumont,dadegrandpre}@deloitte.ca

Abstract. The objective of this research is to investigate how many users are needed in usability testing to identify psychophysiological pain points (PPP) experienced by users during a human-computer interaction (HCI). Fifteen subjects were tested in a new user training context and results show that out of 15 participants, 82% of the total PPP were experienced after 9 participants. Calculations using 1000 trials of random orders were then performed to demonstrate the independence of the order. This research provides guidelines about what could be an ideal sample size for user test using psychophysiological measures.

Keywords: User experience (UX) · Usability testing · Psychophysiological measures · Psychophysiological pain points · Pain points

1 Introduction

Within the field of user experience (UX), pain points are known as user irritants impacting their interaction with digital entities [1]. Identifying pain points can be crucial to improve the usability, satisfactory and adaptability of interactions [2]. The majority of methods currently used in UX evaluation are based on explicit (i.e., self-reported) and observational data [3]. However, previous research suggests that traditional approaches may not capture users' reactions to a new interface in an unbiased way [4]. Hence, psychophysiological measures can be an alternative method to comprehend users' emotional states [2]. This paper is building upon previous work of Giroux-Huppé et al. (2019), which proposes a new method to analyze online user journeys by identifying psychophysiological pain points; hereinafter referred to as PPPs [5]. PPPs are defined as interaction moments for which users experience high emotional arousal and high negative emotional valence [5]. Past research in HCI has provided guidelines for self-reported UX test sample size, but there is no evidence if

T. Ahram et al. (Eds.): IHIET 2019, AISC 1018, pp. 136–142, 2020.
https://doi.org/10.1007/978-3-030-25629-6_22

these apply to PPPs. Therefore, this research focuses on investigating the optimal number of users needed in order to identify most PPPs in a given user journey.

2 Background

2.1 Sample Size in Usability Testing

Usability is the user's ability to use a system, product, or service to perform a given task successfully [6]. On the other hand, UX encompasses all aspects of the user's interaction with the entity, which extend to the emotional and cognitive states, thoughts, and perceptions of the user [6]. Thus, the main purpose of user testing is to evaluate the user interactions with a system, product, or service and to identify usability problems (UPs) and pain points within their individual journey, thereby providing feedback to designers in order to improve the system [3].

As user tests can be very expensive, the benefit of each additional participant must surpass their marginal cost, which emphasizes the need for practitioners to have the optimal sample size [7]. Early research with the thinking aloud method suggests that 5 participants are usually necessary in order to obtain up to 77% to 85% of UPs [8]. Testing additional users increases the number of UPs found, but progressively decreases the marginal gain [8]. Since its publication, "The Magic Number 5" rule and sample size in user testing have induced a long-running debate that has not reached a consensus yet [8–10]. Nevertheless, this number is considered as the reference in usability testing [6].

Moreover, lab-based user research methods, such as usability testing, usually aim to find and resolve problems [11]. Hence, those methods analyze the users' behaviors with a more qualitative approach [11]. Thereby, a smaller sample size suffices as it allows one to gain a deeper understanding of the participants' perception of the experience [12].

2.2 Psychophysiological Measures in Usability Testing

Traditional methods to assess a user's experience throughout experimentation has been proven to render only a portion of the user's feelings toward a new digital product or service, as these methods rely only on explicit and observational measures [4]. Furthermore, users may encounter UPs throughout a user test, but usually only convey their emotional reactions at the end of it, which does not allow one to fully understand each moment-to-moment user reaction [3]. Hence, research shows that self-reported measures represent more of an overall evaluation by the user, which has been proven to be influenced by the Peak-End Effects [13, 14].

Psychophysiological measures provide an unobstructive and implicit manner to ascertain a user's affective and cognitive conditions in HCI [2]. This is a reliable approach to comprehend the user's emotional state in real time during usability testing, as it allows to record physiological manifestations of the user's psychological sentiments [15]. At least two measures need to be simultaneously used to have a rich comprehension of the user's state [14, 16]. For example, facial emotions can be detected and analyzed to fit a range from negative to positive, i.e., emotional valence [18]. Arousal level can be measured with electrodermal activity (EDA), ranging from very calm to neutral to highly stimulated [19].

2.3 PPP

Pain point is a term rooted in the medical domain, in which it refers to the localization of a hostile sensation caused by unbearable, perturbing, or even harmful stimuli [1]. In UX, it is widely known as an emotional irritant for the user in his/her journey [1]. UPs could be considered explicit pain points; users are conscious and aware of those system issues intervening while they execute their tasks [3]. PPPs are more comprehensive since they include automatic, often unconscious, negative physiological reactions of the users. They are defined by high arousal and high negative emotional valence prompted by non-optimal interaction moments [5]. Thus far, to the extent of our knowledge, no research has focused on providing guidelines on the number of subjects required for usability testing with PPPs.

3 Method

3.1 Design, Sample, and Procedure

We conducted a controlled study in the context of the implementation of a new information system in a business. The experimentation was designed to evaluate PPPs for new users in training.

Fifteen participants (3 men and 12 women) were recruited through our institution's recruitment panel. Age ranged from 19 to 39 with a mean of 23.6 years (SD = 4.98). The user journey consisted of 5 tasks. Users had to reproduce the actions that were presented to them once in an instructional video before each task. The multi-step sequence displayed in the videos were representative of actions that new users would have to execute, such as basic data entries. As the tasks followed a linear order, the same sequence was used for every subject. The duration of the test was between 45 and 60 min, including the EDA baseline measures. The participants received a 20$ gift card as a compensation at the end of the experiment. They had to read and sign a consent form before beforehand. This project was approved by our institution's Institutional Review Board (IRB).

3.2 Apparatus

Throughout the study, participants' facial emotions (to assess their emotional valence) and EDA (to assess their arousal) were recorded [2]. Moment-to-moment emotional valence was measured in real-time using Facereader v6.0 (Noldus, Wageningen, Netherlands). This software detects participants' facial movements using the Facial Action Coding System (FACS) developed by Ekman and Friensen [19] to detect the 6 core emotions: happy, sad, angry, disgust, fear and surprised, with the addition of the neutral emotion [17]. The software computes the intensity of those emotions and scores them between 0 and 1 [18]. The emotional valence is then calculated as the intensity of happy (as the only positive emotion) minus the highest intensity between the negative emotions (sad, angry, scared and disgusted) [18]. Thus, the valence score is between 0 and 1, from negative to neutral to positive [18]. The Acknowledge software (BIOPAC, Goleta, USA) was used to measure the arousal with the standardized EDA of the participant [18]. A Tobii eye tracker (Tobii, Stockholm, Sweden) was used to record eye-tracking data in Tobii Studio software, which was also used to record the experiment. Event markers were also positioned manually after the test at the beginning and at the end of each task in Tobii Studio. Those event markers were used to perform the PPP analysis as well as creating a color code in Tableau® (Tableau, Seattle, USA). The Observer XT software (Noldus, Wageningen, Netherlands) and Cube HX (Montreal, Canada) was utilized to synchronize the equipment and event markers.

3.3 Analysis

PPPs were calculated with the statistical software SAS 9.4 using the same thresholds for valence and arousal as Giroux-Huppé et al. [5], i.e., moments where the subject is his ninetieth percentile for standardized EDA as well as in his tenth percentile of valence. Thus, those are moments where, compared to the user baseline state, high arousal coincides with high negative valence [5].

The user journey was modeled from the subtasks displayed in the instructional videos, i.e., a series of actions that the participant had to execute in order to fulfil each task. This user journey allowed to pair the PPPs with subtasks where participants experienced them by using the video replay function in Tobii Studio. Theses results were graphically illustrated afterward as an individual journey map with Tableau®.

4 Results

PPPs experienced by each participant were recorded chronologically. For each participant, we tallied the PPPs experienced, we counted new PPPs, i.e., those that were not experienced by any precedent participant, and the accumulated number of distinct PPPs we observe with each additional participant. Results show that over 15 subjects, 22 distinct PPPs were identified and 82% of those were identified after 9 participants (Table 1).

Calculations using 1000 trials of random orders were then performed to demonstrate the independence of the order [8]. The result shows that on average 80.4% (std = 7.5%) of the identified PPPs were found with the first 9 participants. Those permutations are shown in the figure, in which the x-axis represents the number of participants and the y-axis represents the cumulative percentage of PPPs found (Fig. 1).

Table 1. Details of psychophysiological pain points experienced per participant

Participant number	Number of PPPs	New PPPs	Cumulative PPPs	Cumulative %
1	2	2	2	9%
2	2	2	4	18%
3	5	3	7	32%
4	6	3	10	45%
5	6	4	14	64%
6	5	2	16	73%
7	0	0	16	73%
8	1	0	16	73%
9	5	2	18	82%
10	6	0	18	82%
11	3	1	19	86%
12	0	0	19	86%
13	5	2	21	95%
14	3	0	21	95%
15	5	1	22	100%

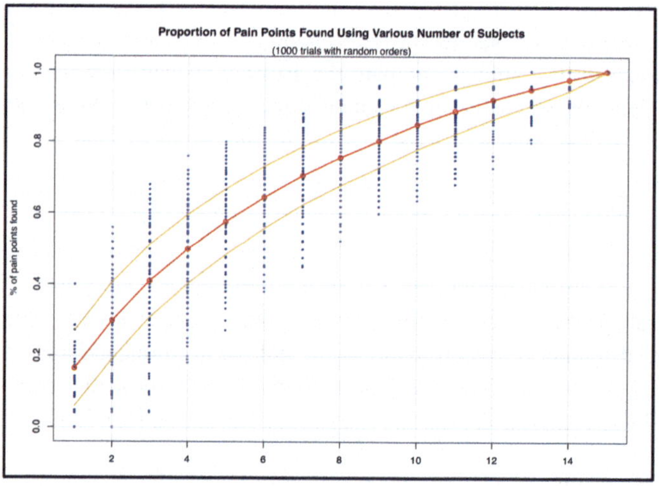

Fig. 1. With 1000 permutations, the average curve (*Accumulated Proportion of Detected Pain Points*) follows a consonant curve to a single permutation, proving its independence.

5 Discussion and Concluding Comments

As user testing with physiological measures in usability is an emerging practice, this research's objective was to provide empirically-based guidelines to UX researchers on the sample size required. Our results show that while employing psychophysiological measures in user testing with 15 participants, more than 80% of PPPs were experienced with 9 participants. Thus far, only guidelines for sample size for explicit pain points were proposed in the HCI literature [8–10].

From a managerial point of view, those results can enhance usability testing planning and ROI, by providing guidelines about what could be a standard sample size to identify PPPs. It can help resolve cost management issues within organization that are transitioning to user testing with psychophysiological measures.

However, some limitations need to be considered. As this was a lab-based experiment and the instructional videos were only watched once by each participant, it did not render a totally natural experience as the participant could not just go back and watch the instructions of the action where he was blocked. Some videos were more complex and had longer duration, so they required more engagement from participants. Furthermore, as the experiment was in a specific context, external validity should be tested by investigating PPPs in other contexts.

Future research should try this approach in a two-phase process, the first one being the same as the one used in this study. The second phase should aim to evaluate if the overall number of PPPs decreased if they were addressed between development phases.

References

1. Platzer, D.: Regarding the pain of users: towards a genealogy of the "pain point". In: Ethnographic Praxis in Industry Conference Proceedings, pp. 301–315 (2018)
2. Dirican, A.C., Göktürk, M.: Psychophysiological measures of human cognitive states applied in human computer interaction. Procedia Computer Science **3**, 1361–1367 (2011)
3. Bruun, A., Heintz, M., Law, L.C., Alkly, L.H.A.: Understanding the relationship between frustration and the severity of usability problems: what can psychophysiological data (not) tell us? In: Proceedings of the 2016 CHI Conference on Human Factors in Computing System, pp. 3975–3987. ACM, New York (2016)
4. de Guinea, A.O., Titah, R., Léger, P.M.: Explicit and implicit antecedents of users' behavioral beliefs in information systems: a neuropsychological investigation. JMIS **30**(4), 179–210 (2014)
5. Giroux-Huppé, C., Sénécal, S., Fredette, M., Chen, S.L., Demolin, B., Léger, P.M.: Identifying psychophysiological pain points in the online user journey: the case of online grocery. In: The HCI International 2019 Conference Proceedings (Forthcoming)
6. Tullis, T., Albert, W.: Measuring the User Experience: Collecting, Analyzing, and Presenting Usability Metrics, 2nd edn. Morgan Kaufmann, Burlington (2013)
7. Lewis, J.R.: Sample sizes for usability tests: mostly math, not magic. Interactions **13**, 29–33 (2006)
8. Nielsen, J., Landauer, T.K.: A mathematical model of the finding of usability problem. In: Proceedings of the INTERCHI 1993 Conference on Human Factors in Computing Systems, pp. 206–213. IOS Press, Amsterdam (1993)
9. Nielsen, J.: Estimating the number of subjects need for a thinking aloud test. IJHCS **41**, 385–397 (1994)
10. Schmettow, M.: Sample size in usability studies. CACM **55**(4), 64–70 (2012)
11. Rohrer, C.: When to use which user-experience research methods. Nielsen Norman Group (2014)
12. Vernette, E., Filser, M., Giannelloni, J.L.: Études Marketing Appliquées: De La Stratégie Au Mix: Analyses et Tests Pour Optimiser Votre Action Marketing. Dunod, Malakoff (2008)

13. Cockburn, A., Quinn, P., Gutwin, C.: Examining the peak-end effects of subjective experience. In: Proceedings of the ACM Conference on Human Factors in Computing Systems (CHI 2015), pp. 357–366 (2015)
14. Ganglbauer, E., Schrammel, J., Deutsch, S., Tscheligi, M.: Applying psychophysiological methods for measuring user experience: possibilities, challenges and feasibility. In: User Experience Evaluation Methods in Product Development (UXEM 2009) (2009)
15. Andreassi, J.L.: Psychophysiology: Human Behavior and Physiological Response. Lawrence Erlbaum Associates Inc, Mahwah (2000)
16. Maia, C.L.B., Furtado, E.S.: A study about psychophysiological measures in user experience monitoring and evaluation. In: Proceedings of the 15th Brazilian Symposium on Human Factors in Computing Systems, pp. 7:1–7:9. ACM, New York (2016)
17. Loijens, L., Krips, O.: FaceReader Methodology Note. Wageningen, Noldus (2018)
18. Dawson, M.E.: The electrodermal system. In: Cacioppo, J.T., Tassinary, L.G., Berntson, G. (eds.) Handbook of Psychophysiology. Cambridge University Press, Cambridge (2007)
19. Ekman, P., Friesen, W.V.: Manual for the Facial Action Coding System. Consulting Psychologists Press, Palo Alto (1978)

Seeking Cognitive Convergence: Small Group Collaborative Visualization in the Library Learning Commons

Deborah A. Middleton(✉)

Department of Design, Effat University, 33293 Jeddah, Saudi Arabia
middleton.deboraha@gmail.com

Abstract. In order to generate a hybrid and ubiquitous approach to integrating multiple visualization modalities within spatial settings, it is essential to understand how small group users select and adapt technology and spatial settings to generate co-located visualization. Insights are needed to guide the design of spatial-visualization hybrid technologies that are ubiquitous, and user intuitive to adjustable to group size as scalable displays interfaces. This study examines the constructed visualization formats of small groups in a library learning commons to understand the visual and social affordances of group generated visualization formats.

Keywords: Human factors · Spatial design · Information display · Social proxemics · Ubiquitous visualization in physical environments

1 Introduction

In order to advance the design of ubiquitous visualization enabling environments there is a need to understand how small groups spontaneously constructs shared visualization (projector, computer display and inscription surfaces) in the collocated setting. Recent innovations such as laptops with articulating and detachable screens and large-scale spatial-technological hybrids such as CoVE settings, and interactive screen surfaces have advanced user capabilities for interacting with shared visualizations. The miniaturization of mobile technology has improved productivity for individuals and 2–3 member teams, yet challenges remain for small groups (4–8 members) seeking to collaborate and share collocated data visualizations. This study examines the proxemics relations that small groups spontaneously organize to collaborate with visualizations relative to the visual configuration properties inherent to the spatial setting they choose to work in.

2 Small Group Co-located Visualization

Small group interact with shared visualizations to enable collaborating members to construct awareness and understanding, categorize content, engage in ideation, and manage the process of information and knowledge integration. (Isenberg et al. 2011;

T. Ahram et al. (Eds.): IHIET 2019, AISC 1018, pp. 143–149, 2020.
https://doi.org/10.1007/978-3-030-25629-6_23

Fischer et al. 2005; Yusoff et al. 2015; Stahl 2006; Jacobsen et al. 2013) One important cognitive process in small group collaboration is the need to achieve cognitive convergence, also referred to as clarification, (Kim and Maher 2008) and correspondence. (Trevesky 2014) Spatial settings structure the social learning behavior of small groups seeking to solve problems, and coordinate learning activities with small groups gravitating to spatial settings with high social density proximity. Previous studies have established how technology-spatial formations support user interactivity for collocated shared visualization. A common visualization format enabling multi-user viewing with more than two members is side-by-side views, yet this method inherently challenges visual tasks. (Alabi et al. 2013) Focal attention theory has been linked to structures for peripheral visualization of single or multiple surfaces. This modality is found to support individual computing, group socialization, and enhance users focal attention, while allowing easy shifting between the periphery and the center of attention. (Juola 2016; Vermeulen et al. 2016) Multiple coordinated displays (MVC) such as large wall displays, CoVes, and 3D holographic imagery are currently being studied to assess how these formats enhance user spatial organization and coordination with spatial hypermedia (2D, white boards, 3D displays and holographic maps using semi transparent layers with 3D points), to generate multiple visualization layers in physical space. (Mahmood et al. 2019; Langner et al. 2018) Studies of small group social engagement with interactive table-tops and wall surfaces (ITSs) supporting multi-dimensional data visualization, and social proxemics interactions (Isenberg et al. 2013; Marquardt et al. 2010) Future research into the design of physical environments to enable intuitive interaction with these future visualization modalities is needed to create a more robust typology of small group interaction and collaboration capability to generate spontaneous layouts of shared visualizations.

3 Data Collection and Analysis

This study examines how small groups engage in collaboration with various shared visualizations modalities in the Library-East (LEC) and 2nd floor West Commons (LWC2) of the Library of the Georgia Institute of Technology (Georgia Tech). The library contains multiple dynamic and varied collaborative settings that are open 24/7 for students, researchers and faculty use. Workstation configurations are designed to support collaboration and individual work-study, with a few offering flexibility for user adaptation. A visual survey into how users organize spatial and social settings to engage with shared visualizations focused on the location of the activity, group size, and user customization of spatial settings to construct shared visualization. Visual graph analysis (VGA), a space syntax method, was used to characterize properties of the physical spatial configuration according to the settings ability to support and extend spatial visibility factors for informational and social affordances.

3.1 Small Group User Spatial Preferences

Users spatial selection preference was measured during different time epochs over a one-week in the middle of the spring semester, following a sequential route through the library. MATLAB was used to generate a three dimensional analysis of data to establish relationships between spatial settings selected by small groups (size 2, 3, 4, 5, 6, 7+) across 26 time epochs. The intensity of library commons space use by groups is displayed in Fig. 1 with the *y* axis reflecting the time of observation in descending order from morning to late evening. The *x* axis establishes the different spatial areas 1–6 (LEC), 7, 8 (LWC) 9–13 (LWC2). Results of users counts reveal that the majority of G2 spatial setting usage concentrates in the LWC2 area. The dominant space used to supporting individual users is the LWC and LWC2, both of which have small footprint table spaces in an open environment. Two areas within LEC are found to support groups with G3 usage clustered in fixed systems furniture. LWC2 areas concentrates group occurrences (G3, G4, G5) observed to collaborate in the early to late evening. Spaces reflecting the highest usage counts are in LEC (3, 4, 5), and LWC2 (2, 3) with intensive and dynamic collaboration seen to occur in the early to late evening (Table 1).

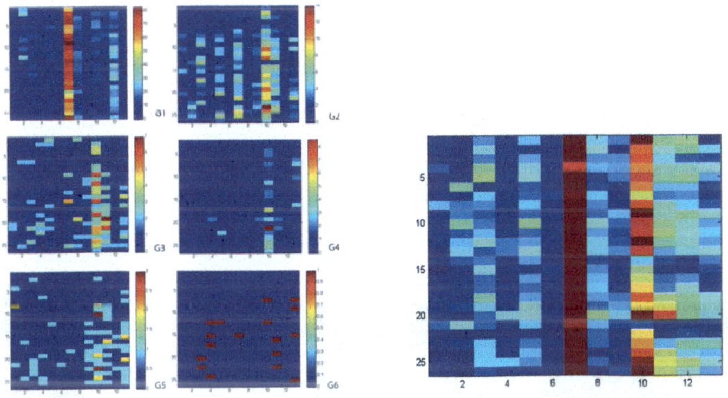

(A) (B)

Fig. 1. (A) Spatial use patterns organized by group size across different time of day. (B) Intensity of space use by all group sizes.

Table 1. Small group spatial preference for collaboration

		LEC = 196						LWC = 149		2LWC = 322				
Group size		1	2	3	4	5	6	1	2	1	2	3	4	5
seats avail		**40**	**20**	**30**	**60**	**24**	**22**	**124**	**25**	**56**	**108**	**77**	**33**	**48**
	1	68	176	232	133	233	143	1794	362	117	309	301	535	61
	2	60	54	142	38	132	28	198	40	98	376	190	26	116
	3	27	24	57	42	54	0	60	57	57	276	153	18	84
	4	12	16	20	20	21	0	28	9	36	212	40	8	80
	5	20	10	23	20	5	5	5	0	40	106	60	15	75
	6	0	0	12	24	6	0	6	0	0	12	18	0	24
	7	7	0	0	0	0	0	0	0	0	21	7	0	14
		7.5	10.8	19.1	10.7	10.2	6.0	80.4	18.0	13.4	50.0	25.7	23.2	17.5
seats avail		**40**	**20**	**30**	**60**	**24**	**22**	**124**	**25**	**56**	**108**	**77**	**33**	**48**
% usage		19	54	64	18	76	31	65	72	24	46	33	70	36

3.2 Visual Experience in Spatial Environments

Observations reveal small groups commonly rely on flexible spatial settings to collaborate in that provide high peripheral social accessibility to peers, and support for visual focal attention to visualization displays. A highly used space, LEC space 3, 5 contains large curved work surfaces and dual monitors, providing users the ability to construct multi-user viewing cones to small scale visualization displays with moderate visual privacy from adjacent spaces and corridors. LWC2 cluster of tables with partial semi transparent dividers offers peripheral whiteboard configuration. The setting is densely designed and users are seen to customize technology configurations for shared display. Table size is narrow enabling user to coordinate multiple vision cones with computing devices and inscription surfaces. Both workstation clusters spaces are highlighted in dark blue in Fig. 2. The visual affordances of these two settings generated strong visual privacy from outside viewers, while enabling a closed environment. Spatial use is dense and noisy due to number of groups situated together in the same space. The VGA reveals the most integrated locations of co-visibility in red with colors progressively decreasing in value from red to darkest blue to identify the least visually permeable spaces. The darkest blue workstation clusters offer limited visualization surfaces real estate as compared to other work table areas in both the floor plans LEC and LWC2.

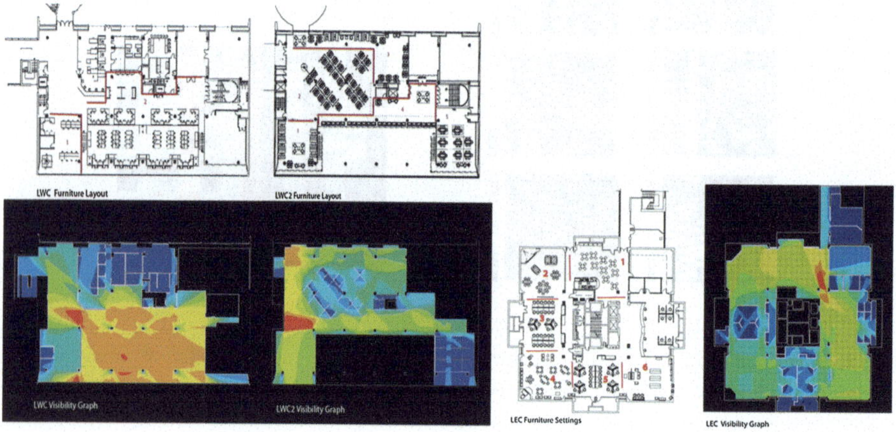

Fig. 2. Visibility graphs of three learning commons LWC, LWC2 and LEC.

3.3 Shared Visualization and Group Proxemics

Small groups establish highly compressed and dense proxemics to achieve accessibility to visualization displays, and they structure the spatial environment for (seating-standing-movement) activity near the visualization surface in tandem with visual cone orientation (depth and cone diameter). Peer to peer visualization activity requires a symbiotic structuring of inscription and views to multiple display modalities. When users manipulate devices and furniture, a layering of visualization planes occurs where small group members can access multiple device views. Chair width dimensions are seen to be an impeding factor that limits users ability to view small surface visualization modalities. Ability to engage in dynamic movement in concert with the display and personal devise is a characteristic behavior (Fig. 3).

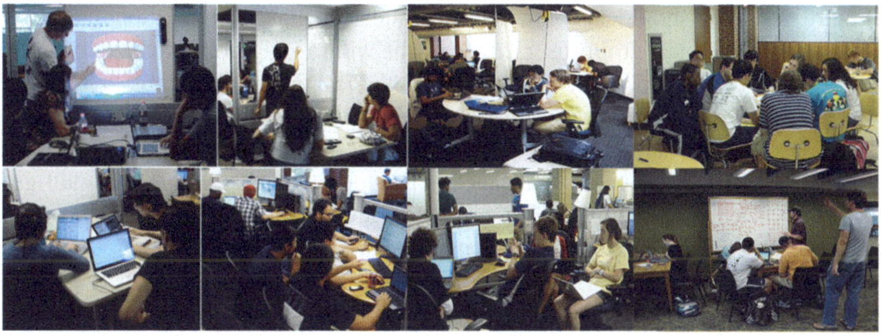

Fig. 3. Small group formations for shared visualization in LEC and LWC2

4 Conclusion

This study into patterns of small groups collaborative activity with visualization highlights the impact of furniture shape (perpendicular or curvilinear work surfaces) ability to enable users to scale up visualization and accommodate individual devices. Spatial setting customization is used to establish small group (4–8 members) cognitive convergence using shared visualizations. Users are found to spend a high percentage of time adapting to or modifying settings to accommodate variable group sizes. Setting inhibitors are identified as dimensions of chair and table surfaces. Narrow table widths, and moderate lengths are preferred to enable sightlines to personal computing devices and a peripheral visualization surface. Library learning commons design was first implemented in LEC, with LWC and LWC2 designed as second generation collaborative spaces. LWC2 removed side-by-side dual display monitor provisions yet this modality was highly sought after by all group sizes making this are in the LEC the second most utilized. Users are seen to manipulate furniture in settings to create personalized workspaces and position the inscription surface towards a shared viewing plane to avoid distractions from moving peers. This occurs even as the group preference is for settings in areas of high social density, and even as nearby settings offer more aesthetic design and quieter ambience. The preference for LEC and LWC2 layouts appears to be due to the settings ability to enable variable group sizes to synchronize views with multiple devices and inscription surfaces, and experience co-presence with surrounding peers. Individual spatial orientation relative to the visualization plane is coordinated to support multiple individual devices and group members while offering the ability to scale up the visualization format. When users collaborate with multiple viewing devices, a layering of visualization displays is seen to occur. This appears to enable multiple screens to be seen by leaders of the group to coordinate work flow in a command/control role. One of the main problems in developing a hybrid spatial-multi-modal and spontaneous small group visualization environment is the construction of a symbiotic inscription and interactive viewing of multiple information modalities. Coordinating furniture design provisions to enable layering of horizontal and vertical devices, with scalable visualization may reduce the density of proxemics in small group collaboration.

Future research should accommodate physical spatial configuration factors into understandings of small group user engagement with a range of visualization modalities for intuitive and spontaneous deployment. Designing ubiquitous settings with multiple types of display modalities will require advancement of projection and sensing parameters, to adjust individual experience to viewing location angles, scales and interactivity differences. The primary need is to rapidly adjust support for small group users proxemics relationships, and coordinate viewing cones and scaling of visualization and space formats aligned to group size and proxemics dynamics.

References

Alabi, O.S., Wu, X., Harter, J.M., Phadke, M., Pinto, L., Petersen, H., Bass, S., Keifer, M., Zhong, S., Healey, C., Raylor II, R.M.: Comparative visualization of ensembles using ensemble surface slicing. Proc SPIE in PMC (2013)

Fischer, F., Mandl, H.: Knowledge convergence in computer-supported collaborative learning: the role of external representation tools. J. Learn. Sci. Taylor Francis Routledge **14**(3), 405–441 (2005)

Isenberg, P., Elmqvist, N., Scholtz, J., Cernea, D., Ma, K.L., Hagen, H.: Collaborative visualization: definition, challenges, and research agenda. J. Inf. Vis. – special issue on state of the field and new research directions **10**(4), 310–326, October 2011. Sage Publisher (2011)

Isenberg, P., Isenberg, T., Lee, B., von Zadow, U., Tang, A.: Data visualization on interactive surfaces: a research agenda. Visualization Viewpoints IEEE Comput. Graph. Appl. 16–24 (2013)

Jacobsen, M., Haile, Y.S., Knudsen, S., Hornbaek, K.: Information visualization and proxemics: design opportunities and empirical findings. IEEE Trans. Vis. Comput. Graph. **19**(12), 2386–2395 (2013)

Juola, J.: Chapter 3 theories of focal and peripheral attention. In: Bakker, S., Hausen, D., Selker, T. (eds.) Peripheral Interaction Challenges and Opportunities for HCI in the Periphery of Attention. Human-Computer Interaction Series, Springer (2016)

Kim, M.J., Maher, M.L.: The impact of tangible user interfaces on spatial cognition during collaborative design. Des. Stud. **29**(3), 222–253. Elsevier, New York, NY (2008)

Langner, R., Kister, U., Dachsett, R.: Multiple coordinated views at large displays for multiple users: empirical findings on user behavior, movement and distances. IEEE Trans. Visual. **25** (1), 608–618 (2018)

Mahmood, T., Butler, E.: Building multiple coordinated spaces for effective immersive analytics through distributed cognition. International Symposium on Big Data Visual and Immersive Analytics (BDVA) (2018)

Marquardt, N., Greenberg, S.: Applying proxemics to mediate people's interaction with devices in ubiquitous computing ecologies. ITS'10 November 7–10, 2010. Saarbrucken, Germany (2010)

Stahl, G.: Analyzing and designing the group cognition experience. Int. J. Coop. Inf. Syst. 15(2), 157–178 © World Scientific Publishing Company (2006)

Tobiasz, M., Isenberg, P., Carpendale, S.: Lark: coordinating co-located collaboration with information visualization. IEEE Trans. Visual. Comput. Graph. **15**(6), 1065–1072, November/December (2009)

Tversky, B.: Visualizing thought. In: Huang, W. (ed.) Handbook of Human Centric Visualization. New York, NY (2014)

Vermeulen, J., Houben, S., Marquardt, N.: Chapter 7 fluent transitions between focused and peripheral interaction in proxemic interactions. In Bakker, S., Hausen, D., Selker, T. (eds.) Peripheral Interaction: Challenges and Opportunities for HCI in the Periphery of Attention. Human-Computer Interaction Series, Springer (2016)
Yusoff, Nor'ian Mohd Salwah, Siti.: A systematic review of shared visualizations to achieve common ground. J. Vis. Lang. Comput. **28**, 83–99 (2015)

Genesis of Attention in the Process of Interaction Weak Visual Person – Work System in a Local Environment

Jorge Gil Tejeda[1(✉)] and Lorena Olmos Pineda[2]

[1] Universidad Autónoma Metropolitana Unidad Xochimilco, Mexico City, Mexico
networkcloud@outlook.com
[2] Universidad Nacional Autónoma de México, Mexico City, Mexico
lolmospi@gmail.com

Abstract. The way in which a person with visual weakness interacts with a device in a local environment provides useful information to study the processes that he requires in the mental construction of the object. The analysis of these processes can originate valuable information about those patterns that promote a sensory equivalence and thereby understand the origin of the attention in the process of interaction with a **Work System (WS)**. A determinant factor is the correct spatial location of the hands of a **Weak visual person (Wvp)** in the WS because each device used by a Wvp implies a dishabituation to the system. Likewise, it has been found that the processes of construction of mental models differ in a Wvp and a **Normal visual person (Nvp)** by the use of equivalent systems (When a damage exist in the motor limbs, there is a spontaneous reorganization. They are replaced by other motor systems that they had not previously associated [1].) however, there is a correspondence of data in the mental models obtained and a variability in levels of attention.

Keywords: Weak visual person · Normal visual person · Process of interaction · Mental models · Motor interaction · Design

1 Introduction

A keyboard in a work environment behaves like an interface of a work system [2]. This interface transfers information to the user through different levels of human interaction in the relationship user - **Keyboard Interface (KI).** The perceived information depends on this relationship, so it becomes an artifact of first necessity for the performance of various activities and fulfillment of objectives.

Practically there are no variations in the design of a keyboard. They are very similar to the mental models created from a typewriter of the 80's. All of this has created a historical memory and habituation in Normal visual persons (Nvp), facilitating their interaction no matter variations in their dimensions, textures, intensity of pressure among other factors. However, any variation of patterns on the keyboard offers a different user experience in a person with visual weakness. Each variation in the patterns of an input device generates dishabituation [3] in the interaction of a Wvp with the device.

T. Ahram et al. (Eds.): IHIET 2019, AISC 1018, pp. 150–156, 2020.
https://doi.org/10.1007/978-3-030-25629-6_24

Studies shown that these factors cause higher levels of attention in the interaction process in the Wvp - K relationship compared to the Nvp - K relationship. However, the interaction process Wvp - K in a local work environment behaved as a continuous task and caused negative effects of additional stress on the user. Likewise, it was observed that a Wvp use equivalent systems that substitute the visual system to interact with the keyboard, which implies a considerable variation of time in the execution of tasks.

2 Context

In a specific context such as the user's work environment, it is observed that keyboards have perceptible differences in patterns such as dimensions, organization, levels of pressure, textures, symmetry, groups of information, separation between sensitive elements, among other factors. And it has been observed that any variation in the patterns cause dishabituation in a Wvp in the interaction with the K.

3 Description of Human Interaction

The specific activities to perform were: 1. Interface location, 2. Enter user information, 3. Enter password information, 4. Error in password data capture, 5. Enter correct information (Tables 1 and 2).

Table 1. Description of the human interaction processes in the Wvp-K relationship

Process	Type of interaction	Function
Physical location of the object	Motor interaction	Movement of spatial location to have physical contact with hands and K. Prolonged process
	Visual interaction	Complementary system to provide more sensory information to Wvp
Habituation process to a new system: K	Motor interaction	Macro and micro exploratory movements of the hand with the K
	Tactil interaction	Locate Keyboard interface. Prolonged process. The recognition of the K interface is done by crossing limits
	Visual interaction	Complementary system to provide more sensory information to Wvp
	Propioception	Spatial location of the keyboard with the hands through the motor and tactile interaction
Process of execution of the action	Motor interaction	Exploratory movement with hands
	Digital pressure	Submit information. Post-security action of spatial location of the hands
WS response	Sound interaction	It generates Dishabituation. Answer given by the WS by an error of entering the information in the password. There is no security of the type of error involved. It generates stress. High levels of atention

(*continued*)

Table 1. (*continued*)

Process	Type of interaction	Function
Emotional response: Wvp	Interoception	Sensation of discomfort and stress, dishabituation and generation of high levels of attention
Habituation process to the K system	Motor interaction	Place hands spatially on the keyboard again
	Tactil interaction	Locate Keyboard interface. Prolonged process. The recognition of the K interface is done by crossing limits
	Visual Interaction	Complement to the sensory equivalence achieved with the motor, tactile, proprioception interaction by Wvp. Prolonged process
	Propio-ception	Placement of the hands sensorially on the keyboard interface
Process of execution of the action	Motor interaction	Delete and enter correct information generally from the last entry field
	Digital pressure	Submit information. Post-security action of spatial location of the hands
WS response	Sound interaction	Wvp is more likely to be wrong again

Table 2. Description of the human interaction processes in the Nvp-K relationship

Process	Type of interaction	Function
Physical location of the object and habituation	Visual interaction	Locate keyboard interface spatially. Immediate response
	Propio-ception	Placement of the hands sensorially on the keyboard interface
Process of execution of the action	Motor Interaction	Movement to have physical contact with the hands and the K
	Digital pressure	Submit information
	Tactil interaction	Place fingers in the correct area
WS response	Sound interaction	It generates Dishabituation. Answer given by the WS by an error of entering the information in the password. There is no security of the type of error involved. It generates stress. High levels of atention
Emotional response:Nvp	Intero-ception	Sensation of discomfort, immediate adaptation to K, high levels of attention
Adaptation and	Visual interaction	Detect the error by sight and receive sensory information of my location

(*continued*)

Table 2. (*continued*)

Process	Type of interaction	Function
Process of execution of the action	Propio-ception	Spatial location of the keyboard with the hands
	Motor interaction	Delete and enter precise information in the entry field
	Digital pressure	Submit information. Action after the placement of the hands on K
	End of the action	There is less chance that person Nvp will get wrong again

Basically the differences in the process are: (A) The execution time in each level of interaction; the greater the number of processes the longer time required. (B) Process of spatial placement of the hands; fundamental factor to execute the task correctly. (C) How to use the senses to solve the problem during the process: directly in the case of the Nvp and by sensory equivalence in the case of Wvp. (D) Dominant system in the processes: Visual system for the Nvp and Motor system for the Wvp. (E) Adaptation and Dishabituation to the system.

4 Methodology

We used a qualitative method [4] linked to the times and activities described below (Tables 3 and 4):

Table 3. The qualitative method used in the work environment is shown.

Factor	Description
Method	1. Application of participant observation in the context of work with a Wvp 2. Assignment of a discrete task to a Wvp and a Nvp 3. Analize the process of interaction
Time:	Observation in real time of the activities carried out to fulfill the discrete task
Activities	1. Set objective: enter to the operative system of a laptop by a Wvp and a Nvp 2. Identify interaction processes 3. Identify subsequent responses to an error in the execution of the task 4. Identify patterns that generate adaptability and dishabituation to the WS
Goals	Detection of the origin in the highest levels of attention in the cycle of human interaction before a discrete task in a Wvp and a Nvp to give an approximation to the genesis of the attention in these processes interactions
Observations	The correct spatial location of the hands in the keyboard interface was found decisive in order to initiate the task execution process

Table 4. Nomenclature used and its description.

Symbol	Description	Symbol	Description
K	Keyboard	Mi	Motor interaction
WS	Work System	Vi	Visual interaction
Wvp	Weak visual person	Si	Sound interaction
WSR	Work System Response	Ti	Tactil interaction
Er	Emotional response	Dp	Digital pressure
Sr	Selective response	Prop	Propioception
Nr	Natural response	Intero	Interoception
1Hi	First level of human interaction	S	Stimulus

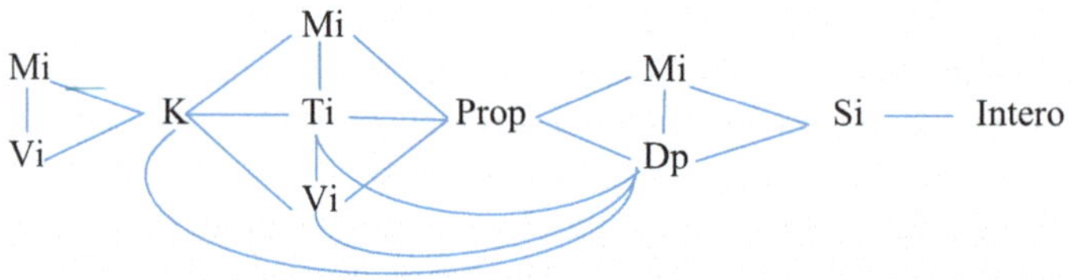

Fig. 1. First cycle: given until the answer given by the WS.

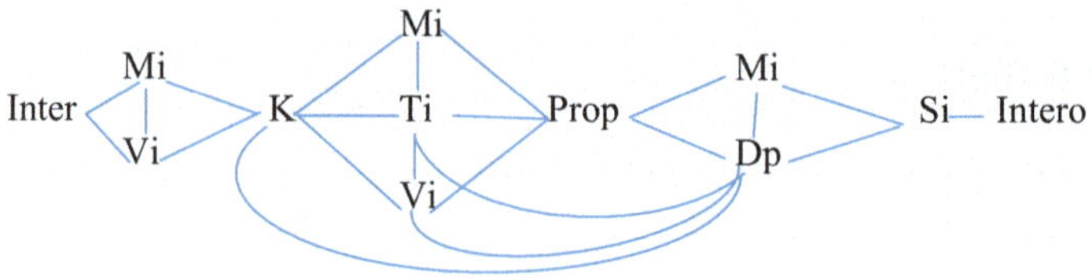

Fig. 2. Second cycle: given until the end of the task

With the analysis of those figures the following observations in the Wvp were obtained (Figs. 1 and 2):

1. It is observed the intervention of 6 systems in the interaction process Wvp - K: 3 systems of motor equivalence, proprioceptive system, audible system, visual system.
2. It is observed that in the interaction process Wvp - K substitute systems are used to complement the information of the damaged system: visual system.
3. There is evidence to think that during the interaction process Wvp -K there is no habituation/adaptation.
4. There is evidence to think that the highest levels of attention are executed during the intervention processes of several systems to solve a problem.
5. There is evidence to think that the highest levels of attention in the Wvp -K interaction processes are carried out while some system of motor equivalence is present.

6. There is evidence to suggest that the higher level of dishabituation, the greater levels of attention
7. Any change in the sensitive patterns of the keyboard generate dishabituation in a Wvp.
8. There is evidence to suggest that the greater of dishabituation with WS, the greater involvement of substitute systems in the interaction process Wvp - K
10. There is evidence to think that the greater dishabituation with the WS, the greater number of processes to solve the problem, which is directly related to the time of interaction with the WS.
11. There is evidence to suggest that Wvp is more likely to give emotional responses during the interaction process.
12. All the process includes: A. Interface location, B. Enter user information, C. Enter password information, D. Error in password data capture, E. Enter correct information.

Based on the same objective, the following relationship diagram is shown in the Human Interaction with the person NvP (Fig. 3):

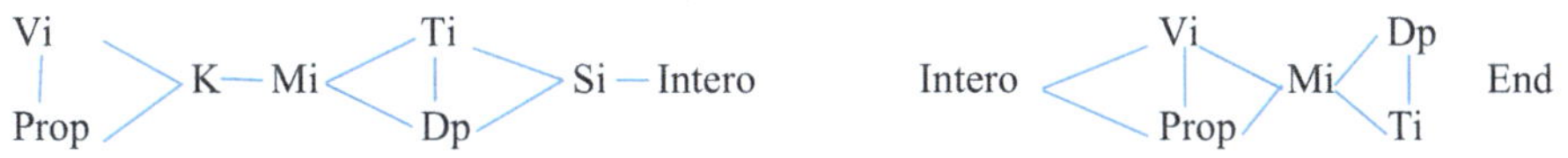

Fig. 3. Left first cycle: given until the answer given by the WS. Right SECOND CYCLE: Given until de end of task

With the analysis of those Figures the following observations in the Nvp were obtained:

1. It is observed that in Nvp - K interaction process, the visual system is used to generate a spatial ubication.
2. There is evidence to think that during the Nvp - K interaction process there is habituation /adaptation to the WS.
3. There is evidence to think that a greater adaptation to the WS modifies the interaction processes.
4. There is evidence to think that a greater adaptation with the WS less involvement of systems in the interaction process in the Nvp – K relation.
5. All the process includes: A. Interface location, B. Enter user information, C. Enter password information, D. Error in password data capture, E. Enter correct information.

5 Conclusions

It is observed that the genesis of the attention in the relationship Wvp - K is given by the following processes:

1. Dishabituation in the interaction generates constant modification in the neuronal states and generates the highest levels of attention in the Wvp.
2. Motor interaction in the relationship Wvp - K causes the construction of the object in the mental processes.
3. However, for the execution of tasks and work efficiency, the dishabituation in the interaction process Wvp - K becomes a continuous task that generates stress in the Wvp.
4. Based on the results for a Wvp, a keyboard must show constant patterns that generates adaptation.
5. The Adaptation is a factor that reduces the level of attention observed in the Nvp - K interaction process.

References

1. Lashley, K.F.: The Neuropsychology of Lashley. McGraw-Hill, New York (1960)
2. Olmos, L., Gil, J. Génesis de la atención en larelación alumno - Objeto de Arpendizaje en un entorno de aprendizaje. Congreso Internacional sobre Aprendizaje, Innovación y Competitividad. Zaragoza (2017)
3. Pribram, K.H.: Languages of the Brain. Prentice Hall, California, Monterrey, United States (1971)
4. Hernández, S.R., Collado, C.F., Baptista, L.P.: Metodología de la Investigación (Tercera, edición edn. Mc Graw Hill, México (2003)

Investigating Educationally Fruitful Speech-Based Methods to Assist People with Special Needs to Care Potted Plants

Dimitrios Loukatos[1(✉)], Konstantinos G. Arvanitis[1], and Nikolaos Armonis[2]

[1] Department of Natural Resources Management and Agricultural Engineering, Agricultural University of Athens, Iera Odos 75, 11855 Athens, Greece
{dlouka, karvan}@aua.gr

[2] Hellas Digital Research and Innovative Products Company, G. Gennimata 119, 16561 Athens, Greece
n.armonis@hellasdigital.gr

Abstract. For elderly or people with special needs, caring plants is a good practice to reinforce an optimistic aspect of view. Unfortunately, similar tasks often require physical strength and senses to work fine. This paper reports exactly on the effort of students of Agricultural Engineering to bridge this gap, through the exploitation of innovative hardware along with speech and voice recognition techniques. Into this context, the paper describes methods to combine speech- based applications, relying on either cloud or local services, with smart phones and similar innovative systems, ranging from arduino to raspberry pi ones, to trigger plant caring actions or to query the values of several plant-related parameters. Plants are converted into speaking entities. The derived software and hardware configurations are evaluated. Furthermore, students "demystify" the potential of the recently appeared "exotic" devices and techniques that have been introduced in the modern agriculture.

Keywords: Speech recognition · Embedded systems · Speaking plants · Disabled people

1 Introduction

Historically, the relation between humans and plants was beneficial for both parties and not only in terms of nutrition. Plants can embellish and perfume the home era and even assist in people's good emotional state [1]. For elderly people or people with special needs, caring plants is a good practice to reinforce an optimistic aspect of view [2]. Unfortunately, many of such tasks require physical strength and senses to work fine, but, not all people can meet these criteria. The World Health Organization estimates that more than one billion of people are exhibiting some form of disability and almost 200 million experiencing considerable difficulties in functioning [3]. Disability will be an even greater concern in the future because of the ageing of populations and/or the increase in potentially dangerous health conditions such as diabetes, cardiovascular disease, and mental health disorders. The technology advances very fast [4], tries to

T. Ahram et al. (Eds.): IHIET 2019, AISC 1018, pp. 157–162, 2020.
https://doi.org/10.1007/978-3-030-25629-6_25

relief similar problems by various ways [5, 6] and considerable motivation is offered [7]. Many solutions are not easily applicable due to constrains in money, processing power or space.

Thankfully, the fast growing mobile phone market has made available devices like credit card - sized computers, typically Arduino Uno [8] and Raspberry Pi [9] units, and various accompanying components, like sensor and radio modules, at very affordable prices. These systems, along with smart phones, can be used to realize many helpful applications, even with cloud based artificial intelligence (AI) features, like speech and voice recognition.

Into this context the paper highlights how specially designed, educationally friendly, software platforms, like the MIT App Inventor [10], can facilitate the programming in order to benefit of the potential that these mobile devices have, provided that supplementary code is written, in python or C, on the corresponding communication end (typically on a Raspberry pi unit). The latter unit is acting as a server near the plants and coordinates typical sensors and actuators, possibly supervising Arduino uno units as well. The case when there is no presence of Internet connection to provide access to a remote speech or voice recognition server is also assessed. In this case, off-line running software tackles with voice recognition issues, as embedded boards are now powerful enough to maintain such tasks, for a limited set of words or phrases. A good example of such off-line software is the SOPARE package [11], which is easily installed and is well documented. For better efficiency, alternatives to Raspberry pi unit are also tested. In most scenarios, the voice interaction process can be triggered whenever the human is shaking its mobile device or getting closer to a specific plant, guided by proximity sensors or even by image recognition software. For this experimental implementation Wi-Fi protocol is used to carry the necessary information. Students of Agricultural Engineering orchestrated these diverse design, implementation and testing efforts, thus gaining educationally fruitful [12] assets, valuable for their forthcoming role in the rapidly evolving agricultural era. The paper concludes with remarks and comments on the use case scenarios and highlights open issues and plans for future work.

2 Design and Implementation

The applications scenarios to be covered are of diverse nature, exactly like peoples' need are, and thus, require increased flexibility in the design of the system that is going to support them. This requirement is assured, at experimental level, if the overall implementation retains a modular nature, based on generic and open components. For simplicity reasons, two ends are assumed: the user's end and the plant's end. The user can speak to the device near to him (at user's end) and the corresponding commands circulate, via a typical network infrastructure, to the plant's end to trigger the necessary actions, like watering it or queering the value of a critical parameter (e.g., of the soil humidity). The acknowledgment/response, typically as a voice message, can be generated directly at plant's end or, indirectly, by the equipment at user's end.

The most apparent variant of the discussed platform architecture to support the abovementioned scenarios exploits the MIT App Inventor environment to create a smart phone application, able to intercept (and forward) the user's voice commands. The voice recognition process may start whenever the phone is shacked. On the other hand, the discussed application is able to handle the plant's replies to the user, by playing the suitable prerecorded messages or by performing simple speech synthesis tasks. The techniques been used by the students to implement these tasks are based on (and extending) the work described in [13].

Inside the App Inventor application, the suitable HTTP requests are generated and are destined towards the corresponding server (typically at the plant's end). This server, namely a Raspberry Pi unit, handles these requests, using features like OS system calls [14]. By this method, the server can generate prerecorded messages [15] or convert text to speech [16], providing further information and guidance at plant's end as well. This server unit coordinates typical sensors and actuators, possibly supervising Arduino Uno units, connected wirelessly or via cable, as well. Many sensors and actuators can be handled directly by the Raspberry Pi as well via the features provided by [17]. This Raspberry Pi, at plant's end, is responsible for the preparation and the delivery to the user's end of all the corresponding reply content.

The case when there is no presence of Internet connection to provide access to a remote speech or voice recognition server is also assessed. A suitable off-line (i.e., locally) running software (e.g., in SOPARE), running on an Raspberry Pi unit (in lieu of the smart phone) is tackling with the voice recognition issues, and forming the necessary commands using HTTP request invocations, through suitable plug-ins, via mechanisms like the one described in [18]. However, interaction through UDP [19] messaging has been implemented as well, to achieve faster response.

According to some other use scenarios, the roles of the two discrete ends (i.e., of the user and of the plant) can be merged and hosted by the same device (typically a Raspberry Pi) which is lying near the plants (e.g., by their pot). There is also provision for scenarios, where the voice interaction process is triggered whenever the human is getting closer to a specific plant, guided by low cost proximity (or PIR) sensors. Such configuration arrangements establish a completely transparent mechanism, converting potted plants into speaking entities, able to talk with their gardeners.

For simplicity reasons, in the discussed experimental implementations, the Wi-Fi protocol is used to carry the necessary information. Nevertheless, more sophisticated network communication scenarios among enhanced nodes (typically the Raspberry Pi units) or nodes of reduced capabilities (typically Arduinos) can be derived but their description is omitted due to space constrains.

In Fig. 1 an extended implementation design supporting human – plant interaction is presented, to better highlight the discussed functionality. The enhanced Raspberry Pi node (here at the plant's end) supports various voice functions on its own and coordinates typical actions. In a typical case, a reduced features set is applied.

Figure 2 depicts an indicative implementation to support human – plant interaction, based on audio communication. Plant's soil humidity levels are reported after a suitable voice-triggered command.

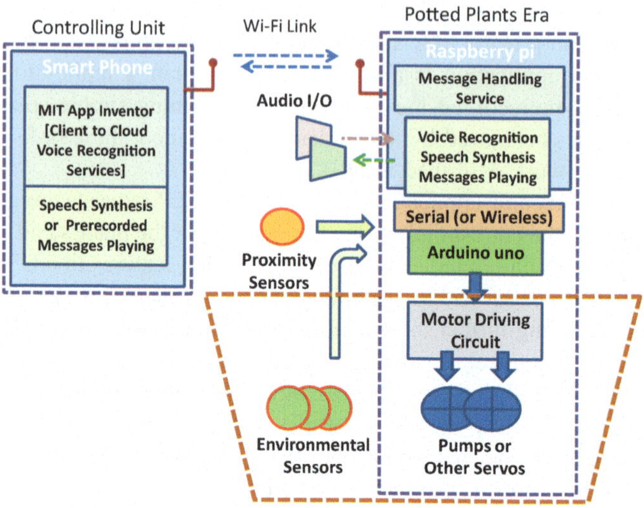

Fig. 1. Extended implementation design supporting human – plant interaction

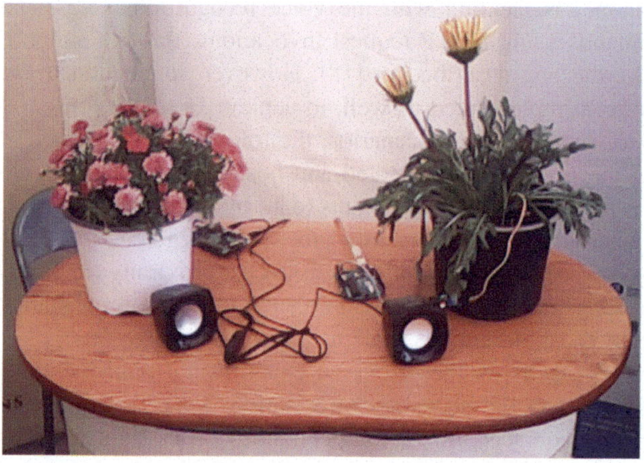

Fig. 2. Indicative implementation supporting human – plant interaction, based on audio. Plant's soil humidity is reported after a suitable voice – triggered command.

3 Results and Discussion

The evaluation tests presented in this work are focusing on highlighting the feasibility of solutions based on generic and cost effective innovative hardware components, along with free software packages, both visual and textual ones, to provide assistance for elderly or people with disabilities while caring potted houseplants.

The voice recognition accuracy when using cloud based services, was better, because well-trained AI engines carried out the voice recognition tasks. In case of the off-line installed engine, the voice recognition accuracy, for a limited set of typical commands, varied, depending on the details of learning and parameterization stages and the potential of the audio device. Matching between 0.5 and 0.9 was achieved.

In terms of delay, the off-line voice recognition engine exhibited faster response. In this case, the total response time varied from below 1 s to 2 s, including both processing and networking delays. In case of cloud-based voice recognition, the response times were slightly longer (between 1 s and 3 s). It should be taken under consideration though that, in the local (off-line) voice recognition scenario, the Raspberry Pi unit was sometimes pushed at its knees, trying to tackle with such a CPU demanding process as the continuous sampling of human's commands or the following pattern matching process. Apparently, problems were more intense when the Raspberry Pi unit had to carry out other "heavy" tasks at the same time, like serving a VNC monitoring session. Experiments performed using more powerful boards, like the ASUS tinker board [20], which has almost identical layout with the Raspberry Pi, achieved better response times (near to half, in duration). For performance reasons, alternative implementations using similar to SOPARE packages (e.g., like the Snips [21]) should be assessed in the future.

In terms of power consumption, the system at high activity (i.e., during voice recognition, speech synthesis, .wav files playing) consumed currents of the order of 1A, while the Arduino component less than 50 mA. As boards like the Raspberry Pi the do not support sleep mode features, the system was modified so as the Arduino components to fire up (i.e., to power on) the Raspberry Pi components, by intercepring triggers caused by the reach of humans, via PIR sensors. This scenario of course, drastically affects the time response of the system and requires further investigation.

4 Conclusions and Future Plans

This paper highlighted the efforts of students of Agricultural Engineering to exploit low cost innovative systems in order to implement speech or voice recognition applications, either cloud or off-line based ones, for assisting elderly or people with special needs to remotely trigger plant caring actions or to query the values of several critical parameters of their potted plants. Plants are converted into speaking entities. These efforts were also beneficial, from educational aspect, for students, which have to adapt in the fast evolving technological environment of the agricultural era.

A balanced mixture of software parts, written ether in textual (Python and C) or visual (MIT App Inventor) environments, was needed to realize the above task. In terms of hardware, Arduino and Raspberry Pi units, connected with typical sensors and actuators and equipped with radio interfaces, were the basis for a pilot implementation. Scenarios involving faster units were also assessed.

In the future, more efficient hardware devices should be used, in order to save energy and achieve faster and more accurate response to voice commands. We also intend to evaluate more software packages performing off-line voice recognition tasks. The further enrichment of sound data with extra parameters provided by machine vision techniques or diverse types of sensors data would assist in better intercepting people's orders. The combination with databases and computational intelligence techniques would be a step towards achieving an ambient intelligent ecosystem, assistive for elderly or people with disabilities.

References

1. Soga, M., Gaston, K.J., Yamaurac, Y.: Gardening is beneficial for health: a meta-analysis. 92–99 (2016). https://doi.org/10.1016/j.pmedr.2016.11.007
2. Detweiler, M.B., Sharma, T., Detweiler, J.G., Murphy, P.F., Lane, S., Carman, J., Chudhary, A.S., Halling, M.H., Kim, K.Y.: What is the evidence to support the use of therapeutic gardens for the elderly? Psychiatry Investig. **9**(2), 100–110 (2012). https://doi.org/10.4306/pi.2012.9.2.100
3. World Health Organization: World report on disability. https://www.who.int/disabilities/world_report/2011/report.pdf (2011). Accessed Apr 2019
4. Krishna, K.R.: Push button Agriculture: robotics, drones, satellite-guided soil and crop management. Apple Academic Press, Oakville, Ontario, Canada (2016). ISBN-13: 978-1-77188-305-4
5. Malik, A.A., Nizamani, F.R.: Speaker identification based home automation system for aging populations through speech recognition. Int. J. Eng. Res. Gen. Sci. **4**(2) (2016). ISSN 2091-2730
6. Busatlik, B., Dogru, N., Lera, I., Sukic, E.: Smart homes with voice activated systems for disabled people. TEM J. **6**(1), 103–107 (2017). https://doi.org/10.18421/tem61-15
7. Agrability, Assistive Technology Program for Farmers with Disabilities funded by the USDA. http://www.agrability.org/about/program/. Accessed Apr 2019
8. Arduino Uno board description on the official Arduino site. https://store.arduino.cc/arduino-uno-rev3
9. Raspberry Pi 3 Model B board description on the official Raspberry site. https://www.raspberrypi.org/products/raspberry-pi-3-model-b/. Accessed April 2019
10. MIT App Inventor Programming Environment. http://appinventor.mit.edu/explore/. Accessed April 2019
11. Sound Pattern Recognition – SOPARE: https://www.bishoph.org/. Accessed April 2019
12. Eaton, E.: Teaching integrated AI through interdisciplinary project-driven courses. AI Magazine **38**(2) (2017)
13. Loukatos, D., Kahn, K., Alimisis, D.: Flexible techniques for fast developing and remotely controlling DIY robots, with AI flavor. In: Edurobotics 2018. Rome, Italy (pending proceedings' publishing by Springer) (2018)
14. OS: Miscellaneous operating system interfaces (Python). https://docs.python.org/3/library/os.html. Accessed Apr 2019
15. mpg321: a simple and lightweight command line MP3 player. http://mpg321.sourceforge.net/. Accessed Apr 2019
16. eSpeak: Speech synthesizer. http://espeak.sourceforge.net/. Accessed Apr 2019
17. RPi.GPIO Module Basics (Python): https://sourceforge.net/p/raspberry-gpio-python/wiki/BasicUsage/. Accessed Apr 2019
18. HTTPie: A command line HTTP client. https://httpie.org. Accessed Apr 2019
19. User Datagram Protocol – UDP: https://en.wikipedia.org/wiki/User_Datagram_Protocol. Accessed Apr 2019
20. ASUS Tinker Board Credit Card Computer: https://www.asus.com/us/Single-Board-Computer/Tinker-Board/. Accessed Apr 2019
21. Snips Voice Recognition Engine: https://snips.ai/technology/. Accessed Apr 2019

Actuarial Models in the Design of Human-Oriented Production Systems and Products

Evgeny Kolbachev and Yulia Salnikova(✉)

Platov South-Russian State Polytechnic University (NPI), Prosveshcheniya, 132, 346428 Novocherkassk, Russian Federation
kolbachev@yandex.ru, yuliasalnikova@gmail.com

Abstract. The article describes an approach to determining the cost characteristics of human-oriented production systems and products (mainly machines) at the conceive stages. The cost characteristics are determined on the basis of an estimate of the probability of a trouble-free operation of the machine during operation. At the same time, actuarial models and the Bayes formula are used, and the cost of ensuring safety in the production system or in the product is assumed to equal to the insurance fund to overcome the consequences of accidents. It has been established that it is expedient to organize work on the design of human-oriented production systems and machines at the stages of conceive, as well as concept design and detailed design, based on the AGILE-ideology.

Keywords: Human-oriented systems · Machine design · Actuarial models · Conceive stage · Concept design · Detailed design · Cost · Design organization · AGILE-ideology

1 Introduction

The desire of researchers and developers of technology to the harmony of man and machine was typical already in the industrial era.

Many works describing the role of the human factor in economy use the key ideas from well-known classical works, for example, from the prominent book by Rowntree [1] that firstly used the term "human-oriented systems" and mentioned their influence on human capital.

New technical capabilities require not only legal and moral discussion and regulation, but also future-oriented assessments of the consequences of scientific and technical progress. This was realized, in particular, by the US Congress, which in 1972 founded the Bureau of Social Appraisal of Technology.

In Germany, for the first time in the 1980s, a special commission of questioning was created on issues of "assessing the use of equipment and its effects," whose powers were extended and further [2].

T. Ahram et al. (Eds.): IHIET 2019, AISC 1018, pp. 163–168, 2020.
https://doi.org/10.1007/978-3-030-25629-6_26

In the seventies of the last century, the terms "engineering ethics", "bioethics", "ethics of managers", etc. began to be widely discussed. Hans Jonas's book "The Principle of Responsibility" [3] sparked a discussion in this thematic area.

It should be noted that special attention to operational safety is typical for all engineering products. Obviously, the priorities are the requirements for operational safety of equipment, which is a potential source of man-made disasters, leading to damage to a significant number of people and the ecosystem. However, in world practice there are no clear boundaries, outlining the scope of just such machines.

In the Industrial Age was worked out another methodology that is close to the concept of human-oriented design. It is ErgoDesign concept that was widely presented from the late 1960th to early 1980th. Well-known authors, such as E. Grandjean [4], D. Azrican [5] and others, described ErgoDesign as the technology of mechanical design that differs from "traditional" ergonomic and artistic design. A declared objective of the ErgoDesign is making human's being successful and thriving basing on three aspects of design, which are inseparably linked with each other. These aspects are the convenience, the comfort and the esthetic perfection of the facilities and conditions for the human being. However, this concept does not pay attention to the social aspects of the human being. That is why, in contrast with the nowadays explorers of the ErgoDesign axiological aspects, we cannot represent ErgoDesign as something similar to human-oriented design.

Working out of the NBIC-technologies and appropriate production systems' development is a reason for human capital's extending. This type of causation exists as an effect of NBIC-technologies' features: their fundamental properties; complexity of required applied researches; many-sided cognitive processes; working out and exploitation of special machinery; importance of technological safety. The said researches and processes are a source of original knowledge's appearance and personnel's development during NBIC-processes.

Development of NBIC-technologies under the reindustrialization conditions is used to be taken as a great prospect for humanity. But numerous researches dedicate their works to risks and threats that may be caused by wide spreading of these technologies [6–9]. The most dangerous thing in this situation is how technologies may affect a human being, and change his biological and psychological essence. Ensuring the safety of production systems and products is declared one of the most important design tasks.

It's one of the reasons why this work is timely and actual.

2 Economic Security Management: The Use of Actuarial Models

Since a person-oriented product is primarily a safe product, a technical system can be considered safe if it works without accidents that are dangerous to human health and do not cause damage to the environment.

This approach is relevant not only in the design of technical systems that prevent accidents and environmental damage. The termination of the operation of any useful object brings potential damage.

An example of such situation is dysfunction of cold-storage chambers at the food manufacturing enterprise. The result is a great amount of spoiled products and economic losses. Alternative is a number of measures (quickly, and that is why, expensive) that give a possibility to relocate products to other storage, or to sell them as fast as possible (and of course, the price will be commercially disadvantageous).

Emergency shutdown of system from the human settlement's life support system complex may cause a social crisis. To eliminate its consequences and find an alternative way of system's parts functioning a number of very expensive measures are to be carried out, etc.

The economic results of risk reduction in the operation of technical systems can be described using insurance (actuarial) models [10]. In this case, risk insurance is considered as an alternative to a technically safe system or product. This kind of insurance covers a great number of subjects and risks, but all these objects are rather homogenous and insurance payments are approximately similar.

Thus, the hypothetical situation that we consider is that any technical system or product in operation gives an economic result similar to the existence of a special insurance fund from which payments are made and the damage from the termination of this technical system/ product is compensated.

The use of the mechanism of actuarial calculations in the design process requires the use of appropriate parameters. Compliance with the insurance and design parameters are given in Table 1.

Table 1. Compliance of insurance and design parameters

Parameter designation	Parameter content	
	For insurance conditions	For design conditions
P	The amount of insurance premiums collected	The total cost of the function "ensure security"
B	Insurance indemnity paid	The amount of costs associated with the elimination of the consequences of a single accident
C	Total insured amount of the insured objects	The amount of costs associated with the elimination of the consequences of accidents for all objects with a permissible probability for Bayes
Cm	Sum Insured per Policyholder	The sum of the costs associated with the elimination of the consequences of accidents on one object with a permissible probability for Bayes ($Cm - C/m$)
m	The number of affected objects as a result of the insured event	The number of accidents involving economic and legal consequences, the likelihood of which is excluded due to the cost of security

(*continued*)

Table 1. (*continued*)

Parameter designation	Parameter content	
	For insurance conditions	For design conditions
L	The number of insurance events	The number of adverse factors that can lead to an accident
n	Number of insurance objects	The number of machines (objects) in the party (in operation)
Kt	The amount of insurance fund required to pay the insurance indemnity by the end of year *t*	The amount of capital investments in work to improve the safety of objects

Certain difficulties for calculations arise in cases where there is a lack of representative statistical information about emergencies and the associated shutdowns in the operation of technical systems and objects. In such cases it is expedient to use a well-known decision-making model with the Bayes formula [11].

This model was used in the engineering and economic substantiation of projects of electric locomotives [12] and equipment for coalmines [13] in order to calculate the costs of ensuring the safety of these technical systems.

Calculated in the described above way, the cost of ensuring the safe operation of the designed technical system serves as the basis for determining its operating costs. This can be done using value engineering [14]. The resulting cost parameters can be used as fundamental in the formation and adoption of engineering decisions relating to the design of the designed object.

3 Experience in the Organization of Design Using Actuarial Models

The said methodology was taken as a basis for working out of complex algorithm. The algorithm may be used during the designing of any human-oriented production system or product [15]. It was successfully used for project engineering during working out locomotives and other railroad engineering, machinery for mine construction, melioration and land reclamation. The feature of algorithm is using designed system's cost parameters as a basis for its constructional perfection on the subsequent levels of design and project engineering. To calculate cost parameters indexes an actuarial method is to be used.

Thus, project engineering is considered to be a step-by-step process of decreasing designed system's or product's entropy, and, in the same time, accumulation of information about it [16]. On practice was used a conditional entropy index, presented by A. Renyi [17]. This index decreases during the process of choosing the best of alternative constructions.

The most efficient way of using presented approach is making it a part of CAx system, such as MCAD, EDA, CAE, CAA [18] and of the Agile ideology-based systems.

4 Conclusion

It has been found that the most effective way to determine the value of human-oriented technical systems and products on the design stage is the use of actuarial models and a probabilistic approach. In this case establishes compliance with the insurance parameters and design parameters of the components of the designed system, ensuring its safe operation. At the same time, the cost of ensuring safety in the production system or in the product is assumed to be equal to the value of the insurance fund for overcoming the consequences of accidents.

The cost of the safety components calculated in this way allows the cost engineering method to calculate the cost of the entire designed system and form design solutions based on it. In this case, the choice of the optimal ones can be carried out using the indicator of conditional entropy of the structure.

It is most expedient to implement this algorithm within the framework of the design support systems for MCAD, EDA, CAE, CAA and Agile ideology.

Some experience has been gained in the application of this approach in the design of railway equipment, equipment for coalmines, and equipment for land reclamation and water management.

References

1. Rowntree, B.-S.: The Human Factor in Business. Longmans Green and Co., London (1921)
2. Lenk, H.: Zur Sozialphilosophie der Technik. Suhrkamp, Frankfurt am Main (1982)
3. Jonas, H.: Das Prinzip Verantwortung. Frankfurt am Main (1979)
4. Grandjean, E.P.: Fitting the Task to the Man: An Ergonomic Approach. Taylor and Francis, London (1969)
5. Azrican, D.A.: ErgoDesign. Problems and Prospects. Technical Aesthetics **3**, 17–23 (1987)
6. Nordmann, A.: Converging Technologies – Shaping the Future of European Societies. European Commission, Brussels (2004)
7. Schmidt, J.C.: NBIC-interdisciplinary? a framework for a critical reflection on inter- and transdisciplinary of NBIC-scenario. Georgia Inst. of Tech. Working Paper (2007)
8. Simondon, G.: Du mode d'existence des objets techniques. Aubier, Paris (2001)
9. Nishimoto, S., An, T.V., Naselaris, T., Benjamini, Y., Ben, Y., Gallant, J.L.: Recon-structing visual experience from brain activity evoked by natural movies. Curr. Biol. **21**(19), 1641–1646 (2011)
10. Trowbridge, C.-L.: Fundamental Concepts of Actuarial Science. AERF, Washington, DC (1989)
11. Kahneman, D., et al.: Judgment under Uncertainty: Heuristics and Biases. University Press, Cambridge (2005)
12. Gorobets, D.G.: Economic features of working out dangerous or responsible products of machine-building. Cost analysis and innovation of the enterprise, pp. 23–24. SRSPU (NPI), Novocherkassk (2010)
13. Liderman, K.M.: Economic instruments to work out a really efficient mining equipment. Economy of the business processes and production system, pp. 25–28. SRSPU (NPI), Novocherkassk (2002)

14. Sharma, A., Belokar, R.M.: Achieving success through value engineering: a case study. In: Proceedings of the World Congress on Engineering and Computer Science, vol. II. WCECS, San Francisco, USA (2012)
15. Kolbachev, E., Zharov, V., Tsukerman, V.: Cost management for PLM systems: a way to improve the competitiveness in digital economy. In: IOP Conference Series: Materials Science and Engineering, vol. 497 (2019)
16. Kolbachev, E.: Management of mechanical engineering design processes based on product cost estimates. SHS Web of Con. **35**, 1–5 (2017)
17. Renyi, A.: Dialogues on Mathematics. Holden-Day, New-York (1967)
18. Saaksvuori, A.: Product Lifecycle Management. Springer, Heidelberg (2008)

Exploration of Product Design Emotion Based on Three-Level Theory of Emotional Design

Tianjiao Zhao(✉) and Tianfei Zhu

College of Intelligence and Computing,
Tianjin University Beiyang Campus, Tianjin, China
zhaotianjiao@tju.edu.cn

Abstract. The three-level theory of emotional design put forward by Donald A. Norman is highly recognized and respected by designers and researchers. Based on this theory, this study uses 2000 design award-winning works as materials. Through the extraction of typical emotional words in product design, the labeling of emotions in design, and the statistical analysis of design emotions, researchers try to explore the method of emotional integration into product design. This research finds that high-level emotions can hardly be decoded and realized in emotional design. It proposes design methods based on five senses, design experience process and human needs to generate high-level emotions.

Keywords: Emotional design · Product design · Design innovation · User psychology

1 Introduction

Emotional design, as a popular design research and development direction, has been well known and widely accepted. More and more product designs begin to pay attention to emotional factors [1]. Emotional ergonomics [2], emotional usability [3], aesthetic emotion [4], emotional products [5] are some examples of this phenomena. Among current theoretical researches, Kansei Engineering [6] and three-level theory [7] can be seen as systematic theories. Donald A. Norman put forward three levels of design emotion in his book Emotional Design, namely instinct level, behavior level and reflection level. Although this theory has been deeply rooted in people's hearts, it has not been systematically mentioned how to exert emotions in design and how to express them accurately. Its application in design practice has certain limitations. Kansei Engineering uses engineering technology to explore the relationship between the sensibility of "human" and the design features of "objects", and transforms the vague emotional needs of people into the form elements of detailed design. It mainly has guiding significance for the first level of emotional design, but seldom explores the second and third levels [8]. Based on emotional design theory, this study reveals the corresponding relationship between design features and design emotions, explores design emotions from the perspective of design features, enriches emotional design theory, Strengthens Design Education and Designer's Self-cultivation and professional Identity, and plays a positive guiding role in design practice.

T. Ahram et al. (Eds.): IHIET 2019, AISC 1018, pp. 169–175, 2020.
https://doi.org/10.1007/978-3-030-25629-6_27

2 Basic Theories

Corresponding to cognitive psychology, the human brain has three different levels of processing: instinctive, behavioral and reflective. Norman put forward the three-level theory of emotional design (Fig. 1).

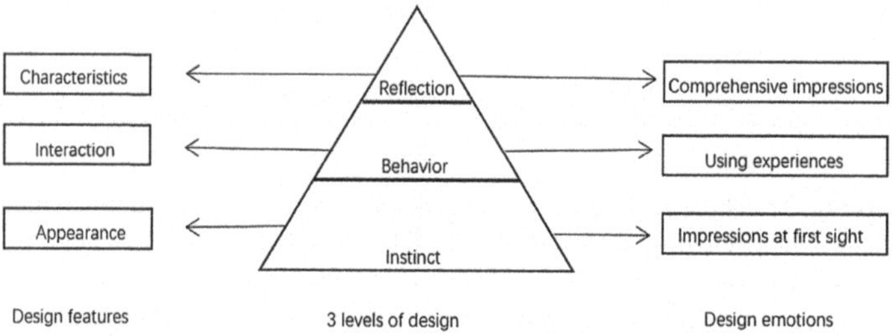

Fig. 1. The 3 levels of design and design emotions

Emotion is first injected by designers and then received by users in the whole process. Smooth and accurate emotional communication inevitably requires designers to grasp the corresponding relationship between emotions and design features in the emotional injection stage, understand which kind of design will stimulate which kind of emotions, decompose the features of the design that may stimulate certain emotions, in order to design emotional products that meet the expectations.

The hierarchical division of emotions is not absolute, and the relationship between design features and emotions in all levels is not one-to-one correspondence. The design features affecting emotions are various and multi-level. But generally speaking, most of the emotions are mainly determined by the design features at corresponding levels. In order to facilitate research, this study uses emotion words as the direct expression of emotions and simplified the meaning of words, distributed them to different levels according to the main meanings. The corresponding relationship between design features and emotions is shown in Fig. 2.

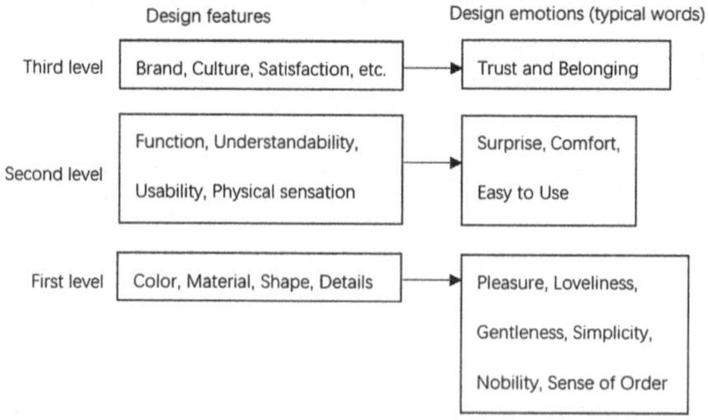

Fig. 2. The corresponding relationship between design features and emotions

3 Experiment

In order to find out what are the main emotions in current product design, what are the similarities and differences among different kinds of products in different fields, and the distribution of emotions at different levels in product design, emotional labeling of 2054 red dots and IF award-winning product pictures is conducted.

First, we collected, classified and numbered 2054 pictures of Red Dot and IF winning products, according to year and category. Second, we selected 65 representative pictures with outstanding emotions. Third, on the basis of learning the three-level theory of emotion, nine experimenters wrote the most prominent three emotion words on 65 typical products pictures, we obtained 1756 effective descriptions and 342 words. After that, 11 emotion words with the most frequent occurrences were obtained after removing repeated and synthesizing the words. Finally, we carried out emotional labeling of 2054 pictures by questionnaires.

4 Discoveries

4.1 Typical Emotion Words in Product Design

The 11 emotion words can be used as a reference for the current typical emotion words of product design. According to the frequency of occurrence, from low to high, the 11 words are shown in Fig. 3 below.

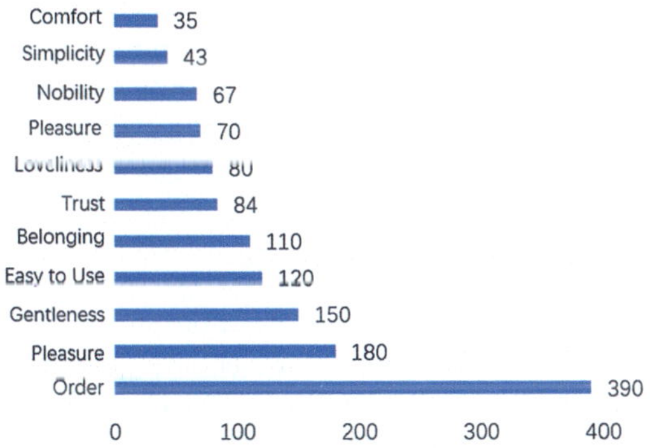

Fig. 3. Words frequency

After classifying these words into 3 levels according to Fig. 2, we found that from the first level to the third level, the number of emotion words is decreasing, and the frequency of being described is also decreasing. This also reflects that the current design emotions are still dominated by the first level of emotions, while the higher level of emotions still need to be further explored.

4.2 Mental Model of Emotion

Different kinds of goods have different explicit emotions and different emotional richness, which forms different emotional mental models of different products. For example, the emotions brought by electronic products are relatively single, mainly Easy to Use, while home and environment products have richer emotions, comfort and softness are more prominent. This is formed gradually in the process of satisfying people's different needs through the ages. It is determined by the functional attributes of products, reflecting people's different emotional demands for different kinds of products. In the process of innovation, we must understand and respect the mental model that people have formed for a long time. When we try to increase or decrease emotions or change emotions, we should make moderate innovation, acceptable innovation and comply with the MAYA [9] principle of design.

4.3 Mono-Emotion Products and Multi-emotion Products

Through the analysis of the questionnaire, it is found that the labeled products can be divided into moto-emotional products and multi-emotional products.

Mono-emotional products refer to products that have one single prominent emotion while other emotions are not obvious. Questionnaire results show that the proportion of moto-emotional products is only about 5%, and that single emotion mainly distributes in the first level.

Multi-emotional products refer to products with multiple prominent emotions coexisting to meet people's growing emotional needs with rich emotions. From the results of the questionnaire, about 95% of the products have multiple emotions. Multiple emotions of multi-emotional products can be distributed in the same level or across levels. Similar to the situation of the moto-emotional products, the emotions of the multi-emotional products are majorly distributed in the first two levels, and very few in the third level.

4.4 Emotion Distributions in Product Design

As shown in Fig. 4, although the number of emotions at the second level is not the largest, the proportion of Easy to Use and comfort at the second level is the highest, and it has become the most prominent emotion words. This also reflects the current trend of emotional design towards the second level, which is determined by the nature of emphasizing practicability in the industrial era, but in the process of using, there are far more emotions to be found and the corresponding design features should not only be functional. From the scarcity of the emotion of surprise, it can be seen that the development of the second level is only limited to the direct functional evaluation of products. The emotions of the third level have the least variety, and the feeling of belonging has the least occurrence.

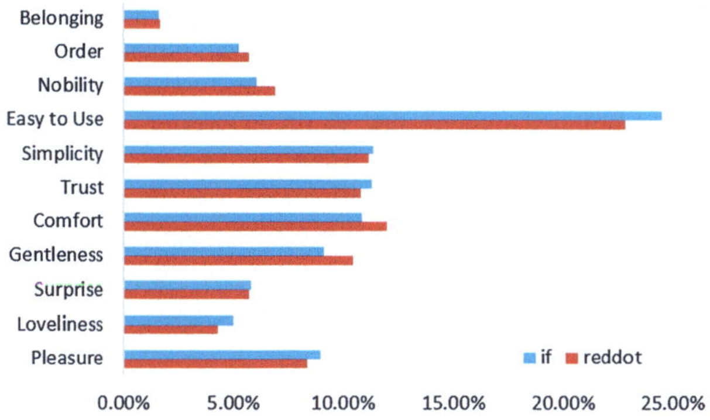

Fig. 4. Overall emotions distribution of the two awards (Percentage)

5 Inspirations

At present, the mainstream of emotional design concentrates on instinctive emotion. High-level emotional design challenges designers to gain a deeper understanding of user psychology. As mentioned above, the qualitative mining of emotions can be transferred to design features based on the corresponding relationship between design features and emotions. Here are some methods that may bring inspirations to designers to generate high-level emotions.

5.1 Five Senses Design Method

God has given human senses - sight, hearing, touch, smell, taste, which are the five senses of human beings. When using different senses, you will have a more comprehensive understanding of the same thing, thus generating new ideas and different experiences. A good designer should use the pleasure of five senses in life and design to create a high-level emotional experience. Even when the sensory stimulation cannot be applied in the design, it can also be shown through synesthesia method [10], through other channels, visible in the invisible, audible in the silent, even "hearing" in the eyes, seeing in the ears, to produce the creative effect of feeling interchange, reality and illusion complementary.

5.2 Emotional Design Based on Experience Process

From the user's overall experience process, emotional design should not only bring good sensory stimulation before use, but also bring excellent experience in use, and leaving a good impression after use.

Before use, the product mainly affects the user's emotion through the instinct and the reflection level. It is necessary to endow the appearance with design features of the reflection level like memories, culture, brand, concept and so on, so that users can feel the high-level design features contained in the product as soon as they touch it, and then generate high-level emotions.

Emotional design in use aims to enhance the user experience in the using process through product features such as function, performance, efficiency, easy to learn, easy to use, which are the current contents of product usability research [11]. However, there are still more rich emotional experiences worth exploring, not only to achieve the intended use, but also to create the fun of using.

Reflection level can not only play an important role independent of the first two levels, say, establishing brand culture, but also can be expressed in the appearance and use process of the product, say, creating stories and memories, conveying excellent ideas. This emotional design mainly plays a role after use.

5.3 Emotional Design Based on Hierarchy of Needs

Hierarchy of needs theory [12], in the form of pyramids, shows the high and low ranking of human needs, each of which has high-level emotions worth exploring, which can bring important inspirations for high-level emotional design.

6 Conclusion

Based on the three-level theory, emotions can be stratified, high-level emotions can more impress users, significantly improve user experience, but its importance has not been paid enough attention to. Through the research, it is found that the high-level emotions generated by design features besides appearance are still scarce in terms of quantity and type. Through the corresponding relationship between design features and emotions, this paper puts forward three design methods to generate high-level emotions, in order to inspire the theory and methods of emotional design and the design work of designers.

References

1. Thackara, J.: In the Bubble: Designing in a Complex World. The MIT Press, Cambridge, MA (2005)
2. Seymour, R., Powell, R.: Emotional ergonomics. Design Week (2003)
3. Leder, H., Benno, B., Oeberst, A., Augustin, D.: A model of aesthetic appreciation and aesthetic judgments. Br. J. Psychol. **95**, 489–508 (2004)
4. Kim, J., Yun Moon, J.: Designing towards emotional usability in customer interfaces trustworthiness of cyber-banking system interfaces. Interact. Comput. **10**, 1–29 (1989)
5. Demirbilek, O., Sener, B.: Product design, semantics and emotional response. Ergonomics **46**(13/14), 1346–1360 (2003)
6. Yamamoto, K.: Kansei Engineering-the Art of Automotive Development at Mazda, pp. 1–24. University of Michigan, Ann Arbor (1986)
7. Norman, D.: Emotional Design: Why We Love (or Hate) Everyday Things. Basic books, New York (2004)
8. Tracey, M.W., Hutchinson, A.: Reflection and professional identity development in design education. Int. J. Technol. Des. Educ. **28**, 263 (2018)

9. Hekkert, P., Snelders, D., Wieringen, P.C.W.V.: 'Most advanced, yet acceptable': typicality and novelty as joint predictors of aesthetic preference in industrial design. Br. J. Psychol. **94**(Pt 1), 111–124 (2003)
10. Cytowic, R.E.: Synesthesia: A union of the senses, 2nd edn. A Union of the Senses, Synesthesia (2002)
11. Yu, D., Wu, X.: Relation between easy to use and emotion in design. Packag. Eng. **27**(6), 308 (2006)
12. Maslow, A.: Deficiency motivation and growth motivation. University of Nebraska, Lincoln (1955)

Co-creation Design Mechanism for the Online Entrepreneur Community Building

Chen Li(✉)

Tongji University, Shanghai, China
lichen0317@126.com

Abstract. In recent years, Innovation and entrepreneurship have been a heatedly discussed topic and become a development philosophy of many cities and regions. Maker spaces and incubators are blossoming all over the world. However, many obstacles emerge from the mechanism, such as lacking vitality, limiting resource sharing and knowledge flow, hindering interdisciplinary collaboration. This paper proposed a hypothesis that online co-creation platform can help bridge these gaps. Then we use qualitative research methods to discuss the issues. A preliminary conclusion was drawn that the online co-creation design method can link stakeholders, establish sharing mechanisms and promote entrepreneurial communities building. This study proposed that an online entrepreneurial community with a co-creation approach has a good effect on breaking through information barriers and improving the full flow of knowledge, technology, human resources, and investment. Finally, based on all the research findings and analysis, a set of design strategies are proposed that the online entrepreneurial community should follow.

Keywords: Co-creation · Entrepreneur community · Interdisciplinary collaboration · Makerspaces · Incubators

1 Introduction

With the fluctuations of the world economy, innovation and entrepreneurship have been a hot topic in various regions of the country. Innovative entrepreneurship is often seen as a weapon to break the economic deadlock and is considered as the core driving force of the new economic growth point by many organizations. Maker spaces and incubators are often set up in universities, governments, and organizations, as well as large commercial groups. They are often equipped with office space, professional equipment and laboratories, providing a friendly living environment for entrepreneurial teams. Although they have shown positive effects on entrepreneurial projects, the conversion rate of entrepreneurial projects remains an issue that not been discussed sufficiently. For innovative entrepreneurship an action that requires resource mobility, the resources and assistance that existing entrepreneur mechanisms can provide are still very limited. As an interactive and inclusive approach, Co-creation has shown effectiveness in solving social or business problems. It can coordinate the relationship between multiple roles and solve problems with high efficiency and high quality through participatory design, flat communication, etc. In this article, we will explore

T. Ahram et al. (Eds.): IHIET 2019, AISC 1018, pp. 176–182, 2020.
https://doi.org/10.1007/978-3-030-25629-6_28

whether the co-creation design approach can be applied in the field of innovation and entrepreneurship and whether it can play a role in the start-up process of entrepreneurial projects.

2 Challenges and Problems

After a series of desktop surveys, we found some challenges and problems in the current state of entrepreneurship in China:

Distribution of Social Resources. The success of an entrepreneurial project is multifaceted. British educator Gibb has proposed the MAIR model; he believes that entrepreneurship is an activity in which entrepreneurs conduct creative practice to make use of these four elements: Motive, Ability, Idea, and Resources. Entrepreneurs, as the primary initiator of entrepreneurial behavior, are restricted by many factors in the process of entrepreneurship. Professor Lin Nan of Duke University (1999) believes that the social status determines the level of social resources people can get in a large extent. Entrepreneurs should play an active role in building social capital and get benefit from it. However, the 2015 China Entrepreneurial Attitude Survey report shows that the social resources that entrepreneurs can get often depend on some of their backgrounds, such as family background, industry experience, human networks, education background and so on.[1] Therefore, how to help entrepreneurs to obtain and develop resources most effectively is an important issue that we need to discuss.

The Dilemma of Entrepreneurs. Nesta's survey shows that many entrepreneurs do not have a complete project structure when they enter the maker space, lacking components such as business model, brand strategy and marketing.[2] It will make it difficult for their products to survive on the market and hard to known by customers. Therefore, how to improve the integrity of the project structure and to create a composite cross-professional team reveal especially important [1].

The Dilemma of Investors. For venture capitalists, logical integrity is the absolute standard in the process of projects screening. Projects with the following four aspects show extremely attraction to the capitalists: 1. Projects that satisfy users' needs indeed. 2. The product or technology is differentiated. 3. Projects with business value. 4. Projects with reasonable team composition. A mature project with a collaborative and well-matched team is necessary for investors [2].[3]

The dilemma of Makerspaces and Incubators. Due to time and space constraints, not all high-quality startup projects can enjoy the benefits of maker spaces and incubators. Limited by information barriers, makers spaces did few in helping entrepreneurs

[1] 2015 China entrepreneurial attitude survey report, http://www.useit.com.cn/thread-10959-1-1.html.

[2] Made in China: Makerspaces and the research for mass innovation, https://www.nesta.org.uk/report/made-in-china-makerspaces-and-the-search-for-mass-innovation/.

[3] Dingee, A.L., Haslett, B. and Leonard, E.S., Characteristics of a successful entrepreneurial management team. Pratts Guide to Venture Capital Sources, Securities Data Publishing, Inc., NY, NY, pp. 23–28 (1995).

to expand their relationships and increase brand awareness. Influenced by the industry of the organizer and the qualification of admission, the existing mechanism of makers spaces limits the flow of knowledge, technology, human resources, and capital. Makerspace should be a gathering place for innovative ideas, but the existing maker spaces are mostly driven by technology and do not play the value of design well [3].

3 Related Works

3.1 Academic Research on Co-creation Approaches

In fact, the practice of collective creative design has existed for nearly 40 years, and research projects on users' participation in system development can be traced back to the 1970s. In Norway, Sweden, and Denmark, a collective resource approach was established to increase the value of industrial production by involving employees in the development of new workplace systems [4]. Co-creation has been widely used to explore business and consumer relationships in the past decade, such as in the process of developing new products [5] by organizing consumer engagement, co-creation, and co-production with the company, to test the profit that consumers care about and gain [6]. Companies that know how to exploit consumer insights will be able to gain a competitive advantage [7]. In this process, Online and digital methods are included. By organizing different people gather and work together to solve a specific problem. The co-creation method can be applied either at the initial stage of the idea or at each node throughout the design process [4]. Participatory design (also known as co-creation design) has the potential to "prevent the escalating problems of the artificial world" [8]. In this case, people rediscovered the role of cooperation in enhancing individual abilities and generated new collaborative organizations to facilitate problem-solving [9].

3.2 Project Analysis of Co-creation Online Entrepreneur Community

IDEAS Website of LEGO Company. LEGO, a famous Danish toy manufacturer, has developed a platform called IDEAS to collect innovative solutions from quality players in order to enhance the participation of users. Players upload their own LEGO bricks model to the platform, where these models could be LIKED and commented by the public. The program will enter the review phase when the number of supporters reaches 10,000 during the specified time, and will have a chance to be put into production. The creator of the program will receive a portion of the proceeds from the later sales of the toy. The most significant advantage of this platform is to create a toy project that is truly user-friendly and has a user base with the number of LIKEs as the evidence. It can give consumers a sense of participation and achievement and mobilize their enthusiasm. This mode has a good efficiency in reducing the cost and the risk of new product development, as well as promoting the brand's popularity (Fig. 1).

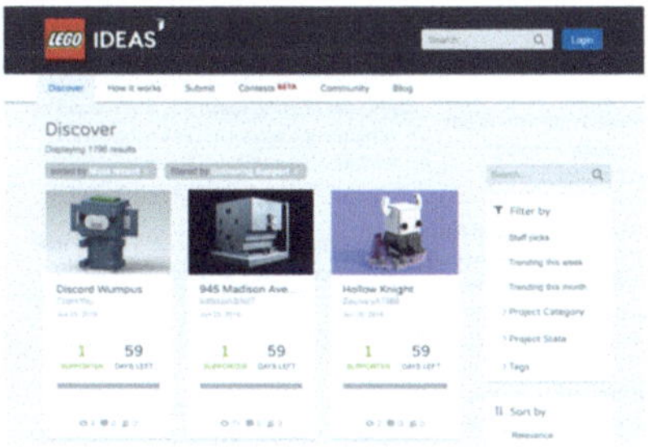

Fig. 1. LEGO online co-creation platform (Source: https://ideas.lego.com/dashboard)

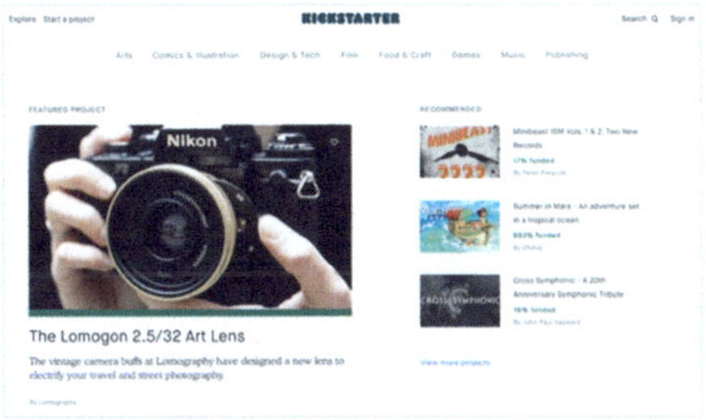

Fig. 2. Kickstarter funding website (Source: https://www.kickstarter.com)

Kickstarter Funding Platform. Kickstarter is a crowdfunding platform for creative projects. Entrepreneurs are able to upload their projects and set a crowdfunding amount. Projects which are fully funded in a particular time will be regarded as a success. Otherwise, the funds will be returned to the payers. The projects then move on to the next phase of development and deliver on their commitment to the payers. In this mode, users' acceptance of new products can be intuitively shown on the platform to reduce the risk of new product development. If the pre-set amount is not raised within the specified time, the project can be stopped to reduce the loss. The data on the platform also provide strong evidence for companies to attract new investments. This platform provides good access for start-ups to increase public attention and social influence. It is not only a platform for financing but also a platform for market research, which shows sufficiency in surfacing those demands that cannot be found in other ways [10] (Fig. 2).

4 User Research

Based on the above problems and assumption, we did semi-structured interviews with investors and different types of entrepreneurs from the following five aspects: problems encountered in the entrepreneurial process, key elements of entrepreneurial success, ways of team formation and investment attraction, project awareness building. Among them, we summarized representative views and analyzed their requirements, as follows (Fig. 3):

From the analysis, it is obvious that the problems we mentioned before are common existed in these three groups of people. Their common requirement is to improve the project conversion rate by improving team composition, reducing the cost of acquiring social resources, and attracting users. If makerspaces and incubators want to help them to the maximum, a new mechanism with a co-creation approach should be considered to build.

Interviewees	Problem and Difficulties	Reasons	Requirements Analysis
Entrepreneurial Designers	It is difficult to further improve and iterate technically. Feel struggling in the commercialization of the project. All of the problems lead to a low conversion efficiency of input and output.	The composition of the team is unreasonable. The understanding of market conditions is not comprehensive and is greatly affected by information barriers.	Need a way to find and examine reliable partners in order to reach out to professionals in different majors such as engineers and marketing talents; Need a way to circulate information and mobilize social resources.
Technical Entrepreneurs	The products are not as popular as they imagined, and sometimes leads to huge losses. Due to the small number of users, it is difficult for them to collect enough feedback. They also feel hard to let more people know their project.	The envisioned product is out of touch with the actual market demand. The founders have insufficient understanding of the market, and the deviation of the investigation leads to the possibility of obtaining false demand.	Need a channel that can be used to test user acceptance. Need a platform that can help projects expand their impact and improve user awareness.
Investors	The observation period for project is long. (A mature project takes 2-3 months, and a less mature project takes 6-12 months). It is prone to deviations in the competitive advantage and commercial evaluation of the product. Investment risks are often unpredictable due to changes in team members.	The cost of tracking and evaluating projects is relatively high, and the projects involved are more dependent on the acquaintance's credit guarantee. The rationality and stability of the team composition are difficult to ensure.	Need a channel to get in touch with good projects. A platform is needed to examine the reliability of startup teams and the integrity of the project logical chain.

Fig. 3. Summary and analysis of semi-structured interviews

5 Findings and Design Strategy

5.1 An Online Entrepreneur Community with the Co-creation Design Method

Based on the above discussion, a hypothesis is proposed: the online co-creation method has a positive effect on breaking the information barriers of innovation and entrepreneurship and promoting the flow of social resources. Firstly, the online co-creation method is able to help team formation and improvement of the entrepreneurial project, as well as cross-professional collaboration. So that designers, product managers, technicians, marketers and other talents in different fields can play a better role in the integrity of project logic-chain. Second, the online co-creation approach allows incubators and investors to have a clearer understanding of the project's development process, which lay the foundation for the project to win investment in the future.

5.2 Implementation Strategy

Startup teams have practical needs for social resources, which include not only e tangible resources such as human resources, material resources, and financial resources, but also intangible resources such as technology, knowledge, organization, and social relations. Based on the above findings, we believe that an online entrepreneurial community that can solve the above problems should follow the following design strategies:

To Solve the Problem of Intangible Resources: Startup projects could upload their project progress situation and publish the dilemmas and problems they encountered on this platform. Through the co-creation mechanism to collect solutions from the whole platform, people who propose high-quality solutions can be recommended to be the project partners. Entrepreneurs from different majors gather together to contribute the project so that the project could find teammates and partners who are needed and authentically knowledgeable and capable.

To Solve the Problem of Tangible Resources: Firstly, Entrepreneurs from different regions and different industries will be gathered in such a community to find suitable collaborators through the screening mechanisms according to labels. Based on the above research, a basic framework for the formation of an entrepreneurial team was proposed: designers, technicians, and marketers. A scientific team needs at least the composition of these three aspects. Secondly, Online entrepreneur community should be linked with offline entrepreneur communities. Maker spaces and incubators should provide application portals to projects and track the progress online to screen the most suitable projects. By offered priority to enter and provided office spaces and basic facilities, the projects will be given much support to grow. The online entrepreneur community should provide a path for the startup team to get in touch with the capital. Those online co-creation data could be strong support for the investment. The development track on the platform could also be a window for investors to look into the project, and give them more opportunities to discover reliable projects. The online entrepreneur community should be a bridge in breaking through information barriers and flattening projects and capital resources.

6 Conclusions

Through literature review, desk research and case study, we identified some common issues in current entrepreneurial environment of China. Through fieldwork and interviews of stakeholders, this research proposes a new collaboration modality for the entrepreneur community in the new context. Based on the new modality, we propose a series of design strategies and action guides for building online communities, not only including improving approaches for existing entrepreneurial communities, but also the application of online co-creation methods on entrepreneurial teams building and entrepreneurial projects improvement. This study provides a solution for the entrepreneur communities which facing the dilemma of activeness.

References

1. China entrepreneurial attitude survey report. http://www.useit.com.cn/thread-10959-1-1.html (2015)
2. Dingee, A.L., Haslett, B., Leonard, E.S.: Characteristics of a successful entrepreneurial management team, pp. 23–28. Pratts Guide to Venture Capital Sources Securities Data Publishing Inc, NY, NY (1995)
3. Kingsley, J., Saunders, T.: Made in China: makerspaces and the research for mass innovation. https://www.nesta.org.uk/report/made-in-china-makerspaces-and-the-search-for-mass-innovation/
4. Sanders, E.B.-N., Stappers, P.J.: Co-creation and the new landscapes of design. Codesign **4** (1), 5–18 (2008)
5. Sawhney, M., Verona, G., Prandelli, E.: Collaborating to create: the internet as a platform for customer engagement in product innovation. J. Interact. Mark. **19**(4), 4–17 (2005)
6. Nambisan, S., Baron, R.A.: Virtual customer environments: testing a model of voluntary participation in value co-creation activities. J. Prod. Innov. Manag. **26**(4), 388–406 (2009)

7. Williams, A.D.: Wikinomics. Portfolio, London (2006)
8. Cross, N. (ed.): Design participation: proceedings of the design research society's conference 1971. Academy Editions, London, UK (1972)
9. Manzini, E.: Design, when everybody designs: an introduction to design for social innovation. MIT press, Cambridge (2015)
10. Anderson, C.: Makers. Nieuw Amsterdam (2013)

Use of Robotics Laboratory Programs in Improving STEAM Outcomes in India

Jagannath Venkoba Rao Kallakurchi(✉) and Pradipta Banerji

Center for Urban Science and Engineering, IIT Bombay, Powai, Mumbai 400076, India
jagan@choice-solutions.com, pbanerji.iitb@gmail.com

Abstract. In the digital era, Information-Technology (IT) based learning tools have gained prominence to capture the interest of the millennial generation. Their thirst for knowledge has increased multifold due to IT tools in K-12 education. India has over 250 million children in the age group of 6 to 18 years. The industry has been working on developing educational robotics laboratory programs, to help in STEM outcomes in grades 6 through 10. However, this study shows that the robotics laboratory programs have an unintended effect of improving skills in the Arts domain too, possibly due to group activity and communication skills being integral to the robotics program. The skills have been quantitatively measured through marks improvement in the robotics program group. The control group against which this improvement is studied are students that have no or less than 6 months exposure to the robotics program. Thus a new term is coined here - STEAM (Science, Technology, Engineering, Arts and Mathematics) as against STEM, with Arts also included as a considered domain. Data also shows that students exposed to the robotics laboratory program experience improved motivation towards overall studies, causing significant improvement in grades, and learning outcomes.

Keywords: Educational robotics lab · School programs · STEAM outcomes

1 Introduction

In recent years growth in use of technology is gaining its popularity among the students due to increased specialized job opportunities in the fields of STEM, entertainment, and medicine. There is a general acceptance among the educationalists that an advanced technology curriculum will be useful in all level of K-12 education [1]. The impact was studied and stated that there is a clear correlation to robotics labs to STEM subjects [2, 3].

The robotics lab course is not a core subject in any curriculum as part of the school educational system. All robotics lab courses are still run by private organizations, who choose to partner with a school or any educational institution. "The main teachings and experiments involving robotics activities are not part of regular classroom activities; they take place separately either after-school programs, in weekends or summer camps" [3]. Technology educators, of course, recommend that robotic labs be part of technology curricula for all students interested in STEM education for complementing their science and math courses [4].

T. Ahram et al. (Eds.): IHIET 2019, AISC 1018, pp. 183–188, 2020.
https://doi.org/10.1007/978-3-030-25629-6_29

Robotics lab participation has helped students to learn new skills with relevance to subjects they study both in the classroom and laboratories [5, 6]. Those students involved in their robotics lab classes did their projects with enthusiasm by learning teamwork, project management, time management, technical concepts, and relevant programming software. Everyone in academia knows the value and impact of the robotic lab in K-12 education. However, a report from OECD remarked: "technology is everywhere, except in schools" [7].

Robotics programs in India are in a nascent stage at the present time. They are currently developed by individual companies in exactly the same manner as elsewhere in the world, and are neither structured nor governed by any education regulatory body. The program is available only in a few private schools and registering for the program is optional and left to an individual student's choice. The fee to get access to the robotic lab is paid by the student.

This paper presents the impact of the robotic lab not only in correlation with STEM subjects, but based on some previous conjectures [5, 6] in correlation with arts (humanities and languages) subjects.

2 Background of Study

Unfortunately, current school science labs do not seem appropriate for fostering critical thinking, problem-solving, creativity, teamwork, and communication skills since their focus is on rigorous, disciplined, and scripted experiences [8] in which students are working through recipe-style predefined concepts.

A robotic lab is a place where students are familiarized with components used in robots like sensors, motors and LED's. They are then exposed to robots' future applications, artificial intelligence, problem-solving techniques while constructing robots. They are also introduced to microcontrollers and to developing humanoid robots. When a student has multiple year exposure to the robotics lab, the student will be exposed to building robot hand assemblies, motion and other forms of robots other than humanoid. The robotic labs are equipped with allied technical devices like 3D printers to design and create objects to use as part of robotic experiments. The design and creation increase in difficulty as a student's experience improves. Apart from learning concepts of physics, mathematics, electronics, and computer science, the design and group activity elements are key aspects that provide soft learning skills that is so important for arts subjects.

The participating students are assigned to teams consisting of 3 to 4 students. Each team is assigned different tasks during every practical class during an academic year. Working in groups, the students learn life skills such as time management, project management, teamwork and knowledge sharing with different perspectives during the program.

Robotic labs help students to get first-hand experience of multidisciplinary functions and tasks. An example is a student, while designing a functional stage, will learn concepts such as the center of gravity, flowchart for activities, technical vocabulary in English, introduction to current, chemical compositions, logic building and programming in information technology, GUI, algorithms, use-cases, data collection, and electronic storage.

3 Results and Analysis

To study the effects of the current robotics program in Indian schools, a questionnaire was created using google forms to be filled by students from schools that have a robotics programs. Each respondent is a student between 6th and 10th grade, in schools where the robotics program has been adopted.

The questionnaire had seven questions with multiple options that related to measuring the impact of the robotics program. The schools are distributed over four states spread across India. The questions could be filled using either a mobile phone or a computer. The initial part of the information was related to the student such as name, class, section, school name, city, and state (These were just for aggregation and spatial distribution purposes only). The seven questions were 1. How long have you been enrolled in the robotics lab classes? (Five options were given based on the length of enrolment). 2. What have you learned during this period of attending classes? (Six options were given with the allowance for multiple options allowed). 3. What kind of practicals are you doing? (Five options were given with the allowance for multiple options allowed). 4. Have robotics labs classes had any connection with the studying subjects? (Six options were given with the allowance for multiple options allowed). 5. In which of the following subjects your present grades/marks had improved as compared to past? (Five subjects with three marks improvement intervals). 6. What are the reasons for the improvements? (Five options were given with the allowance for multiple options allowed). 7. Why did you enroll in a robotics lab course? (Six options were given with the allowance for multiple options allowed).

There were 408 respondents from all schools currently enrolled in the robotics program – a significant sample were obtained across all four states of India. Among the four states, two states are progressive states and the other two states are upcoming given educational technologies adoption. This allowed for a spectrum analysis. Among students who responded 261 students were enrolled for between six months to one year, 53 were enrolled for between one year to two years are at, and 78 were enrolled for more than two years and 16 were enrolled for below six months. This data is presented in percentage form in Fig. 1.

The survey results to question two indicate that 303 students mentioned that their key learning is working in a group, 302 students said learned components of robot and 287 said learned basics of electronic components. Thus, for students working in a group, which is a soft skill, was considered to be as important, if not more, as learning the basics of robotic components, which is a hard skill.

While trying to establish a direct co-relation with STEM-related subjects at school level it is observed that 330 students responded for science and 180 students for mathematics. However, surprisingly 274 students said it has co-relation to arts subjects – such as English, social studies and allied subjects. Thus, it is found that the correlation to arts subjects are significantly greater than the correlation for mathematics, a STEM subject. This highlights the STEAM nomenclature used in this study.

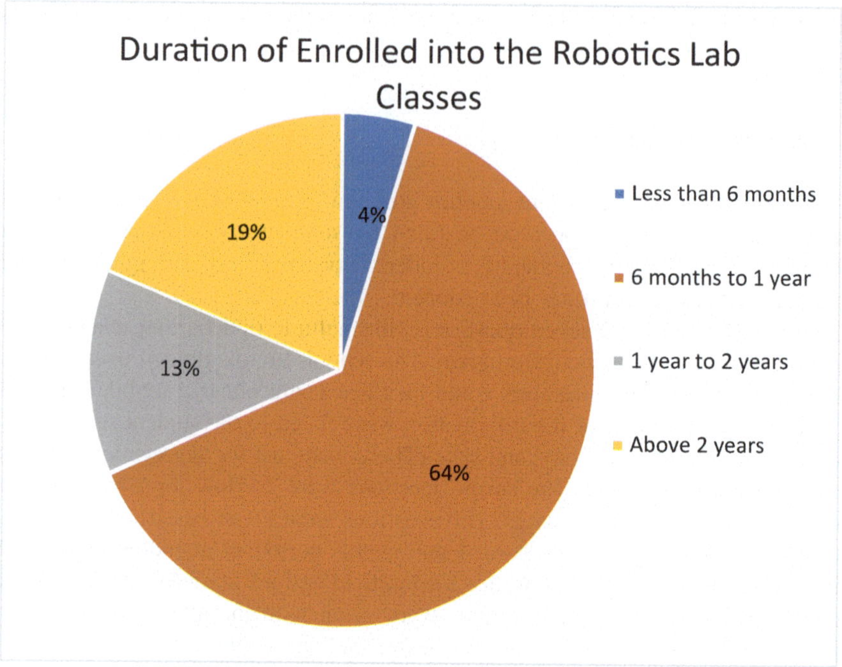

Fig. 1. Duration of student enrollment into the robotics lab classes

It is evident from Fig. 2 that over 250 respondents said that 20 marks and above and an average of 165 respondents said ten marks and above improved in their performance as compared to the prior period in Science, the corresponding numbers for English are more than 200 and 165, respectively. It is followed 10 to 20 marks in Mathematics, Social sciences, and other subjects. This again highlights the fact that while the robotics program does obviously improve the performance in science and technology subjects, it has an equal emphasis on communication and arts subjects, possibly more than the improvement in math courses.

When further analyzed for key reasons in the improvement in students marks in the examinations as compared to prior periods, opting for robotics lab course stood second with 255 respondents only after 343 respondents attributed credit to teacher. The other significantly lower influencing factors are parents, friends and school environment. Thus the robotics program came in second to the teacher, although even the teacher for the robotics program obviously helps ignite the initial interest in the robotics program. Thus, it can be said that the robotics program does have a significant roll to play in the improved performance of students.

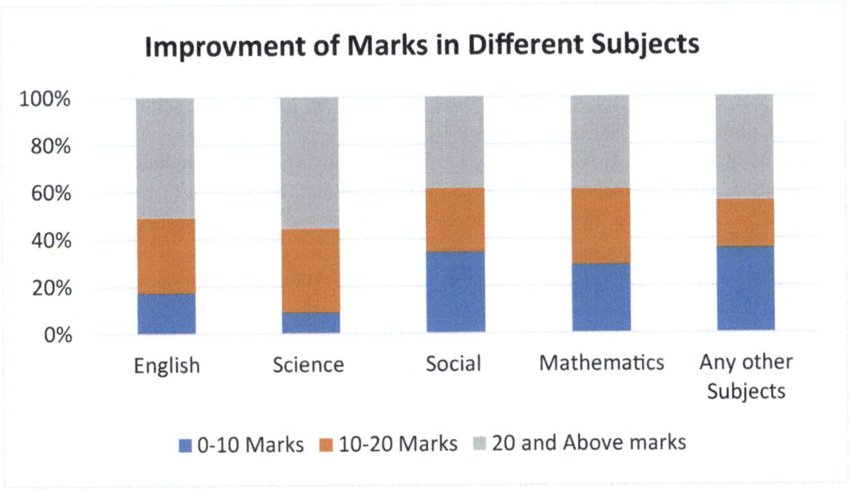

Fig. 2. Marks improvement of the students in different discipline.

4 Conclusions

In this paper, it has been shown that the impact of a robotics program in secondary school does not only improve understanding of science and technology subjects, but also improves the understanding of the arts stream of subjects. Thus, a robotics program can be considered to be important for STEAM outcomes, as opposed to STEM outcomes. It is an important factor to note that the open-ended curriculum of the robotics program helps in raising curiosity levels to know more about technology in students, and helps them improve critical thinking and directly correlates to their improvement in examination outcomes across subjects. The evidence is strong that the robotics program in India has helped students to not only gain experience in multi-disciplinary functions and tasks, but also gain experience in teamwork, project and time management skills. It can be concluded that the key factor behind improved learning in overall student performance across subjects are due to the very nature of the design of robotics programs in India. It is, therefore, important that such a program is available not only in private schools, but also in public schools to improve the outcomes for a larger percentage of secondary school students in India.

References

1. Kolberg, E., Orlev, N.: Robotics learning as a tool for integrating science technology curriculum in K-12 schools. In: 31st Annual Frontiers in Education Conference. Impact on Engineering and Science Education. Conference Proceedings (Cat. No. 01CH37193), vol. 1, pp. T2E–12. IEEE (2001)

2. Eguchi, A.: What is educational robotics? theories behind it and practical implementation. In: Society for Information Technology & Teacher Education International Conference, pp. 4006–4014. Association for the Advancement of Computing in Education (AACE) (2010)
3. Benitti, F.B.V.: Exploring the educational potential of robotics in schools: a systematic review. Comput. Educ. **58**(3), 978–988 (2012)
4. Wright, M.D., Washer, B.A., Watkins, L., Scott, D.G.: Technology education: beyond the technology is applied science paradigm. J. Technol. Educ. **8**(1), 7–15 (1996)
5. Detsikas, N., Alimisis, D.: Status, and trends in educational robotics worldwide with special consideration of educational experiences from Greek schools. In: Proceedings of the International Conference on Informatics in Schools: Situation, Evolution, and Perspectives, pp. 1–12 (2011)
6. Litinas, A., Alimisis, D.: Planning, implementation and evaluation of lab activities using robotic technology for teaching the phenomenon of motion. In: Proceedings of the 3rd Pan-Hellenic Conference "Integration and Use of ICT in Educational Process." HAICTE & University of Piraeus (in Greek), Piraeus (2013)
7. Pedró, F.: New millennium learners: a project in progress. Paper preparado para el CERI, OECD Governing Board. Documento utilizado sólo para la presente propuesta: no-citar (2008)
8. Blikstein, P.: Digital fabrication and 'making' in education: the democratization of invention. FabLabs Mach. Mak. Inven. **4**, 1–21 (2013)

Designing a Pleasant Waiting Area for the Gastrointestinal Endoscopy Unit Based on Subjective Experiences and Needs of the Japanese People

Nermin Elokla[1(✉)] and Harumi Kagawa[2]

[1] Faculty of Applied Arts, Helwan University, Cairo, Egypt
nelokla@hotmail.com
[2] Faculty of Architecture and Civil, Kyushu Sangyo University, Fukuoka, Japan

Abstract. An endoscopy unit refers to a dedicated area where medical procedures are performed with endoscopes, which are cameras used to visualize structures within the body, such as the digestive tract. There is a lack of studies about designing such a unit. Therefore, this study attempted to evaluate the waiting space design of the endoscopy unit, and identify the problems which the patients and the medical staff meet there. We focused on what the patients hope from their endoscopy experience. For care to be patients centered, we should respect patients' views on how they wish to be managed, see them as partners in shared healthcare decision making—the basis of "no decision about me without me". The authors discussed the following: usability and attractiveness of space. To carry out this study, different design methods were used to capture people's subjective experience, including an emotional evaluation method which is called Kansei sheet.

Keywords: Healthcare · Japanese people · Needs and emotions · Waiting area · Gastrointestinal endoscopy unit

1 Introduction

In the world, the needs of endoscopic exam are growing year by year due to increasing of the incidence of colorectal and gastric diseases [1]. Endoscopy unit usually located within a hospital. Based on the survey, there are rare studies discussing the design of this unit [2]. This means that designers produce their own designs with or without consulting endoscopists working in such a unit. According to the phrase of" enter the patient's world, see the situation through the patient's eyes" [3], the authors evaluated the present design of endoscopy unit, and identify its main problems through the subjective experiences of both Japanese patients and staff too. We focused on the design of waiting area of endoscopy unit, as the patients spend an average from one hour to 4 h before their examinations. With patients spending a large portion of their visit in waiting areas, it is important they have a pleasant, and comfortable space that fosters their mental, emotional, and physical health.

T. Ahram et al. (Eds.): IHIET 2019, AISC 1018, pp. 189–195, 2020.
https://doi.org/10.1007/978-3-030-25629-6_30

2 Methods

To carry out this research, one of the largest an endoscopy unit in the Fukuoka city (Japan) was selected as a case study. Two groups of Japanese people (3 females and 3 males- in various ages) were selected to evaluate the waiting space design of this unit. First group includes two different cases of outpatients (patient A “male”- colonoscopy case, and patient B “female”- an upper endoscopy case), second group includes 4 medical staff who are working in this unit (two doctors and two nurses). We captured people subjective experiences, and identify their problems and needs by using; Kansei sheet, and face-to-face interviews. Kansei sheet is an evaluation method which presents 14 distinct emotional responses [3]. Each person can select from it the image/s that best express his or her emotional responses to a design. We captured from each person three levels of experience. These experiences have been elicited by three different design levels; visceral design, behavioral design, and reflective design [4]. All groups were asked to use Kansei sheet in each design level. Afterwards, interviews were conducted with all in order to have complete and clear views about their experiences. The following are the questions used to evaluate the design of waiting space.

A. Physical attractiveness (visceral design)

Q.1 What do you feel about the color (including furniture, wall paint, and the staff’s uniform colors)? Q.2 What do you feel about the form furniture, and art objects? Q.3 What do you feel about the materials, including surface texture and finish? Q.4 Overall design evaluation, what do you feel about the physical attractiveness of space?

B. Design and usability (behavioral design)

Q.1 What do you think about circulation spaces, including walkways, and entrances?

Q.2 Does a waiting space offer you with relaxation and de-stress? Q.3 What do you think about the space safety? Q.4 What do you think about space ventilations (including space air, smell and temperature)? Q.5 What do you think about the space lighting? Q.6 What do think about the space privacy? Q.7 Do you think that the waiting area is comfortable (a state of physical ease and freedom from pain)? Q.8 Overall design evaluation, what do you think about the space usability?

C. Design value and its notable memories (reflective design)

Q.1 Does the space evoke a personal remembrance?

3 Results and Discussions

3.1 Patients’ Types and Procedures

Based on the survey, this endoscopy unit receives about 100 patients in a day. However, the number of seats available for the patients is 53 chairs. About 40 people are working there, including 20 doctors, 12 nurses, 2 technical staff and 6 Lavage (endoscope) staff. This unit receives 2 categories of patients; inpatients and outpatients. Outpatients include the following: a colonoscopy, and an upper endoscopy, and a patient who needs a rapid diagnosis and receiving a medicine (Fig. 1).

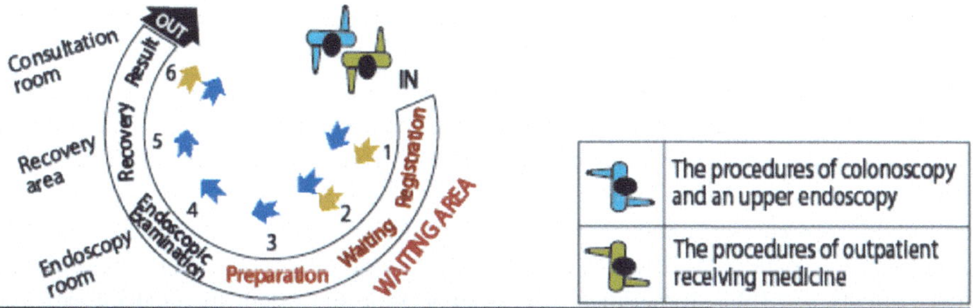

Status (Waiting Area)	Colonoscopy	Upper endoscopy	Outpatients receive the medicine
▪Waiting time	**About 4 hours** prepartation before the examination	**About an hour and a half** due to many examinations	**30 mintues ~ an hour** due to many patients
▪Preparation before the endoscopic examination	Patient is asked to drink a special solution (called oral Lavage) to clean their bowel	Topical and intravenous anesthesia	None
▪Walking exercise	Slow walking improves bowel preparation before the examination	None	None
▪Patient safety after the endoscopic examintion	For the patient safety, being accompanied by relative is better due to the anesthesia effects.		None

Fig. 1. The examination rules and procedures for the outpatients

3.2 Space Design Evaluation from the Outpatients' Points of Views

A. Physical Attractiveness (Visceral Design)

The results of Kansei sheet and interviews with 2 outpatients (A and B) revealed that the design of waiting area was not pleasant. They had negative feelings due to the following; old fashioned furniture and its unattractive color, and the black color of some doctors' clothes. The space is planned like a bus- couches organized in line. Patients want a design that makes the space itself pleasant and inviting. They want "a waiting area patient-friendly", in which relieves anxiety and tension. It is better to use modern furniture, natural colors, pleasant art works, natural plants, free WiFi, and light music. Overall, the design of waiting area should make the waiting time part of the treatment so that gives patients gift of relaxation, nature, and interest [5].

B. Design and Usability (Behavioral Design)

Regarding the space usability, the patients' emotional experiences were a mix of discomfort and dissatisfaction due to the problems of circulation spaces and safety, uncomfortable couches, a lack of privacy, and unpleasant smell. About the first problem, patient (A) said that walking exercise is needed before the examination. However, there is no enough space to walk. As for people safety, there is a problem related to the main entrance. This unit has two entrances. However most of the staff and patients (including patients with different conditions) use the main one. Also, doctors use it to transport the medical equipment from and to the unit. The reason is that the second entrance (for emergency cases) is smaller, manual operated, and locates far from the emergency room of hospital. Thus, the main entrance is usually crowded and obstructing people movement. So it might expose both patients and staff to a risk to their health or safety (Fig. 2). Regarding the problem of couches, the design is not comfortable. Patients complained about a lower back of couch and its height. About the patient privacy, patient (B) dislikes to discuss her symptoms with the nurses in front of other patients. And this sometimes drives her to hide important medical information. Therefore, we have to consider the patients' needs, and protect their confidentiality. Generally, it is better to design a various levels of privacy, such as, creating a space for groups, and a quiet area for individuals. As for the last problem, it is related to the space ventilation and unpleasant smell near the toilet area.

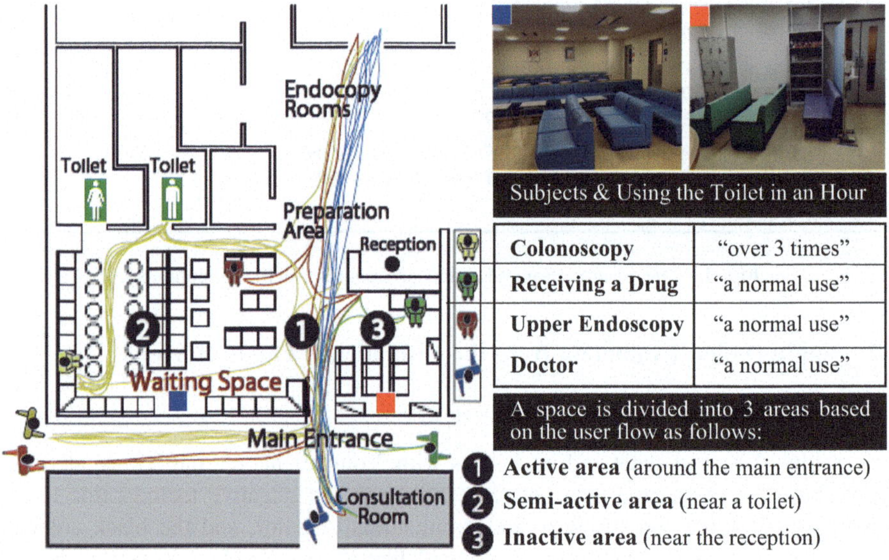

Fig. 2. Space usage intensity and user flow in the waiting area

C. Design Value (Reflective Design- Reflecting on Past Experiences)

Patient (B) mentioned that the design of this unit is open space, in which lets many patients to see preparation and examination procedures. The layout of waiting area triggers her emotions, as it sometimes allows her to see the endoscopic examinations of other patients. It awakens most negative emotions and thoughts caused during her past endoscopic examination. In other words, it reminds her with a panic attack that occurred to her before, during and after her last examination (Fig. 3). At this level of design, the patient said that the layout of this unit evokes unpleasant personal remembrance to her. Therefore, in such a case, it might be better to use partitions to divide the floor plate into different settings that support a range of activities.

Separating examination area from the waiting space is better also for the first-time patient who has no experience with the endoscopic exam, as a study found that most people would not want to know their future. People would rather avoid the suffering that knowing the future could cause [6]. From the mentioned complaints, this study pays attention to the impact of building design on our emotions. Building brings memories, and memories bring the scene of building as well. Architecture has an effect on one's mood. It becomes a matter of how a particular place is designed to arouse an emotional response in its occupants. People often say the phrase "innovative building." But what about saying "emotional building?" Generally, the design of building takes its occupants into its journey, and this experience might be described by unforgettable emotional and sensory experiences [7].

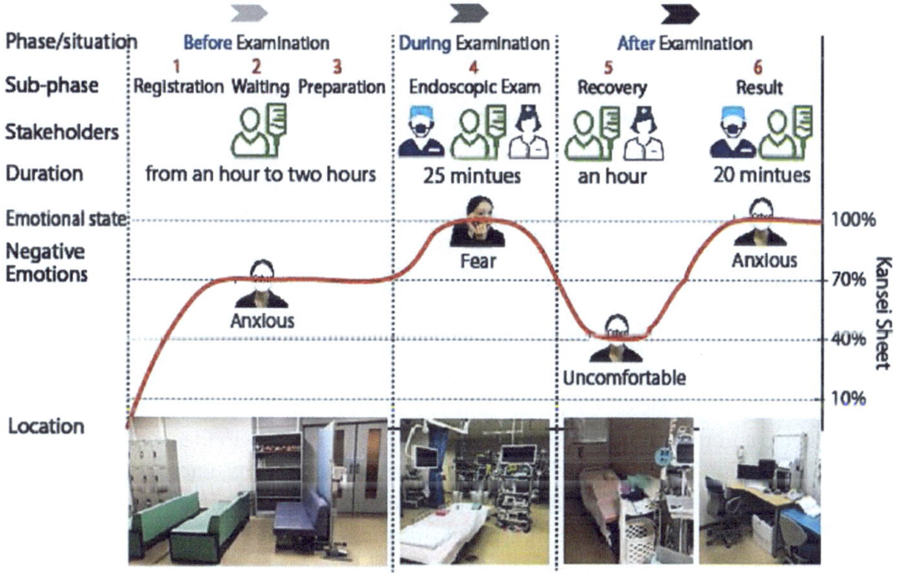

Fig. 3. Emotional journey of patient B in the endoscopy unit

3.3 Space Design Evaluation from the Medical Staff's Points of Views

The results of kansei sheet and interviews with 4 staff revealed that their impressions about physical attraction of waiting area were somewhat positive. As for the space usability, they were a little annoyed due to the following problems; the circulation spaces and safety, and uncomfortable design. The first problem has been explained in the patients' part. About the second problem, using partitions (near the main entrance) impede doctors to see the patients easily. Also, there is no partition to hide the female toilet from view. And, changing the space layout is difficult due to heavy-weight furniture. Furthermore, there is no space for greater numbers of patients.

From the above, we found that the two groups have different perceptions, views and analysis for the same design. The difference between both is that the patients took into account subjective characteristics of the design more than the staff who obviously focused on the design objective and usability. This might be due to the following; (A) People have different beliefs. Every people has its own way on how they view certain things. Patients believe that waiting area should be adaptable, attractive and pleasant to provide them with better healthcare experiences. In contrast, the staff thinks that this space is just for a work, and it is no matter to be appealing or pleasant. They believe that since the design of the waiting area fulfills its role well (such as, clean and safe), so it is good. (B) Patients usually happen to be highly sensitive to everything around them, including their surrounding environments. This might be due to their physical pain, or negative life experiences. Highly sensitive people often feel too much and feel too deep. They are more emotionally reactive. Sensitive people are more detail-oriented than less sensitive people. They are the first ones to notice the details of space design [8]. This might be one of the reasons why our patients have evaluated the space design more acute than other group. (C) The medical staff has adapted to the design of waiting space due to the following: familiar place, routines, and predictable patterns of interaction. So they did not notice any significant problem regarding the attractiveness of space design. Overall, from the endoscopists' opinions, there are design tips to create a better waiting area as follows; (1) Priority seats is required. The couches in the waiting space should be arranged according to the patient physical abilities. For example, older people (colonoscopy cases) cannot reach to the toilet quickly. So the most nearest seats to the toilet should be designated for them. (2) Making building inclusive, safe, and easy to use. Entrance should be automatically operated by sensors. (3) Regarding the colonoscopy cases, design an enough space for a slow walking. (4) Endoscopy rooms and preparation space should be invisible from waiting areas, and not face the entrance. We must add a privacy to the examination area by using a partition which allows the staff to observe the patients, and in the same time conceals this area from view (5) Add privacy to the toilet area. Toilet should be hidden from view. (6) Use compact and lightweight furniture for easy moving.

4 Conclusions

According to the phrase of "designing with people in mind", this study aimed at evaluating the waiting space design of endoscopy unit based on people's subjective experience. We focused on design usability, and the physical attractiveness of space. Healthcare experiences are made up of more than moments of care—they also include the time we usually spend in transition between those moments. Our study revealed that the transitional space where the outpatients wait is uncomfortable and not inviting, so that it increases feelings of stress and negative mood. Therefore, the present study suggested some design tips to create a pleasant waiting area which enhances patients' healthcare experience, and makes time pass quickly.

References

1. World Health Organization. https://www.who.int/news-room/fact-sheets/detail
2. Guidelines for designing a digestive disease endoscopy unit: Report of the World Endoscopy Organization. https://www.ncbi.nlm.nih.gov/pubmed/23701732
3. James, A.M., Yasuyuki, H.: The Bloomsbury Companion to Contemporary Philosophy of Medicine. An imprint of Bloomsbury publishing. ISBN: 9781474233002, UK (2017)
4. Nermin, E., Yasuyuki, H.: Evaluation of assistive mobility product for the Japanese elderly by the Kansei sheets. Elsevier, Procedia Manufact. **3**, 2205–2212 (2015)
5. Norman, D.: Measuring emotion. Des. J. **6**(2) (2003)
6. Susan, M.: 5 ways to improve the hospital waiting room experience. http://www.healing-health.com/improve-hospital-waiting-room-experience/
7. Harry, P.: No spoilers! 90% of people Don't want to know what their future holds. https://www.dailymail.co.uk/sciencetech/article-4248960
8. Maria, L.: How emotion impacts the perception of architecture. https://marialorenalehman.com/post/how-emotion-impacts-architecture
9. Amanda, L.C.: 16 habits of highly sensitive people. Life Wellness (2017)

Natural Human-Robot Interaction Toolkit

Ruslan Gaifullin(✉), Mikhail Ivanou, and Rustem Gazizov

Innopolis University, Universitetskaya. 1, 420500 Innopolis, Russia
{r.gayfullin,m.ivanov,r.gazizov}@innopolis.ru

Abstract. Conventional human-robot interaction is usually limited to a set of commands a professional human operator is supposed to use, and/or teleoperation capabilities. The paper explores capabilities a robot could use to communicate more naturally with a human, support for a range of hardware configurations is provided. The capabilities developed for interaction toolkit include speech and face recognition. Finally, a use case for such a toolkit and performance with respect to different hardware configurations are discussed.

Keywords: Human-robot interaction · Robotics · Interaction infrastructure · Human-centered design

1 Introduction

Conventional interaction between human and a robot is limited to straightforward "master-slave" communication with a predefined set of possible input commands for a human to use (i.e., set a specific goal/task according to specifications). Thus, the majority of human-robot interaction (HRI) has been limited to teleoperation with an interface which comprises a video feed from a robot to an operator and some means of controlling the robot operations directly. To put it another way, the interaction model is one-way - the human "commands", while the robot "obeys" [1]. These HRI capabilities were primarily developed for people who have a specific set of skills to operate the robot, specialists. Considering the introduction of commercially available robots for wider audiences and increase in robots' capabilities and autonomy, we need to reshape the way humans and robots interact and come up with new solutions to operating a robot to accommodate human-in-the-loop.

A robot could be designed to clean a house, take aerial shots (a camera drone) or drive (a vehicle that has some degree of autonomy can be considered a robot). The tasks that robots are designed to solve can vary wildly, which impacts the way one would usually design the HRI solution.

The objective of the paper is to study how more natural human-robot interactions can be achieved in relation to an autonomous robot with or without a stable connection to computational assistance. The most attention is given to processing and constructing interaction in the form of a human-friendly dialog. This way of interaction has numerous advantages: it is similar to how humans interact to achieve common goals, which means less qualified people will be able to interact with a robot and achieve results; learning curve for working in such a way is less burdensome; it is also extendable which means it can be tailored for any specialization a robot could have;

T. Ahram et al. (Eds.): IHIET 2019, AISC 1018, pp. 196–200, 2020.
https://doi.org/10.1007/978-3-030-25629-6_31

interactions with a robot with any level of autonomy can benefit from a more human-centered way of shaping communications.

2 Human-Robot Interaction System

A human-robot interaction toolkit project aims to enhance the experience people get when interacting with a robot. The proposition of the paper is to increase the convenience of interaction with robots by adding human-centered capabilities to the robot. So that robot communication has more in common to ordinary human to human communications.

The solution builds on top of several major components that provide the following functionalities:

1. Human face recognition and identification.
2. Speech recognition, or speech-to-text (STT).
3. Text-to-speech system (TTS).

Several robotics-related cases for those technologies have been explored:

- Identify people and greet them when have not seen them in a long time.
- Find a person—recognize faces "seen" by the robot and report success when a specified person is recognized.
- Orient the robot towards a human face to mimic a natural dialogue between people.

A UML execution diagram showing a detailed description of how a human face is tracked is shown on Fig. 1. A more detailed description of modules and their interaction is described further.

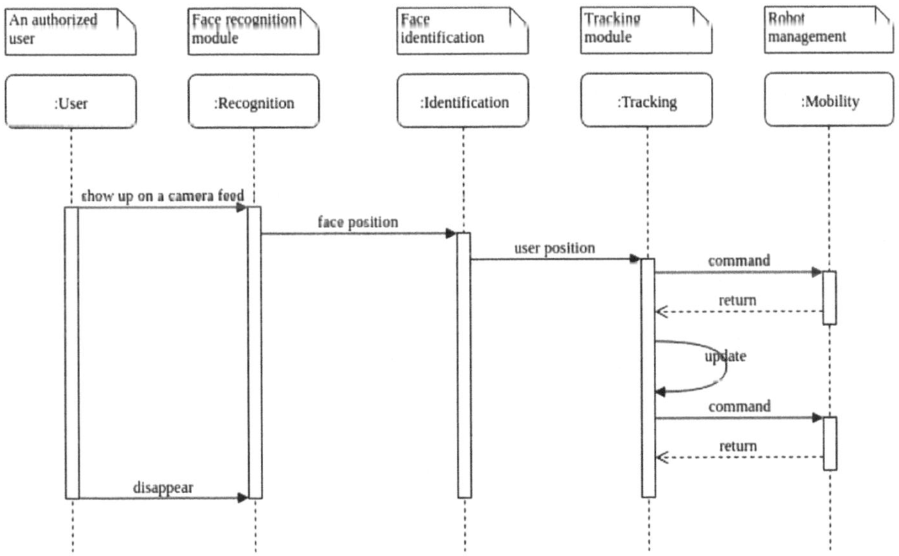

Fig. 1. UML execution diagram for the case of tracking a person's head.

2.1 Software

Concerning software, the toolkit is primarily being built upon the previous researches in human face recognition and uses the following frameworks: TensorFlow [2], openVINO [3] and Kaldi [4].

Typically for each functionality needed, we have tested several models. There are several requirements imposed by the domain that have guided our choice in every aspect of software development:

1. Portability across devices, both hardware compatibility, and performance portability.
2. Memory consumption within constraints of a single board computer (SBC).
3. Reasonable framerate on several devices with wildly varying performance including GPU, desktop and mobile CPUs (both x86 and ARM).

Face Recognition. Face recognition is split into identification and recognition. We have tested several face identification techniques for the project. The best model currently in use uses an approach similar to that used by FaceBoxes [5] – it is a single-shot detector. The choice is driven by the need to find and align several faces on a single frame without considerable performance penalties.

The identification itself is done in two stages:

1. Facial feature extraction.
2. Face identifications.

The facial feature extraction module uses an implementation of the neural network architecture described in a FaceNet paper. Identification is done easily via any available classification algorithm, such as k-NN, thanks to a direct mapping from face images to Euclidean space where distances directly correspond to a measure of face similarity [6].

Speech Recognition. Speech recognition uses Kaldi toolkit, the architecture of the currently used acoustic model is a TDNN. GStreamer [7] and Kaldi GStreamer plugin [8] multimedia framework are used as a medium for transporting voice data.

2.2 Hardware

The toolkit is purposely being built to be used in mobile robots, thus, it needs to support a range of hardware.

Set of devices capable of running the toolkit includes a range of single board computers using ARM CPU and standard x86 computer.

Computer vision tasks are compute-intensive, thus, it is required to provide means of acceleration for face recognition tasks on single board computers. For those purposes, there are two options:

1. GPU acceleration.
2. Neural Compute Stick (NCS) [9] – an application-specific integrated circuit (ASIC) for running compatible neural networks in the openVINO framework.

In our implementation, two tasks were shown to take the most compute: face recognition and facial feature extraction; an average performance for different devices in those tasks is presented in Table 1. Table 1 data show sequential processing performance, with no batch processing applied as that better represents our case – analysis of a live video feed.

Table 1. Computer vision tasks performance.

Device	Recognition	Feature extraction	Full frame
NCS	70 ms	30 ms	N/A
SBC	90 ms	150 ms	280 ms
Desktop	20 ms	31 ms	75 ms
GPU	5 ms	7 ms	N/A

"Full frame" column depicts the time it typically takes to process the whole frame sequentially – only a single frame is processed at a time, processing also includes other stages, such as displaying results, etc. NCS and GPU are accelerators, thus have no data in "Full frame" column.

3 Case Study

To better describe capabilities let's focus on a single demonstrative case. This case expands on what is shown on Fig. 1. And it adds the missing functions developed for the project on top, thus it uses speech and face recognition, and voice feedback. Interaction happens in the following manner:

- Face recognition acts as a locking mechanism – voice recognition works only when a specific person is identified.
- Voice recognition is used to recognize what has been said.
- TTS is used to repeat everything that follows an 'echo' command.

The case proved that natural interaction capabilities might be integrated together to a robot in tandem to build up capabilities towards natural communications.

4 Future Work

There is a lot of room for potential improvements, including:

1. Recognition models' improvement.
2. Study other cases.
3. Develop new capabilities.

The focus of further development shall be centered around using the toolkit to explore other cases and study how the way interaction happens affects the performance of a human-robot team. Human-robot team system performance [10] is of special interest, as the topic of the paper is expected to mainly affect human perception of a robot, while not altering capabilities of robots it integrates with. Thus, other common human-robot interaction metrics might not be as applicable.

5 Conclusion

We have developed and tested an extendable and portable set of tools for human-robot interaction and demonstrated them in a use case. Rich user-centered interactions in robotics could be built even for a robot with little computational and energy potential when using ASICs for compute-heavy parts of the interaction tasks.

Acknowledgements. This work has been supported by the Ministry of Science and Higher Education of the Russian Federation with the project "Development of anthropomorphic robotic complexes with variable stiffness actuators for movement on the flat and the rugged terrains" (agreement: № 075-10-2018-010 (№ 14.606.21.0007), ID: RFMEFI60617X0007).

References

1. Fong, T., Nourbakhsh, I., Kunz, C., Fluckiger, L., Schreiner, J., Ambrose, R., Burridge, R., Simmons, R., Hiatt, L., Schultz, A., Trafton, J.G., Bugajska, M., Scholtz, J.: The peer-to-peer human-robot interaction project. In: Space 2005. American Institute of Aeronautics and Astronautics (2005)
2. Abadi, M., Agarwal, A., Barham, P., et al.: TensorFlow: large-scale machine learning on heterogeneous systems. In: arXiv e-prints (2015)
3. OpenVINO deep learning computer vision toolkit. https://software.intel.com/en-us/openvino-toolkit
4. Povey, D., et al.: The Kaldi speech recognition toolkit. In: Proc. ASRU, Hawaii, US, pp. 1–4 (2011)
5. Zhang, S., Zhu, X., Lei, Z., Shi, H., Wang, X., Li, S.Z.: FaceBoxes: a CPU real-time face detector with high accuracy. In: 2017 IEEE International Joint Conference on Biometrics (IJCB). IEEE (2017)
6. Schroff, F., Kalenichenko, D., Philbin, J.: FaceNet: a unified embedding for face recognition and clustering. In: 2015 IEEE Conference on Computer Vision and Pattern Recognition (CVPR). IEEE (2015)
7. GSteamer multimedia framework. https://gstreamer.freedesktop.org/
8. Alumäe, Tanel: Full-duplex speech-to-text system for Estonian. FAIA **268**, 3–10 (2014)
9. Introducing the Intel Neural Compute Stick 2. https://software.intel.com/en-us/neural-compute-stick
10. Steinfeld, A., Fong, T., Kaber, D., Lewis, M., Scholtz, J., Schultz, A., Goodrich, M.: Common metrics for human-robot interaction. In: Proceeding of the 1st ACM SIGCHI/SIGART Conference on Human-Robot Interaction - HRI '06. ACM Press (2006)

Research and Improvement of Enterprise Safety Behavior Based on SEM

Yuqing Tong, Shaochuan Xu, and Xuebo Chen(✉)

School of Electronics and Information Engineering,
University of Science and Technology, Anshan 114051, Liaoning, China
xuebochen@126.com

Abstract. Recently, many catastrophic accidents are becoming more and more frequently. In order to reduce the incidences of accidents in an enterprise, studies have shown that behavior-based safety (BBS) is closely related to people's safety awareness. In order to improve the overall safety awareness of enterprise employees, this paper adopts the form of questionnaire to interview employees in Shandong oilfield, and uses the knowledge learned in complex systems to model and study. To study the behavioral enterprise security system by using Structural Equation Model (SEM), SPSS.19 and LISREL software are used for data processing and path simulating, so as to reduce the incidences of accidents.

Keywords: Behavior-Based Safety (BBS) · Safety awareness · Structural equation model · Soft simulation

1 Introduction

With the repaid economic development of China, more and more enterprises of all sizes are emerging. Nevertheless, more and more safety accidents happen frequently. On 14th Nov. 2018, carbon 9 leakage caused the water pollution in Guangzhou, Fujian [1], on 12th Aug the explosion of dangerous goods warehouse caused casualties in Tianjin [2] and so on. All of the occurrence of the enterprise dangerous incidents, we must pay more attention to the latent risk factors of major dangerous events of enterprise safety. At present, many people have studied many researches the in the enterprise safety. Safety was firstly put forward by the International advisory group on nuclear safety (INSAG) of the International Atomic Energy Agency (IAEA) because of the accident of Chernobyl nuclear power plant in the former Soviet union in 1986 [3]. The awareness of safety within groups is mainly due to the summation of the awareness and attitudes of the personnel within the organization, that is, on the one hand, the necessary system within the unit and the hierarchical system of responsibility of the management departments, and on the other hand, the personal attitudes at all levels respond to and benefit from the above systems [4]. In the aspect of safety principles, we should have a deeper understanding of the problem of human factors, so as to have a better understanding of the solution to safety problems [5].

T. Ahram et al. (Eds.): IHIET 2019, AISC 1018, pp. 201–206, 2020.
https://doi.org/10.1007/978-3-030-25629-6_32

2 Design the Scheme of Investigation Sample Size and Reliability

2.1 Sample Selection

The investigation was conducted in Shandong oilfield, with employees in the third, fifth and sixth districts as the investigation respondents. There were 284 employees participating this investigation. The surgery participants were local workers, including employees, team leaders, junior mangers and government functionaries. The numbers are one hundred and ninety-nine, twenty-two, twenty-five and two. The fan distribution diagram is shown in Fig. 1.

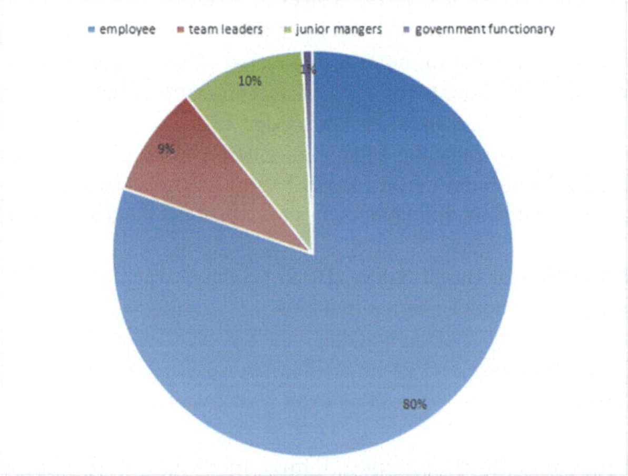

Fig. 1. The number of people in different positions.

2.2 Questionnaire Design

By using SEM method to analyze the safety factors of employees in the enterprise among people, things and environment, the safety awareness is divided into external environment coefficient and personal safety literacy, personal physical quality and leadership management. Personal safety literacy, personal physical quality and leadership management are internal factors, external environment coefficient is used as an external factor. It shows in Table 1.

2.3 Reliability of Statistical Data

Reliability refers to the degree of stability or consistency of the measurement results. If the reliability coefficient is above 0.8, we will believe this data credibility is high 0.7–0.8 can be accepted; 0.6–0.7 can be accepted reluctantly and under 0.6 the data can not be valid. Reliability can be obtained by SPSS software by KMO and Bartley sphere

Table 1. Observation variables and measurement factors

Symbol	Classifications of potential factors	The factors affects staffs safety
C_1	Personal safety literacy	Knowledge of safety rules
C_2		Current work experience
C_3		Familiarity with safety work
C_4		Work environment safety risks and dangers
C_5		Approval of safety operations regulations
C_6	Personal physical quality	Physical fitness
C_7		Level of fatigue at work
C_8		Attentions of working
C_9		Personal psychological quality
C_{10}	External environment factor	Leaders' emphasis on safety production
C_{11}		Performance of colleagues on safety production
C_{12}		Comfort level of working environment
C_{13}		Enterprise security atmosphere
C_{14}		Abrasion of production machines
C_{15}	Management factors	Reasonableness of plan
C_{16}		Level of consummation of enterprise safety productions systems
C_{17}		Reward and punishment of enterprise safety production
C_{18}		Degree of investment in safety productions
C_{19}		Enterprise safety production supervision
C_{20}		Frequency and strength of enterprise safety production

test. If the KMO value is above 0.5 and the significant level is below 0.05, we believe the factor analysis is suitable for the analysis.

The results obtained by factor analysis with SPSS software are shown in the Table 2.

Table 2. Results of KMO test and Bartlett test.

KMO and Bartlett test		
Kaiser-Meyer-Olkin measures sample adequacy		0.863
Bartlett's spherical test	Chi-square	2173.311
	df	190
	Significant	0.000

3 The Establishment of SEM

3.1 Initial Establishment of SEM Model

According to the latent variables and the observation index variables in paper [6], the initial model of the data is set up and the structure equation is

$$\begin{bmatrix} \eta_1 \\ \eta_2 \\ \eta_3 \end{bmatrix} = \begin{bmatrix} 0 & 0 & \beta_{13} \\ \beta_{21} & 0 & 0 \\ 0 & 0 & 0 \end{bmatrix} \begin{bmatrix} \eta_1 \\ \eta_2 \\ \eta_3 \end{bmatrix} + \begin{bmatrix} \gamma_1 \\ \gamma_2 \\ \gamma_3 \end{bmatrix} \xi + \begin{bmatrix} \varsigma_1 \\ \varsigma_2 \\ \varsigma_3 \end{bmatrix} \quad (1)$$

In the equation above, ξ is the exogenous variable of the observation index, η_i are the exogenous latent variables of the observation indexes. And β_{21} are β_{13} the interactions between endogenous latent variables. $\gamma_i (i = 1, 2, 3)$ are the influences of exogenous latent variables on endogenous latent variables. $\varsigma_i (i = 1, 2, 3)$ are the error terms of the endogenous latent variables that cannot be measured by the model.

The formula of endogenous latent variables measurement is as follows:

$$\begin{bmatrix} A_{10} \\ A_{11} \\ A_{12} \\ A_{13} \\ A_{14} \end{bmatrix} = \begin{bmatrix} 1 \\ \alpha_1 \\ \alpha_2 \\ \alpha_3 \\ \alpha_4 \end{bmatrix} \xi + \begin{bmatrix} \delta_1 \\ \delta_2 \\ \delta_3 \\ \delta_4 \end{bmatrix} \quad (2)$$

Among them, $A_i (i = 10, \cdots 14)$ are exogenous observation indicator variables $\alpha_i (i = 1, 2, 3)$ are the path coefficient between the exogenous latent variables and the exogenous observation indexes $\delta_i (i = 1, 2, 3, 4, 5)$ are the error term of the exogenous observation indexes.

3.2 Results of SEM Model Fitting

Obtaining observation equation and structural equation from SEM equation, we use LISREL to build the model. By using the method of maximum likelihood estimation, the coefficients are normalized. The SEM simulation result is shown in Fig. 2.

3.3 Model Results Analysis

Among many observation variables that affect personal safety literacy, current work experience (C_2) is the most affecting safety, the second factor is work environment (C_4), approval of safety operations regulations (C_5), familiarity with safety work(C_3), knowledge of safety rules(C_1) in personal safety literacy is 0.79, 0.57, 0.49, 0.79, 0.34.

Among many observation variables that affect personal physical quality, the coefficients from big to small is that, attentions of working (C_8), level of fatigue at work (C_7), physical fitness (C_6), personal psychological quality (C_9) is 5.89, 3.38, 0.65, 0.61.

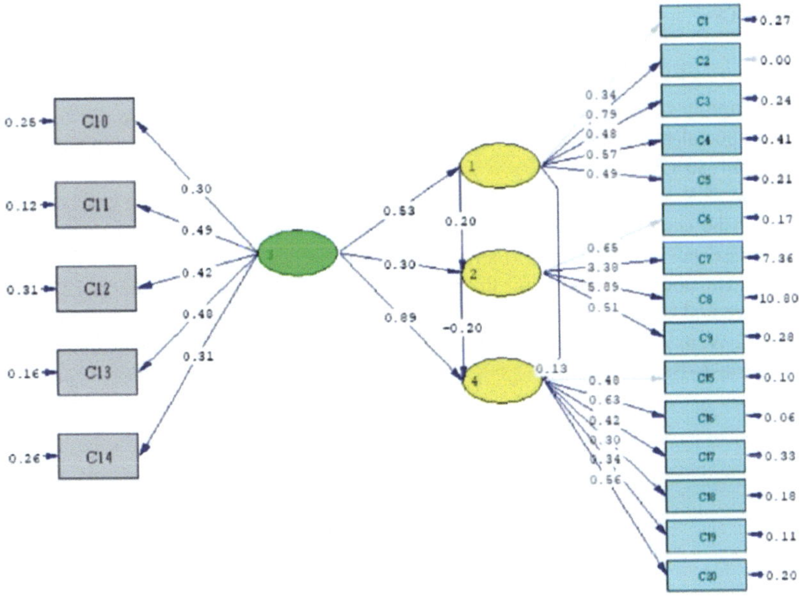

Fig. 2. SEM simulation results

Among many observation variables that affect leadership management, level of consummation of enterprise safety productions systems (C_{16}), frequency and strength of enterprise safety production(C_{20}), reasonableness of plan (C_{15}), reward and punishment of enterprise safety production (C_{17}), enterprise safety production supervision (C_{19}), degree of investment in safety productions (C_{18}) is 0.63, 0.56, 0.48, 0.42, 0.34, 0.30.

4 Suggestions

From the above analysis, there are the following suggestions to improve enterprise security:

1. For the external environment created by the enterprise, it should try to pay attention to the expression form of safe production.
2. Enterprises should pay attention to the health of employees, attention is the ultimate guarantee of enterprise security.
3. For enterprise managers, levels of consummation of enterprise safety productions systems are the top priority of enterprise safety.
4. Work experience is also important, so before-work training is a must.

Acknowledgments. This research reported herein was supported by the NSFC of China under Grants No. 71571091 and 71771112.

References

1. Huang, P.P.: Risk communication in sudden environmental events-a case study of the carbon-nine leakage in Quangang [J]. Media Today, 2019, **27**(3): 41–43 (2019)
2. Feng, Y: Social work services were carried out in the relief work for the Tanjin port explosion disaster, 14–15 (2005)
3. Schwatka, N.V., Hecker, S., Goldenhar, L.M.: Defining and measuring safety climate: a review of the construction industry literature, 537–550 (2016)
4. Wu, T.: Use safety psychology to strengthen enterprise safety management, 61–62 (2006)
5. Li, X.Y.: The countermeasures for the high-risk society – reflections on the "8.12" especially serious fire and explosion accidents in Tianjin port, 63–64 (2015)
6. Hou, J.T., Wen, Z.L., Cheng, Z.J.: Structural Equation Model and Its Application. Education Science Press, Beijing (2004)

Towards the Linguistic Gender Differentiation in Dictionaries: A Perspective of Human Interaction in Languages

Pingfang Yu, Jiali Du(✉), and Xinguang Li

Guangdong University of Foreign Studies,
Baiyun Avenue North 2, Guangzhou 510420, China
{201310051,201310039,200311088}@oamail.gdufs.edu.cn

Abstract. There's an intimate link between language and ideology, and social relations are mediated through language. The lexicographical treatment of cultural loaded lexical item has a direct influence on the dictionary users' perception of the world, the conceptualization of categories in that world and how the user will act in future. This paper seeks to analyze how gender differences are presented in learners' dictionaries from a society-oriented cross-linguistic perspective, and finally we find there is an observable "anthropological turn" in the treatment of the example sentences in some distinguished English learners' dictionaries.

Keywords: Human factors · Linguistic anthropology · Cross-cultural interaction · Dictionary

1 Introduction

Language ideologies have emerged in recent years and attracted the attention of linguistic anthropologists. The term "ideology", as a social construct, denotes belief systems such as communism, racism or feminism; and the term "language ideologies" refers to sets of representations through which language is imbued with cultural meaning for a certain speech community [1–3]. The speech community living in different cultural circumstances develop cultures of various kinds. Culture is deeply rooted and recorded in human languages. What is desirable in language are always systematically related to other areas of cultural discourse such as the nature of persons, of power, and of a desirable moral order [4–7]. A language is to some degree a mirror of the culture, including the gender differences. Scholars, especially the feminist linguists identify the centrality of language in the routine maintenance of social inequality. The normal linguistic behavior of women and men will be represented in ways congruent with the community's more general representation of the essential natures of the two groups [8–12]. Lexicographers have agreed that except for some scientific and technical vocabularies, many general lexical units, except for the pure scientific and technical vocabularies, are culture-specific or culture bound in a language. This paper seeks to analyze how gender differences are presented in learners' dictionaries from a society-oriented cross-linguistic perspective. The purpose of the present research is to

T. Ahram et al. (Eds.): IHIET 2019, AISC 1018, pp. 207–212, 2020.
https://doi.org/10.1007/978-3-030-25629-6_33

investigate if there exist a biased treatment of sex discrimination in example sentences in learners' dictionaries; and what kinds of strategies should be adopted to delimit the imbalance of gender representation.

2 Sex, Gender and Language

Linguistic dictionaries, as well as being a scholarly record of the whole language and large information set, are regarded as a cultural phenomenon, even "an ideological weapon" which are large mirrors to reflect the cultures of a society without distortion. Dictionaries can be used as a means of access to the mainstream values of a society. Among all the lexicographic elements, example sentences of a headword occupies a particular position to reflect the culture and social value of a society.

The relation between sex and gender is a hot topic in sociolinguistics. It's argued that sex is based on an individual's physical body which is determined by primary sexual characteristics at birth and it's connected with genital appearance. Gender, however, is the combination of constantly changing associations, attitudes and practices prescribed by human social groups for their members according to their sexed bodies. To put it in a simple way, gender, constructed by the human society, is a sort of social correlate of sex. In this view, biological males and biological females possess certain "culturally" imbued characteristics which fall neatly into the same two biologically determined categories. Men and women are instructed to "learn" appropriate sex roles. To be short, sex is biological-based; while gender is culture-bound. Therefore, language and gender are closely related.

According to linguistic anthropologists, people are perceived through a "lens" of gender polarization [13], which are extremely obvious in dictionary examples. There's a strong tendency for gender stereotyping in dictionary examples. Stereotyping focus obsessively on certain characteristics, real or imagined, and exaggerate them. For example, the stereotype of women is often an empty-headed chatter and that of men a strong-minded speaker. This kind of gender stereotypes is "closely lined with and support gender ideologies.

Three frameworks are identified in the research into language and gender: "deficit", "dominance", and "differences. The deficit model are approached in terms of male norm and female deficiency; In what is often called the dominance framework, language patterns are interpreted as manifestations of a patriarchal social order; asymmetries in the language use of mean and women are thereby seen as enactments of male privilege. In some learners' dictionaries, there is likely to be a hint of sexist stereotypes. We are interested in the following questions: Does the gender orientation shown by the examples in learners' dictionaries truly reflect the sex images prescribed by the society? Or do lexicographers deliberately choose the "right" or "appropriate" sentences as dictionary examples, trying to make an ideal state of gender equality in their dictionaries?

3 Sex Discrimination in English and Non-English Dictionaries

The anti-sexist climate is widespread and becomes more and more prevailing in our times, and lexicographers should not reinforce the sexist stereotypes in their word-books. And the examples in dictionaries should be neural, not deliberately showing the stereotypes imposed on the two sexes by the society.

We collect data of some dictionaries published between 1970s–2000s, and conduct a survey of the use of sexually biased pronouns in example sentences of some English learners' dictionaries, trying to find out if there is a tendency of avoidance of these kind of pronouns.

According to Table 1, we can see that there are fewer examples with *she* than those with *he* in Oxford Advanced Learners' Dictionary (abbreviated as OALD) (1974). While in the edition of OALD in 1989 and 1995, the frequency gap of examples with *she* and *he* is narrowing down, and finally the number of examples with *she* outweighs that of examples with *he* in the 2006 edition of OALD. It's obvious that OALD is always trying to capture the social changes of its time, mirroring the cultural revolution and the philosophical movement and proclaiming its awareness of the social issue of the time. In later editions of OALD, male dominance and female subordination are consciously minimized and the compilers of OALD honestly try to take account of the changing state of affairs in the dictionary examples. That's a good idea that a dictionary should be up-to-date both in linguistic, philosophical and cultural information.

Table 1. Pronouns used in some English learners' dictionaries

Dictionaries	OALD		LDOCE		CCALD		CALD	
	F	M	F	M	F	M	F	M
70 s	15	61	10	10	/	/	/	/
80 s	33	41	36	33	30	51	/	/
90 s	37	38	46	58	30	80	65	70
00 s	56	42	39	61	28	59	54	53

Longman Dictionary of Contemporary English (LDOCE, 1987) is the only one which has more examples with female pronouns than those with male pronouns, and in other editions, there's still man predominance in example sentences. In spite of this, we can find some examples of Political Correctness (PC). For example. In the 1st edition of LDOCE, one sense of "chair" has the example "She holds the chair of Chemistry at that university"; and at "buzz", an example is "She buzzed for her secretary"; And at the headword "bathe", we can find the example "He's bathing the baby" in LDOCE1. From the perspective of prototype theory, the prototype of holding professorships or buzzing for a secretary should be a man instead of a woman. It's self-evident that the afore-mentioned example sentences in LDOCE1 is a kind of intentional subversion of the traditional stereotypes.

The first edition of Cambridge Advanced Learners' Dictionary (CALD) has an equal share of female and male examples. Its policy is clearly to give both a female and a male example in each individual entry. It's obvious that CALD has consciously adopted the principle of politically correct. In the later edition of CALD, there appear more and more examples which describe a female playing an important role in society.

When there are more than two examples of a headword, the compilers of CALD try to consciously balance the ratio of the both sexes in examples. For example, the headword "chef" has two examples, which are "He is one of the top chefs in Britain" and "She is head-chef at the Waldorf-Astoria". Some headwords in CALD have a few example sentences to portray an image of a powerful woman. One sense of "acknowledge" has the examples "……Historians generally acknowledge her as a genius in her field" and "She is usually acknowledged to be one of our best artists"; at the headword "aid", an example is "She went to the aid of a man trapped in his car" and "A woman in the street saw that he was in trouble and came to his aid", etc.

Collins-Cobuild Advanced Learners' Dictionary (CCALD) has much more example sentences with male pronouns than those with female pronouns. That's not surprising. Sinclair, the chief editor of CCALD, claims that CCALD is a totally corpus-based dictionary, and all the example sentences come from the corpus and thus represent real language. Even more, the whole of the Cobuild dictionary is based on evidence derived from real language, providing true-to-life examples. And in human discourse, the society is man-dominant, which is naturally reflected in human's discourse and also in Sinclair's corpus.

It's safe to say that as a kind of "ideology", language ideology is in some way oppose to truth. OALD and CALD adhere to the principle of PC, therefore a lot of socially "progressive" while scientifically "untrue" examples are chosen and the two dictionaries are challenging established ideologies of language. We can see that some English dictionary-makers, for example, the compilers of OALD and CALD, are willing to react to new developments in language and society, which can be seen as a compiling policy——in order not to be thought as sexists. Lexicographers consciously increase the active and positive images of women in example sentences, although the linguistic data is sometimes contrary to the social fact that women are still inferior to men in many aspects. CCALD, however, chooses to record the "real English" as it is, without any modification to avoid the usage of so called "sexism". LDOCE, however, is not as radical as OALD and CCALD, nor is it as conservative as CCALD. It lies in between: sometimes describing the linguistic reality; sometimes using modified sentences to be regarded as politically correct.

Whether does the sex discrimination exist in the non-English dictionaries? We conduct a survey of the use of sexually biased pronouns in example sentences of some non-English learners' dictionaries, trying to find out if there is a tendency of avoidance of these kind of pronouns.

It's clear that in the Japanese dictionaries in Table 2, when denoting people, the pronouns of example sentences are mainly neural or plural such as "children" "prisoner" "leader" and "audience", etc., which can be found almost on every page of these dictionaries. That proves to be an effective way to avoid saying whether a person is a male or a female, fading the gender orientation in Japanese dictionaries. Occasionally the Japanese dictionaries surveyed in our research show the woman or girl in active and positive roles.

Table 2. Pronouns used in some non-English learners' dictionaries

Dictionaries	Male	Female	Neural	Plural
MingJing Japanese dictionary	11	6	29	36
New Mingjie Japanese dictionary	10	3	20	13
Digital Japanese dictionary	22	27	29	33
Japanese-Chinese dictionary	51	27	39	42
Robert French dictionary	106	87	90	39
Larousse French dictionar	35	13	24	6
Chinese learners' dictionary	39	17	17	8
Chinese pedagogical dictionary	29	8	31	20
English-Chinese multi-functional dictionary	26	10	2	9
New English-Chinese dictionary	59	29	6	6

In the French dictionaries, we can find the fixed gendered stereotypes in the example sentences such as "Elle se rongeait fébrilement les ongles" (She bites her fingernails restlessly) and "Il a été fait maréchal" (He got promoted and he is a marshal now). There are also some examples of stereotype derivation such as "Il est trop faible pour prendre une décision" (He's irresolute and hesitant) and "Il fait de la neurasthénie" (He was suffering from nervous exhaustion), etc. The pronouns are chosen randomly, and therefore we can also find such example sentences as "Il est devenu fataliste" (He became a fatalist) and "Elle s'est fait mordre par un chien" (She was bitten by a dog).

The Chinese learners' dictionaries have more example sentences with male pronouns. These kinds of sentences are in line with the stereotypes in human cognition. We can also find the examples of stereotype derivation. Besides, we can find much more example sentences with a randomly chosen pronoun such as "His eyesight is failing" and "He is fair at physics", which, we think, result from the fact that a few Chinese lexicographers may be apt to "invent" or "make up" a sentence as a dictionary example, instead of selecting a sentence from a large balanced corpus.

4 Conclusion

Dictionaries do not exist in a vacuum, and the information in dictionaries are clearly shaped by the social issues circulating within particular societies. With regard to the role of dictionaries in presenting cultures, two kinds of methods are available. The first one is that, lexicographers should truly record the culture facts of a given speech community and in this way, dictionaries are a mirror; the other is that, lexicographers should not only reflect social and ideological change but also tailor the cultural and ideological aspect of a society and exert a progressive influence in furthering these views. Lexicographical treatment of cultural loaded lexical item will have a direct influence on the dictionary users' perception of the world. Some English dictionary-makers have realized that an intimate link between language and ideology exists and social relations are mediated through language, and these dictionaries consciously abandon sexism—women being linguistically inferior to men. But in non-English learners' dictionaries, we haven't found a hint of Political Correctness in example sentences. We argue that dictionaries should try to be up-to-date both in linguistic, philosophical and cultural information, and take account of the changing state of the society.

Acknowledgments. This article is sponsored by "Thirteen-Five Major Project" for National Science and Technology Terminology Validation Committee (ZD2019001), China Social Science Fund (2018FYY006), China Natural Science Fund (61877013), and Guangdong Science and Technology Department Project (2018A070712032).

References

1. Cameron, D.: Gender and language ideologies. In: Holmes, J., Meyerhoff, M. (eds.) The Handbook of Language and Gender. Blackwell, Oxford (2003)
2. Eckert, P., Mcconnellginet, S.: Think practically and look locally: language and gender as community-based practice. Annu. Rev. Anthropology. **21**(1), 461–490 (1992)
3. Stokoe, E.H.: Gender and discourse, gender and categorization: current developments in language and gender research. Qual. Res. Psychol. **1**(2), 107–129 (2004)
4. Holmes, J.: Politeness and postmodernism–an appropriate approach to the analysis of language and gender. J. Sociolinguistics. **9**(1), 108–117 (2010)
5. Mavisakalyan, A.: Gender in language and gender in employment. Oxf. Dev. Studies. **43**(4), 403–424 (2015)
6. Yu. B.: Language and gender in Congressional speech. Lit. & Linguist. Comput. **156**(15), 2986–3004 (2013)
7. Mahmud, M.: Language and Gender in English Language Teaching. Teflin J. **21** (2010)
8. Nguyen, H.T.: What role do race, ethnicity, language and gender play in the teaching profession? Race Ethn. Educ. **15**(5), 653–681 (2012)
9. Darani, L.H., Darani, H.H.: Language and gender: a prosodic study of Iranian speakers' talks. Procedia - Soc. Behav. Sci. **70**, 423–429 (2013)
10. Jack, S.: Language and gender in the Caribbean. J. Pidgin Creole Lang. **27**(1), 141–157 (2012)
11. Du, J.L., Alexandris, C., et al.: Controlling interaction in multilingual conversation revisited: a perspective for services and interviews in Mandarin Chinese. In: International Conference on Human-Computer Interaction, pp. 573–583. Springer, Cham. 10271 (2017)
12. Hacohenkerner, Y., Hagege, R.: Language and gender classification of speech files using supervised machine learning methods. Cybern. Sys. **4**, 1–26 (2017)
13. Bem, S.L.: The lenses of gender: transforming the debate on sexual inequality. Am. J. Sociology. **6**, 92 (1993)

Computation and Intelligent Design

Data-Driven Arithmetic Fuzzy Control Using the Distending Function

József Dombi and Abrar Hussain(✉)

Institute of Informatics, University of Szeged, Szeged 6720, Hungary
{dombi, hussain}@inf.u-szeged.hu

Abstract. Data-driven fuzzy control techniques suffer from the flat structure problem, i.e. the number of fuzzy rules grows exponentially as the input dimension increases. The consequence is greater complexity and poorer interpretability. In this article, we present a solution to the above-mentioned problem by proposing a novel data-driven fuzzy controller. Its unique features are: (1) A new type of membership function is used; (2) It helps to identify few and important fuzzy rules; (3) These rules cover the whole input space; (4) Dombi operators (usually the conjunctive) are employed to generate a higher dimensional control surface; (5) The designed fuzzy controller is based on fuzzy arithmetic operations; (6) Defuzzification is single step calculation. Due to the small number of fuzzy rules, the complexity of the fuzzy model decreases and it becomes interpretable. The effectiveness of the proposed scheme is demonstrated using the data-driven based control of vehicle lateral dynamics.

Keywords: Data Driven fuzzy control · Distending function · Fuzzy arithmetic

1 Introduction

The traditional fuzzy inference engine consists of a fuzzifier, a rule base system, fuzzy operators and defuzzification. The fuzzy rules describe the dependencies between the input and output variables. As the number of input variables increases, the required number of rules and the system complexity increases exponentially. In most of the cases, expert knowledge is not available. If the working data of the process is available then a data driven design is an attractive option. In this case, the problem reduces to identifying a suitable fuzzy model, which fits the given data [1].

The data-based identification of a fuzzy model consists of qualitative and quantitative identification. Qualitative identification focuses on the number and description of fuzzy rules, while quantitative identification is concerned with the identification of parameter values. In the case of qualitative identification, soft computing methodologies are used [2]. In quantity identification, neural networks are mostly used. Combining these two leads to the development of Neuro-Fuzzy Inference systems [3].

The above-mentioned approaches, however, have some drawbacks. They are:

1. **Qualitative identification.** The identified rule base has a so-called flat structure (curse of dimensionality) problem. In most cases, triangular membership functions are used and the support of these functions covers a limited area of the input space

T. Ahram et al. (Eds.): IHIET 2019, AISC 1018, pp. 215–221, 2020.
https://doi.org/10.1007/978-3-030-25629-6_34

(the grade of membership is zero outside this area). If the input falls in these uncovered areas, then the identified rule base does not generate any action. Even if some sort of interpolation technique is applied, the computation complexity will increase [10]. To cover the input space completely, a huge number of rules are required.

2. **Quantitative identification.** The computation complexity of the identified fuzzy model also increases exponentially with the number of rules.
3. **Interpretability.** If the number of rules grows exponentially, then it is not possible to predict the response of the model. The model tends to be more like a black box.
4. **Complexity of control design.** The Mamdani or TS techniques are computationally expensive due to the implication, the aggregation requirements and the defuzzification step.

In this article, we propose a new methodology for a data-driven fuzzy control design. This new method has the following unique features: (1) A new type of membership function called the Distending function is used. The grade of membership always has a non-zero value and the whole input space is covered; (2) The Distending function has only three parameters. Usually two parameters can be kept constant and one parameter is used for tuning. A single step calculation is required to calculate this parameter; (3) The interpretability of the model increases due to the significant decrease in number of fuzzy rules; (4) Arithmetic-based fuzzy controller is used to generate the control signal. There is no implication operator involved. Defuzzification is a single step calculation.

The rest of the paper is organized as follows. In Sect. 2, we describe the Distending function and its properties. In Sect. 3, we explain the data-driven fuzzy control design. In Sect. 4, we outline the benchmark systems, simulations and the results. Lastly, in Sect. 5, we draw some conclusions.

2 The Distending Function and Its Properties

Zadeh proposed various membership functions [4] and based on these, we define a more general parametric function called the Distending function.

Definition 1. The Distending function (DF) is a symmetric membership function (Fig. 1), defined as

$$\Delta_{\epsilon,v}^{(\lambda)}(x-a) = \frac{1}{1+\frac{1-v}{v}\left|\frac{x-a}{\epsilon}\right|^{\lambda}}, \tag{1}$$

here, $\Delta_{\epsilon,v}^{(\lambda)}(x-a) : \mathbb{R} \to [0,1]$, $\lambda > 1$, $\varepsilon > 0$ and $v \in (0,1)$. $\in$ is the error/tolerance and v is the threshold parameter. The threshold v separates the truth and false regions in the membership grade interval (i.e. $[0,1]$). When $-\epsilon < x < \epsilon$, the input value is treated as true; otherwise it is false. In Eq. (1), the notation $x-a$ means that the function has a peak value at $x=a$. The DF is continuous from $-\infty$ to ∞. The λ parameter changes the shape of the distending function. If $\lambda \to \infty$ then DF approaches the classical characteristic function. The DF can take different shapes such as rectangular, close to Gaussian and triangular depending on λ. As $\Delta(x)$ is an even function, the coordinate of the Centre of Gravity (COG) of $\Delta(x-a)$ is a).

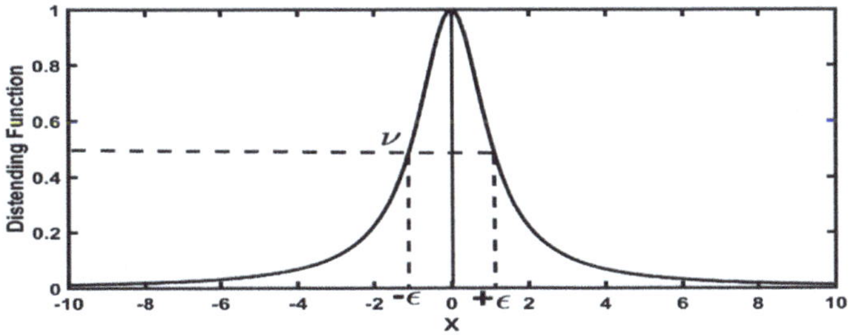

Fig. 1. Distending function ($\nu = 0.5$, $\varepsilon = 0.5$, $\lambda = 2$, $a = 0$)

2.1 The Distending Function in Higher Dimensions

We will represent the inputs and outputs using the DFs. If the number of input variables (i.e. input dimensions) increase then the output is generated in the higher dimensional space. We give an expression for the higher dimensional output DF using the input DFs. Let

$$\Delta_{x_i} = \Delta^{(\lambda_i)}_{i(\epsilon_i,\nu_i)}(x_i - a_i) = \frac{1}{1 + \frac{1-\nu_i}{\nu_i}\left|\frac{x_i - a_i}{\epsilon_i}\right|^{\lambda_i}}, \tag{2}$$

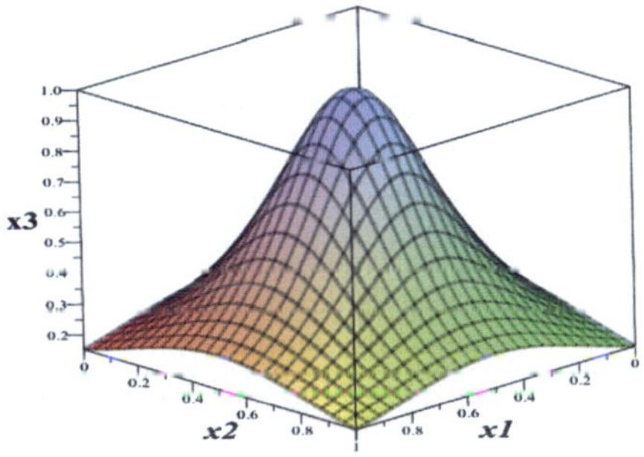

Fig. 2. The 3-dimension distending surface of two variables ($x_1$andx_2)

If we apply the Dombi conjunctive operator on these n input DFs [5], then the resultant output DF $\Delta_{x_{n+1}}$ in higher dimension (Fig. 2) is

$$\Delta_{x_{n+1}} = \frac{1}{1 + \frac{1-\nu}{\nu}\left(\left|\frac{x_1 - a_1}{\epsilon_1}\right|^{\lambda} + \ldots + \left|\frac{x_n - a_n}{\epsilon_n}\right|^{\lambda}\right)}, \tag{3}$$

3 Data Driven Based Control

The proposed algorithm is motivated by our previous work, where fuzzy arithmetic was used [6]. A Multi-input single output (MISO) system has the following form:

$$\begin{aligned} &\text{if } x_1 \text{ is } U_1^i \text{and} \ldots\ldots \text{and } x_n \text{ is } U_n^i \\ &\text{then } y_t \text{ is } V_t^i, \end{aligned} \tag{4}$$

Let us now assume that the input and output training data has the following form:

$$\boldsymbol{U} = \left[a_j^i\right]; \boldsymbol{V} = \left[b^i\right];\ \boldsymbol{i} = 1, .., \boldsymbol{l}\ \boldsymbol{and}\ \boldsymbol{j} = 1, .., \boldsymbol{n}, \tag{5}$$

where U contains the l data points of each input and V contains the corresponding l output data points. The data points $a_1, a_2, \ldots, a_n$ correspond to the input fuzzy subsets $U_1, U_2, \ldots, U_n$ and b corresponds to the output fuzzy subset V. We can now divide our proposed method into following three key steps:

Construction of Estimated Control Surface and Rule Base. From the given data of Eq. (5), an estimated control surface G' can be constructed. The columns of the training data matrix U are transformed to the $[0, 1]$ interval. Next, we extract a few rows from U that contain the key (boundary and average) values of the input variables. These rows and the corresponding elements in V are used to construct the rule base. The antecedent part contains a row of U and the consequent part contains an element of V. The antecedent part of the *ith* fuzzy rule has the fuzzy logical expression which may contain logical operators. We can use a general class of parametric fuzzy operators [7].

Generation of Fuzzy Control Surface and Error Surface. In the second step we generate the fuzzy control surface $\hat{G}$ using the DF. We construct DFs for all the different input variables of the antecedent part. The value of parameter a of the DF is equal to the corresponding input value in the database. Set the values of λ to 2 and ε to 0.3 (Other values can be chosen depending on distance between selected input values). The same value of v is used for all the DFs of the same rule. This v value will be set so that it minimize the influence of higher dimensional DFs. Each rule is evaluated using Eq. (3).

For all the l rules, l output DFs will be generated. All these output DFs form a fuzzy control surface $\hat{G}$. The new v value of the output DFs will be calculated based on the minimum influence principle i.e. each of the l output DFs should not influence any other DF. We can construct an error surface E as

$$E_{(x1,\ldots,x_n)} = G'_{(x1,\ldots,x_n)} - \hat{G}_{(x1,\ldots,x_n)}, \tag{7}$$

we want to decrease the magnitude of E to a given threshold by adding new rules in the rule base. The coordinates of the maximum error in E are used to select new entries from the database. We include this new output DF in $\hat{G}$ and as a result the maximum error in E will decrease. This process is repeated iteratively until the error surface E lies within the given threshold.

Designing the Arithmetic-Based Controller Using the Rule Base. The fuzzy rule has two parts, namely the antecedent and consequent part. We will deal with the these parts separately to design a fuzzy controller based on arithmetic operations.

The antecedent part of the *ith* fuzzy rule can be described by the expression

$$\mathcal{L}(\delta_1(x_1)^i, \delta_2(x_2)^i, \ldots, \delta_n(x_n)^i) = \hat{w}_i(x), \tag{8}$$

where $\hat{w}_i(x)$ is the rule applicability function. For a specific set of input values x^*, Eq. (8) leads to a single numeric called the strength of the *ith* rule $\hat{w}_i(x^*)$. We normalize these strengths to get the firing strength $w_i(x^*)$ of the *ith* rule.

$$\boldsymbol{w}_i(\boldsymbol{x}^*) = \frac{\hat{\boldsymbol{w}}(\boldsymbol{x}^*)}{\sum_{i=1}^{l} \hat{\boldsymbol{w}}(\boldsymbol{x}^*)}, \text{ where } \sum\nolimits_{i=1}^{l} \hat{\boldsymbol{w}}(\boldsymbol{x}^*) = 1. \tag{9}$$

The consequent part of the *ith* fuzzy rule is a numeric value and it is an element of the matrix V given in Eq. (5). The crisp output control C of the fuzzy controller is

$$\boldsymbol{C} = w_1(\boldsymbol{x}^*)\boldsymbol{b}^1 + \ldots + w_l(\boldsymbol{x}^*)\boldsymbol{b}^l. \tag{10}$$

4 Benchmark Systems, Simulations and Results

The effectiveness of the proposed data-driven based control strategy is verified using a simulation study on vehicle lateral dynamics.

To simulate the vehicle lateral dynamics, we used an open access package [8] with the Matlab environment. The whole simulation model consists of a tire model and a vehicle model [8]. The nonlinear tire model for the simulations is derived by modeling the relationship between the vehicle lateral forces and the slip angle using the Pacejka empirical formula [9].

Control Scenario (Lateral Position Control). First, a large training data set is generated using a working vehicle lateral position control system. The training data consists of the steering control signal δ and the four inputs i.e. error 'e' in the lateral position y, the yaw angle ψ, velocity v_T and the side slip angle α_T. The training data set is used to generate the estimated control surface G'. Then the training data set is used to identify the actual control surface $\hat{G}$. The threshold is set to .07. The control and error surfaces for two inputs (e and ψ) are shown in Fig. 3. 16 fuzzy rules are identified. The response of the data-driven fuzzy controller for modifying the path of the vehicle by adjusting its lateral position is shown in Fig. 4.

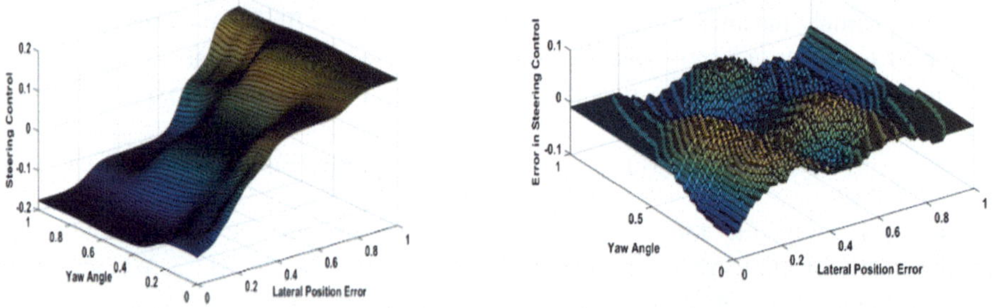

Fig. 3. Control surface $\hat{G}$ (left) and error surface (right) for Y and ψ

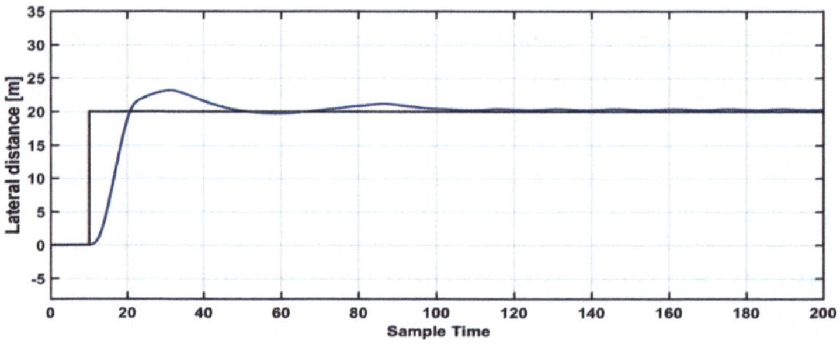

Fig. 4. Reference signal and the actual lateral position of the vehicle

5 Conclusion

In this study a Data-driven fuzzy controller is designed which solves the so-called flat structure problem. Instead of the classical membership functions, DF is used. The DF covers the input space using a few fuzzy rules. The complexity of the qualitative and quantitative parts of the data-driven fuzzy model is reduced. A control surface is generated by applying Dombi operator on DFs. The derived rule base is used to generate a fuzzy controller based on arithmetic operations. The effectiveness of the proposed approach was demonstrated by controlling the lateral dynamics of a vehicle.

Acknowledgments. This research work was supported by the European Union and co-funded by the European Social Fund (EFOP-3.6.3-VEKOP-16-2017-0002).

References

1. Tsai, S.H., Chen, Y.W.: A novel identification method for Takagi-Sugeno fuzzy model. Fuzzy Sets Syst. **338**, 117–135 (2018)
2. Zhang, R., Tao, J.: A nonlinear fuzzy neural network modeling approach using an improved genetic algorithm. IEEE Trans. Ind. Electron. **65**(7), 5882–5892 (2018)
3. Piegat, A.: Fuzzy Modeling and Control. Springer Physica, Heidelberg (2013)

4. Zadeh, L.A.: Outline of a new approach to the analysis of complex systems and decision processes. IEEE Trans. Syst. Man Cybern. **1**, 28–44 (1975)
5. Dombi, J.: A general class of fuzzy operators, the De Morgan class of fuzzy operators and fuzziness measures induced by fuzzy operators. Fuzzy Sets Syst. **8**(2), 149–163 (1982)
6. Dombi, J., Szepe, T.: Arithmetic-based fuzzy control. Iran. J. Fuzzy Syst. **14**(4), 51–66 (2017)
7. Dombi, J.: Towards a general class of fuzzy operators for fuzzy systems. IEEE Trans. Fuzzy Syst. **16**(2), 477–484 (2008)
8. MATLAB Central. https://ch.mathworks.com/matlabcentral/fileexchange/58683-vehicle-dynamics-lateral
9. Pacejka, H.: Tire and Vehicle Dynamics, 2nd edn. Elsevier, Oxford (2005)
10. Kóczy, L., Hirota, K.: Ordering, distance and closeness of fuzzy sets. Fuzzy Sets Syst. **59**(3), 281–293 (1993)

A Heuristic Fuzzy Algorithm for Hardware Engineers Assignment in University Sectors

Agniraj Senthilrajan(✉)

Alagappa University, Karaikudi, Tamilnadu, India
directorccalu@gmail.com

Abstract. The assignment of hardware computer engineers to the various departments is often done manually in most universities. An efficient software is needed for scheduling the hardware computer engineers and system technicians to reach the High quality satisfaction. A newly proposed algorithm is implemented for scheduling the hardware computer engineers for satisfy the professors over the time window. This paper suggest a heuristic fuzzy algorithm for hardware engineer's assignment in university sectors. By taking the advantage of the group structure of the given problem the proposed algorithm uses the genetic approach across the hardware engineer's schedules and within each hardware engineers and technicians in a university. The proposed approach shows the effective experimental results.

Keywords: Fuzzy algorithm · Hardware computer engineers · Technicians · University departments

1 Introduction

The scheduling the hardware engineers should satisfy as much as possible, the expectations of the professors and students as well as the university management. The hardware engineers schedule should be the actual times are close to the desired time needed for the users of the systems. The use of conventional method such as linear programming and basic dispatching techniques such as slack and first in first out is limited. The other methods also involve very difficult to implement because of rigid structure. The computer hardware engineers assignment problem characterised by the following features:

(a) The preferences of assigning the hardware engineers the fuzzy logic will be satisfied by the professors
(b) The expectations of the hardware engineers by the professors will depends upon the time windows
(c) Need to find out the solution for conflicting goals of the problem

The purpose of this research is to develop a fuzzy approach to assign a work to the hardware engineers in a university in an efficient way.

This article has been written with the financial support of RUSA - phase 2.0 grant sanctioned vide Letter No. F. 24-51/ 2014-U, Policy (TNMulti-Gen), Dept. of Edn. Gov. of India, Dt.09.10.2018.

T. Ahram et al. (Eds.): IHIET 2019, AISC 1018, pp. 222–227, 2020.
https://doi.org/10.1007/978-3-030-25629-6_35

2 Computer Hardware Engineers Assignment Problems

2.1 Problem Description

The Computer Hardware Engineers Assignment Problem (CEAP) is concerned with the allocation of a set of Hardware Engineers to the various departments in the university in an efficient manner. The essence of the problem in that all the tasks must be assigned, so that the nature of the tasks and their precedence relationships should satisfy. Normally the work assigned to the hardware engineers is often carried out manually using the excel sheets. The assignment task may be Internet Connectivity problem, System problem, Printer problem, sharing resource problem and Video conferencing setup can be categorised. The job assignment is classified into soft and hard constraints.

2.2 Problem Definition

Assigning the work to the hardware engineers by issuing the daily worksheet is called as hardware constraints, whereas by attending the service call from various departments in university is called as software constraints. The hardware constraints are connected with the parameters like task priority, hardware service engineer's availability at a particular time etc. The problem definition is following below

a index for A activities, a = 1, 2 …A; t index for T_t tasks in activity a, t = 1, 2………T; d_a Desirable due date of activity a; rt_a Release time of activity a;

t_{at} Starting time for hardware engineer t activity of a; $ct_{t1,t2}$ Change over time from task t1 to t2; P_{at} Expected processing time of task t of activity a.

Release Time Condition. The release time of a task for the hardware engineers to the earliest time when that particular task is ready for execution.

$$t_{at} \geq rt_a,\ \forall_{a,a} = 1,2.\ldots\ldots A;\ \forall_{t,t} = 1,2.\ldots\ldots T_t. \tag{1}$$

Precedence Condition. The precedence condition relates to the structural sequence of tasks that should be observed when executing specific tasks. It follows the succeeding hardware engineers service tasks that cannot be handled until their predecessors are finished.

$$t_{at-1} + p_{a,t-1} < t_{at},\ \forall_{a,a} = 1,2.\ldots\ldots A\ ,\ \forall_{t,t} = 1,2.\ldots T_a. \tag{2}$$

Capacity Condition. The capacity conditions limit the number of tasks that an h/w engineer can perform at any given time. In this case the h/w engineer can perform only one task at a time.

$$t_{a1,t1} + p_{a1,t1} + ct_{t1,t2} \leq t_{a2,t2}.$$

where t1 and t2 represent any two tasks from any activity to be performed by a specific h/w engineer.

The three type of software conditions are with due date to complete the assign work, task to change from one position to other and time taken to finish the work (Daily work sheet).

Precedence Condition. Precedence condition where the h/w engineer task cannot take the assign work until the previous task of the same h/w engineer work is finished.

Due date to complete the work. The due date condition ensures that the end time of each work is close to the desirable due date of activity. The due date restriction is expressed by

$$t_{at} + p_{at} \leq d_a, \; \forall_{a,a} = 1, 2.\ldots\ldots A \;, \; \forall_{t,t} = 1, 2.\ldots\ldots\ldots t_a.$$

Task to change from one position of work to another (change over time). These condition ensure that the task change from one position so another position of assigned work. There will be time gap between the succeeding assigned work and predecessor's assigned work.

$$t_{at2} \approx t_{at1} + p_{at1} + \text{change overtime a1a2}.$$

$$\forall_t, \forall_{t1}, \forall_{t2}.$$

Where v_1 and v_2 are same work assign to the h/w engineer a, and work t_2 can only start after t_1 is completed.

Daily worksheet condition

The daily worksheet condition shows that the assigned work to h/w engineer should be within the desired time which is stated in the work sheet condition. Time stated in the daily work sheet are T_a^1, T_a^2 where T_a^1 and T_a^2 are the lower and upper bounds on the expected execution time for the assigned work a

$$t_{at} \geq T_a^1 \text{ and } t_{at} + p_{at} \leq T_a^2, \; \forall_a \forall_t.$$

2.3 Problem Objectives

The objective is to maximise fairness in the work load assigned to the h/w engineer.

To minimize violation of software condition.

The proposed algorithm is an interactive decision making for the given problem.

3 Genetic Algorithm Approach for Grouping

Genetic grouping algorithm (Gga) is used to grouping genetic values (or) members. It uses the fuzzy theory to evaluate the performance of the alternative solutions. The grouping algorithm includes representation, Initialisation, Genetic operators and membership functions.

3.1 The Genetic Grouping Scheme

A coding scheme is developed to explore the group structure of the problem.

G = {1, 2, 3, 4, 5…….V} be the chromosome representing a set of V tasks to be performed by J h/w engineers. The calculation of G involves partitioning tasks along G into groups g such that all conditions should satisfied both the s/w and h/w conditions.

Let's assume that there are 10 departments in the university, given 10 tasks (V = 10) and assume that h/w engineers (I = 4). The grouping is shown below

$$(1, 2, 3, 4) \text{ - - - - - } y1 (5, 6) \text{ - - - - - - - - - - - - } y2 (7, 8, 9, 10) \text{ - - - - - - - } y3$$

3.2 Setting the Initial Value

Setting the initial value is assigned by either ascending order or priority basis. Normally the ascending order will be initiated to the hardware engineers and their expected start time. Unassigned tasks may also be initiated first for the hardware engineers.

3.3 Crossover Chromosome

The selection operator selects the best performing chromosomes in to a mating pool called tbest. Among various selection process each chromosome g is selected and stored in best according to its expected count e_c

$$e_c = \frac{Ft\ (s)}{1/ps \sum_{s=1}^{ps} F_t(s)}$$

Where p_s is the population size.

F_t (S = 1 P_s) is the fitness function of the Sth chromosome. Each chromosome receives copies equal to the integer part of e_c, plus additional copies obtained by using the fractional part of e_c as a success probability of getting an additional copy of chromosome S. The best performing candidates are selected with higher probability in to the best. The selection mechanism enables to explore unassigned task in the task table. Crossover point between 1 and g is randomly generated, where g is the number of groups. The groups on the right of the crossover points are interchanged. The offspring are repaired as necessary. The process is repeated till the desired pool size. Pool size is achieved the goal. After cross over some of the chromosomes may appear in more than one group while others may be missing. Offspring is used to repair the eliminating duplicated chromosomes on either side of the cross point.

3.4 Mutation

Mutation is applied to every new chromosome in two forms: interchange mutations and change mutations or shift mutations. Interchange mutation exchanges the genes between the two groups in an individual chromosomes, while change mutations moves a randomly chosen between two groups by shifting the variables one step to right or to the left.

3.5 Inversion

The population for the algorithm may prematurely converge to a particular result, thus the given population should be controlled. Inversion restructure the genes of a chromosome in the reverse order.

3.6 Heuristic Fuzzy Algorithm (HFA)

The overall algorithm combines the different operators, starting from the selecting the appropriate variables. The three main selected variables are cross over, mutation and inversion probability. The initial assigned variables are 0.25 to cross over, 0.01 to the mutation and 0.02 to the inversion probability. The algorithm starts with the taking the random variables for the assigning the hardware engineers. The HFA algorithm proceeds into a continuous loop structure which involves the three main variables cross over, mutation and inversion until condition satisfied for assigning the hardware engineer tasks.

4 Experiments and Results

4.1 Experiments

The algorithm was coded in IDL and R programming. Windows 10 Professional operating system, on an intel core I7-7700 processor (3.6GHZ up to 4.20GHZ), 8 MB L3 Cache, 32 GB DDR4. The performance of HFA algorithm was compared with genetic algorithm (GA) and particle swarm optimization (PSO) [1, 2].

4.2 Results

The below shows a transcription of the fitness values for a maximum of 300 iterations. The comparative performance of HFA against the PSO and GA shows that HFA outperforms the two competitive algorithms in terms of efficiency and the final fitness value (Table 1).

Table 1. Comparison of HFA, PSO and GA

No	Algorithm	CPU time seconds	Search success rate
1	HFA	3.6	95%
2	PSO	4.5	90%
3	GA	5.2	80%

The algorithm was tested for search success rate based on a hypothetical problems that consists of 10 hardware engineers and 40 departments with a known optimal solutions. HFA has a higher potential for efficient and effective performance. Hence this approach can be used efficiently assigning the staff and nurses in hospitals [3–6].

5 Conclusion

Higher the task achievement by the hardware engineers, the higher the task schedule be achieved. This problem demands the interactive method for fuzzy logic. By using the exploiting permutations of group of tasks across candidate task schedules and within each candidate schedule, using enhanced heuristic operators, the algorithm can address the problem efficiently. This approach provides useful contributions to researches and hardware engineers in universities.

References

1. Paulussen, T.O., Jennings, N.R., Decker, K.S., Henzl, A.: Distributed patient scheduling in hospitals. In: Proceedings of the 18th International Joint Conference on Artificial Intelligence, pp. 1224–1229 (2003)
2. Chang, M., Ozaku, H.I., Ota, J.: Nursing care scheduling problem. In: Proceedings of the 2007 IEEE International Conference on Systems and Cybernetics, SMC, pp. 1681–1687, October 2008
3. Bard, J.F., Purnomo, H.W.: Real-time scheduling for nurses in response to demand flutings and personnel shortages. In: Proceedings of the 5th International Conference on Scheduling: Theory & Applications (MISTA), pp. 397–406 (2005)
4. Vermeulen, I., Bohte, S., Somefun, K.: İmproving patient activity schedules by multi-agent Pareto appointment exchanging. In: Proceedings of the 8th IEEE Conference on E-Commerce Technology (CEC 06) (2006)
5. Aiken, L.H., Clarke, S.P., Sloane, D.M.: Hospital staffing organization and quality of care. Int. J. Qual. Health Care **14**(1), 5–13 (2002)
6. Chang, M., Ozaku, H.I., Ota, J.: Simulated annealing algorithm for scheduling problem in daily nursing cares. In: Proceedings of the IEEE International Conference on Robotics and Biometrics, Saniya, china, 15–18 December 2007

Research on Enterprise Security Early Warning System Architecture Based on Internet of Things

Liyun Lan, Yunjiang Liu, and Xuebo Chen(✉)

School of Electronic and Information Engineering,
University of Science and Technology Liaoning,
Anshan, Liaoning 114051, People's Republic of China
xuebochen@126.com

Abstract. Safety in production is the premise of sustainable development of enterprises. To better protect the safety of employees in enterprises, the enterprise security early warning system is established. Internet of things technology is introduced into the enterprise security early warning system. The connection between employee groups and enterprise safety early warning system can be realized by making employees wear the safety card. In this paper, the early warning rules of unsafe behavior are set up, the early warning processes of unsafe behavior are established. The enterprise safety early warning system is used to monitor and analyze employees' unsafe behavior, so as to give warning to employees before accidents occur. Therefore, the safety card undertake the function of warning employees. Based on three aspects of human, material and environment, the enterprise safety early warning system can minimize the occurrence of accidents and ensure the personal safety of enterprise employees.

Keywords: Internet of Things · Staff unsafe behavior early warning system · Behavior monitoring · Behavior analysis · Safety card

1 Introduction

The productive process of enterprises is complex, the productive line is long and has strong continuity. In some productive processes, there are not only the characteristics of high temperature, high pressure and high energy, but also the toxic, harmful, inflammable and explosive substances. Meanwhile, there are mechanical injuries such as falling objects and striking objects in the working environment of high building and mechanical processing [1, 2]. With the acceleration of modernization in China, enterprises have developed rapidly, but at the same time, the probability of major accidents such as fire, explosion, poisoning and leakage is increasing year by year. Starting from the law of accident occurrence, effective early warning of accident symptoms has become an important means to reduce accident losses [3].

With the rapid development of science and technology, Internet of Things has attracted more and more attentions. It has been listed in the national "Twelfth Five-Year Plan" technology development plan [4]. It has played an active role in demonstration projects in the fields of national defense, military, smart grid, intelligent

T. Ahram et al. (Eds.): IHIET 2019, AISC 1018, pp. 228–233, 2020.
https://doi.org/10.1007/978-3-030-25629-6_36

transportation, smart home, medical and health [5, 6]. Introducing Internet of Things technology into the enterprise accident early warning system will certainly give full play to its technological advantages [3, 7–9]. At present, the enterprise accident early warning system has become more and more mature, but most employees' unsafe behaviors are still in the post-event analysis stage. The design of the safety card makes the post-event analysis turn into in-event analysis and early warning. It can alert employees more accurately and in real time, in order to reduce the probability of accidents.

2 Construction of Enterprise Security Early Warning System

2.1 Enterprise Accident Early Warning System Architecture Based on Internet of Things

This section briefly introduces the architecture of enterprise security early warning system based on Internet of Things technology. Safety early warning system is a timely prediction and early warning of accident omen. It can take countermeasures to solve the danger and prevent the eventual occurrence of accidents. Internet of Things (IOT) is a product of the information age, which provides new ideological guidance and strong technical support for enterprise security early warning system.

The architecture of enterprise security early warning system based on the Internet of Things takes the Internet of Things framework as the model. The framework of enterprise accident early warning system based on Internet of Things technology is shown in Fig. 1.

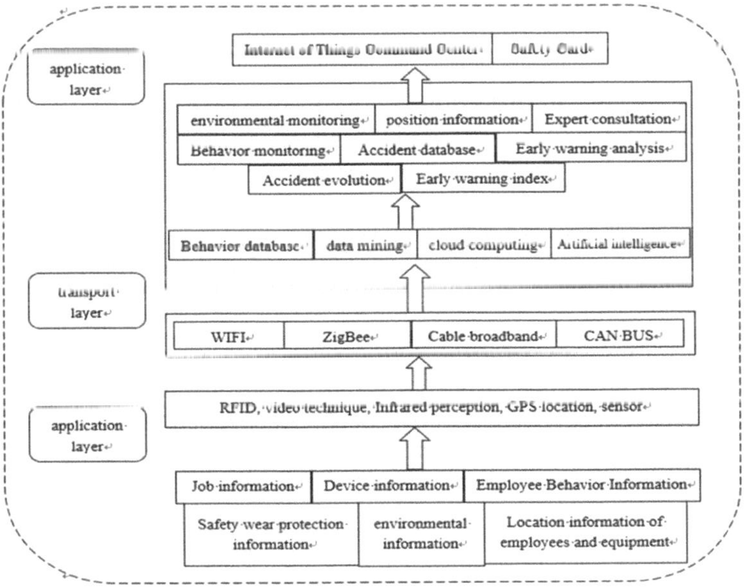

Fig. 1. Enterprise accident early warning architecture based on Internet of Things

2.2 Three Kinds of Unsafe Behaviors of Employees in Enterprises

Safety production is the premise of sustainable development of enterprises. Hein Hilary believes that more than 88% of safety accidents in enterprises are caused by people's unsafe behavior [10]. A large number of accident investigation results also show that the vast majority of safety accidents are caused directly by people's unsafe behaviors. Therefore, relying on the construction of enterprise accident early warning system, the establishment of employees' unsafe behavior early warning subsystem, focusing on employees' unsafe behavior early warning [11].

In view of unsafe behaviors, the Classification Criteria of Casualty Accidents for Employees in GB6441-86 Enterprises gives a simple definition: unsafe behaviors refer to human errors that can cause accidents [12].

This paper divides the unsafe behaviors of enterprise safety production into three categories.

(1) The use of protective articles is not regulated and operation without personal safety protector.
(2) Close to dangerous areas; Work in an unsafe place; Unauthorized access to non-post area; Do not keep safe distance.
(3) Illegal operation; Erroneous operation; An act of inattention.

2.3 Early Warning Rules and Procedures for Unsafe Behaviors

According to the type of unsafe behaviors, the corresponding early warning rules are formulated.

(1) Non-standard early warning rules for safety protector

①Input the information of employees' rights and safety protector into the system in advance.

②By reading and calculating the data of the tags worn on the employees and the tags assembled on the safety equipment through the tag recognizer set at the entrance and exit of the production area, the positions of the employees can be identified and determine whether the employees have the right to enter the area.

③Judge the safety protector that the employee needs to wear according to the position of the employee, and check whether the employee wears the safety articles required by symbols according to the regulations. The non-standard warning process for safety supplies is shown in Fig. 2.

(2) Early warning rules for approaching dangerous areas

Through GPS positioning and tracking technology, the location information of employees is searched in real time, and the distance between employees and dangerous areas is calculated whether it exceeds the safe range, so as to judge whether the location of workers is appropriate, and timely alarm.

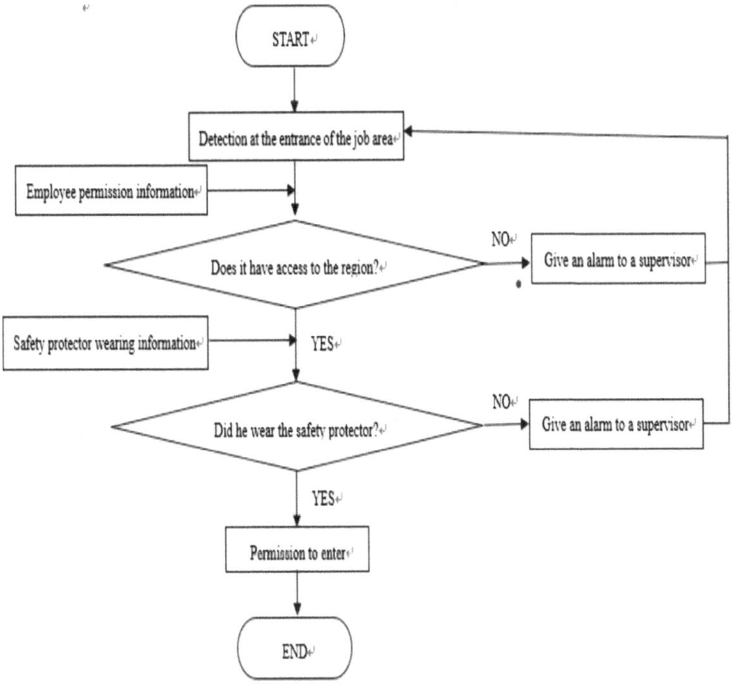

Fig. 2. Flow chart of nonstandard warning for safety supplies

(3) Early warning rules for illegal operations

Firstly, according to the operation criteria of safety production in enterprises, the type of operation behavior is defined, and according to the object characteristics and behavior characteristics designed by various types of operation behaviors, the corresponding illegal operation model library is established. Secondly, through video surveillance, by means of video analysis technology, the operator's operation can be analyzed whether it conforms to the operation specification. Then which are in accordance with the rules and regulations of safety and which are not can be further defined. In the process of safety production in the future, the model base is improved by machine intelligent learning, so as to realize early warning of illegal operations.

The process of early warning for illegal operations is shown in Fig. 3.

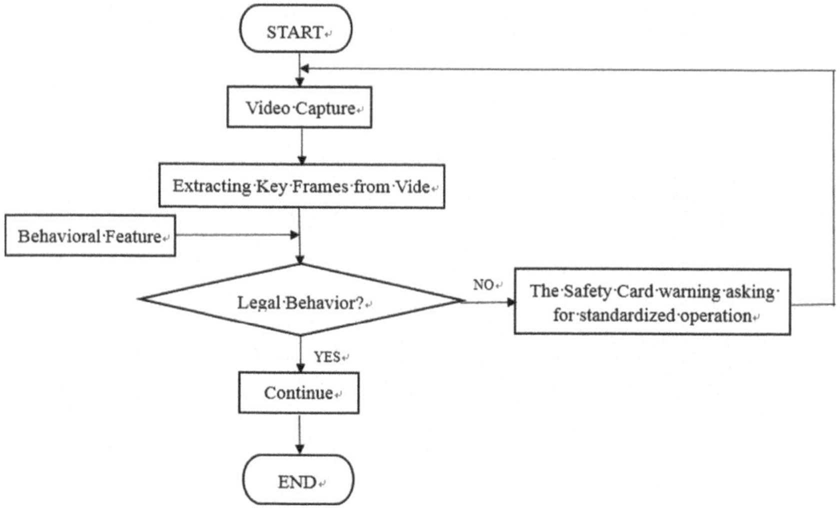

Fig. 3. Flow chart for early warning of illegal operations

3 Conclusions

With the development of science and technology, Internet of Things technology is also gradually improving. The application of Internet of Things technology in behavioral safety management system will continue to deepen. The application of Internet of Things technology in the early warning system of accidents, real-time dynamic monitoring of enterprise production, and reasonable control measures for early warning accident symptoms will be adopted, so as to reduce the occurrence of accidents, achieve "feeling-perception-control" —— the scientific and procedural management and ensure the rapid growth of enterprises.

The construction of the early warning system based on Internet of Things is a long-term system engineering, and many problems still need to be faced in the construction project [6]. Therefore, these need enterprises and relevant research institutions to constantly explore in production.

Acknowledgments. This research reported herein was supported by the NSFC of China under Grants No.71571091 and 71771112.

References

1. Wang, S.M.: Management of major hazard sources in China's safe production. J. Jin Ling Inst. Technol. **32**(2), 48–51 (2016). (in Chinese)
2. Hang, M.G.: Research on control and management of production risk source in thermal power plant. J. Telecom World **11**, 158–159 (2017). (in Chinese)

3. Xu, Y.G., Chen, X.B., Sun, Q.B.: Construction of the early warning system of employee unsafe behavior. J. Process. Autom. Instrum. **38**(6), 56–58 (2017). (in Chinese)
4. https://baike.baidu.com/item
5. Hu, D.T.: Study on non-coal underground mine safety monitoring early-warning and decision platform based on IOT. In: School of Resources and Environmental Engineering, Wuhan University of Technology (2014). (in Chinese)
6. Ma, J.: Focus on internet: application of mobile terminal plentiful Internet of things. J. World Telecom **7**, 44–49 (2011). (in Chinese)
7. Liu, Z.D., Li, P.F.: Research on accident early warning system for metallurgical enterprises based on internet of thing. J. Saf. Environ. Eng. **22**(2), 88–91 (2015). (in Chinese)
8. Shi, J.Z., Wang, L.L.: Research on the application of the internet of things in the field of safety production. J. Energy Technol. Manag. **6**, 99–100 (2010). (in Chinese)
9. Zhang, Y.: Target recognition and abnormal behavior modeling and analysis in intelligent video monitoring. In: Institutes of Image Processing and Pattern Recognition Shanghai Jiao Tong University (2010). (in Chinese)
10. Xie, Y.H.: Misunderstandings and countermeasures for the prevention of unsafe behavior. J. Mod. Occup. Saf. **3**, 20–23 (2016). (in Chinese)
11. Liu, M., Sun, X.H., Yang, W.Y.: Analysis and control of unsafe behavior. J. Environ. Prot. Xinjiang **1**, 60–61 (2008). (in Chinese)
12. Liu, T.S.: The discuss of unsafe behavior in safety management. J. West-China Explor. Eng. **17**(6), 226–228 (2005). (in Chinese)

An Optimal Real-Time Solution for Limited-TSP: Using Smart Algorithms to Find an Optimal TSP Real-Time Solution Over Limited Destinations

Hatem F. Halaoui(✉)

Computer Science, Haigazian University, Beirut, Lebanon
hhalaoui@haigazian.edu.lb

Abstract. TSP, the Traveling Salesman Problem is a famous hard problem in computer science. Finding an optimal solution for TSP in a map consisting of huge number of locations will take huge amount of time (possibly years). A traveller (salesman) needs to visit a limited number of locations out of these thousands locations (each building is an address or location). It is desirable to solve TSP efficiently with real-time factors (traffic, distance, real-time delays). Online applications like Google maps, Yahoo maps, and many others do not give efficient solutions for a multiple-destinations queries. Minimizing the number of locations to exactly the number of destinations asked in the query (by the traveller) will make the optimal hard solution time-acceptable. This paper uses smart heuristics, intelligent algorithm A*, traditional graph Hamilton circuit algorithm, as well as efficient data structures to finding an efficient cycle path between multiple addresses, and hence finding and optimal solution for TSP in real-time. The main idea is to build a virtual graph VG built from a minimized list of vertices (equals exactly to desired list of destinations) and a list of virtual edges that are computed using the smart algorithms A*.

Keywords: A* algorithm · Traveling Salesman Problem · Intelligent navigation algorithms · Hamilton circuit

1 Introduction and Background

Navigating multiple locations is one common task for many users. In many cases, these users desire to visit them in a single trip. The proposal in this paper offers a real-time optimal solution for such queries. The main topics behind the proposed approach are presented in this section: The Travelling Salesman Problem (TSP), heuristics and navigation with heuristics.

1.1 Tsp

The Travelling Salesman Problem (TSP) [11], was defined by the Irish mathematician Hamilton and by the British mathematician Kirkman in the 1800s. It presents the problem of a traveler (salesman) who needs to navigate between a certain number of

T. Ahram et al. (Eds.): IHIET 2019, AISC 1018, pp. 234–239, 2020.
https://doi.org/10.1007/978-3-030-25629-6_37

locations (in any order) in one trip starting and ending back at the start location taking the shortest path. Finding the optimal solution for the TSP, with high number of map vertices, using traditional algorithms is time consuming (exponential) and not applicable in real-time problem. To solve the problem, the number of vertices in the graph has to be limited to the number of desired destinations.

1.2 Heuristics in Navigation and Hamilton Circuit

Heuristics is the process of gaining knowledge by intelligent guess [3]. Daily people activities involve heuristic solutions. When using maps, moving from one location to next location and finally reach a destination, the algorithm guesses the next move intelligently using an evaluation function. This paper presents a real-time optimal solution for TSP. Moreover, calculating the shortest or fastest path with algorithms like Hamilton path [1] is exponential time (high complexity) for real-time large graphs. Hence, use heuristic smart algorithms like A* to minimize the graph size which hence minimizes running time.

The paper is organized as follows: Sect. 2 presents related work and used applications. Section 3 presents the main proposal of this paper.

2 Related Work and Background Algorithms

This section presents some definitions, notations, and algorithms, used in the solution.

2.1 Artificial Intelligent Heuristic Algorithm A*

A* [2] is an Artificial Intelligent graph algorithm proposed by Pearl. A* aims is to find an optimal efficient graph path between two locations in a graph using a smart heuristic function. The heuristic evaluation function's main goal to minimize the problem next choices according to intelligent criterion. The heuristic function is H (V1, V2) is defined as follows:

Input: a source vertex V1 and a destination V2.
Task: evaluate V1 based on the Destination V2 using the following heuristic function:
Travelled_So_Far + Stright_Line_Distance (V1, V2) Where,
Travelled_So_Far = Real distance taken so far to reach the vertex V1
Stright_Line_Distance (V1, V2) = straight line distance from V1 to destination V2 calculated by using their coordinates.

The A* Algorithm
A*(Graph G, Source S, Destination D)
Task: takes a Graph G, Source S and Destination D and returns the optimal path solution from S to D.

- If S = D, then return solution
- Else expand unvisited neighbours (Ni) of S

- Mark S as visited
- For each Ni
  - Get Vi = H (Ni, D)
  - Add all (Ni, Vi) to the Fringe (list of all expanded Vertices)
  - From the Fringe, Choose an Unvisited Vertex V with Least Vi
  - If no more Unvisited, return Failure
  - Else Apply A*(V, D)

The time complexity is O(n^2) [2].

Figure 1 is an example of the A* behaviour finding a path from "Arad" to "Bucharest" in Romania [2]. First, start at Arad and go to the next neighbour with the best heuristic function (Sibiu). Then, explore all neighbour of Sibiu based on the heuristic function. The algorithm continues until it reaches Bucharest.

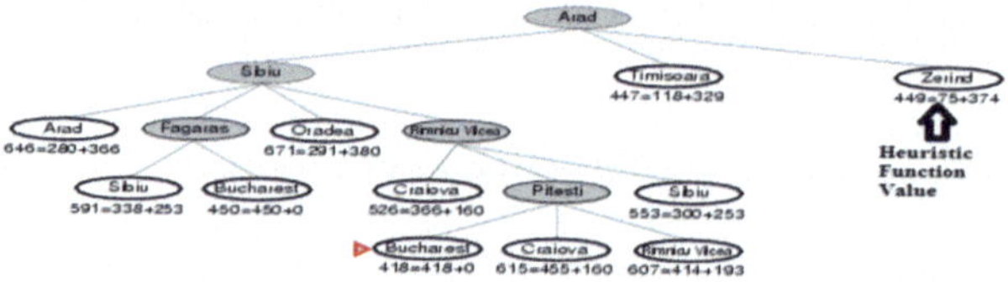

Fig. 1. Calculating the path from Arad to Bucharest

Russell and Norvig [2] present the proof of A* optimality.

2.2 Definitions

Graph definitions, algorithms, and related work are presented in this section. For, each algorithm, the time-complexities is briefly stated.

Hamilton Circuit [1]: A path (presented in red in Fig. 2) that passes over all the graph vertices once returning back to the source node. The source is the only vertex that is visited twice.

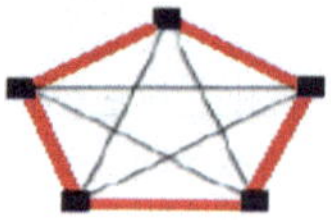

Fig. 2. Hamilton circuit

A*Multiple [10] is a previous work aims to find the shortest path (least time) to visit a desired list of destinations in one trip. Each step, the algorithm uses a smart heuristic function to find the next destination (move).

Algorithm 1. **A*Multiple (Source, Destinations)**

Task: returns an efficient path from source passing over all in Destinations array.
Returns: a list of destinations (VSL) and a list of paths (PSL).

VSL: An ordered list of vertices that the desired path follows in the trip.
PSL: Path Solution List PSL, which is the list of paths to take each time to each destination (vertex) from a vertex in the list VSL to another in the same list.

How does A*Multiple Work?
This section presents the execution of A*Multiple. To present the proposed approach better, consider the following problem: Suppose the user is at Nice Airport and want to visit the following destinations in Nice: Promenade des Anglais, Grande Corniche, Notre-Dame de Nice and Port Lympia. As time or distance, means that visitng them in any order with efficient time. In this case, choosing the next destination (at each step) shall be done smartly. The A*Multiple will return the following:
VSL: Nice Airport, Promenade des Anglais, Port Lympia, Notre-Dame de Nice, Grande Corniche
PSL: Path1 (orange), Path2(blue), Path3(pink), Path4(yellow). See Fig. 3

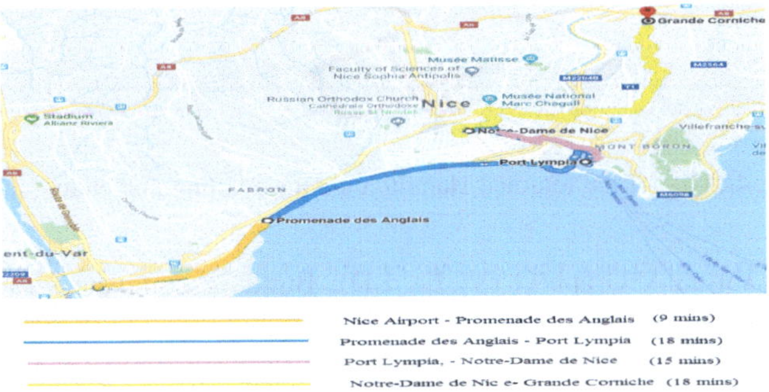

Fig. 3. Paths for multiple destinations (Nice Airport, Promenade des Anglais, Port Lympia, Notre-Dame de Nice, Grande Corniche)

3 SmartA*TSP

SmartA*TSP presents the solution to navigate a multiple destinations path starting and ending at the same location. The approach runs as follows:

- Given: Graph G, destination list DL repressing, and Source S.
- Build a new virtual complete Graph VG1 with vertices V1 = DL + S and virtual edges VE = {(xi, yi),..}. Edges (xi, yi) are paths computed using A*.
- For each valid Hamilton Circuit starting and ending at S, check its validity.
- Choose the shortest Valid Hamilton Circuit.

VG, the virtual graph, is a dramatically minimized version of V (much less number of vertices and edges of the graph) where Hamilton path algorithm is to be applied. In order to present a formal algorithm of the proposed approach, SmartA*TSP, the following algorithms are presented:

Algorithm 2. HamiltonCircuit (G (V, E), S): returns the shortest Hamilton circuit in graph G starting and ending at the same given Source location S ($\in$V).

Returns OL: An ordered list of vertices which is Hamilton Circuit starting and ending at the starting location S.

1. Get all possible permutations (LSP_i) of n vertices in V.
2. SP = Select all permutations that start with S.
3. Add S to the end of each list in SP
4. Choose the valid permutations from SP (valid edges)
5. Choose the shortest one from step 4

Algorithm 2 time Complexity: Step1: n! (n is the number of vertices), Step2: n!, Step3: n!, Step4: n^2 * n!, and Step5: n. Total time is approximately (n^2 + 4) n! which is exponential-time algorithm O(n!). For Large n's it is time consuming. Figure 4 presents one of the results (out of many).

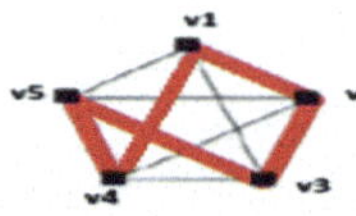

Fig. 4. One of the returned Hamilton circuits starting and ending at v1

Algorithm 3. VirtualA*Graph(G (V, E), LD): Builds a complete virtual graph VG using A*.
G: Graph (vertices V, Edges E), LD: Desired list of destinations ($\in$ V)
Returns VG (V1, VE): a virtual complete graph (list of vertices V1, List of virtual edges VE). Each virtual edge in VE refers to a path returned by the A* algorithm.

1. For each Vi in LD.
2. Use A* to compute the paths from Vi to all other vertices. Add them to VE.
3. Finally, LD and VE are used to build the VG (V1, VE).

Step1: O (m*n^2), where m is the number of vertices LD and n^2 is A* time complexity, Step2: O (m^2), and Step3 is constant. As a result, it will be O (n^2).

The edges in Fig. 5 (left) are built using A*. Edge (v1, v5) with weight 45 in Fig. 5 (left) represents a real path p1 calculated using A* algorithm. Figure 5 (right) is an example of the virtual complete graph with edges representing paths calculated with A*. There will be another 24 options. The shortest will be chosen.

Algorithm 4. SmartA*TSP (Graph G (V, E), LD, S): returns the shortest Path from a starting location S travelling over all requested destinations in LD. Algorithms 2 and 3 are used to build the virtual graph (algorithm 3) and then apply Hamilton Circuit (algorithm 2) on it.

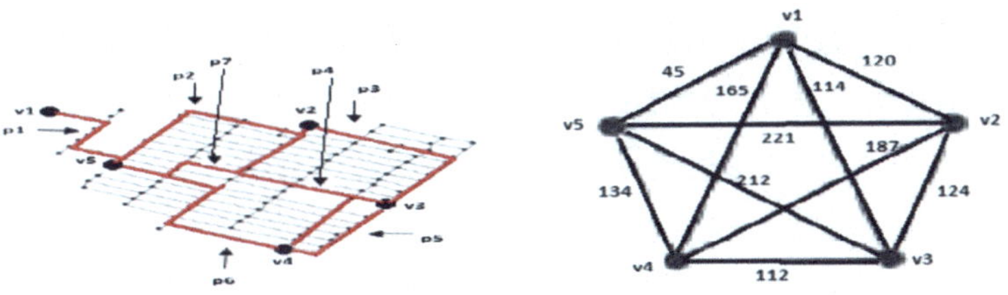

Fig. 5. Paths calculated using A* and Transformed into complete virtual graph

G: Real Graph representing real map with list of vertices V and list of edges E
S: Starting source Vertex (∈V)
LD: Desired destinations list (LD subset of V)

1- Build the virtual graph VG (Vi, VE) using VirtualA*Graph(G, LD) (Algorithm 3)
2- HPath = HamiltonCircuit (VG, S) (Returns the shortest Hamilton Circuit in VG that start with source S∈Vi)

Algorithm 4, time complexity is in O (n^2 + m!).
For small m's (<= 9), its maximum time will be around 1 s (9! = 3,628,80 steps). Accordingly, SmartA*TSP time complexity is real-time acceptable.

References

1. Ross, K., Wright, C.: Discrete Mathematics. Prentice Hall, Upper Saddle River, New Jersey (2003)
2. Russell, S., Norving, P.: Artificial Intelligence a Modern Approach. Prentice Hall, Upper Saddle River, New Jersey (2003)
3. Pearl, J.: Heuristics: Intelligent Search Strategies for computer Problem Solving. Addison Wesley, Reading, MA (1984)
4. Halaoui, H.: Smart Traffic Online System (STOS): Presenting road networks with time-weighted graphs. In: IEEE International Conference on Information Society (i-Society 2010) London, UK, June 2010, pp. 349–356
5. Google Earth Blog Google Earth Data Size, Live Local, New languages coming. http://whatis.techtarget.com/definition/Google-Maps. Accessed September 2015
6. Halaoui, H.: Smart traffic systems: dynamic A*Traffic in GIS driving paths applications. In: Proceeding of IEEE CSIE09, IEEE, Los Angeles, USA. March 2009, pp. 626–630
7. Halaoui, H.: Intelligent traffic system: road networks with time-weighted graphs. Int. J. Infonomics (IJI) **3**(4), 350–359 (2010)
8. Google Maps. https://www.google.com/. Accessed September 2015
9. Halaoui, H.: Spatial and spatio-temporal databases modeling: approaches for modeling and indexing spatial and spatio-temporal databases. VDM Verlag (2009)
10. Halaoui, H.: SMART navigation: using artificial intelligent heuristics in navigating multiple destinations. In: Proceedings of SOTICS 2015 (The Fifth International Conference on Social Media Technologies, Communication, and Informatics). Barcelona, Spain. November 2015
11. Lawler, E.L., Lenstra, J.K., Rinooy Kan, A.H.G., Shmoys, D.B. (eds.): The Traveling Salesman Problem, pp. 145–180. Wiley, Chichester (1985)

The Impact of Different Levels of Creative Thinking Members in Group Collaboration Based on Semantic Link

Zhengyu Wang(✉), Meiyu Zhou, and Xiangyu Liu

East China University of Science and Technology, No. 130, Meilong Road, Xuhui District, Shanghai, People's Republic of China
753501966@qq.com

Abstract. Based on the analysis of the semantic information in the process of team design task and its internal link representation, this paper makes a visual analysis of the performance of members with different creativity and evaluates them from multiple dimensions, so as to provide a visual reference basis for fuzzy and complex design tasks.

Keywords: Semantic link · Design cognitive · Creative thinking · Group collaboration

1 Introduction

Most of the traditional design activities of innovation and insight from the design of the long-term accumulation [1], nowadays, Some scholars have discovered the importance of the relationship between design information to design innovation [2], Yang, K. & Li proposed a theory of design knowledge network construction, data mining and knowledge reuse based on complex network theory, Xu, J. & Wang, X.Y. established a multidimensional cognitive model integrating data link, process link and concept link from the perspective of cognitive semantic inference design and linkography structure theory, however, these studies only focus on innovative itself, but ignore the influence of members' creativity, Although many researchers have explored the influence of personal ability on team design, such as the difference between the analogical reasoning creativity of novice designers and experts [3], and the influence of personal ability on team design [4], However, there are few researches on creativity and team design, and most of them focus on qualitative research [5]. Based on the qualitative research method, this study mines, analyzes and evaluates the semantic information of members with different creativity in team design through semantic link and its internal link representation, and evaluates team members from multiple dimensions, providing visual reference basis for fuzzy and complex design tasks.

T. Ahram et al. (Eds.): IHIET 2019, AISC 1018, pp. 240–246, 2020.
https://doi.org/10.1007/978-3-030-25629-6_38

2 Creativity Assessment and Semantic Information Network

TTCT scale was used to evaluate the subjects' creativity in three dimensions: fluency, creativity and originality. Semantic information linkography, link structure coding and C-K coding were used to build the semantic information network, and the complex link situation of each node in the semantic information network was analyzed through the deterministic information t-code theory, so as to obtain the node data information.

2.1 Creativity Assessment

The Torrance creative thinking test (TTCT) is the most widely used and most frequently cited creativity test scale [6]. Compared with other scales, TTCT has a larger span of target population [7] and can greatly reduce subjective errors [8]. Besides, TTCT has been proved to be applicable in China [9].

2.2 Linkography

Linkography was first put forward by Goldschmidt [10] and other scholars have suggested that the evaluation of designer and his team is an effective means of design thinking level [11]. To build the linkography, the non-social semantic data should be sequentially coded, these separate coding to represent the dynamic evolution of the concept of design in the process of design, through the design concept of correlation to determine whether there is a correlation between nodes, correlation degree is higher, if the two links the attachment, and according to the order of design node labeled with in turn (Fig. 1).

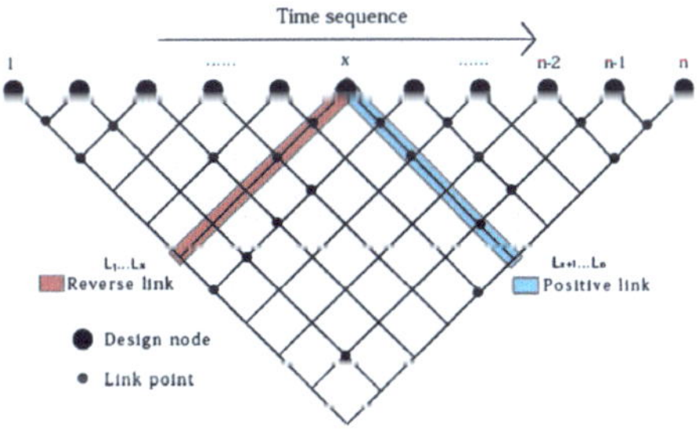

Fig. 1. Linkography

2.3 C - K Coding

Concept-Knowledge theory is a theory that studies the reasoning process of design. Used to distinguish C (concept space) and K (knowledge space) in the process of design [11]. The inspiration of new concepts in the design task process requires continuous learning of knowledge and selection of feasibility knowledge until the end of the design, By adding C-K theory, it can distinguish the nature of nodes, understand the evolution of node design concept, expand the content space of linkography, and to delve the hidden data through analysis.

3 Design Cognitive Information Analysis Methods

In this study, the deterministic information theory T-code [12] is adopted to process the data, and computes the number of steps required to build the string (which is composed of the reverse link and positive link), so as to calculate the complexity (T_c), information content (T_i) and entropy (T_e) in the data.

$$T_c = \sum_{i=1} \log_2(k_i + 1) \tag{1}$$

$$T_i = l_i^{-1}(T_c) \tag{2}$$

$$T_e = T_i/\|x\| \tag{3}$$

In the formula, i represent the number of decomposition, K_i represent the repetitions of string pattern, ||x|| represents the length of the string, T_c is mainly used to calculate the complexity of nodes and links to other nodes, T_i is used to characterize the complexity of the design process, the higher value represents the more complex the character pattern characterized by T_e, high entropy value node usually indicates the transition concept or turning the formation of the concept, or design concept developed to a new stage; However, low-entropy node is a concept of aggregation or a new concept generated. Potential new concepts may be obtained through the mining of this node, and the difference between extreme points of entropy value represents the difference between former and late concepts [2].

4 The Experiment

There are two experiments in the experiment section. The TTCT creative thinking test is mainly carried out on the subjects in experiment 1, Its main purpose to screen subjects with different levels of creative thinking for the experiment 2 team collaborative design task.

4.1 Experiment 1

55 subjects (41 male 14 female, aged 22–25) of the same background (industrial design, first-year graduate) were tested using the same TTCT test, get effective 48 questionnaire, through the TTCT manual scoring criteria for grading [9], through overall arrangement and the determination of the expert group, the subjects were divided into A (high), B (middle), C (lower), three different creativity level interval, and 2 subjects were selected from each level, and a total of 6 subjects formed a design group to participate in experiment 2.

4.2 Experiment 2

6 subjects (2 male, 4 female, aged 23–24) to form the design team, design the elderly flushing toilet, drawing and language communication were adopted to discuss the specific solution of the design task. The experiment time was set at 90 min, reflect on the design until a complete design is achieved. The voice data was collected with recording device and converted into text data. The dialogue related to the design task was processed and coded, and 128 semantic nodes were obtained.

5 Analysis of Experimental Results

The data of node link was quantified into matrix $L_{(128\times128)}$, the linkography was drawn, and the node complexity T_c, information content T_i and entropy T_e were calculated and analyzed, and the data fluctuation chart was derived. As shown in Figs. 3, 4, With the transition the design stage, the overall value shows a trend of fluctuation, but the overall trend is stable, It can be seen that the design process has better fluency, integrity and less backtracking, the node N_5 entropy value of 0.32, N_5 presents the design of toilet should focus on the process of the elderly security and sat down (Fig. 2).

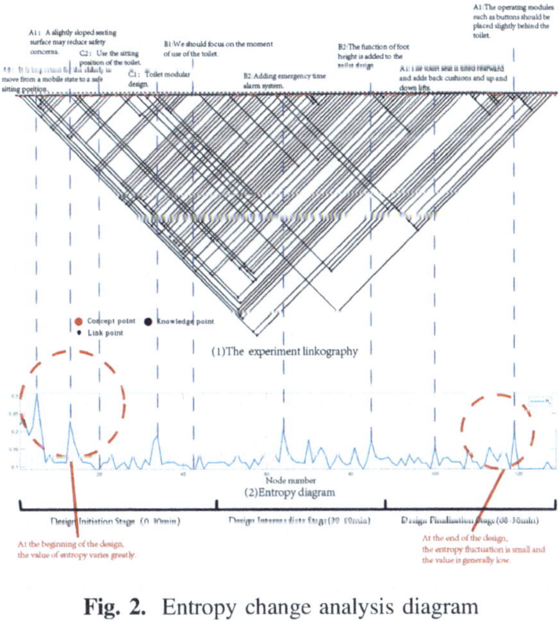

Fig. 2. Entropy change analysis diagram

This node provides a lot of thinking guidance for the subsequent design development, node N_{20}, N_{27}, N_{30}, N_{54}, N_{99} minimum entropy, are less than 0.1, the node entropy is low and has no link, N_{64} node is an important node in the middle stage of

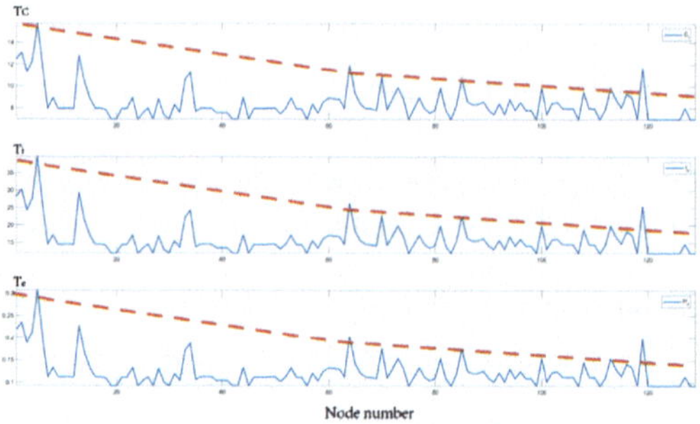

Fig. 3. Data wave pattern

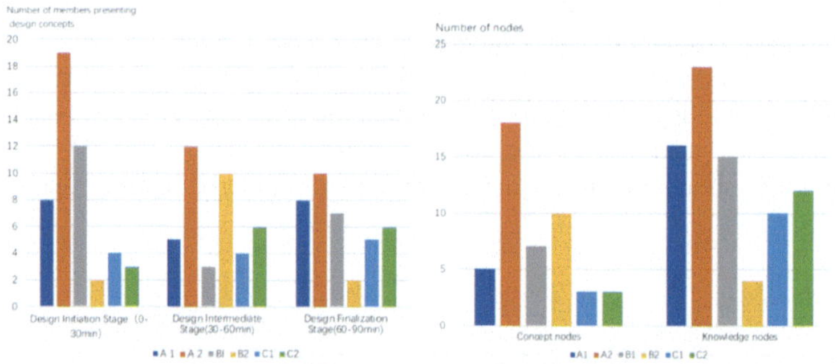

(1) Conceptual quantity diagram of different members in each stage

(2) C-K Numbers for different members

Fig. 4. Node information comparison diagram for different members

design. This node proposes to add the toilet emergency system. Although there is no node in the reverse link of this node, it has great inspiration for the subsequent design and plays a role of local innovation and connecting the preceding and the following in the overall design.

In the number of concept nodes, Group A was basically higher than group B, C and the trend of overall data appear the phenomenon of decline, shows that with the development of design, the amount of design information provided by group A gradually decreased, but the overall number was still higher than the other two groups, the number of concepts provided by group B is in the middle and the overall data showed A trend of contrary, in the intermediate stage of design, the number of concepts provided by B1 decreased obviously, while B2 increased obviously, by analyzing the information provided by B1 in the intermediate stage of design, found that even though the number information is less, but the quality of information coding node is higher, with more node links and larger tribute provided at this stage, the overall data of the subjects in group C showed a trend of gradual increase. The team members provided less information at the initiation of the design phase and gradually increased in the intermediate and finalization stages. In terms of the number of C-K nodes, the analysis showed that the subjects in group A had the highest number of concept nodes, followed by group B and group C, at the knowledge node, the subjects in group A are the highest, followed by group C and group B are the lowest, indicating that group C is superior to group B in providing knowledge information. On the concept of innovation, according to the comprehensive analysis of Figs. 2, 3 and 4, and the judgment of the entropy value and c-k code of the nodes proposed by different team members, it is found that the subjects in group A are more active in team design, and there are more critical creative ideas and creative ideas proposed, such as N_2, N_6, N_{13}, N_{33} etc, from the perspective of the performance of group B, this group plays a key role in inspiring key ideas in team design, for example, the proposal of N_{64} or other nodes can provide great inspiration for subsequent design and promote the development of design, the nodes proposed by group C members in the team design are mostly distributed around the innovation concept, and the contents are mostly complementary to the innovation concept, and the number of knowledge nodes is large, which can provide knowledge supplement for concept nodes and promote the development of design concepts.

6 Conclusion

This paper makes a visual analysis of the performance of members with different levels of creativity in team collaborative design tasks, and by using a new design cognition research method to obtain the complexity, formation content and entropy of the design nodes and then capture the tacit knowledge in the design process, Promote the scientific composition of design teams with the same background, improve the efficiency of design cognitive computing research, and provide visual reference for complex design tasks.

References

1. Yang, K., Li, Y., Xiong, Y., et al.: Product innovation design driven by knowledge based on complex network. Comput. Integr. Manuf. Syst. **21**(9), 2257–2269 (2015). (in Chinese)
2. Xu, J., et al.: Design cognitive complexity calculation method based on deterministic information theory. China Mech. Eng. **28**(5), 596–602 (2017). (in Chinese)
3. Ozkan, O., Dogan, F.: Cognitive strategies of analogical reasoning in design: differences between expert and novice designers. Des. Stud. **34**(2), 161–192 (2013)
4. Tindale, R.S., Larson, J.R.: Assembly bonus effect or typical group performance? a comment on Michaelsen, Watson, and Black (1989). J. Appl. Psychol. **77**(1), 102–105 (1992)
5. Vasconcelos, L.A., Crilly, N.: Inspiration and fixation: questions, methods, findings, and challenges. Des. Stud. **42**, 1–32 (2016)
6. Lissitz, R.W., Willhoft, J.L.: A methodological study of the torrance tests of creativity. J. Educ. Meas. **22**(1), 1–11 (1985)
7. Fishkin, A.S., Johnson, A.S.: Who is creative? identifying children's creative abilities. Roeper Rev. **21**(1), 40–46 (1998)
8. Kim, K.H., et al.: Can we trust creativity tests? a review of the torrance tests of creative thinking (TTCT). Creat. Res. J. **18**(1), 3–14 (2006)
9. Wu, J.J., Gao, Q.D., Wang, J.R., et al.: The Torrance tests of creative thinking norms-technical manual figural forms, pp. 1–64. Yuan Liu Publishing, Taiwan (1981). (in Chinese)

10. Goldschmidt, G., Anat, L.S.: Inspiring design ideas with texts. Design Studies **2**(2), 139–155 (2011)
11. Xu, J., et al.: Design cognition multidimensional modeling method based on semantic link. Chin. J. Mech. Eng. **53**(15), 32–39 (2017). (in Chinese)
12. EL-Khouly, T.: Creative discovery in architectural design processes: an empirical study of procedural and contextual components. London University, London (2015)

Solving Game Theory Problems Using Linear Programming and Genetic Algorithms

Marwan Abdul Hameed Ashour[1,2,3(✉)], Iman A. H. Al-Dahhan[1,2,3], and Sahar M. A. Al-Qabily[1,2,3]

[1] College of Administration and Economics University of Baghdad, Baghdad, Iraq
dr_marwan2012@yahoo.com, Iman.Saeed@dcec.uobaghdad.edu.iq
[2] Continuing Education Center/University of Bagdad, Baghdad, Iraq
[3] Business Economics College Al-Nahrain University, Baghdad, Iraq

Abstract. In this paper, we proposed an efficient genetic algorithm that will be applied to linear programming problems in order to find out the Fittest Chromosomes. This paper aim to find the optimal strategy of game theory in basketball by using genetic algorithms and linear programming as well as the comparison between traditional methods and modern methods being represented in artificial intelligence, Genetic algorithms as applied in this paper. A new method was adopted in finding the optimal game strategy for player (A) and player (B) through the application of linear programming and finding solutions by using (GA) in MATLAB. The final results confirmed the equivalent of linear programming and genetic algorithms as the model was in the linear approach, and in the case of nonlinearity, genetic algorithm will be in favor definitely. The Matlab program in the calculation of the results for great possibility optimization should also be adopted.

Keywords: Game theory · Genetic Algorithm · Linear Programming · Optimal strategy

1 Introduction

The internal consistency and mathematical foundations of game theory make it a prime tool for modeling and designing automated decision-making processes in the interactive environments [11]. As a mathematical tool for the decision-maker, the strength of game theory is the methodology which provides structuring and analyzing problems of strategic choices [3]. The process of formally modeling a situation as a game requires the decision-maker to enumerate explicitly the players and their strategic options, and to consider their preference smooth reactions [7].

The beginning of the 20th century could be considered as the inception of the extensive use of mathematical models and optimization fields. Optimization consists of numerous fields, such as operations research, artificial intelligence, and even computer sciences [11]. Therefore, these fields together could help us to improve the efficiency of

T. Ahram et al. (Eds.): IHIET 2019, AISC 1018, pp. 247–252, 2020.
https://doi.org/10.1007/978-3-030-25629-6_39

industries, especially practical ones. Holland introduced the Genetic Algorithm (GA) as the first evolutionary algorithm for global optimization using chromosomes and their genes [2].

In this paper, we're going to introduce an optimization algorithm based on team game strategies involving basketball. Team games have to follow several straight forward rules which are vital for them to succeed. Genetic Algorithm (GA) mimics all the processes based on the concept of natural evolution to find the optimum solution to the given problem residing in the search space. The GA pool contains a number of individuals called chromosomes.

2 Game Theory

The term game represents competition or conflict between two or more different players, each of which has a specific or an unspecified number of strategies [12]. Each opponent tries to maximize his decision at the expense of the other opponent and his decision affects the value of return of the other opponent [2]. Basketball is one of the teamwork games which each individual player plays a strategic role in generating and choosing the most winning sets of strategies that will enable them achieve the main aim of the game [12].

Strategy: A plan (decision) taken by a certain party, according to scientific rules that believe that the follow-up mechanism will automatically increase its profits or reduce its losses.

Payoff matrix: A matrix whose elements represent the results obtained by each player as a result of applying the different strategies available to him.

3 Genetic Algorithm

The beginning of the 20th century could be considered the inception of the extensive use of mathematical models and optimization fields [13]. In this respect, evolutionary computations as one of the sub-categories of artificial intelligence have been utilized to address those particular problems [1, 3]. This idea is based on a multi-point search instead of one-point that was originally introduced by Rechenberg [6].

Later, Holland introduced the Genetic Algorithm (GA) as the first evolutionary algorithm for global optimization using chromosomes and their genes [10].

A genetic algorithm is a heuristic search method used in artificial intelligence and computing. It is used for finding optimized solutions to search problems based on the theory of natural selection and evolutionary biology [5]. Genetic algorithms are excellent for searching through large and complex data sets [9].

Genetic Algorithms were invented to mimic some of the processes observed in natural evolution [4]. The father of the original Genetic Algorithm was John Holland who invented it in the early 1970's [10].

4 Mathematical Programming Model

In Linear Programming (LP), all of the mathematical expressions for the objective functions and the constraints are linear. The term programming as used in linear programming is an archaic word "Programming" to mean "Planning" [5].

We can consider linear programming as "Planning with linear models. The minimum and maximum problems in this corollary are so-called linear programming (LP) problems [8]. The common minimum/maximum is called the value of the LP, and x and y achieving the value are called optimal solutions [11].

Linear programming was used to solve the match theory and its results were compared with the algorithm to make sure it reaches the optimal solution by using MATLAB R2016.

Data

A matrix of potentials for two matches between Karkh and Minaa teams was established for the Iraqi Basketball League 2017–2018 through the adoption of the form in the International Federation as shown in Fig. 1 and filled by experts accredited to the Iraqi Federation of basketball.

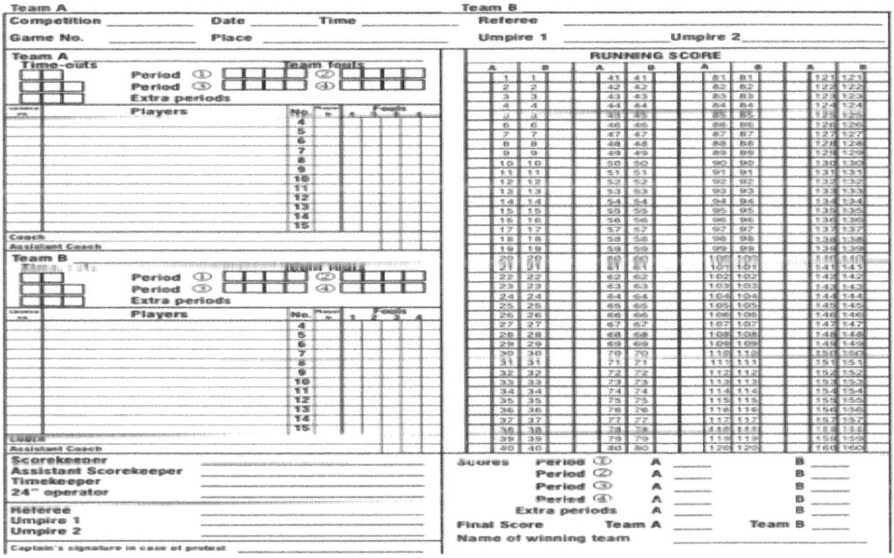

Fig. 1. International Basketball Federation Iraq Basketball Association Scoresheet

Build the matrix

(3, 4, 3, 3, 4, 3, 4, and 3). The probability values of the matrix are calculated based on the results of the experts. The form is shown in Fig. 1 and the probability of scoring goals in each period for the winning team and the form in Fig. 1 for previous matches.

The first match and Second match

The first match was held in 2016/2/12 and the win was for the benefit of the port team who scored 79 points against the Karkh team, who scored 74 points.

The second match was held in 2016/19/19 and was expected to be in the favor of the Karkh team who scored 79 points against the port team, which scored 72 points.

The matrix of the first and second match was built as follows

A	B							
	A				B			
	Period 1	Period 2	Period 3	Period 4	Period 1	Period 2	Period 3	Period 4
Point 1	1	0.8	0.5	0.6	0.8	0.7	0.6	0.6
Point 2	0.5	0.2	0.7	0.8	0.8	0.5	0.8	0.7
Point 3	0.5	0	0.3	0	0	0	0.5	0

Solution

The results of the Two games solution using programming and algorithm are as follows:

The first and second game

The linear model was solved using WINQSB (Fig. 2).

	Decision Variable	Solution Value	Unit Cost or Profit c(j)	Total Contribution	Reduced Cost	Basis Status	Allowable Min. c(j)	Allowable Max. c(j)
1	X1	0.6250	0	0	0	basic	-0.6000	0.2000
2	X2	0.3750	0	0	0	basic	-0.2000	0.6000
3	X3	0	0	0	-0.3500	at bound	-M	0.3500
4	X4	0.5750	1.0000	0.5750	0	basic	0	1.0000
	Objective	Function	(Max.) =	0.5750	(Note:	Alternate	Solution	Exists!!)

	Constraint	Left Hand Side	Direction	Right Hand Side	Slack or Surplus	Shadow Price	Allowable Min. RHS	Allowable Max. RHS
1	C1	-0.2375	<=	0	0.2375	0	-0.2375	M
2	C2	0	<=	0	0	0.2500	-0.3000	0.2714
3	C3	0	<=	0	0	0.7500	-0.5000	0.1000
4	C4	-0.1000	<=	0	0.1000	0	-0.1000	M
5	C5	1.0000	=	1.0000	0	0.5750	0	M

A

	Decision Variable	Solution Value	Unit Cost or Profit c(j)	Total Contribution	Reduced Cost	Basis Status	Allowable Min. c(j)	Allowable Max. c(j)
1	X1	0.6667	0	0	0	basic	0	0.5000
2	X2	0.3333	0	0	0	basic	-0.2500	0
3	X3	0	0	0	-0.5000	at bound	-M	0.5000
4	X4	0.5000	1.0000	0.5000	0	basic	0	1.0000
	Objective	Function	(Max.) =	0.5000	(Note:	Alternate	Solution	Exists!!)

	Constraint	Left Hand Side	Direction	Right Hand Side	Slack or Surplus	Shadow Price	Allowable Min. RHS	Allowable Max. RHS
1	C1	0	<=	0	0	0	-0.1600	0.2000
2	C2	-0.1333	<=	0	0.1333	0	-0.1333	M
3	C3	0	<=	0	0	1.0000	-0.2000	0.0727
4	C4	-0.2333	<=	0	0.2333	0	-0.2333	M
5	C5	1.0000	=	1.0000	0	0.5000	0	M

B

Fig. 2 Result of optimal solution for Game One and Game Two

A		B	
Decision variable	Solution value	Decision variable	1 Solution value
X_1	0.625	X1	0.6667
X_2	0.375	X2	0.333
X_3	0	X3	0
X_4	0.575	X4	0.5
Objective function (Max) = 0.575		Objective function (Max) = 0.5	

The Optimal solution for player A and B strategies are as follows:

	A	**B**
The Optimal solution for strategy probability number one is	0.62	0.66
The Optimal solution for strategy probability number two is	0.37	0.33
The Optimal solution for strategy probability number three is	0	0
The Optimal solution for strategy probability number four is	0.575	0.5

Game value =0.57

Solution using genetic algorithm

Results of the solution using MATLAB program are as follows:

A		B	
0.575	**F**	0.5	**F**
0.62	$\mathbf{X_1}$	0.66	$\mathbf{X_1}$
0.37	$\mathbf{X_2}$	0.33	$\mathbf{X_2}$
0	$\mathbf{X_3}$	0	$\mathbf{X_3}$
0.57	$\mathbf{X_4}$	0.5	$\mathbf{X_4}$

Analysis of the results

	A	**B**
The score of one point in the game was	62%	67%
The score of two points in the game was	37%	33%
The score of three points in the game was	0%	0%
The goal function, which represents the percentage of scoring goals in the game is	57%,	50%

Analysis of the results

The results of the solution are shown by matching the results of the linear programming and the genetic algorithm, indicating the efficiency of both methods. Therefore, the first, second and fourth strategies were adopted.

5 Conclusion

I. Stabilization results match linear programming and genetic algorithm because the linear model and in the case of nonlinearity will be a better genetic algorithm for sure

II. The best strategy for the game is to adopt the one-shot strategy and the second and not to adopt the three-point shot

III. Adopt the method of matches in determining the best strategy for each team to achieve the best results

IV. The Matlab program in the calculation of the results for the greatest possibility of optimization

References

1. Guo, C., Yang, X.: A programming of genetic algorithm in Matlab7.0, China (2011)
2. Lee, C.: Multi-objective game-theory models for conflict analysis in reservoir watershed management. Chemosphere **87**, 608–613 (2012)
3. Sadiq, S., Zhao, J.: Money Basketball: Optimizing Basketball Player Selection Using SAS®, paper China (2014)
4. Ismail, I.A., El Ramly, N.A., El Kafrawy, M.M., Nasef, M.M.: Game theory using genetic algorithms. Proceedings of the World Congress on Engineering (2007)
5. Datta, S., Garai, C., Das, C.: Efficient genetic algorithm on linear programming problem for fittest chromosomes. J. Global Res. Comput. Sci. 1 (2012)
6. Sivaraj, R., Ravichandran, T.: An efficient grouping genetic algorithm. Int. J. Comput. Appl. **21**(7), 0975–8887, May (2011)
7. Singh, A.P.: Optimal solution strategy for games. Int. J. Comput. Sci. Eng. **2**(9), 2778–2782 (2010)
8. Linear programming and game theory by Chakravorthy, J.G., University of Calcutta and Ghosh, P.R., University of Calcutta
9. Goldberg, D.E.: Genetic algorithms. Addison-Wesley (1989)
10. Gen, M.: Genetic Algorithms and Engineering Optimization. John Wiley and Sons, Inc. (2000)
11. Peters, H.: Game Theory: A Multi-Leveled Approach, p. 1989. Springer- Verlag, Berlin (2008)
12. Schecter, S., Gintis, H.: Introduction to Game Theory. North Carolina State University, January 17 (2012)
13. Shi, Y., Xing, Y., Mou, C., Kuang, Z.: An optimization model based on game theory. J. of Multimedia **9**(4), 583, April 2014, Genetic algorithms. Sci. Am 267, 66e72 (1992)

Augmented, Virtual and Mixed Reality Simulation

A Validated Failure Behavior Model for Driver Models to Test Automated Driving Functions

Bernd Huber[1(✉)], Christoph Sippl[1], Reinhard German[2], and Anatoli Djanatliev[2]

[1] Simulation Electric/Electronic, AUDI AG, 85045 Ingolstadt, Germany
{bernd2.huber, christoph.sippl}@audi.de
[2] Computer Networks and Communication Systems, Friedrich-Alexander Universität Erlangen, Martensstr. 3, 91058 Erlangen, Germany
{reinhard.german, anatoli.djanatliev}@fau.de

Abstract. This contribution proposes a failure behavior model for driver models, which is validated by findings from accident research. Our concept is based on the five-step-method which is used in accident research. Based on this concept, we present a prototypical implementation of an information processing failure and validate the implemented failure model on the basis of a real traffic accident. In conclusion, we discuss and interpret the validation results.

Keywords: Human modeling · Failure behavior modeling · Simulation

1 Introduction

Automated driving will change futures mobility, especially for private transport. On the one hand, this is due to economic considerations, e.g., new sales concepts [1]. On the other hand, road safety is expected to increase due to the automation of the driving task. This assumption is based on evaluation of accident researchers, who are able to assign the accident cause to the human being in over 90% of all analyzed accidents [2].

Automated driving functions (ADFs) are carried out in open traffic areas, consequently the systems have to cope with countless situations involving any other road user. Thus, the validation of ADFs poses enormous challenges for academia and industry. The challenge of validating ADFs is linked to the unfeasibility of statistical proof of safety. Therefore, alternative validation techniques are necessary [3]. Ulbrich et al. [4] describe the systematic application of simulation methods for testing during the development phase. The authors validated a lane changing function of an automated vehicle. Therefore, the experts developed simulation scenarios to validate the functionality of the system. The manual creation of simulation scenarios is time-consuming and complex, since the behavior of each individual entity in the simulation must be described. To overcome this problem, different researchers presented the automated generation of simulation scenarios [5, 6]. Using combinatorial approaches for scenario generation result in countless simulation scenarios. Hence, generated scenarios must be reviewed whether they represent physically correct scenarios for an efficient validation process [7]. Another possibility to determine the behavior of road users in the

T. Ahram et al. (Eds.): IHIET 2019, AISC 1018, pp. 255–261, 2020.
https://doi.org/10.1007/978-3-030-25629-6_40

simulation is the use of driver behavior models. Numerous driver behavior models for various purposes and different levels of detail have been presented in the literature. Near crash behavior models are suitable for the efficient validation of ADFs. These models are able to describe very rarely occurring situations in road traffic. Near crash behavior models that have already been introduced are not validated accordingly, so that they can be used for the validation of ADFs [8].

2 Concept

Human failure behavior is the main cause for accidents in road traffic. Therefore, we propose a failure behavior model for driver models, which is based on the analysis of real traffic accidents. The accidents were analyzed by an interdisciplinary accident research team called Audi Accident Research Unit (AARU)[1]. In addition to technical and medical examinations, the AARU also conducts a psychological assessment of traffic accidents. Based on these analyses, the AARU is able to provide data about the circumstances of a crash, a reconstructed simulation, interviews with the persons involved and an error classification according to the five-step-method [9]. Thereby, the five-step-method associates human cause factors with the human decision-making process (cf. Table 1).

Table 1. Detailed description of the error classification defined within the five-step-method, based on [9].

Category	Description
(1) Information access	Was the driver able to objectively perceive the relevant information?
(2) Information reception	Was the driver's information reception impaired?
(3) Information processing	Was the perceived information correctly interpreted depending on the situation?
(4) Objective	Has a hazard prevention intention adapted to the situation been formed?
(5) Action	Has the intended objective been translated into a corresponding action?

In our approach, the failure classification of the five-step-method provides the database for the failure behavior models. Since the failure classification is derived from the human decision-making process, it is necessary to use a driver behavior model that considers the human decision-making process in its implementation. Such models are categorized by Michon [10] as motivational models or cognitive (process) models. Hence, the findings of the AARU can be used to implement corresponding failure behavior models in respective layers of a cognitive driver behavior model.

[1] Audi Accident Research Unit (AARU): https://www.aaru.de/.

The implementation of the failure behavior model is relying on the results of the five-step-method, as it describes the human failure behavior according to psychological reports of the AARU. Additionally, the interviews with involved persons support the failure modelling process. Subsequently, the failure behavior model is validated by comparing simulation results with real traffic accidents.

3 Application of the Methodology

3.1 Database

For this proof of concept, we used the assessment of the five-step-method of real accidents. According to the AARU accident researchers, a possible cause of the traffic accidents is due to a driver failure in the information processing layer [9]. More precisely, the driver's misjudgment about the distance and/or speed of another road user is a typical cause of traffic accidents.

3.2 Implementation

Prior to demonstrating the implementation of the failure behavior model, see the mode of operation of the driver behavior model in [11]. The driver's failure behavior during the information processing was implemented in the driver model's situation awareness layer. The information processing is derived from the perceived objects over time. This includes the estimation of distance and speed of perceived objects. Especially as the Time-to-Collision (TTC) is computed from the speed and distance of other objects, the result of this value is manipulated. Furthermore, the situation awareness layer receives perceived objects categorized by their lane position. The following algorithm presents the implemented failure behavior:

```
for all obj ∈ objlist do
  if obj on left_lane then
  // the TTC is calculated as if the obj is projected
  // on the same lane as the drivers vehicle set TTC to 1000
  else
      calculate correct TTC
  endif
endfor
```

In consequence of the high value of the TTC, distance and speed of another objects are underestimated. Conclusions based on the TTC, e.g., whether a lane is free, are defective.

The effects of the failure behavior model are demonstrated in a typical situation on an autobahn access road. Therefore, a simulation scenario with manipulated information processing is compared with the identical simulation scenario without manipulation. Figure 1 illustrates the simulation scenario. The driver behavior model controls the blue vehicle on the autobahn access road. At the same time, another road user is driving in the left lane of the autobahn at 150 km/h (cf. left picture, Fig. 1), as well as a truck that travels in the right lane at 80 km/h. Both vehicles are controlled by the driver model of the traffic simulation and both vehicles drive at their desired velocity. At the end of the acceleration lane, the blue vehicle changes to the left lane of the autobahn (cf. right picture, Fig. 1). The effect of the failure behavior model in this situation is illustrated by the two upper pictures in Fig. 2.

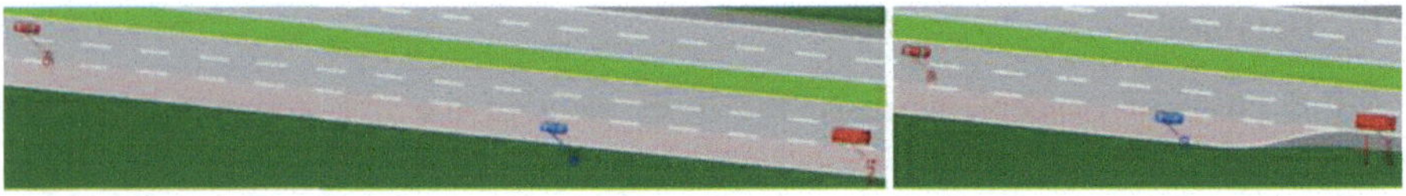

Fig. 1. The left figure illustrates the scene at timestamp 0. The right figure shows the scene at timestamp 1.

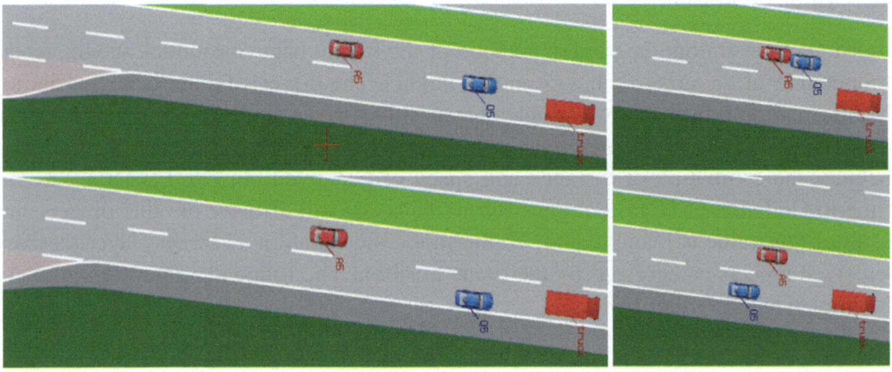

Fig. 2. Pictures on the left side illustrate the scene at timestamp 3. Pictures on the right side displays the scene at timestamp 4. The upper pictures show the situation with activated failure behavior model, while the lower pictures present the situation without manipulation.

The blue vehicle changes to the overtaking lane of the autobahn. However, the red vehicle can not decelerate sufficiently, resulting in an accident. This behavior by the blue vehicle is explainable due to the failure in the information processing layer. The driver behavior model perceived the red vehicle, but assumed, based on the high TTC value, that sufficient space was available to overtake the truck safely. The results of the simulation with deactivated failure behavior model show, that the blue vehicle does not perform a second lane change (cf. lower pictures of Fig. 2). Without the manipulation of the information processing, the driver behavior model considers a lane change to be potentially unsafe and stays behind the truck. Consequently, the situation does not evolve into a traffic accident.

4 Validation of the Failure Behavior Model

After the effect of the failure behavior model on the driver behavior model is demonstrated, we compare the virtually generated situation with situations from a real traffic accident database. In this database, we identified a similar accident, whose main cause also lies in the information processing layer. The reconstructed traffic accident is illustrated in Fig. 3.

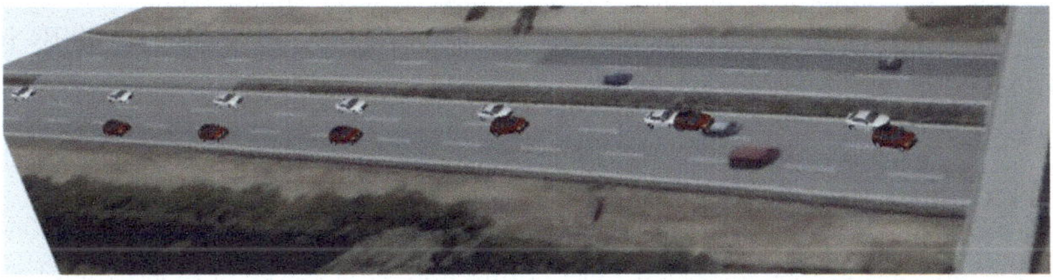

Fig. 3. Reconstruction of an analyzed traffic accident by the AARU.

The reconstruction shows a double lane change by the red vehicle starting from the acceleration lane. Simultaneously, the white vehicle approaches at high relative speed. The driver of the white vehicle attempts to deaccelerate, but cannot avoid the traffic accident. The results of the five-step-method identify an information processing failure by the driver of the red vehicle. Similar as in the simulation with activated failure behavior model, the accident perpetrator does perform a double lane change maneuver starting from the acceleration lane. According to the accident type catalogue of the insurers' accident research department, both traffic accidents are assigned to the identical accident type [12]. The accident type classifies both accidents in longitudinal traffic and the cause of the accident is a lane change maneuver to the left lane. Therefore, the failure behavior model is able to reconstruct accident situations with the same accident cause. For better comparability, the real accident was simulated in our traffic simulation framework. The lane markings were used as reference points to reconstruct the behavior of the vehicles (cf. Fig. 4).

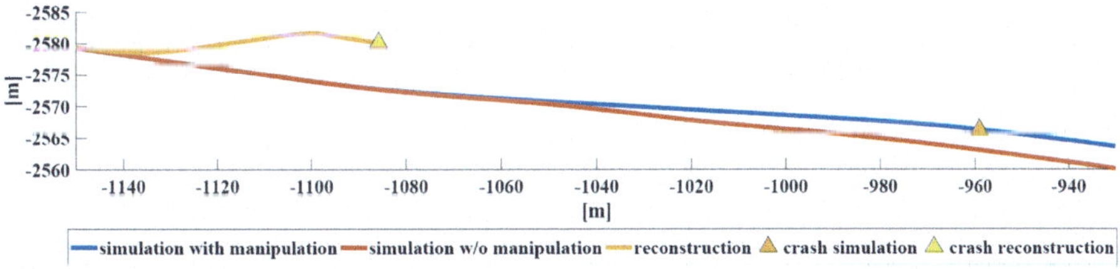

Fig. 4. Plot of the trajectory of the accident perpetrator in each simulation setup.

The red line illustrates the behavior of the driver with deactivated failure behavior model. The blue line presents the trajectory of the car with activated failure behavior model. The crash is indicated with the orange triangle. The behavior of the reconstructed traffic accident is shown in yellow. Here, the crash is indicated by the yellow triangle. The main difference is the position of the crash visualized by the triangles. The difference is explainable due to two factors. First, in the reconstruction of the AARU the driver leaves the autobahn access road in the middle of the acceleration lane. This behavior is not implemented in our driver behavior model. Second, the driver model is not aggressive enough to perform such a lane change maneuver. Although this behavior may be reconstructed by altering the driver type and the driver skills in the driver behavior model parametrization.

5 Discussion and Future Work

This contribution presents a concept for a failure behavior model, which is validated by findings from accident research. Additionally, a prototypical implementation of an information processing failure is provided. Subsequently, the failure behavior model is validated on the basis of a real accident. The validation shows, that a very precise reconstruction of the accident depends on further factors next to the human failure behavior. However, the result show that the five-step-method is an adequate indicator of human accident causes.

In future work we will implement further human failure behavior models on the basis of the five-step-method and validate it on the evidence of real accidents. The driver behavior model with the ability of human failures will be used to define the behavior of road users when virtually testing automated driving functions.

References

1. McKinsey & Company: Automotive revolution – perspective towards 2030: how the convergence of disruptive technology-driven trends could transform the auto industry. Report, Advanced Industries (2016)
2. Singh, S.: Critical reasons for crashes investigated in the national motor vehicle crash causation survey. Report, Traffic Safety Facts – Crash (2015)
3. Winner, H., Wachenfeld, W., Junietz, P.: Validation and introduction of automated driving. In: Winner, H., Prokop, G., Maurer, M. (eds.) Automotive Systems Engineering II, pp. 177–196. Springer, Cham (2018)
4. Ulbrich, S., Schuldt, F., Homeier, K., Steinhoff, M., Menzel, T., Krause, J., Maurer, M.: Testing and validating tactical lane change behavior planning for automated driving. In: Watzenig, D., Horn, M. (eds.) Automated Driving, pp. 451–471. Springer, Cham (2017)
5. Schuldt, F., Reschka, A., Maurer, M.: A method for an efficient, systematic test case generation for advanced driver assistance systems in virtual environments. In: Winner, H., Prokop, G., Mauerer, M. (eds.) Automotive Systems Engineering II, pp. 147–175. Springer, Cham (2017)

6. Bagschick, G., Menzel, T., Maurer, M.: Ontology based scene creation for the development of automated vehicles. In: 2018 IEEE Intelligent Vehicles Symposium (IV), pp. 1813–1820 (2018)
7. Lotz, F.G.O.: Eine Referenzarchitektur für die assistierte und automatisierte Fahrzeugführung mit Fahrereinbindung. Doctoral dissertation (2017)
8. Markkula, G., Benderius, O., Wahde, M.: Comparing and validating models of driver steering behaviour in collision avoidance and vehicle stabilization. In: 52th Vehicle systems dynamics, pp. 1658–1680 (2014)
9. Weber, S., Ernstberger, A., Donner, E., Kiss, M.: Learning from accidents: using technical and subjective information to identify accident mechanisms and to develop driver assistance systems. In: Dorn, L., Sullman, M. (eds.) Driver Behaviour and Training, vol. VI, pp. 223–230. Ashgate, Surrey (2013)
10. Michon, J.A.: A critical view of driver behavior models: what do we know, what should we do? In: Human Behavior and Traffic Safety, pp. 485—524. Plenum Press, New York (1985)
11. Human Factor Consult Driver Modeling. https://human-factors-consult.de/en/services-and-products/driver-modeling/
12. Gesamtverband der Deutschen Versicherungswirtschaft e. V.: Unfalltypen-Katalog. https://udv.de/sites/default/files/tx_udvpublications/unfalltypen-katalog_udv_web_2.pdf

Virtual Reality-Based Simulation of Age-Related Visual Deficiencies: Implementation and Evaluation in the Design Process

Christina Zavlanou[1(✉)] and Andreas Lanitis[1,2]

[1] Visual Media Computing Lab, Department of Multimedia and Graphic Arts, Cyprus University of Technology, 31 Archbishop Kyprianos Street 3603, Limassol, Cyprus
cg.zavlanou@edu.cut.ac.cy

[2] Research Centre on Interactive Media, Smart Systems and Emerging Technologies, Nicosia, Cyprus
andreas.lanitis@cut.ac.cy

Abstract. Age-related changes significantly affect elderly users' interaction with specific products and services. Nevertheless, the challenges experienced by elderly users are difficult to be perceived and understood, especially by younger people. Inspired by the concept of aging suits, we propose a Virtual Reality-based approach, where age-related visual impairments are simulated in virtual environments. The aim is to provide an approximation of the experience of viewing and interacting with a product, from the perspective of elderly persons with specific age-related visual problems. The effectiveness of the proposed approach is examined through an experiment involving package design evaluation. The experimental results demonstrate that Virtual Reality can play an important role on understanding the challenges that elderly users face, thus support the design of elderly-friendly products.

Keywords: Virtual reality · Simulation · Elderly-friendly design

1 Introduction

Age-related changes introduce increased levels of difficulty, but not necessarily incompetence, despite the general perception that elderly people are weak and cannot be self-dependent [1]. When it comes to products and services, difficulties faced by elderly people are often attributed to insufficient design [2], which fails to consider the characteristics of a large portion of end users and adequately address their needs.

Considering the United Nations' prospects for world population, in about 30 years, in almost all regions of our planet, one in four people will be over 60 years old [3]. Therefore, it becomes increasingly important to place more emphasis on elderly population in terms of product-service accessibility.

Inspired by the concept of aging suits, we propose a Virtual Reality (VR) based approach, where age-related visual impairments are simulated in virtual environments. The aim is to provide an approximation of the experience of viewing and interacting

T. Ahram et al. (Eds.): IHIET 2019, AISC 1018, pp. 262–267, 2020.
https://doi.org/10.1007/978-3-030-25629-6_41

with products, from the perspective of elderly persons with specific age-related visual problems.

Albeit associated with an age group, the term "elderly" is relative and there is no precise age, over which someone is clearly considered an elderly person [4]. In the context of this research, we refer to "elderly" as people over 75 years old, as this age group is characterized by the greatest demand in medical and social care [5]. Since the process of aging is unique for different individuals [6] and depends on many factors apart from age, for the needs of this paper we refer to elderly people who experience age-related problems, but who can live an autonomous life.

2 Related Work

Various methods have been employed to facilitate and optimize the design of elderly-friendly products and services and various method classifications exist in the literature [7]. In the context of this research, the approaches to address elderly-users' needs in the design process are categorized into two types: the non-simulated and the simulated approaches.

With the term "non-simulated", we refer to analytical methods based mainly on data collection to record and understand the needs of the elderly users. Non-simulated approaches include, among others, Field Research, Participatory Design and User Personas. Concerning elderly users, the use of non-simulated methods raises difficulties, such as achieving targeted conversation and receiving specific feedback [2], partly due to the experiences of short-term memory loss encountered by the elderly [8]. Moreover, compared to the simulated, non-simulated methods do not provide a visualization of the problems faced by the elderly, thus the designers find it difficult to provide sufficient feedback during the evaluation stage of the design process [9].

The simulated approaches involve more applied methods in which the designers are using various accessories to simulate age-related changes and thus "take the role" of elderly users. There are several approaches for simulating age-related problems, including both physical [10] and VR-based aging simulators [11].

2.1 Physical Aging Simulation

Physical age simulators usually come in the form of "aging suits", such as the Age Gain Now Empathy System (AGNES), developed at the Massachusetts Institute of Technology (MIT) [10], which is used by students and professionals, to experience the difficulties that accompany old age.

While physical aging suits are capable of simulating aging effects, there are some weaknesses related to their use. The inability to easily customize the intensity of the effects of aging and the amount of the time required for the users' preparation to wear the accessories, are two of the most considerable ones. Cost is yet another factor that should be considered, as aging suits are expensive and are dedicated for the sole purpose of the aging simulation.

2.2 VR-Based Aging Simulation

Instead, VR technology is more affordable and has a multipurpose use, so the cost corresponding to the simulation part is lower.

There are several reports on the simulation of age-related problems and visual impairments using VR technologies [9, 11–13]. In [12], a VR headset along with a PlayStation camera were used to create an environment that simulated visual problems, through live streaming videos on which appropriate filters were applied. This work bears similarities with our approach, but in our case the experience is fully virtual. Similarly, but dedicated to architectural and space design, [13] implemented a VR environment to simulate specific visual disabilities and support the understanding of the difficulties that visually impaired people encounter.

3 Methodology

Aging is a multidimensional phenomenon, affecting many aspects of a person's life, from physical changes [14] to complex mental disorders [15]. In the context of this research, we focus on two common visual impairments associated with aging.

Cataract. Cataract is one of the most prevalent eye disorders associated primarily with age [16]. Over time, cataract causes an increase in lens density, hindering the clarity of vision. Cataract disease can be associated with a series of symptoms such as yellowing of the lens, blurry vision, fainted colors symptom, difficulty in differentiating colors [16] and need for extra lighting [14]. In the virtual environment, the clouding of the lens was achieved using the blur image effect with the intensity amounted to 30%. For the simulation of toneless vision, image contrast was reduced to 20%. Finally, for the reduction of the lighting reaching the retina to one-third [14], image brightness was proportionally reduced.

Macular Degeneration. Nearly one in three people aged over 75 years old suffers from macular degeneration [14]. Macular degeneration mainly affects central vision and is associated with symptoms such as dark spots in the center of the field of view. To simulate the symptoms of this eye disease in the virtual environment, overlay textures were applied in the center of the viewport (Fig. 1, right).

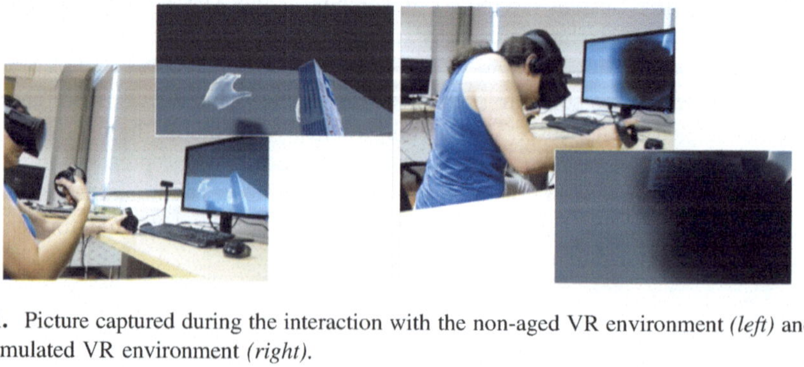

Fig. 1. Picture captured during the interaction with the non-aged VR environment *(left)* and the age-simulated VR environment *(right)*.

To test the efficacy of the proposed VR-based aging simulation, we carried out an experiment involving a pharmaceutical package design. The purpose was to investigate whether by using an age simulated VR environment, it is feasible to detect design faults on packages that could prevent the correct use of products by the elderly.

The experiment was conducted using the Oculus Rift CV1 VR headset along with the Oculus Touch controllers for the interaction in the virtual environment and the manipulation of the virtual pill box (see Fig. 1).

The virtual environment used in this experiment consisted of a three-dimensional object – the virtual representation of a real pill box, and a grey background with depth perception (see Fig. 1). For the modeling of the virtual box, scanned images of the six sides of the actual pill box were used. Using image editing software, two alternative virtual pill boxes were modelled using identical graphic elements to avoid the case where the participants remembered the information from the first trial.

The experiment was assessed by 23 young adults – 9 males and 14 females – aged between 18 and 34 years old. The participants were separated into two equal groups: the first group (group A) started the experiment using the aging simulated environment and then carried on with the non-aged virtual environment, while the second group (group B) performed the experiment in the opposite order. Thereby, previous knowledge and/or familiarity did not factor into the overall performance of the tasks and the results of the questionnaires.

During the experiment, the participants were requested to locate and read aloud: the name of the medicine (Q1), the expiry date (Q2), the amount of the active ingredient of each pill (Q3) and the indications about the medicine (Q4).

After the interaction with each of the two environments, participants were given a questionnaire (see Table 1) related to the ease of completion of the four requested tasks and were asked to provide answers on a 5-point Likert scale (1: the task was not easy at all, and 5: the task was extremely easy to perform). Moreover, they were asked to quote their perceived age in each of the two variations of the virtual environment.

4 Results

According to the experimental results, reading the information on the pill box was clearly more difficult in the age-simulated than in the non-aged virtual environment (Table 1). P-values were calculated with Fisher's exact test to compare the responses given after trying the non-aged and after trying the age-simulated virtual experience. There was a significant difference in all scores ($p < 0.05$) concerning the reading part of the info. The results imply that the difficulty encountered could have been avoided if designers were able to visualize the packaging from the perspective of elderly people, effortlessly detect design defects and design a more elderly-friendly packaging.

Regarding the design elements that one would change in the package, while in the non-aged environment the answers were distributed, in the aging environment, most of the participants concluded that the main defect was the size of the fonts.

Given that virtual prototyping techniques are often used along with VR technology [17] to impart greater efficiency to the design process; the additional feature that the VR-based aging simulation can provide, namely the visualization of age-related problems, could help in identifying design weaknesses related to elderly users.

Table 1. The questions regarding the easiness of the completion of the tasks along with the P values from the Fisher's exact test.

Questions	Name (Q1)		Expiry date (Q2)		Quantity (Q3)		Indications (Q4)	
Environment	Non-aged	Aged	Non-aged	Aged	Non-aged	Aged	Non-aged	Aged
Median	5.00	4.00	4.00	3.00	5.00	4.00	4.00	1.00
Deviation	0.00	1.00	1.00	1.00	0.00	1.00	1.00	0.00
P-value	0.01		0.00		0.00		0.00	

Regarding the perceived ages in the two variations of the virtual environment compared to participants' actual age, paired samples t-test was conducted between (1) the perceived age in the non-aged environment and participants' actual age ($p = 0.1056$), (2) the perceived age in the aged environment and participants' actual age ($p = 3.201e{-}05$) and (3) the perceived age in the non-aged environment and the perceived age in the aged environment ($p = 5.966e{-}05$). The results indicated that participants realized that the experiment concerned age-related effects, even without having prior information about the aim of the experiment.

5 Conclusion

An investigation into the development and an evaluation of VR-based simulation of age-related visual impairments in the product design process, were presented. The aim was to investigate whether by using an age simulated VR environment, it is feasible to detect design faults on pharmaceutical packages that could prevent the correct use of medicines by elderly people. The results indicated that VR-based simulation can highlight the difficulties that elderly people, suffering from age-associated problems face during a seemingly easy process, such as reading pill package's information and support the design of elderly-friendly products and services. Similar applications could be used by designers to take the role of elderly consumers to facilitate the accessibility of products. Compared with other methods used for aging simulation, VR can be easily applied to many scenarios under highly controlled settings.

In the future, the incorporation of additional age-related factors is planned. A configuration could be made to enable the adjustment of the intensity and type of simulated aging effects based on different variables such as age, sex and lifestyle allowing in that way the customization of virtual aging simulators at various circumstances.

Acknowledgments. This research is part of the project that has received funding from the European Union's Horizon 2020 research and innovation programme under grant agreement No 739578 (RISE – Call:H2020-WIDESPREAD-01-2016-2017-TeamingPhase2) and the Government of the Republic of Cyprus through the Directorate General for European Programmes, Coordination and Development.

References

1. Adams-Price, C.E., Morse, L.W.: Dependency stereotypes and aging: the implications for getting and giving help in later life. J. Appl. Soc. Psychol. **39**(12), 2967–2984 (2009)
2. Lindsay, S., Jackson, D., Schofield, G., Olivier, P.: Engaging older people using participatory design. In: Proceedings of the SIGCHI Conference on Human Factors in Computing Systems, pp. 1199–1208. ACM (2012)
3. United Nations, Department of Economic and Social Affairs, Population Division. World Population Prospects: The 2015 Revision, Key Findings and Advance Tables. Working Paper No. ESA/P/WP.241 (2015)
4. Guzmán, J.M., Pawliczko, A., Beales, S.: Ageing in the twenty-first century: a celebration and a challenge (2018)
5. Sixsmith, A.J.: An evaluation of an intelligent home monitoring system. J. Telemed. Telecare **6**(2), 63–72 (2000)
6. Kowal, P., Dowd, J.E.: Definition of an older person. Proposed working definition of an older person in Africa for the MDS Project. World Health Organization, Geneva (2001). https://doi.org/10.13140/2.1.5188.9286
7. Sankowski, O., Krause, D.: User-centered product design for older adults – comparison and applicability of methods. In: Design for X, Beiträge zum 29. DfX-Symposium, Tutzing, pp. 25–36 (2018)
8. Joshi, S.G., Bratteteig, T.: Designing for prolonged mastery. On involving old people in participatory design. Scand. J. Inform. Syst. **28**(1), 3–36 (2016). http://aisel.aisnet.org/sjis/vol28/iss1/1
9. Zavlanou, C., Lanitis, A.: Product packaging evaluation through the eyes of elderly people: personas vs. aging suit vs. virtual reality aging simulation. In: IHSED: Future Trends and Applications, pp. 567–572. Springer, Cham (2018)
10. Osawa, H., Imai, M.: Enhancing empathy toward an agent by immersive learning. In: International Conference on Human-Agent Interaction (2013)
11. Zavlanou, C., Lanitis, A.: An age simulated virtual environment for improving elderly wellbeing. In: XIV Mediterranean Conference on Medical and Biological Engineering and Computing, pp. 891–896. Springer, Cham (2016)
12. Ates, H.C., Fiannaca, A., Folmer, E.: Immersive simulation of visual impairments using a wearable see-through display. In: Proceedings of the Ninth International Conference on Tangible, Embedded, and Embodied Interaction, pp. 225–228. ACM (2015)
13. Väyrynen, J., Colley, A., Häkkilä, J.: Head mounted display design tool for simulating visual disabilities. In: Proceedings of the 15th International Conference on Mobile and Ubiquitous Multimedia, pp. 69–73. ACM (2016)
14. Payne, V.G., Isaacs, L.D.: Human Motor Development: A Lifespan Approach. Routledge, Abingdon (2017)
15. Geerligs, L., Renken, R.J., Saliasi, E., Maurits, N.M., Lorist, M.M.: A brain-wide study of age-related changes in functional connectivity. Cereb. Cortex **25**(7), 1987–1999 (2014)
16. Asbell, P.A., Dualan, I., Mindel, J., Brocks, D., Ahmad, M., Epstein, S.: Age-related cataract. Lancet **365**(9459), 599–609 (2005)
17. Choi, S., Jung, K., Noh, S.D.: Virtual reality applications in manufacturing industries: past research, present findings, and future directions. Concurr. Eng. **23**(1), 40–63 (2015)

Designing Technologies for Neurodiverse Users: Considerations from Research Practice

Vivian Genaro Motti[1(✉)] and Anna Evmenova[2]

[1] Volgenau School of Engineering, George Mason University, Fairfax, VA 22030, USA
vmotti@gmu.edu

[2] College of Education and Human Development, George Mason University, Fairfax, VA 22030, USA
aevmenov@gmu.edu

Abstract. This paper presents and discusses the perspectives of ten investigators experienced with design of technologies for and with neurodiverse users. Although the advances on emerging technologies improved their potential to assist users with neurodiverse needs, existing methods for participatory design, usability tests and evaluation have been created for, and validated with, able-bodied users. User-centered design methods are not always well-suited to meet the unique needs of neurodiverse individuals. Therefore, to involve neurodiverse users iteratively in the design process, investigators need to adapt traditional methods from HCI to successfully conduct user studies. Through an online questionnaire, we identified the experimental designs commonly adopted and the major problems investigators face during recruitment, data collection, analysis and design. Based on the analysis of the investigators' experiences, we provide nine recommendations to conduct studies with neurodiverse users, aiming at engaging them as active participants front and center in the research and design process.

Keywords: Accessibility · Inclusive design · Assistive technologies · Neurodiverse users

1 Introduction

Extensive research on accessibility has been conducted in the past decades, however most efforts focus on technologies for users with visual, hearing, and motor impairments. The involvement of neurodiverse users in scientific research is limited. Frameworks [2], guidelines [5], principles and tools dedicated to create accessible technologies for neurodiverse users are lacking. Still, cognitive disabilities stand out as the second most frequent disability [14]. Also, the number of users with cognitive impairments, intellectual and developmental disabilities has been growing, thanks to better diagnostic techniques, more assistive services, and also due to the aging of the human population. Even though the research and development efforts of the accessibility community often overlook neurodiverse users, this user population could largely

T. Ahram et al. (Eds.): IHIET 2019, AISC 1018, pp. 268–274, 2020.
https://doi.org/10.1007/978-3-030-25629-6_42

benefit from innovative technologies that carefully consider and address their unique needs, including smart objects, mobile and web applications.

To understand design considerations for the development of assistive technologies for neurodiverse users, this paper reports the perspectives of ten scientific investigators studying accessible technologies for neurodiversity. The research questions that drive the data collection focus on design methods and engineering considerations, cutting across three major themes: (1) recruitment of participants for user studies, retention and attrition throughout the research project, (2) methodological approaches for accurate data collection and scientifically-rigorous analysis, and (3) accessibility considerations and inclusive design practices to propose, implement and evaluate technologies striving to involve neurodiverse users as active participants in the research and design process and also to achieve ecological validity, large scale adoption and sustained engagement with novel technologies.

The investigators selected for the study have extensive experience working with neurodiverse users, including individuals with intellectual and neurodevelopmental disabilities, such as: Down syndrome, Autism Spectrum Disorders, Attention Deficit and Hyperactivity Disorder and Dyslexia. The participants in the studies considered include children as well as young and older adults. The technological artifacts proposed, implemented and evaluated in the research projects encompass tangible interfaces, online tools, games, mobile applications, and wearable devices.

The methodological approaches employed involve mixed-methods, including interviews with end users and caregivers, ethnographic studies, usability tests, evaluation and observation sessions in the field or in controlled settings. The data has been collected manually (through written notes) or automatically (through sensors), using questionnaires, audio and video recordings, as well as annotations from observation sessions. The data sets include objective measures from sensors and logs, and subjective measures self-reported in questionnaires, provided by caregivers or assistants, or annotated from observations. The data sets have been subject to quantitative and qualitative analysis of participants' responses and behaviors, including statistical methods, coding from annotations and transcripts, and thematic analysis.

The findings from the study contribute to advance the state-of-the-art in the domain by: (1) informing investigators on how user studies with neurodiverse users have been successfully conducted, and (2) providing best practices and recommendations for designing novel solutions that take into account the needs of neurodiverse users. By shedding light into the design of accessible technologies for neurodiversity, we pave the way for scientific foundations aimed at providing better support for designers, investigators and practitioners. The ultimate goal of this analysis is to encourage stakeholders to involve neurodiverse users front and center in the design process, to enable large-scale adoption of accessibility practices and implementation of technological solutions that are more inclusive for individuals with neurodiverse needs.

2 Related Work

Neurodiversity is broader than autism and learning difficulties [1], covering intellectual and developmental disabilities and cognitive impairments [2]. Seeking to positively reframe neurological conditions concentrating on their strengths [2] and in line with the neurodiversity movement, this paper focuses on research methods for inclusive design solutions for neurodiverse users. Gifted users with diverse needs are "at risk of growing frustrated or bored with technologies because their needs are not well understood" [2]. For Frauenberger, "the disabled experience is arguably richer and often more complex as can be projected from the functional limitations of people" [7].

As Table 1 lists, advances on smart technologies enable new forms of assistive technologies to support social interactions, self-regulation, skill training, among others. Assistive technologies allow people with disabilities to become more able to complete tasks that would be difficult, or even impossible, to complete without technology [12].

Table 1. Examples of seven smart technologies designed for neurodiverse users.

Category	Method	Purpose
Smart objects	Participatory design	Involve neurodiverse users in the design process to create smart objects (e.g. games, smart toys, and tangible interfaces [8] and fidgets [10])
Mobile app (Tablet)	Deployment study Lab study, experiment	Emotion regulation [9] Cooperation [13]
Video games	User study, semi-structured interviews, co-design	Neurofeedback training for attention [11]
Wearable	Interviews, focus groups, usability tests	Self-regulation, interventions, reminders. checklists [3, 4]
	Interviews and experiments	Offer proximity awareness [6]

Wearable solutions can aid children with ASD in interpersonal communication skills [6], and smartwatch applications can provide in-class assistance [3, 4]. Mobile apps can help with self-regulation of affective states [9] and cooperation training [13], whereas video games with brain-computer interfaces can provide neurofeedback training to sustain attention [11].

Concerning experimental design, prior work has mainly employed qualitative methods, such as interviews, observations, and questionnaires, targeting at children with ASD and/or ADHD. While investigators rely on traditional HCI methods, they highlight some adaptations needed, including the need to desensitize participants when wearable sensors are used [11], to account for high attrition rates [13], and to adapt study settings to ensure participants are comfortable and engaged in the study sessions [11].

3 Method

In this paper we report the findings of an online survey applied with researchers of the HCI community. The participants have been recruited through purposeful sampling, by email, and word of mouth. The study received IRB approval upon data collected. Ten participants responded to the survey. It included 20 questions, being 5 demographics (age, gender, years of experience, and research interests), 10 on research experience (recruitment, data collection, analysis, participants' profiles, age, conditions, location of the study, sample size, attrition and problems faced), and 5 on design recommendations, considerations, risk mitigation and error prevention.

For the analysis of the results, we quantified users' responses, and categorized the qualitative responses of open questions.

4 Results

4.1 Demographics

The investigators who responded the survey were mostly young adults with age ranging from 28 to 69 years old (AVG = 36.2, SD = 12). Most respondents were female (n = 6) and had at least 4 years of experience working in the domain (AVG = 11, SD = 13). They were mostly academics, except for two participants who were working in a research center or working as accessibility consultant. Most respondents were faculty members (n = 6) or researchers (n = 4) working as graduate students, postdoctoral research fellows or independent consultants. As research interests most respondents investigated assistive technologies (n = 9), users with special needs (n = 8), accessibility (n = 7) and universal design (n = 6). A few of them were interested in Ubiquitous Computing (n = 4), game design and wearables (n = 3), and mobile development (n = 2). Additional research interests, mentioned only once each, included: ethnography, speech technologies, critical approaches on technologies for aging and dementia, and interaction log analysis.

4.2 Research Experience

Concerning the user population, most respondents studied Autism Spectrum Disorders (n = 6), Neurodiversity (n = 5), and few respondents investigated Intellectual and Developmental Disabilities (n = 4), Dyslexia (n = 3), or other conditions including ADHD, Down Syndrome, Complex Communication Needs and Dementia (n = 1).

Most of the respondents recruited children as study participants (n = 6) with age ranging from 3 to 16 years old, two respondents focused on older adults (older than 50 years).

For recruitment, most respondents used word of mouth (n = 7), and phone calls (n = 5). Few participants used email and flyers (n = 4), email lists (n = 3), social media posts (n = 2), in person (n = 1) or specialized clinics (n = 1).

Concerning methodological approach, respondents mostly used interviews (n = 9), questionnaires and observations (n = 8), usability tests and log analysis (n = 5). Few respondents employed focus groups and ethnography (n = 4), and experiments with cognitive psychologists and neuroimaging (n = 1). All respondents reported to use at least two methods, and most of them employed at least three methods (n = 8).

In terms of location, all respondents conducted the studies at the field, in users' homes, schools, workplaces and specialized centers, whereas few respondents conducted studies in controlled settings such as a laboratory (n = 4).

Most users involved multiple participants' profiles in their research, mainly users with diverse needs (n = 9), and caregivers (guardians, relatives) or practitioners (medical doctors, instructors) (n = 7).

On average respondents recruited 30 participants for the studies, ranging from 5 to 100.

To collect data, most respondents relied on video recordings and written annotations (n = 8), audio recordings (n = 7), sensors (n = 6) and logs of the user interaction (n = 5). All respondents combined multiple methods for data collection.

For data analysis, coding was the most common method (n = 80), followed by descriptive statistical analysis and qualitative content analysis (n = 6), few respondents used thematic analysis (n = 4), advanced statistical analysis (n = 3), and grounded theory (n = 1).

Half of the respondents reported no attrition rates in their studies, whereas the other half of respondents noticed it a few times, depending on the method, but not significantly (n = 5).

Recruitment was the most common problem faced by the investigators (n = 6), followed by limited adherence (n = 3) and cooperation (n = 3). Other issues mentioned included: the heterogeneity of study participants (n = 1), difficulties with a proper method (n = 1), and informed consent (n = 1).

4.3 Design Considerations

The recommendations respondents proposed to address the problems encountered and improve the success of a study were:

- **Oversampling.** in the recruitment phase, to oversample the number of participants selected to account for attrition, limited adherence and incomplete data;
- **Simplify communication.** to facilitate consent, emphasize the communication with participants using plain language and request for short answers to keep the scope;
- **Prefer depth instead of broader studies.** to conduct in-depth studies with more cooperative participants, minimizing attrition risks associated with larger studies;
- **Refer to existing community services.** relying on established social networks facilitates the recruitment of participants; conducting studies in locations already familiar to participants ensures their comfort;
- **Triangulate stakeholders' perspectives.** refer to caregivers and parents to collect data in addition to observing the participants for cross-validation and to reduce bias;
- **Desensitize.** to conduct a desensitization process for participants to get used to devices and prototypes, and training sessions with practitioners involved to learn how to use the technologies;

- **Know the user population.** to become more familiarized and acquainted with the study population prior to the study to facilitate trust building, anticipate potential problems and cope with those appropriately;
- **Learn from prior literature.** and also from experts (psychologists and therapists) to prevent additional stress during the studies;
- **Question your own potential biases.** to increase validity.

Concerning shortcomings in the domain, respondents highlighted the lack of well-established, validated, and scientifically rigorous methods for conducting research with neurodiverse users, and the need of a community to establish a network of partners for cooperation.

5 Conclusion

This study sheds light in to current design practices involving participants with neurodiverse needs. The key findings indicate challenges in the recruitment and retention of participants, and in the data collection. The main recommendations of investigators include relying on a community network to facilitate recruitment, on familiarizing oneself with the study population to foster engagement and build trust, on simplification of the research process to facilitate communication with participants and desensitization of participants with novel technologies prior to data collection. The triangulation of participants' perspectives as well as research methods for data collection and analysis stood out. Most investigators emphasized the importance of a holistic approach in which perspectives from the community, including caregivers, instructors and therapists, are also taken into account to facilitate the study and cross-validate findings.

Acknowledgments. We thank all the respondents of the survey who contributed to this study sharing their experiences and recommendations.

References

1. Brosnan, M., Holt, S., Yuill, N., Good, J., Parsons, S.: Beyond autism and technology: lessons from neurodiverse populations. J. Enabl. Technol. **11**(2), 43–48 (2017)
2. Benton, L., Vasalou, A., Khaled, R., Johnson, H., Gooch, D.: Diversity for design: a framework for involving neurodiverse children in the technology design process. In: Proceedings of the Sigchi Conference on Human Factors in Computing Systems, pp. 3747–3756. ACM, April 2014
3. Evmenova, A.S., Graff, H.J., Genaro Motti, V., Giwa-Lawal, K., Zheng, H.: Designing a wearable technology intervention to support young adults with intellectual and developmental disabilities in inclusive postsecondary academic environments. J. Spec. Educ. Technol. **34**(2), 92–105 (2019). https://doi.org/10.1177/0162643418795833
4. Zheng, H., Genaro Motti, V.: Assisting students with intellectual and developmental disabilities in inclusive education with smartwatches. In: Proceedings of the 2018 CHI Conference on Human Factors in Computing Systems, p. 350. ACM, April 2018

5. Britto, T., Pizzolato, E.: Towards web accessibility guidelines of interaction and interface design for people with autism spectrum disorder. In: ACHI 2016: The Ninth International Conference on Advances in Computer-Human Interactions, pp. 1–7 (2016)
6. Benssassi, E.M., Gomez, J.C., Boyd, L.E., Hayes, G.R., Ye, J.: Wearable assistive technologies for autism: opportunities and challenges. IEEE Pervasive Comput. **17**(2), 11–21 (2018)
7. Frauenberger, C.: Disability and technology: a critical realist perspective. In: Proceedings of the 17th International ACM SIGACCESS Conference on Computers and Accessibility (pp. 89–96). ACM, October 2015
8. Frauenberger, C., Spiel, K., Makhaeva, J.: Thinking outsideTheBox-designing smart things with autistic children. Int. J. Hum.–Comput. Interact. **35**(8), 666–678 (2019)
9. Fage, C.: An emotion regulation app for school inclusion of children with ASD: design principles and preliminary results for its evaluation. ACM SIGACCESS Access. Comput. **112**, 8–15 (2015)
10. Hansen, A.K., Hansen, E.R., Hall, T., Fixler, M., Harlow, D.: Fidgeting with fabrication: students with ADHD making tools to focus. In: Proceedings of the 7th Annual Conference on Creativity and Fabrication in Education, p. 13. ACM, October 2017
11. Mercado, J., Espinosa-Curiel, I., Escobedo, L., Tentori, M.: Developing and evaluating a BCI video game for neurofeedback training: the case of autism. Multimed. Tools Appl. 1–38 (2018)
12. Boyd, L.E., Day, K., Stewart, N., Abdo, K., Lamkin, K., Linstead, E.: Leveling the playing field: supporting neurodiversity via virtual realities. Technol Innov. **20**(1–2), 105–116 (2008). https://doi.org/10.21300/20.1-2.2018.105
13. Sobel, K., Rector, K., Evans, S., Kientz, J.A.: Incloodle: evaluating an interactive application for young children with mixed abilities. In: Proceedings of the 2016 CHI Conference on Human Factors in Computing Systems, pp. 165–176. ACM, May 2016
14. Kraus, L., Lauer, E., Coleman, R., Houtenville, A.: 2017 Disability statistics annual report. University of New Hampshire, Durham, NH (2018)

Investigating the Relationship Between Students' Preferred Learning Style on Their Learning Experience in Virtual Reality (VR) Learning Environment

Shiva Pedram[1(✉)], Sarah Howard[2], Ken Kencevski[3], and Pascal Perez[1]

[1] SMART Infrastructure Facility, Faculty of Engineering and Information Sciences, University of Wollongong, Wollongong, Australia
spedram@uow.edu.au

[2] School of Education, Faculty of Social Science, University of Wollongong, Wollongong, Australia

[3] Devika, University of Wollongong, Wollongong, Australia

Abstract. This study aims to investigate the effects of a virtual reality (VR)-based learning environment on learners with different preferred learning styles by measuring various dimensions of technology mediated approach. The learning outcomes were measured through academic performance, and affectively through "learning experience" and "perceived learning". "Learning experience" in VR was measured through perceived realism, immersion, interaction, presence, engagement, enjoyment, ease of use, usefulness, technology functionality, task-technology fit and attitude towards using the technology. A pretest-posttest design was employed for this study. Students were categorized based on their preferred learning style and their responses were compared. Results presented here are based on data collected from 130 students (grade 5–11) in NSW, Australia. As the result of our analysis indicates, regardless of students' preferred learning style, students similarly benefited from VR and their learning experience and learning outcome did not differ significantly.

Keywords: Virtual Reality · Experiential learning · Learning style · Education · STEM · Technology-mediated · Learning

1 Introduction

Advanced technologies such as Virtual Reality (VR) have gained renewed popularity as a teaching platform among educators and schools, allowing students to learn and experience dangerous, expensive and inaccessible events. Even though virtual reality as a training and teaching platform has proven useful over the years in different industries (flight, surgery, and driving simulators to name a few), these three-dimensional virtual environments are currently not widely utilized in the education sector [1]. However, the trend is changing and the use of computer simulations as learning environments, has progressively embraced technological innovations from chart-based interfaces to fully immersive environments [2].

T. Ahram et al. (Eds.): IHIET 2019, AISC 1018, pp. 275–281, 2020.
https://doi.org/10.1007/978-3-030-25629-6_43

As educational technologies are pushing their ways into the schools, there have been few studies investigating the relationship between different individual's preferences for learning on how they interact with VR environment. Hwang [4] and Lee et al. [3] investigated the effects of a virtual reality (VR) based learning environment on learners with different learning styles. In both studies, they confirm that VR-based learning environment offers promise in accommodating individual differences pertaining to learning styles and there was no difference between students' "cognitive knowledge gain". To complement previous studies, in this study we are focusing on students' "learning experience" and we are going to investigate the relationship between students' preferred learning style and their "learning experience" in VR. Students' perceived "learning experience" in VR is going to be measured through: their perceived "realism", "immersion", "interaction", "ease of Use", "usefulness", "functionality", "task technology fit", "attitude towards the technology", "presence", "engagement", "enjoyment", "stress and worry", "task characteristics". Then students learning experience will be compared based on their preferred learning style.

2 Experiential Learning and VR as a Teaching Platform

Dewey [5] believed learning best occurred through direct experience with the learning environment and content. Effective learning experiences are characterized as active experiential, situated, problem-based, capable of providing immediate feedback [6] and high level of engagement [7]. Realistically, true experiential learning is difficult in many cases and/or significantly limited. VR technologies allowing direct interaction with environments and content through virtual spaces and objects, and it is predicted to enhance the possibility of delivering experiential learning [8].

The greatest capability of VR is in creating "experiences" close to real life events. Mikropoulos [8] defined VR learning environment "as a virtual environment that has one or more educational objectives, pedagogical metaphors, provides users with experiences they would otherwise not be able to experience in the physical world and leads to the attainment of specific learning outcomes" (p. 198). To capture students' learning experience in VR, the factors affecting the learning experience in VR environment are extracted from the body of knowledge.

The objective characteristics of VR is "Immersion" [9] and immersion is what makes it possible to experience and be included in. Skarbez et al. [10] stated that immersion enables presence in VR environment. Sense of "Presence" enhances the students' firsthand experience [11] and first-hand experience happens when students' can directly "Interact" with the virtual or real world. Sense of presence encourage trainees to "Engage" and transform them to be active participants of virtual world [8]. Besides to that, based on Technology Acceptance Model (TAM) and Task-Technology Fit (TTF) technology must be "Easy to use", "Useful" and "Fit the task (Task Technology Fit)" in order for users to "Enjoy" their interaction and experience to ultimately engage with the task to achieve the expected outcome. Contrary, if students feel excessively "Distress and Worry" due to finding the technology hard to use or the learning material hard that would adversely affect their learning process.

Having said that, Kolb [15] argues that people learn in different ways according to their preferred learning style. The 'learning-style' of every learner indicates his/her cognitive trends [12]. This is supported by constructivism where constructivists believe that learning is dependent upon the learner's ability to analyze, synthesize and evaluate information to create meaningful, personalized knowledge [13]. Since learners vary in their cognitive or learning styles, they also benefit from those teaching techniques that appeal to their individual styles [14]. Experiential Learning Theory (ELT) defined nine different learning styles as: (1) Initiating, (2) Experiencing, (3) Imagining, (4) Acting, (5) Reflecting, (6) Deciding, (7) Thinking, (8) Analyzing and (9) Balancing [15]. ELT emphasizes that learning style is not a fixed psychological trait but a dynamic state resulting from synergistic transactions between the person and the environment [15]. The stability and endurance of these states in individuals comes from consistent patterns of transaction between the individual and his or her environment. This highlights the importance of learning environment. This study aims to investigate the relationship between students' "learning preferences" and their "learning experience" in VR. Therefore, firstly students' "learning experience" and the "outcomes" of, Virtual Reality (VR) teaching session will be measured and then students' responses will be compared based on their preferred learning style.

3 Methodology

3.1 Participants

The participants of this study were 130 students from five different public and private schools in NSW, Australia. The participants were boys and girls and they were in grade 5 to 11 (Table 1). The students were randomly selected by their teachers and researcher had no control over selecting the participants.

Table 1. Sample distribution

Year	# Students	Schools participated in this study
Year 5	38	(28 students from school 1, 10 students from school 2)
Year 6	18	(18 students from school 3)
Year 8	10	(5 students from school 4 and 5 students from 5)
Year 9	15	(11 students from school 5 and 4 students from St 4)
Year 10	40	(20 students from 5 and 20 students from school 4)
Year 11	9	(9 students from school 4)

3.2 Scenario

In this study students experienced the Antarctic and learnt how to interact with penguins (Fig. 2). The content was developed by Australian Company (Devika) and delivered via the virtual reality headset HTC VIVE (Fig. 1). The scenario is extracurricular and mapped to the Australian school curriculum. The Antarctic scenario

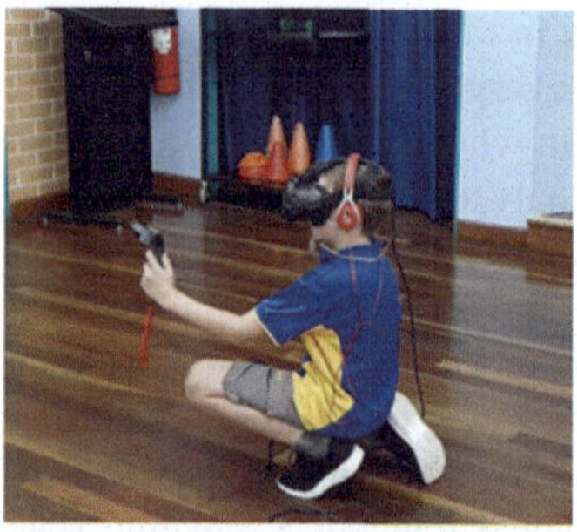

Fig. 1. Student experiencing VR

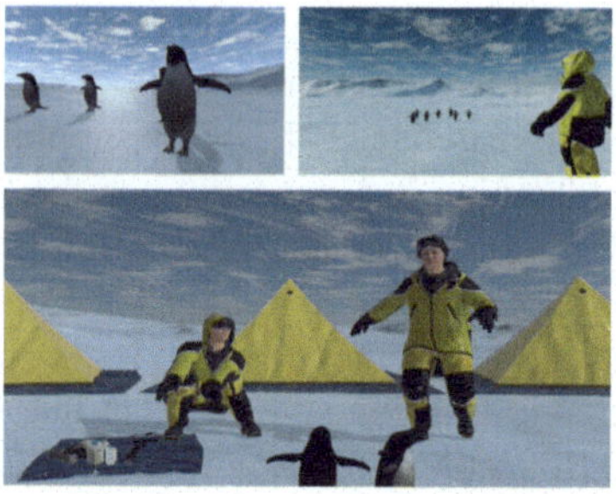

Fig. 2. Antarctic scene in VR

begins where a scientist will introduce the topic and explain the reasoning for their presence, their significance with the ecology, and some of the activities that take place. The scenario teaches students about Antarctica by placing them in a VR experience that requires them to listen to a scientist in Antarctic. This is done by having the students complete a series of tasks such as photographing penguins with the aid of a narrator.

3.3 Procedure

A pretest-posttest design was employed for this study.

Pre-test Phase

(i) Prior to the experience content related questions were distributed: The aim is to assess students' knowledge level about penguins, Antarctic and climate change prior attending the learning session in VR. They were asked to answer six questions related to the scenario, such as: "What is the average temperature in Antarctic?" Or "What is the effect of climate change on penguins?" The total score of each content related test was 6.

(ii) Prior to the experience KLS v4 [7]. Inventory was distributed: The aim is to assess students' preferred learning style prior exposure to VR. A participant who took this test needed to complete 12 sentences that described learning. Each item had four endings and the participants were required to rank these endings according to how well he or she thought each ending described the way he or she learned. The scores were calculated to determine the dominant type of learning style for each participant.

Post-test Phase

(i) After the experience post-experience questionnaire was distributed: 5–10 min After the learning experience in VR, a post-training questionnaires was distributed (10-likert scale where 0 was highly disagree, 10 was highly agree and 5 in middle was neutral), to measure students experience in VR. The items in this questionnaire are taken from standard questionnaires.

(ii) After the experience, Content related questions were distributed again: in order to measure students' knowledge gain the content related questions were repeated within one-hour timeframe of the first test.

4 Result and Discussion

4.1 Gain Score and Preferred Learning Style

From the survey result (subjective analysis), 74% of students (95 students out of 124) reported that they have learned from VR experience and they know more about penguins, Antarctic and climate change after VR experience (perceived learning score was 7, 8, 9 or 10 out of 10). Additionally, the result of content related (pre and post test) reveals that students' performance enhanced by 37%. Moreover, one-way ANOVA was performed to see whether statistically there is a significant difference between students' gain score with respect to their preferred learning styles. As the result of analysis indicated there was no significant difference between the mean scores ($p > 0.05$) and regardless of students' preferred learning style they have opportunity to benefit from a VR experience.

4.2 Learning Experience in VR and Preferred Learning Style

Correlation between factors measured after the VR learning experience indicates that the measured factors are statistically significant and correlated with perceived learning, also there is a correlation within these factors which is going to be discussed in our next paper. In Table 2, ATU is (Attitude Toward Use), TTF is (Task Technology Fit) and TC is (Task characteristics).

Then, one-way ANOVA was performed to see whether students' who have different preferred learning styles are having different learning experience in VR. The result of analysis indicated that statistically there were no significant difference ($P > .05$) between students and it is safe to claim there is no relationship between students' preferred learning style and "learning experience" in VR.

Table 2. Correlation table between learning and factors affecting learning experience

	Realism	Immersion	Interaction	Ease of use	Usefulness	Function-ality
Learning	.536	.575	.663	.563	.771	.815
p value	.000	.000	.000	.000	.000	.000

	ATU	TTF	Presence	Engagement	Enjoyment	Stress	TC
Learning	.653	.789	.646	.672	.717	-.545	.724
p value	.000	.000	.000	.000	.000	.000	.000

5 Discussion and Conclusion

Game play provides learners the opportunity to learn by doing and though role-play, enhancing students' learning outcome (e.g. [16]), our findings also suggest this view. In this study, students played the role of scientists in VR, and as our subjective (perceived learning) and objective (results of content related questions) analysis revealed, students' knowledge level enhanced. Our knowledge test was short and there was not enough time lag between two tests, but hat being said, the result of our analysis indicated that there was no relationship between students' preferred learning style and students' knowledge gain. Lee et al. [3] also, reported the same findings that, there was no significant difference in the cognitive and affective learning outcomes for students with different learning styles in the VR-based learning environment.

Moreover, the result of correlation indicated that there is a relationship between students' knowledge gain in VR and students' "learning experience" through perceived sense of presence, immersion, realism, interaction and affective factors including perceived sense of enjoyment, engagement, usefulness and attitudes towards using technology. However, our findings indicates that there is no relationship between students' "preferred learning style" and their "learning experience" in VR. Therefore, based on our findings and the trend we observed in students' performance after VR session and their positive perception of "learning experience" in VR, educators and decision makers are encouraged for future investigation in VR integration into classrooms.

References

1. Dholakiya, N.D., Ferjencik, M., Schofield, D., Kubík, J.: Virtual learning for safety, why not a smartphone? Process Saf. Prog. **38**(2) (2019)
2. Bell, P.C., Taseen, A.A., Kirkpatrick, P.F.: Visual interactive simulation modeling in a decision support role. Comput. Oper. Res. **17**, 447–456 (1990)
3. Lee, E.A.L., Wong, K.W.: Learning with desktop virtual reality: low spatial ability learners are more positively affected. Comput. Educ. **79**, 49–58 (2014)
4. Hwang, G.J., Wu, P.H., Chen, C.C.: An online game approach for improving students' learning performance in web-based problem-solving activities. Comput. Educ. **59**(4), 1246–1256 (2012)
5. Dewey, J.: Democracy and Education. Macmillan Company, New York (1916)
6. Ketelhut, D.J., Schifter, C.C.: Teachers and game-based learning: improving understanding of how to increase efficacy of adoption. Comput. Educ. **56**(2), 539 (2011)
7. Park, B., Plass, J.L., Brünken, R.: Cognitive and affective processes in multimedia (2014)
8. Mikropoulos, T.A., Natsis, A.: Educational virtual environments: a ten-year review of empirical research (1999–2009). Comput. Educ. **56**(3), 769–780 (2011)
9. Slater, M.: Measuring presence: a response to the witmer and singer presence questionnaire. Presence: Teleoper. Virtual Environ. **8**(5), 560–565 (1999)
10. Skarbez, R., Brooks Jr., F.P., Whitton, M.C.: A survey of presence and related concepts. ACM Comput. Surv. (CSUR) **50**(6), 96 (2018)
11. Winn, W., Jackson, R.: Fourteen propositions about educational uses of virtual reality. Educ. Technol. **39**, 5–14 (1999)

12. Nawaz, A., Kundi, G.M.: From objectivism to social constructivism: the impacts of information and communication technologies (ICTs) on higher education. Int. J. Sci. Technol. Educ. Res. **1**(2), 30–36 (2010)
13. Phillips, P., Wells, J., Ice, P., Curtis, R., Kennedy, R.: A case study of the relationship between socio-epistemological teaching orientations and instructor perceptions of pedagogy in online environments. Elect. J. Integ. Technol. Educ. **6**, 3–27 (2008). http://ejite.isu.edu/. 6 (1). Accessed 10 Apr 2007
14. Cagiltay, N.E., Yildirim, S., Aksu, M.: Students' preferences on web-based instruction: linear or non-linear. J. Edu. Technol. Soc., **9**(3): 122–136 (2006). http://www.ask4research.info/. Accessed 10 Apr 2007
15. Kolb, D.A.: The kolb learning style inventory 4.0: guide to theory, psychometrics, research and applications (2013)
16. Annetta, L.A., Minogue, J., Holmes, S.Y., Cheng, M.T.: Investigating the impact of video games on high school students' engagement and learning about genetics. Comput. Educ. **53** (1), 74–85 (2009)

AugmentedBook: A Collaborative E-Learning Augmented Reality Platform

Nouf M. Alzahrani[1(✉)] and Sonia Lajmi[1,2(✉)]

[1] Information Technology Department, Faculty of Computer Science and Information Technology, Albaha University, Albaha, Saudi Arabia
{noufalzahrani, slajmi}@bu.edu.sa

[2] MIRACL: Multimedia InfoRmation Systems and Advanced Computing Laboratory, University of Sfax, Technological Pole of Sfax, Sakiet Ezzit, 3021 Sfax, Tunisia

Abstract. This paper introduces an augmented reality-based framework (called AugmentedBook) for e-learning that allows the creation of collaborative notes, illustrative media (i.e. video, 2D or 3D image, audio) for mobile devices or Google glass. The augmented content can be added to real-world educational support to make it more comprehensive, interactive and collaborative. In this platform, students and teachers can add collaborative notes to any part of the educational support system. They can also find illustrative media and indicate the pertinence of the result. Using our AugmentedBook platform, students can also download the enriched support using a mobile device. Our framework solves the problem of standard integration of augmented reality applications in education, offering a distributed framework which is e-learning compliant.

Keywords: Augmented reality · E-learning · Collaborative annotation · Mobile device

1 Introduction

The augmented reality (AR) domain has shown widespread growth in recent decades. This is not surprising given the scale of use of advanced mobile devices containing cameras that record reality and add different types of metadata (2D images, 3D images, text, audio or video) in real time. The application of AR can be useful in several areas: for example, in the field of medicine this technology could allow the surgeon to have a more detailed, real-time and 3D view of the organs when operating, which could also be an effective way to improve diagnosis.

As we show, the use of such technology is paramount in many areas. Indeed, we increasingly need to align knowledge and create a new reality in which connectivity, interactions and visualization of all activities are not centralized but distributed, collaborative and interactive.

The field of education can take advantage of this scientific progress to improve educational process. Nowadays, the use of computer tools to support education, known as e-learning, optimizes teaching and learning processes. According to [1], e-learning must go beyond platforms such as Learning Management Systems (LMS) to allow the

T. Ahram et al. (Eds.): IHIET 2019, AISC 1018, pp. 282–288, 2020.
https://doi.org/10.1007/978-3-030-25629-6_44

students to work collaboratively using computer resources. In addition, AR could benefit e-learning processes through an intuitive way of interacting and collaborating between real and augmented objects.

According to [2], including AR technologies in educational settings improves learner outcomes, allows pedagogical contributions and allows more interaction. It can enhance learning achievement and motivation; improve satisfaction, confidence, comprehension and attitude; and decease cognitive load. It can provide the following interaction opportunities: student-student, student-material and student-teacher. Finally, AR can enable the visualization of invisible and abstract concepts and events. We propose a promising AR framework for e-learning called AugmentedBook.

One of the main ideas in our AugmentedBook framework is to provide collaborative and illustrative media (i.e. text, video, image) related to a target in the educational support system. This framework allow the students and teachers to work together for rich educational support. To the best of our knowledge, there is no previous work in AR applied in the e-learning domain that allows collaborative work on the educational support itself. Our system proposes to add various explanatory multimedia on any target without requiring a plug-in.

The rest of this paper is organized as follows: the literature review is described more in depth in Sect. 2, the AugmentedBook architecture is detailed in Sect. 3, experimental setup and results are presented in Sect. 4, and in Sect. 5 we conclude with a summary and perspective of our work.

2 Literature Review

Thanks to the development of mobile devices, AR technology has responded quickly. In fact, nowadays, mobile devices integrate all the functions necessary to launch AR applications, such as a broadband internet connection, excellent computing power, cameras and sensors such as GPS, accelerometer and fingerprint reader.

As a result, the use of AR has received a lot of attention in several domains and especially in education [3]. There is no doubt about the potential of AR content to improve motivation and learning as shown in studies such as [3] and [4], but a lack of standardization delays integration into educational environments. Currently, AR-based education systems still do not offer a standard solution that groups all the features mentioned earlier, according to [2].

In the last few decades, several AR e-learning frameworks have been proposed. One of the first approaches is described in [5]. They took advantage of the first versions of Web3D technologies to introduce a web-based editor for creating 3D content and a viewer for educational purposes. Although the idea was innovative, specific plug-ins were required and it was intended for a tabletop environment. Some developments use AR for a particular educational application. For example, one study [6] proposes a simple interface for examination applications that allows user interaction with one finger. This approach limits the user to response either yes or no, and there are still no standards for integration with an LMS. A system described in [7] uses an authoring tool to develop AR applications for industrial sequential procedures. Although sequential application is a considerable improvement, it requires specific hardware and software.

An AR-based mobile software that provides 3D and multimedia e-learning material for complementing books or other educational support is presented in [8].

According to [9], mobile devices offer an ideal platform for AR applications as they are very cost-effective and easy to use, especially for younger students [10]. Desktop computers can support AR applications, but they are not portable due to hardware limitations [11]. In contrast, mobile devices provide many advantages, such as portability and encouragement of high social interactivity [12]. They are also beneficial to students who engage in outdoor observations and learning activities [13]. Furthermore, location-based AR on mobile devices enables students to immerse themselves in the learning process [11] and increases their collaboration skills [14]. The 2010 Horizon Report [15] indicated that users would no longer need to be tethered to their desktop computers thanks to wireless mobile technology.

To the best of our knowledge, there is no work in the field of AR e-learning that allows the teacher and students to add class notes related to the textbook. Videos and explanatory audio can be added to the course material itself, which allows students and teachers to interact and collaborate (in the same way as social media comments) by adding notes in real time and overlaying it directly on the course material. There is no similar mobile device application available that does not require installation of a plug-in.

3 AugmentedBook Architecture

As illustrated in Fig. 1, the AugmentedBook e-learning platform allow students and teachers to add collaborative comments on any target from the educational support. The system also recommends illustrative videos to a given target. The recommended videos and audio can help students to better understand the content of the educational support.

AugmentedBook has a distributed architecture, using Cloud and mobile devices to create AR applications. The architecture of the education platform is n-tier. In the following sections, the different tiers and layers of the AugmentedBook are explained.

3.1 The Client Tier

The mobile device constructs our client tier and the Android engine communicates with sensors like the camera and accelerometer. The user event via GUI (Graphical User Interface) are listened and the target is tracked. The tracked target can be an image or text from the educational support, and is transmitted to the AR engine via the Android engine. We adopted Vuforia[1] as the AR engine because there is no plug-in to install. The last part of client tier constructs local storage. An SQlite database is used to store the last used target, to avoid sending a recognition query to the target management system each time.

[1] www.vuforia.com.

3.2 The Application Tier

The second tier in our architecture is the application tier. It includes a Data Access Object layer which is responsible for getting/setting data from the data source. The second layer is a business layer responsible for processes like recognizing the target and video retrieval. The recognition of the target (text or image) is executed by the target management system. The last layer of the application tier is the web service layer, which can contain several technologies or types of communication such as Rest, Corba and SOAP. Communication is via Restful web service, which was chosen over other kinds of web services due to its popularity, simplicity, its perfect adaptation to the client-server architecture and because communication is independent of the state of the client. Communication with the wider web services is via http/JSON. The application communicates with three different services:

- The first service is dedicated to recognition of the image targets. For this purpose, the Target Image Recognition service of Vuforia is used which is based on a machine-learning algorithm.
- The second service is dedicated to recognition of the text target. For this purpose, the Target Text Recognition service of Vuforia is used. For the moment, the service supports only the English language.
- The third service takes as input the result of the second service, with the objective of returning a video that is relevant to the recognized text. The YouTube API is used for this purpose and proposes the five most relevant videos. If the user validates the relevance of the video to the selected context, it is stored in a tree structure in the Firebase database (explained in Sect. 3.4). In this way, potential viewers of the same text will see the same videos judged relevant by the user. They can likewise appreciate the video, comment or add other videos.

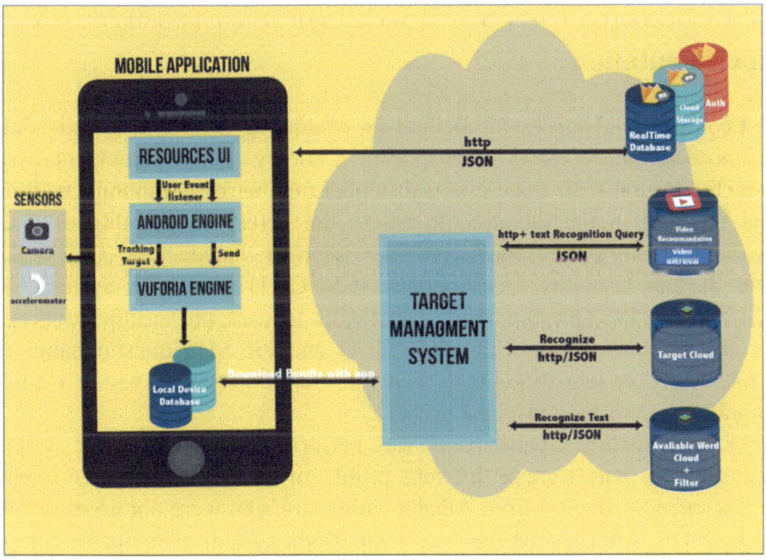

Fig. 1. Overview of the AugmentedBook framework

3.3 The Data Tier

The last tier in our AR framework is the data tier, which establishes communication with the authentication service, Firebase storage and Firebase real-time database. These services are used as follows:

- Storage: Firebase storage is dedicated to storing and retrieving user-specific large files such as photos or videos.
- Authentication: allows easy creation and management of various means of authentication (such as Google, Facebook or email) for easy and secure access to AugmentedBook.
- Real-time database: data is stored as JSON and synchronized in real-time to every connected client. This allow us to rapidly receive updates with the latest data and manage concurrent users more easily.

3.4 Firebase Real-Time Tree Data Structure

The two types of collaboration (student-student and teacher-student) help to create rich educational support. To allow collaboration between different participants (teachers and students), a real-time Firebase tree structure is used to store targets as well as all the associated metadata. Indeed, as illustrated in the JSON structure, each target is associated with an identifier, a type, a value and an idOwner (which is the identifier of the person who has marked this target). In addition, the target can be associated with different multimedia documents such as video, text, audio or image. In the same way, these multimedia documents are identified by identifiers, idOwners and popularity. For each multimedia document, a response can be associated, which constitutes social interactions between participants around the multimedia document that enriches the target. The documents themselves are stored in the Firebase Storage Service.

4 Experimentation

The most common and successful method for evaluating an HCI is to carry out a user study. This technique consists of proposing a survey to the participants, who can answer each question with a score. A substantial number of questionnaires have been used and reported in the literature to assess the perceived usability of interactive systems, namely the Questionnaire on User Interface Satisfaction (QUIS) [16], the Computer System Usability Questionnaire (CSUQ) [17] and the System Usability Scale (SUS) [18, 19] Questionnaire. The QUIS focuses on specific aspects of the human-computer interaction, while the CSUQ and the SUS questionnaires revolve around interactive system usability in general. Our proposed survey to evaluate our AugmentedBook system is inspired by [17].

A user study with 25 participants was performed to evaluate our system. The participants taking part were a different profile of students (computer science, IT, literature, science, medicine) from Albaha University who were not necessary familiar with Android OS. After testing the AugmentedBook system, participants completed a form containing the following questions. Scores range from 1 to 7 where 1 represents 'strongly disagree' and 7 'strongly agree'. The first eight questions assess system usefulness. Questions 9–15 assess participants' satisfaction with the quality of the information associated with the system. Questions 16–18 allow the participant to rate the interface quality.

Subsequently, we provide a graphical representation (in the form of a chart) of these answers. The histogram (Fig. 2) shows that the majority of scores are between 5 and 7. Based on the result of this experiment, we conclude that using our AR system does not entail any major drawbacks. Nevertheless, there is a need to improve certain points such as detecting text written in Arabic in the system.

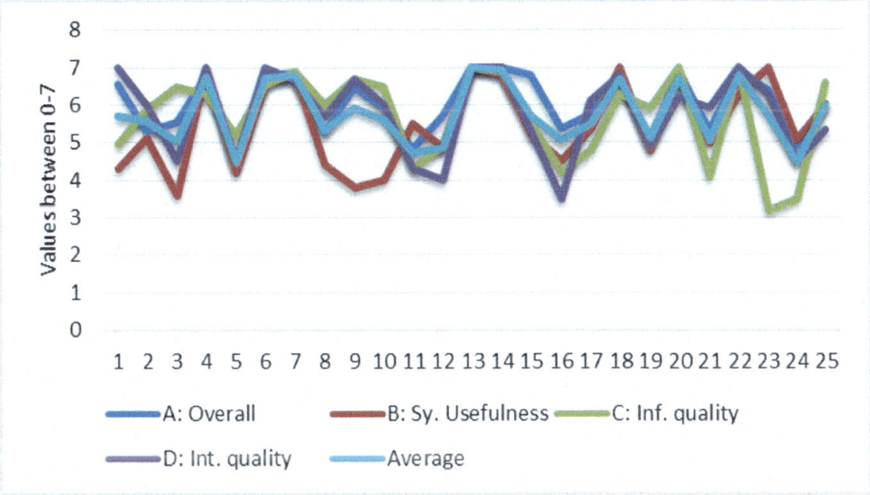

Fig. 2. Average score of AugmentedBook from 25 participants from different profiles

5 Conclusion

In this paper, we propose a new AR framework called AugmentedBook. We also collected and classified AR applications based on several criteria, and through these comparisons found that AugmentedBook is the first educational application that combines the most important features and characteristics needed by both student and teacher in the educational environment and learning process.

Nevertheless, it remains to improve several aspects in our AugmentedBook system. We plan to extend the evaluation from 25 students to at least 25 teachers and 100 students from different profiles (computer science, literature, science, medicine). We plan to integrate a multimodal search starting from the text target. For the moment, our platform supports only explanatory video suggestions to the text recognized in the educational medium. We plan also to recognize Arabic text since the educational support system in our university is in both the English and Arabic languages.

References

1. Dalsgaard, C.: Social software: E-learning beyond learning management systems. Eur. J. Open Dist E-Learn. (2006). http://www.eurodl.org/materials/contrib/2006/Christian_Dalsgaard.htm
2. Akçayır, M., Akçayır, G.: Advantages and challenges associated with augmented reality for education: a systematic review of the literature. Educ. Res. Rev. **20**, 1–11 (2017)
3. Wu, H.-K., Lee, S.W.-Y., Chang, H.-Y., Liang, J.-C.: Current status, opportunities and challenges of augmented reality in education. Comput. Educ. **62**, 41–49 (2013)
4. Di Serio, A., Ibáñez, M.B., Kloos, C.D.: Impact of an augmented reality system on students' motivation for a visual art course. Comput. Educ. **68**, 586–596 (2013)
5. Liarokapis, F., Mourkoussis, N., White, M., Darcy, J., Sifniotis, M., Petridis, P., Basu, A., Lister, P.F.: Web3d and augmented reality to support engineering education. World Trans. Eng. Technol. Educ. UICEE **3**(1), 11–14 (2004)
6. Wang, M.-J., Tseng, C.-H., Shen, C.-Y.: An easy to use augmented reality authoring tool for use in examination purpose. In: Forbrig, P., Paternó, F., Mark Pejtersen, A. (eds.) HCIS 2010. IFIP AICT, vol. 332, pp. 285–288. Springer, Heidelberg (2010)
7. Orduña, J.M., Fernández, M., Gimeno, J., Morillo, P.: An advanced authoring tool for augmented reality applications in industry. In: XXIII Jornadas de Paralelismo, pp. 586–591 (2010)
8. Kose, U., Koc, D., Yucesoy, S.A.: An augmented reality based mobile software to support learning experiences in computer science courses. VARE Proc. Comput. Sci. **25**, 370–374 (2013)
9. Henrysson, A., Billinghurst, M., Ollila, M.: Face to face collaborative AR on mobile phones. In: ISMAR 2005 Proceedings of the 4th IEEE/ACM International Symposium on Mixed and Augmented Reality, pp. 80–89, IEEE, Washington (2005)
10. Furio, D., GonzáLez-Gancedo, S., Juan, M.-C., Seguí, I., Costa, M.: The effects of the size and weight of a mobile device on an educational game. Comput. Educ. **64**, 24–41 (2013)
11. Chiang, T.H., Yang, S.J., Hwang, G.-J.: Students' online interactive patterns in augmented reality-based inquiry activities. Comput. Educ. **78**, 97–108 (2014)
12. Hwang, G.-J., Tsai, C.-C., Chu, H.-C., Kinshuk, K., Chen, C.-Y.: A context-aware ubiquitous learning approach to conducting scientific inquiry activities. Aust. J. Educ. Technol. **28**(5), 931–947 (2012)
13. Chiang, T.H., Yang, S.J., Hwang, G.-J.: An augmented reality-based mobile learning system to improve students' learning achievements and motivations in natural science inquiry activities. J. Educ. Technol. Soc. **17**(4), 352–365 (2014)
14. Bressler, D., Bodzin, A.: A mixed methods assessment of students' flow experiences during a mobile augmented reality science game. J. Comput. Assist. Learn. **29**(6), 505–517 (2013)
15. Johnson, L., Laurence, F., Smith, R., Stone, S.: The 2010 horizon report. The New Media Consortium, Austin, Texas (2010)
16. Chin, J.P., Diehl, V.A., Norman, K.L.: Development of an instrument measuring user satisfaction of the human-computerinterface. In: Proceedings of the SIGCHI Conference on Human Factors in Computing Systems, CHI 1988, pp. 213–218. ACM, New York (1988)
17. Lewis, J.R.: IBM computer usability satisfaction questionnaires: psychometric evaluation and instructions for use. Int. J. Hum.-Comput. Interact. **7**(1), 57–78 (1995)
18. Brooke, J.: SUS-a quick and dirty usability scale. Usability Eval. Ind. **189**(194), 4–7 (1996)
19. Brooke, J.: SUS: a retrospective. J. Usability Stud. **8**(2), 29–40 (2013)

The Effects of Virtual Reality Learning Environments on Improving the Retention, Comprehension, and Motivation of Medical School Students

Neil Gomes[1,2(✉)], Yiping Lou[2], Viraj Patwardhan[1], Timothy Moyer[1], Victoria Vavala[1], and Cacilda Barros[1]

[1] Thomas Jefferson University, 925 Chestnut Street, Philadelphia, PA 19107, USA
neil.gomes@jefferson.edu
[2] University of South Florida, 3202 E Fowler Avenue, Tampa, FL 33620, USA

Abstract. As Virtual Reality (VR) technologies have become affordable, portable, and realistic, the use of VR for education is becoming a reality. However, while VR environments are novel and interesting, this project studies if learning medical concepts in a VR environment truly improves the retention, comprehension, and motivation of medical school students. This paper presents the key results of a literature review of the current corpus of studies on these topics. The review revealed a modest number of peer-reviewed studies that assessed the retention, comprehension, and motivation of adult learners using VR in medical education. However, these studies presented several insights summarized in this paper. Additional research needs to be done on this topic to prove the efficacy and validity of this new medium for medical training and instruction. This paper also presents avenues for future research and describes a study that the researchers plan to conduct following this literature review.

Keywords: Virtual Reality · Medical education · VR · Retention · Comprehension · Motivation · Augmented Reality · AR · Medicine · Education · Learning · Literature review

1 Introduction

"We live here, in the OASIS. For us, this is the only reality that has any meaning". Wade Watts makes this statement in the book and movie Ready Player One by author Ernest Cline [1]. The OASIS, in the sci-fi epic Ready Player One, is a virtual reality environment that all our future counterparts immerse themselves in as their reality is a bleak existence and the OASIS their escape.

Fortunately, we are not there yet! However, virtual reality is increasingly being recognized as the next frontier for communication, collaboration, and learning. Healthcare and medical education are also turning to this new and exciting medium to engage and motivate learners. Virtual reality technology has frequently been seen in the news and discussed in areas of medicine ranging from opioid addiction to surgical training.

T. Ahram et al. (Eds.): IHIET 2019, AISC 1018, pp. 289–296, 2020.
https://doi.org/10.1007/978-3-030-25629-6_45

At Thomas Jefferson University (TJU), the home of Sidney Kimmel Medical College, high-quality medical education is one of the core components of our institution. The Digital Innovation and Consumer Experience (DICE) Group at TJU and Jefferson Health designs, develops, and implements value-driven and consumer-focused solutions that transform healthcare and education by focusing on Jefferson Health's mission: We Improve Lives. Over the past two years, the XR (Extended Reality) Lab, within the DICE Group, has worked to create a collaborative environment where healthcare meets XR technology. Our team studies the potential benefits of augmented reality and virtual reality for education and patient health and wellness. Our work is also informed by the experiences of healthcare providers who help us create and run IRB (Institutional Review Board)-approved studies utilizing XR technology.

2 The Research Question

The current landscape of medical education is ripe for innovative approaches to enhance learning and outcomes for upcoming physicians. For decades the structure of medical education has remained largely unchanged. As the amount of information and delivery of specialized care grows in complexity and volume [2], future physicians are asked to comprehend and retain more material in shorter periods of study. To account for this exponential growth in expected knowledge, medical education needs to adapt. Thus, new modalities of andragogy need to be explored. Emerging technologies, such as virtual reality, present possibilities for engaging students with medical content in immersive environments.

At DICE, it is our goal to find new and innovative ways to leverage technology. As part of TJU and Jefferson Health, we see firsthand the importance of developing new learning tools for educating current and future medical professionals. To explore how the emerging medium of virtual reality can positively impact the growing needs of medical educators and their students, it is essential to start broad, evaluating learning outcomes using global criteria. The College of Education at University of South Florida (USF) is an institution that is equally interested in studying the effects of Virtual Reality (VR) environments on learning and so we collaborated with Dr. Yiping Lou, the major professor of one of our co-authors, to conduct this study. After preliminary searches, we determined that comprehension, retention, and motivation were key outcomes in evaluating the efficacy of virtual reality as a learning modality in medical education and, therefore, our research question focused on: Does learning medical concepts in a VR environment improve the comprehension, retention, and motivation of medical school students and in what contexts?

It is important to note that while there are countless published works regarding the efficacy of evaluating learning tools, our goal was to limit our scope to studies conducted utilizing head-mounted displays (HMDs). Frequently the term "virtual" in the context of education studies refers to "digital" teaching, but not virtual reality as it is currently recognized. Additionally, as the industry has grown and HMDs have become more accessible, the technology has continued to exponentially improve. We decided to limit our scope to the past ten years, with the understanding that the majority of virtual reality hardware currently on the market is only five years old or newer.

While there are studies evaluating VR that were published more than ten years ago, we determined that – much like comparing a computer running Windows 95 to a current PC – technology used in studies earlier than 2009 is largely obsolete and not indicative of what current VR technology can achieve.

In this paper, we present the key results of a literature review of the current corpus of peer-reviewed studies that assessed the retention, comprehension, and motivation of adult learners using VR in medical education. This paper also describes a study that we plan to conduct following this literature review.

3 Comprehension

With any learning tool, it is first vital to determine if it effectively teaches students – do they comprehend the information they have learned? Do learners develop an understanding of the intended topic? How does their level of understanding compare to their comprehension via typical methods of learning? The majority of contemporary studies that incorporated comprehension as a measurement did so in relation to patients accurately understanding abstract or dense medical concepts [3–6].

A study published in 2019 measured comprehension related to how physicians learn anatomy and surgical procedures using VR [7]. In this study, a virtual reality environment that visualizes three-dimensional patient-specific models was displayed through a mobile head-mounted display. Thirty-three medical practitioners and trainees participated in the study and completed a six-question/statement, five-point Likert-type scale survey. Of the six questions/statements, the one most relevant to our inquiry was: "It allows a better comprehension of anatomy compared with medical imaging datasets (anatomy comprehension)" [7].

After conducting the study, the researchers concluded that "our approach, based on open-source software and mobile hardware, proved to be a valid and well-appreciated system to visualize 3D patient-specific models, paving the way for a potential new tool for teaching and preoperative planning" [7].

In another study, published in 2009 on, *Testing the effects of educational strategies on comprehension of a genomic concept using virtual reality technology* [3], researchers examined the effect of learning mode on comprehension of a genomic concept. 156 individuals aged 18–40 were randomly assigned to either a Virtual reality learning or didactic learning condition and were measured for:

- Recall (how much presented information participants remembered)
- Transfer (if participants could apply what they had learned)
- Mental models (change in mental models in response to learning activities).

The researchers in this study concluded that "increases in comprehension were greater with didactic learning, while motivation, interest and enjoyment were rated more highly for active learning", [3].

The studies noted above suggest a variety of methods for assessing comprehension of adult medical school learners. Surveys or questionnaires seem to be the most feasible for simplifying study design measurements, however, comprehension is a complex facet of learning and often difficult to measure.

4 Retention

For any student, it can be tempting to learn new information simply for an examination, but for a learning modality to be truly useful, learners must be able to hold onto that information for future use as well. Similar to comprehension, it is important to understand if learners retain the information they learn via a new mode of learning as compared to traditional learning methods. In studies conducted over the last decade, the primary goal was to compare existing 2D mediums (TV, Desktops, PowerPoint presentations) with immersive 360-degree virtual reality, delivered via the medium of head mounted displays (HMDs).

In a recent multi-site study [8], 197 nursing students were exposed to disaster decontamination training through one of three modalities: traditional written instructions, simulated scenes on a PC, and virtually simulated scenes on an Oculus Rift HMD. Students were evaluated using a traditional paper-and-pencil 20-question cognitive learning test based on the *FEMA IS-346: An Orientation to Hazardous Materials for Medical Personnel*, as well as a practical exam on a manikin. The same examinations were conducted again six months later to evaluate retention. At this point, no discernable differences were found between all three groups regarding their retention, though the learners using both the computer and VR simulated training modules reported more enjoyment.

In a different study, investigators attempted to evaluate the concept of virtual memory palaces for adult learning and retention [9]. Forty participants were introduced to a virtual mind palace, both on a PC and in a VR HMD. Conducted in a cross-over design, participants experienced both displays in succession, with a break in between mediums. Participants were asked to memorize the locations of 21 face-name pairs in each scene in the course of five minutes. For the two minutes immediately following, investigators asked participants questions designed to take the place of short-term memories. After, participants were asked to recount the face-name pairs, now from their long-term memory. The results showed that "participants were able to recall better in the HMD condition as compared to the desktop condition" and that the overall recall of HMD users was 8.8% higher than those using the desktop version. The authors suggest that using spatial awareness is an important part of the immersive quality of virtual reality.

While these are only a sampling of the research covering the area of VR and learning retention, they suggest some key points for understanding the relationship between the two. First, as with any learning modality, repetition is important. Learners cannot be expected to try something once and retain it six months later without practice. Second, immersive interactions are more engaging to students. Finally, creating virtual learning environments that take advantage of the "space" in the virtual world – promoting learners' spatial awareness – are vital to fully taking advantage of virtual reality as a medium.

5 Motivation

While comprehension and retention are vital to evaluating effective learning tools, they are not the only key concepts to consider. Learner motivation, or how driven students are to learn, is a vital part of any learning experience. If students are not motivated, then regardless of how effective a tool may be, students may not use it. Learner motivation can often be considered subjective, but it is important to review in conjunction with comprehension and retention to get a fuller picture of virtual reality as a learning tool.

In 2018, a randomized controlled study of 66 medical students attending the University of Saskatchewan examined "the impact of immersive virtual-reality neuroanatomy training and compare[d] it to traditional paper-based methods" [10]. Though retention is suggested as a primary measure for the study, the results of this study "suggest that integration of virtual-reality into neuroanatomy training may improve knowledge retention [and] increase study motivation," as well as that "the novelty and potential for increased motivation to learn is an asset for virtual-reality technology in the medical curriculum that may enhance students' incentive to study" [10].

Another neuroanatomy study published in 2017, [11] by Stepan et al. evaluated the motivation of medical students via a randomized controlled study, also of 66 participants. Students reviewed neuroanatomical structures "using either online textbooks or the VR interactive model" [11]. The researchers used the *Instructional Materials Motivation Survey* [IMMS], a previously-validated assessment as a method of measurement. The study showed mixed results between the two groups, but reported that "the VR group…scored significantly higher on the motivation assessment" [11].

Based on our analysis of the studies conducted over the past decade, form factors and presentation of virtual content have significant bearing on learner motivation. Perceived ease of use and perceived usefulness are other factors that affect learner engagement along with the type of content and the learners' comfort with new and emerging technology [12].

6 Additional Research

The majority of studies we surveyed did not incorporate dynamic interaction with content or virtual subject matter. Most studies compared traditional 2D learning mediums (TV, Desktop, PowerPoint presentation) with immersive 360-degree media. We would like to encourage other researchers to conduct more studies that incorporate dynamic interaction with content or virtual subject matter as the cost and time required to create such content is reducing. Moreover, dynamic interaction with content in immersive virtual reality environments will truly test what appear to be the greatest advantage of such environments.

Our literature review analysis revealed two key variables for measuring effectiveness of learning in virtual reality environments – retention and motivation. Comprehension, we found, was a very fluid concept in terms of definition between studies and a variable that was hard to objectively measure. Based on our literature review and practical expertise in the field of AR/VR research and development, we think it would be beneficial to the field of healthcare and medicine to conduct a study that analyzes if retention and motivation of medical students is improved by using immersive and dynamic VR environments for learning. We plan to conduct such a study as the next step in the evolution of our research. In this study, we will measure the following:

- Motivation: Measured via qualitative and quantitative questions that will assess if the material was engaging and ask participants to rate their desire to use such a form of learning again to study similar concepts.
- Retention: Measured via a quantitative test on specific material covered when participants engaged in the VR simulation. There will also be a quantitative pre-test to measure existing knowledge of the subject being taught.

This VR study design will follow the criteria listed below:

- Content selection: The content will be based on a medical education topic and will be succinct.
- Type of medium: The study will use both immersive VR and traditional online 2D learning media to objectively compare retention and motivation.
- Self-contained: Each participant will traverse the study individually and in one session.
- Environment: The research environment for the study participants will be similar to avoid having any extraneous variables (noise, smell, comfort, etc.) affecting the learning outcomes.

The study results will help researchers compare the benefits of both environments and better understand if medical students are able to retain their learning better in one environment over the other or if either of the environments provided more motivation to learn the existing content and future content. The study will also inform researchers, learning designers, and faculty about how motivated medical students are to adopt and embrace new learning technologies.

7 Conclusion

As new learning technologies are discovered and developed and start to enter the mainstream, researchers need to review and study these technologies to measure their effect on retention, comprehension, and motivation to learn. We turned our attention to immersive virtual reality (VR) environments presented via head mounted displays (HMDs) in this study as this is a medium of learning that is becoming quite popular. We specifically wanted to examine the research already conducted to determine *if learning medical concepts in a VR environment truly improves the comprehension, retention, and motivation of medical school students*.

What we found is that there are some studies that answer this research question, but more research needs to be conducted to better understand the effect of this new medium of learning on students' comprehension, retention, and motivation; especially in the field of medical education. We also found that comprehension is defined very differently between studies and is a variable that was hard to objectively measure. However, we did find studies that indicate that retention and motivation among medical students improved when learning was presented in VR environments.

We also outlined a study that we plan to conduct as a next step in our research journey that will gather primary data that will help us better answer the modified question of whether *learning medical concepts in a VR environment truly improves the retention and motivation of medical school students.*

We also highly encourage researchers to conduct more studies that incorporate dynamic interaction in VR environments and objectively measure the effect of such environments on retention and motivation in medical learning scenarios.

References

1. Cline, E.: Ready Player One. Crown Publishers, New York (2011)
2. Wartman, S.A., Combs, C.D.: Reimagining medical education in the age of AI. AMA J. Ethics **21**(2), E146-152 (2019). https://journalofethics.ama-assn.org/article/reimagining-medical-education-age-ai/2019-02
3. Kaphingst, K.A., Persky, S., McCall, C., Lachance, C., Loewenstein, J., Beall, A.C., Blascovich, J.: Testing the effects of educational strategies on comprehension of a genomic concept using virtual reality technology. Patient Educ. Couns. **77**(2), 224–230 (2009). https://doi.org/10.1016/j.pec.2009.03.029
4. Thompson-Butel, A.G., Shiner, C.T., McGhee, J., Bailey, B.J., Bou-Haidar, P., McCorriston, M., Faux, S.G.: The role of personalized virtual reality in education for patients post stroke-a qualitative case series. J. Stroke Cerebrovac. Dis. **28**(2), 450–457 (2019). https://doi.org/10.1016/j.jstrokecerebrovasdis.2018.10.018
5. Palanica, A., Docktor, M.J., Lee, A., Fossat, Y.: Using mobile virtual reality to enhance medical comprehension and satisfaction in patients and their families. Perspect. Med. Educ. (2019). https://doi.org/10.1007/s40037-019-0504-7
6. Parkhomenko, E., O'Leary, M., Safiullah, S., Walia, S., Owyong, M., Lin, C., James, R., Okhunov, Z., Patel, R.M., Kaler, K.S., Landman, J., Clayman, R.: Pilot assessment of immersive virtual reality renal models as an educational and preoperative planning tool for percutaneous nephrolithotomy. J. Endourol. (2018) https://doi.org/10.1089/end.2018.0626
7. Vertemati, M., Cassin, S., Rizzetto, F., Vanzulli, A., Elli, M., Sampogna, G., Gallieni, M.: A virtual reality environment to visualize three-dimensional patient-specific models by a mobile head-mounted display. Surg. Innov. (2019) https://doi.org/10.1177/1553350618822860
8. Smith, S.J., Farra, S.L., Ulrich, D.L., Hodgson, E., Nicely, S., Mickle, A.: Effectiveness of two varying levels of virtual reality simulation. Nurs. Educ. Perspect. **39**(6), E10-E15 (2018). https://journals.lww.com/neponline/Abstract/2018/11000/Effectiveness_of_Two_Varying_Levels_of_Virtual.21.aspx
9. Krokos, E., Plaisant, C., Varshney, A.: Virtual memory palaces: immersion aids recall. Virtual Reality (2018). https://doi.org/10.1007/s10055-018-0346-3
10. Ekstrand, C., Jamal, A., Nguyen, R., Kudryk, A., Mann, J., Mendez, I.: Immersive and interactive virtual reality to improve learning and retention of neuroanatomy in medical students: a randomized controlled study. CMAJ Open. **6**(1), E103–E109 (2018). https://doi.org/10.9778/cmajo.20170110

11. Stepan, K., Zeiger, J., Hanchuk, S., Del Signore, A., Shrivastava, R., Govindaraj, S., Iloreta, A.: Immersive virtual reality as a teaching tool for neuroanatomy. Int. Forum Allergy Rhinol. **7**(10), 1006–1013 (2017). https://doi.org/10.1002/alr.21986
12. Huang, H.-M., Liaw, S.-S., Lai, C.-M.: Exploring learner acceptance of the use of virtual reality in medical education: a case study of desktop and projection-based display systems. Interact. Learn. Environ. **24**(1), 3–19 (2013). https://doi.org/10.1080/10494820.2013.817436

Design of Virtual Manikins in Spaces with Complex Topology and High Density of Occupation

Eusébio Conceição[1,2(✉)], João Gomes[2], Maria Conceição[3], Maria Lúcio[1], and Ángel Álvarez-Corbacho[4]

[1] FCT-Universidade do Algarve, Campus de Gambelas, 8005-139 Faro, Portugal
econcei@ualg.pt
[2] CINTAL, Campus de Gambelas, 8005-139 Faro, Portugal
[3] Instituto Superior Técnico, Av. Rovisco Pais, 1049-001 Lisbon, Portugal
[4] Instituto Universitario de Arquitectura y Ciencias de la Construcción, Av. R. Mercedes 2, 41012 Seville, Spain

Abstract. This work presents a software developed to design virtual manikins inside spaces with complex topology and high density of occupation. The software is used to design 330 typical seated occupants in a roman theatre or in an adapted auditorium. The virtual manikins are used by a numerical software in the evaluation of the occupants' thermal comfort level. This software simulates the human body and clothing thermal responses and analyses simultaneously several persons inside a space. The human body is divided into 1 spherical and 34 cylindrical elements. These elements consider the height and the weight of the occupants and have dimensions and angles similar to the human body. In the theatre and auditorium, all fundamental elements are considered.

Keywords: 3D design · Numerical software · Roman theatre · Thermal comfort · Virtual manikin

1 Introduction

Greek and Roman theatres are public buildings of great importance in the History of Western culture. Many of these spaces are still used today for their original function with minor adaptations or none at all. The exceptional achievement of the former designers to provide such spaces has attracted architects and, in this framework, acoustics and other facilities play an essential role [1].

In every building, the existence of a good level of thermal comfort contributes to the improvement of the performance of their occupants in the work they develop, in terms of their learning or in terms of the enjoyment of a musical or theatrical performance. In this sense, it is also justified to develop a study that analyzes the level of thermal comfort of Roman and Greek theatre occupants. Although classical antiquity theatres are open buildings, it is possible to numerically assess their level of thermal comfort taking into account parameters such as solar radiation, air temperature, mean radiant temperature, air velocity and air relative humidity.

T. Ahram et al. (Eds.): IHIET 2019, AISC 1018, pp. 297–302, 2020.
https://doi.org/10.1007/978-3-030-25629-6_46

According to Fanger [2], the level of thermal comfort that occupants of an enclosure are subjected to depends, among other factors, on the levels of physical activity and clothing and on the heat exchange between the human body and the surrounding environment. The thermal comfort model, presented in [2] and [3], is based only on the body's thermal equilibrium (mass and heat exchanges) with the surrounding environment, and the body internal temperature is maintained through some physiological responses. In order to evaluate the level of thermal comfort, the Predicted Mean Vote (PMV) and the Predicted Percentage of Dissatisfied (PPD) indexes, developed by Fanger in 1970 [2] and presented in ISO 7730 [3], are used.

The radiative exchanges may be done between the sections of the same body, between sections of different bodies and between the sections of the bodies and the surrounding surfaces of the building interior. These radiative heat exchanges are obtained from the resolution of the system of radiosity equations [4], and depend on the shape factors, temperatures and emissivity of the body and the building surfaces.

The heat flux from the solar radiation, which enters through the glass and that affects the bodies of the occupants, depends on the intensity of the solar radiation and how it affects the occupants. To do this calculation, the parallel ray method is used (please, see details in [5]).

The calculations of the above radiations depend strongly on the position of the human body and its location in the occupied space. In this calculation, the shadings of the different sections of the human body and of the surrounding surfaces in the occupied compartment are also considered. It is therefore necessary to have a three-dimensional mesh defining the limits of the outer surfaces of the occupants' bodies and the interior surfaces of the compartment (please, see details in [6]).

This work presents a software developed to design virtual manikins in spaces with complex topology and high density of occupation. The software is used to design 330 typical seated occupants in a roman theatre or in an adapted auditorium. These virtual manikins are used in the numerical software for the evaluation of the occupants' thermal comfort level.

2 Numerical Models

In this study, a coupling between a building thermal behavior (BTB) numerical model and a human thermal response (HTR) numerical model is used. The BTB model estimates the opaque and transparent surfaces temperatures, the indoor air temperatures, the average thermal comfort and indoor air quality (IAQ) [7]. This information is used by the HTR model to calculate, simultaneously, each occupant's body, clothing temperatures and thermal comfort level [8]. In order to obtain these values, it is necessary to have detailed virtual manikins with thermal and thermoregulatory systems well defined.

The human body model (please, see Fig. 1) is divided into 35 elements (34 cylindrical and 1 spherical): head, neck, chest, abdomen (upper and lower areas), arms (upper and lower areas), forearms (upper and lower areas), hands, fingers, thighs (upper and lower areas), legs (upper and lower areas) and feet. The arms and legs are made up of 4 cylinders, the neck, hands, fingers and feet are made up of 1 cylinder and the trunk is made up of 3 cylinders. In turn, each element is sub-divided into 64 infinitesimal areas. That is, the outer surface of each person has a total of 2240 infinitesimal areas, which are used in the incident radiation calculus. In the thermal comfort determination, each element is sub-divided into 12 cylindrical (or spherical) layers.

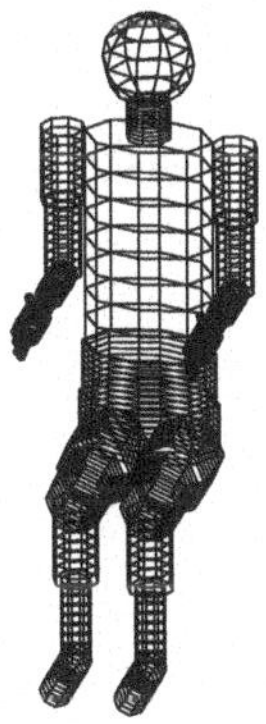

Fig. 1. Virtual manikin (human body model).

In the calculation of the radiation level that each person element receives, trigonometric relations between the incident solar radiation and the person are used.

In the thermal comfort level evaluation, it is used the PMV index [2]. The PMV index depends on air temperature, air relative humidity, mean radiant temperature, air velocity, activity level and clothing level. In the IAQ evaluation, it is used the dioxide carbon concentration.

3 Numerical Methodology

The virtual Roman theatre used in the simulations, presented in Fig. 2, is constituted by 718 opaque surfaces. In turn, each surface is sub-divided into several infinitesimal areas with 20 × 20 cm dimensions. The virtual adapted auditorium, presented in Fig. 3, is obtained from the Roman theatre envelopingit by 58 transparent surfaces (in a total of 776 surfaces).

In the numerical simulations, it is considered that the roman theatre and the adapted auditorium are occupied by 330 persons, equally distributed by 15 rows and 22 columns. Each occupant is numbered from the bottom to the top of the column; the first column is located on the far right side of the theatre. Each occupant is considered to have a height of 1.7 m, a weight of 70 kg and an activity level of 1.2 met.

In this work, the carbon dioxide concentration, air temperature, PMV and solar radiation, for a winter typical day, are numerically calculated using the BTB software. The clothing level is considered to be 1.5 clo inside the auditorium and 1.5 or 3.0 clo inside the theatre. The PMV distribution and solar radiation level, to which each person is subjected at 12:00 p.m., are calculated using the HTR software.

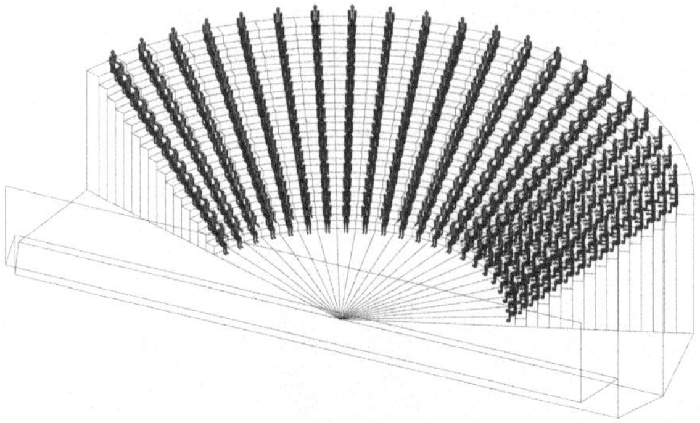

Fig. 2. Virtual Roman theatre.

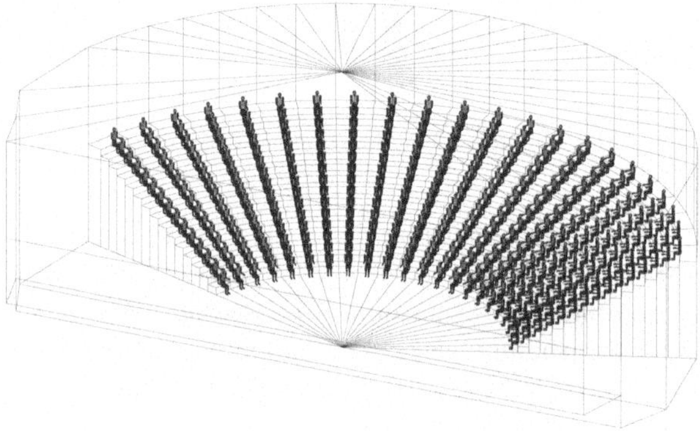

Fig. 3. Virtual adapted auditorium.

4 Results and Discussion

In this section, for a typical winter day conditions of a Mediterranean climate type, the carbon dioxide concentration results, the air temperature evolution (Fig. 4a) and the auditorium and theatre PMV evolution (Fig. 4b), are calculated by the BTB. The solar radiation flux on each human body sections (Fig. 5a) and PMV distribution (Fig. 5b) to which each person is subjected at 12:00 p.m., calculated by the HTC, are presented. In Fig. 4b), the clothing level is identified.

The carbon dioxide concentration obtained results show that its values, during all day, are below the standard value of 1800 mg/m^3 [9], meaning that the adapted auditorium has good IAQ. The results show that the auditorium air temperatures are between 20 and 22 °C around noon and in the beginning of the afternoon. This is achieved only by solar radiation. In the auditorium, the persons are comfortable around noon and in the beginning of the afternoon, by negative PMV values, according to category C [3], at least. In the theatre, the persons are comfortable by PMV values within category C [3], at least, but only if dressed with a high clothing level of 3.0 clo.

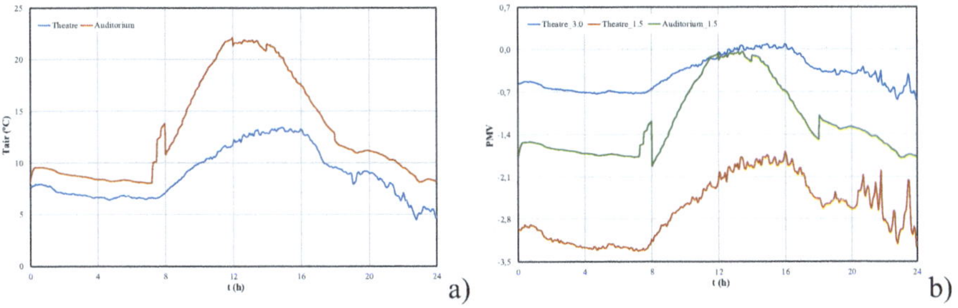

Fig. 4. BTB results for the theatre and auditorium: (a) air temperature and (b) PMV.

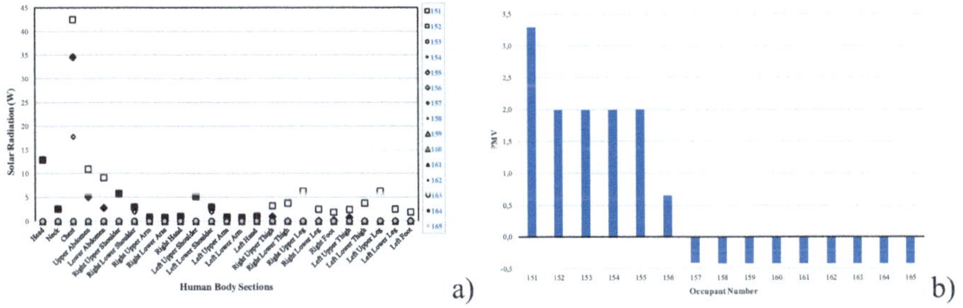

Fig. 5. HTR results in the auditorium: (a) solar radiation values on the human body sections of 15 occupants; (b) PMV index distribution for each selected occupant.

The results of the solar radiant flux on the occupants' body sections show that their levels depend on the occupant location inside the auditorium and it is affected by the shading that occurs between them. As an example, in Fig. 5b, the solar radiation levels on the occupants' body sections of the column 11 are presented. It can be seen that occupants with numbers 158 to 165 receive no solar radiation, and, for example, occupants with numbers 151 to 155 receive high values of solar radiation, mainly in the head and trunk. Only those that are not subjected to solar radiation are thermally comfortable, by negative PMV values, according to category C [3].

5 Conclusions

In this work, a software developed to design virtual manikins in spaces with complex topology and high density of occupation is presented. The virtual manikins are used by a numerical software to evaluate each occupant thermal comfort level.

The BTB numerical results, for a typical winter day, show that the adapted auditorium presents good IAQ and good thermal comfort levels during the period of greatest sun exposure. The Roman theatre occupants, in winter conditions, are only comfortable when highly dressed. The individual occupant thermal comfort level, calculated by the HTR, is acceptable and is near the space average thermal comfort, but only for those not subjected to solar radiation. The occupants that are subjected to solar radiation have unacceptable thermal comfort levels.

These results reveal the importance of using virtual manikins in this kind of study, because allow to identify the thermal comfort levels and to suggest some improvements. In this case, it is suggested to introduce an opaque roof in the auditorium.

As future work, it is also suggested to evaluate the importance of these shading elements on the thermal comfort levels of the auditorium and theatre occupants.

Acknowledgments. The authors would like to acknowledge the support of the research project, financed by the Ministry of Economy, Industry and Competitiveness of Spain with reference BIA2017-85301-P.

References

1. Bo, E., Astolfi, A., Pellegrino, A., Pelegrin-Garcia, D., Puglisi, G., Shtrepi, L., Rychtarikova, M.: The modern use of ancient theatres related to acoustic and lighting requirements: stage design guidelines for the Greek theatre of Syracuse. Ener. Build. **95**, 106–115 (2015)
2. Fanger, P.: Thermal Comfort. Danish Technical Press, Copenhagen (1970)
3. ISO 7730: Ergonomics of the thermal environments – analytical determination and interpretation of thermal comfort using calculation of the PMV and PPD indices and local thermal comfort criteria. International Standard, Switzerland (2005)
4. Ozisik, M.: Transferência de calor: um texto básico. Editora Guanabara, Rio de Janeiro (1990)
5. Ozeki, J., Konishi, M., Narita, C., Tanabe, S.: Effective radiation area of human body calculated by a numerical simulation. In: 6th International Conference on Air Distribution in Rooms – RoomVent 1998, Stockholm, Sweden, 14–17 June 1998
6. Conceição, E.: Geração de malha em torno de ocupantes e em compartimentos com topologia complexa. In: VII Congresso de Mecânica Aplicada e Computacional, Évora, Portugal, 14–16 April 2003
7. Conceição, E., Lúcio, M.: Numerical simulation of the application of solar radiant systems, internal airflow and occupants' presence in the improvement of comfort in winter conditions. Buildings **38**, 1–20 (2016)
8. Conceição, E.: Evaluation of thermal comfort and local discomfort conditions using the numerical body of the human and clothing thermal system. In: Proceedings of the 7th International Conference on Air Distribution in Rooms – RoomVent 2000, Reading, UK, 9–12 July 2000
9. ASHRAE Standard 62.1: Ventilation for acceptable indoor air quality. American Society of Heating, Refrigerating and Air-Conditioning Engineers, Atlanta, GA, USA (2010)

Augmented Reality and 3-D Visualization Effects to Enhance Battlefield Situational Awareness

Chia-Chi Mao(✉) and Fei-Yi Chen

Department of Applied Arts, Fu Hsing Kang College, National Defense University, No.70, Sec. 2 Zhongyang N. Rd. Beitou Dist., Taipei, Taiwan
Chia-ChiMao@gmail.com, Fei-YiChen@gmail.com

Abstract. This study presents the augmented reality technology and 3D information visualization for Army's military education to realize the interactive tactical course teaching and consider the user center research and human-computer interaction architecture as a solution to improve the common operational picture. The purpose is to improve the Army's command and general staff officers in tactical operations to learn battlefield situational awareness to enhance interest in learning and effective decision support. We constructed a prototype augmented reality program, the traditional tactical image and symbols of war games into 3-D virtual images, Which includes military equipment, urban architecture and geography scenes and other models, teaching applications to import tactical operations, not only to break through the limitations of a traditional 2 D image, enhanced visual effects and digital technology information, revealing a more complete battlefield scene. At the same time, through virtual operation, students are more interactive. In order to verify and collect the utility and data of learning, quasi-experimental research has been used. Experiments have shown that using 3-D information Visualization for better understanding of military tasks and space environments can enhance learning interest and perception of situation awareness.

Keywords: Situation awareness · Augmented Reality · 3-D animation · Information visualization · Human-computer interaction

1 Introduction

Battlefield Situational Awareness was the core of military tactics, and the purpose of fostering military trainees' effective command and control. The main instructional tool in military tactics courses is the common operational picture (COP). At present, military units around the globe place military maps under acetate tablets to form operation overlays, and mark military tactic images and symbols on the overlays to engage in military simulations. Commanders use COP to instruct staff officers about limitary plans, and staff officers produce various operation overlays to suit different situation needs, with the aid of post-it notes, thick paper boards [1, 2].

T. Ahram et al. (Eds.): IHIET 2019, AISC 1018, pp. 303–309, 2020.
https://doi.org/10.1007/978-3-030-25629-6_47

Recent studies on command and staff operations in Taiwan [3–5], have focused on procedures and steps in military operations. However, experts in Army Tactics indicate insufficient information presented by COP, pointing to the fossilization of the operation methods. The existing problems include (a) an over-reliance on texts and forms, leading to the lack of visualization effects, (b) a reliance on personal experiences and perceptions for interpreting images on COP and limited situation awareness, and (c) over-standardization of operation procedures that lead to low interest and attention.

Studies point out that AR has proven to be able to provide great impact on affect and create better perceptions and learning experiences [6]. This is because AR permits learners to interact with real-world and virtual objects. In addition, the effectiveness of AR-based learning activities [7] show that AR can foster basic knowledge, flexibility, creativity [8], and increase motivation among learners [9].

The current study investigates the incorporation of virtual technology into tactics instruction at a military academy in Taiwan, and discusses interactional flow and visual aesthetics in order to produce more effective learning and heightened learning interest among commanders and staff trainees under low cost and high efficiency.

2 Related Work

The application and design of AR in education, with the use of mobile and situation awareness technology in outdoor settings, has been proven beneficial in real-world language and experiential learning [10]. AR systems can also improve learning content and interaction. For instance, in Chemistry courses, AR allows invisible substances or chemical reactions to be visualized and guides learners through operations, reducing dangers involved in real Chemical experiments [11].

Since 1992, the U.S. military has been developing AR systems for training the army, including the earliest virtual devices to help the air force carry out long distance operations with wearable devices. Later developments include devices for different service and force characteristics. One example is the Battlefield Augmented Reality System (BARS) developed by the naval research laboratory for instant situation understanding [12] and Military Operations on Urban Terrain (MOUT) for supporting army tactic training in urban warfare [13]. One important theme in common for military AR systems is the enhancement of situation awareness. The basic features include rapid understanding about the battlefield in terms of time and space. Such affordances for predicting future events are paramount in warfare [1, 12, 14, 15].

3 Method

According to the above problems, the present study the construction of tactical teaching system based on augmented reality. The system contains AR scene, 3D objects, and target recognition make up the content of the current system architecture, and the operation mode as Fig. 1. 3D Unity, with its easy-to-use 3-D animation creation procedure, was used to construct the AR operation along with immediate rendering techniques and drive event script editing. Pairing with Vuforia (https://developer.vuforia.com/) allowed the AR camera to recognize images and build cross-platform AR application procedures. The 3-D model object for the AR system was made in Maya based on the physical environment, major landscapes, and troop equipment described in the course.

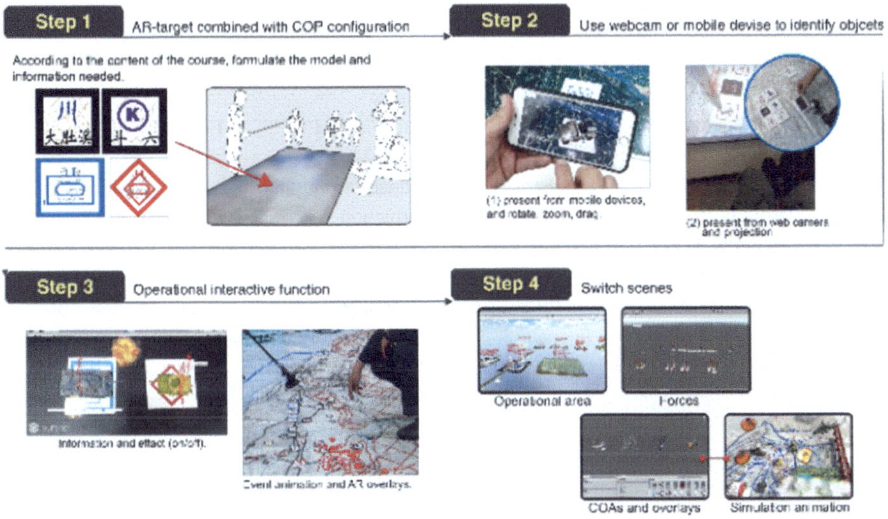

Fig. 1. Operate process of ARTCOP system

The participants were 40 students from Army Command and Staff College in Taiwan Army, including 37 males (M = 35) and 3 females (M = 32), aged between 31 and 40 years old, from across Taiwan. All the participants met the eligibility criteria for the expert level, which are: serving in the Army units over 10 years, participated at least one task such as war chess deduction and training exercise. All participants have completed tactical course before the experiment. The operating environment is the same classroom as the tactical course and retains the original equipment and material.

The technology acceptance model (TAM) model is one of the most popular theories used to explain the information systems. Davis (1989) proposed TAM to depict external variables on internal beliefs, attitudes, and subjective norms, and behavioral willingness influence. In order to explore the external variables for perceived usefulness and perceived ease of use of influence for explaining the cause-effect relationships, the use of potential factors. Table 1 presents the definition of the research facet and related theoretical sources.

The hypothesis in this research encompasses three external variables: information visualization, situational awareness, and interaction design. According to the variable term is the construct of intention to use. The constructs are discussed along with its research hypothesis architecture (see Fig. 2). For the consideration of external variables, in previous military-related studies, it was stated that the understanding of the battlefield situation has an important influence on the use of tactical systems [13, 16, 17].

Table 1. Operational definitions and measurement of variables.

Construct	Operational definition	Source of the measurement
IV	It has a good visual effect, only a graphical way to communicate clearly and effectively convey the message [16]	Yu et al. (2009)
PU	Technology tools can help with tactical courses, enhance the understanding of the curriculum, and influence the satisfaction of the students with the tools [17]	Davis (1989)
PEU	It means that technology tools can be easily operated without any burden on the tactical courses for trainees	
SA	The user's perception of the situation awareness and understanding of the mission [18]	Endsley (1995)
ID	Information transfer between users and feedback from the use of tools, emphasis is on "sensory and information richness" [19]	Manzari and Trinidad-hristensen (2006)
ITU	Understand user's intention to use new technology [20].	Mathieson (1991)

IV = information visualization; PU = perceived usefulness; PEU = perceived ease of use; SA = situational awareness; ID = interaction design; ITU = intention to use

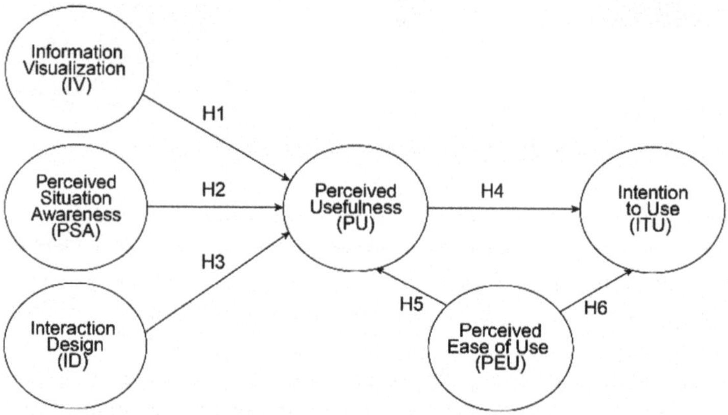

Fig. 2. A revised TAM model

The measurement items in the model are all reflection facets, and each facet item is revised according to the actual field study and interpretation meeting and is fully reviewed by experts to determine the validity of the content. 21 questions were asked for each aspect. The facet item SA4 was a reverse question, which was to avoid the subjects from thinking about rigid and disorderly filling. The measurement scale used in the questionnaire was measured by Likert scale ranging from 1 (strongly disagree) to

5 (strongly agree). There are 6 research hypotheses (H1 to H6), the following research hypotheses were formulated based on the research model:

H1. Information visualization (IV) will positively affect perceived usefulness (PU).
H2. Perceived situation awareness (PSA) will positively affect perceived usefulness (PU).
H3. Interaction design (ID) will positively affect perceived usefulness (PU).
H4. Perceived usefulness (PU) will positively affect intention to use (ITU).
H5. Perceived ease of use (PEU) will positively affect perceived usefulness (PU).
H6. Perceived ease of use (PEU) will positively affect intention to use (ITU).

4 Results

This research employed path analysis with the Structured Equation Modeling approach [24] to describe the effects of independent variables and correlated factors (see Fig. 3 and Table 2). The values revealed by the path coefficient and R2 provide adequate explanatory power to account for the structure of the AR system its adaptation relationship with the observed data. The model has 13.5–16.0% square difference (R2 = 48 square multiple correlation). The predictive power of the pattern can be explained from the path, the overall predictive power of the three potential variables of IV, PSA and ID on the usefulness of the variable in use is 67.0%; the usefulness and ease of use on the destination path are 58.5% for the usage intention. The total effect of displaying the potential strain item procedure and the self-variable path coefficient is good. In the path of external factors, H1, H2, and H3 solve the structural relationship between visual information, battlefield situational awareness, and interactivity to PU. The effects of IV ($b = 0.579$, $p < 0.001$) and PSA ($b = 0.286$, $p < 0.05$) have statistically significant contributions to PU. However, the ID facets had no significant effect on the PU ($b = -0.096$, $p > 0.05$) was found.

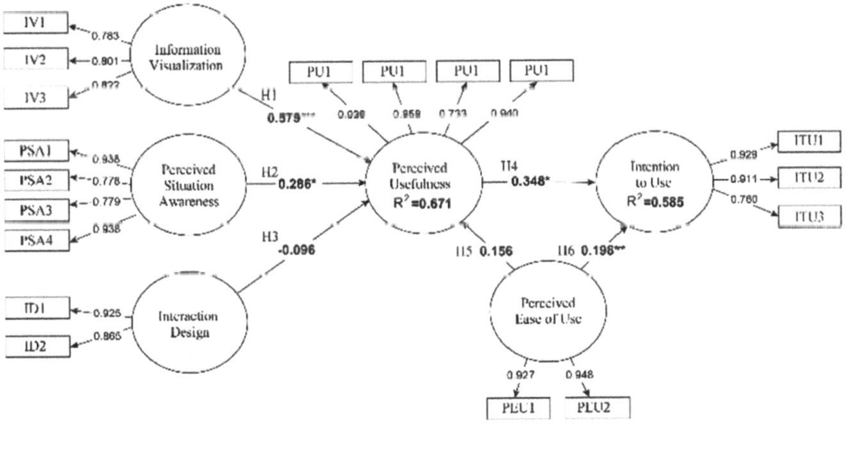

Fig. 3. Results of SEM analysis

Table 2. Standardized structural estimates and hypotheses tests

Hypothesis	Path	Estimates	t-value	Results
H1	Information visualization -> perceived usefulness	0.579	4.169	Supported
H2	Perceived situation awareness -> perceived usefulness	0.286	2.533	Supported
H3	Interaction design -> perceived usefulness	−0.096	0.636	**Not**
H4	Perceived usefulness -> intention to use	0.348	2.255	Supported
H5	Perceived ease of use -> perceived usefulness	0.156	1.097	**Not**
H6	Perceived ease of use -> perceived intention to use	0.498	3.264	Supported

5 Discussion and Conclusion

The study set out to improve the instructional tool for army tactics courses. Results show high usability and acceptance of AR technology among the participants during the stages of the case analysis. The system effectively enhanced situation awareness and focus during the learning process, achieving the objectives of this research.

In summary, the current AR and VR technologies have become the mainstream of military education and training. However, research on the use of VR technology in military research has focused on situation awareness and operation capabilities instead of a user-centered and HCI approach, resulting in a lack of user feedback and evaluations. The current study employed a needs-based investigation on the evaluation stages of the experiment using the proposed learning system. The effectiveness identified with regards to AR and 3D animation techniques combined with the COP operation mode could serve as a reference for future research development.

References

1. Briggs, R.O., Adkins, M., Kruse, J., Nunamaker Jr., J.F.: Lessons learned using a technology transition model with the US navy. In: Proceedings of the 32nd Annual Hawaii International Conference on Systems Sciences, HICSS-32, p. 10 (1999)
2. Kim, Y.J., Hoffmann, C.M.: Enhanced battlefield visualization for situation awareness. Comput. Graph. **27**, 873–885 (2003)
3. Jhen-Fu, H.: A study of intelligence preparation of the battlefield. Army Acad. Bimon. **48**, 56–73 (2012)
4. Sun, C., Peng, Z.-L.: How to improve military decision making process for system thinking. WHAMPOA - Interdiscip. J. **66**, 89–108 (2014)
5. Huang, R.X.: Improve military decision making process of my opinion. Army Acad. Bimon. **425**, 1–13 (2001)
6. Mao, C.C, Sun, C.C, Chen, C.H: Evaluate learner's acceptance of augmented reality based military decision making process training system. In: Proceedings of the 2017 5th International Conference on Information and Education Technology, pp. 73–77. ACM (2017)

7. Nicolau, S., Soler, L., Mutter, D., Marescaux, J.: Augmented reality in laparoscopic surgical oncology. Surg. Oncol. **20**, 189–201 (2011)
8. Chang, H.Y., Wu, H.K., Hsu, Y.S.: Integrating a mobile augmented reality activity to contextualize student learning of a socioscientific issue. Br. J. Educ. Technol. **44**, E95–E99 (2013)
9. Mao, C.-C., Chen, C.-H., Sun, C.-C.: Impact of an augmented reality system on learning for army military decision-making process (MDMP) course. In: Advances in Intelligent Systems and Computing (2017). https://doi.org/10.1007/978-3-319-41685-4_58
10. Chen, C.H., Chou, Y.Y., Huang, C.Y.: An augmented-reality-based concept map to support mobile learning for science. Asia-Pacific Educ. Res. **25**, 567–578 (2016)
11. Wojciechowski, R., Cellary, W.: Evaluation of learners' attitude toward learning in ARIES augmented reality environments. Comput. Educ. **68**, 570–585 (2013)
12. Livingston, M.A., Ai, Z., Karsch, K., Gibson, G.O.: User interface design for military AR applications. Virtual Real. **15**, 175–184 (2011)
13. Ting, S.P., Zhou, S., Hu, N.: A computational model of situation awareness for MOUT simulations. In: Proceedings - 2010 International Conference on Cyberworlds, CW 2010, pp. 142–149 (2010)
14. Golberg, S.: Human factors issues in the use of virtual and augmented reality for military purposes – USA. Security (2005)
15. Lindberg, B.D., Mccauley, M.: Panoramic augmented reality for persistence of information in counterinsurgency environments (2010)
16. Yu, S.Y.S., Deng, L.D.L., Zhang, Y.Z.Y.: Visualization user interface for decision support systems. In: 2009 Ninth International Conference on Hybrid Intelligent Systems, vol. 1, pp. 63–66 (2009)
17. Davis, F.D.: Perceived usefulness, perceived ease of use, and user acceptance of information technology. MIS Q. **13**, 319–340 (1989)
18. Endsley, M.R.: Measurement of situation awareness in dynamic systems. Hum. Factors J. Hum. Factors Ergon. Soc. **37**, 65–84 (1995)
19. Manzari, L., Trinidad-christensen, J.: User-centered design of a web site for library and information science students: heuristic evaluation and usability testing. Inf. Technol. Libr. **25**, 163–169 (2006)
20. Mathieson, K.: Predicting user intentions: comparing the technology acceptance model with the theory of planned behavior. Inf. Syst. Res. **2**, 173–191 (1991)
21. Campbell, T., Armistead, L.: Information operations: warfare and the hard reality of soft power. Int. J. **60**, 868 (2005)
22. Balfour, R.E.: Next generation emergency management common operating picture software/systems (COPSS). IEEE Syst. Appl. Technol. Conf. **2012**, 1–6 (2013)
23. Rummukainen, L., Oksama, L., Timonen, J., Vankka, J.: Visualizing common operating picture of critical infrastructure. In: Next-Generation Analyst II, p. 912208. International Society for Optics and Photonics (2014)
24. Keller, J.M.: Motivational Design for Learning and Performance: The ARCS Model Approach. Springer, Heidelberg (2010)

Visual Attention Convergence Index for Virtual Reality Experiences

Pawel Kobylinski[1](✉) and Grzegorz Pochwatko[2]

[1] Laboratory of Interactive Technologies, National Information Processing Institute, al. Niepodleglosci 188b, 00-608 Warsaw, Poland
pawel.kobylinski@opi.org.pl

[2] Virtual Reality and Psychophysiology Lab, Institute of Psychology, Polish Academy of Sciences, ul. Jaracza 1, 00-378 Warsaw, Poland
grzegorz.pochwatko@psych.pan.pl

Abstract. The paper introduces a novel quantitative method in the domain of eye tracking (ET) for virtual reality (VR). The method might be of interest to researchers on the human factor in VR, behavioral psychologists, and designers of VR experiences. Several mathematical formulas describing a novel index quantifying convergence of visual attention are introduced. The index is based on recently developed distance variance [1], a function of distances between observations in metric spaces. An aggregated version of the visual attention convergence index introduced in the paper allows to measure the effectiveness of any system of attentional cues employed by a designer to guide the attention of VR experience participants along an intended narration line. An individual version of the index allows to capture individual differences in the convergence of visual attention across participants. Possibilities for real-life and academic usage of the index are discussed and example results of application to real VR ET data are summarized.

Keywords: Virtual Reality · Eye tracking · Positional tracking · Attention · Behavior · Narration · Energy statistics · Distance variance · Human-technology interaction · User experience · Research methodology · Social sciences · Psychology

1 Introduction

Users love good narratives [2, 3]. Classic, computer-generated graphic and cinematic virtual reality (VR) environments, to be effective and/or attractive, should be immersive, create the illusion of spacial and social presence, and "tell" a good story. Effective narration is required equally in games, training and therapeutic environments, as well as in cinematic VR experiences. Presence and good narrative lead to motivation, engagement, better memory, and/or persuasion [4–6]. Presence involves treating virtual environment as a primary reference frame and ignoring distraction from outside, flesh reality. Effective narration keeps users' attention focused during a virtual experience, helps following the storyline and improves performance [7, 8].

T. Ahram et al. (Eds.): IHIET 2019, AISC 1018, pp. 310–316, 2020.
https://doi.org/10.1007/978-3-030-25629-6_48

Cinematic VR, a new kind of VR experiences, has recently emerged and is growing in popularity. In such an environment a video surrounds a viewer, which brings new challenges for creators, who need to narrate in a different way to keep the viewer's attention in the right place of the scene. It also creates new possibilities of applications other than art or entertainment. Persuasive or training (educational or vocational) cinematic VR experiences are the best examples.

If a designer of a VR experience employs any system of attentional cues (e.g. spatial sounds) to guide participants' attention along an intended narration line, they might be interested in measuring the system's effectiveness [9]. This is why we have devised and introduce in this paper an aggregated version of the visual attention convergence index (denoted as *VRCa*). In simple words, *VRCa* tells us if several participants looked at the same or rather different virtual objects/areas during a VR experience.

In the paper we also put stress on individual differences in responses to VR experiences. Some users look around a lot to explore the virtual space, whereas others do not execute visual exploration at all. In order to measure such differences in the visual exploration, we have devised an individual visual convergence index (denoted in this paper as *VRCi*).

During the first 30 s of a given experience different patterns of visual attention may occur. This initial pattern of visual convergence may influence the way the narrative is experienced later on. In the paper we present example results of a study in which participants experienced an educational cinematic VR. The material contained different kinds of attention-grabbing stimuli, both visual and auditory. Both aggregated data and individual behavior were analyzed with the usage of *VRCa* and *VRCi*.

The *VRC* indices are calculated from eye tracking (ET) data. Application of the *VRC* indices requires prior knowledge in the ET domain and, of course, a VR headset equipped with an eye tracker. Though ET in three- or six-degree-of-freedom VR environments [10] may pose a challenge to researchers, we believe it is worth the effort.

A mathematical method harnessed to construct the indices is based on recently developed distance variance [1], a function of distances between observations in metric spaces [11].

2 Mathematical Method

Let us consider a set of n gaze fixations $F = \{f_1, f_2, \ldots, f_n\}$ detected from eye tracking data recorded during a VR experience for a chosen time interval. The fixations may originate from either a number of participants of the VR experience (in this case, F is a union of many individual subsets) or a single participant (in this case, F equals a single subset). We will discuss both the aggregated and individual variants later.

Three coordinates x_i, y_i, and z_i are identified for every fixation f_i. Thus, for the chosen time interval of interest, we obtain a three-dimensional discrete variable with n values. This variable can be represented as a matrix $\boldsymbol{T}$ with n rows and three columns.

In the first step, $\boldsymbol{T}$ is transformed into matrix of Euclidean distances between rows treated as three-dimensional vectors of observations (square matrix $\boldsymbol{D}$ with n rows and n columns).

2.1 Distance Variance Coefficient (*dVar*)

Let $\boldsymbol{D}'$ denote a $n \times n$ matrix obtained by double-centering the distance matrix $\boldsymbol{D}$ (i.e. the row and column means of $\boldsymbol{D}$ are subtracted and the grand mean added). The distance variance *dVar* is defined as follows [1, 9]:

$$dVar = \frac{1}{n}\sqrt{\sum_{i,j=1}^{n}\left(\boldsymbol{D}'_{ij}\right)^2}. \tag{1}$$

The distance variance *dVar* constitutes the basis for further calculations. *dVar* is nonnegative and $dVar_{min} = 0$ represents a situation in which the spatial coordinates for all fixations $f_i \in F$ are equal:

$$\begin{bmatrix} x_1 \\ y_1 \\ z_1 \end{bmatrix} = \begin{bmatrix} x_2 \\ y_2 \\ z_2 \end{bmatrix} = \cdots = \begin{bmatrix} x_n \\ y_n \\ z_n \end{bmatrix}. \tag{2}$$

The more the coordinate vectors differ from each other, the greater the value of *dVar*. *dVar* can be easily calculated with the usage of the R package energy [12].

2.2 Visual Attention Convergence Index (*VRC*)

Let *VRC* denote the most basic form of the visual attention convergence index:

$$VRC = 1 - dVar. \tag{3}$$

$VRC_{max} = 1$ represents a situation in which the spatial coordinates for all fixations $f_i \in F$ are equal (Eq. 2) and implies maximal possible level of the visual attention convergence. The more the coordinate vectors differ from each other, the smaller the value of *VRC*. Though neither $VRC = 0$ nor $VRC < 0$ imply any convenient interpretation, the basic form of the index suffices for experimentally controlled comparisons of visual attention convergence levels measured with regard to the same virtual reality environment.

2.3 Scaled Visual Attention Convergence Index (*sVRC*)

Let *sVRC* denote a scaled version of the visual attention convergence index:

$$sVRC = 1 - \frac{dVar}{dVar_{max}}. \tag{4}$$

$sVRC \in [0, 1]$, so interpretation of its values becomes convenient. $sVRC_{max} = 1$ implies maximal possible level of the visual attention convergence. Depending on the choice between theoretical (mathematically derived for a chosen virtual reality environment) and empirical (ever observed for a chosen virtual reality environment) value of $dVar_{max}$, $sVRC_{min} = 0$ implies either minimal theoretically possible or minimal empirically observed level of the visual attention convergence. In the first and preferred case scenario, though carefully, $sVRC$ can be used to compare visual attention convergence levels not only within but also between virtual reality environments.

The basic form of the visual attention convergence index requires double-centering the distance matrix $\boldsymbol{D}$ (Eqs. 1 and 3), which is a way to deal with the central tendency in the set of distances between the gaze fixations. This complication is however unnecessary when we choose to explicitly scale the values of the index into the $[0, 1]$ interval. Thus, in the case of the scaled index, Eq. (1) takes the following form:

$$dVar = \frac{1}{n}\sqrt{\sum_{i,j=1}^{n}\left(\boldsymbol{D}_{ij}\right)^2}. \tag{5}$$

As soon as a theoretical value of a maximal possible distance d_{max} between positions of gaze fixations in a virtual reality environment of choice is established, it is possible to calculate the theoretical value of $dVar_{max}$, based on Eq. (5):

$$dVar_{max} = \frac{1}{n}\sqrt{(n^2 - n)d_{max}^2} = \sqrt{\frac{n-1}{n}}d_{max} \approx d_{max}. \tag{6}$$

Based on Eqs. (4) and (6), the scaled version of the visual attention convergence index is calculated as follows:

$$sVRC = 1 - \frac{dVar}{d_{max}}. \tag{7}$$

In the case of the cinematic VR, a 360-degree video is displayed on a virtual sphere (or twin spheres in the case of stereoscopic cinematic experience). Let r denote the radius of the sphere. Then:

$$d_{max} = 2r. \tag{8}$$

Thus, in the case of cinematic VR experiences, Eq. (7) takes the following form:

$$sVRC = 1 - \frac{dVar}{2r}. \tag{9}$$

2.4 Aggregated Visual Attention Convergence Index (*VRCa*, *sVRCa*)

For reasonably short time intervals, if the set F contains fixations originating from more than one participant of a VR experience, VRC conveys information about similarity in the visual attention distribution across participants. To simplify the interpretation: a value of the aggregated visual attention convergence index (let us denote it as $VRCa$ and $sVRCa$) tells us if several people looked at the same or rather different virtual objects/areas during a chosen, short time interval. It is only natural that a participant of a VR experience can choose freely where to look and/or in which direction to move. This is why VR experience designers devise systems of attentional cues based on gaze, motion, sound, context, and perspective [13]. *VRCa* and *sVRCa* allow us to measure the effectiveness of any system of attentional cues employed by a designer to guide the attention of VR experience participants along an intended narration line.

Figure 1 originates from an empirical study and illustrates changes in *VRCa* calculated for half-second intervals over 96 participants of the same educational cinematic VR experience. As we can see, at the beginning of the 360-degree video subjects clearly differed as to the areas of interest. During the first 30 s of the projection the areas of interest steadily converged and then over the next 30 s, subjects steadily followed the intended narrative.

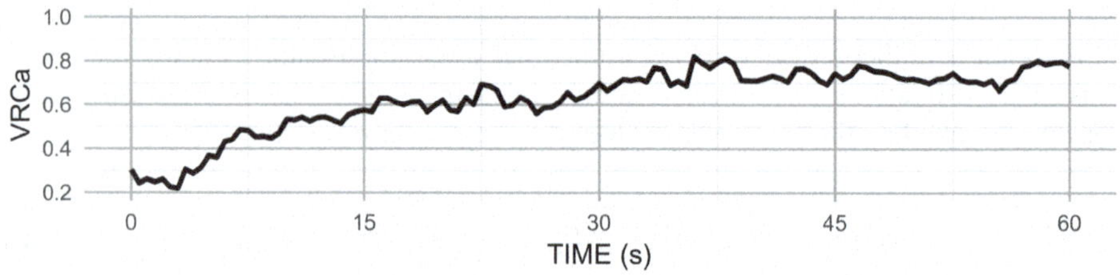

Fig. 1. Changes in the aggregated visual attention index (VRCa) calculated for half-second intervals over 96 participants of an educational cinematic VR experience.

2.5 Individual Visual Attention Convergence Index (*VRCi*, *sVRCi*)

While *VRCa* tells us something about the narration in a VR experience, we also might want to capture individual differences in the visual attention convergence. In order to achieve it, *VRC* must be calculated separately for each participant of a VR experience, for any chosen time interval. Let us denote the individual visual attention convergence index as *VCRi* (and *sVRCi* for the scaled version).

Figure 2 illustrates data originating from the empirical study already mentioned. For the sake of the example, we calculated *VCRi* for six ten-second intervals, for each viewer of the educational 360-degree video. The figure shows *VCRi* values averaged for two groups of subjects. In this simple example viewers belonging to the "red group" exhibited less visual exploration (more visual convergence) during the first 30 s of the educational cinematic VR experience.

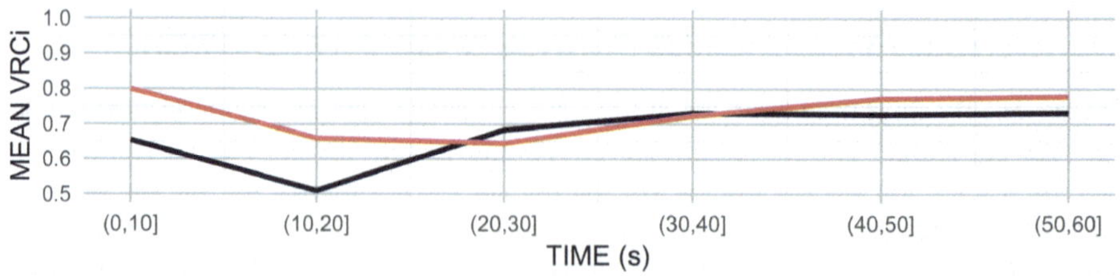

Fig. 2. Differences in the mean individual visual attention index (VRCi) calculated for 10-s intervals for two groups (red and black) of participants of an educational cinematic VR experience.

3 Conclusion

We believe that the novel method described in the paper might be of interest to researchers on the human factor in VR, behavioral psychologists, and – last but not least – designers of VR experiences. Effectiveness of a system of attentional cues employed in a VR experience, especially in cinematic VR, can be examined *ex post* with the usage of the aggregated version of the visual convergence index. This possibility may help creators of VR content to better understand how to build cohesive narration. On the other hand, the individual visual attention convergence index may be employed both in real-time and offline. Real-time application may be linked to a feedback system that reacts to lack of visual focus. *Ex post* application of *VRCi* may give behavioral psychologists insight into individual differences in the way people react to VR experiences. *VRCi* can be used in combination with other psychological (questionnaire) or psychophysiological measures (e.g. heart rate) to dive into mechanisms of attention, presence, and immersion.

The scope of research in which the method may find its applications is not limited to the ET for VR field. Research involving augmented reality (AR), standalone, and mobile 2D ET may benefit from usage of the methodology described in this paper. It is also conceivable to apply *VRC* to positional tracking data in virtual, augmented and real-space setups [9].

References

1. Szekely, G.J., Rizzo, M.L.: Brownian distance covariance. Ann. Appl. Stat. **3**, 1236–1265 (2009)
2. Napiorkowski, N.: Mitologia wspolczesna (Modern Mythology). Wydawnictwo Naukowe PWN, Warsaw (2018)
3. Danilicheva, P., Klimenko, S., Baturin, Y., Serebrov, A.: Education in virtual worlds: virtual storytelling. In: 2009 International Conference on CyberWorlds, pp. 333–338. IEEE Press, New York (2009)
4. Lin, J., Duh, H.B.L., Parker, D.E., Abi-Rached, H., Furness, T.A.: Effects of field of view on presence, enjoyment, memory, and simulator sickness in a virtual environment. In: Proceedings IEEE Virtual Reality, pp. 164–171. IEEE Press, New York (2002)
5. Baylor, A.: Promoting motivation with virtual agents and avatars: role of visual presence and appearance. Philos. Trans. R. Soc. Lond. B Biol. Sci. **364**, 3559–3565 (2009)
6. Tussyadiah, I.P., Wang, D., Jung, T.H., tom Dieck, M.C.: Virtual reality, presence, and attitude change: empirical evidence from tourism. Tour. Manage. **66**, 140–154 (2018)
7. Hsu, C.L., Lu, H.P.: Why do people play on-line games? An extended TAM with social influences and flow experience. Inform. Manage.-Amster. **41**, 853–868 (2004)
8. Gorini, A., Capideville, C.S., De Leo, G., Mantovani, F., Riva, G.: The role of immersion and narrative in mediated presence: the virtual hospital experience. Cyberpsychol. Behav. Soc. Netw. **14**, 99–105 (2011)

9. Kobylinski, P., Pochwatko, G., Biele, C.: VR experience from data science point of view: how to measure inter-subject dependence in visual attention and spatial behavior. In: Karwowski, W., Ahram, T. (eds.) Intelligent Human Systems Integration, IHSI 2019. Advances in Intelligent Systems and Computing, vol. 903, pp. 393–399. Springer, Cham (2019)
10. Duchowski, A.T.: Eye Tracking Methodology: Theory and Practice. Springer, Berlin (2007)
11. Szekely, G.J., Rizzo, M.L.: The energy of data. Ann. Rev. Stat. Appl. **4**, 447–479 (2017)
12. Rizzo, M.L., Szekely G.J.: energy: E-statistics: multivariate inference via the energy of data. R package version 1.7-5 (2018). https://CRAN.R-project.org/package=energy
13. Godde, M., Gabler, F., Siegmund, D., Braun, A.: Cinematic narration in VR - rethinking film conventions for 360 degrees. In: Chen, J., Fragomeni, G. (eds.) VAMR 2018. LNCS, vol. 10910, pp. 184–201. Springer, Cham (2018)

Exploration of Underinvestigated Indoor Environment Based on Mobile Robot and Mixed Reality

Aydar Akhmetzyanov(✉), Rauf Yagfarov, Salimzhan Gafurov, Mikhail Ostanin, and Alexandr Klimchik

Center for Technologies in Robotics and Mechatronics Components, Innopolis University, Innopolis, Russia
{a.akhmetzyanov, r.yagfarov, s.gafurov, m.ostanin, a.klimchik}@innopolis.ru

Abstract. Mobile robots allow human to explore impassable or unsafe indoor locations remotely. There are a large number of scenarios where the implementation of mobile robots is the only way to successfully complete them. Herewith, human-robot interaction is the key factor that determines the efficiency of overall mission accomplishment. This paper presents a real-time approach for remote exploration of underinvestigated indoor environment conducted by human-robot interaction. The approach is based on the mobile robot and mixed reality. We have chosen a differential drive mobile robot platform called Plato and mixed reality glasses Microsoft Hololens for experimental investigation of the proposed approach. Our paper demonstrates the results of experimental investigations of the proposed approach. The results have shown that the proposed approach is helpful, intuitive and convenient for spatial understanding and improves natural interaction both with a mobile robot and remote environment. Moreover, our approach is able to significantly increase the speed of indoor environment exploration.

Keywords: Human-robot interaction · Mixed reality · Mobile robots

1 Introduction

Mobile robots have run the gamut from simple devices to highly sophisticated autonomous vehicles. Autonomous mobile robots have become hugely popular, largely driven by their technical fit-out and overall performances. Mobile robots are capable to reconnoitre locations which are impassable or dangerous for humans. Such scenarios include rescue missions, intelligence operations, inspections, path-finding or explorations in civilian and military spheres. All of these scenarios have a common feature: navigation inside an indoor environment are accompanied by a number of uncertainties. Real-time exploration of an uncertain indoor environment by means of mobile robots requires intuitive and convenient methods for communication with a robot [2]. Collaborative work of human and mobile robot increases the accomplish efficiency of various exploration scenarios providing additional capabilities for human. This so-called human-robot interaction can be provided by means of various methods. Research

T. Ahram et al. (Eds.): IHIET 2019, AISC 1018, pp. 317–322, 2020.
https://doi.org/10.1007/978-3-030-25629-6_49

[2] showed that Mixed Reality (MR) is one of the best approaches to provide HRI. MR technology provides an intuitive way to control objects and visualise scenes increasing informativeness of the operator with simultaneous reducing of cognitive load.

A considerable amount of HRI realization based on head-mounted displays. One of the examples is shown in research [3] where the handheld display was used to show images to the user from fixed surveillance cameras overlaid on a camera image of the current environment. Showed approach has been using extensively in a number of investigations. However, it has a significant disadvantage: it cannot be implemented for exploration of the environment in real-time as it is assumed to perform pre-processing procedures to evaluate the raw data from sensors.

Discussed above extreme situations dictate that interaction with a mobile robot should be considered through a navigation problem, the problem of objects detection, their labelling to provide operator information about the remote location in real-time. Such interaction should provide the instant aggregate picture of the location. Despite the fact that there are two viewing modes to control the robot: egocentric and exocentric, only exocentric viewing mode is suitable for exploration of an underinvestigated indoor environment. Exploration in egocentric viewing mode is a challenging task as it does not provide an instant aggregated picture of the environment. However, the indoor environment limits the application of exocentric mode.

Our paper introduces effort in improvement current technics in MR-based control and exploration of remote areas in combination with mobile robots. The goal of the paper is to develop a method for underinvistigated areas exploration with map generation in real-time, MR-based obscured objects visualisation.

The novelty of the research consists in improvement of the latest MR approaches for human-robot interaction for remote areas exploration in real-time. Our goal is to outperform current limitation of the pre-loaded maps requirement as well as runtime limitations.

2 System Architecture

2.1 System Overview

The approach developed in our paper is based on three main parts: user interface, controller and mobile robot. User interface is realized by means of Microsoft HoloLens MR glasses and responsible for the communication between the user and mobile robot, and also for visualization of environment and objects. The controller performs all calculations, transfers commands between the interface and robot. It is also responsible for robot control and local navigation. Global path-planning is conducted by the user in our approach. After receiving the commands from a user by means of user interface, the controller performs local planning and navigate by means of the SLAM algorithm.

2.2 Hardware and Software

MR environment was used to provide human-robot interaction. We used Microsoft HoloLens as a hardware platform. We used Unity 2017.4 game engine and MRTK (Mixed Reality Toolkit) to develop a human-robot interface. Interaction between HoloLens and ROS was realized by means of a modified RosSharp package for UWP (Universal Windows Platform). Modifications include message types used in ROS.

The developed system is able to work with various mobile robots. A differential drive mobile robot called "Plato" was used in our project for experimental investigations. Plato is equipped with the onboard computer NVIDIA Jetson TX2, bumper sensors, sonars, Troyka IMU module, Velodyne VLP-16 3D Lidar, HD-camera and wheel encoders for wheel odometry. Wheel motors are controlled by Arduino Mega. Ubuntu 18.04 LTS and ROS Melodic software were installed into the onboard computer.

2.3 System Flowchart

Detailed block diagram of the system architecture is shown in Fig. 1. HoloLens provides the MR Interface and Virtual Environment. Robot control and interaction between robot and user are conducted by ROS Melodic.

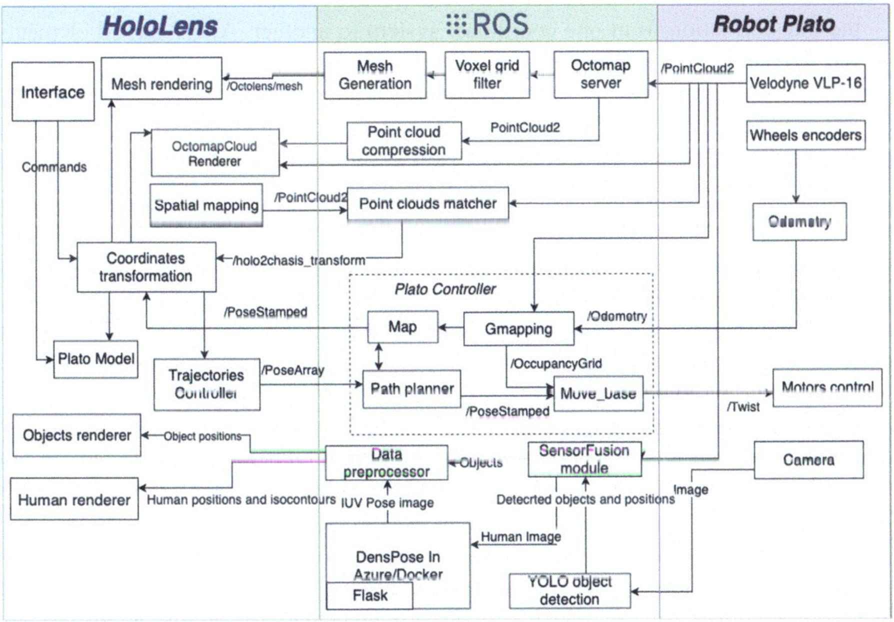

Fig. 1. System flowchart

"Spatial mapping" and "Velodyne VLP-16" blocks send points clouds to "Points clouds matcher" where calculations of transformation between them are performed.

"Spatial mapping" represents the HoloLens environment and Velodyne real environment. Commands from HoloLens Interface block are sent to the robot by means of "Coordinates transformation" and "Trajectories controller" blocks. Plato has software modules for mapping, localization and control that are realized by means of ROS Melodic. A 2D space map-based localization was used for mobile robot navigation. We used Gmapping algorithm for SLAM [4]. This algorithm was shown in research [5] to be accurate and fast enough for indoor exploration scenarios in comparison with other popular algorithms available in the ROS presented in [6, 7]. Gmapping algorithm takes raw laser range and odometry data as inputs and outputs an occupancy grid map. Occupancy grid map consists of cells that correspond to the state in the physical space and they can be either free or occupied. As far as the robot has an environment map, it is necessary to build a motion trajectory. "Move base" ROS node is intended for this, which takes a point in 2D space and starts global and local planning. Move base node also produces two cost maps: global and local.

3 Implementation

The pipeline of the system:

(1) Initialization and matching of the coordinate systems: the mobile robot and HoloLens send clouds points to the Points clouds matcher node, which calculates the transformation from one coordinate system to another. After that, all elements can operate in one overall area.
(2) A pose or a sequence of poses are established using the MR interface and then are transmitted to the control unit (Fig. 2, a).
(3) The main calculations are performed by the control unit: construction of a map and trajectory planning for the mobile robot.
(4) The control unit sends control commands to the robot and exploration is executed.

Exploration of underinvestigated indoor environment based on our proposed approach is presented on the video [8].

HoloLens initializes T-HoloLens coordinate system when starts, it is located in started position. It allows the virtual objects (Fig. 2, a) to have coordinate relative to T-HoloLens. The mobile platform has its own coordinate system for mapping and localization. For the connection between the Plato and HoloLens, we match two points clouds: the first one is a lidar frame relative to T-Map and the second one is Spatial Mapping to T-HoloLens. As a result, we obtain a transformation T-Plato. Thus, we gain all the necessary transformations in our system.

Comparison of HoloLens' and Plato's coordinate systems is based on the comparison of corresponding points clouds and is conducted according to the following steps: (i) HoloLens scans the room and builds a points cloud; (ii) Points cloud from one scan is obtained by using robot onboard 3D LIDAR (Fig. 2, b); (iii) Points clouds are compared by using a modified ICP (Iterative Closest Point) algorithm [9]. In such a manner we obtain the transformation matrix of one coordinate system to another.

We visualized remote locations by means of the octomaps representation. The initial point cloud for map generation was obtained by means of 3D LIDAR sensor Velodyne VLP-16 (Fig. 2, b). We used a number of approaches for map generation using obtained points cloud. A map also can be represented by means of mesh structure [10] (Fig. 2, c). This technique implements voxel grid filter [10] for decreasing of data features from octomap. Mesh structure implementation also required smoothing of generating mesh After that we were able to implement the greedy projection triangulation algorithm for mesh generation [10].

Another approach for map visualization is based on octomap native map representation with octotree node centres by means of points cloud. However, the density of this point cloud is too high for Microsoft Hololens glasses to represent separately each object of the environment. We developed an algorithm for controlled reducing of the dense of obtained point cloud [10].

The final approach for map generation is based on explicit lidar's point cloud visualisation. Here we also implemented voxel grid filter for decreasing of data features obtained from of lidar.

The developed approach also provides the detection of such objects as doors, chairs, tables and peoples (Fig. 2, d). They are visualised as 3D objects. We implemented DensePose algorithm to recognize poses of detected humans. To decrease the hardware requirements for the mobile robot we used cloud service MS Azure as it proposes unlimited computational resources. We send data from onboard camera to Azure cloud where we create Docker-based microservice with DensePose algorithm. We used the https protocol to send data. It requires using of python web-framework

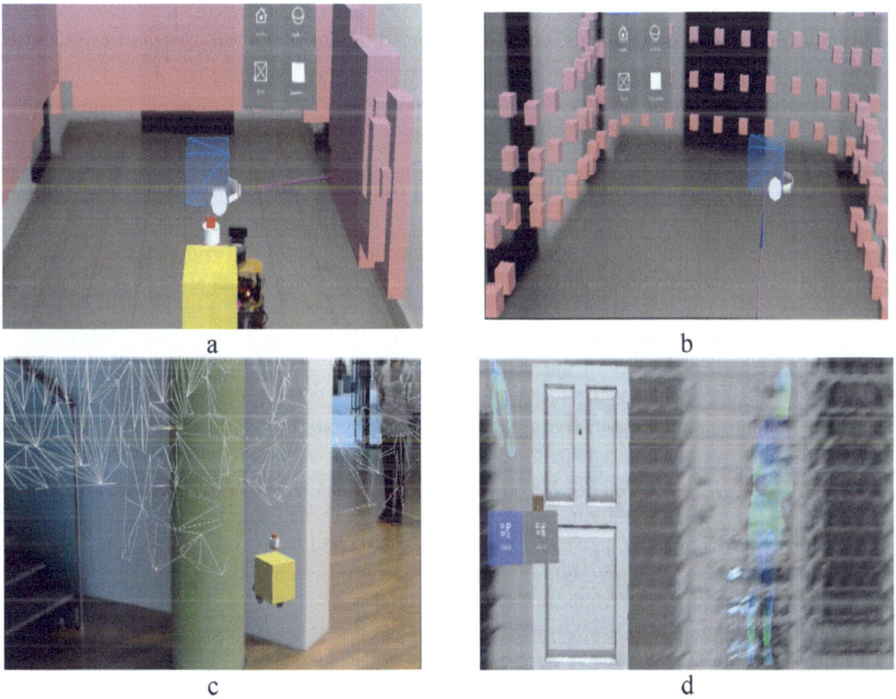
a b c d

Fig. 2. Indoor environment exploration. a – Real and virtual representations of the Plato robot. User interface is also shown here; b – LIDAR point cloud visualization; c – visualization by means of mesh structure; d – objects and human pose detection

Flask on the microservice side. Recognized humans' poses are rendered in a 2D plane which is always looking at the user. Dense pose output converted to isocontours which are 2D images which looks like 3d object from a user point of view.

4 Conclusion

Developed in our paper approach is intended to be implemented for user's x-ray vision during exploration scenarios in real-time. It depicts objects, shows their simplified virtual models for better understanding of remote locations. The approach is based on the implementation of both MR and mobile robot. Our study has shown that the proposed approach extends the user's possibilities for indoor environment exploration and increases his informativeness about remote locations. System accuracy has been increased by using of SLAM algorithm allowing the mobile robot to avoid obstacles which are cannot be observed by the user.

Acknowledgments. This research was supported by the Russian Education Ministry under the Agreement No. 075-10-2018-017 on granting a subsidy from 11.26.2018 "Development of a commercial urban transport with the intellectual driver assistance system "City Pilot". The customer is a federal target program. The unique identifier of the project RFMEFI60918X0005. Industrial partner - KAMAZ

References

1. Terrence, F., Nourbakhsh, I., Dautenhahn, K.: A survey of socially interactive robots. J. Robot. Auton. Syst. **42**(3–4), 143–166 (2003)
2. Goodrich, M., Schultz, A.: Human–robot interaction: a survey. J. Found. Trends Hum.–Comput. Interact. **1**(3), 203–275 (2008)
3. Avery, B., Piekarski, W., Thomas, B.: Visualizing occluded physical objects in unfamiliar outdoor augmented reality environments. In: the 6th IEEE and ACM International Symposium on Mixed and Augmented Reality. IEEE Computer Society, (2007)
4. Grisetti, G., Stachniss, C., Burgard, W.: Improved techniques for grid mapping with rao-blackwellized particle filters. J. IEEE Trans. Robot. **23**(1), 34–46 (2007)
5. Yagfarov, R., Ivanou, M., Afanasyev, I.: Map comparison of lidar-based 2D SLAM algorithms using precise ground truth. In: 15th International Conference on Control, Automation, Robotics and Vision, ICARCV (2018)
6. Hess, W., Kohler, D., Rapp, H., Andor, D.: Real-time loop closure in 2D lidar slam. In: IEEE International Conference on Robotics and Automation (ICRA), pp. 1271–1278. IEEE Press (2016)
7. Kohlbrecher, S., Von Stryk, O., Meyer, J., Klingauf, U.: A flexible and scalable slam system with full 3D motion estimation. In: IEEE International Symposium on Safety, Security, and Rescue Robotics (SSRR), pp. 155–160. IEEE Press (2011)
8. Presentation of the Research. https://www.youtube.com/watch?v=DDF83pcj5gY
9. Besl, P.J. McKay, N.D.: Method for regis- tration of 3-D shapes. In: Sensor Fusion IV: Control Paradigms and Data Structures, vol. 1611, pp. 586–607. International Society for Optics and Photonics (1992)
10. Algorithms for Human-robot Interaction. https://github.com/AydarAkhmetzyanov/plato_hololens

Wearable Technologies, Social and Affective Computing

Use of Wearable Technologies with Machine Learning to Understand University Student Learning Behaviours to Predict Students at Risk of Failing

Aidan McGowan(✉), Phil Hanna, Des Greer, John Busch, Neil Anderson, Matthew Collins, David Cutting, Darry Stewart, and Andrew McDowell

Queens' University, Belfast, Northern Ireland
aidan.mcgowan@qub.ac.uk

Abstract. The challenges of effective teaching in mass education environments are well documented. The cohorts of large size generally means that identification of struggling students is usually only at a point when meaningful interventions are too late. This paper reports on the use of novel technologies to provide insights into areas of learner behaviour in large-scale computer programming modules. Accordingly, this paper brings together a previous series of investigative studies of student key engagement points during a typical programming module (1) seat position tracking during programming lectures, (2) Video Lecture Capture viewing behaviours and (3) Student Heart Rate monitoring during lectures. The paper combines the significant findings of each investigation to provide a variety of analysis using Machine Learning (ML) classification modeling. The purpose of the MC study is to create models that could identify students that are likely to pass and those that may be at risk of failing the module.

Keywords: Wearable technologies · Social and affective computing · Human factors programming learning third level education

1 Introduction

The digital and creative industries contribute almost nine per cent of total UK gross value added (GVA) and employ 2.1 million people. The labour force backbone of these industries are Computer Science (CS) graduates with the subject discipline providing the UK Exchequer with the most net benefits after Medicine and Dentistry, Law and Architecture [1]. Evidence continues to point to the constant and vital need for a strong supply of CS graduates for future innovation, productivity and growth [2].

The challenges of effective delivery in these mass education environments are well-documented [3]. Although university education generally requires much self-learning, class size remains solidly at the top of the policy agenda and concerns for both faculty and students [4]. One of the major recurring concerns of increasing larger class sizes are high attrition rates. This is especially prevalent in computer programming based

T. Ahram et al. (Eds.): IHIET 2019, AISC 1018, pp. 325–331, 2020.
https://doi.org/10.1007/978-3-030-25629-6_50

courses, which already suffers badly in that regard, with attrition rates being reported as around 11% in the UK universities [5].

This paper gathers the significant findings from a series of previous investigative studies by the authors into student key engagement points during a typical programming module, (1) seat position tracking during programming lectures, (2) Video Lecture Capture viewing behaviours and (3) Student Heart Rate monitoring during lectures.

The first study [6] sought to track students' seating positions in lectures to investigate student behaviour in terms of seating position and particularly in relation to their final grade performances. Unlike most previous studies in this area, it did not control the students' seating arrangements enabling an unrestricted study of the effects of lecture theatre seating choices on assessment performance. It found that the best assessment results were achieved by the students in the front row and that assessment score degraded the further students sat from the front.

The Video analytics study [7] sought to investigate and assess the impact on learning of recording lectures in a programming module. The study considered behavioural trends of the students towards watching recorded lectures, such as when, frequency, duration, repeat views and an in depth study of video viewing behaviours including dropout, rewind and replay and relates all of these factors to academic impact, especially focusing on academic attainment. It found that there were some significant measureable factors that could be correlated with student attainment.

The measurement of cognitive activity using physiological means such as heart rate activity is a well-established mostly clinical research practice. The majority of previous studies have concluded that elevated heart rate occurs when an individual is cognitively engaged. This study [8] considered students' heart rate (HR) activity during a series of computer programming lectures measured using wearable devices. It benchmarked student heart rate patterns during lectures and concluded that there is a significant correlation between elevated heart rates and module scores.

1.1 Machine Learning (ML)

The paper brings together the significant findings of each these investigations to provide a variety of analysis, using Machine Learning (ML) classification modeling. It provides models to classify students as Passing and At Risk, using common classifier algorithms including Naive Bays, Decision Trees, Support Vector Machines, Artificial Neural Networks and K Nearest Neighbour (KNN) algorithms. The purpose of the ML strand of the study is to create models that could identify students that are likely to pass and those that may be at risk of failing the module.

Machine learning (ML) is an extensive area, which incorporates a vast number of classification approaches, each lending themselves to a range of different applications. Classification is an essential task in Machine Learning analysis and is used to predict unknown class labels. Classification is the act of looking for a model that describes a class label in such a way that the model can be used to predict an unknown class label [9]. For instance, a classification model could be used to classify an email message as either spam or otherwise, based on attributes, such as number of recipients, message body length or key words within subject message title or body.

There are different techniques and algorithms that may be engaged with to build a classification model. The performance of techniques such as Decision Trees, Rule Induction Probability function, Neural Networks and Support Vector Machine classifiers is used to analyse and provide alternative classification models. The classifiers chosen for this study (Table 1) are notably the most commonly used within MC analysis and represent the majority of the major categories currently employed.

Table 1. Classifiers used in the study

Classifier name	Classifier category
Naive Bays	Naive Bays
J48	Decision tree
SMO	Support vector machine
MPL (multi-layer perception)	Artificial neural network
IBk	KNN (k nearest neighbour)

While statistical based modeling such as linear regression may be used to predict student module scores the following ML analysis seeks to classify students that are at risk of failing the module based on their various electronic footprints and demographic attributes. For the purposes of training the classifiers in this study an At Risk boundary was set at a module score of 59% or less achieved. This boundary is relatively close to the 50% pass mark for the module and also considers that a student that eventually scored in the range 50–59% was still at risk of failing if their performance in the final heavily weighted assessment was weak. Recall that a stated investigative aim of this study was to potentially provide warning indicators of struggling students. Thus, module scores at or less than this boundary were considered in this nominal At Risk category to potentially help identify struggling students.

2 Methodology

The study was conducted over two years with two separate cohorts of postgraduate students (n = 201) taking a compulsory programming module on a conversion Masters course. The previous studies mentioned above found that there were some key and statistically significant electronic markers that could be related to over module score. The electronically measured factors identified from the previous studies that have statistical significance to module score were (1) Frequency of repeat views of LC videos (2) Engagement (including attendance) (3) Seating in lectures and (4) Percentage variance between the resting HR and lecture HR of students. In addition, there were a number of demographic factors that were recorded for each student and are included in some of the models. Each of the variables used in the various MC models are detailed in Table 2. Inclusion of the demographic features has the potential to enrich the analysis and enable a comparison of prediction of module performance between purely demographic information attained before the course about a student versus the electronic measurements recorded for the students during the course.

The suitability of the nominated classifiers was evaluated using WEKA data mining software [10]. To facilitate this, the electronic and demographic features in the dataset were recoded into ARFF files. The module scores were categorized into At Risk (0%–59%) or Pass (60%–100%). Other attributes were selectively recoded to enable a more intuitive model reporting, for example Gender 0 and 1 to Male and Female. Each file was then loaded into the WEKA environment and tested against the nominated classifiers using a standard 10-fold stratified cross validation as described in [11].

Table 2. Significant electronic and demographic markers used as classifiers for MC

Variable	Description	Value
Engagement	Engagement based on attendance, weekly test activity and online accessing of resource	(0–5) 0 non engagement - 5 high engagement
Repeat views videos	Actual number of average repeat views of LC videos	(0 to …)
Seating	General area of seating during the course	0 front - 1 seating elsewhere
Heart rate	Based on difference between RHR and average LHR	Percentage increase
Previous degree	Based on declared previous degree type	0 arts - 1 STEM
Previous programming	As indicated by the students before stating the course	0 none - 1 some
Previous degree classification	Based on declared previous degree classification	0 non 1st class - 1 1st class)
Gender		0 male – 1 female
Part-time work	Average part time hours worked during the course per week	0–40

3 Results

Summary results for the various models are presented in Table 3. The summary outputs include the models based on 1. All Attributes, 2. All electronic, 3. Demographic Attributes and 4. Best subset. The Best subset combination (evaluator CfsSubsetEval and Greedy Stepwise) produced a best subset list as: HR, Engagement, Previous Degree Type and Repeat Views.

3.1 Feature Set Analysis

In terms of correctly identified cases the Demographic attributes feature set performed worst, with an average of correctly identified cases of 59.64% between all classifiers. With considerable variance of performance between and within the other sets depending on classifiers, but averaging overall as: Electronic (72.41%), All attributes (70.45%) and Best subset (68.97%). The accuracy of FP Rate passing also showed considerable varied performances between each dataset, with the best overall performance coming from the Electronic measures (0.304) with the worst performer being the Demographic feature set (0.500).

Table 3. MC Results for the datasets

		All attributes	Electronic attributes (only)	Demographic attributes (only)	Best subset (all attributes)
Naive Bayes	Correctly classified	72.41%	65.52%	56.90%	70.69%
	F score	0.725	0.653	0.565	0.708
	Precision	0.728	0.653	0.563	0.709
	Recall	0.724	0.653	0.569	0.707
	FP rate (passing)	0.208	0.440	0.462	0.320
J48	Correctly classified	72.41%	72.41%	53.49%	67.24%
	F score	0.772	0.725	0.530	0.672
	Precision	0.723	0.728	0.528	0.671
	Recall	0.724	0.724	0.534	0.672
	FP rate (passing)	0.360	0.280	0.498	0.400
SMO	Correctly classified	76.41%	74.14%	65.51%	74.14%
	F score	0.725	0.739	0.650	0.741
	Precision	0.728	0.740	0.651	0.740
	Recall	0.724	0.741	0.650	0.741
	FP rate (passing)	0.280	0.360	0.480	0.320
MPL	Correctly classified	68.97%	75.86%	63.68%	58.62%
	F score	0.691	0.759	0.623	0.588
	Precision	0.707	0.777	0.620	0.596
	Recall	0.690	0.759	0.637	0.586
	FP rate (passing)	0.240	0.160	0.622	0.400
IBk	Correctly classified	62.07%	74.14%	58.62%	74.14%
	F score	0.618	0.742	0.588	0.741
	Precision	0.618	0.743	0.591	0.740
	Recall	0.618	0.741	0.586	0.741
	FP rate (passing)	0.480	0.280	0.440	0.320

3.2 Ranking the Classifiers

The best case identifier was the SMO classifier with on average 72.55% success rates. The other classifiers returned comparable averages IBk (67.24%), MPL (66.78%), J48 (66.39%) and Naïve Bayes (66.38%). The best FP Rate was the 0.160 returned by MPL using the Electronic feature set.

4 Discussion and Conclusion

While the best performing classifier was SMO it is of interest to note the high accuracy FP Rate returned using the Electronic feature set using MPL. Both have potential in predicting academic performance in relatively small datasets that include HR attributes. Overall, MPL and Naïve Bayes and a lesser extent SMO classifiers appear well suited to academic performance prediction using electronic attribute based data. However, as with all classifiers there is the potential with overfitting, in this case there were more Passing than At Risk students and therefore other dataset optimisations, such as the use of wrapper classes would be of benefit to enhance the models.

Using the MPL model in a real world implementation, from the given sample of 201 students (127 Passing and 74 At Risk students) would have resulted in 114 correctly predicted as Passing; additionally 47 At Risk students would have been correctly identified, with an overall accuracy of 80.1%. Conceptually the At Risk students could be invited to attend an intervention, for example extra tuition or one to one sessions. The model would also have resulted in 13 Passing students (6.5% of the total students) unnecessarily invited to the same intervention. This may be inconvenient or potentially wasteful of resources but unlikely to be harmful to the individual student's progress. This leaves 27 At Risk students (13.4% of all students and 36.9% of all At Risk students) that would not have been included in the intervention. Overall if implemented early enough in the programme that has the potential to reduce the At Risk percentage from 36.8% to 23.4% and likely follows that the eventual fail rate in the module would be lower.

If the goal to is identify those At Risk and subsequently to help these students then MC classification using electronic measurements presents an informed model to potentially target interventions. However, it must be acknowledged that even the best performing model is by no means perfect, with slightly over a third of At Risk students not being identified.

Mass education environments are now commonplace at third level education for programming courses. Having readily accessible electronic tracking that may be leveraged to target meaningful academic interventions has the potential to improve the learning experience and attainment. Considering the relatively high dropout rate in programming courses and the worldwide demand for programmers then this is likely no bad thing.

References

1. The Returns to Higher Education Qualifications, London Economics (2011). https://assets.publishing.service.gov.uk/government/uploads/system/uploads/attachment_data/file/32419/11-973-returns-to-higher-education-qualifications.pdf
2. Shadbolt, J.: Shadbolt review of computer sciences degree accreditation and graduate employability (2017). https://dera.ioe.ac.uk/16232/2/ind-16-5-shadbolt-review-computer-science-graduate-employability_Redacted.pdf
3. Mulryan-Kyne, C.: Teaching large classes at college and university level: challenges and opportunities. J. Teach. High. Educ. **15**(2), 175–185 (2010)
4. Bandiera, O., Larcinese, V.: The impact of class size on the performance of university students (2010). https://voxeu.org/article/impact-class-size-performance-university-students#fn
5. UK Performance Indicators: Non-Continuation Rates HESA (2017). https://www.hesa.ac.uk/news/07-03-2019/non-continuation-tables
6. McGowan, A, Hanna, P, Greer, D., Busch, J.: Learning to program – choose your lecture seat carefully? Paper Presented at Innovation and Technology in Computer Science Education, Bologna, Italy, 03–07 July 2017
7. McGowan, A, Hanna, P., Anderson, N.: Teaching programming: understanding lecture capture YouTube analytics. In: ITiCSE 2016 Proceedings of the 2016 ACM Conference on Innovation and Technology in Computer Science Education, pp. 35–40. ACM (2016)
8. McGowan, A., Hanna, P., Greer, D., Busch, J.: Lecturing to your students: is their heart in it? FTC **880**, 1005–1016 (2018). https://doi.org/10.1007/978-3-030-02686-8_75
9. Jiawei, H., Micheline, K., Jian, P.: Data Mining: Concept and Techniques, 3rd edn. Elsevier, Amsterdam (2011)
10. Hall, M., Frank, E., Holmes, G., Witten, I.: The WEKA data mining software. ACM SIGKDD Explor. Newsl. **11**(1), 10 (2009)
11. Longadge, R., Dongre, S.: Class imbalance problem in data mining review. **2**(1) (2013). www.ijcsn.org. ISSN 2277-5420

Innovative Wearable Systems for Improving Workers' Safety

Alessandro Ledda(✉) and Raffaele Palomba

Department of Technological Innovations, Italian National Institute for Insurance against Accidents at Work, Via Roberto Ferruzzi 38, 00143 Rome, Italy
{a.ledda, r.palomba}@inail.it

Abstract. The innovations introduced by industry 4.0 and the Internet of Things have allowed the development of new and more efficient technologies. These innovations, if applied to Personal Protective Equipment, make it possible to improve efficiency and make work safer. The high-tech developed PPE are known as Smart PPE. These use wireless technologies, intelligent textiles and advanced electronics to transform a traditional PPE into an object with advanced and innovative features. Italian National Institute for Insurance against Accidents at Work wants to give its contribution to increase worker safety by exploiting the latest technologies and making them available to a wide public.

Keywords: Personal Protective Equipment · Smart PPE · Workers' safety · Industry 4.0 · Internet of Things · Innovative wearable technologies

1 Introduction

The prevention of accidents at work often is linked to a quick and correct perception of the hazard, while the protection of workers is mainly achieved using Personal Protective Equipment (PPE). The Department of Technological Innovations (DIT) of the Italian National Institute for Insurance against Accidents at Work (INAIL) has been involved to developing both these issues for years [1]. The widespread digitization, the 4.0 industry and the Internet of Things (IoT) has allowed to open new ways to connect "prevention" with "protection", creating an integrated approach for workers' safety [2].

The use of smart PPE is one of the most interesting ways to increase PPE's protection standards. Smart PPE can be defined as "*Intelligent personal protective equipment, which integrate materials, components and ICT solutions enhancing product multi-functionality*". They are designed using industry 4.0 technologies: sensors for body functions and environmental monitoring; wireless communication; personal localization (GPS) and geographic information system (GIS); cooling heating elements; active PPE; smart textiles; devices wireless tracking and identification; physical security information management; augmented/virtual reality.

T. Ahram et al. (Eds.): IHIET 2019, AISC 1018, pp. 332–337, 2020.
https://doi.org/10.1007/978-3-030-25629-6_51

2 Standard PPE

The basic steps in occupational safety management planning are the identification of the hazards in the workplaces, the safety risk assessment, the choice of the best control, the implementation of the chosen control, the evaluation of the effectiveness of the control adopted [3].

Once workers' hazards are highlighted they should be removed or substituted with less hazardous ones. Then, in the traditional hierarchy of controls, should be adopted engineering controls to reduce the source of exposure. In a subordinate position should be used administrative controls, reducing the risks through a different work organization. PPE should be adopted as a last solution when all other methods are not possible of efficient. PPE are equipment worn to reduce exposures such as chemical contact or noise (Fig. 1).

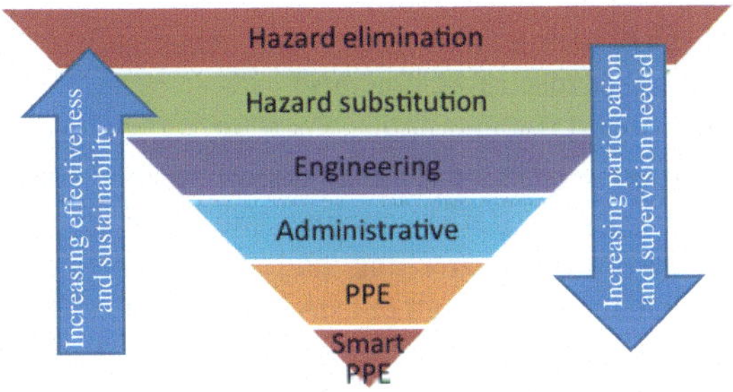

Fig. 1. Hierarchy of risk controls

According to Regulation 2016/425/EU, personal protective equipment means "… *equipment designed and manufactured to be worn or held by a person for protection against one or more risks to that person's health or safety*; …". PPE has the limitation that it does not eliminate the hazard at the source.

PPE are classified according to three risk Categories: "I" protecting exclusively the minimal risks; "II" includes PPE protecting the risks other than those listed in Categories I and III; "III" protecting exclusively the risks that may cause very serious consequences such as death or irreversible damage to health. Each PPE is subject to the conformity assessment procedure. PPE includes respiratory protective equipment (RPE) (full/half-face mask, self-contained breathing apparatus), protective clothing (jackets, trousers, apron, coveralls and suits), gloves (chemical resistant, heavy-duty, cuts and abrasions or heat/cold resistant), safety helmet (hits or falls protection), footwear (covers, shoes, half-boots, boots), ear (earplugs, earmuffs), eye protection (safety glasses, goggles, face shield).

3 Smart PPE

The main objective of Industry 4.0 applied to occupational safety can be summarized as the introduction of intelligent systems during the management and execution of the operations carried out in each work phase finalized to increase workers' safety. Other objectives are the collection of operational data, the development of highly adaptable and modular systems, the integration of sustainable and advanced management technologies and the promotion of automation technology and human-machine interaction.

The interest in innovative PPE is highlighted for example by an EU programme basing on Industry 4.0 devices to improve health and safety protection for workers and population [4] and by many European projects on smart PPE (e.g. smart@fire [5]) or smart textiles.

The use of smart PPE is one of the most interesting way to increase PPE's protection standards, and secondarily to improve workers productivity and reduce costs. Smart PPE can be defined as "Intelligent personal protective equipment, which integrate materials (e.g. technical textiles and smart materials), components and ICT solutions enhancing product multi-functionality".

Smart PPE use industry 4.0 technologies such as: sensors for body functions and environmental monitoring; wireless communication; personal localization (GPS) and geographic information system (GIS); cooling and heating elements; active PPE functions; smart textiles; wireless tracking and identification of devices; physical security information management; augmented/virtual reality. The IoT give limitless opportunities for workers' protection. The most common applications of wearable and sensors in PPE, but not the only ones, are: locating systems; smart communication systems; safer equipment; protection from invisible risks; improve efficiency/safety through remote management; app alerts; augmented/virtual reality protective equipment (Fig. 2).

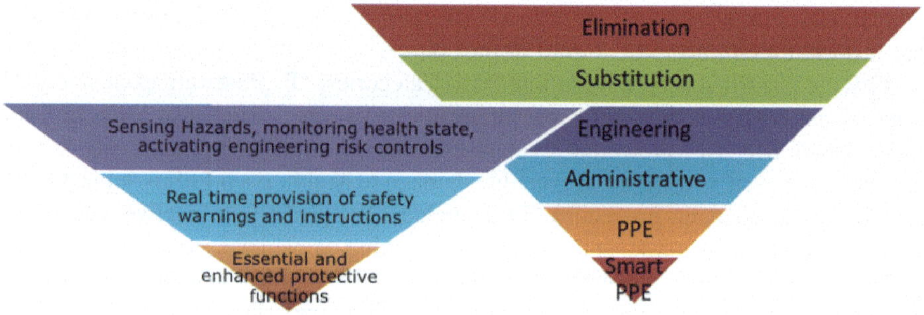

Fig. 2. Functions of smart PPE in relation to the hierarchy of risk controls

It is possible to highlight the main advantages and disadvantages in the use of smart PPE, not exhaustively summarized in Table 1.

Table 1. Comparison between main advantages and disadvantages in using smart PPE.

Advantages	Disadvantages
• Health monitoring; • Real time environmental monitoring; • Wireless communication Device to Device (D2D); • Wireless communication Device to Other (D2X); • Checking correct use of PPE; • Real time positioning in case of emergency; • Authorized access based on GPS/wireless technology; • Reacting to adverse climate conditions; • Active reaction to hazards; • Additional features linked to smart textile; • Hazards forecast and warning; • Additional information on working activities/workplace	• Complex training and use; • Respect of privacy rules; • Failures of complex technological devices; • Failures due to extreme environmental conditions (temperature, humidity, contaminants, etc.); • Uncertainty of environmental and health measures; • Wireless communication depending on 3G/4G network; • Production of electromagnetic fields; • Reliability on wireless communication; • Low resolution of positioning GPS based; • High costs

4 Existing Smart PPE

Existing smart PPE have been tested in some work activities to prevent and protect workers from accidents. The most popular smart systems are based on the communication between PPE and smartphones or special receivers, using Bluetooth or RFID TAGs applied to PPE. The activities that can be carried out with this type of smart PPE are: checking the foreseen PPE and in case inhibits the beginning of the work; alarm in case of non-detection of PPE; an emergency button for the operator (indicating the GPS position); sending real time alarms events.

A further system uses Radio Frequency IDentification (RFID) sensors to authorize access in areas considered at risk, to verify and certify the correct use of PPE and to define "no trespassing" areas.

Some systems perform Area control and Face recognition operations to control access/transit in specific areas and to verify the identity and authorization of workers, also connected with smart PPE.

An innovative system provides to anticipate possible accidents or near misses using Physical Security Information Management (PSIM), SW platforms able to receive and manage data coming from smart PPE and collective protection systems, to analyze them and to avoid the occurrence of potentially hazardous situations (Situation Awareness).

4.1 Inail's Project

Industry 4.0 is an equal opportunity for innovation, but it often differentiates between companies of varying resources and experience. Adopting smart PPE is complicated, expensive and needs of IoT and IT experience. Smaller companies may have difficulty acquiring the resources and teams necessary to manage and use a smart product [6]. For this reason, Inail is developing a new smart PPE with few and relatively cheap components. The system is still pending patent, so all the details of the project will not be specified.

The project concerns the use of a specific software and hardware in order to transform any standard PPE to a "smart PPE". The project includes a small CPU connected, via physical or wireless connections to sensors for detecting different environmental parameters with some associated risks. Thanks to other sensors can be correlated the environmental data with those of the worker's health. It is possible to add some accessories that allow the system to "react" to the risk. The reaction is decided on the basis of the information obtained and of the "risk assessment" calculated by the control unit. The system will merge different sensors and technologies to create a strong ecosystem that provide a full suite of solutions for workers' safety. At the end of the research and experimentation, both the software and the hardware will be available free of charge.

5 Conclusions

Many activities, such as remediation of contaminated sites, waste management, chemical industry/laboratories, etc. present high risks to workers than other activities [7, 8], for this reason the aspects of prevention of injuries and workers' protection, through the use of PPE, are fundamental. Industry 4.0 applications and IoT allow employers and workers to improve operational efficiency, to optimize productivity and to increase workers' safety [9]. The use of smart PPE, in compliance with EU regulations, may guarantee a better protection, new "smart" features, "active reactions" to hazards and more information on many parameters. Using smart PPE ensure a sustainable workplace in terms of health and safety.

The new "smart" technologies are spreading very quickly and their use in PPE is one of the most recent, with interesting applications. IoT is changing how we think about PPE, as the introduction of ABS led to new standards about driving safety, smart technologies applied to occupational safety will increase the standards of workers' safety.

References

1. INAIL Statistical data. https://www.inail.it/cs/internet/attivita/dati-e-statistiche.html
2. Badri, A., Boudreau-Trudel, B., Saâdeddine, A.S.: Occupational health and safety in the industry 4.0 era: a cause for major concern? Saf. Sci. **109**, 403–411 (2018)
3. European Union information agency for occupational safety and health. https://osha.europa.eu/en

4. EU CORDIS, Reducing the risk of injury in complex systems through advanced personal protective equipment. https://cordis.europa.eu/project/rcn/98866/factsheet/en
5. Integrated ICT Solutions for Smart Personal Protective Equipment for Fire Fighters and First Responders Smart@fire. https://cordis.europa.eu/project/rcn/105991/factsheet/en
6. EU Eurofound, Sixth European Working Conditions Survey – Overview report, Publications Office of the European Union, Luxembourg (2017). ISBN 978-92-897-1597-3
7. Eurostat Labour Force Survey, Accidents at work and other work related health problems. https://ec.europa.eu/eurostat/data/database
8. Rushton, L.: Health hazards and waste management. Br. Med. Bull. **68**(1), 183–197 (2003)
9. Frost & Sullivan, Innovations Enabled by Industrial IoT Accelerate the Shift to Manufacturing 4.0 (2017)

Applying Oculography and Biosignals Measurements to Gameplay Modes Analysis

Iwona Grabska-Gradzińska, Leszek A. Nowak(✉), and Jan K. Argasiński

Faculty of Physics, Astronomy and Applied Computer Science, Jagiellonian University, Kraków, Poland
{iwona.grabska, leszek.nowak, jan.argasinski}@uj.edu.pl

Abstract. In this paper we present results of an experiment designed to measure correlation between Galvanic Skin Response – GSR (also: Electrodermal Activity – EDA) and Oculographic (Eye Tracking) data. In the experiment we analyze the participants reactions on changing gameplay modes (changing dynamic and pace of user interaction with the game mechanics). The goal of the analysis is to demonstrate what influence of changing gameplay modes have on physiology (especially spontaneous body response). The gameplay modes used in experiment were chase mode (dynamic) and sneak mode (satisfying). In the experiment we have used Pupil Lab eye-tracker and EDA sensor based on BITalino platform. The game Serial Cleaner by iFun4all was used to conduct the experiment. The experiment resulted in multiple observations. Substantial correlation between participant failure and change of EDA pattern were observed as well as over 10% change in fixations durations.

Keywords: Affective computing · Biosignals analysis · Oculography · Eye Tracking · Gameplay analysis

1 Introduction

The aim of this study is to present the application of physiological measurements to distinguish between two modes of gameplay in a videogame. The "gameplay" is defined as the specific way in which player interacts with the videogame. Thus the "gameplay modes" can be various and changing depending on the game.

In this paper, the game *Serial Cleaner* (iFun4all, 2017) was used to conduct the experiment. In the game, the player is tasked with series of simple objectives that need to be completed without being detected. It requires careful observation and acting in accordance to movement patterns of AI (Artificial Intelligence) opponents. This will be called "sneak mode". If the player was spotted, he enters the "chase mode", where he must as fast as possible move out of the AI opponents' field of view to avoid being caught (see Fig. 1). If the player is captured by AI opponent, the level is reset, and the game starts over.

T. Ahram et al. (Eds.): IHIET 2019, AISC 1018, pp. 338–343, 2020.
https://doi.org/10.1007/978-3-030-25629-6_52

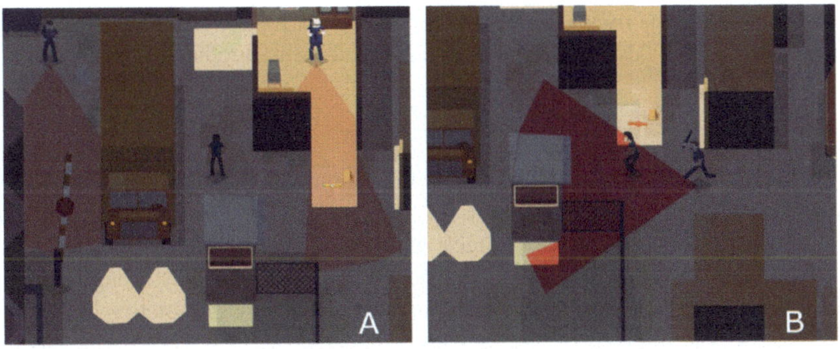

Fig. 1. Sneak mode (A, left side) and Chase mode (B, right side) in the game *Serial Cleaner* by iFun4all, 2017

2 Methodology

In the following section software and hardware means of conducting the experiment are presented.

Oculography. The eye tracker outputs a sequence of time-stamped spatial coordinates, representing momentary gaze points, which can be subsequently analyzed. Base on the output, gaze paths and heat maps describing the area of interest on the screen can be prepared [1]. Both are popular in Human Computer Interaction research and evaluation. The heat maps are used especially for game evaluation with static maps [2]. Gaze paths can be converted into gaze fixations information and is used in this research, where correlation between Electrodermal Activity and oculographic data was analyzed. We used both sequences of fixations and gaze distance measurement. Every fixation point correlate with focus of attention and show region of player's interest [3].

Electrodermal Activity. EDA (also: Galvanic Skin Response – GSR) refers to the variation of electrical properties of the skin surface as result of the arousal-induced secretion. The activity is generated by the sweat glands as a spontaneously body response. Usually signs of increased electrodermal activity occur in presence of stimuli such as loud sounds, stress, surprise. Response is measured using electrodes connected to dedicated device. Electrodes are usually placed on the fingers, inner side of the hand or inner part of the wrist (regions with largest accumulation of glands). The EDA is commonly used in experimental psychology as indicator of autonomic arousal/response [4].

The goal of conducted study was to ascertain if the observed changes in participant's electrodermal activity translate to changes in gameplay modes.

EDA measurements were already been used in games related studies [5].

3 Conducted Study

In our experiment we have used Pupil Lab head-mounted 120 Hz eye-tracker [6], with camera resolution of 1920 × 1080 px. For the fixation detection the Dispersion-Based Algorithm [7] and Pupil Capture software were used. For the measurement of EDA,

BITalino platform was used [8]. Players the game via mouse and keyboard. External display was 24" Dell Monitor. Data was registered using another PC laptop.

3.1 Participants

Eighteen subjects, differing in experience with computer games were invited to participate in the experiment. The time of the gameplay varied from 5.38 min to 21.39 min. The shortest and the longest gameplay was taken into further detailed consideration, with the results presented below. The shortest playthrough was completed by experienced player and concluded with challenge completion. The longest playthrough was terminated by the user after repeated failures. The player was unexperienced with this kind of game.

3.2 Procedure

Experimental procedure was conducted as follows:

- participant was introduced to procedure by investigator and asked to read description of experiment and sign the consent to participate;
- EDA sensor were placed on the participant's middle and index finger;
- the eye tracker was placed on the participant's head;
- the eye tracker was calibrated and BITalino connected;
- the experiment started with calming neutral introductory video;
- participant was asked to go through two levels of the game;
- after finishing the play participant was debriefed and all his/her questions about procedure was answered;

The recording of eye movement and EDA initiated automatically after starting the game. Game starts in sneak mode where the player gets familiar with level objectives. The sneak mode continues until the player finishes the challenge or the chase mode is triggered. At the start of the chase mode the timestamp is recorded. The chase mode can end if player is either captured or escapes. In both cases the timestamp of the end of the chase mode is recorded again. Eye-tracker generates high-resolution recording of the camera view, supplemented by various metadata (pupil position, gaze position, fixations occurrences, fixations duration, pupil diameter, etc.). The recording allowed to verify the start and ending of each chase mode and helped to recognize any anomalies in the gameplay.

4 Results

4.1 Electrodermal Activity

The EDA changes in comparison to chase mode occurrences were analyzed and some interesting correlations were found.

As mentioned before, the chase mode ends either with player capture (followed by level reset) or with player escaping. Player capture resulted in the short but noticeable growth of EDA value (see Fig. 2). The EDA value growth can be noticed within 4–5 s after the end of chase mode event. Player escape on the other hand, resulted in steady decline of the EDA value.

Figure 3 illustrates EDA of most inexperienced player; whose gameplay was the longest (almost 22 min). In the beginning, we can see that arousal is medium due to the novelty of the experience (none of the participants has played Serial Cleaner before).

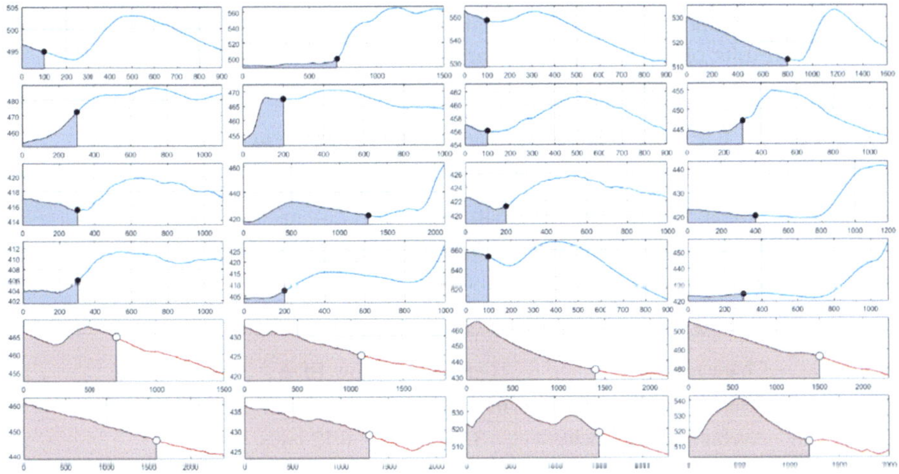

Fig. 2. EDA plots of the chase mode events followed by additional 8 s of recording. In blue are the plots representing chase mode that ended in player capture. In red are the plots of chase mode that ended in escape.

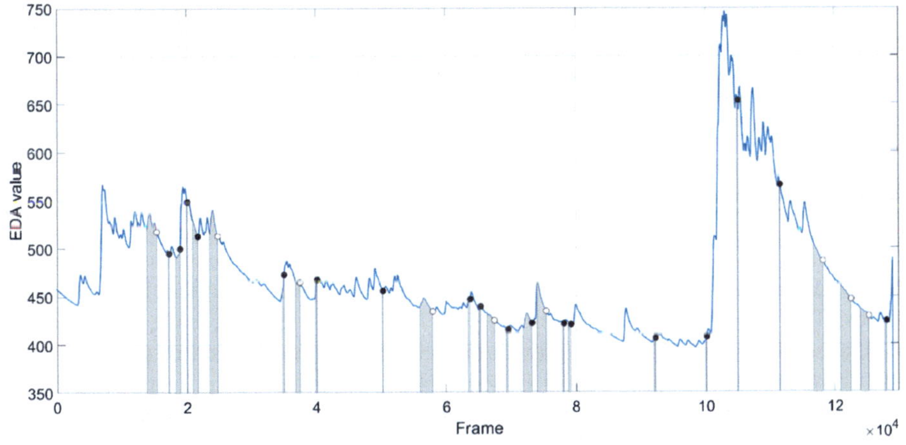

Fig. 3. EDA plot of the least experienced player. Gray color illustrates chase mode events. Around 16-min mark, a significant increase in EDA readings indicate great player disappointment followed by termination of the game.

We can observe that the arousal falls as a result of player getting used to the situation. There is the moment in the gameplay when, after few failures, the player was very close to the success, but failed and was set back to the beginning. As a result, rapidly growing arousal induced by stress and overwhelming frustration is observed.

4.2 Oculography

The two main aspects of eye-tracker research are fixations measurement and gaze path analysis. The research aim was to compare duration of fixations in two specific divisions: gameplay aspect (chase mode/sneak mode) and affective aspect (high EDA/low EDA). The results of the measurement are shown in the tables below.

Table 1. Eye movement pattern characteristic in relation to gameplay modes.

Characteristic	Chase mode	Sneak mode	Variation
Average fixation duration	640.40 ms	577.38 ms	9.84%
Average gaze velocity	5.05 cm/s	4.25 cm/s	15.84%

Table 2. Eye movement pattern characteristic in relation to EDA value.

Characteristic	High EDA	Low EDA	Variation
Average fixation duration	625.02 ms	487.44 ms	22.01%
Average gaze velocity	3.73 cm/s	6.12 cm/s	39.05%

Gameplay Aspect. It can be noticed, that there is the difference in the players eyes behavior in the state of the alert, in opposition to the state of no pressure.

Affective Aspect. The most interesting result of the experiment is significant different distance of saccades in correlation with high value of EDA associated with very short fixation durations. There was no amplification of the effect of the chase mode when occurred simultaneously with the high EDA, despite there is some coincidence with the high EDA following the chase episode.

5 Discussion

As shown in Tables 1 and 2 we have registered significant changes in oculographic data in relation to chase modes events, as well as oculographic data in relation to EDA values. This proved our initial assumptions. Not surprisingly we have observed the correlation between EDA value growth and chase mode that ended in player failure. The correlation on average occurred within 4–5 s after the chase event. This delay agrees with usual reaction of EDA measurements that are delayed between 3–10 s. Although the reaction of chase mode event can vary greatly within the game, as many aspects of the gameplay can be predicted by the player. The experience plays great role. Contrary to our previous research [9] we have noticed inverted influence of experience on player gaze movement. Previously in game where information processing plays stronger role than reflex and situational averseness. More experienced player had lower average gaze velocity than inexperienced one. In this research on the other hand, we have registered exactly opposite results, as the experienced player was able to process more information from the environment than the inexperienced one. This fact suggests the need for further research on player behavior in relation to type of challenge placed before him.

References

1. Kiili, K., Koivisto, A., Finn, E., Ketamo, H.: Measuring user experience in tablet based educational game. In: Felicia, P. (ed.) Proceedings of the 6th European Conference on Games-Based Learning, ECGBL 2012, Cork, Irleand (2012)
2. Almeida, S., Mealha, O., Veloso, A.: Interaction behavior of hardcore and inexperienced players: "call of duty: modern warfare". In: Proceedings of SBGames 2010 – IX Brazilian Symposium on Computer Games and Digital Entertainment (2010)
3. Duchowski, A.: Eye Tracking Methodology: Theory and Practice. Springer, New York (2003)
4. Benedek, M., Kaernbach, C.: Physiological correlates and emotional specificity of human piloerection. Biol. Psychol. **86**(3), 320–329 (2011)
5. Nalepa, G.J., Gizycka, B., Kutt, K., Argasiński, J.K.: Affective design patterns in computer games. Scrollrunner case study. In: FedCSIS Communication Papers (2017
6. Pupil Labs. https://pupil-labs.com
7. Salvucci, D., Goldberg, J.: Identifying fixations and saccades in eye-tracking protocols. In: Proceedings of the 2000 Symposium on Eye Tracking Research and Applications, ETRA 2000, pp. 71–78. ACM (2000)
8. Batista, D., da Silva, H.P., Fred, A., Moreira, C., Reis, M., Ferreira, H.A.: Benchmarking of the BITalino biomedical toolkit against an established gold standard. Healthc. Technol. Lett. **6**, 32–36 (2019)
9. Argasiński, J., Grabska Gradzińska, I.: Patterns in serious game design and evaluation application of eye-tracker and biosensors. In: Proceedings Artificial Intelligence and Soft Computing: 16th International Conference, ICAISC 2017. LNCS. LNAI, pp. 367–377. Springer, Cham (2017)

Integrating Trust in Automation into Driver State Monitoring Systems

Jaume Perello-March(✉), Christopher Burns, Mark Elliott, and Stewart Birrell

Warwick Manufacturing Group, The University of Warwick, Coventry, UK
{Jaume.Perello-March, C.Burns.2, M.T.Elliott, S.Birrell}@warwick.ac.uk

Abstract. Inappropriate trust in highly automated vehicles (HAVs) has been identified as one of the causes in several accidents [1–3]. These accidents have evidenced the need to include a Driver State Monitoring System (DSMS) [4] into those HAVs which may require occasional manual driving. DSMS make use of several psychophysiological sensors to monitor the drivers' state, and have already been included in current production vehicles to detect drowsiness, fatigue and distractions [5]. However, DSMS have never been used to monitor Trust in Automation (TiA) states within HAVs yet. Based on recent findings, this paper proposes a new methodology to integrate TiA state-classification into DSMSs for future vehicles.

Keywords: Trust in Automation · Driver State Monitoring Systems · Highly automated vehicles · Machine learning

1 Introduction

Highly Automated Driving will change the manner in which we drive, will place new demands of their users, and as a consequence, new human factors such as Trust in Automation (TiA) will arise. TiA is an attitude that leads to a behaviour - reliance - [6] from which several behavioural outcomes can result including correct use, misuse, disuse and overuse of automation [7]. In addition, TiA is a multidimensional construct [8], implying that TiA may have many states. The taxonomy proposed here for Driver State Monitoring System (DSMS) would classify them as Appropriate TiA, Over-TiA and Distrust in automation.

The current standardised methodology to evaluate TiA uses self-reporting tools [9, 10]. These tools have proven to be valid and feasible but are limited to experimental scenarios and post-hoc data analysis, and do not allow active real-time measurement. Therefore, a different methodology in accordance with DSMSs capabilities needs to be developed. Recent findings in the TiA literature have suggested a promising alternative for this problem – using psychophysiology [11, 12]. Using the existing TiA scales [9, 10], this review will focus on identifying the aforementioned TiA states and their psychophysiological correlates, and investigate the use of DSMS data to train a TiA classifier using machine learning algorithms.

T. Ahram et al. (Eds.): IHIET 2019, AISC 1018, pp. 344–349, 2020.
https://doi.org/10.1007/978-3-030-25629-6_53

2 TiA Decision-Making Processes

It has been proposed that TiA is an attitude involving both affective and cognitive decision-making processes [6, 13–15]. Following the proposal by Lee and See [6], these can be classified as:

- Analogical: trust judgements based on rules and heuristics, making use of previously known solutions for similar current problems, other individuals' experiences, societal norms, etc. Analogical decisions are less cognitively demanding than analytic judgements, allowing faster decision-making.
- Analytical: a judgement based on active evaluations of risks and benefits of trusting an automated system. It relies on knowledge about the automated system's characteristics and performance. Analytical decision-making is more cognitively demanding and time-consuming.
- Affective: This mechanism bases trust judgements on impressions, feelings and emotions regarding the trustee. Often users may not trust automation only because they feel uneasy, lacking any kind of reasoning. Affective processes are used when time pressure is high or when cognitive resources are not available to make a judgement [6].

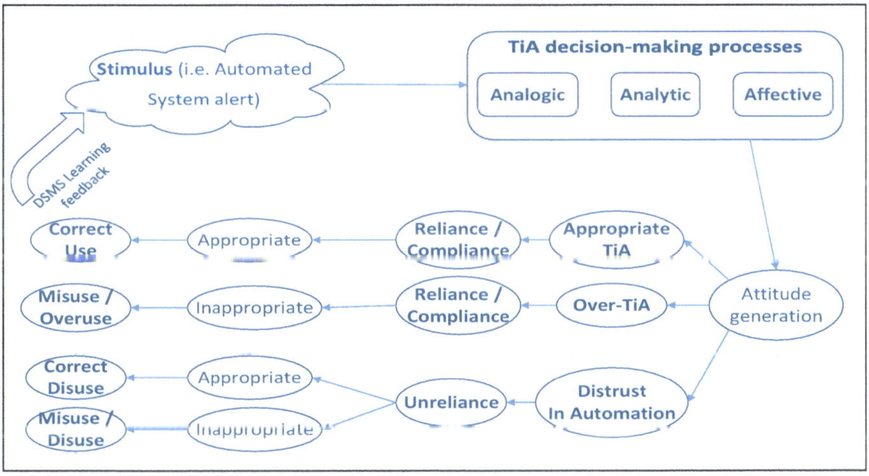

Fig. 1. Model of TiA process

The use of each mechanism depends on the cognitive resources available (knowledge about the system, similar past experiences, cognitive workload, etc.) and time pressures [6]. For example, the user may rely on analytic processing when there is sufficient time and cognitive resources available but when cognitive resources are limited and time is constrained, the user may instead rely on faster, more subconscious analogical and affective processes [15]. Building upon the existing models of TiA, this paper proposes that attitudes generated may represent particular psychophysiological patterns, which importantly for DSMS could be evaluated in real-time. To enable future research in this area this paper presents a diagrammatic representation of the initial decision-making, to final behavioural outcome, process (see Fig. 1). Importantly for our research this enables a controlled stimulus (or automated vehicle scenario) to be created, and physiological responses evaluated, leading to a greater understanding of the TiA decision-making process which results in an attitude being formed.

3 Modelling Trust in Automation

Previous authors have already proposed mathematical models to classify TiA [16, 17]. However these models are grounded on TiA frameworks [18, 19] which have been updated [6] and [15]. Recent developments in the Human-Robot interaction domain suggest that mathematically modelling TiA in HAVs based on mental workload and affective states is achievable [20, 21]. Therefore, it is worth considering updating and adapting these newer models to the present state-of-the-art for HAVs. The following section proposes a new methodology, building on Fig. 1, which could be used to classify TiA into three states using machine-learning algorithms:

1 - Appropriate Trust in Automation. An appropriate level of TiA means that the user's trust is calibrated accordingly with the automated system's reliability [22] – i.e. the user is aware of the system limitations and capabilities, and of the current traffic situation and uses the automated system appropriately. This is the desired state as it leads to a correct and safe use of the HAV. Appropriate TiA means that a user will be ready to take manual control when the systems requires by being aware that the system's capabilities are limited in certain situations [6]. Another example is that the user will rely upon and activate automated driving when suggested. Under such a scenario, it can be assumed that the user will be aware of the situation, engaged in the driving task and is confident about the automated system's capabilities. This raises the possibility of classifying appropriate TiA as an expected state of relaxation (i.e. positive valence and low arousal) with mental engagement. Previous studies have successfully classified relaxation states using Support Vector Machine (SVM), Regression Tree (RT), K-Nearest Neighbour (KNN) and Bayesian Network (BN) classifiers based on a Heart Rate Variability (HRV) decrease, an increase of Heart Rate (HR), Respiration Rate (RR) and Electro-Dermal Activity (EDA) [23, 24]. A similar method to that used in [24], could be also implemented for Electroencephalography (EEG), EDA and eye-tracking signals to classify emotional states. Mental engagement or increased mental workload has also been successfully classified using SVM [25, 26] and Artificial Neural Networks (ANN) [27–29]. These classifiers were based on an increase in pre-frontal activity via Event-Related Potentials from EEG, blood oxygenation increases from functional Near Infrared Spectroscopy (fNIRS), increased pupil size, fixations, saccades and reductions in blink-ratio. In addition, identification by Random Forest (RF) has been used for eye-tracking metrics [30].

2 - Over-Trust in Automation. This occurs when TiA is not properly calibrated due to e.g. higher expectations regarding the automated system's capabilities [6]. Over-trust is probably the most undesirable and hazardous state and some of the accidents reported in the introduction are good examples [1, 2]. In this case, the user lacks knowledge regarding the actual system reliability and therefore tends to believe that the automated system will be able to appropriately contend with situations that it cannot. For example, users may not be expecting a request to take-back control and may miss or ignore this, as they are not aware of the current situation and the vehicle's performance. Therefore, over-TiA could be related to low arousal emotional states (from bored to sleepy) and a relative lack of cognitive engagement with the driving task which could be classified using SVM, RT, KNN and BN [23] based on reduced RR, EDA, HR and increased HRV. A lack of situational awareness, complacency, automation bias and even a state of drowsiness can be classified using Extreme Learning Machine (ELM) and SVM methods based on reduced pre-frontal activity via EEG or fNIRS. RF may also be used for eye-tracking parameters [30] such as increased blink ratios, reduced pupil size, reduced fixation ratio and saccadic rates [25].

3 - Distrust in Automation represents the state in which a user's self-confidence is higher than the expectations of system performance, and can be due to previous negative or inferior experiences with other, similar automated systems. Distrust may also be motivated by excessive system performance expectations that do not match the system's real capabilities, resulting in user dissatisfaction. Ultimately, the outcome of distrust usually leads to Automated System disuse [7]. Such as [3], where the HAV operator took manual control and turned right when approaching a leading vehicle, consequently colliding with an approaching motorbike on the right side. The HAV was about to reduce the speed when approaching the leading vehicle, and if the operator had not taken control, the crash would not have occurred. High-distrust situations could be associated with increased alertness or monitoring behaviours and can be classified using ELM [25], based on an increase on pre-frontal activity, pupil size, fixations, saccades and reduced blinking ratio, and RF for these visual parameters [30]. Increased mental workload can be classified using SVM [26] and ANN [27, 28], based on an increase on pre-frontal activity, increased HR, increase of tonic EDA responses, increased RR, increased pupil size, and reduced eye blinking ratio. Finally, affective states with high arousal and negative valence such as fear, distress or frustration can be expected and classified using SVM, RT, KNN and BN [23] based on increases in HR and RR, reduced HRV and increase in EDA as inputs.

4 Further Research and Conclusions

Logically, future research should focus on finding correlations between physiological data and TiA scales ([9, 10]) to identify basic TiA states (appropriate trust, distrust, and over-trust). The first study following up this paper will focus on testing whether the-expected psychophysiological tendencies suggested in Sect. 3 are confirmed. Automation reliability expectations will be generated on naïve HAV users in order to build up different TiA among them. Using WMG's 3xD driving simulator, participants will be driven along scenarios of increasing complexity. We expect that their TiA will develop depending on the pre-administered system reliability expectations. We hypothesize that psychophysiological patterns associated with participants who trust the HAV will be statistically different from those who distrust the system. These results may serve as a TiA baseline for further related studies and as a pool of data to feed the DSMS through machine learning techniques.

References

1. NTSB: Collision between a Car Operating with Automated Vehicle Control Systems and a Tractor-Semitrailer Truck. NTSB/HAR-17-XX (2016)
2. NTSB: Preliminary Report HWY18MH010, p. 4 (2018)
3. Waymo: The very human challenge of safe driving, 5 November 2018. https://medium.com/waymo/the-very-human-challenge-of-safe-driving-58c4d2b4e8ee. Accessed 10 Dec 2018
4. Melnicuk, V., Birrell, S., Crundall, E., Jennings, P.: Towards hybrid driver state monitoring: review, future perspectives and the role of consumer electronics. In: Proceedings of the IEEE Intelligent Vehicles Symposium, pp. 1392–1397, August 2016
5. Ledezma-Zavala, E., Ramrez-Mendoza, R.A.: Towards a new framework for advanced driver assistance systems. Int. J. Interact. Des. Manuf. **12**(1), 215–223 (2018)
6. Lee, J.D., See, K.A.: Trust in automation: designing for appropriate reliance. Hum. Factors J. Hum. Factors Ergon. Soc. **46**(1), 50–80 (2004)
7. Parasuraman, R., Riley, V.: Humans and automation: use, misuse, disuse, abuse. Hum. Factors **39**(2), 230–253 (1997)
8. Spain, R.D., Bustamante, E.A., Bliss, J.P.: Towards an empirically developed scale for system trust: take two. In: Proceedings of the Human Factors and Ergonomics Society Annual Meeting, vol. 52, no. 19, pp. 1335–1339 (2008)
9. Jian, J.-Y., Bisantz, A.M., Drury, C.: Foundations for an empirically determined scale of trust in automated systems. Int. J. Cogn. Ergon. **4**(1), 53–71 (2000)
10. Körber, M.: Theoretical considerations and development of a questionnaire to measure trust in automation. In: 20th Triennial Congress of the IEA, pp. 1–20, March 2018
11. Morris, D.M., Erno, J.M., Pilcher, J.J.: Electrodermal response and automation trust during simulated self-driving car use. In: Proceedings of the Human Factors and Ergonomics Society Annual Meeting, vol. 61, no. 1, pp. 1759–1762 (2017)
12. Waytz, A., Heafner, J., Epley, N.: The mind in the machine: anthropomorphism increases trust in an autonomous vehicle. J. Exp. Soc. Psychol. **52**, 113–117 (2014)
13. Jan De Visser, E.: The World Is Not Enough: Trust in Cognitive Agents. George Mason University, Fairfax, VA (2012)
14. Madsen, M., Gregor, S.: Measuring human-computer trust. In: Proceedings of the Eleventh Australasian Conference on Information Systems, pp. 6–8 (2000)
15. Hoff, K.A., Bashir, M.: Trust in automation: integrating empirical evidence on factors that influence trust. Hum. Factors **57**(3), 407–434 (2015)
16. Itoh, M., Tanaka, K.: Mathematical modeling of trust in automation: trust, distrust, and mistrust. In: Proceedings of the Human Factors and Ergonomics Society Annual Meeting, vol. 1, no. 1994, p. 9 (2000)
17. Lee, J., Moray, N.: Trust, control strategies and allocation of function in human-machine systems. Ergonomics **35**(10), 1243–1270 (1992)
18. Muir, B.M.: Trust in automation: Part I. Theoretical issues in the study of trust and human intervention in automated systems. Ergonomics **37**(11), 1905–1922 (1994)
19. Muir, B.M., Moray, N.: Trust in automation. Part ii. Experimental studies of trust and human intervention in a process control simulation. Ergonomics **39**(3), 429–460 (1996)

20. Wang, X., Shi, Z., Zhang, F., Wang, Y.: Mutual trust based scheduling for (semi) autonomous multi-agent systems. In: Proceedings of the American Control Conference, pp. 459–464, July 2015
21. Wang, Y., Shi, Z., Wang, C., Zhang, F.: Human-robot mutual trust in (semi)autonomous underwater robots. In: Koubaa, A., Khelil, A. (eds.) Cooperative Robots and Sensor Networks. Studies in Computational Intelligence, vol. 554, pp. 115–137. Springer, Heidelberg (2014)
22. Khastgir, S., Birrell, S., Dhadyalla, G., Jennings, P.: Calibrating trust through knowledge: introducing the concept of informed safety for automation in vehicles. Transp. Res. Part C Emerg. Technol. **96**(July), 290–303 (2018)
23. Rani, P., Liu, C., Sarkar, N.: An empirical study of machine learning techniques for affect recognition in human-robot interaction. In: 2005 IEEE/RSJ International Conference on Intelligent Robots and Systems, IROS, pp. 2451–2456 (2005)
24. López-Gil, J.-M., Virgili-Gomá, J., Gil, R., García, R.: Corrigendum: method for improving EEG based emotion recognition by combining it with synchronized biometric and eye tracking technologies in a non-invasive and low cost way. Front. Comput. Neurosci. **10** (November), 9–10 (2016)
25. Chen, L.L., Zhao, Y., Zhang, J., Zou, J.Z.: Automatic detection of alertness/drowsiness from physiological signals using wavelet-based nonlinear features and machine learning. Expert Syst. Appl. **42**(21), 7344–7355 (2015)
26. Hogervorst, M.A., Brouwer, A., Van Erp, J.B.F.: Combining and comparing EEG, peripheral physiology and eye-related measures for the assessment of mental workload. Front Neurosci. **8**, 1–14 (2014)
27. Wilson, G.F., Russell, C.A.: Real-time assessment of mental workload using psychophysiological measures and artificial neural networks. Hum. Factors J. Hum. Factors Ergon. Soc. **45**(4), 635–644 (2003)
28. Wilson, G.F., Russell, C.A.: Performance enhancement in an uninhabited air vehicle task using psychophysiologically determined adaptive aiding. Hum. Factors **49**(6), 1005–1018 (2007)
29. Wilson, G.F., Russell, C.A., Force, A., Base, A.F.: Operator functional state classification using multiple psychophysiological features in an air traffic control task. Hum. Factors **45**(3), 381–389 (2003)
30. Zemblys, R., Niehorster, D.C., Komogortsev, O., Holmqvist, K.: Using machine learning to detect events in eye-tracking data. Behav. Res. Methods **50**(1), 160–181 (2018)

Research on the Netizens Trust Model in Social Network Dissemination

Yunqi Dong, Tao Chi, and Xuebo Chen(✉)

School of Electronic and Information Engineering,
University of Science and Technology, Liaoning,
Anshan 114051, Liaoning, People's Republic of China
xuebochen@126.com

Abstract. Traditional media has always been the main medium of information dissemination. In order to solve the negative effects on information flooding, truth and falsehoods in social network communication, a trust model of netizens is proposed. The Deffuant model is analyzed and the trust network is constructed according to the interaction behavior between the netizens and the government and the characteristics and definitions of the trust relationship. Netizens trust model describes the trust degree between netizens and the government. Then the simulation is carried out under different degrees of trust through MATLAB. The influence of the trust degree on social network dissemination is observed by changing the step size. Based on the analysis of the simulation results, we can conclude that when the trust between the netizens and the government is large, it's easier to reach a consensus. It plays a positive role in promoting dissemination.

Keywords: Netizen trust model · Trust degree · MATLAB · Network dissemination

1 Introduction

Trust is a complex concept on different understandings and definitions in different research areas. A typical representative of the sociological theoretical trust model is the Marsh model. The model is based on the attributes of trust society. By referring to the thought of computational trust in psychology and sociology, a computable trust model in distributed artificial intelligence environment is proposed [1]. In computer science, trust represents the contract and commitment of the object based on identity, password, password system and so on. The network hot spot event discovery system is improved based on the K-means algorithm [2]. In the statistical principle, to overcome the shortcomings of the existing trust model, a trust model based on statistics is proposed by taking the trust model of eBay as an example. After further improvement, an iterative trust calculation model was proposed [3]. In the reference to the concept of trust in the disciplines of psychology and sociology, many probabilistic-based trust calculation models are proposed by using the probabilistic method. Taking Beth's trust model as an example, this model plays a certain role in the demonstration of trust and trust derivation [4]. But the trust federation algorithm is too simple. The Deffuant model is a classic continuous viewpoint evolution model. The researches of scholars at

T. Ahram et al. (Eds.): IHIET 2019, AISC 1018, pp. 350–355, 2020.
https://doi.org/10.1007/978-3-030-25629-6_54

home and abroad include Grauwin are based on the Deffuant model. When the difference of the individual viewpoint is greater than the trust threshold, the viewpoint is corrected with a certain probability. It's good for consensus finally [5]. Therefore, based on the theory of complex networks, this paper improves and constructs the Deffuant model, and uses MATLAB software to program and simulate, and analyzes the influence of the degree of trust between netizens and the government on the information dissemination process.

There are usually various social relationships (netizens, governments, opinion leaders, mainstream media, and authoritative experts) in social networks. In the trust network topology, there are connections among different nodes. Figure 1 shows a schematic diagram of a trust network structure, where A to F represent netizens, and the connection between netizens indicates that there is an interaction between netizens. The numbers such as t1, t2, and t3 represent the degree of trust in the interaction between nodes.

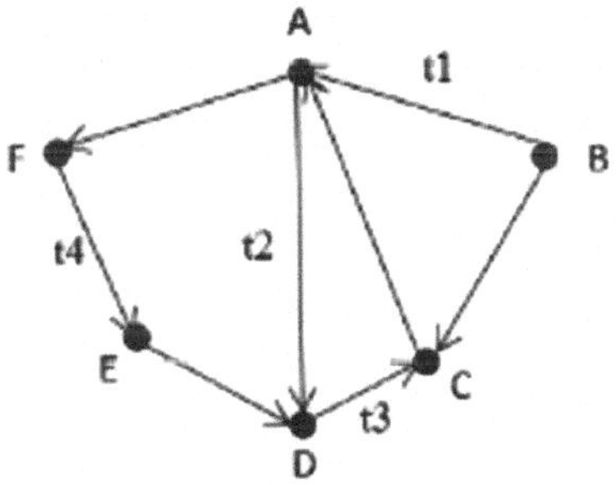

Fig. 1. Trust network diagram

With the rise of complex network research, it is found that the real world and the individual interaction structure in the Internet community satisfy the characteristics of complex networks, especially small world networks, scale-free networks and networks containing communities [6]. Therefore, the viewpoint dynamics on complex networks and the adaptive co-evolution of complex networks and viewpoints (the interaction between network structure and individual perspective evolution) have gradually become the hot spots of viewpoint dynamics research. In real life, the credibility of the opinion provider is considered. For example, the government, mainstream media and authoritative experts have higher credibility, while the average individual's opinion is less credible. Therefore, this paper comprehensively considers the trust, evolution and consensus of the views in the trust degree between netizens and governments in social groups.

2 Model Construction

Assume that there be a subject $n \in N$ in the network, and the subject's $S \in R^d$ opinion space. Introduce the distance relation matrix xi and xj, where $i \neq j$, set the initial value of the system $x(0) \in S^n$, the trust threshold of each subject $\varepsilon 1, , \varepsilon 2, \ldots, \varepsilon n > 0$, and the initial normal form is $\|\bullet\|_2$. The subject-based Deffuant model process is defined as a random process related to time $x(t), t \in N$. At each time step $t \in N$, two arbitrary subjects i and j will perform the following processes: Similarly, the same exchange process is performed. Similarly, The formula $xj(t+1)$ performs the same exchange process [7].

$$\begin{cases} xi(t+1) = (xj(t) + xi(t))/2, & \|xi(t) - xj(t)\| \leq \varepsilon i; \\ \qquad\qquad xi(t), & else \end{cases} \tag{1}$$

Deffuant model is a classic continuous viewpoint interaction model. It is assumed that when two individual viewpoints interact with each other, only the trust degree can conduct viewpoint interaction within a specific range of difference values, and the different value is the interaction threshold, generally expressed by d. The group is composed of N individuals, each individual will produce a value of Opinion $Ox(x = 1, 2, 3, \ldots, N)$, between [0, 1]. There are only two random interactions at a time [8]. Assuming that individual x and individual y meet at time t, when their Opinion value is less than or equal to the initial set interaction threshold ($|Ox - Oy| \leq d$), the interaction rules between x and y are as follows:

$$\begin{aligned} Ox(t+1) &= Ox(t) + \mu(Oy(t) - Ox(t)) \\ Oy(t+1) &= Oy(t) - \mu(Oy(t) - Ox(t)) \end{aligned} \tag{2}$$

Among them, μ is the trust degree of netizens' opinions, $\mu \in [0, 0.5]$. Otherwise, the values of both views remain the same at the next point in time. From the above interaction rules, it can be seen that the trust degree of netizens' opinions μ plays an important role in the process of opinion interaction. When μ is small, it means that netizens in the internet populations have low trust in the government in the interactive process, it will not easy to accept the views of the government,holding a stubborn attitude. When μ is large, it indicates that netizens in the network group have high trust in the government, easily accept the government's views and are more likely to compromise [9].

By improving the Deffuant model, this paper proposes netizens trust model. This model divides the network group into netizens and the government and describes the trust degree of netizens among social network communicators through the influence degree of the government on netizens.

In the real network group, the degree of trust of netizens in the information conveyed by the government varies more or less when they communicate with each other. In this paper, the step size of simulation is used to express the degree of trust between two related individuals, and T is used to represent the value range of T is [0, 1]. Every moment can interact randomly with every other two individuals except itself. Among them, a higher value indicates the higher trust between netizens and the government, besides the value range is between (0.5, 1]. The medium grade trust value is between (0.05, 0.5], Finally, the value of low trust is between (0, 0.05]. Therefore, the interactive rules of the netizen trust model are:

$$\begin{aligned} & when\ |Ox - Oy| \leq \varepsilon, \\ & Ox(t+1) = Ox(t) + T * \mu(Oy(t) - Ox(t)) \\ & Oy(t+1) = Oy(t) - T * \mu(Oy(t) - Ox(t)) \end{aligned} \tag{3}$$

3 Simulation

Under ideal conditions, in order to study the influence of netizens' trust in government opinions on the evolution process of opinions, this paper conducts simulation experiments with MATLAB. Each netizen is regarded as an individual with random distribution of initial coordinates. Think of the government as an individual whose coordinates are always the same. The number of simulation individuals is selected as N, and the number of interrelated ones is K = 29. The coordinate of a fixed point is defined as (5, 5, 5). The model simulation runs for 5000 time points. Observe the evolution of views in individual interactions by changing the step size. As can be seen from the figures, the small black dots represent netizens, and the initial coordinates of netizens are randomly distributed. The red five-pointed stars represent the government, whose coordinates are always fixed. The colored lines represent the trajectory of the movement of ideas. With the increase of simulation step size, the degree of viewpoint aggregation changes obviously.

As can be seen from Fig. 2, when the trust degree between individuals is 0 at the same time point, individual opinions are randomly distributed in the coordinate axis. As shown in Fig. 3, when the level of trust between individuals is 0.05, individual views tend to converge, but their views are scattered, and their views are not unified within 5000 steps. As can be seen from Fig. 4, when the individual trust degree is 0.5,

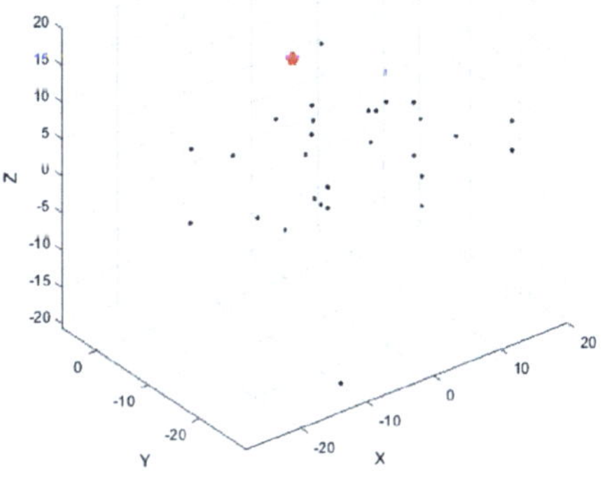

Fig. 2. Trust level is 0

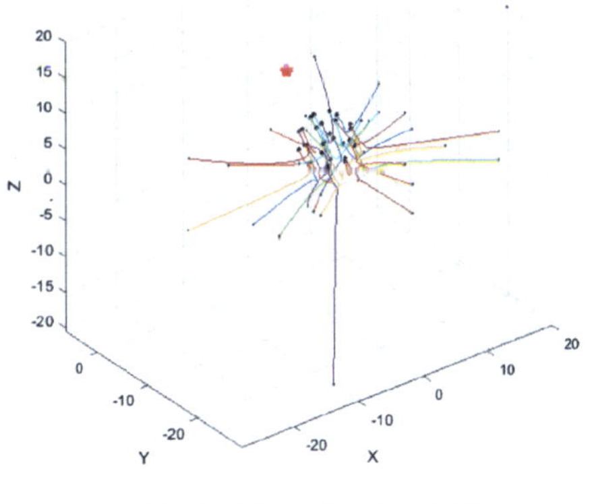

Fig. 3. Trust level is 0.05

the individual's viewpoint aggregation is relatively concentrated and basically consistent. As can be seen from Fig. 5, when the degree of individual trust is 1, the individual views closely surround the fixed point and the degree of aggregation is the closest. It can be concluded that the greater the degree of individual trust is, the faster and closer the aggregation of individual views is, and the easier it is to reach a consensus.

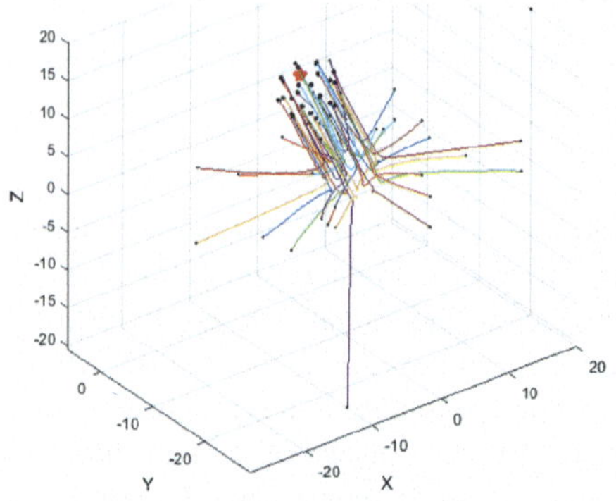

Fig. 4. Trust level is 0.5

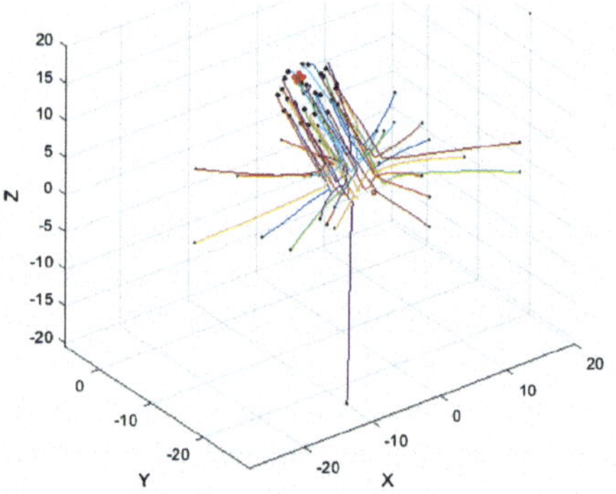

Fig. 5. Trust level is 1.0

4 Conclusion

Through the comparative analysis of the above multiple sets of simulation images and data, it can be concluded that in the evolution process of opinions, the degree of trust of netizens will converge to the direction of the government's opinions. When there is greater trust between netizens and the government, it is easier to reach a complete consensus of views. Therefore, in the context of social network, it is necessary to establish a high degree of trust in the group, because this can make the right guidance in the shortest time. Only when people believe that the information with a high degree of trust will they form a tendency to spread, and then spread. Therefore, improving the trust between netizens and the government will play a positive role in promoting dissemination.

Acknowledgments. This research reported herein was supported by the NSFC of China under Grants No. 71571091 and 71771112.

References

1. Qiao, W.: Micro-blog information personalized recommendation system based on trust relationship. Xi'an University of Architecture and Technology (2014)
2. Wei, L.: Dynamics and stability of trust model in e-commerce. Comput. Mod. (2014)

3. Beth, T., Borcherding, M., Klein, B.: Proceedings of the European Symposium on Research Security. LNCS, vol. 875, pp. 3–18 (1994)
4. Zhang, L.H.: On China's public policy and network public opinion. Guangxi Soc. Sci. (07), 96–99 (2009)
5. Ma, Y.J., Du, Y.Y.: Research on the evolution of public opinion based on the complex network Deffuant model. J. Intell. **37**(06), 91–95+159 (2018)
6. Gandica, Y., Charmell, A., Villegas-Febres, J., Bonalde, I.: Cluster-size entropy in the axelrod model of social influence: small-world networks and mass media. Phys. Rev. E **84**(4), 046109 (2011)
7. Huang, T.: Cluster self-organizing motion control of swarm robot system. Dalian University of Technology (2015)
8. Li, G.Q., Luo, Y.Y., Zang, X.L.: Research on the evolution of public opinions in online communities based on bounded trust model. Inform. Sci. **35**(6), 63–68 (2017)
9. Zhu, Y.H., Zhang, C.Q.: Simulation research on the evolution and propagation of online public opinions based on influence model. J. Intell. **34**(2), 28–37 (2015)

Human–Computer Interaction

Simulation of a New Airport Security Design Concept

Martin Jung[1(✉)], Axel B. Classen[1], André Castro[2], and Catarina Ferreira[2]

[1] Institute of Air Transport and Airport Research, Linder Hoehe, German Aerospace Center, 51147 Cologne, Germany
{m.jung, axel.classen}@dlr.de
[2] Almadesign, Rua Armando Cortez, Ed. Interface, nº 1C R/C D, 2770-233 Paço de Arcos, Portugal
{andre.castro, catarina.ferreira}@almadesign.pt

Abstract. Airport Security is a complex and important task directly affecting airports' operational performances and passenger comfort. As part of the EU Horizon 2020 project PASSME, passenger centric airport and airplane interiors were redesigned in order to meet passengers' needs and reducing door-to-door travel time. This paper will describe how simulation was used to provide early feedback as part of the security design process and for evaluating the outcome while avoiding high implementation cost and without disturbing operational processes. We will also describe the new developed security design concept as well as the simulation approach with Anylogic software. The simulation output – effects of the new design concept – will be discussed at the end of the paper along with an outlook on further research opportunities.

Keywords: Airport · Simulation · Security · Design process

1 Introduction

Passengers consider the airport security process as one of the most stressing times in door-to-door travel [1]. Security screening must run smoothly in order to allow faster processing and improve passenger experience. Queuing management systems, real time information and enough physical space for passengers to pack and repack are usually important aspects in the process. One of the key performance indicators is waiting time. As part of the project PASSME, co-funded by EU's Horizon 2020 Research and Innovation Programme, passenger centric airport and airplane interiors were redesigned in order to meet passengers' needs and to reduce door-to-door travel time. Principally it is acceptable to have queues as passengers are used to long process times, but in order to reduce stress and waiting time PASSME partners developed an alternative security together with a Cart concept which could potentially help to improve the passenger experience. PASSME interior design solutions aim at improving passenger flow at the airport, optimize the use of space and make the travel experience more seamless and enjoyable for the passengers. The security area and process has been identified as the major passenger stress touch-point and was chosen as one of the intervention areas.

T. Ahram et al. (Eds.): IHIET 2019, AISC 1018, pp. 359–364, 2020.
https://doi.org/10.1007/978-3-030-25629-6_55

But implementation of design changes at airports is difficult, time consuming and costly. This is even more the case for changes of airport security concepts. Exactly here is where the strengths of simulation can be ideally used both to support design development as well as for evaluation purposes.

In this paper we will show how simulation was used to provide early feedback as part of the design process and for evaluating the outcome while avoiding high implementation cost and without disturbing operational processes. We will describe the new developed security design concept and as well our simulation approach. The simulation is created with the simulation software Anylogic. Anylogic is a multi-methods simulation software that supports system dynamic, discrete events and agent based modeling. It is also capable of mixing these simulation methods within one model. We show how we combined an existing pedestrian social force model simulation with the agent-based modelling approach to have a more specific behavior of the simulated passengers in the security area.

2 Security Concept Design Development

The layout of the PASSME security area has been redesigned in order to reduce passenger stress and processing times. Through new process layouts and a Cart design, the system is potentially capable of accommodating different passenger segments and reducing process times, specifically during peak hours.

To make queuing time in the security area more productive, PASSME partners developed a Cart to allow passengers to unpack at an earlier stage of the process. When picking up the Cart or during queuing waiting time, passengers are able to unpack and keep their personal belongings close to them. The Cart includes a tablet support, where different information about the security process can be presented to passengers through the PASSME API which provides personalized real-time information. Figure 1 shows a prototype of the Cart. Passengers with specific needs and expectations (e.g. Families, Seniors, First Time Travelers) can benefit from the system due to more information available and more comfort in use.

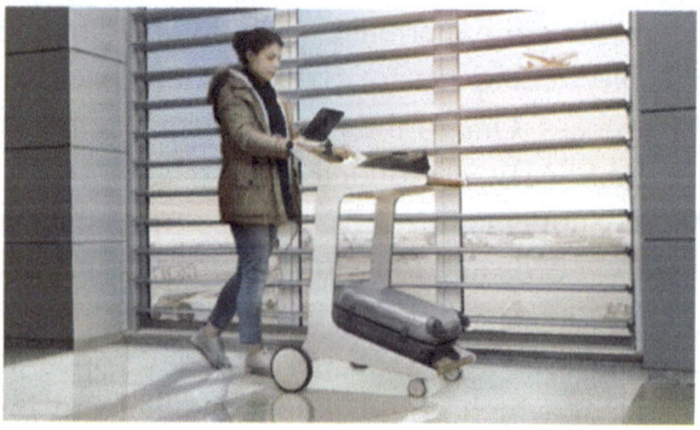

Fig. 1. Visualization of prototype of the security Cart

The main innovations in the PASSME proposal address both the queuing area - by allowing passengers to store their luggage and personal items in the Cart – and in the screening area, with two separate lanes: passenger screening and Cart x-ray. As the unpacking process is done as passengers collect their Cart or even during queuing, the concept allows for a better use of time. The Cart is designed "stackable" and includes an area to stow luggage, a top tray to place personal items, a holder for the jacket and extra space for another jacket/personal belongings. The use of composite polymer materials without almost any metallic elements could allow the Cart to be scanned in a standard technology X-ray machine using only small changes to fit the cart. The luggage and personal items would be X-rayed together with the cart on the dedicated lane.

The use of a clear graphic interface can be customized with relevant information for specific passenger segments (i.e. universal pictograms, minimum text) or the possibility to adjust the information according to the passenger´s native language.

Two 1:5 scale models were developed for design evaluation and two 1:1 scale prototypes were built for preliminary testing and validation. Due to security restrictions at airports real life implementation and testing at PASSME partner airports was not possible. Hence, simulation was used to provide early feedback as part of the security design process and for evaluating the outcome while avoiding high implementation cost and without disturbing operational processes.

3 Simulation Development

Technical core of the simulation is build with Anylogic, and combines the social force model with the agent based modelling to gain more specific behaviors of the simulated passengers.

As a baseline scenario we extended an existing security simulation that we developed in an earlier project together with a European international airport serving around 12 million passengers per year (2017). The baseline scenario was therefore already validated well together with the airport's practitioners (see [2]). We also already tailored and extended the behavior of the Anylogic pedestrian library for our specific needs. For example we applied a queue selection algorithm for the security lanes as well as to the simulated passenger behavior in the waiting queues and before the security checks.

The main impact parameters for the security check simulation are the flight plan stating the schedule of the flights, the number of passengers booked on every flight, opening periods of every security lane and the process times per security lane. This input data was received from the European airport described above. Also the terminal layout is based on this real airport. Prior to a simulation run all these parameters are imported from an Excel sheet. The arrival distribution for the passengers for each flight is based on reservation details, passenger survey data and historical observed patterns. The process parameters, e.g. details of the hand luggage handling, conveyer speed and also re-inspection rates, are based on [3].

4 Simulation Results and Evaluation

In this section we describe the scenarios we used in our simulation and also the results that show the effects of the new security design concept that we used for the interaction and feedback-loops with the design team. We used two scenarios to simulate the impact of the PASSME security design concept.

- Scenario I is the baseline scenario which represents a common security process. This scenario is based on a real operational medium sized European international airport. It represents one terminal and security area which is serving around 18,000 passengers a day.
- Scenario II is based on scenario I with implementation of the PASSME security concept design. For this purpose the security lanes in the layout of the simulation model were reshaped and placed to scale in the given airport terminal. Also the Cart collection and Cart retrieval isles were placed in this virtual terminal. The procedures also had to be adapted to match the innovative security design concept, especially incorporating the Cart concept with the separate Cart stream. Due to using Carts the space requirements for the passenger agents with Carts needed to be adapted in this scenario as well.

For validation of Scenario I we used data records from the airport, real world observations as well as feedback meetings with the airport and security employees (see also [2]).

As a direct output the simulation provides waiting times for economy and business/first class passengers, overall process times, a cost summary for security lanes, amount of checked passengers, maximum waiting times and the number of passengers having to wait more than 35 min.

Figure 2 shows a comparison of the total process times (from entering the queue until leaving the security area) of the simulation runs of scenario I with the measurements of scenario II. It illustrates the total average results of 30 Monte Carlo simulation runs with a small standard deviation of 1.6. The baseline scenario shows two typical waiting time peaks between 5:00–7:30 and 9:30–11:00. This matches well the experience of the airport employees during real operations. Main improvement of the latest design concept of PASSME over the baseline scenario can be observed exactly during those peak phases. Whereas during time of lower demand the effect is rather negligible and sometimes even slightly negative.

As an average over the whole simulated and evaluated period passengers can save 8.5% waiting and process times with the new PASSME security concept design. However, when looking at the critical phases of peak demand the effect is much higher. During peak 1 (5:00–7:30) the improvement is at 14.1% and during peak 2 (9:30–11:00) we see an average overall procedure time which is 21.9% shorter than in the baseline scenario. The simulation provided valuable visual feedback already at an early stage during the design process which helped the design team also in defining the procedures and to cover all relevant aspects of the security requirements in a viable way.

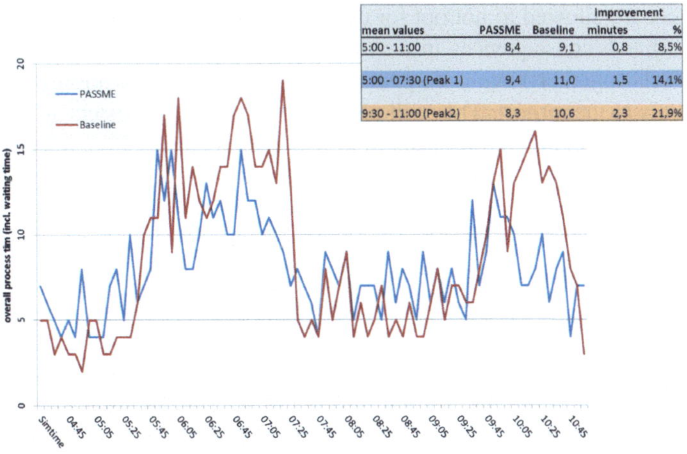

Fig. 2. Comparison of overall process times

5 Conclusion

Although Security areas are of great interest to address in terms of design improvements, changes are extremely difficult to be implemented since they are mostly operated and owned by federal police or security companies, which have an enormous responsibility regarding security of the passengers at airports while maintaining punctual traffic flows. This presented a great challenge for the implementation within the PASSME project's timeframe, budget and context. The simulation described above was therefore a great opportunity to provide early feedback to the design team as well as to help evaluating the effect, the design concept would have on an airport's operation and the passenger's journeys.

Design feedback was not just provided by the simulation results but even more by the process of modeling beforehand. The questions asked to gain the detailed input needed for a realistic and working simulation urged the design team to think even more into depth of process design in specific aspects and to complete the design in a more precise and viable way.

Comparing the results of the PASSME security design concept simulation with the baseline scenario shows a positive effect of the developed design on the overall process time of airport security checks. Average time saving is at 0.8 min (or −8.5%) in average over the whole simulated time period. However, this value alone seems not to be of peculiar significance. Even more interesting is the fact that the largest positive effect of the design concept is at peak times. This is exactly where it hurts and where the relief is needed the most. During peak 1 time saving is at 1.5 min (−14.1%) and during peak 2 improvement is at 2.3 min (−21.9%).

In phases of low waiting times and short queues, however, overall process time values are a bit worse than in the baseline scenario. This is due to a minimum of time consumption which is calculated for using the cart and the process of unpacking without being able to use this time during a waiting and queueing phase. However, as the passengers are allowed to not opt for the cart in low traffic phases, this effect would not have too harsh consequences in real operations.

Both effects together have a de-peaking impact on the utilization of the security check channels at the airport. This will also lead to a more consistent workload of the deployed resources and therefore leads to new potentials in resource management. For the passengers this means an improvement of the service quality and a reduction of unwanted waiting times.

As we only simulated against one baseline scenario with a given number of passengers and resources it would be interesting to examine the full potential and limits of the design concept e.g. in more adverse conditions by using another baseline scenario where waiting times are higher. The question would then be whether the improvement would scale with the average process time or whether there are limits to the time savings of this concept. Another question could be to what extent a different resource management would change the results and whether there are interdependencies – positive or negative. Future refinement could also be achieved in extending the simulation by the cart management which was not modeled in the simulation work so far. Another step could be to incorporate stress levels in the simulation by augmenting the agent based approach described above with situational stress components like waiting times and time to boarding etc. Stress levels could then also be evaluated based on the simulation. This leaves space for further research and testing.

The results so far show that the PASSME security concept could allow for a more productive queuing time. This adds up in reducing stress by allowing for a less stressful unpacking process and reduced waiting times by enabling passengers to store their luggage and personal items on specific Carts during queueing and dividing the screening process in two processing lanes.

Acknowledgments. The project PASSME has received funding from the European Union's Horizon 2020 research and innovation programme under grant agreement No 636308. The opinions expressed in this document reflect only the author's view and reflects in no way the European Commission's opinions. The European Commission is not responsible for any use that may be made of the information it contains.

References

1. Blekxtoon, F.J.: Innovation of the schiphol departure hall based on the passenger experience. Master thesis, Product Innovation Management, TU Delft, Delft (2010)
2. Jung, M., Classen, A.B., Rudolph, F.: Creating and validating a microscopic pedestrian simulation to analyze an airport security checkpoint. In: Yilmaz, L., Chan, W.K.V., Moon, I., Roeder, T.M.K., Macal, C., Rossetti, M.D. (eds.) Proceedings of the 2015 Winter Simulation Conference, pp. 904–905. Institute of Electrical and Electronics Engineers, Inc., Piscataway (2015)
3. Alers, T., Classen, A.B., Kellner, S.: More input - generic data for microscopic airport simulation. In: AIAA Aviation, Los Angeles (2013)

Leading Diverse Teams to Success: What Are the Factors that Can Make a Difference?

Renate Motschnig(✉) and Seyhan Güver

Faculty of Computer Science, CSLEARN - Educational Technologies, University of Vienna, Währinger Straße 29, 1090 Vienna, Austria
renate.motschnig@univie.ac.at, seyhanyilmaz@gmail.com

Abstract. Rapidly increasing globalization and international, often virtual communication require – besides intercultural competencies of people - thoughtful and well-designed strategies and tools for managing diversity. Interestingly, studies on the relationship between diversity and performance of teams have yielded inconsistent results. This is why in our research we want to find out what can be done to contribute to a positive relationship between diversity and team outcomes and thus pose the guiding research question: Which features tend to influence the relationship between diversity and team processes/outcomes? Once identified through a systematic literature analysis, our research goal is to arrange and visualize these features in a systematic way such as to provide an online visual aid to help practitioners and researchers to see at a glance which features to consider for a positive difference in managing team-diversity.

Keywords: Diversity · Heterogeneity · Teams · Workgroups · Moderators · 3Ts-MAC taxonomy · Systematic literature review · Team outcome · Team leadership

1 Introduction

Over the past decades, the workforce has become increasingly diverse in demographic characteristics and new organizational forms have brought together people with different backgrounds. Moreover, the increasing focus of project-based work has catapulted the team paradigm to an unprecedented level of importance. Hence, organizations need to accommodate an increasing number of teams and workgroups, many of which are heterogeneous. To manage and lead these teams effectively, knowledge about how various diversity-features and project/task characteristics impact project/task outcome is indispensable [1].

This study assumes that achieving effectiveness is significantly facilitated by a thorough *understanding* of the features influencing the dynamics and impact of diversity. This understanding is destined to help developing *attitudes* and employing the right *approaches and actions* while managing and working in diverse teams. Thus, an up-to-date comprehensive review of the impacts of diversity and its management on team dynamics and outcomes was found to be essential. Research on the relationship between team/work group diversity and performance has yielded inconsistent results

T. Ahram et al. (Eds.): IHIET 2019, AISC 1018, pp. 365–370, 2020.
https://doi.org/10.1007/978-3-030-25629-6_56

(e.g. [2–5]). Hence, the main focus of this work is an investigation of *moderators* being most relevant for leadership, organizational behavior, and teamwork. *Diversity moderators* are factors having an influence on or intervening in the relationship between team diversity and team processes and outcomes. For example, extreme time pressure can turn the benefits resulting from diversity, such as increased creativity, into the drawback of not finishing in time. In the study, *diversity is* defined as "differences between individuals on any attribute that may lead to the perception that another person is different from self" [6, p. 517].

In this paper, we pursue a direction that is in tune with several recent diversity researchers who respond to the question "Is a diverse team an advantage or a hindrance?" with "It depends!" and suggest to study moderators of the diversity-performance relationship (e.g. [7, 8]). Hence, we pay particular attention to *moderating factors* and are suggesting a *moderator taxonomy* to increase transparency and open-up the field for further systematic investigation. Our study differs from previous studies, reviews, and meta-analysis by systematically arranging moderators in a taxonomy and covering literature until 2018. In the current study, a systematic literature review served as the method of choice. The data collection was followed by a qualitative analysis of the 131 laboratory and field studies selected for analysis as well as 19 review studies on diversity in teams, conducted between 1959 and 2018. Furthermore, the moderators we identified are arranged in a taxonomy and tagged with annotations indicating the direction of the modification. The results from this work are intended to point managers to issues that matter in leading diverse teams to success, whereby factors concerning human interaction are given special attention.

2 Research Method

Based on the inconsistent results and zero relationships found between diversity types and team outcomes in meta-analytic review studies, we chose to interpret the existing literature descriptively. We based our investigation on Fink's [9] procedure for a systematic review and defined the following research questions:

1. Which factors moderate the impact of diversity in team processes and outcomes?
2. In how far is a taxonomy of moderators a helpful representation of the field?

As the second step, we researched more than 100 databases that were available through remote access of the Vienna University of Economy and the University of Vienna including JSTOR, SSCI-Social Science Citation Index, EconLit (EBSCO), ABI/Inform Global (T&I ProQuest), and EBSCO Business Source Premier. Thirdly, we determined search terms and searched databases and bibliographies by using a combination of the search terms "diversity", "heterogeneity", and "faultline" with "team", "workgroup" and "working group" (e.g. diversity team). Since the preliminary literature searches yielded too many articles, we set the criteria for inclusion such that we included studies which (i) were empirical (laboratory or field), (ii) explicitly researched effects of diversity on group processes and outcomes (excluding, for example, studies on organizational diversity), and (iii) were reviews of previous empirical studies. We also performed a manual search for studies referenced in the selected articles. As a next step, we synthesized the resources focusing on studies that addressed moderating factors in the diversity-team functioning linkage. These were 69 laboratory and field studies and 9 meta-analytic review studies. We first elaborated a list of diversity moderators and started to design a taxonomy as depicted in Fig. 1. After three iterations between the (multi-cultural) authors we converged toward a fairly balanced structure with 6 top-level categories. It is worth pointing out that some features, for example *time pressure,* fitted into more than one category, namely "time" as well as "management". In these cases we decided to choose one category and refrain from multiple categorizations for simplicity.

Furthermore, we needed to propose criteria to decide whether to include or dismiss a feature. For transparency and practicability, we decided to include a feature if there was at least one study that found (statistical) evidence of the moderating effect of that feature. Figure 1 sketches the proposed taxonomy representing the six moderator-categories of: *task, time, team, management-leadership, atmosphere, and context*, and the moderating factors under these categories.

3 Findings

The core goal of the subsection is to systematically depict those features that need to be attended to in order to facilitate the potential positive effect of diversity and reduce the potential negative one. The review by [2] confirmed that diversity is a highly complex phenomenon. Similar to the concept of risk, it depends on a multitude of factors, some of which are determined in advance and others that can be influenced by stakeholders. Knowing these factors can help to navigate teams towards success. This is why we focus on diversity moderators and investigated them systematically. Ideally, project managers and teams would engage in a diversity analysis guided by the moderators to get a handle on effective diversity management [1].

Among the moderators identified in the review, *time, task,* and *team* (3Ts) are the most researched and sensitive moderators for diversity. Looking beyond the 3Ts, some scholars studied other moderating factors that we suggest to categorize as *managerial/leadership-related* (e.g. leadership style, conflict management), *atmosphere-based* (e.g. team climate, cohesion), and *contextual* (e.g. country, organizational features) moderators (MAC). In the taxonomy displayed in Fig. 1, the "+" tag means that the factor moderates the team functioning-diversity association in a way in that it has a positive influence on team processes and/or team outcomes. The "−" tag, conversely, indicates a negative influence, the small circle a mixed (both positive and negative) influence and the dow-headed arrow stands for a differentiated effect, as discussed in more detail in [2].

3.1 The 3Ts: Time, Task, and Team

Time. The first T, *time*, refers to temporal factors such as tenure, longevity, and duration of the team, and time pressure within the team. *Team tenure* refers to the length of time a team member has been with the team, while *team longevity* refers to

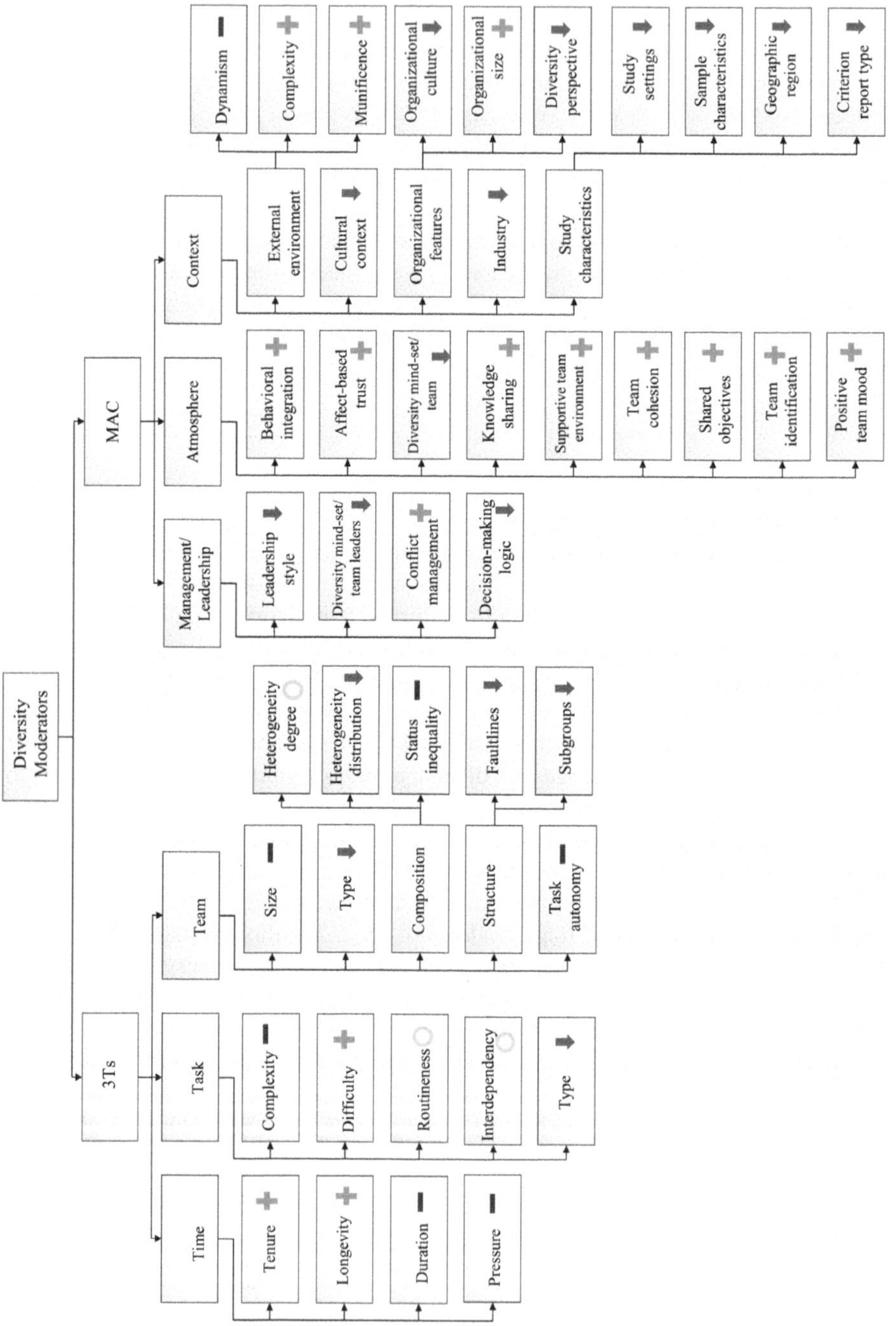

Fig. 1. 3Ts-MAC: a new taxonomy of diversity moderators

the length of time a team has existed [10]. *Team duration* indicates "the length of time a team was expected to exist" [11, p. 617]. *Team-tenure, longevity, and duration* are among the most important moderating factors of the association between diversity and team functioning (e.g. [11]).

Task. The second T, *task*, refers to the task-characteristics such as difficulty, complexity, routineness, interdependence, and type of the task. *Task interdependence* refers to "the extent to which team members rely on each other to complete their tasks" [11, p. 610].

Team. The third T, *team*, refers to team-characteristics such as size, type (e.g. co-located, dispersed; product development, project, top management), composition, and structure (subgroups and faultlines) as well as the task autonomy of team members.

3.2 The MAC Factors: Management, Atmosphere, Context

Management/Leadership. Recent studies exhibited that management- and leadership-related factors such as *leadership style* (e.g. [12]), *diversity mind-set of team leaders* [13], *conflict management* [14], and *decision-making logic* [15] moderated the relationship between diversity and team functioning.

Leadership style refers to "the assumption of leadership role and responsibility by the entire team" [16, p. 2]. In line with the general notion of the performance-leadership interaction, diversity-leadership studies demonstrated that leadership style moderates the association between diversity and team performance through its effects on group processes such as creativity and satisfaction. For example, [12] demonstrated that positive effects of cognitive diversity on team creativity and intrinsic motivation increased as the level of transformational leadership rose. Studies on the *diversity mind-set* [13] showed that pro-diversity beliefs of team leaders mitigated the negative impact of socio-demographic faultlines on team functioning.

Atmosphere. Recent studies (see [2] for discussion) established the following atmosphere-based factors as moderators: *cohesion, behavioral integration, affect-based trust, knowledge sharing, diversity mind-set* within the team, *shared objectives, team identification, supportive team environment*, and *positive team mood.*

Context. Contextual moderators address organizational and environmental characteristics such as *external environment, cultural context, organizational features, industry*, and *study characteristics*. Moreover, *diversity perspectives of organizations* have an influence on team/workgroup functioning.

4 Discussion and Conclusions

The "zero-relationship" and inconsistent results in previous review studies led us to acknowledge that there is no generally valid direct effect of diversity on team processes and outcomes. This insight had motivated us to systematically research diversity moderators and to arrange them into a taxonomy, aimed to provide a systematic knowledge base that can be exploited to approach leading diverse teams to success.

On a practical basis, our research confirms that in order to positively influence features of the *"management-leadership"* and *"atmosphere"* moderator categories, knowledge *and* social- and communication skills as well as attitudes of team leaders and members are of utmost importance [2, 17].

References

1. Böhm, C., Motschnig, R.: Developing diversity awareness of software engineers - a diversity framework and its application in an academic and life-long learning context. In: Proceedings of 46th ASEE/IEEE Frontiers in Education Conference. IEEE, Erie (2016)
2. Güver, S.: Communication in multicultural project teams: developing a communication model. Ph.D. thesis, Faculty of Business, Economics and Statistics, University of Vienna (2017)
3. Schneid, M., Isidor, R., Li, C., Kabst, R.: The influence of cultural context on the relationship between gender diversity and team performance: a meta-analysis. Int. J. Hum. Resour. Manag. **26**(6), 733–756 (2015)
4. Stewart, G.L.: A meta-analytic review of relationships between team design features and team performance. J. Manag. **32**(1), 29–55 (2006)
5. Meyer, B.: Team diversity: a review of the literature. In: The Wiley Blackwell Handbook of the Psychology of Teamwork and Collaborative Processes. Wiley-Blackwell, Chichester (2017)
6. van Knippenberg, D., Schippers, M.C.: Work group diversity. Ann. Rev. Psychol. **58**(1), 515–541 (2007)
7. van Knippenberg, D., Dawson, J.F., West, M.A., Homan, A.C.: Diversity faultlines, shared objectives, and top management team performance. Hum. Relat. **64**(3), 307–336 (2011)
8. van Knippenberg, D., van Ginkel, W.P.: The categorization-elaboration model of work group diversity: wielding the double-edged sword. In: Crisp, R. (ed.) The Psychological of Social and Cultural Diversity. Wiley-Blackwell, Malden (2010)
9. Fink, A.: Conducting Research Literature Reviews: From the Internet to Paper. Sage, Thousand Oaks (2013)
10. Schippers, M.C., Den Hartog, D.N., Koopman, P.L., Wienk, J.A.: Diversity and team outcomes: the moderating effects of outcome interdependence and group longevity and the mediating effect of reflexivity. J. Organ. Behav. **24**(6), 779–802 (2003)
11. Joshi, A., Roh, H.: The role of context in work team diversity research: a meta-analytic review. Acad. Manag. J. **52**(3), 599–627 (2009)
12. Wang, X.H.F., Kim, T.Y., Lee, D.R.: Cognitive diversity and team creativity: effects of team intrinsic motivation and transformational leadership. J. Bus. Res. **69**, 3231–3239 (2016)
13. Schölmerich, F., Schermuly, C.C., Deller, J.: How leaders' diversity beliefs alter the impact of faultlines on team functioning. Small Group Res. **47**(2), 177–206 (2016)
14. Mello, A.L., Delise, L.A.: Cognitive diversity to team outcomes: the roles of cohesion and conflict management. Small Group Res. **46**(2), 204–226 (2015)
15. Kristinsson, K., Candi, M., Sæmundsson, R.J.: The relationship between founder team diversity and innovation performance: the moderating role of causation logic. Long Range Plann. **49**, 464–476 (2016)
16. Gupta, V.K., Huang, R., Niranjan, S.: A longitudinal examination of the relationship between team leadership and performance. J. Leadersh. Organ. Stud. **17**(4), 335–350 (2010)
17. Motschnig, R., Ryback, D.: Transforming Communication in Leadership and Teamwork Person-Centered Innovations. Springer, Switzerland (2016)

Towards Visual Data Science - An Exploration

Marina Tropmann-Frick and Jakob Smedegaard Andersen(✉)

Department of Computer Science, Hamburg University of Applied Sciences, Hamburg, Germany
{marina.tropmann-frick, jakob.andersen}@haw-hamburg.de

Abstract. Visual perception is one of the most essential abilities for humans. This ability allows us to discover the world around us and to understand interdependencies with regard to both global context and particular concrete problem statement. We present in this paper an exploration of visualization and visual analytics approaches. Thereby, we focus on the field of data science with data-centric analytic methods and applications. Data science is closing the gap between visualization techniques, traditional hypothesis-driven methods and processing of mostly huge, heterogeneous and noisy data. A combination of smart visualization, advanced analytical methods and additional (domain) knowledge, mostly provided by humans, makes it possible to gain insights and discover new opportunities for problem solving.

Keywords: Data science · Visualization · Visual analytics · Visual interaction

1 Introduction

Data science is a relatively new rapidly developing field dealing mostly with big data. The goal of data science applications is to analyse and to extract knowledge from data, which can be used for simulation, decision making, process optimization, innovation support, etc. The process of knowledge discovery comprises data preparation techniques, statistical modeling, computational methods, visual analysis, and domain-driven problem solving. Data science relies on methodology developed in such fields as statistics, data mining, machine learning, big data, or human–computer interaction. Visualization and visual analytics build an essential part of data science.

Although both domains are dealing with visual representation, their scope and impact are different. Visualization provide techniques for presentation of data or relationships for the purpose of explanation, interpretation, communication etc. Visual analytics encompasses a process of knowledge discovery by supporting the analyst to discover patterns in data, building formal models that can be processed by machines, and developing new hypothesis. Visual analytics strongly relies on effective interaction of a human and a machine. The *Human in the Loop (HiL)* concept is characteristically for the continuous support of machine processing by human feedback. In the context of Visual Analytics, *HiL* stands for providing continuous feedback, correcting algorithmic approaches and selecting appropriate techniques during the analytical process.

We present in this work a survey on visual analytics in data science. The next section describes the main visualization aspects. Then we discuss the domain of visual

T. Ahram et al. (Eds.): IHIET 2019, AISC 1018, pp. 371–377, 2020.
https://doi.org/10.1007/978-3-030-25629-6_57

analytics and take a closer look on the *HiL* concept as well as present a comparison of visual analytics tools developing by experts and described in scientific publications in computer science journals.

2 Visualization and Visual Analytics

The design space of visualization is enormous ranging from aesthetic aspects to structural organization that affect perception. Many proven techniques have been developed to present information. These include various types of diagrams for graphical representation of proportions or numerical values as well as structures for mapping relationships and set affiliations. Visual processing pursues several different objectives such as the recognition of contexts, patterns and trends, finding outliers and clusters, classification or examining structures. Data objects can be integrated in a visualization in different ways, such as points, lines or areas as a representation object over the visual properties such as colour, shape, size and position, and the layout of the presentation.

Visualization should always be done very carefully. It is easy to misinterpret or to get misleaded by charts and graphs. Misleading data visualizations are often designed by violating standard practices. People are used to the fact that pie charts represent parts of a whole or that timelines progress from left to right. When those rules get violated, we would very likely misinterpret such a visualization. Nonetheless, a non-standard technique can make a visual representation more expressive and give it an outstanding position. Such visualizations draw our attention and make us aware of the subject representing.

Visual analytics is an interdisciplinary approach to support exploratory knowledge discovery especially regarding large and complex data sets [1–3]. The subject of visual analytics is the effective obtaining, extending and generation of knowledge. The central concept of visual analytics is to combine automated analysis techniques with interactive visualization in order to improve the overall analysis [2]. Through combining these fields, more challenging problems can be solved, which cannot be addressed by using only pure analytical or visual approaches. On the one hand, the data is often too large for pure visual approaches and therefore requires an automated pre-processing step. On the other hand, many problems are too exploratory in nature for purely automated analysis, which demands for the integration of human cognition.

Visual analytics is primarily concerned with the needs of exploratory data analysis [1]. Problems, which are solved by visual analytics, are initially unknown or vaguely formulated and presume a specific background knowledge, which the machine does not possess [4]. Through the integration of the user in an early stage of the analysis process, the user gets into the position to interactively learn the data and thus to specify and set up hypotheses. The exploratory orientation of visual analytics assists the analysts in unveiling unexpected connections and phenomena [3]. The analyst can follow various intentions in different sections of the analysis like overlooking the data, the exploratory search for new insights or the testing of hypotheses. In addition, the analysis process ranges from high level analytical tasks which strongly depend on background knowledge and expertise of the user to low level activities like the selection of the underlying data sets.

2.1 Human in the Loop

One of the main concepts regarding interactive analysis is the *HiL* concept. *HiL* emerged from the observation that some machine approaches require analytical judgement, others can be significantly improved or accelerated by interacting with humans. Characteristically for *HiL* is the continuous support of machine processing by human feedback. In the context of visual analytics, this concept occurs in terms of providing continuous feedback and correcting algorithmic approaches within the analysis. There is no general accepted definition of *HiL* and it remains open, which loop is finally meant. The optimization of learning behaviour in machine learning is a field of application for *HiL* in visual analytics, which is often used. The user is hereby directly integrated in the train-tune-phase as the user implicitly or explicitly alters the parametrization. For instance, the user extends the underlying training data, corrects them or might provide additional information.

The combination of analytical reasoning and computational models can result in usability problems. Problems arise for instance if interactions are not intuitive. Often users have to express their expectations through a variety of parameters and configurations. Users are confronted with the issue to communicate their knowledge and expertise with the machine, which affects the overall process negatively. Therefore, Endert et al. argues for a shift towards a *Human is the Loop* perspective to focus more on a seamless integration of interactions [5]. There is a demand for orientating interactions more on analytical cognitive processes in order to reduce cognitive burdens.

Nonetheless, human reasoning, decision making and knowledge generation processes are essential for the effectiveness of *HiL* and should have a central role in the process. We consider the loop as part of the computational sense making by means of adjustable environments. In our opinion *HiL* describes a machine environment that is managed by human knowledge in order to conduct continuous analytical discourses.

3 Comparison

As we mentioned above, visualization and visual analytics represent two different approaches to gain insights from data. Visualization is concerned with the depiction of data to assist the perceiving of patterns, structures and coherences. The objective hereby is to gain insights in order to comprehend data, make decisions and to build trust in the underlying data. Data as well as models are depicted through visual artefacts or diagrams. In order to visualize data effectively, it has to be in a structured form. In this context pre-processing steps like data cleaning and wrangling are applied on the raw data. Visualizations are not just static, but also provide interactions to change views.

The main focus of visual analytics is on the solving of problems. Visual analytics uses the techniques and methods provided by visualization to close the gap between algorithmic processes and human factors. Visualization is primarily concerned with the selection of optimal visual forms and interactions for a given problem, whereas visual analytics deals with the integration of analytical approaches into the entire knowledge generation process. The challenges of visual analytics are to find the best analytical approaches for a given problem, automate them as much as possible and finally provide an integrated tool, which considers human factors [2].

Since finding the right models and parameters for a given problem can be a difficult task, this task can also be shared with the user. In comparison to visualization, visual analytics includes a structured reasoning process to gain knowledge out of data [6]. The user plays an active role by steering the underlying processes and models via interactive interfaces. Visualization is used to continuously clarify the state of the analysis, to visualize data and to communicate new knowledge mutually. The combination of data-centric methods with user-centric interactions through visual interfaces is an object of visual analytics. Whereas visual representations without reference to analytical approaches are the subject of visualization.

Table 1. Comparison of visual analytics tools from (top down) [7–26]

	Why				Who			What						How		
Visual Analytics Tools	Exploring Data	Interpretability & Explainability	Debugging & Improving Models	Comparing & Selecting Models	Model Developers & Builders	Model User	Non-Experts	Relationships	Similarities	Time	Subsets	Aggregated Information	Distribution	Points	Lines	Areas
Kwon et al., 2018	x	x		x		x			x			x	x	x	x	x
Stasko et al., 2007	x	x					x	x			x	x		x	x	x
Cavallo and Demiralp, 2019	x	x	x	x	x	x			x		x	x	x	x	x	x
Park et al., 2018	x	x				x			x	x	x	x		x		x
Gotz and Stavropoulos, 2014	x	x				x	x	x	x	x	x	x	x	x	x	x
Höferlin et al., 2012		x	x	x	x							x		x		x
Jeong et al., 2009	x	x	x		x	x			x		x	x	x	x	x	
Brown et al., 2012	x	x	x		x	x			x			x	x	x		x
Alsakran et al., 2011	x	x	x				x		x	x	x		x	x		
Soo Yi et al., 2005	x						x		x		x			x		
Krause et al., 2014	x	x	x	x	x	x					x	x	x			x
Strobelt et al., 2018	x	x				x			x	x	x	x			x	x
Bögl et al., 2013		x		x		x				x	x	x	x	x	x	x
Krause et al., 2016	x	x					x	x			x	x	x	x	x	x
Chandrasegaran et al., 2017	x	x					x			x	x		x		x	x
Du et al., 2016	x	x					x		x	x	x	x	x	x	x	x
Kim et al., 2017	x						x		x		x	x		x		
Kwon et al., 2017	x					x			x		x	x			x	x
Pezzotti et al., 2018		x	x		x					x		x		x	x	x
Bailey et al., 2018	x						x	x		x	x	x			x	x

Visual Analytics focuses on exploratory analysis and is not limited to visualization and automated analysis. It also includes the entire infrastructure for creating visual analytics tools. By connecting machine processing power and capacity, visual analytics is also applicable to huge amounts of heterogeneous and dynamic data, where visualization cannot be used. Several visual analytics tools were developed in the last years. The purpose and effectiveness of those tools varies depending on utilization scenarios, provided visualization techniques and user knowledge. Table 1 presents our comparison of visual analytics tools developed by experts and described in scientific publications. Each row in the table is the main publication corresponding to one visual analytics tool. The references are listed below the table in a chronological order of the publications (top down). Each column of the table corresponds to a subsection from four interrogative questions - why, who, what and how. Each question serves as a category for classifying the tools by:

- Why - Why is it appropriate to use the particular tool, for what reason?
- Who - Who should use or is able to use the tools?
- What - What are the main features that can be analysed and visualized?
- How - How the visualization can be done, what techniques can be used? For this category we distinguish only between three general techniques.

4 Conclusion

This survey is dedicated towards reviewing the state-of-the-art in visualization and visual analytics in data science. We presented both topics separately and compared well-known visual analytics tools based on four categories presented in Sect. 3. Several times we underlined the importance of visualization and visual analytics in data science. Data are more than just numbers and words. Analysing data is similar to storytelling. The stories in this process are dealing with the real world and can be simple and straightforward as well as complex and uncontrollable. We intend to focus our further research on development of a platform for visual data science. Our vision is to allow a flexible and dynamic interconnection of analytical methods and visual techniques with automatic adaptation to data and possible problem statements.

References

1. Thomas, J.J., Cook, K.A.: Illuminating the path. National Visualization and Analytics (2005)
2. Keim, D., Andrienko, G., Fekete, J.-D., Gorg, C., Kohlhammer, J., Melançon, G.: Visual analytics: definition, process, and challenges. In: LNCS, pp. 154–176 (2008)
3. Mansmann, F., Ellis, G.: Mastering the Information Age Solving Problems with Visual Analytics. Taylor & Francis Group, Abingdon (2010)
4. Pohl, M., Smuc, M., Mayr, E.: The user puzzle - explaining the interaction with visual analytics systems. IEEE Trans. Vis. Comput. Graph. **18**(12), 154–176 (2012)

5. Endert, A., Hossain, M.S., Ramakrishnan, N., North, C., Fiaux, P., Andrews, C.: The human is the loop: new directions for visual analytics. J. Intell. Inf. Syst. **43**(3), 411–435 (2014)
6. Sacha, D., Stoffel, A., Stoffel, F., Kwon, B.C., Ellis, G., Keim, D.: Knowledge generation model for visual analytics. IEEE Trans. Vis. Comput. Graph. **20**(12), 1604–1613 (2014)
7. Kwon, B.C., Eysenbach, B., Verma, J., Ng, K., De Filippi, C., Stewart, W.F., Perer, A.: Clustervision: visual supervision of unsupervised clustering. IEEE Trans. Vis. Comput. Graph. **24**(1), 1604–1613 (2018)
8. Stasko, J., Gorg, C., Liu, Z., Singhal, K.: Jigsaw: supporting investigative analysis through interactive visualization. In: IEEE Symposium on Visual Analytics Science and Technology, pp. 131–138 (2007)
9. Cavallo, M., Demiralp, Ç.: Clustrophile 2: guided visual clustering analysis. IEEE Trans. Vis. Comput. Graph. **25**(1), 267–276 (2019)
10. Park, D., Kim, S., Lee, J., Choo, J., Diakopoulos, N., Elmqvist, N.: ConceptVector: text visual analytics via interactive lexicon building using word embedding. IEEE Trans. Vis. Comput. Graph. **24**(1), 361–370 (2018)
11. Gotz, D., Stavropoulos, H.: DecisionFlow: visual analytics for high-dimensional temporal event sequence data. IEEE Trans. Vis. Comput. Graph. **20**(12), 1783–1792 (2014)
12. Höferlin, B., Netzel, R., Höferlin, M., Weiskopf, D., Heidemann, G.: Inter-active learning of ad-hoc classifiers for video visual analytics. In: IEEE Conference on VAST, pp. 23–32 (2012)
13. Jeong, D. H., Ziemkiewicz, C., Fisher, B., Ribarsky, W., Chang, R.: iPCA: an interactive system for PCA-based visual analytics. In: Computer Graphics Forum. (28)3, pp. 767–774. (2009)
14. Brown, E.T., Liu, J., Brodley, C.E., Chang, R.: Dis-function: learning distance functions interactively. In: IEEE Conference on VAST, pp. 83–92 (2012)
15. Alsakran, J., Chen, Y., Zhao, Y., Yang, J., Luo, D.: STREAMIT: dynamic visualization and interactive exploration of text streams. In: IEEE Pacific Visualization Symposium, pp. 131–138 (2011)
16. Yi, J.S., Melton, R., Stasko, J., Jacko, J.A.: Dust & magnet: multivariate information visualization using a magnet metaphor. Inform. Vis. **4**(4), 239–256 (2005)
17. Krause, J., Perer, A., Bertini, E.: INFUSE: interactive feature selection for predictive modeling of high dimensional data. IEEE Trans. Vis. Comput. Graph. **20**(12), 1614–1623 (2014)
18. Strobelt, H., Gehrmann, S., Pfister, H., Rush, A.M.: LSTMVis: a tool for visual analysis of hidden state dynamics in recurrent neural networks. IEEE Trans. Vis. Comput. Graph. **24**(1), 667–676 (2018)
19. Bögl, M., Aigner, W., Filzmoser, P., Lammarsch, T., Miksch, S., Rind, A.: Visual analytics for model selection in time series analysis. IEEE Trans. Vis. Comput. Graph. **19**(12), 2237–2246 (2013)
20. Krause, J., Perer, A., Stavropoulos, H.: Supporting iterative cohort construction with visual temporal queries. IEEE Trans. Vis. Comput. Graph. **22**(1), 91–100 (2016)
21. Chandrasegaran, S., Badam, S.K., Kisselburgh, L., Peppler, K., Elmqvist, N., Ramani, K.: VizScribe: a visual analytics approach to understand designer behavior. Int. J. Hum. Comput. Stud. **100**, 66–80 (2017)

22. Du, F., Plaisant, C., Spring, N., Shneiderman, B.: EventAction: visual analytics for temporal event sequence recommendation. In: IEEE Conference on VAST, pp. 61–70 (2016)
23. Kim, M., Kang, K., Park, D., Choo, J., Elmqvist, N.: TopicLens: efficient multi-level visual topic exploration of large-scale document collections. IEEE Trans. Vis. Comput. Graph. **23** (1), 151–160 (2017)
24. Kwon, B.C., Kim, H., Wall, E., Choo, J., Park, H., Endert, A.: AxiSketcher: interactive nonlinear axis mapping of visualizations through user drawings. IEEE Trans. Vis. Comput. Graph. **23**(1), 221–230 (2017)
25. Pezzotti, N., Höllt, T., Gemert, J.V., Lelieveldt, B.P.F., Eisemann, E., Vilanova, A.: DeepEyes: progressive visual analytics for designing deep neural networks. IEEE Trans. Vis. Comput. Graph. **24**(1), 98–108 (2018)
26. Bailey, S.M., Wei, J.A., Wang, C., Parra, D., Brusilovsky, P.: CNVis: a web-based visual analytics tool for exploring conference navigator data. Electron. Imaging **1**, 1–11 (2018)

Joystick versus Mouse in First Person Shooters: Mouse Is Faster than Joystick

Hilde Pedersen[1], Rein Frimannslund Refvik[1], Johnnadel Salita Uy[1], and Frode Eika Sandnes[1,2](✉)

[1] Oslo Metropolitan University, Oslo, Norway
frodes@oslomet.com
[2] Kristiania University College, Oslo, Norway

Abstract. Many gamers use desktop or laptop computers with a mouse when gaming, instead of a special purpose gaming input device such as a joystick. This study compared the hitting speed and success rates of mouse and joystick for a simple first-person shooter. A between-subjects experiment with n = 22 participants using a tailor-made game task was conducted. The results show that the mouse only takes 68.8% of the time compared to the joystick in hitting targets. No significant differences were found in terms of success rate with the two methods.

Keywords: Computer games · First person shooter · Target-hitting · Mouse · Joystick · Game controller

1 Introduction

Computer gaming are used on many platforms including dedicated consoles, mobile consoles and general-purpose computers. Computer game sales shows that many gamers use general purpose computers. Many of these rely on the standard input devices such keyboards and mice and may not have dedicated gaming controllers.

This study therefore set out to explore the difference between using a conventional mouse and a dedicated joystick game controller in terms of computer gameplay, or more precisely, target hitting in a first-person shooter. Klochek and MacKenzie has pointed out that there is relatively little research into the performance of computer game input devices [1]. Although studies have compared various types of game controllers there are only a few comparisons of joystick and mouse in gaming specifically. However, mice [2, 3] and joysticks [4, 5] have been studied extensively in their own right. The use of touch display devices in computer games have also been investigated [6]. Previous studies have contrasted the mouse to joysticks and the Wii controller [7] and the results showed that the mouse gave best performance, while the Wii controller was preferred by the users.

Trackball [8], thumb-stick, thumb-pad and gyro-sensors [9], gestures [10], tangible designs [11, 12] and exercise promoting input devices in games [13–15] has also been explored for controlling games.

T. Ahram et al. (Eds.): IHIET 2019, AISC 1018, pp. 378–382, 2020.
https://doi.org/10.1007/978-3-030-25629-6_58

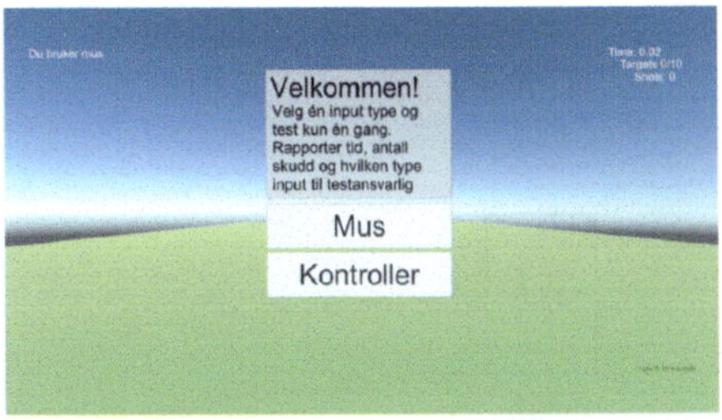

a) Start screen

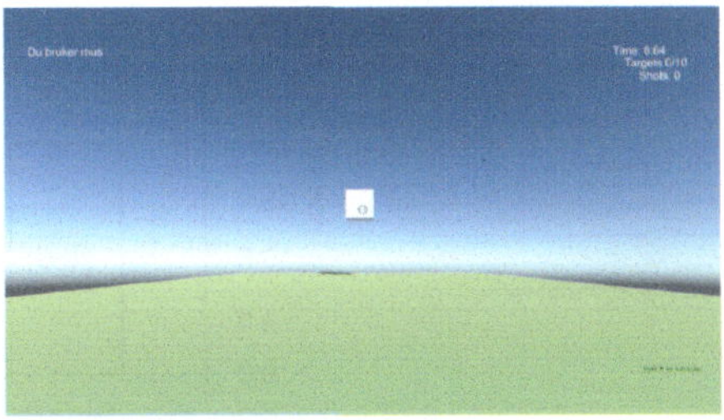

b) Gameplay using mouse

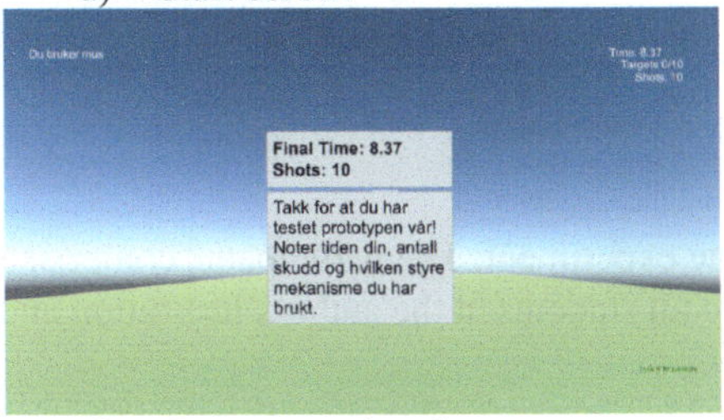

c) Game completed screen

Fig. 1. Screenshots of experiment software.

Our first hypothesis was that the mouse will lead to faster target hitting compared to the joystick, as reported in [7]. The mouse offers a larger movement range compared to the analogue joystick. The mouse allows the user to move the pointer directly towards the target in one continuous motion which can be modelled using Fitts' law [16], while the joystick needs to be held in the desired direction until the aim has reached the target. The second hypothesis is that the mouse also will be associated with a higher success rate than the joystick as one may be more likely to overshoot the target while waiting to for the aim to reach the target.

2 Method

2.1 Experimental Design

A between-subjects design was chosen for this study. The time to complete the task and number of shots fired was used as the two dependent variables and the input device was the independent variable. The between-subjects factor input device had two levels, namely joystick and mouse.

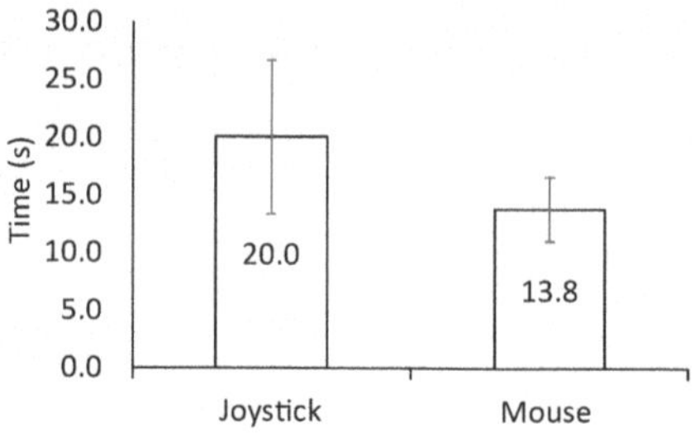

Fig. 2. Task completion times (seconds). Error bars show standard deviation.

2.2 Participants

A total of 22 participants were recruited for the experiment. The participants comprised 18 males and 4 females. The participants were all students at the authors institution and reported to be regular gamers.

2.3 Procedure

A simple first-person shooter was created using the Unity Game Engine (https://unity3d.com/) see Fig. 1. A standard Xbox360 controller was used for the experiments.

The participants were asked to hit 10 targets presented sequentially. The participants were not given any time constraints and could shoot as many times as they liked. The game finished once the participant had successfully hit 10 targets.

The participants were tested individually in a quiet meeting room with two of the authors present. The time from when the participant pressed start to when 10 targets had been successfully hit was measured as well as the total number of shots fired. Each test took less than one minute. Statistical analyses were conducted with JASP version 0.8.6.0.

3 Results

Figures 2 and 3 show the results of the experiment. The mean completion time (in seconds) plotted in Fig. 2 was shorter for mouse ($M = 13.8$, $SD = 2.8$) than for joystick ($M = 20.0$, $SD = 6.6$) and a Welch t-test shows that this difference was significantly different ($t(13.356) = 2.873$, $p = .006$). A Welch test was used since a Levine test showed that the t-test assumptions of equal variances where not satisfied. A Shapiro-Wilk tests confirmed that the measurements were normally distributed.

The success rates plotted in Fig. 3 shows that the mouse is associated with slightly higher success rates ($M = 0.95$, $SD = 0.10$) than the joystick ($M = 0.88$, $SD = 0.17$). However, this difference is not statistically significant ($U = 80.5$, $p = .083$). A Mann-Whitney test was used as a Shapiro-Wilk test revealed that the measurements were not normally distributed.

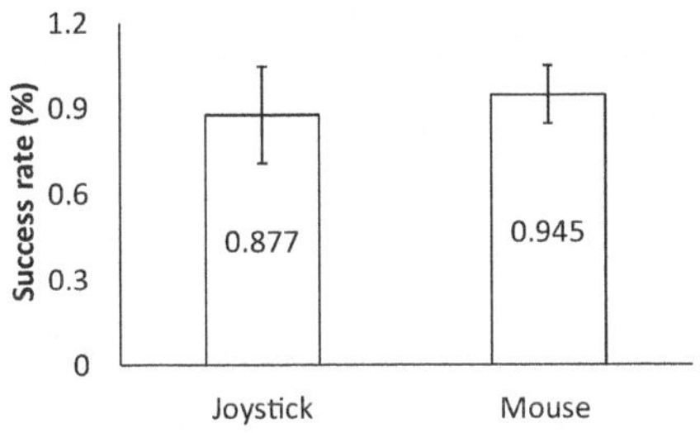

Fig. 3. Success rate. Error bars show standard deviation.

4 Discussion

The results support the first hypothesis that the mouse leads to faster target hitting, and the difference is quite large as the mouse only took 68.8% of the time of the joystick. Clearly, with the mouse the user can hit the target in one continuous motion, while with the joystick the user must hold the joystick in the desired direction until it hits the target. However, the second hypothesis is not supported, namely that the mouse leads to better accuracy. This may not necessarily translate to other game tasks such as steering a car in a driving game as experiments have shown no difference between joysticks and keyboards for such tasks [17].

5 Conclusion

The target hitting performance of regular mouse and a dedicated joystick game controller were compared for a simple first-person shooter. The results show that the mouse leads to faster target hitting taking 68.8% of the time of the joystick. This time difference can be critical in some games and the results are thus in favor of the mouse for games involving first person shooters compared to just joysticks. No differences were found in terms of success rate between the two methods.

References

1. Klochek, C., MacKenzie, I.S: Performance measures of game controllers in a three-dimensional environment. In: Proceedings of Graphics Interface 2006, pp. 73–79. Canadian Information Processing Society, Toronto (2006)
2. Hourcade, J.P., Bederson, B.B., Druin, A., Guimbretière, F.: Differences in pointing task performance between preschool children and adults using mice. ACM Trans. Comput.-Hum. Interact. **11**(4), 357–386 (2004)
3. Ahlström, D., Hitz, M.: Revisiting PointAssist and studying effects of control-display gain on pointing performance by four-year-olds. In: Proceedings of the 12th International Conference on Interaction Design and Children, pp. 257–260. ACM, New York (2013)
4. Sandnes, F.E., Aubert, A.: Bimanual text entry using game controllers: relying on users' spatial familiarity with QWERTY. Interact. Comput. **19**(2), 140–150 (2006)

5. Wobbrock, J.O., Myers, B.A., Aung, H.H., LoPresti, E.F.: Text entry from power wheelchairs: edgewrite for joysticks and touchpads. In: Proceedings of the 6th International ACM SIGACCESS Conference on Computers and Accessibility, pp. 110–117. ACM, New York (2003)
6. Baldauf, M., Fröhlich, P., Adegeye, F., Suette, S.: Investigating on-screen gamepad designs for smartphone-controlled video games. ACM Trans. Multimed. Comput. Commun. Appl. **12**, Article 22 (2015)
7. Natapov, D., Castellucci, S.J., MacKenzie, I.S.: ISO 9241-9 evaluation of video game controllers. In: Proceedings of Graphics Interface, pp. 223–230. Canadian Information Processing Society, Toronto (2009)
8. Natapov, D., MacKenzie, I.S.: The trackball controller: improving the analog stick. In: Proceedings of the International Academic Conference on the Future of Game Design and Technology, pp. 175–182. ACM, New York (2010)
9. Ramcharitar, A., Teather, R.J.: A Fitts' law evaluation of video game controllers: thumbstick, touchpad and gyrosensor. In: Proceedings of the 2017 CHI Conference Extended Abstracts on Human Factors in Computing Systems, pp. 2860–2866. ACM, New York (2017)
10. Geurts, L., Woensel, A.V., Abeele, V.V.: No sweat, no fun: large-gesture recognition for computer games. In: Proceedings of the 4th International Conference on Fun and Games, pp. 109–112. ACM, New York (2012)
11. Nagy, G.M., Young, J.E., Anderson, J.E.: Are tangibles really better?: keyboard and joystick outperform TUIs for remote robotic locomotion control. In: Proceedings of the Tenth Annual ACM/IEEE International Conference on Human-Robot Interaction Extended Abstracts, pp. 41–42. ACM, New York (2015)
12. Kajiyama, H., Inoue, A., Hoshi, T.: SHAPIO: shape I/O controller for video games. In: Proceedings of the 2015 Annual Symposium on Computer-Human Interaction in Play, pp. 565–570. ACM, New York (2015)
13. Park, T., Lee, U., MacKenzie, S., Moon, M., Hwang, I., Song, J.: Human factors of speed-based exergame controllers. In: Proceedings of the SIGCHI Conference on Human Factors in Computing Systems, pp. 1865–1874. ACM, New York (2014)
14. Gerling, K.M., Dergousoff, K.K., Mandryk, R.L.: Is movement better?: comparing sedentary and motion-based game controls for older adults. In: Proceedings of Graphics Interface, pp. 133–140. Canadian Information Processing Society, Toronto (2013)
15. Zhang, D., Cai, Z., Chen, K., Nebel, B.: A game controller based on multiple sensors. In: Proceedings of the International Conference on Advances in Computer Enterntainment Technology, pp. 375–378. ACM, New York (2009)
16. MacKenzie, I.S., Buxton, W.: Extending Fitts' law to two-dimensional tasks. In: Proceedings of the SIGCHI Conference on Human Factors in Computing Systems, pp. 219–226. ACM, New York (1992)
17. Astrup, B.K., Danielsen, V., Grønvold, K.L., Hals, A.W.I., Klophmann, A., Sandnes, F.E.: Car steering in a racing game: game controller is not better than keyboard. Manuscript in Preparation (2018)

Digital Technology as a Significant Support for the Teaching Process

Petr Svoboda([✉])

Masaryk Institute of Advanced Studies, Czech Technical University in Prague, Kolejní 2637/2a 160 00 Praha 6, Prague, Czech Republic
Petr.Svoboda@cvut.cz

Abstract. The aim of the paper is to highlight the importance of digital technologies as a support and complement in education. The reason is that there are currently many questions about what influence and impact to education represents digital technology, and whether its use in teaching is directed towards learning objectives. The paper attempts to define goals and visions for the future, its main advantages and also the barriers to integration into the teaching process are mentioned. It is possible to name the positive and negative aspects of new technologies, overcome contradictions and see the positive and negative impacts on the young generation. It is especially important to show the importance of mutual learning when using digital technologies. It is particularly important to compare the views of teachers and students.

Keywords: Digital technologies · New trends in education · Teacher's digital competences · Education 4.0 · Industry 4.0 · Research

1 Introduction

The young generation is intensively using digital technologies. The dynamic transformation of society is reflected in the demands for changes to the education system, in which teachers must prepare pupils even for professions, that currently do not exist. This fact is also reflected by the European Commission [1], which issued recommendations for member countries on how to define teachers' necessary digital competences. These recommendations are built on previously developed Digital Competence Framework for Citizens (DigComp) and on a definition of a digitally functioning educational organization (DigCompOrg). In the information society, which is based on knowledge economy and where ideas and knowledge become commodities, a tumultuous development of digital technologies, that affect most of human life spheres, takes place. Especially serious impact is reflected in the new possibilities of industry, which is called Industry 4.0. A new generation of digitally literate workers must be trained for the needs of this industry. Very important role is played by teachers who must prove sufficient digital competences. Increasing attention focused on the competences required by the information society leads individual schools and the entire education system to introduce necessary changes within their curriculum. The aim of the current education is to develop digital literacy (digital thinking) and computer science thinking of pupils, to improve their competence to work with digital technologies, and to introduce new

T. Ahram et al. (Eds.): IHIET 2019, AISC 1018, pp. 383–389, 2020.
https://doi.org/10.1007/978-3-030-25629-6_59

learning methods. Teachers' digital competences are thus the key to streamlining the existing processes and tasks of teaching work, as well as a ticket to qualitatively new ways of managing the learning process of pupils and students. The change in the content of education, accompanied by expanding demands on teachers' competences, is reflected by the amount of scientific studies, research plans and scientific literature.

The methodology of the paper is based on an analysis of the current situation in the teaching of vocational subjects at Czech secondary schools and research in this field. The paper is also based on the currently implemented research and development project in support of applied social and humanitarian research, experimental development and innovation of ETA TACR (Technological Agency of the Czech Republic) at Czech Technical University in Prague, Masaryk Institute of Advanced Studies (research grant, project number TL01000192 - Developing digital competences of teachers of social sciences and secondary vocational schools).

2 New Objects Focused on Digital Technologies in Education

Virtualization and gamification have become increasingly popular, with dynamic growth in recent years. This is reflected in the emergence of a range of objects applicable to the education reality. New objects in teaching enable more efficient use of teaching methods and thus more effectively achieve the set goals for example remote laboratories, **virtual laboratories** with applets, e-technology park with remote and virtual laboratories.

Access to these remote laboratories is now via a web browser. Virtual laboratories with applets, simulations, and models are emerging technologies in the natural sciences. We can compare real data with virtual or vice versa virtual to import into real-time measuring software. **E-technology park** with remote and virtual laboratories – Internet access is provided not only to finished laboratory tasks (including text and methodology), but also allows free access to the technological basis of their own remote tasks. We are facing the task of creating our own laboratory role (text, tasks, methodology) for this engagement [2].

There are currently being used **virtual class** (classroom) – it is an interactive web tool; including software to the mediation of communication, cooperation, and exchange of experience, meetings without necessity personal presence of participants through a computer connected to the Internet, tablet or PC headphones, so-called on-line access. We can use e-textbooks, educational videos, 3D virtual objects, an interactive encyclopedia, hypermedia.

Nowadays **virtual and augmented reality** (education in 3D virtual reality) expands. The possibilities of using 3D virtual reality and 3D multi-user virtual environments provide students and teachers with a sense of social community and virtual social relationships. It was created by the convergence of 3D virtual simulations, online computer games, and social networks. It allows you to create social interactions between users through virtual avatars that meet in the environment and can communicate in a manner very similar to real-world communication (including non-verbal means). Here we can mention game-oriented gameplay and story-based, role-playing. It uses methods of experiential learning and simulation learning. It uses the principles of connectivity and constructivism - requiring active collaboration of people in manipulating 3D virtual objects (working in groups), using virtual simulations of real professions (experimental learning, simulator). A lot of researches suggest that in the recent years there has been a growing interest in introducing AR, mixed reality and 3D models into teaching. They pointed out to the effectiveness of augmented reality in education. It was the most widely applied in elementary schools and led to the improvement of learning outcomes. 95% of pupils approach the augmented reality positively, better remember, learn and understand the new substance [3].

Personal assistants expand as well. Personal assistant (Virtual Assistant, ChatBot, Digital Assistant, using **artificial intelligence**). Smart application generating automatic answers that can communicate with the user completely autonomously. Chatbot has a database of predefined responses to respond to users, plus learning how artificial intelligence helps. Chatbots are useful in education, for example, when enrolling and registering for educational events, when collecting input questionnaires. Communication can help draw students into online education, especially MOOC courses, where it is difficult for a large number of participants to get a teacher's answer. Some questions are asked again and again.

Current trends in teaching emphasize the development of computer science thinking. The first steps are most often realized through specialized miniature robots. It is an interactive toy that develops creativity and logical thinking. It is a didactic tool that represents the path to true **programming and robotics**. In the classroom, students draw different paths that robots (Ozobot, mBot) tracks and adds first commands and monitors his behavior.

These new objects in teaching enable more effective use of teaching methods and thus achieve the set goals more effectively. Students are not only dependent on the perception of transmitted knowledge but are offered the opportunity to manipulate objects or imitations and display them using virtual environments. The most effective use is in multimedia classrooms. Bloom's digital taxonomy can help. Bloom's digital taxonomy (remember, understand, apply, analyze, evaluate, create) was devised by Andrew Churches in connection with the preparation of pupils for life in the 21st century.

3 Digital Competences and Trends in Education Using Digital Technologies

Digital competences of educators are based on the European Digital Competence Framework of Educators, which is divided into five core areas: information literacy, data literacy, communication and collaboration, digital content creation, security and problem solving. It is necessary to create curriculums for teachers to build and develop the digital competences so that they can prepare pupils for life in the 21st century, the world of digital technology, which is a natural micro-environment for emerging generations that use it naturally for own entertainment and communication. These means of digital technologies also fundamentally interfere in the field of forming and personal (self) development, i.e. generally in education and (self) education. While respecting the fundamental links between the digital competences of the European framework, we assume that the curriculum is modular in three levels of competence, including a defined standard that ensures an adequate quality of the educational process [1, 8]. The individual modules relate to the selected topics: professional competences of teachers, pedagogical competences of teachers and support of pupils' (students') digital competences.

Being a digitally competent teacher also means tracking current trends in education with a focus on digital technologies and being able to use the learning potential of these technologies. Virtual reality, augmented virtual reality, 3D multi-user virtual environments, robotization, gamification, artificial intelligence, and the internet of things enter the forefront. Self-education and personal development of teachers – existing communication programs, on-line courses, blogs, professional community of teachers, webinars, MOOC courses and their combinations allow teachers to take a variety of forms personal and professional growth, collaboration through professional communities (creating Personal Learning Environment - PLE).

Current trends in education in the coming years will focus on blended learning, flipped classroom, m-learning, adaptive learning technologies, learning analytics, the Internet of Things, the new generation of LMS, re-designing learning spaces, learning to support innovation culture, the development of in-depth learning, artificial intelligence, natural interface [3–5]. Let us focus on selected trends in education and their benefits now.

Blended Learning - the advantage is adapting teaching to educational needs, engaging more senses, multimedia, encouraging flexibility and individualization of education, encouraging students to think and self-study.

Flipped Classroom - the advantage is that students can prepare for the lesson in advance (for example, to watch a video tutorial, animations or a new substance) and then to apply key concepts with feedback (the student has questions and performs active tasks). Subsequently, students check their understanding and extend their learning.

M-Learning - the advantage of using mobile technologies in education is the ability to learn anywhere and anytime. The equipment is always available. 70% of users are motivated to learn via mobile devices. This is because learning is faster by 45% than by PC [5], but courses and tutorials need to be adapted to mobile technologies. Another advantage of m-learning is the combination of **gamification** and **microlearning** (i.e., any short-term training for 5–10 min, such as a 4 min repetition). M-learning also combines extended virtual reality such as learn languages in augmented reality. We can use adaptive learning technology, virtual tutor and ChatBot to learn. We must not perceive mobile devices as a substitute for education, but only as an add-on or support. The purpose of "mobile learning" is not to replace classroom instruction, classroom lectures or classical computers, but to increase its efficiency [6].

Another trend is to share materials in the cloud, work in the cloud and video conversation. **Cloud solutions** offer a whole range of new sharing and collaboration options. Sharing of documents and media content, storing and sharing of individual versions in the work phase, data synchronization, virtual space, web conferences, lectures and training [7]. These tools enable online learning. Students or teachers work together in groups or peer-to-peer activities, thus developing social constructivism, international collaboration, collaborative learning, student-centered learning, highlighting interactions, working in groups, and solving real problems. It is precisely the emphasis on greater interconnection of people (so-called shared learning) that is an important trend in on-line education and informal education. Cloud services are also used in education to improve teamwork among students and educators, the school head and other staff. Research surveys have proven in practice that the use of cloud services in education is clearly more effective than traditional practices [3, 7].

Learning Analytics – tools for analyzing learning outcomes and learning failures. Research in seven European countries shows the results of student assessment of teaching. What competences and evaluations they acquired at the end of their studies [8, 9]. The trend will be the transition from summative to formative [10]. Education 4.0 will change society and create new professions. Wearable devices are also related to the trend of learning analytics: biometric sensors measuring emotions, stress, pressure, facial expressions, voice. These sensors are in smart watches, bracelets, smart glasses, cars or pens. Joining the **IoT (Internet of Things)** will measure all classroom learning not only online (trend around 2025). Experts estimate that the Internet of Things will include some 30 billion devices in 2020. Such smart devices communicate with each other via the Internet, Bluetooth, RFID, NFC, but also with QR code, barcodes or digital watermarks. Smart devices use these channels to send data to each other to interact with each other. Smart homes, smart schools, smart cities and smart regions will be created. Obviously, IoT is expanding into both our homes and our cities and will affect each of us. Therefore, attention needs to be paid in this area and in our schools to include the IoT in teaching. The development of empathic thinking will also be very important according to the report of the Economic Forum [11]. There is talk of changing LMS from a curriculum management tool to support adaptive learning and the use of special data analysis and visualization tools for improved student design and student progress recording [11].

Redesign of Educational Spaces and Libraries. Spaces that support flexibility (customization and modification). Necessary to customize for project-based learning and the ability to use multiple devices simultaneously (e.g. cameras, tablets, touch screens, interactive displays, multiboards, 3D glasses) [12]. Can be connected with clouds and touch walls and cameras, use 3D printers, scenery, moving furniture (hybrid classes and laboratories such as laser cutting, CNC machining, metalworking). The learning space can be a classroom and after a lab. Different classrooms may have the same interpretation. Classic classroom layout is no longer enough. Libraries will become coworking centers with the ability to build robots, electrical circuits, use gaming consoles.

In-depth Learning - learning based on experience and authentic fact-based learning. Use of internet encyclopedia, blogs, involvement in project work by students from all over the world (learning by doing).

4 Barriers in Using Digital Technologies

On the one hand, digital technologies can effectively help and support educational process can, on the contrary, be complicated, unclear and for someone even a useless and dangerous area in the form of barriers. Barriers in the use of new technologies in education are associated with dynamic developments in the world of technology, some of which are out of date and replaced more recent, often incompatible. Among the weaknesses are according to professional publications, different forms of addiction, the occurrence of negative socialization effects, digital dementia, growth of child aggression and new forms of social pathology such as cyberbullying. Technologies from the point of view both of pedagogues and experts should be perceived as a tool, that can find a suitable fulfilment in some spheres of teaching and on the contrary in others it could be less efficient than classical methods and sometimes it could be even counterproductive [12].

5 Conclusion

The acquired knowledge of technologies may be reflected in the international curriculum in the reforms of school education systems, especially of models of approaches to the acquisition and further development of teachers' digital competences. The changes in society caused by the development of science and technology act as accompanying signs of the transition to the information society. At the same time, it should be borne in mind that the development of teachers' digital competences must be accompanied by the development of non-digital competences and, especially, by their transfer to pupils and students. Besides the work with information and communication technologies, it is necessary to develop a whole complex of skills for the work with information resources.

Innovative methods and forms of teaching are important means that put emphasis on the use of information and communication technologies and elements of practice learning. Actually, we should rather speak about a society of intensive knowledge processes instead of a knowledge society. Indeed, everything that can be observed is a huge and unprecedented dynamic of processes connected with the knowledge. Permanent innovation becomes a necessary condition for the survival of a firm on the market, the lifelong learning is an unavoidable prerequisite of employment, the continual recombination of a huge quantity of findings produces new and new knowledge. It all corresponds to Education 4.0.

References

1. The European Commission's science and knowledge service. https://ec.europa.eu/jrc/en
2. Lustig, F.: Problematika Vzdálených a Virtuálních Laboratoří. https://www.pf.ujep.cz/cs/
3. New Media Consortium, Horizon Report. https://www.nmc.org/nmc-horizon/
4. Open University Inovation Report. http://www.open.ac.uk/
5. Gartner. https://www.gartner.com/en
6. Lynda. https://www.lynda.com/
7. Svoboda, P.: M-learning - use of mobile technologies in teaching. http://journals.vstecb.cz
8. Svoboda, P.: Assumptions and reasons for the use of digital technologies in education. Studia Pedagogiczne **50**(1), 195–206 (2017). Polska Academia Nauk, Poland
9. Eurashe. https://www.eurashe.eu/

10. EUA. https://eua.eu/
11. The world Economic Forum. https://www.weforum.org/
12. Svoboda, P.: Innovative didactic tools in education. In: Proceedings of the 10th International Conference on Education, Training and Informatics, ICETI 2019. International Institute of Informatics and Systemic, Orlando (2019)

The Interplay of Artificial and Human Intelligence in Radiology – Exploring Socio-Technical System Dynamics

Uta Wilkens[1(✉)] and Marc Dewey[2]

[1] Institute of Work Science, Chair for Work, Human Resources and Leadership, Ruhr-University Bochum, Universitätstr. 150, 44801 Bochum, Germany
uta.wilkens@rub.de

[2] Institute of Radiology, Charité – Universitätsmedizin Berlin, Charitépl. 1, 10117 Berlin, Germany
marc.dewey@charite.de

Abstract. Workplaces with increasing interaction between individual and artificial intelligence (AI) have to face socio-technical system dynamics resulting from the interplay between technology and human behavior. The paper specifies the key characteristics and moderating factors for these dynamics for the use case of radiology. Radiology gives a good example because of its central role in the initiation of integrated clinical care processes. The structurational model of technology with its recent outlines on the materiality of technology serves as theoretical framework. It specifies the system dynamics between technology, human agents and institutional properties. Closing remarks are related to implementation challenges aiming at better understanding drivers and inhibitors in socio-technical system change.

Keywords: Artificial intelligence · Socio-technical system · Technology enactment · Social acceptance of technology · Radiology

1 Introduction

More than 3.6 billion radiological imaging procedures are performed worldwide every year [1]. This data has mostly been neglected for the digital transformation of health care yet could bring in fundamental change in diagnostic processes for patients. It becomes obvious that artificial intelligence (AI) can play an increasingly important role in healthcare, especially in radiology where the further use of AI tools has a considerably high implementation potential [2, 3].

Value-based radiology aims at better outcomes at lower costs through higher proficiency and better integration of diagnostic imaging in clinical care processes which avoid ambiguity and vagueness in diagnosis and related overuse of services [4]. The focus relies on digital solutions in terms of validated clinical prediction rules for individual disease probabilities [5], artificially augmented human image analysis [6],

M. Dewey—Heisenberg Professor of Radiology at the German Research Foundation.

T. Ahram et al. (Eds.): IHIET 2019, AISC 1018, pp. 390–395, 2020.
https://doi.org/10.1007/978-3-030-25629-6_60

and structured radiology reports [7]. It is proposed that an intensified use of AI tools may lead to better decision making about which radiological testing, if any, should be done; the quantification of disease on diagnostic imaging; and the integration of radiology findings into subsequent clinical care pathways [2]. In order to take advantage from this potential it is important to understand and cope with the socio-technical system dynamics as this is crucial for the successful implementation. The further outline first gives emphasis to the characteristics and potential of AI in radiology by explaining the concept of the *Bionic Radiologist.* Building on these explanations the succeeding paragraph faces implementation challenges and frames the use case as socio-technical system with distributed intelligence. The structurational model of technology serves as theoretical basis. The contribution ends up with an agenda for coping with implementation challenges.

2 The Future of Radiology: The Bionic Radiologist

The *Bionic Radiologist* is an integrative concept of humanity and digitalization and follows three objectives for adding value to clinical care: (1) more consistent decisions about diagnostic test choices in individual patients based on disease probabilities; (2) augmented human radiologist image analysis enhanced using digital automated image analyses; and (3) integrating imaging information with other medical data for a close linkage with therapy recommendations [2].

There are relevant barriers to the implementation of the *Bionic Radiologist*: radiologists' being reluctant to jointly interpret radiology images with 'machines', resulting possible reduction in satisfaction at work, lowering of image reading knowledge of future radiologists, and perceived increase in patients being at risk when human involvement is reduced.

We suggest that the implementation of the *Bionic Radiologist* will be facilitated using: (1) visualization tools for the interpretation of automated decisions, (2) radiologists' involvement in shared decision making with patients and maintenance of expertise with automatic feedback loops, and (3) and evolvement of the role of radiologists towards moderators of clinical care processes.

This implies a transformation of the work system with a shift from individual expertise to artificial expertise augmenting or possibly even replacing human decision making for certain tasks [3]. It becomes obvious that AI in healthcare challenges socio-technical system design and leads to socio-technical system dynamics. The next paragraph aims at a deeper understand.

3 Understanding Distributed Intelligence and Socio-Technical System Dynamics in Radiology

Emerging work systems as exemplified for radiology can be characterized in terms of distributed intelligence between the individual actor and the AI technology [8, 9]. The development is challenging with respect to tool development but also with respect to individual skills and role definition [10]. Different scenarios co-exist and there is potential that a symbiotic interplay of artificial and individual intelligence leads to a win-win constellation with high social acceptance for new technologies in the workplace [11]. However, counterproductive work behavior cannot be excluded as long as the definition of the individual expert role is not clear and social acceptance might suffer. It becomes obvious that technology acceptance is not a pure function of perceived usefulness of a technology and its ease of use as originally described in the technology acceptance model [12] but that there is a need to reflect on individual behavior and attitudes [13, 14]. In this regard the consideration of perceived justice [15] has already been outlined for healthcare.

In order to better understand socio-technical systems dynamics and especially the interplay between individual and artificial intelligence the Structurational Model of Technology [16] can be considered as helpful. This is especially the case when combining the original concept with considerations on the materiality of technology [17, 18] in the course of analysis. The model allows exploring the dualistic and dialectic development between AI tools, individual behavior and institutional properties in order to find out how technology is enacted in a specific context of implementation.

Radiology serves as a good example for deeper analysis because of its central role in the initiation of integrated clinical care processes [19, 20]. Referring the Structurational Model of Technology to the use case of radiology the following components are in the center of analysis.

(1) There is a social construction of the technology in use which means that it is not just treated as a proficient tool but enacted in a manner that there are trade-offs in how to really make use of the tool according to individual needs, attitudes and skills in how to work with the tool [16]. The efficiency of tool implementation also depends on organizational properties, e.g. whether there is interoperability of the systems in terms of shared standards on conceptual, organizational and technological level [21]. The interoperability moderates both, the social acceptance of AI technology and the performance conditions for the use of the technology with respect to work standards. Facing the characteristics of the technology itself it makes a difference whether the software is adaptive and based on self-learning mechanisms that work without further support from individual intelligence or adaptable in the meaning that the individual can redirect machine action [22]. The latter means that the AI remains under individual control and that the role definition in terms of 'machines serve the individuals' and not the other way round is an accepted principle in the work system.

(2) Referring to the individual characteristics the way of coping with and enacting a technology depends on individual skills and competencies in terms of digital competencies and system regulation, e.g. coping with a certain level of complexity [23, 24]. Moreover, the social acceptance can depend on perceived justice and other categories of organizational behavior [10, 15] which make the difference when considering productive or counterproductive work behavior. Moreover, in addition to the individuals who make use of new technologies there is a second group of agents, the experts who develop and create AI tools. In most cases they are outside the work system and it is even not clear whether there are feedback-

loops from the users to the developers of AI tools beyond machine-based records of actions. If socio-technical system development aims at a higher level of system learning [25] in a mutual development between the individual and the technological learning process the overall feedback system needs to be reflected.

(3) The measurement of outcomes needs to address different levels as well. The direct outcome of the technical system can be explored by the appropriateness, completeness, and timeliness of radiology imaging procedures for different levels of integration [26]. This shows the overall potential for further proficiency. A second measurement could give emphasis to the design trade-offs made in order to make a technology adaptable in a specific work system [27].

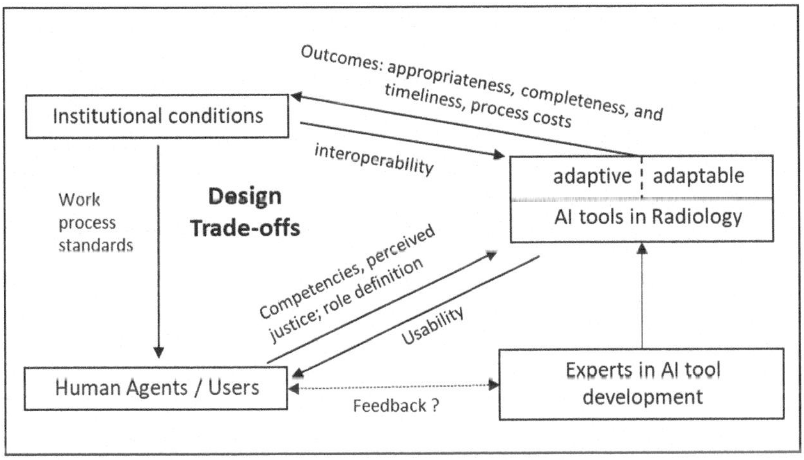

Fig. 1. Adapted structurational model of technology for radiology

Figure 1 gives a brief summary of the described characteristics explaining socio-technical systems dynamics and underlining the interplay between individual and artificial intelligence.

4 Outlook: Coping with Implementation Challenges

In order to face the implementation challenges in a sufficient manner there is a need for empirical based process analysis in order to better understand drivers and inhibitors on the pathway to better integrated clinical care.

It also becomes obvious that facing the digital tool is a too narrow view for a beneficial development in the field of AI. The interplay with the individual actors and the feedback-loops need high attention in implementation processes.

Moreover, institutional properties for moderating between the technology in use and the individual actors should also be considered as crucial for technology acceptance.

Finally, understanding which design trade-offs come out from the implementation process is of high value for other fields aiming at making higher use of AI tools in the workplace. Design trade-offs entail information about how to create technology from the actors' perspective.

References

1. UNSCEAR 2008 Report: Sources and effects of ionizing radiation, Volume I. http://www.unscear.org/unscear/en/publications/2008_1.html
2. Dewey, M.: The future of radiology: adding value to clinical care. Lancet **392**(10146), 472–473 (2018)
3. Forsting, M.: Artificial intelligence with radiology as a trailblazer for super-diagnostics: an essay. RöFo **191**(1), 73–78 (2019)
4. Boland, G.W., Duszak Jr., R., McGinty, G., Allen Jr., B.: Delivery of appropriateness, quality, safety, efficiency and patient satisfaction. J. Am. Coll. Radiol. **11**(1), 7–11 (2014)
5. Genders, T.S., Steyerberg, E.W., Hunink, M.G., Nieman, K., Galema, T.W., Mollet, N.R., Laule, M.: Prediction model to estimate presence of coronary artery disease: retrospective pooled analysis of existing cohorts. BMJ **344**, e3485 (2012)
6. Brink, J.A., Arenson, R.L., Grist, T.M., Lewin, J.S., Enzmann, D.: Bits and bytes: the future of radiology lies in informatics and information technology. Eur. Radiol. **27**(9), 3647–3651 (2017)
7. Pinto Dos Santos, D., Scheibl, S., Arnhold, G., Maehringer-Kunz, A., Duber, C., Mildenberger, P., Kloeckner, R.: A proof of concept for epidemiological research using structured reporting with pulmonary embolism as a use case. Br. J. Radiol. **091** (2018)
8. Cobb, P.: Learning from distributed theories of intelligence. MCA **5**(3), 187–204 (1998)
9. Fischer, G.: Communities of interest: learning through the interaction of multiple knowledge systems. In: IRIS'24, Ulvik, Norway, pp. 1–14. Department of Information Science, Bergen (2001)
10. Wilkens, U., Artinger, F.: Design components of clinical work environments with computerized decision support systems. In: Karwowski, W., Ahram, T. (eds.) Intelligent Systems Integration 2019. IHSI Conference Proceedings, pp. 137–141. Springer, Wiesbaden (2019)
11. Wilkens, U.: Distributed intelligence in the workplace – a matter of hr policy. Full paper Accepted for International Interdisciplinary Conference on HRM, Gothenburg, April 2019
12. Davis, F.D.: User acceptance of information technology: system characteristics, user perceptions and behavioral impacts. Int. J. Man. Mach. **38**(3), 475–487 (1993)
13. Venkatesh, V., Davis, F.D.: A theoretical extension of the technology acceptance model: four longitudinal field studies. Manag. Sci. **46**(2), 186–204 (2000)
14. Marangunić, N., Granić, A.: Technology acceptance model: a literature review from 1986 to 2013. UAIS **14**(1), 81–95 (2015)
15. Karsh, B.T.: Beyond usability: designing effective technology implementation systems to promote patient safety. Qual. Saf. Health Care **13**(5), 388–394 (2004)
16. Orlikowski, W.J.: The duality of technology: rethinking the concepts of technology in organizations. Organ. Sci. **3**(3), 398–427 (1992)
17. Leonardi, P.M., Barley, S.R.: What's under construction here? Social action, materiality, and power in constructivist studies of technology and organizing. Acad. Manag. Ann. **4**(1), 1–51 (2010)

18. Orlikowski, W.J.: Managing and designing: attending to reflexiveness and enactment. In: Boland Jr., R.J., Collopy, F. (eds.) Managing as Designing, pp. 90–95. Stanford University Press, Stanford (2004)
19. Maskell, G.: The practice of radiology needs to change. BMJ **358**, j4102 (2017)
20. Rimmer, A.: Five minutes with … Nicola Strickland. BMJ **359**, j4675 (2017)
21. Chen, D., Vallespir, B., Daclin, M.: An approach for enterprise interoperability measurement. MoDISE-EUS **341**, 1–12 (2008)
22. Fischer, G.: Shared knowledge in cooperative problem-solving systems – integrating adaptive and adaptable components. In: Schneider-Hufschmidt, M., Kuehme, T., Malinowski, U. (eds.) Adaptive User Interfaces – Principles and Practice, pp. 49–68. Elsevier Science Publishers, Amsterdam (1993)
23. Wilkens, U., Sprafke, N.: Micro-variables of dynamic capabilities and how they come into effect – exploring firm-specificity and cross-firm commonalities. Management International Accepted (2019)
24. Süße, T., Wilkens, U., Hohagen, S., Artinger, F.M.: Digital competence of stakeholders in product-service systems (PSS): conceptualization and empirical exploration. Procedia CIRP **73**, 197–202 (2018)
25. Argyris, C.: A life full of learning. Organ. Stud. **24**(7), 1178–1192 (2003)
26. Ethics approval EA1/297/16 Charité - Universitätsmedizin Berlin
27. Fischer, G.: Identifying and exploring design trade-offs in human-centered design. In: Proceedings of the Conference on AVI, Article no. 22 (2018)

Making Mobile Map Applications Accessible for Visually Impaired People

Alireza Darvishy(✉), Hans-Peter Hutter, and Jasmin Frei

InIT Institute of Applied Information Technology, ZHAW Zurich University of Applied Sciences, Technikumstr. 9, P.O. Box, 8401, Winterthur, Switzerland
{alireza.darvishy,hans-peter.hutter}@zhaw.ch, freijasl@students.zhaw.ch

Abstract. Mobile map applications have become a ubiquitous and important tool for navigation and exploration. However, existing map applications are heavily based on visual information, and are targeted towards persons with normal vision. Users with visual impairments face significant barriers when using these apps – currently, no major map app offers an accessible, intuitive or understandable presentation of map data in a non-visual format. The goal of this ongoing research project is to explore how mobile map application data can be displayed in an accessible and understandable way for visually impaired persons. As a first step, existing solutions were researched, identified and analysed. It was found that information retention is highest when a combination of different output modalities is used. Three major non-visual modalities were identified: Voice output (speech synthesis), ambient sounds (e.g. running water, birdsong, etc.), and vibration patterns. An initial prototype was created which combines all of these modalities, and first user tests were performed. Based on the test results, new iterations of the app are being developed. These will be tested and improved, after which a proof of concept will be developed, and ultimately a functioning app will be created and tested by target users.

Keywords: Visual impairment · Accessible maps · Accessibility · Output modalities

1 Introduction

According to a study by the Swiss Central Association for the Blind (SZB) in 2012, there are about 325,000 visually impaired persons in Switzerland [1]. Persons with visual impairments encounter many major obstacles, one of which is the difficulty in navigating and exploring unknown areas independently. In order to explore an unknown area, they can not easily resort to maps, since the target group of commercially available maps are people with normal vision.

One solution is tactile maps, which are maps on which the information can be felt with the fingers. These are made using a special paper printing process which causes printed areas to swell upwards. However, these maps have significant disadvantages: They are expensive to produce, take up a lot of space, and generally present very little information on one page, since small details would be too difficult to distinguish by touch.

T. Ahram et al. (Eds.): IHIET 2019, AISC 1018, pp. 396–400, 2020.
https://doi.org/10.1007/978-3-030-25629-6_61

In recent decades, the presentation of geographical information has moved away from printed formats in favour of more convenient digital formats. Mobile map applications have become a ubiquitous and important tool for navigation and exploration. They have the advantage of being size-adjustable, meaning that the user can decide on the scope and level of detail they wish to be shown.

However, existing map applications are still heavily based on visual information, and, like most printed maps, are targeted towards persons with normal vision. Users with visual impairments face significant barriers when using these apps – currently, no major map app offers an accessible, intuitive or understandable presentation of map data in a non-visual format. This makes it essentially impossible for persons with visual impairments to quickly get a sense of a given environment, something which is particularly important before travelling to a new or unknown destination.

The goal of this research project is to explore how mobile map application data can be displayed in an accessible and understandable way for visually impaired persons in such a manner that it offers a quick and intuitive overview of a location and its surroundings.

1.1 Existing Research

In 2011, Zeng et al. [2] examined existing mapping systems for visually impaired persons. In their investigations, they distinguished between desktop and mobile solutions. Desktop solutions were defined as those used in a fixed location, whereas mobile solutions are GPS-based and are mainly used on smartphones. The authors concluded that, at the time the paper was published, there were still few mobile applications suitable for persons with visual impairments, but that many different solutions were expected for the future. They note that the possibilities of audio output offer great potential, but also a combination of mobile application and braille output is conceivable, as this distracts the user less from the everyday sounds around him.

In a study by Poppinga et al. in 2011 [3], it was examined whether a digital map using speech and vibration provides better accessibility than standard digital maps. The test subjects were instructed to use their finger to detect a network of streets and then attempt drawing them on paper. The result showed that it is generally possible to provide a visually impaired person with an overview of a map using this output method. These findings are very promising and serve as a basis for this work. Given that smartphone technology has improved continuously since 2011, it is expected that even better results can be achieved today.

2 Methods

A smartphone-based prototype app was created, offering the user simplified maps of fictional places. To explore the area, the user must move their finger across the screen. The map elements are presented as rectangles for maximum clarity and simplicity. In future prototypes, the concept will be expanded so that more complex shapes can be represented.

The initial prototype presents a sample scenario: the user has been invited to a birthday party in a forest cabin (Fig. 1). The user's task is to use the app to get an overview of the location and its surroundings. In the app, the cabin appears in the center of the screen; near it and around it are a forest, a lake, and one road. Using their finger to explore on the map, the user encounters different vibration patterns, sounds, and/or speech synthesis for each of these different elements.

Four different output methods were used for the first prototype (Table 1). These were chosen to enable all important information to be displayed as clearly as possible. In the case of forests and waters, names and exact boundaries are not of primary significance – it is more important that the user knows where a forest or body of water are located relative to other elements. Therefore, only audio clips were used as output, without additional vibration or voice output. This allows users to explore the area without being distracted by less relevant information. It is conceivable that the name of the water body or the forest could be output via an additional user action. For streets, the name and direction are of highest importance. As such, when touching the street, the device starts to vibrate and the name of the street is output once by voice. Vibrations emitted through continuous finger contact with the screen offers users a sense of the street's path. The street name is reissued every time the street is touched again, allowing different streets to be more easily distinguished.

The forest cabin is in the center of the map. If it is touched, the cabin name is heard in an endless loop. This form of output may not be an option for real maps, as few buildings have a name.

Table 1 serves as a legend to Fig. 1. It also describes which output modalities were used for the corresponding elements when the user touches them with their finger.

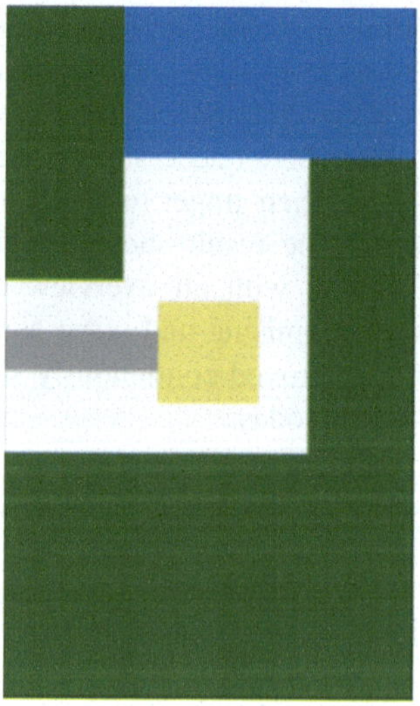

Fig. 1. Visual representation of the map for the sample scenario, as implemented in the initial prototype interface.

Table 1. Overview of the map elements in the initial prototype.

Colour	Element type	Output
Green	Forest	Plays audio recording of birdsong
Blue	Body of water	Plays audio recording of water splashing
Grey	Street	1x speech output of street name, plus continuous vibration
Yellow	Building	Continuous speech output of building name

This initial prototype was first tested with a group of people who have normal vision. In order to be able to test the prototype with sighted persons, the map elements were hidden so that only a white screen could be seen. This ensured that the subjects could not see the map elements.

Since this was a first attempt, the user survey was conducted without any measurable or comparable criteria. It was based on the question of what the subjects were able to perceive and how they rated the experience.

3 Results

The subjects were able to recognize and distinguish all elements while operating the app. They were able to find their way around, and in a follow-up conversation they were able to remember which elements could be found on the map.

There was initially some difficulty in deciding whether the water was a lake or a river. However, most of the subjects were able to determine that it was a lake upon further exploration of the map, based on the shape of the water. They also expressed the desire to be able to learn the name of the lake through a user action.

The repetitive speech output for the cabin turned out to be less than optimal. Although it was possible to identify where the cabin was located, it was difficult to determine its outline or boundaries. In addition, difficulties arose in finding the way leading to and from the cabin.

For the subjects, it quickly became clear that the vibrating line was supposed to be a road. This realization was supported by the spoken street name every time the line touched. Because the finger repeatedly left and returned to the defined area of the road during touch exploration, this repeatedly led to the app speaking out the street name.

The subsequent discussions with the test subjects showed that the persistent vibration for the road was perceived as too strong and disturbing. A lighter vibration pattern with accompanying sound reproduction would help determine the type of road. In addition, it would be sufficient if the street name were only issued by an additional user action, since the name of a street may not be relevant in every case.

4 Discussion and Future Work

The first prototype has shown that it is possible to explore a simple map just by outputting vibration, sounds and speech. In future iterations, the selected output options for the lake and forest will be maintained. For the output of the street, a concept with a combination of vibration pattern and audio output will be explored. It will also be important to examine the possibilities of additional user actions with the map which could offer more detailed information on certain elements when desired, such as the names of bodies of water.

Based on the experience gained with the initial prototype, the next one is currently being implemented with improvements and a new scenario. In addition to the prototypes, isolated analyses of individual details will be carried out, and the collected findings will be summarized. Finally, a concept will be developed for how to present map data in a mobile app, and a proof of concept will be implemented and usability tested with selected users. Based on the test results a map application will be developed and will then be field tested with a larger group of target users.

References

1. Sehbehinderung und Blindheit: Entwicklung in der Schweiz: Unpublished study by the Swiss Association for the Blind (SBZ) (2013)
2. Zeng, L., Weber, G.: Accessible maps for the visually impaired. In: Proceedings of IFIP INTERACT 2011, Workshop on ADDW, pp. 54–60 (2011)
3. Poppinga, B., Pielot, M., Magnusson, C., Rassmus-Gröhn, K.: TouchOver map: audio-tactile exploration of interactive maps. In: MobileHCI 2011, pp. 545–550 (2011)

Towards a Toolbox for the Development of Intercultural User Interfaces

Rüdiger Heimgärtner(✉)

Intercultural User Interface Consulting (IUIC), R&D HMI,
Lindenstraße 9, 93152 Undorf, Germany
ruediger.heimgaertner@iuic.de

Abstract. In this paper, a method-mix (cultural dimensions, intercultural variables, user interface characteristics and human machine interaction (HMI) dimensions) for intercultural user interface design (IUID) is explained and discussed based on application examples. These examples elucidate why and how cultural aspects play a role in HMI design and usability/UX engineering. Implications for the consideration of variables such as speed and frequency of information/interaction for dialogue design in the cultural context are also added. The readers are sensitized to the challenges of intercultural usability/UX engineering and intercultural HMI design and will be equipped with methodological knowledge relevant to the derivation of design recommendations for user interface design for and in their desired cultural contexts.

Keywords: Culture · Human factors · UX · Usability engineering · Intercultural user interface design · Toolbox · HMI dimensions

1 Introduction

Intercultural user interface design (IUID) is a prerequisite for improving the intercultural usability of software, which in turn is a prerequisite for global sales opportunities. Using methods of intercultural usability engineering, further design guidelines can be iteratively derived from the results of the tests and the feedback of potential users from all over the world for intercultural user interface design. Hence, the perception and consideration of the customs and requirements of other cultures by the developers of intercultural user interfaces is one of the main tasks within intercultural user interface design. Based on feedback from tutorials and workshops on IUID (M&C, Interact, IHCI, SouthCHI, ICCHP, HCII) and the revised summary of the state of research on IUID in [1], the author reviewed the synopsis of well documented IUID methods in academic literature to construct a toolbox for IUID. This method-mix approach as an initial toolbox for the development of intercultural user interfaces will be presented, explained and exemplified using an application example.

T. Ahram et al. (Eds.): IHIET 2019, AISC 1018, pp. 401–406, 2020.
https://doi.org/10.1007/978-3-030-25629-6_62

2 Related Work

Differences between cultures can be found by analyzing critical interaction situations between people [2]. [3] made this method available for cultural differences in Human-Machine Interaction (HMI). Critical interaction situations that arise due to problematic user interfaces or are based on the given system functionality have been analyzed. The internal model of the user about the system is shaped by the culture of the user, his expectations about the characteristics of the system and his interaction experience with the system. [4] found that e.g. Hofstedes "Individualism Index" (cf. [5]) is related to user satisfaction and usability of the product and has a significant influence on intercultural usability. [6] proposed the "Method for Culture-Oriented Design" (MCD), which integrates the factors of new concepts of culture-oriented HMI design and the knowledge of cultural differences into existing concepts of HMI design. Relevant cultural variables for intercultural HMI design must be determined analytically based on literature and requirement studies. Their values represent culture-dependent variations that occur at all levels of HMI localization (interface, functionality and interaction) and can be used for intercultural user interface design (IUID). Similarly, [7] focus on culture-oriented design. Further methods are applying the user interface characteristics by [8] or the cultural markers by [9]. Other approaches, e.g. by [10] or [11], are based on semiotic theory. One of the most promising methods to preserve cultural differences in HMI is the observation and analysis of user interaction with the system (cf. [12]). The results of these observations in the form of cultural variables and their manifestations serve as a basis for guidelines in intercultural HMI design and for intercultural usability engineering (e.g. cultural interaction indicators, cf. [12]) and a model (cf. [13], cf. also Fig. 1 in this paper in Sect. 3).

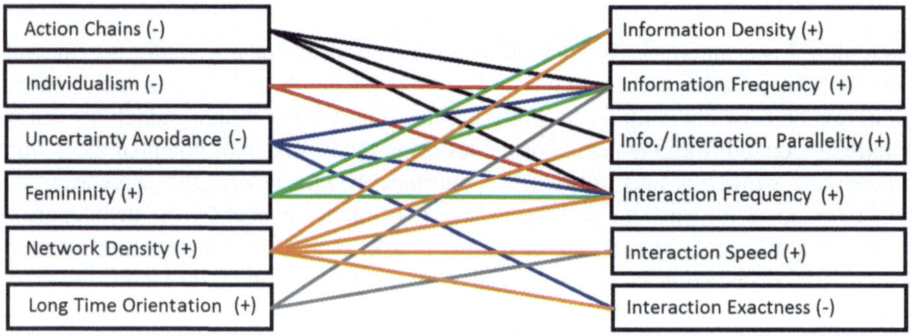

Fig. 1. Hypothetical relationship between cultural and HMI dimensions [13].

3 Path to the IUID Toolbox

At the moment, the IUID toolbox consists of a combined and hybrid use of:

- Cultural dimensions,
- Intercultural variables,

- User interface characteristics,
- HMI dimensions,
- Method of culture-oriented design.

3.1 Cultural Dimensions

Cultural dimensions and cultural standards serve to describe and compare cultural systems (cf. e.g. [2, 5, 14]). The characteristics of cultural dimensions influence the user experience and provide orientation for the usability engineering process. Differences between cultures can be found by analyzing critical interaction situations between people [2]; The mental model of the user about the system depends on the culture of the user, his expectations about the characteristics of the system and his experience of interaction with the system. The cultural aspects and their manifestations can be empirically determined using qualitative and quantitative methods.

3.2 Intercultural Variables

Cultural dimensions are too rough for intercultural user interface design. For this reason, additional cultural variables are necessary which – in relation to user interface design – divide the cultural aspects into smaller units (cf. [6]). Intercultural variables describe the differences in HMI design with respect to the preferences of users from different cultures. Direct intercultural variables are most important because they have a direct and essential influence on the HMI design. "Visible" intercultural variables (VIVs) are immediately perceptible at a certain time (font, color, window size, navigation, etc.). In contrast, "invisible" (or "hidden") intercultural variables (NVIVs) are only recognizable over a certain period (interaction speed, information display duration, dialogue display frequency, use of the navigation bar, etc.).

3.3 User Interface Characteristics

The user interface characteristics "Metaphor", "Mental Model", "Navigation", "Interaction" and "Presentation" are linked to five of Hofstede's cultural dimensions [5, 6, 8]. User interface characteristics can be used in conjunction with empirical surveys on their characteristics for the corresponding cultural target context to derive recommendations for the development of intercultural user interfaces.

3.4 HMI Dimensions

There are correlations between the user's interaction behavior and his culture or between the cultural dimensions and information science variables such as information density or interaction frequency at the interaction level [12]. Information science values such as information speed (speed of dissemination and frequency of occurrence of information), information density (number and distance of information units) or information order (sequence of occurrence and arrangement of information), also correlate with culturally different basic patterns of behavior at the information level [12]. HMI dimensions describe the behavior of a user (HMI style) with an interactive information processing system [13]. Moreover, HMI dimensions represent classes of HMI variables (expressions of HMI dimensions) useful for HMI design, which are operationalized by means of (interaction) indicators in HMI metrics.

3.5 Method of Culture-Oriented Design

[6] proposed the “Method for Culture-Oriented Design”, which integrates the factors of new concepts of culture-oriented HMI design and the knowledge of cultural differences into existing concepts of HMI design. Relevant cultural variables for intercultural HMI design must be determined analytically based on literature research and requirement studies. Their values represent culture-dependent variations that occur at all levels of HMI localization (surface, functionality and interaction) and can be used for intercultural user interface design (IUID).

3.6 Hybrid Approach: Integrated Use of the Concepts

A hybrid approach integrates the concepts described above (cf. [13, 15]). Based on the method of the culture-oriented HMI design (MCD, see [6]), cultural differences are identified based on cultural dimensions and cultural variables are derived for the project. With this knowledge of cultural differences and affected aspects of the HMI system, further effects on the HMI design have been determined and supported by hypothesis-driven data transmission using user interface characteristics (see [8]) and HMI dimensions (see [12]) leading to a toolbox for IUID consisting of reasonably arranged methods. The values of these concepts represent the HMI style of the user in the respective cultural context [13].

First, the application, main use cases and the desired target culture is chosen. Depending on the use case, the respective UI elements (e.g. layout, buttons, text fields) have been determined and mapped to the category of the cultural variables (direct, indirect, visible, hidden) as well as to the user interface characteristics (presentation, interaction, navigation, mental model and metaphor). Using this information, the time and space related HMI dimensions concerned are analyzed (such as information density or interaction frequency). Via the explanatory model for culturally influenced HMI (Fig. 1), the detected HMI dimensions are related to the cultural dimensions in order to derive cultural interaction indicators as well as design recommendations for the design of intercultural user interfaces.

Table 1 shows the outcome of the applied IUID methods for four examples of applications representing the characteristics of decisive variables for the development of intercultural user interfaces. For example, the higher density of the information network (e.g. as in China according to [14]), the stronger the values of the HMI dimensions (such as information density and interaction frequency) according to [13], cf. Fig. 1. The value of the cultural dimensions can be looked up in the literature of culture experts (such as [5] or [16]). For example, if individualism in a culture is low (e.g. for China in contrast to Germany according to [5]), then information frequency and interaction frequency tends to be high (e.g. for China in contrast to Germany according to [13]). Application details using several examples can be found in [17].

Table 1. Results of the application of the IUID methods (extract from an IUID workshop by the author).

Application/Use case	Cultural aspect/Cultural dimension	Cultural variable	UI characteristics	HMI dimension	Cultural interaction indicator	IUID implication
Word processing/Filling in a form	Language	Direct (word length), layout	Presentation, Interaction	Information density, Interaction frequency	Average number of chars per word, page	Resizing, calculate size of display according to language
E-learning system/Learning content	Communication speed, power distance, uncertainty avoidance	Visible (character set, buttons)	Presentation, Navigation	Information presentation speed	Dialogues per minute, Number of breaks in interaction	Adapt speed of guided dialogues (wizards) and button size
Phone/Looking up dialing via name or number	Communication speed, density of the information network	Indirect (online operating manual)	Interaction, Mental model	Interaction speed and interaction style	Number of buttons pressed per task	Choose appropriate input method editor (IME) and sorting algorithms

4 Discussion

There must be at least one potential indicator as a measurement variable in order to represent the character of an HMI dimension. For real use, however, several empirically proven indicators should be used. Moreover, the localization of hidden intercultural variables is very difficult to realize because the contextual relation to the cultural background as well as to the product is very strong for interaction and dialogue design. However, it is precisely this culturally distinct context and consequently the cultural dependency thereupon that these patterns and non-visible intercultural variables are so important for information architecture as well as for interaction design and, hence, for the resulting dialogues ([6]). Although cultures are constantly changing, at least for a product life cycle of a few years, trends can be determined, and for special cases of application even selective parameters can be determined, which serve the intercultural user interface design. If HMI dimensions are consistently represented based on cultural variables, one can use "(Inter-)Cultural HMI Dimensions", which express a culturally influenced HMI style. The HMI style coefficient describes the culturally influenced HMI style of users, thereby representing the average information density, information frequency, interaction frequency and interaction speed expected by members of a certain cultural group.

5 Conclusion and Outlook

The IUID method-mix represents a hybrid approach integrating several cultural methods [1]. Using the hybrid IUID method-mix is a reasonable approach towards an IUID toolbox integrating the methods and the explanatory model for culturally influenced HMI, where areas such as intercultural usability engineering and intercultural user interface design (IUID) can benefit to the extent that the model is further developed and empirically validated in order to be successfully applied to new examples, use cases or products to allow predictive design recommendations.

References

1. Heimgärtner, R.: Intercultural user interface design. In: Blashki, K., Isaias, P. (eds.) Emerging Research and Trends in Interactivity and the Human-Computer Interface (2013)
2. Thomas, A., Kinast, E.-U., Schroll-Machl, S.: Handbook of Intercultural Communication and Cooperation. Basics and Areas of Application. Vandenhoeck & Ruprecht, Göttingen (2010)
3. Honold, P.: Intercultural usability engineering: barriers and challenges from a German point of view. In: Day, D., Galdo, E.D., Prabhu, G.V. (eds.) Designing for Global Markets 2. Second International Workshop on Internationalisation of Products and Systems, pp. 137–147 (2000)
4. Vöhringer-Kuhnt, T.: The Influence of Culture on Usability, M.A. master thesis, Freie Universität Berlin (2002)
5. Hofstede, G.H., Hofstede, G.J., Minkov, M.: Cultures and Organizations: Software of the Mind. McGraw-Hill, Maidenhead (2010)
6. Röse, K.: Model of culture and their applicability for designing user interfaces. Paper presented at the Conference WWDU 2002-World Wide Work, Berchtesgaden (2002)
7. Shen, S.-T., Woolley, M., Prior, S.: Towards culture-centred design. Interact. Comput. **18**, 820–852 (2006)
8. Marcus, A.: Cross-cultural user-experience design. In: Barker-Plummer, D., Cox, R., Swoboda, N. (eds.) Diagrammatic Representation and Inference, vol. 4045, pp. 16–24. Springer, Heidelberg (2006)
9. Badre, A., Barber, W.: Culturability: the merging of culture and usabilty. In: Proceedings of the 4th Conference on Human Factors and the Web, Basking Ridge, NJ, USA (1998)
10. Castro Salgado, L., Leitão, C., Souza, C.: Semiotic Engineering and Culture. In: A Journey Through Cultures, pp. 19–42. Springer, London (2013)
11. Pereira, R., Baranauskas, M., Liu, K.: The value of values for HCI: an informed discussion beyond philosophy. In: Proceedings of the 14th Brazilian Symposium on Human Factors in Computing Systems, pp. 1–10. ACM, Salvador (2015)
12. Heimgärtner, R.: Cultural Differences in Human-Computer Interaction. Oldenbourg Verlag (2012)
13. Heimgärtner, R.: Reflections on a model of culturally influenced human computer interaction to cover cultural contexts in HCI design. Int. J. Hum.-Comput. Interact. (2013)
14. Hall, E.T., Hall, M.R.: Understanding Cultural Differences: Germans, French and Americans. Intercultural Press, Boston (2009)
15. Heimgärtner, R.: IUID Method-mix: towards a systematic approach for intercultural user interface design. J. Comput. Commun. (2019)
16. Schwartz, S.H.: Mapping and interpreting cultural differences around the world. In: Vinken, H., Soeters, J., Ester, P. (eds.) Comparing Cultures, Dimensions of Culture in a Comparative Perspective, pp. 43–73. Brill, Leiden (2004)
17. Heimgärtner, R.: Method-mix for the development of intercultural user interfaces - exemplified. Int. Hum.-Comput. Interact. (2019)

Using Dynamic Real-Time Haptic Mediation in VR and AR Environments

Ahmed Farooq(✉), Patrick Coe, Grigori Evreinov, and Roope Raisamo

Tampere Unit of Human Computer Interaction (TAUCHI),
Faculty of Information Technology and Communication,
Tampere University, Tampere, Finland
{Ahmed.Farooq, Patrick.Coe, Grigori.Evreinov, Roope.Raisamo}@TUNI.fi

Abstract. As VR, and AR become more popular forms of interaction with standalone and wearable computing systems, there is an inherent need to redefine the role of haptics in virtual environments. Complex virtual environments require more comprehensive tactile information. For this reason, primitive tactile signals currently being used in most commercial systems, need to give way to more precisely calibrated actuation, which is specifically designed for various applications. In this research we have extended the "Haptic Mediation" concept to test and improve haptic actuation for virtual interaction by developing a Dynamic Self-sensing and Actuation Architecture (DSAA) using Autonomous Haptic Devices (AHD). We have developed autonomous mobile versions of small haptic devices with embedded actuators, sensors, power sources as well as a radio communication channel (transceiver). These haptic devices can be attached to any part of the body to perform sensing and actuation. Our testing shows that this approach can improve users' overall experience in VR games and that AHDs can create reliable, perceivable actuation signals even when the user is actively moving around.

Keywords: Human-system integration · Multimodal interaction · Haptics

1 Introduction

Our ability to learn and adapt, creates the basis of our interaction in new virtual environments. However, these are limits on how much the mechanics of a virtual system can vary, to still be considered usable reliable and similar to the physical space. When an external system utilizes commonly used real world interaction techniques (i.e. door knob being rotated clockwise or anticlockwise to open a door), the user of the system is easily able to transition into this interaction paradigm, even if the environment or its surroundings vary considerably. Current virtual environments are now pushing the boundaries of what is physical and what is virtual. These environments have more complex and enriching 3D worlds that are governed by intricate laws of interaction, perhaps even slightly different from the physical world (random spawning, teleporting etc.). These visually enhanced 3D environments should increase user

T. Ahram et al. (Eds.): IHIET 2019, AISC 1018, pp. 407–413, 2020.
https://doi.org/10.1007/978-3-030-25629-6_63

immersion but in some case they do not. In fact, users identify a clear disconnect [4] between the 3D enhanced virtual and physical environments. This is because these virtual environments may have photo-realistic visual interfaces and 3D surround audio, but fundamentally come into conflict with our imagination and physical experiences due to the lack of meaningful haptic feedback. Thus, although users may be interacting with these environments directly (using their hands) or indirectly (using intermediate controller), the absence and immersive haptic feedback creates the fundamental gap.

Studies have shown that haptic feedback increases performance over visual only feedback in a wide range of tasks [1]. In fact, research by Cheng et al. [2] shows that by the addition of simple vibrotactile feedback it is possible to significantly improve task completion times in virtual environments. Similar research by Moehring and Froehlich [3] illustrates that addition of vibrotactile actuation signals with reference to grasping and manipulating virtual object can greatly increase system immersion. However, addition of haptic feedback does not always improve system interaction. As identified by Pawar and Steed [4], natural feedback cues are critical in creating immersive environment mechanics. Moreover, delays and inconsistent force feedback [5] parameters can negatively impact user perception. Furthermore, large heavy tethered wearable devices [6] can also reduce the immersive effect. Therefore, it is essential to provide context specific vibrotactile and kinesthetic actuation signals without using large heavy mechanical devices that need to be tethered to control and power sources for effective visualization and actuation [7].

2 Dynamic Self-sensing and Actuation Architecture

To achieve more complex and precise actuation signals it is important to calibrate and control not only the actuation signals but the actuation itself in real time. For this reason, we developed a self-encompassing actuation setup. Using the Haptic Mediation concept [7], we developed a Dynamic Self-sensing and Actuation Architecture (DSAA). This architecture consists of an actuator, a battery, driving circuitry, a wireless transceiver and an onboard 6-axisgyroscope. The onboard gyroscope provides real time actuation feedback, which is needed to dynamically adjust the actuation signals and to over-come environmental noise. While the transceiver and battery ensure that the system can provide tether-less actuation yet still be controllable, if needed.

To test the DSAA and its efficiency we created two Autonomous Haptic Devices (AHD). To keep the size as small as possible we utilize components that would be useful for mobile wearable devices or addons. We utilized an 8-Ω nominal Techtonic TEAX09C005-8 miniature voice coil actuator, which is optimized for electrodynamic transducer and has wide bandwidth and wide directivity. To drive the actuator, we used an Adafruit Feather M0 Bluefruit with onboard Bluetooth Low Energy (BTLE) and built in USB and battery charging. Driving signal from the M0 was amplified using an L298N high voltage, high current dual full-bridge driver. For dynamic actuation and motion sensing we used the UM6 r2 ultra-miniature orientation sensor as it has onboard gyro, accelerometer, magnetic sensor as well as a 32-bit ARM Cortex processor to compute sensor orientation up to 500 times per second. Powering the setup was a

PKcell LP503035, 3.7 v (1200mAh) Lithium polymer battery which was be recharged using the M0 Bluefruit main board (Fig. 1).

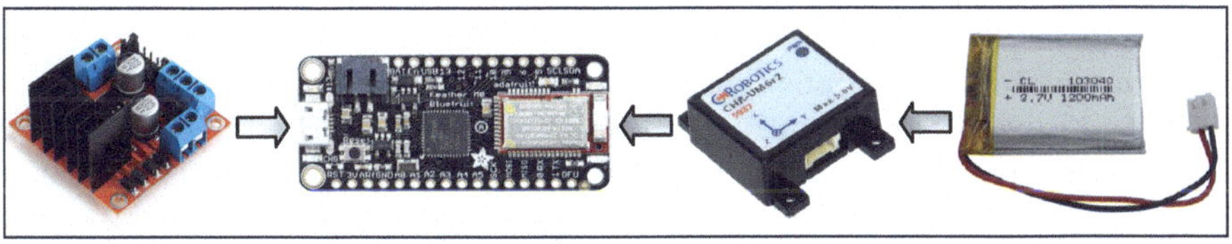

Fig. 1. (left to right) L298 N signal amplifier, M0 Bluefruit Microcontroller with BTLE, UM6 r2 IMU and a LiPo battery.

2.1 Dynamic Actuation Signals

The two AHD devices use an onboard signal simulator which have preprogrammed haptic signals. These signals were designed to simulate a gunshot effect to the user. The signal was similar to the Immersion SDK actuation signal (Weapon_87 and Weapon_88), with an absolute value of 10 Hz applied for 175 ms. Using this as a base signal, we developed 6 variations of the amended signals (S_F1 to S_F6) altering the frequency by a measure of 20% from the base signal. This meant that the application signal frequency varied from 4 Hz to 18 Hz.

2.2 VR System Integration

The VR environment chosen for this research was a game, Overdrive. This is a popular shooting game that requires the player to avoid being struck by bullets and shoot the non-playing characters (NPCs). For the purpose of this research participants were instructed to not shoot at the NPCs but to simply avoid the bullets fired at them. This ensured that the participants did not have to use the Oculus controllers and were provided visual feedback in the game. The HMD used for VR interaction was the Oculus Rift (1st generation), with no onboard audio feedback. The game was powered using an Alienware Laptop with a GTX 1070 mobile graphics card. The haptics feedback was generated using the audio feedback through the laptop system. The attachment was such that if the user was shot in the VR environment, the auditory feedback was used as a trigger to send a Bluetooth signal to the AHD devices (worn on the chest and back). Once the AHD devices were triggered, they either provided the 'Base application Signals' or a version of the 'Amended Actuation' depending on the experiment condition and user movements detected from the onboard motion sensor.

3 User Study

3.1 Testing Methodology

We conducted a basic user study with 24 student participants (10 male 14 female). The participants played 'OverDrive' using the Oculus Rift HMD without any controllers or audio feedback. Two AHDs were attached to the participants, one on the chest at the 'Sternum' and one at the back at on the 'Dorsum'. There were three separate conditions in which the participants were asked to play the game; sitting on a rotating chair; standing normally and jogging in a standing position. Each condition was completed once the participants were shot 14 times, twice for every actuation signal. Once the participants perceived the haptic signal of being shot, they were asked to press a force sensitive resistive (FSR) button strapped (using a SEN-09375 ROHS sensor) to the palm of their dominant hand. Using this information researchers identified the response time and pressure & force of the response of the participants, to each feedback signal in the three conditions like Kim et al., [8]. After each condition the participants were asked to specify how many times they were shot in the game. They were also asked to rate the 7 signals according to their perceptual force or strength and how pleasurable each signal was within the specific condition.

3.2 Results and Discussion

If we look at the time it took the users to press the FSR button on their palm (Fig. 2), we see that there is a clear trend for condition C between S1, S2, S3 and SB. As expected, lower frequency actuation signals took longer to be recognized by the users in condition C. Moreover, we see the same trend with amount of force by which the participants press the button, where lower frequency signals were followed by greater force presses of the FSR button, however, this trend evens out for the higher frequency actuation signals for all three conditions. Results also show that participants' response times did not vary through the seven actuation signals and the remaining two conditions (A & B). This would suggest that the participants' response times and force applied to the button were not affected by the variations in frequency between the tested actuation signals, either positively or negatively, but by the jogging condition (C) (Fig. 3).

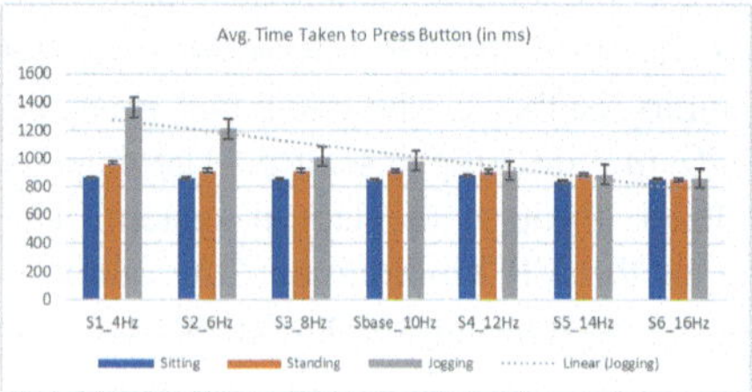

Fig. 2. Time taken to press the FSR button for all 3 conditions.

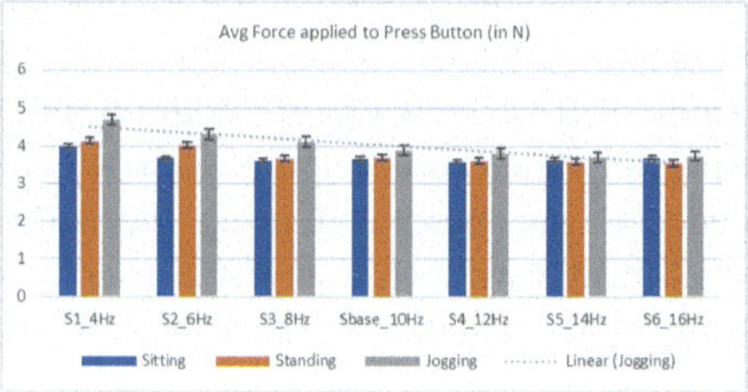

Fig. 3. Average force applied to the FSR button for all 3 conditions.

More interestingly when comparing the results of the recorded errors across the three conditions and seven actuation signals (Fig. 4), we see that the errors were much higher for condition C overall and specifically for signals with lower frequencies. This meant that the users either did not sense the applied signal or the signal was so weak

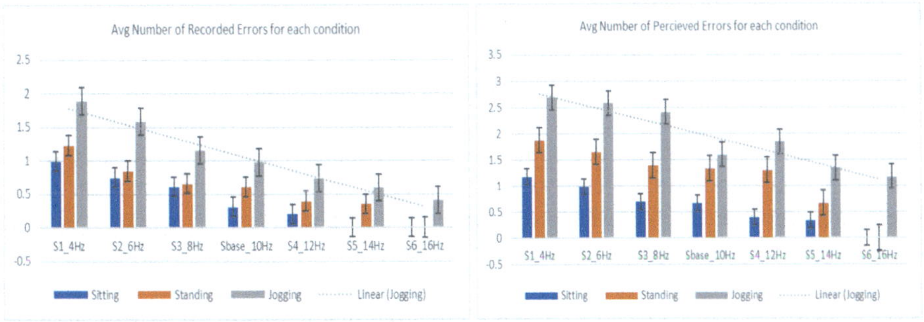

Fig. 4. Average number of recorded errors (left) compared to perceived errors (right) while pressing the FSR button for all 3 conditions.

that they did not identify it w.r.t the 'shooting event' in the VR environment. Moreover, if we compare the recorded errors with the participants perceived error rate, we see that on average the participants felt they performed more poorly than recorded. In fact, this can be seen throughout the results of condition C, which points to the fact that participants were unsure of the signal while jogging and felt the haptic feedback was unreliable.

Looking at the perceived sensitivity of the actuation signals over the three condition, we can again see from the result (Fig. 5) that lower frequency signals were felt less sensibly as a whole, specifically in condition C. On the other hand, pleasantness results suggest that user perceived the lower frequency signals to be felt more pleasant yet less sensible in different conditions. This trend is visible for all three conditions, however the variations for condition A and B is greater than for condition C for the same signals. This would mean that once the applied signal was sensible, the users preferred the lower frequency feedbacks over the higher frequency signal (Fig. 6).

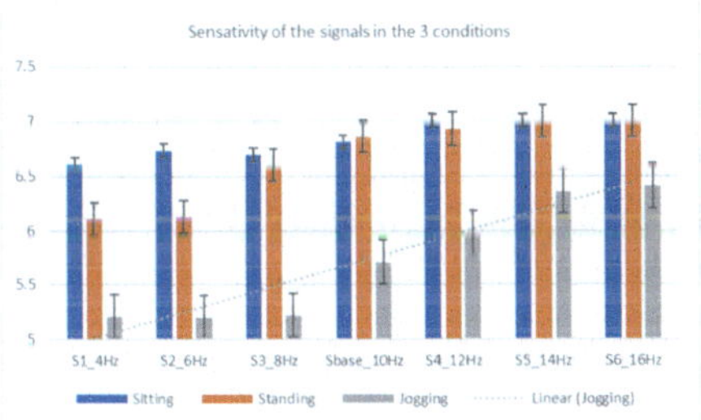

Fig. 5. Average Sensitivity rating for each applied signal over the 3 conditions.

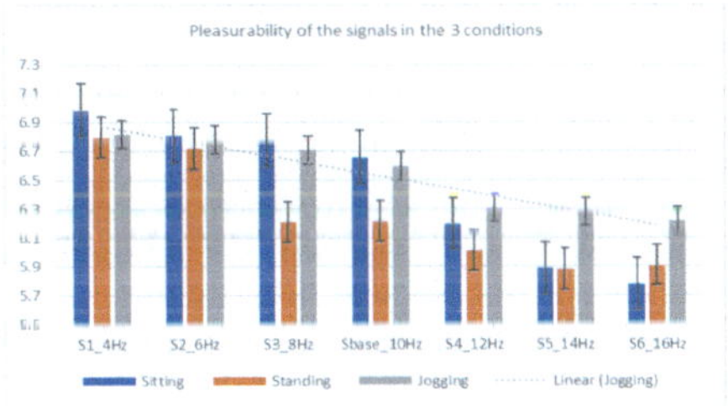

Fig. 6. Average Pleasantness rating for each applied signal over the 3 conditions.

4 Conclusions

In this research we have extended the dynamic haptic mediation technique to test and improve haptic feedback for virtual interaction by developing a Dynamic Self-sensing and Actuation Architecture (DSAA) using Autonomous Haptic Devices (AHD). Instead of using traditional techniques of having a single actuation signal for a VR based interaction event the AHDs can provide a larger scope of actuation signals depending on the environmental noise or movement of the user. To test the AHDs, we conducted a user study with 24 participants who played "OverDrive", a VR game using the Oculus Rift headset. Once the AHDs recognized that the participants were moving around the frequency of haptic feedback provided to the participants was adjusted according to their movements. Results demonstrate that dynamic haptic mediation improved the users' overall experience in the VR game and created a larger scope of haptic actuation rather than what is possible using current techniques. AHDs enhanced the actuation signal and increased the area of sensibility when the participants were actively moving around. Moreover, the variation of the signal did not create any adverse effects and ensured that when needed, the users could be provided the most pleasant actuation signal as possible. Similarly, in haptically noisy environments, the AHDs can provide a slightly altered signal to increase perceptual strength and reliability of the haptic feedback. Furthermore, this technique can filter out fringe frequencies generated by environmental vibration-noise (movement) and reduce the audio-component of the attached actuators. In our future research, we plan to explore how it may be possible to combine multiple AHDs over a range of actuation signals within a complex haptic stimulus yet keeping the signal perceptual integrity [7].

Acknowledgments. The research was supported Finnish Culture Foundation's Post-Doctoral mobility grant awarded to the PI and was also partially funded by Business Finland (MIVI Project, decision 8004/31/2018), and was carried out in collaboration with the Haptic Interface Research Lab (HIRL) at Purdue University, Indiana.

References

1. Burke, J.L., Prewett, M.S., Gray, A.A., Yang, L., Stilson, F.R.B., Coovert, M.D., Elliot, L.R., Redden, E.: Comparing the effects of visual-auditory and visual-tactile feedback on user performance: a meta-analysis. In: Proceedings of the 8th International Conference on Multimodal Interfaces, pp. 108–117. ACM (2006)
2. Cheng, L.-T., Kazman, R., Robinson, J.: Vibrotactile feedback in delicate virtual reality operations. In: Proceedings of the Fourth ACM International Conference on Multimedia, pp. 243–251. ACM (1997)
3. Moehring, M., Froehlich, B.: Effective manipulation of virtual objects within arm's reach. In: 2011 IEEE Virtual Reality Conference, pp. 131–138 (2011). https://doi.org/10.1109/VR.2011.5759451
4. Pawar, V.M., Steed, A.: Evaluating the influence of haptic force-feedback on 3D selection tasks using natural egocentric gestures. In: Virtual Reality Conference, VR 2009, pp. 11–18. IEEE (2009)

5. Berg, D.V.D., Glans, R., Koning, D.D., Kuipers, F.A., Lugtenburg, J., Polachan, K., Venkata, P.T., Singh, C., Turkovic, B., Wijk, B.V.: Challenges in haptic communications over the tactile internet. Access IEEE **5**, 23502–23518 (2017)
6. Blake, J., Gurocak, H.B.: Haptic glove with MR brakes for virtual reality. IEEE/ASME J. Trans. Mechatron. **14**(5) (2009). https://doi.org/10.1109/tmech.2008.2010934
7. Farooq, A.: Developing technologies to provide haptic feedback for surface based interaction in mobile devices, Ph.D. thesis, University of Tampere, Faculty of Communication Sciences (2017). http://tampub.uta.fi/handle/10024/102318
8. Kim, J.H., Aulck, L., Bartha, M.C., Harper, C.A., Johnson, P.W.: Differences in typing forces, muscle activity, comfort, and typing performance among virtual, notebook, and desktop keyboards. Appl. Ergon. **45**(6), 1406–1413 (2014)

E-Coaching as a Persuasive Support in Self-management Programs for Health

Robbert Jan Beun(✉)

Department of Information and Computing Sciences, Utrecht University, Princetonplein 5, 3584 CC Utrecht, The Netherlands
R.J.Beun@uu.nl

Abstract. In this paper, we discuss the characteristics of a smartphone system that behaves as an automated e-coach that supports behavior change. To mimic the behavior of a human coach and to build a relationship with the end-user, the system offers a conversational experience and behaves as an active virtual coach that discusses various aspects with the coachee about the therapy. For that, the system provides two types of integrated interfaces that we call the 'Talk-and-Tools' paradigm. Talk provides the functionality for the conversational experience, while various Tool-interfaces form a coherent structure of input and output facilities that enable the user to get access to and manipulate relevant information. Currently, the system supports cognitive behavior therapy for insomnia, but its generic design targets at a broad range of application domains. Various types of tests and user evaluations were performed, ranging from expert analysis to a randomized controlled trial with insomnia patients.

Keywords: E-coaching · Persuasive technology · Talk-and-tools paradigm · Conversational experience · Cognitive behavior therapy · Insomnia

1 Introduction

In parallel with contemporary technological and health care developments, a new field of interaction technology has emerged: so-called 'persuasive technology' [1]. On the basis of motivation and behavior models from psychology and social sciences, technological systems are introduced that support users in changing behavior through technology. Relatedly, a new terminology was adopted: not only are computer systems user-friendly, they must be cooperative, trustful, and able to build a relationship with users [2].

In this paper, we discuss the characteristics of an electronic system called SleepCare that behaves as an automated e-coach that supports behavior change. The system currently supports cognitive behavior therapy for insomnia on a smartphone. To mimic the behavior of a human coach and to build a relationship with the end-user (the 'coachee'), the system offers a conversational experience and behaves as an active virtual coach that discusses various aspects with the coachee about the therapy. Basically, the system gives tailored advice to the coachee to do certain exercises, makes appointments for consultation, and gives feedback with respect to the current state of the coachee and progress in the therapy. In addition, it includes a variety of persuasive

T. Ahram et al. (Eds.): IHIET 2019, AISC 1018, pp. 414–420, 2020.
https://doi.org/10.1007/978-3-030-25629-6_64

strategies targeted at improving the coachee's adherence. The system does not only respond to interactional activities of the coachee, but also operates proactively to take the initiative to interact.

The SleepCare-system provides two types of integrated interfaces that we called the 'Talk-and-Tools' paradigm. Talk provides the functionality for the conversational experience in a WhatsApp-style interface structure, while various Tool-interfaces form a coherent structure of input and output facilities that enable the user to get access to and manipulate relevant information (e.g., electronic sleep diary, exercise schedule, relaxation exercise). In what follows, we will briefly discuss the application of e-coaching in the domain of insomnia therapy, some of the applied persuasive strategies and the system's user-interface. Finally, we discuss the type of testing that was conducted to show the system's acceptability and effectiveness.

2 E-Coaching for Insomnia Therapy

Coaching is considered as a goal oriented activity to help people enhance aspects of their personal and professional lives by fostering self-directed learning through collaborative goal setting, action planning and feedback [3]. In the coaching process two types of learning are essential: a. learning through individual experience and b. learning as a social practice. The first dimension refers to the experiential and action oriented process of the coachee; the second refers to the idea of a collaborative dialogue that unfolds between the coaching parties and where the coachee learns in interaction with the coach [4].

2.1 E-Coaching

In this paper, the electronic version of a coach will be called the 'e-coach'. E-coaching systems exist in many forms and functions, may include sophisticated avatars, and may be targeted at a variety of health domains. Here, we focus on fully automated mobile systems (i.e., without human interference) that aim at a form of sustainable behavior change.

Examples of automated e-coaches range from obesity to depression treatment (e.g., [5]). In line with [6], we aim at developing a reusable mobile framework based on generic coaching principles. Our perspective starts from communication and cybernetics theory, and is based on concepts such as alignment, evaluation, feedback and adaptation. This enables us to include various persuasive strategies such as tunneling, adaptation, negotiation and increase of motivation. The domain of insomnia will be applied as a proof of concept.

2.2 Cognitive Behavior Therapy for Insomnia

Insomnia is a sleep disorder with a high prevalence (about 10% of the population) and can have severe individual and societal consequences (e.g., concentration problems, increased risks of accidents, depression); people with insomnia have difficulty initiating and/or maintaining sleep. Today, it is widely accepted that behavior change treatments such as Cognitive Behavior Therapy produce sustainable positive changes in the condition of insomnia (CBT-I) [7].

CBT-I offers a wide variety of exercise types [8]: sleep restriction (i.e., curtailing the time spent in bed), stimulus control (i.e., restoring the coachee's positive association with the bed and bedroom), cognitive therapy (i.e., changing dysfunctional beliefs and attitudes), sleep hygiene (i.e., making the person aware of practices and environmental factors that influence sleep) and various relaxation exercises. The actual intervention is usually preceded by a one- or two-week alignment period.

3 Persuasive Strategies

Basically, the e-coach offers evidence based behavior change techniques that should be experienced for a particular period of time. Activities are introduced or changed in the coachee's daily life such as filling in a sleep diary, performing relaxation exercises or going to bed at a particular time. The coach 'tunnels' these type of activities: it determines the exercise types and, in collaboration with the coachee, determines the properties of the exercises. To cope with the many uncertainties in the therapy and the coachee's daily life, a frequent feedback loop is included to reshape and personalize the offered techniques.

In general, adherence rates to the exercises are an ever present problem in CBT-I, in particular when the human coach has been replaced by a self-help book or, as in our case, an automated system [9]. We, therefore, designed the e-coach as a cooperative partner who not only helps to set therapy related goals, but who also uses persuasive strategies to improve adherence to the exercises.

A persuasive strategy is considered as a collection of coherent activities that support the process of behavior change. In line with [10], we assume that persuasive strategies aim at two dimensions with respect to the intended behavior change: increasing the ability and/or the motivation of the coachee. Loosely speaking, improving ability implies that the coachee may decrease the amount of effort that should be put into the therapy; improving motivation, on the other hand, implies that the coachee is willing to put more effort into the therapy. In practice, the distinction between the two concepts is not always that clear, however.

To improve ability, exercises and interaction are personalized and adapted to the circumstances. For that, the explicit alignment phase of one week and frequent feedback loops were included (usually after one week of practicing). Moreover, some therapy related activities that do not have to be experienced individually are supported by specialized tools or automated; examples are tools for handling sleep data (e.g., registration, overviews), activity scheduling and relaxation. To improve motivation, strategies were included such as showing (non-)adherence, performance and progress, shared decision making, explicit user commitment, explanation of therapy and exercise rationale, and expectation management.

4 The System's User-Interface

From an interaction point of view, persuasive strategies can be classified into two categories: a. strategies that polish the road to the desired situation and b. meta-level strategies that add a symbolic level to the previous category [11]. Examples of the first one correspond with direct manipulation interfaces from dedicated tools such as the electronic sleep diary or relaxation exercise; examples of the second one correspond with what is often called 'social interaction'. Social interaction is inspired by the periodic consults with a human coach and considerably increases the expressive power of the e-coaching system. It enables the designer to incorporate conversational moves such as explanation, negotiation and building commitment and may be represented by the language of, for instance, an embodied character.

In line with these two interaction categories, we distinguish between so-called 'Talk' and 'Tool' interfaces [12]. The Talk-interface provides the functionality for the conversational component (currently in Dutch) in a WhatsApp-style interface structure, while the Tool-interface provides coherent structures of input and output facilities for direct manipulation and observation of the insomnia and other related domains (e.g., registration and observation of sleep data, scheduling). To cover the main interaction needs for a 6-week CBT-I training program, 18 different conversational types were included (e.g., introduction, planning and commitment, and evaluation) [13] (Fig. 1).

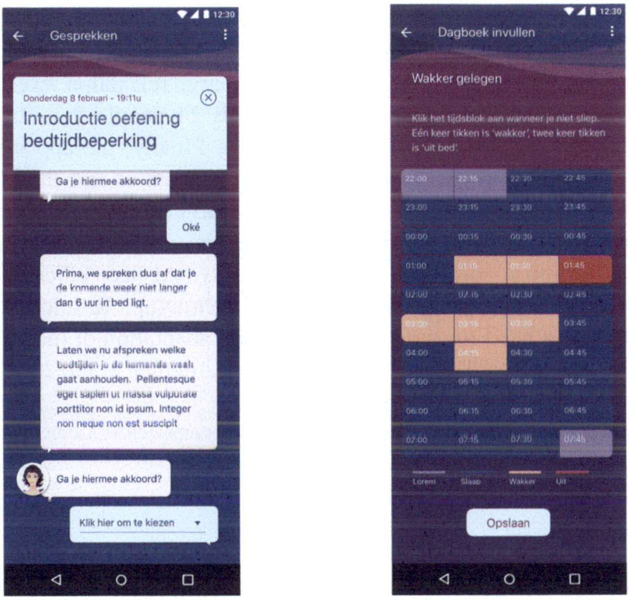

Fig. 1. Left picture: A conversation represented by the Talk-interface (*Gesprekken*). Right picture: The sleep diary represented by a Tool-interface (*Dagboek invullen*).

One of the conversational meta-level strategies that is applied in the e-coaching system is *negotiation*. Negotiation enables coachees to be involved in a shared decision making process of the attributes of their treatment. An important advantage of negotiation is the support of the coachee's autonomy and commitment to the therapy plan. It was therefore expected that negotiation may have a positive effect on the coachee's adherence to the therapy. Negotiation was applied to CBT-I's most intensive exercise: sleep restriction. During a negotiation round, a limited number of proposals can be exchanged to reach agreement about the bedtime duration. Usually the system puts forward a very restricted bedtime duration on the basis of the first week of alignment. Both e-coach and coachee may then put forward a number of less restricted bedtime durations in a number of counter-proposals until a particular proposal is mutually accepted or rejected by the coachee. The content of the various proposals (i.e., the so-called negotiation space) depends on the stage of the therapy, on the actual sleep behavior and on general constraints posed by the CBT-I guidelines [14].

5 Testing and Evaluation

To evaluate the acceptability of the system various tests and user evaluations were performed. First, an automated testing environment was developed that simulated the coachee's interactive behavior [15]. In total 32 scenario's were designed and tested in cooperation with an insomnia expert. Running these simulations resulted in minor adjustments, such as additional warnings in case the coachee's diary showed an average sleep time of less than five hours. In addition to these simulations, various tools were evaluated separately (e.g., filling in sleep diary, relaxation exercise) with 10 people and a pilot experiment was conducted with 24 people that started using an Android version of the SleepCare-app in daily life. Finally, the app was tested in a randomized controlled trial (RCT) with insomnia patients to test the efficacy of the whole system. In the trial, the app condition (74 participants) was compared with a wait-list group (77 participants). In general, the results showed significant interaction effects favoring the app condition on insomnia severity and sleep efficiency [16]. These improvements were also retained in a 3-month follow-up. Results from the RCT showed that there is a need for interaction about and adaptation of the attributes of the behavior change (i.e., shared decision making), in particular in those cases where the behavior change requires strong perseverance.

6 Conclusions

In this paper, we briefly discussed the design and implementation of an automated e-coaching system that applies persuasive strategies in the domain of cognitive behavior therapy for insomnia. Strategies pertained to the increase of the coachee's ability and motivation. By means of conversations (or so-called 'Talk') the system enables the designer to incorporate social elements, such as personalized explanations and shared decision making. So-called 'Tools' were included to simplify particular activities, such as sleep and wake registration, and activity scheduling. From various tests and evaluations it followed that the system is acceptable as an e-coaching system and effective with respect to its coaching goal. Currently, we are transforming the SleepCare-system into a commercial version called 'Lyla Coach'.

Acknowledgments. The research was supported by Philips and Technology Foundation STW, Nationaal Initiatief Hersenen en Cognitie NIHC under the Partnership program Healthy Lifestyle Solutions.

References

1. Fogg, B.J.: Persuasive Technology: Using Computers to Change What We Think and Do. Morgan Kaufmann Publishers, Amsterdam (2003)
2. Bickmore, T.W., Picard, R.W.: Establishing and maintaining long-term human-computer relationships. ACM Trans. Comput.-Hum. Interact. **12**(2), 293–327 (2005)
3. Grant, A.M.: The impact of life coaching on goal-attainment, meta-cognition and mental health. Soc. Behav. Personal **31**, 253–264 (2003)
4. Greene, J., Grant, A.M.: Solution-Focused Coaching: Managing People in a Complex World. Momentum Press, London (2003)
5. Both, F., Cuijpers, P., Hoogendoorn, M., Klein, M.: Towards fully automated psychotherapy for adults: BAS - behavioral activation scheduling via web and mobile phone. In: 3rd International Conference on Health Informatics, pp. 375–380 (2010)
6. Bickmore, T.W., Schulman, D., Sidner, C.L.: A reusable framework for health counseling dialogue systems based on behavioral medicine ontology. J. Biomed. Inform. **44**, 183–197 (2011)
7. Morin, C.M., Bootzin, R.R., Buysse, D.J., Edinger, J.D., Espie, C.A., Lichstein, K.L.: Psychological and behavioral treatment of insomnia: update of the recent evidence (1998–2004). Sleep **29**, 1398–1414 (2006)
8. Morin, C.M., Espie, C.A.: Insomnia: A Clinical Guide to Assessment and Treatment. Springer, New York (2003)
9. Horsch, C.H.G., Lancee, J., Beun, R.J., Neerincx, M.A., Brinkman, W.P.: Adherence to technology-mediated insomnia treatment: a meta-analysis, interviews with users, and focus groups with users and experts. J. Med. Internet Res. **17**(9), e214 (2015)
10. Fogg, B.J.: A behavioral model for persuasive design. In: Persuasive 2009, Claremont, California (2009)
11. Beun, R.J., Brinkman, W.P., Fitrianie, S., Griffioen-Both, F., Horsch, C., Lancee, J., Spruit, A.G.L.: Improving adherence in automated e-coaching: a case from insomnia therapy. In: Meschtscherjakov, A., De Ruyter, B., Fuchsberger, V., Murer, M., Tscheligi, M. (eds.) Persuasive 2016. LNCS, vol. 9638, pp. 276–287. Springer, Berlin (2016)
12. Beun, R.J., Fitrianie, S., Griffioen-Both, F., Spruit, A.G.L., Horsch, C., Lancee, J., Brinkman, W.P.: Talk and tools - the best of both worlds in mobile user interfaces for e-coaching. Pers. Ubiq. Comp. **21**(4), 661–674 (2017)
13. Fitrianie, S., Griffioen-Both, F., Spruit, S., Lancee, J., Beun, R.J.: Automated dialogue generation for behavior intervention on mobile devices. Procedia Comp. Sci. **63**, 236–243 (2015)
14. Beun, R.J., Griffioen-Both, F., Lancee, J.: Negotiation in automated e-coaching: an application in mobile insomnia treatment. In: Proceedings of 32nd International BCS HCI Conference (2018)

15. Griffioen-Both, F., Spruit, S., Fitrianie, S., Lancee, J., Beun, R.J.: Testing for mobile e-health interventions. In: Proceedings of the 31st Annual ACM Symposium on Applied Computing, SAC 2016, pp. 137–142 (2016)
16. Horsch, C.H.G., Lancee, J., Griffioen-Both, F., Spruit, S., Fitrianie, S., Neerincx, M.A., Beun, R.J., Brinkman, W.P.: Mobile phone-delivered cognitive behavioral therapy for insomnia: a randomized waitlist controlled trial. J. Med. Internet Res. **19**(4), e70 (2017)

Task Identification Framework to Automatically Detect Anomalies in Users' Interactions with Mobile Application to Support Usability Evaluation

Kateryna Sergieieva(✉), Thierry Martial Ngondji Bitchou, and Gerrit Meixner

Usability and Interaction Technology Laboratory, Heilbronn University, Max-Planck-Straße 39, 74081 Heilbronn, Germany
{kateryna.sergieieva, thngondj, gerrit.meixner}@hs-heilbronn.de

Abstract. Nowadays usability is a crucial factor for mobile applications to retain users. However, its traditional methods are still expensive and time-consuming. To overcome these disadvantages and support the automated approach to usability evaluation, current research offers a framework for automated detection of anomalies in users' interactions with mobile applications. It first uses sequence detection with regular expressions to perform the correct user's task identification and a Long Common Subsequence algorithm to identify tasks with anomalies and locate them in the user's interaction sequences. For the framework evaluation, the usage data from the trade fair "DOMOTEX" was taken. It consists of user interface interaction sequences of 24 unique users (163 sessions). The results indicate that by considering the main constraint of the framework: its dependability on the initial baseline, the system can show high accuracy on task and anomaly detection and deliver detailed insight on users' behavior with the application.

Keywords: Usability task identification · Anomaly detection · Pattern matching · Automated usability evaluation

1 Introduction

When consumers have to make a choice between two similar applications, they will rather select the one, that they understand, are comfortable with, and they can benefit most from [1]. As a result, investing more resources in usability will increase the chance for an application to stay in the market. Usability evaluation is defined by Nielsen as a set of methodologies measuring usability attributes of a system user interface [2].

Many usability testing approaches have been developed to the current date. Although traditional usability evaluation methods (Focus Groups, Cognitive Walkthrough, etc.) provide insight in usability problems, they require tedious manual work and are mostly based in a laboratory environment, and hardly scalable in real settings to

T. Ahram et al. (Eds.): IHIET 2019, AISC 1018, pp. 421–427, 2020.
https://doi.org/10.1007/978-3-030-25629-6_65

cover all users' interactions. Moreover, the analysis is mostly based on experts' opinions that can influence the results through different interpretations [3].

To overcome these limitations, the automated approach to usability evaluation was introduced. However, according to Ivory and al. only 33% of usability evaluation methods have automation support [4]. Current statistics show big potential for automation integration, especially based on the high availability of different logging systems and data trackers that can collect user interface events. This information can give a good insight into users' behavior inside an application. Moreover, evaluation should take place in a real environment in order to exclude the influence of evaluators and to keep the experience of all users included. But this can be reached only by the means of automation.

In specific, the automation of task identification gives a development team a clear understanding of the discrepancies between their vision on how a specific task should be performed and how users actually execute it. Additionally, it can address usability metrics such as task efficiency, error rates and effectiveness [5]. All of it provides a solid background for usability analysis and a further improvement in the quality of the application.

The purpose of this paper is to present a prototype framework that performs task identification. The framework is able to automatically identify correct users' tasks and afterward identify user tasks with anomalies and locate them to show the deviation from the expected performance.

2 Related Work

There are many approaches to the analysis of clickstream data. One of them is the metric-based methods, that uses log data to derive several metrics or measurements like navigational errors, task completion, etc. Lettner et al. [6] proposed a toolkit monitoring interaction with any mobile interface with the aim of providing statistics related to the collected data such as navigational errors to help designers and developers to improve their user interfaces. In contrast, the current research is task-centered and intends to focus on how users actually performed the tasks.

However, some other studies use the task-based approach as well. Saadawi et al. [7] for instance, developed a method of automated detection of usability problems from client user interface events. Their method divides tasks into sub-goals and checks if the user actions match the sub-goals. A usability problem is found when the sub-goal has not been completed or the completion took more than 2 min or took three or more steps to fulfill the task. Another researcher Ma et al. [8] developed a toolkit for usability testing of a mobile application. They used a finite state machine method for the task-sequence comparison. The predefined reference sequences with the user interaction clickstreams were used to identify how the user deviated from the baseline. Both approaches give good insight on discrepancies that exist between expected and actual task performance, but they were made in a laboratory environment with already predefined tasks. In contrast, our approach uses real-world usage data and consider the automation of task identification process together with anomaly detection.

The most promising related approach is made by Lettner et al. [5], who developed a task-based concept with sequence mining. To define the final similarity between expected users' behavior and the actual one, they use three similarity scores: task sequence comparison score, time spent on task score and number of interactions in each state score. Although they use a similar approach as in this paper, they consider only states (screen, page, view) and a summary of interactions in this state. This approach doesn't cover situations when different tasks might be performed in the same states with the same number of interactions. Such situations might be misleading for task identification. Moreover, when anomalies lay in the interactions, but not in the states themselves, these cases might also be undiscovered. To overcome these limitations, we assume that adding enough interactions as well as states in the string sequence will give us long and distinguish sequences to identify users' tasks and avoid unstable results.

3 Approach

The proposed approach consists of three main phases. First is a data preparation phase that includes data collection and preprocessing. Two others are a technical realization of the framework itself and cover the main goals of our approach: the automated detection of users' tasks and the location of anomalies in users' interactions. Figure 1 presents the overall design of the framework.

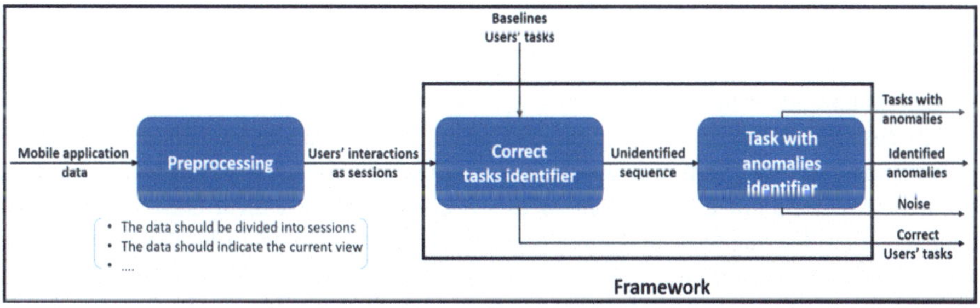

Fig. 1. Framework design structure. It takes as an input preprocessed mobile usage data and gives as an output identified correct and anomaly tasks

3.1 Data Collection

Data were collected as a part of the research project Opti4Apps[1] by the partner organization Heidelberg Mobil International GmbH. They developed and integrated a tracking system inside the trade fair mobile application, called DOMOTEX and performed the data gathering before and during fair time. Tracking system integrates a set of trackers for different mobile activities. For the current research the data from 3 main

[1] The research described in this paper was performed in the project Opti4Apps - Optimization for mobile applications (grant no. 01FJ15133) of the German Federal Ministry of Education and Research.

trackers was taken: device information tracker that collects the data about mobile phone characteristics; life cycle tracker that collects information of the view screens, every time they appear to the user; touch event tracker that gathers information about every interaction user make with a system. The collected data represents a based-on timestamp sequence of tracking records, that forms the user's path in the application.

3.2 Data Preprocessing

Before being eligible for analysis, raw data from the trackers had to be preprocessed. The current solution required the next preprocessing steps:

1. Division of the data into user sessions. Based on Device Information Tracker that marks the start of the application, all the data was divided into 163 sessions.
2. Data cleaning and filling data missing. Original raw data contained some unnecessary system views records, that had to be excluded. Additionally, data didn't contain the tracking of some system buttons.
3. Data encoding. The transformation of the user interaction sequence into the string sequence, where application screens were replaced with letter characters and interactions with number characters.

The preprocessed data represents a set of user sessions interactions, that are encoded into string sequences.

3.3 Correct Tasks Identifier Module

The framework was built with two modules: the correct task identifier and the anomalous task identifier.

The first module gets as an input actual users' interaction sequences and compares them to the baselines, that are represented as regular expressions (RegExp). RegExp defines a development team vision on user's correct actions on a concrete task. All sequences or subsequences, that match baseline, are considered to be the correct task. Others go to the second submodule.

3.4 Anomalous Tasks Identifier Module

The algorithm, that is designed to solve the problem of identifying users' tasks with anomalies, uses the longest common subsequence (LCS) concept. Considering the deviated user task as the task with unwanted interactions, the incomplete task or the task with both problems, the LCS algorithm will extract the flow of interactions that belong to a baseline. During this comparison, we fill a table of correspondence of the current sequence to the different baselines. Based on this table, the filtering mechanism associates sequence (subsequence) with the identified task, based on two main rules: higher matching accuracy and longer length of the matched trajectory. Only situations, when sequences match their baseline at least to 75%, are taken into consideration, but the threshold can vary.

The second module gives as output 3 main results: the tasks with anomalies, the location of discrepancies, and sequences identified as noise.

4 Evaluation

4.1 Evaluation Settings

We used a subset of the dataset from DOMOTEX application, collected prior to and during the trade fair in 2017 – till January 2018. It contains 16649 tracking records for a total of 24 random users. The data collection took place in a real-life environment with the users using the application without been instructed to do anything specific. 17 user tasks were selected for identification in usage data and anomaly analysis.

4.2 Results and Findings

The main goal of the framework is to identify correct and anomaly tasks. Altogether there were 241 tasks execution identified, from them 143 as correct and 98 as an anomaly. Most of the tasks happened to be the "search for the exhibitor", that might be obvious for the trade fair application. Other tasks have a much lower representation.

To validate the quality of task identification, the manual analysis of the results was done, and the confusion matrix was calculated. It is presented in Table 1.

Table 1. Users' tasks validation results.

Task identification confusion matrix	
TP	86.7%
FP	4.9%
FN	8.3%
Accuracy	86.7%

TP (true positive) were considered tasks and noise sequences that were identified correctly. FP (false positive) includes tasks that were classified wrong. FN (false negative) belongs to the tasks that were interpreted as noise.

The current approach showed a result of 86.7% of accuracy. This is a good result for such type of usage data analysis. Compared to Banerjee et al. [9], who analyzed interaction sequences of users that bought products in online shop and achieved 66,67% accuracy (33.33% are mistakenly identified as the wrong task) [5], we reached higher results, and confirmed that solutions based on interaction sequences and their trajectory are more sufficient.

However, we still didn't make 94.44% of Lettner et al. [5] method. Although we changed his technique for interaction similarity detection, that, from our perspective, should support better task detection, we didn't count time information in our study, that we consider evaluating in future work and identify if it influences our results.

At the same time, the algorithm misclassified 4.9% of tasks. The main reason for that is: some tasks have a lot of similar interactions and trajectories, and in a situation when user's behavior is different from expected whether he is doing a task differently or does not complete it, that might become ambiguous to the framework.

In the case of 8.3% of sequences that are false negatives, these are the actual tasks that were mistakenly classified as noise. It happens, mostly because of the framework main limitation, that it heavily relies on the baseline for task identification and in cases where the baseline is inaccurate, it can result in inaccurate "cutting" user session sequence into tasks, that might leave some meaningful data unnoticed in the noise.

5 Conclusion

We presented an approach for finding user tasks from users' interactions with mobile applications. The approach uses sequence mining techniques to extract users' tasks from the flow of users' interactions, collected while using the mobile application. The task identification was achieved by the implementation of a framework made of two modules: correct and anomaly task identification.

To evaluate our approach, we selected the trade fair DOMOTEX application. We considered a dataset of 24 users randomly selected and focused the task identification on 17 relevant users' tasks. The current approach is assessed by comparing the results generated from the framework with the result of manual analysis. The computed accuracy of the task identification is 86.7%. It is an adequate result for such systems. However, it can be improved by dealing with two main constraints: dependability on the baseline of user tasks and the big similarity of tasks.

The current study analyzed just one application and can be tested with other applications and larger datasets. However, the research does not guarantee the same results for every other application.

Acknowledgments. We are grateful for the support provided by Heidelberg Mobil International GmbH in collection and access to the data for the current research.

References

1. Nael, M.: Design issues for usability of residential multifunction terminals. IEEE J. Sel. Areas Commun. **9**, 518–523 (1991)
2. Nielsen, J.: Usability Engineering. Morgan Kaufmann Publishers Inc., San Francisco (1993)
3. Kjeldskov, J., Skov, M.B., Stage, J.: Instant data analysis: conducting usability evaluations in a day. In: Proceedings of the Third Nordic Conference on Human-computer Interaction, pp. 233–240. ACM, Tampere (2004)
4. Ivory, M.Y., Hearst, M.A.: The state of the art in automating usability evaluation of user interfaces. ACM Comput. Surv. **33**, 470–516 (2001)
5. Lettner, F., Grossauer, C., Holzmann, C.: Mobile interaction analysis: towards a novel concept for interaction sequence mining. In: Proceedings of the 16th International Conference on Human-Computer Interaction with Mobile Devices & Services, pp. 359–368. ACM, Toronto (2014)
6. Lettner, F., Holzmann, C.: Automated and unsupervised user interaction logging as basis for usability evaluation of mobile applications. In: Proceedings of the 10th International Conference on Advances in Mobile Computing & Multimedia, pp. 118–127. ACM, Bali (2012)

7. Saadawi, G.M., Legowski, E., Medvedeva, O., Chavan, G., Crowley, R.S.: A method for automated detection of usability problems from client user interface events. In: AMIA Annual Symposium Proceedings 2005, pp. 654–658 (2005)
8. Ma, X., Yan, B., Chen, G., Zhang, C., Huang, K., Drury, J.: A toolkit for usability testing of mobile applications. In: Mobile Computing, Applications, and Services, pp. 226–245. Springer, Heidelberg (2012)
9. Banerjee, A., Ghosh, J.: Clickstream clustering using weighted longest common subsequences. In: Proceedings of the Web Mining Workshop at the 1st SIAM Conference on Data Mining', Chicago, USA, p. 144 (2001)

Human-Machine Interaction

Hermann Kaindl(✉)

Institute of Computer Technology, TU Wien, 1040 Vienna, Austria
hermann.kaindl@tuwien.ac.at

Abstract. Usually, courses are given on *human-computer interaction*, while in recent years there was a major shift towards (mobile) devices and *machines*, with new human interfaces. Of course, they include embedded computers and software, but their interaction with users poses many new challenges and offers new solutions. This tutorial shows manifold *usability problems* as observed by the presenter in daily life, beyond those usually known from graphical user interfaces (GUIs) of traditional PCs (including laptop computers). It explains them by *human factors* usually unknown to embedded engineers and motivates *user experience*. *User*-centered and *Usage*-centered Design are compared with the result that they typically overlap but have a different focus each on *Interaction Design*. Usability *Test* and Usability *Study* are explained and contrasted as well. In addition, this tutorial explains key properties of *Multimodal Interfaces* and UIs of *Mobile Devices*. Finally, it culminates in a sketch of specific challenges of *Human-Robot Interaction*.

Keywords: User experience · Interaction design · Multimodal interfaces · Mobile devices · Human-Robot interaction

1 Introduction

This paper sketches all the topics addressed in this tutorial. In particular, it shows the thread of how these topics build on one another. References to related work, especially of work by the presenter are included as well.

2 Usability/User Experience

While *usability* already has a long tradition in the computing field, see e.g., [9], the notion *user experience* was introduced much later. We think that it is important to explain both, but also to contrast them in this tutorial.

Usability: First and foremost, we find it important to let the participants directly see and possibly feel real problems in daily life, rather than confronting them with a rather dry definition upfront. So, most of the first part is dedicated to a number of problems, where the selection below is typical.

Heating System: This example was actually a key motivation of this author to create and hold a new lecture course and related tutorials. In a nutshell, he was asked by his parents in law to help with changing their new heating system to summer mode. Since

T. Ahram et al. (Eds.): IHIET 2019, AISC 1018, pp. 428–433, 2020.
https://doi.org/10.1007/978-3-030-25629-6_66

its display as shown in Fig. 1 did not have a related menu, he consulted the user manual. It actually deals with this topic, but in a way that he still could not perform the task successfully. In fact, it pointed to the right menu for the water temperature, but did not clearly tell what to do there.

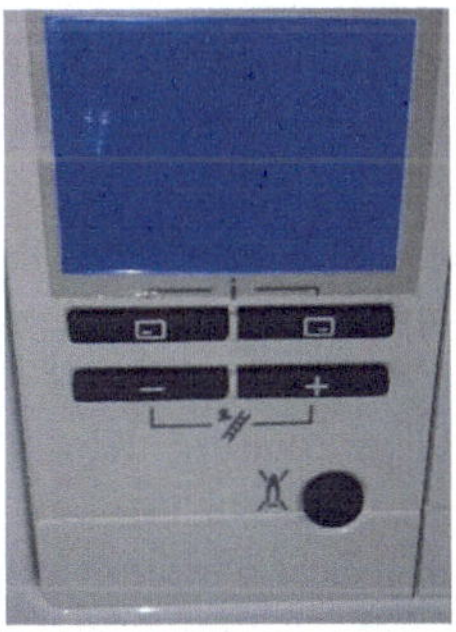

Fig. 1. Display and buttons of heating system.

So, service personnel was called, and being curious, this author attended as well. Since this person was not familiar with this particular device either, he gave up after a few minutes and placed a phone call to a service hotline, where someone familiar with this device was available. In this way, the task was finally achieved.

Coffee Machine: At the institute of this author, there is a coffee machine in operation that seems to be in wide-spread use also in Germany, for instance. It prepares good coffee and is very reliable, but sometimes it runs out of coffee beans, of course. Then its display is as shown in Fig. 2. It requests something like filling the container for beans (abbreviated in German here as "Bohnenbeh.") and displays that it is ready for operation. Actually, it is not, as no coffee is being prepared in this mode. So, whoever sees this message and wants coffee, he or she is motivated to get new beans, to open the container and to fill in beans. Simply pressing the button for requesting a cup of coffee as usual does still not work, however, as it is dark. None of the usual tricks like switching the machine off or unplugging it help, either. In this case, the user manual is of help, and the solution is to press this button for at least six seconds! Then it becomes active again and can be used for requesting coffee. We have not heard yet from anyone who would have found that out without the user manual or asking someone.

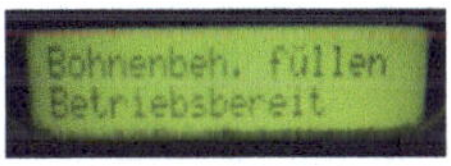

Fig. 2. Display and buttons of heating system.

Other real-world examples include Garage Entry (How to open the door for walking in?), Car Key (How to close (the doors of) the car?), and finally Web-pages (for eShopping, and railway connections and tickets). After having presented these examples of usability problems currently arising with embedded devices and a few Web-pages, time is ripe to present human factors:

3 Human Factors

Hopefully, the examples will have opened up the minds of participants with more technical background by that time, possibly (in part) through introspection in the role of potential users. Still, they need a better understanding of *human factors*, even though this cannot be an in-depth treatment in this tutorial. Primarily, they have to understand that humans are very different from machines, and some key properties of humans as potential users of embedded devices.

From a UI perspective and for motivating them, these participants have to understand that problems or errors during use are through 'bad' UIs in the first place, that such UIs are often a reason for non-use of a system and, that such a system (software or embedded device) as a whole is often judged based on its UI rather than its functionality. That is why design and implementation of UIs should take human factors into account.

With respect to human cognitive abilities, it is important to teach that humans are not all the same. This is also true in terms of their preferences (e.g., graphics vs. text). Still, there are limits that no human can surpass, in principle, such as the well-known limits of short-term memory and reaction time. Another important lesson to be learned is the increasing frequency of errors under stress, but there is, again, a difference between humans.

So far, the focus was just on problems and limitations. However, technology is mature now for more than using systems for work, for serving *human motives* more generally, be it at work or privately. While this author has some caution for contrived messages in this regard, he shows and explains the so-called "Wheel of Joy in Life" [6].[1] *Accomplishment*, *connection*, *identity* and *sensation* are certainly important concepts from psychology to take into account.

The relevant aspects can also be named *empowerment*, *sharing*, etc. An interesting discussion unfolds in class when contrasting Google Glass[2] with Head Camera[3] from such a perspective.

Finally, human factors are related to challenged people, with a focus on blind people. Related points like *accessibility* through barrier-free Web-pages, haptics and special smartphones for blind people are sketched and briefly discussed.

It is also interesting to compare that with special phones for elderly people (including the problem that these people often do not want to admit they are old). Such phones take Presbyopia into account, as well as reduced hearing and motoric abilities. The key point of this discussion is that there is something like being or becoming *gradually* challenged, which concerns close to everyone at a certain age!

---

1 http://www.incontextdesign.com/innovationincool/core-principles/.

2 https://de.wikipedia.org/wiki/Google_Glass.

3 http://shop.gopro.com/EMEA/shopbyactivity/ski/session-ski-bundle-eu.html#/start=1.

4 Interaction Design

Of course, approaches to *user*-or *usage-centered* design are forms of *interaction design*, but what actually is the latter? This important question is, unfortunately, only partly answered by the definition in the most widely sold book on this topic [11]:

"designing interactive products to support the way people communicate and interact in their everyday and working lives"

This definition leaves open with whom people will communicate and interact: some software or embedded system, or with other people? The latter option is certainly important by itself and covered by *Computer-supported Cooperative Work* (CSCW), yet another discipline. Still, it seems as though the book is much more concerned about interaction with technical systems in the first place. In this regard, the importance of repeating design steps and, in particular, of designing alternatives is emphasized.

Avoiding commitment to specific user interfaces during interaction design first is a key feature of an approach to interaction design developed by this author and his team for about a decade, see, e.g., [2, 3, 5, 8, 10, 14]. Its modeling focus is on high-level design representations in the form of models building on *speech acts* and other theories. From such models, GUIs can be automatically generated and tailored to the screen size of a given device.

5 Usability Test/Study

After this design material, a sketch of *evaluation* approaches was deemed to be useful, including the related techniques Usability Inspection, Questionnaire and Usability Test. Especially the latter's restriction to find usability problems can be easily explained by analogy, e.g., to testing software (for systematically detecting bugs).

While these approaches will be largely sufficient for practice at today's state of the art, for scientific evaluations the participants should also be aware of *usability studies*. Again, work of this author is included here, more precisely a study comparing GUIs tailored in two different ways for smartphones [12] and another one comparing GUIs tailored for smartphones and Tablet PCs, respectively [13].

6 Multimodal Interfaces

Since GUIs are more or less ubiquitous, also on smartphones and Tablet PCs, more or less everyone familiar with such devices or PCs has some familiarity with GUIs as well. Also many embedded devices have at least displays, as shown for a heating system and a coffee machine above. However, touchscreen input is fundamentally different from, e.g., input through buttons or mouse and keyboard. It has clear advantages by being more 'natural' and avoid the indirection and cognitive overhead of using a mouse, but for typing, a physical keyboard has its advantages.

None of that poses any problem to understand for the participants, but they may be often unaware of the intricacies of other modalities like speech. In particular, they need to be advised about the difficulties of speech input as compared to output.

It is also important to understand the potential advantage of a multimodal user interface compared to a unimodal user interface, that often a weakness in one modality can be compensated by the strength of another modality. This requires, however, well-designed coordination of different modalities. For giving an idea of related principles, we chose the CARE properties from [4]: *equivalence*, *assignment*, *redundancy*, and *complementarity*.

7 Designing UIs of Mobile Devices

Including computers and applications into mobile devices created a major break-through in the applicability of computing systems and in the impact this had on users. In particular, such devices often provide context-sensitive/context-aware mobile applications and location-based services, with special requirements for their UIs.

This tutorial uses GPS-driven navigation systems as the example for explaining and discussing many of the special features of a mobile device with location-based services. It also helps to connect again with the earlier topic of multimodal user interfaces, where certain modalities like sound and speech output are advantageous over screen output for informing the user of an event that occurred, like having arrived at the target destination. This example also allows contrasting special-purpose embedded hardware, possibly installed in a car, with an App for a smartphone.

8 Human-Robot Interaction

Based on all the previous topics, (communicative) interaction of humans with robots culminates the intricacies of human-machine interaction (unless the robots are simple industrial robots like robot arms for manufacturing). While this is an open-ended topic with many interesting examples, this tutorial primarily builds on previous work by this author (and several other people involved).

One example is to use robot body movements for communication [1]. They can serve as yet another modality employed in multimodal communication. This work can also be used for discussing human-robot interaction 'on the move', which poses even further intricacies for the user and the UI.

Another example is *Robot-Supported Cooperative Work* (RSCW) [7], which extends CSCW in certain ways. In particular, it can involve location-based aspects, including the locations of the users involved.

9 Conclusion

The primary objective of this tutorial is to provide the participants with a better understanding of issues involved in human-*machine* interaction (in addition to traditional human-computer interaction) and how to address them. (Mobile) devices and machines, with new human interfaces include embedded computers and software, but their interaction with users poses many new challenges and offers new solutions.

References

1. Bogdan, C., Ertl, D., Hüttenrauch, H., Göller, M., Green, A., Severinson-Eklundh, K., Falb, J., Kaindl, H.: Evaluation of robot body movements supporting communication: towards HRI on the move. In: New Frontiers in Human-Robot Interaction, John Benjamins Publishing Company, pp. 185–210 (2011)
2. Bogdan, C., Falb, J., Kaindl, H., Kavaldjian, S., Popp, R., Horacek, H., Arnautovic, E., Szep, A.: Generating an abstract user interface from a discourse model inspired by human communication. In: Proceedings of the 41st Hawaii International Conference on System Sciences (HICSS 2008) (2008)
3. Bogdan, C., Kaindl, H., Falb, J., Popp, R.: Modeling of interaction design by end users through discourse modeling. In: Proceedings of the 2008 ACM International Conference on Intelligent User Interfaces (IUI 2008), Maspalomas, Gran Canaria, Spain. ACM Press (2008)
4. Coutaz, J., Nigay, L., Salber, D., Blandford, A., May, J., Young, R.M.: Four easy pieces for assessing the usability of multimodal interaction: the CARE properties. In: Proceedings of International Conference on Human-Computer Interaction (INTERACT 1995) (1995)
5. Falb, J., Kaindl, H., Horacek, H., Bogdan, C., Popp, R., Arnautovic, E.: A discourse model for interaction design based on theories of human communication. In: Extended Abstracts on Human Factors in Computing Systems, CHI 2006, New York, NY, USA, pp. 754–759. ACM Press (2006)
6. Holtzblatt, K., Beyer, H.: Contextual Design: Evolved. Morgan & Claypool Publishers (2014)
7. Kaindl, H., Popp, R., Raneburger, D., Ertl, D., Falb, J., Szep, A., Bogdan, C.: Robot-supported cooperative work: a shared-shopping scenario. In: Proceedings of the 44th Hawaii International Conference on System Sciences (HICSS 2011), pp. 1530–1605 (2011)
8. Mukasa, K., Kaindl, H.: An integration of requirements and user interface specifications. In: Proceedings of the 16th IEEE International Requirements Engineering Conference (RE 2008) (2008)
9. Nielsen, J.: Usability Engineering. Morgan Kaufmann Publishers Inc., San Francisco (1993)
10. Popp, R., Raneburger, D., Kaindl, H.: Tool support for automated multi-device GUI generation from discourse-based communication models. In: Proceedings of the ACM SIGCHI Symposium on Engineering Interactive Computing Systems (EICS 2013) (2013)
11. Preece, J., Sharp, H., Rogers, Y.: Interaction Design: Beyond Human-Computer Interaction, 4th edn. Wiley, New York (2015)
12. Raneburger, D., Alonso-Ríos, D., Popp, R., Kaindl, H., Falb, J.: A user study with GUIs tailored for smartphones. In: Proceedings of the 14th IFIP TC 13 International Conference on Human-Computer Interaction - INTERACT 2013, Part II, LNCS, vol. 8118, pp. 505–512. Springer (2013)
13. Raneburger, D., Popp, R., Alonso-Ríos, D., Kaindl, H., Falb, J.: A user study with GUIs tailored for smartphones and tablet PCs. In: Proceedings of the 2013 IEEE International Conference on Systems, Man and Cybernetics (SMC 2013), pp. 3727–3732 (2013)
14. Rathfux, T., Thöner, J., Kaindl, H., Popp, R.: Combining design-time generation of web-pages with responsive design for improving low-vision accessibility. In: Proceedings of the ACM SIGCHI Symposium on Engineering Interactive Computing Systems (2018)

Exploring Gesture-Based Tangible Interactions with a Lighting AI Agent

Milica Pavlovic[1,2(✉)], Sara Colombo[1], Yihyun Lim[1], and Federico Casalegno[1]

[1] Design Lab, Comparative Media Studies and Writing, Massachusetts Institute of Technology, 20 Ames Street, Cambridge, MA 02142, USA
{milicap, scolombo, yihyun, casalegno}@mit.edu
[2] Interaction and Experience Design Research Lab, Politecnico di Milano, Via Durando 38/a, 20158 Milan, Italy

Abstract. The paper explores a gestural and visual language to interact with an Artificial Intelligent agent controlling connected lighting systems. Six interaction modalities (four gestural and two visual) were designed and tested with users in order to collect feedback on their intuitiveness, comfort and engagement level. A comparison between traditional voice-based interaction modalities with AI and the proposed gesture-based language was performed. Preliminary results are discussed, including the importance of cognitive metaphors in gesture-based interaction, the relation between intuitiveness, innovation, and engagement, and the advantages provided by gesture-based interactions in terms of privacy, subtleness, and pleasantness, versus the limited options and the need to learn a codified language. Insights will help designers in the development of seamless interactions with AI agents for ambient intelligent systems.

Keywords: Ambient UX · Tangible interactions · AI agent · Hybrid materials

1 Introduction

Ambient Intelligence (AmI) [1] system technologies are sensitive, responsive, adaptive, transparent, ubiquitous, and context-aware environments. These systems can be embedded with artificial intelligent (AI) agents, which perform front-end communication with the user. We are observing the rise of different kinds of AI agents designed to communicate with humans through different languages [2].

Finding new languages to communicate with AI agents beyond voice interaction, leaning towards multimodal interactions that engage diverse senses, is a wide and prominent research area. We faced this topic in a project for a lighting AI agent. The study presented in this paper is part of a concluded project aimed at designing a 10-year future vision of a lighting AI agent, Phil. We crafted specific interaction modalities as the communication language between Phil and the user, based on touch inputs rather than the audio channel (used in current well-known personal AI assistants).

Touch-based interactions are perceived by users as natural and seamless [3]. Multi-touch interactions have been analyzed for diverse applications, also in terms of user performance and ergonomics, and design strategies have been proposed in this field [4].

T. Ahram et al. (Eds.): IHIET 2019, AISC 1018, pp. 434–440, 2020.
https://doi.org/10.1007/978-3-030-25629-6_67

Design strategies for gestural inputs also bring up considerations on interacting with diverse media and surfaces, like, for example, on-body interactions [5].

The aim of this explorative work is to investigate the potential of gesture-based interfaces as an alternative to voice interactions in the design of AI agents. We tested our proposed communication language with a group of potential users. We discuss users' responses and provide preliminary insights that can guide further research on the design of new types of communications with AI agents.

1.1 Phil: The Lighting AI Agent

Phil is an artificial intelligent agent controlling ambient lighting systems. By connecting with light sources, it communicates with users and assists them in diverse outdoor and indoor environments, both private and public, supporting activities at home, at work, in leisure, and on the move. Phil is able to understand the context in which the user is, by accessing their biometrics, calendar, as well as by understanding the social dynamics taking place. It is capable of learning user's needs and daily routines, their preferences and interests. After learning, Phil provides the user with desired ambiance lighting, lighting social triggers, wayfinding, and notifications.

We designed a tangible language for the interaction with Phil based on gestural inputs and visual outputs. In our vision, such interactions will be allowed by the development of smart materials enabling projected capacitive touch sensitive surfaces [6]. Such materials can be embedded into everyday surfaces such as furniture, walls, as well as clothing, thanks to electroactive fabrics [7] enabling seamless interactions.

Interaction Modalities. In this paper, we describe and assess six interaction modalities with Phil: four user's gestural inputs, and two visual communications to the user. The interaction language is based on a circular shape, which represents Phil. The user can play with it in different ways, in order to input specific commands. Following are the four gestural interactions and two visual communications (Fig. 1):

1. *Calling Phil*, i.e. activating him by drawing a circle with one finger. After drawing a circle, a visual feedback would show that Phil is active in that particular ambient.
2. *Dismissing a notification* by touching a surface with one finger and swiping the visual circle. Notifications consist of personal messages such as "remember to take your medicine", conveyed through ambient light changes. In this case, the person just wants to confirm the reception of a message, but does not require any further action from Phil.
3. Confirming the reception of a notification and *telling Phil to execute a connected activity*, e.g. saving a suggested event to the calendar. In order to do this, the user engages two fingers on the surface. While one is stable on the visual dot, the other finger starts to draw a larger circle. When the large circle closes by making a full round, it indicates that Phil has finalized the required activity.
4. *Turning Phil off*, i.e. deactivating him in a particular ambiance. This interaction is performed by using three hands and swiping the visual circle towards the users' body. The visual would gradually decrease in intensity and finally disappear from the surface.

5. *Phil showing its presence* to the user by two circles that change sizes and rotate. The same movement is used to indicate that Phil is working in the background, this time by making the two circles spinning faster.
6. *Phil providing spatial directions* for users, when guiding them in the environment. In this case, a number of circles move dynamically towards the intended direction.

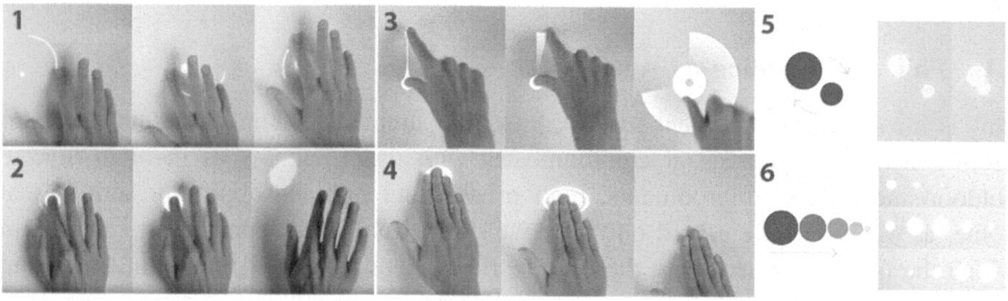

Fig. 1. Six interaction modalities, four based on hand gesture input and two on visual feedback.

2 User Tests

In order to evaluate the proposed tangible interactions, we conducted a user study involving 12 participants (7 females), in a setting within our research lab. Participants' age ranges between 19 and 35, and they all work or study in design and/or engineering fields. They have a high level of tech-savviness (average of 6 on a 7-point Likert scale) and 75% were familiar with AI agents (e.g. Google Home, Alexa, Siri).

Participants were asked to sign a consent and were provided with an overview of the design vision and the elements of the Phil system. As part of the introduction, two video use cases were shown, in order to give users examples of everyday contexts for the interaction with Phil. In one video, a 20-year-old student was guided by Phil in social interactions with her peers, within a co-working environment. The second video showed a young mother being supported and motivated by Phil in her daily workout activities.

After the introduction, users were shown six tutorial videos (see Fig. 1) describing the proposed interaction modalities. After each video, they were asked to repeat each gesture and to assess its intuitiveness, easiness to perform, and level of fun/engagement on a 5-point Likert scale. Additional qualitative questions were asked on each response. For each interaction, we also invited participants to propose alternatives and to indicate if and where they would perform the same interaction on the body (i.e. through smart clothing). Finally, participants were asked if they would prefer interacting with AI agents through voice or gestures.

3 Results

Intuitiveness. Most participants interpreted the set of interactions as intuitive (Table 1), particularly when they could associate them with *cognitive metaphors* or *well-known* *interaction modalities* with existing gestural systems (e.g. gestures on the Mac touch-pad). For instance, gesture 4 was metaphorically associated to the movement performed on the light switch to turn the light off. Similarly, a participant stated that gesture 4 was intuitive because the downward movement is usually associated to the idea of "reducing" or "turning off". Relying on cognitive metaphors helped participants to interpret the gestures correctly. Users assessed as neutral or little intuitive interactions that lacked any reference to existing systems or that were associated to metaphors not consistent with the gesture meaning (e.g. gesture 1 was associated to controlling the volume by one user, who gave a score of 3). Even when assessed less than 5, all interactions but gesture 3 were described as easy to learn even if not immediately understandable.

Table 1. Average scores for each of the six interaction modalities according to their Intuitiveness (I), Comfort (C), and Engagement (E), based on the 5-point Likert scale.

Interaction modalities	1	2	3	4	5	6
I	3.92	4.25	3.25	4.17	4.25	4.65
C	4.67	4.67	4.00	4.75	/	/
E	4.00	4.25	3.67	3.92	4.5	5.00

Comfort. Participants were asked to repeat the gestures and to assess how easy they were to perform. Gesture 3 was assessed as the less comfortable one (with an average score of 4, compared to the others assessed 4.67 and higher). A negative comment regarded the need to use two fingers asymmetrically, which made the participant "impatient". Another participant complained about the need to twist the wrist, which made the gesture unnatural and difficult to perform.

Engagement. The two visual communications were evaluated as very fun, pleasant and engaging, with 100% of participants strongly agreeing on communication 6 being fun/engaging. Gestures received lower scores, with gesture 3 being the less engaging one. Surprisingly, the more intuitive the interaction, the more engaging it was assessed (e.g. in interactions 6, 5, and 2). Similarly, less intuitive interactions were also assessed as the less engaging ones (i.e. gesture 1 and 3). Users U3 U5 and U10, who assessed gesture 3 as little intuitive (with a score of 3), also gave low scores on engagement (3), even if comfort received the highest score (5) in all three cases.

These results may suggest that engagement is more influenced by intuitiveness than comfort when it comes to a new interactions language. Indeed, higher levels of engagement and pleasure might depend on reduced cognitive load instead of the easiness to perform a movement, at least when approaching a new set of gestures for the first time. This outcome is also confirmed by the fact that, during the interviews, gestures assessed as fun were connected to the use of well-known gestures: "it's like saying 'nope, don't like you' on a dating app" (U2 commenting gesture 2, which was rated 5 in engagement).

Alternative Interactions. When asked to suggest alternative interactions to the ones experienced, participants heavily relied on the use of cognitive metaphors. A user proposed a "double tap almost like knocking" to call Phil. As an alternative to gesture

3, one participant suggested wrapping the hand "as to tell I'm closing it", or "I'm saving this information". Some participants proposed gestures more similar to human interactions. For instance, one respondent suggested a "soft touch holding for some seconds to say 'goodnight'" as an alternative to gesture 4. Another stated "I would like to use the whole hand as to closing or opening something, to make the intelligence appear or disappear."

Bodily Interactions. Participants were asked to indicate if they would use on-body interactions in alternative to the proposed on-surface ones. Certain areas kept repeating as the most natural or convenient ones (see Fig. 2), such as palm (voted 26 times), upper wrist (voted 21 times), thigh (voted 18 times), and forearm (voted 13 times). For gestural interactions, the most convenient three areas were palm, thigh and outer wrist, while for visual communications, the three highest ranked areas were palm, outer wrist and forearm. These three areas are indeed in the periphery of the visual field, but still visible. Seven participants observed that they would prefer having a private gestural communication with Phil and not having other people in the surrounding seeing it. The majority of them chose to interact with the palm for this particular reason.

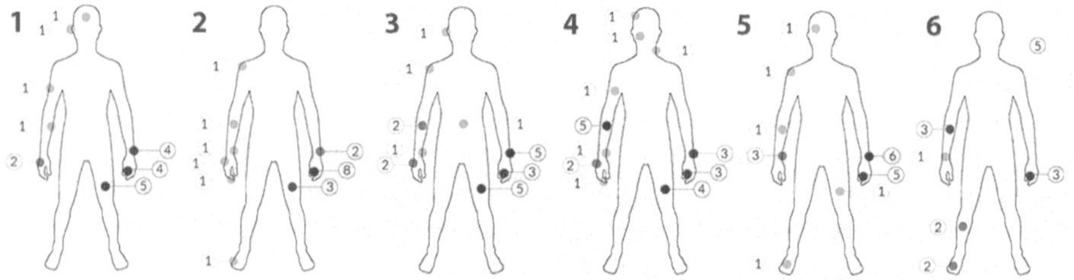

Fig. 2. On-body zones indicated by the study participants for the six interaction modalities; numbers in circles indicate how many times the same zone repeated.

3.1 Advantages of Gestural Interactions

67% of respondents stated they would use a gestural interaction system in public spaces, because it provides more privacy. "Tactile has limitation but it's better for public spaces". "I was suggesting my thigh because no one can notice what I'm doing". Tangible interactions also eliminate the issue of AI listening to private conversations: "I like that it is tangible, a vocal interaction means it always has to listen…".

Voice interactions were described as not suitable for public spaces also because in such environments people do not want to disturb others. As opposite to voice-based AI, Phil was assessed as "less annoying and invasive, also in public contexts". Gestural interactions, being a codified language, were evaluated as a more efficient way to interact with an AI agent than vocal language. "The tangible interface is way more efficient […] the AI doesn't have to interpret what you are saying, so less possibility for misunderstanding, because each input corresponds to a specific output."

3.2 Disadvantages of Gestural Interactions

Compared to voice-based interactions, gestural interfaces were assessed as more effortful: “when I’m home I want to be lazy and this [making a gesture] takes energy”. The need of touching surfaces was assessed as potentially negative in certain contexts. A user stated: “there are considerations for dirty surfaces, I wouldn’t touch [...] the kitchen with dirty hands or outdoors, where billions of people touch the same surface.” Gesture-based interactions are simplified forms of communication, and provide less flexibility compared to voice interactions: “With talking you can say so many things... tactile has limitation”. However, in some cases simple gestures were considered a preferable option: “If it’s an interaction that contains few steps/commands, then I would rather have a conversation; if it’s one step, touch is good.”

4 Conclusion and Future Work

Gestural interfaces do not provide the same advantages of text and voice communication, because they require users to learn a new codified language. However, it emerged that the use of cognitive metaphors can increase intuitiveness and engagement. Though reference to existing interactions (e.g. the ones performed on the phone) was appreciated, users also pointed out the need for novel interaction modalities when communicating with an AI agent. Users much appreciated simple and easy-to-remember gestures. When more than one finger was involved, symmetry was preferred (as in twisting or pinching). Tangible interactions were considered very suitable for office and public spaces, while voice was considered convenient at home. Privacy was seen as one of the main advantages of gestures, especially thanks to the use of on-body gestures, which give an extra layer of intimacy and make the interaction less noticeable.

We tested a limited number of interaction modalities, therefore the preliminary insights on the use of gesture-based interactions with AI agents cannot be considered comprehensive. Additional gestures and visual communications will be tested, especially based on the alternatives provided by users. More detailed analysis through statistical methods will be performed on the collected data, in order to confirm the correlation between elements such as intuitiveness and engagement. This work sets the basis for further investigations on new communication languages in the interaction with AI agents.

Acknowledgments. This research is a result of collaboration between MIT Design Lab and Signify. Doctoral research of the author M. Pavlovic has been funded by TIM S.p.A., Services Innovation Department, Joint Open Lab Digital Life, Milan, Italy.

References

1. Cook, D.J., Augusto, J.C., Jakkula, V.R.: Ambient intelligence: technologies, applications, and opportunities. Pervasive Mob. Comput. **5**(4), 277–298 (2009)
2. Boukricha, H., Ipke W.: Modeling empathy for a virtual human: how, when and to what extent? In: The 10th International Conference on Autonomous Agents and Multiagent Systems, vol. 3, pp. 1135–1136. International Foundation for Autonomous Agents and Multiagent Systems (2011)

3. O'hara, K., Harper, R., Mentis, H., Sellen, A., Taylor, A.: On the naturalness of touchless: putting the "interaction" back into NUI. ACM Trans. Comput. Hum. Interact. (TOCHI) **20**(1), 5 (2013)
4. Ingram, A., Wang, X., Ribarsky, W.: Towards the establishment of a framework for intuitive multi-touch interaction design. In: Proceedings of the International Working Conference on Advanced Visual Interfaces, pp. 66–73. ACM (2012)
5. Mujibiya, A., Cao, X., Tan, D.S., Morris, D., Patel, S.N., Rekimoto, J.: The sound of touch: on-body touch and gesture sensing based on transdermal ultrasound propagation. In: Proceedings of the 2013 ACM International Conference on Interactive Tabletops and Surfaces, pp. 189–198. ACM (2013)
6. Barrett, G., Omote, R.: Projected-capacitive touch technology. Inf. Disp. **26**(3), 16–21 (2010)
7. Syduzzaman, M., Patwary, S.U., Farhana, K., Ahmed, S.: Smart textiles and nano-technology: a general overview. J. Text. Sci. Eng **5**, 1000181 (2015)

InData Envisioning and Prototyping Informed by Data. A Data Scraping and Visualization Tool to Support Design Scenarios

Laura Varisco(✉), Ilaria Mariani, Stefano Parisi, Mila Stepanovic, Michele Invernizzi, and Patrizia Bolzan

Dipartimento di Design, Politecnico di Milano, via Durando 38/A, 20158 Milan, Italy
laura.varisco@polimi.it

Abstract. Acknowledging the roles and potentials of data as activators of the design process within the fields of speculative design and prototyping, we are running a study to foster collaboration between the fields of speculative design, smart materials, digital fabrication, and interactive artifacts. This paper presents the first outcomes from InData, an ongoing research project that investigates how envisioning and prototyping can be informed by data. In this paper, authors present the first research outcome: an interactive tool that scrapes and visualize data from IMDb.com to support designers in envisioning future scenarios outlining the design and testing of the tool through an iterative process that allowed improvements. The purpose of InData Scraping Tool is not limited to the mentioned applications, but rather they have been a pilot of a flexible tool and methodology applicable to other fields and scalable in larger experimental and applied actions.

Keywords: Data · Design tool · Envisioning · Creative process · Research-through-design

1 Introduction

InData is an ongoing research project that investigates how envisioning and prototyping can be informed by data. In particular, it digs into roles and potentials of data as activators of design processes within the fields of speculative design and prototyping. The objective of the research is to produce a theoretical and practical framework and an online platform, which starting from open access data fosters the construction of scenarios which contextualize and legitimize the existence of what is designed, by triggering possible innovations that take advantage of hybrid and smart materials and new interaction modalities. The entire creative process is approached through critical thinking, investigating the complexity of social, cultural, ethical and environmental terms. The research relies on a multidisciplinary approach aimed at activating the transverse dialogue able to stimulate creativity and innovation, as well as reflection on the use and role of data [1]. In this paper, we present the first of research outcomes: the interactive tool that scrapes data from Internet Movie Database (IMDb) [2] and

T. Ahram et al. (Eds.): IHIET 2019, AISC 1018, pp. 441–447, 2020.
https://doi.org/10.1007/978-3-030-25629-6_68

visualizes them to support designers in envisioning future scenarios. Furthermore, the research project will employ a selection of the data-informed scenarios created during the use of the scraping tool, as starting point for the concept design of interactive and smart materials-based artifacts in further experimental activities (i.e. a Hackathon session). We report the first results regarding the use of the tool in the educational context of the Politecnico di Milano, School of Design, pointing out how these activities provided feedback for improving the tool, identifying weak points, and insights for future iterations.

2 InData Scraping Tool

In the area of experimenting with interactive artifacts [3], intelligent materials and digital fabrication, both design fiction and speculative design [4] are performing a key role in enabling designers to better imagine the future taking advantage of the collective knowledge that comes from online open database [5]. The InData Scraping Tool [6] represents one of the outcomes of the research project. It is a web platform designed to support the envisioning of scenarios [7, 8] for students from various design disciplines. The tool takes advantage of online repositories with contents related to storytelling artifacts, and related user-generated metadata. It uses suggestions and inspirations coming from the collective intelligence [9] so to nourish the designers' creativity lessening individual biases and limits of knowledge – that come their subjective perspective that relies on socio-cultural backgrounds as source of knowledge.

2.1 The Tool's Design Iterations

The design process of the scraping tool started from a series of assumptions coming from previous knowledge of the authors about design students' needs in terms of functionalities, interactions and results that the tool necessarily has to present in its first version. Such knowledge comes from authors' expertise gathered through several years of lecturing and conducting design studios, and it highlights the importance of extending designers' perspective by feeding the creativity with references stemming from the realms of the collective imagination. In the light of this reasoning, we drafted the scraping tool, object of this article. The design of the tool follows an iterative process [10] that counts upon our empirical research ran at the Politecnico di Milano, School of Design educational context. During the testing phase, we conducted rapid ethnographies (participant observation), online questionnaires (10 answers received) and some informal interviews. The tool in-use has been tested on 98 students (40 from the Game Design course, 58 from Concept Design Studio) during the first phases of the design concept, namely during the initial desk research. This first version has been developed as a basic prototype and then, as a first test phase, it has been used by students during the two design courses so to: (i) prove its overall usefulness in different design contexts and processes (concept design and game design); (ii) test and validate functionalities, interactions and results, and; (iii) improve them collecting feedback and suggestions from the students and from the observation during the use. The insights extracted led the authors to re-design and develop the second version of the tool. We planned further iterations and test phases during courses, workshops and research activities, in order to collect additional feedback necessary for developing and releasing the final version of the scraping tool. In this paper we present the first test phase reporting both the feedback and suggestions extracted, and some of the results obtained by students using the tool in the didactic context.

2.2 The First Version of the Tool

Through the submission of a query, the web platform scrapes and visualizes data from the IMDb.com results. Starting from the queried keyword, the tool collects the first 50 resulted titles and their metadata (title, IMDb link, keywords associated). Once collected, the web platform calculates: (i) the number of keywords associated to each of the 50 titles; (ii) all the titles among the 50 that has been associated to each of the keywords. When the calculation is complete, the scraping tool visualizes the results on a list and a cluster. The visualization reports on the left side the list of all the keywords ordered by recurrence among the titles, and on the right side a map of connected circles representing the titles. The map shows the first title resulted from the query (according to IMDb.com) in the center of the cluster, and all the other titles are displayed around it, dimensioned according to the number of keywords assigned to them, and spaced according to the number of common keywords (the closer a title is to the center, the more keywords it has in common with the first one). Each circle can be dragged so to facilitate the reading in case of superimpositions of labels. A double click on a title opens the corresponding IMDb page in which the user can explore visual suggestions, plots, quotes and other contents, and watch videos and trailers (Fig. 1).

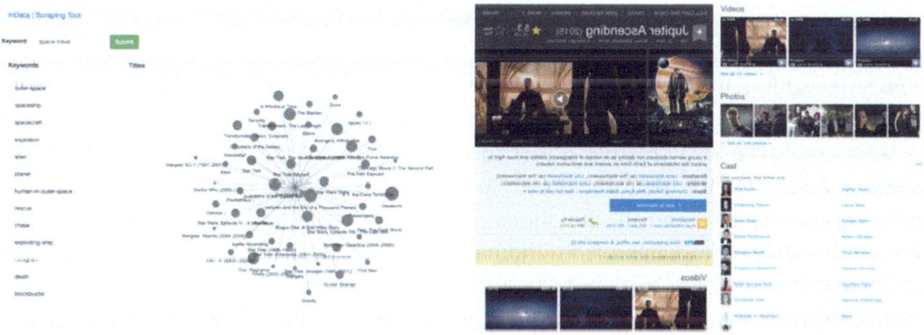

Fig. 1. First version of the tool showing the results of the query "space-travel": the list of keywords ordered by recurrence and the map of titles (*left*). Example of contents in an IMDb.com title page [11] (*right*).

3 Test and Collection of Feedback During Design Courses

The direct observation in two different courses with a varied population of users, allowed us to conduct usability tests, collect insights, identify technical problems, and gather suggestions from in-field experimentation.

Case Study 1: Concept Design Studio. The Concept Design Studio is a course of the M.Sc in Integrated Product Design. Within this course, its initial 5-week unit 'Product Cultures Polimi Futures' Fiction' intends to lead student in the exploration of frontier topics and future perspective, aiming at the definition of speculative product concepts and scenarios. The unit adopted a Research through Design method, following the steps of trends research, scenarios building, concept generation, rough prototyping finalized into 'diegetic prototypes', and design fiction, i.e. short movies to unfold and inquire the concepts' critical dimension. The tool has been tested during the first stages of this didactic unit to refine previously created scenarios. The test involved a total amount of 58 postgraduate product design students divided in 11 groups. We first introduced the web app to the students declaring it as an ongoing project that has the need to be tested and verified through its use so to collect users' opinions and feedback. Then we presented a brief explanation of its purpose, the data it uses, its functionalities and obtainable results. We observed and discussed in a think-aloud process with the students while they were using the tool as a support for the refinements of their scenarios (Fig. 2 – *left*). Furthermore, at the end of the class, we asked the students to fill an online survey to understand how they used it, what kind of information they find more useful to explore and collect opinions and immediate feedback on the tool's usefulness, and additional suggestions for improvements.

Case Study 2: Game Design Course. The Game Design course is a MSc elective course open to designers and computer scientists. It involves a total amount of 40 students with different backgrounds: from communication, product, interior, service and engineering designers, to programmers. The course deals with the development of working prototypes of games, in so doing it carries out in parallel the analysis of the game studies literature and the best practices in the field, and the actual design of a game, from the conception to the development as a working prototype [12]. The tool has been used in the initial phase of the design, namely when students started to identify possible narrative worlds of reference, outlining their possibilities and implications – technological, ethical, socio-cultural, and so on. For this case study, the tool has been employed as a creative starter to foster divergent thinking for the creation of narrative scenarios for board games. As for the previous case study, we briefly explained the purpose and the functions of the tool. Then, starting from sets of keywords previously extrapolated from the narrative or movie they chose as reference for the games, the students explored the results provided by the tool in an inferential journey through the contents related to storytelling artifacts. They investigated and extracted related keywords, visual suggestions and settings. Also, in this case, we observed the students while they were using the tool (think-aloud and participant observation) and collected insights and suggestion through informal interviews on the moment and online questionnaire afterwards. Then we asked them to analyze the results provided by the tool and generate scenarios' mood boards merging their previous research with the inspiration provided by the exploration content supported by the tool. As a consequence of this step, students elaborated inspirational insights and started expanding some initial reasoning, including reference to further fictional imaginaries and developing coherent and consistent storyworlds [13].

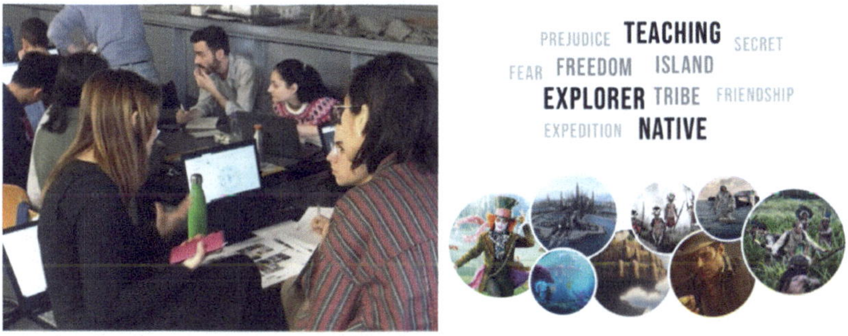

Fig. 2. Students of Concept Design Studio using the tool to refine scenarios (*left*). Scenario's mood board resulted from using the tool in Game Design course (*right*).

4 Refinement of the Tool: Version 2

The observation and collection of insights during case studies, verified the usefulness of the tool as an instrument able to promote divergent thinking and stimulate creativity. While designing (or refining) scenarios, the students (i) enjoyed and took advantage of the inferential exploration allowed by the tool; (ii) found interesting content related to the tool's results to analyze; (iii) revised and implemented their scenarios with the knowledge gathered using the tool and its visualizations. However, some critical elements emerged from the test: both our direct observation and the students' feedback identified some refinements for the second version of the tool. In order to improve the overall experience of the inferential exploration, we recognized the following goals as the most relevant: allow the user to refine the results; have a preview of the contents related to the results so to better address the further in-depth navigation on IMDb. In order to achieve these goals, we implemented: the filtering function according to IMDb categories (Type, Genre, Rating) including these metadata in the scraping; and the possibility to navigate glimpses of the results' content visualizing the number of recurrences of each keyword and, when a title is clicked, reporting the related plot in a separate section so to be immediately readable. To further refine results, we defined a formula to calculate the relevance of each keyword, adding the possibility of keep only the relevant ones in the visualization. The formula (1) uses the votes that IMDb users assign to title keywords. Taking into account the number of total votes (T) and positive votes (P), we consider as relevant only the keywords that has Rel > 0

$$P \quad (T \quad P) = Rel \tag{1}$$

We noticed that when the "keep relevant only" option is selected, the keywords and titles change considerably, and the results are more meaningful. However, we are aware that the refined version of the tool (Fig. 3) cannot be considered as a final one. More tests and improvements of both functions and UI have been planned to eventually create a more seamless and meaningful exploration experience of the tool.

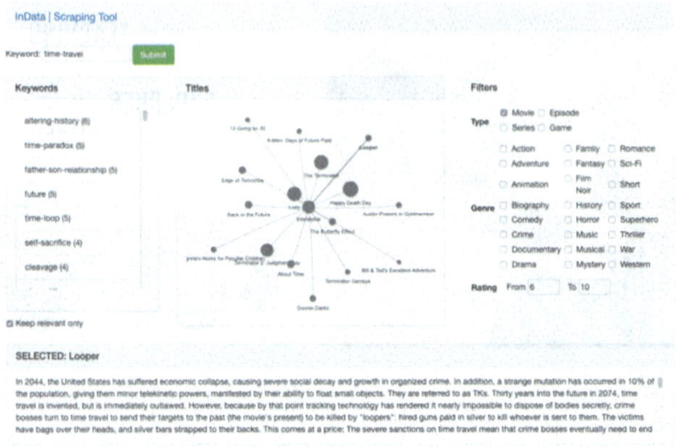

Fig. 3. Refined version of the tool: visualization of the query results filtered by type, genre, rating and relevance (*top*), and the plot related to a selected movie (*bottom*).

Acknowledgment. The work of Laura Varisco has been partially funded by TIM S.p.A., Service Innovation Department, Joint Open Lab S-Cube, Milano, Italy (PhD Scholarship). The work of Stefano Parisi has been partially funded by Fondazione F.lli Confalonieri (PhD Scholarship). The InData project has been funded by the Department of Design of Politecnico di Milano. The InData Scraping Tool has been developed by DeepGlance according to the authors' directions. We thank Manuela Celi and Maresa Bertolo, respectively leading professors in Concept Design Studio and Game Design course. We thank all the students who participated in the tests.

References

1. Arslan, P., Casalegno, F., Giusti, L., Ileri, O., Kurt, O.F., Ergüt, S.: Big data as a source for designing services (2017)
2. IMDb: Internet Movie Database. https://www.imdb.com/
3. Ryan, M.-L., Thon, J.-N.: Storyworlds across media: toward a media-conscious narratology. U of Nebraska Press (2014)
4. Bernabei, R., Power, J.: Hybrid design: combining craft and digital practice. Craft Res. **9**, 119–134 (2018)
5. Manovich, L.: Trending: the promises and the challenges of big social data. In: Gold, M.K. (ed.) Debates in the Digital Humanities, pp. 460–475. University of Minnesota Press (2012)
6. InData Scraping Tool (2019). www.indata.polimi.it/scraping_tool
7. Rosson, M.B., Carroll, J.M.: Scenario-based design. In: Human-Computer Interaction, pp. 161–180. CRC Press (2009)
8. Dzida, W., Freitag, R.: Making use of scenarios for validating analysis and design. IEEE Trans. Softw. Eng. **24**, 1182–1196 (1998)
9. Malone, T., Laubacher, R., Dellarocas, C.: Harnessing crowds: mapping the genome of collective intelligence (2009)
10. Gevers, M.: A decade of progress in iterative process control design: from theory to practice. J. Process Control **12**, 519–531 (2002)

11. IMDb.com title page. https://www.imdb.com/title/tt1617661/
12. Bertolo, M., Mariani, I.: Game Design. In: Gioco e giocare tra teoria e progetto. Pearson, Milano (2014)
13. Wolf, M.J.: Building Imaginary Worlds: The Theory and History of Subcreation. Routledge (2014)

A Proposal of Human Interface for Evacuation Support System on Smartphone

Shohei Taga[1(✉)], Munehiro Takimoto[1], and Yasushi Kambayashi[2]

[1] Department of Information Sciences, Tokyo University of Science, 2641 Yamazaki, Noda 278-8510, Japan
6318702@ed.tus.ac.jp, mune@rs.tus.ac.jp

[2] Department of Computer and Information Engineering, Nippon Institute of Technology, 4-1 Gakuendai Miyashiro-machi, Minamisaitama-gun, Saitama 345-8510, Japan
yasushi@nit.ac.jp

Abstract. We propose a human interface for a smartphone application. The application is an evacuation support system that recommends safe evacuation routes when a natural disaster occurs. In a large-scale disaster occurs, the Internet communication may be difficult due to communication congestion and break down of communication base station. Since our system consists of only smartphones and communicate with each other using ad hoc network without depending on the communication base station, our system is free from the above problems. Evacuees share information by using multi-agent system among them. The main purpose of the evacuation support system is to guide its owner even in a panic situation. Therefore, our system's user interface must be simple. The proposed design consists of the main screen, agent management screen that configures agents, and the guidance screen that display an evacuation route. In this paper, we present the human interface and the background philosophy of the system.

Keywords: Mobile ad hoc network · Mobile software agent · Multi agent · Contingency plan · Risk management · Human interface

1 Introduction

We propose a human interface for a smartphone application. The application is an evacuation support system that recommends safe evacuation routes when a natural disaster occurs. When a large-scale disaster occurs, evacuees have to evacuate to safe areas. It is important for them to collect information and select an appropriate evacuation route. The users must select the route dynamically because the usual route may be unpassable due to fire or collapse of buildings. Even though the current high-performance smartphones let people obtain various information anywhere and anytime through Internet, in a large-scale disaster, the Internet communication may be difficult due to communication congestion and break down of communication base station. Even in such cases, our smartphone base system must provide necessary information to avoid dangerous places and must lead evacuees to the safe places. Since we cannot depend on the communication infrastructure (the Internet), the smartphones that participate in our

T. Ahram et al. (Eds.): IHIET 2019, AISC 1018, pp. 448–453, 2020.
https://doi.org/10.1007/978-3-030-25629-6_69

system have to have some means of information sharing without any central control. Then the interface must provide its owner a simple way of diffusing useful information to other users. The main purpose of the evacuation support system is to guide its owner even in a panic situation. Therefore, our system's user interface must be extremely simple.

The current smartphones have enough capabilities to handle the above requirements. They are already full-scale computing systems, and they let us have implemented a multi-agent system for this evacuation support system in order to collect and diffuse information without depending on the communication infrastructure [1]. They have large memories; they can store detailed map that shows not only distance but also altitude. The altitude information is important in cases of a tsunami and high tide. They have GPS receivers so that they can sense quite precise locations and trajectories. They have acceleration sensors; people unconsciously tend to choose descendent routes rather than ascendant routes because of easiness. The system must prevent such users' choosing descendent route in case of high tide.

The rest of this paper is organized as follows. In Sect. 2, we describe related works. In Sect. 3, we describe our proposed evacuation support system. In Sect. 4, we propose the interface of our system. In Sect. 5, we conclude our discussion.

2 Related Works

Wang et al. proposed an evacuation routing method using artificial bee-colony optimization algorithm [2]. The artificial bee-colony optimization is a swarm intelligence algorithm inspired by the foraging behavior of bees. Ikeda et al. proposed safety evacuation route planning using a method that applies a genetic algorithm to the multi-objective optimization problem [3]. An evacuee's handset records GPS data and acceleration data, and then sends them to a crowd server. The server calculates an evacuation route considering evacuation distance, evacuation time and the safety degree of evacuation route, and then provides the optimal route to evacuees. Avilés et al. proposed an evacuation support system using MANET and ant colony optimization (ACO) for indoor environments [4]. In their study, they implemented ACO by using mobile agents so that the ACO algorithm can take the evacuees' trajectories and speed of evacuees into consideration. Then the evacuation support system constructs an optimal evacuation route for each user.

3 Evacuation Support System

Our evacuation support system aims to provide appropriate evacuation routes for the system users (evacuees). People need to evacuate while avoiding dangerous places such as fires and collapsing buildings. Such dangerous places may increase as time elapses; therefore, it is necessary to collect such information and to respond dynamically during evacuation. In addition, in a large-scale disaster, it may be difficult to collect information using the Internet due to paralyzed communication infrastructure. To address this problem, we have proposed an evacuation support system using a mobile ad hoc network (MANET) and multi-agent system (Fig. 1). The main functions of this system related to the human interface are as follows.

(1) Construction of MANET. MANET is a network constructed by direct wireless communication between portable terminals. The portable terminals on the network relay the communication data to other portable terminals so that portable terminals can send and receive messages with each other without communication infrastructure. Since the network consists of only portable terminals, it is possible to avoid problems we have mentioned in the first section. Our system constructs MANET using smartphone possessed by evacuees.
(2) Information sharing between system users. Our system provides information sharing among system users using mobile software agents. The system generates mobile software agents as needed, and they operate autonomously. Mobile software agents perform their tasks while moving between smartphones connected in the MANET. People with smartphones that make up MANET move constantly, therefore, it is hard to maintain perpetual link between them. If there is no other communicable smartphone, the mobile software agent waits until communicative smartphones appear. We have implemented two types of mobile software agents: diffusion agents and scout agents. When a system user discover a dangerous point, he or she generates the diffusion agent with that information. Then the diffusion agent duplicates itself by the number of smartphones in the vicinity and make them migrate to the smartphones. Upon arrival, they pass the information to the destination smartphones. The discovered information is diffused by repeating this operation certain times. The scout agent is generated at regular time intervals and searches for useful information. When a scout agent finds a dangerous place on the evacuation route, the scout agent obtains the information, and returns to the source smartphone and passes the information to the system. The system then use the information to revise the evacuation route.
(3) Construction of evacuation routes. The system constructs an appropriate evacuation route based on the information collected by the function (2) and presents it to the system user. The evacuation route is the shortest route to the safe area that does not include dangerous places. If the system finds a new dangerous place on the current evacuation route, the system updates the evacuation route accordingly. Thus, the system users can dynamically change their behavior as new damages appear after the disaster occurs. In addition, in the affected areas of tsunamis and high tide, the system considers altitude information and constructs evacuation routes with high altitude. Although this evacuation route may not be the shortest route, it may be safer one by avoiding inundations. Our system calculates an evacuation route based on the Dijkstra method [5]. The Dijkstra method calculates the shortest distance between two nodes in a graph composed of edges with cost and nodes connecting. In our system, the intersection in the evacuation area is the node, the passable road between the intersections is the edge, and the distance of the road is the cost. Our system calculates the shortest distance between the current location of the evacuee and the safe area excluding the edges and nodes that include dangerous places. If our system needs to consider altitude information, the system reflects that information and preferentially selects a high altitude route if there are multiple routes with the same distance.

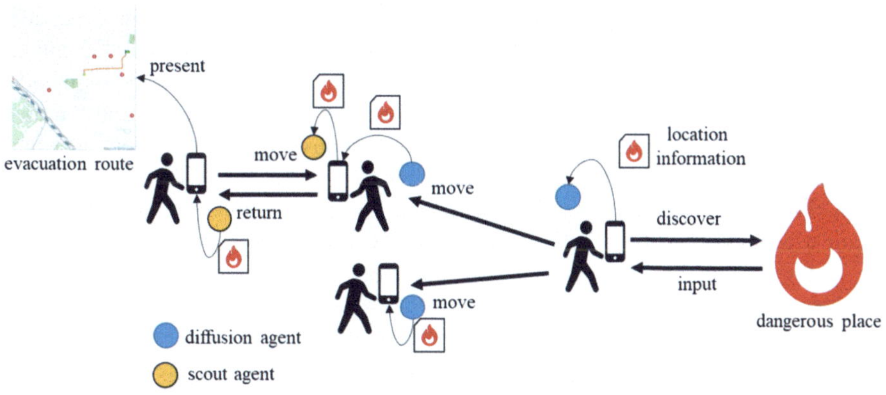

Fig. 1. Evacuation support system.

4 Human Interface

Upon considering the requirements and the capability of the current smartphones, we have designed the following human-computer interfaces in addition to the main screen; they are the agent management screen and the guidance screen.

The agent management screen provides the system user to select what direction and how frequently he or she dispatches scout agents and diffusion agents (Fig. 2a). "How often to send agents" in the figure means how often the system dispatches the scout agent. If the system user selects the "Low," the frequency of the scout agent transmissions will be low and save the battery consumption of the smartphone. On the other hand, if the system user selects the "High", the number of the scout agent transmissions will be high and the smartphone consumes more energy of the smartphone. The "Direction to send agents" in the figure indicates the direction the system dispatches the scout agent. If the system user selects the "One direction", the system dispatches the scout agent to one direction. If the system user selects the "Multi direction", the system concurrently dispatches the scout agent to multiple directions. In the former, the smartphone can keep the battery consumption low because the system transmits only one agent at regular intervals. In the latter, the system can collect more information, but it consumes more energy because the system transmits many agents. The system user selects one of the levels according to the remaining battery power of the smartphone. The system should not make the evacuees perform complicated operations while evacuating. Complex operations can lead them to accidents and dangerous situations. Therefore, the system displays this screen immediately after startup and requests the system user to make settings once. After completing the setting, the screen changes to the guidance screen by pressing the button arranged at the lower left in the figure. Even during an evacuation, the system user can display the agent management screen according to the situation by pressing the button arranged at the same position, but this is not good idea because of the problems just mentioned.

The guidance screen provides the system user a map that describes the evacuation route to the safe area (Fig. 2b). The system displays the map around the current location of the system user (the green circle icon), and shows the recommended evacuation route (the orange line), the destination (the green flag icon), and the locations of the known dangerous places (the red circle icons). When the system user finds a dangerous place, he or she can press the button located at the lower right of the screen. When the button is pressed, the system registers the current position of the system user as the position of the dangerous place. Thereafter, the system places an icon at the current location on the map indicating a dangerous location as well as generates a diffusion agent to diffuse the information. The system also displays the locations of dangerous places that other systems users find on the map. Such information comes from other smartphones and given by other diffusion agents. The system updates the evacuation route when the system obtains information of the dangerous place and if it is on the current evacuation route. It also updates the evacuation route if the system user fails to follow the recommended evacuation route.

In this design, system users need only follow the evacuation route recommended by the system and press one button when a dangerous place is found during evacuation. Our simple design makes sense, as it should be a good idea for the evacuees to reduce the smartphone operations as much as possible during the evacuation.

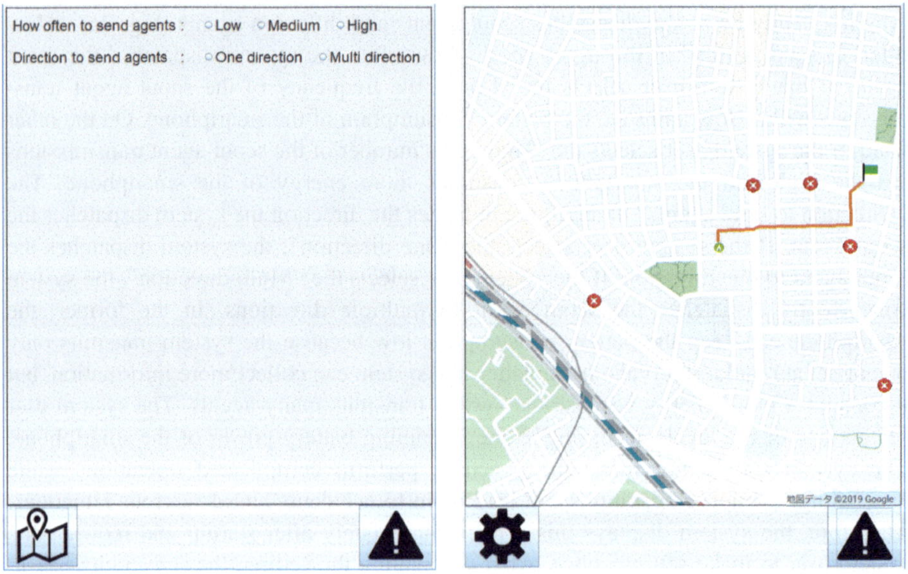

(a) (b)

Fig. 2. The human interface. (a) shows the agent management screen. (b) shows the guidance screen.

5 Conclusion

We proposed a human interface for the evacuation support system. We have made the human interface design as simple as possible in order to reduce the burden on evacuees during and after disasters. We are implementing the evacuation support system using the proposed human interface on an actual portable terminal. In the future, we will transplant the system on popular smartphones. When using this evacuation support system at the time of a disaster, the battery consumption of a portable terminal becomes a serious problem. In this paper, we have designed multiple levels with different battery consumption at the agent setting screen. In order to define exactly how much battery consumption is tolerated at each level, we need to verify with real portable terminals and smartphones.

Acknowledgments. This work is partially supported by Japan Society for Promotion of Science (JSPS), with the basic research program (C) (No. 17K01304 and 17K01342), Grant-in-Aid for Scientific Research (KAKENHI).

References

1. Taga, S., Matsuzawa, T., Takimoto, M., Kambayashi, Y.: Multi-agent base evacuation support system using MANET. Vietnam J. Comput. Sci. **6**(2), 177–191 (2019)
2. Wang, C., Wood, L.C., Li, H., Aw, Z., Keshavarzsaleh, A.: Applied artificial bee colony optimization algorithm in fire evacuation routing system. J. Appl. Math. **2018**, 17 (2018). Article ID 7962952
3. Ikeda, Y., Inoue, M.: An evacuation route planning for safety route guidance system after natural disaster using multi-objective genetic algorithm. Procedia Comput. Sci. **96**, 1323–1331 (2016)
4. Avilés, A., Takimoto, M., Kambayashi, Y.: Distributed evacuation route planning using mobile agents. In: Transaction on Computational. Collective Intelligence XVII, LNCS, vol. 8790, pp. 128–144 (2014)
5. Dijkstra, E.W.: A note on two problems in connexion with graphs. Numer. Math. **1**, 269–271 (1959)

Sonify: Making Visual Graphs Accessible

Safinah Ali[1(✉)], Laya Muralidharan[2], Felicia Alfieri[2], Monali Agrawal[2], and Jacob Jorgensen[2]

[1] MIT Media Lab, 77 Massachusetts Avenue, E14/E15, Cambridge, MA 02139, USA
safinah@mit.edu
[2] Human Computer Interaction Institute, Carnegie Mellon University, 5000 Forbes Avenue, Pittsburgh, PA 15213, USA
laya.muralidharan@gmail.com, felicia.alfieri@gmail.com, monali.r.agrawal@gmail.com, jacobpjorgensen@gmail.com

Abstract. Data visualizations are an essential strategy for summarizing and comprehending large datasets. However, it is challenging for visually impaired people (VIP) to access visual representations of data. Current accessibility solutions fall short in providing comprehensive access to such visualizations. Most VIP must listen to datasets one cell at a time with a text-to-speech tool, which does not allow the user to gather the "gist" of the dataset. To address this gap, we designed and evaluated Sonify. Sonify is a sonification tool that makes data visualizations accessible to VIP through audio and tactile interactions on a mobile app. VIP use Sonify's scrubbing interaction to explore patterns in data through pitch changes in sound. We evaluated Sonify's interactions through contextual inquiries, with (n = 8) VIP. Through Sonify, we demonstrate how a novel scrubbing interaction technique makes 2-variable linear graphs accessible to a broader range of people, including VIP.

Keywords: Human computer interaction · Accessibility · Assistive technology · Iterative design · Human centered design · Sonification · Usability testing · Assistive technology for persons with disabilities

1 Introduction

The ability to collect, interpret, and analyze data has long been integral to professional fields such as science, technology, engineering, mathematics (STEM), finance, and marketing. This has become even more important in recent years due to the increased availability and usage of large datasets. Professionals dealing with data analysis often make use of data visualization techniques such as charting and graphing, but visualizations are often inaccessible for visually impaired people (VIP) [8]. In initial research for this project about accessibility at large, we conducted contextual inquiries with 8 VIP, and found that a common pain point was the inability to understand visually complex interfaces such as graphs and charts. All 8 people with visual impairments reported that they struggle with 'getting the gist' of complex data.

T. Ahram et al. (Eds.): IHIET 2019, AISC 1018, pp. 454–459, 2020.
https://doi.org/10.1007/978-3-030-25629-6_70

The population of blind and VIP constitute 6.8 million adults in the United States [16], which has led to an increase in the amount of assistive technology to help VIP access computers [10]. Despite improvements in general accessibility, data visualizations remain relatively inaccessible for people with visual limitations. At present, screen-readers like JAWS [10] allow VIP to access content via text-to-speech technology (TTS). However, screen-readers often skip over graphs or read only the title and axes labels. If a VIP has access to the dataset, they can manually tab through each cell in a spreadsheet to try to find and understand trends in the data.

Existing technologies in data accessibility utilize tactile and haptic feedback as well as auditory interpretations of chart data, which are prevalent methods for representing visual knowledge in alternative modalities [13, 17]. Tactile solutions have been integrated as standard tools for VIP [11] and sonification of visual information has been used in tools ranging from TTS to blood oxygen monitors [15, 17]. Sonification of data, graphs, and other visual content allows VIP to understand visual content using audio patterns [8]. The Web Sonification Sandbox, a tool developed by the Sonification Lab at Georgia Institute of Technology [14] takes in a static dataset and returns customizable audio output of a single line chart. Sonification can also be used in data representations that are compelling to sighted people, like the work of the Data Driven DJ [5].

While our solution is scalable to all fields that make use of data visualizations, we chose to focus on VIP working in the field of finance, which includes traders and analysts. Prior research reports that, of individuals willing to work, 79% of those with severe visual difficulty and 64% of those with extreme visual difficulty were employed, but only 2.2% of these professionals fell under the category of "Technician or Associate Professional (inspector, finance dealer, etc.)" [9].

We followed an iterative design and testing process over 4 months, which resulted in Sonify, a sonification tool that makes 1 or 2 line graph visualizations of stock price data accessible to VIP. In this paper, we outline details about Sonify and the iterative design cycle we followed while developing the product, and the qualitative evaluation of interactions with (n = 8) users with visual limitations. Through Sonify, we demonstrate how a novel scrubbing interaction technique makes 2-variable linear graphs accessible to a broader range of people, including those with visual limitations.

2 Iterative Design

In this iterative design process, we went through 4 phases of designing and evaluating prototypes of increasing fidelity. To evaluate our prototypes in different stages of the product, we recruited 8 VIP, who constitute potential users, 14 accessibility experts, and 13 finance experts. VIP included 5 VIP with complete blindness, and 3 VIP with partial (mild to severe) visual impairments. In order to gain meaningful user insights, we kept several potential users involved through each stage of design [6]. Methods include varying combinations of contextual inquiries [3], think aloud sessions [20], and cognitive task analysis [19].

2.1 Design Phase 1

In Phase 1, we conducted think-aloud sessions with 10 finance experts in which participants were presented with a static line graph of the NASDAQ stock price graph, and asked to evaluate it in 1 min. Financial professionals reported that, when quickly reading a financial line chart, they look for: (1) overall pattern or trend, (2) high/low price of the stock for that day, (3) the current price of the stock, (4) graph labels and units, and (5) any spikes in the price over time. They may compare the chart with another related one or with relevant news events. After establishing this key information, we designed 5 low-fidelity prototypes and tested them with accessibility and financial experts. While we observed that both tactile and auditory solutions showed promise, tactile interfaces typically require a separate piece of custom hardware that is expensive and cumbersome. Thus, we chose to pursue a combined auditory and tactile solution that could be built into users' current workspace.

2.2 Design Phase 2

We chose to test pitch variation in Phase 2 based on well-documented research on pitch perception indicating that people are able to connect changes in information with changes in pitch [4, 12, 16]. Beyond audio, we recognized that the interactive aspect of tactile interfaces was compelling and effective. And existing sonification tools allow the user to play the audio version of a graph by pressing a button [14]. We sought to combine auditory and tactile interfaces to provide greater interactivity and understanding of the data. We developed and tested 3 prototypes:

1. Trackpad Scrubbing: A desktop application that allowed users to interact with an audio graph via scrubbing (dragging your finger left and right) on a computer trackpad. With X-values (dates) on the horizontal axes and Y-values (prices) corresponding with the pitch.
2. Keyboard Audio Navigation: An application that allowed people to use keyboard shortcuts to play the trend of a line and reveal important summary information such as highest, lowest, and current price.
3. Sound Preference: A system to test sound preferences using an open-source tool built by the Sonification Lab at Georgia Tech [14] to experiment with different sounds for line graphs.

Participants who used the scrubbing prototype were more successful at quickly drawing the "gist" of the graph. While participants who used the keyboard prototype took longer but drew more detailed and refined graphs. We then combined the positive elements from the two interactive prototypes: (1) interactive "scrubbing" control for line audio and (2) key data values from the keyboard shortcuts. Four out of the six participants agreed that they were able to gather the trend of the graph using the scrubbing and keyboard shortcuts. As a participant stated, "I would periodically press the spacebar as I moved through to have a more exact understanding." To address the problem of trackpad disorientation, we chose to switch from using a desktop trackpad to using a touchscreen. The absolute spatial mapping of smartphone and tablet devices would allow users to drag their finger across the graph without losing their place. We specifically chose devices with iOS over Android because our VIP participants emphasized that iOS is widely used by VIP given the accessibility friendly features.

2.3 Design Phase 3

In phase 3, we assigned a set of gestures to provide relevant pieces of information in an iOS application. For sonification of the line, we mapped values to pitches between the data points [2, 7, 17]. Participants were able to correctly describe the general movement of the line graph and identify spikes in the data. All the participants were able to identify changes in data patterns such as crests and troughs. When participants were first given the prototype, there was some confusion on what gestures they should use. We tested on both an iPhone and a larger iPad. While we had hypothesized that using a larger device would provide more granular insight, we found that participants preferred the smaller device because they could constantly feel the edges of the phone and understand where their finger was relative to the edges of the graph.

2.4 Design Phase 4

Based on results in Phase 3, we redesigned the gestures intended for gaining data insights through the GUI to match VoiceOver (iOS built-in screen reader) [1] for improved discoverability and fluidity. We divided the screen so that the top ½ would recognize VoiceOver gestures to provide supplementary info and controls for the graph while the bottom ½ would support scrubbing through the graph and single taps to read out values for that specific point (Fig. 1).

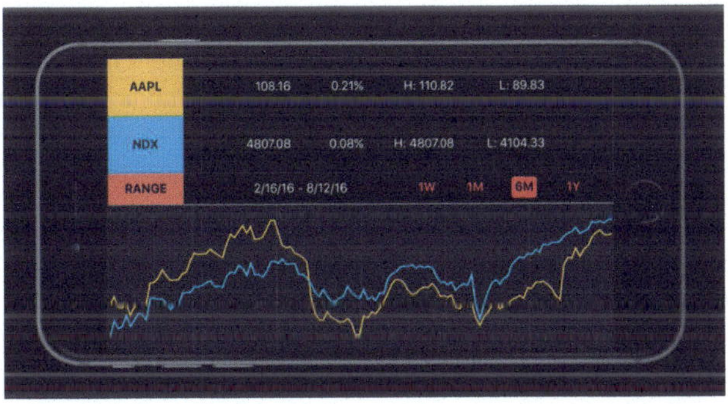

Fig. 1. This is the final design of Sonify, displaying the two stocks with the current, high and low stock prices. The interface also displays the current date range of the data and options to switch between date ranges. Finally, it includes dual stock graphs.

To compare the stocks to the market trends, we added a second line to the graph to allow for VIP to have access to similar data points. The hypothesis was that less complex sounds would be easier to distinguish while listening simultaneously, so we used sine (pure) and square (rougher) wave sounds. One line plays into the left ear audio with a sine wave sound while the second line plays into the right ear as a square wave sound. The user can swipe up and down in the graph section of the screen to switch between playing line 1, line 2, or both. If both lines are selected, Sonify plays both tones corresponding to the user's finger position as they scrub; if they tap, it reads out the current value for each line. We sought to test users' ability to distinguish between the lines and identify points where they cross/diverge, which is an important use case in analyzing stock price charts.

Based on our tests (1) users were able to pick up the Voice-Over gestures well, (2) users were able identify when the 2 lines intersected or spiked, and (3) users were able to gather a gist of the dataset. Finally, we built a barebones visual graphical user interface (GUI) for the application because our VIP participants revealed how important it is to be able to collaborate with sighted peers. We tested this UI to ensure accessibility for people with color blindness and/or low vision.

3 Discussion

In Sonify, we introduce a novel interaction technique that allows VIP to quickly build an understanding of data represented on a line graph, which was previously near difficult or impossible. Sonify's scrubbing interaction combined with standard Voice-Over interactions allows VIP to quickly gather the gist of a line graph, describe its movement, and access key values about the graph. These interactions set the groundwork for interactive data sonification and lay guidelines for designers wanting to expand to other types of graphs or datasets. We exhibit that playing two pitches of different sound quality simultaneously in either ear, when combined with tactile scrubbing, enables VIP to describe movement and crossing points of two different lines on a graph. We also demonstrate the importance of iterative design and working closely with the target users when designing for accessibility, which led us to make key design decisions like focusing on mobile phones over tablets for the VIP audience specifically. We make Sonify an open-source technology, to democratize this technology in the larger spirit of accessibility. Further, we advance the field of comprehending complex data to alternative modalities besides data visualization, and make graphs accessible to users who could not access graphs in the past.

4 Limitations and Future Work

In this paper we outline how we used user-centric iterative design methods to design Sonify, making visual graphs accessible to VIP. While we did multiple rounds of usability evaluations with potential users, there were some stages in which we could not work with VIP. As very few individuals with visual disabilities work in finance, we were not able to recruit individuals who meet both criteria.

While we qualitatively validated the design and accessibility of Sonify, the tool can also be made useful across non-finance domains. We must allow users to upload their own datasets. Sonify can also allow greater dimensions of data to be conveyed by using more complex sound interactions such as loudness, pitch, and frequency, as opposed to the current version, which only uses pitch. The current version of Sonify can be downloaded from the Apple app store found with this link.

References

1. Apple Accessibility (2014). https://www.apple.com/accessibility/ios/
2. Walker, B.N., Ehrenstein, A.: Pitch and pitch change interact in auditory displays. J. Exp. Psychol. Appl. **6**(1), 15–30 (2000). https://doi.org/10.1037/1076-898X.6.1.15
3. Beyer, H., Holtzblatt, K.: Contextual Design: Defining Customer-Centered Systems. Morgan Kaufmann, San Francisco (2009)
4. Chew, Y.C., Davison, B., Walker, B.N.: From design to deployment: an auditory graphing software for math education. In: Proceedings of the 29th Annual International Technology & Persons With Disabilities Conference, San Diego (2014)
5. Data-Driven DJ: An Introduction to Data-Driven DJ. datadrivendj.com
6. Allen, C.D., Ballman, D., Begg, V., Miller-Jacobs, H.H., Muller, M., Nielsen, J., Spool, J.: User involvement in the design process: why, when & how? pp. 251–254 (1993). https://doi.org/10.1145/169059.169203
7. Chew, Y.C.: Assessing the use of auditory graphs for middle school mathematics. Dissertation. https://www.cc.gatech.edu/~ychew3/assets/ChewDissertation.pdf
8. Summers, E., Langston, J., Allison, R., Cowley, J.: Using SAS/GRAPH® to Create Visualizations That Also Support Tactile and Auditory Interaction, SAS Institute Inc., Cary, North Carolina. https://analytics.ncsu.edu/sesug/2012/RI-15.pdf
9. Bell, E.C., Mino, N.M.: Employment Outcomes for Blind and Visually Impaired Adults. https://nfb.org/images/nfb/publications/jbir/jbir15/jbir050202.html
10. Freedom Scientific. BLINDNESS SOLUTIONS: JAWS®. Freedom Scientific. www.freedomscientific.com/Products/Blindness/JAWS
11. Hersh, M., Johnson, M.A.: Assistive Technology for Visually Impaired and Blind People. Springer, London (2014)
12. Flowers, J.H., Buhman, D.C., Turnage, K.D.: Cross-modal equivalence of visual and auditory scatterplots for exploring bivariate data samples. Hum. Factors **39**, 341–351 (1997)
13. Batterman, J.M., Martin, V.F., Yeung, D., Walker, B.N.: Connected cane: tactile button input for controlling gestures of iOS voiceover embedded in a white cane. Assist. Technol. **30**(2), 91–99 (2018). https://doi.org/10.1080/10400435.2016.1265024
14. Kondak, Z., Liang, T., Tomlinson, B., Walker, B.N.: Web sonification sandbox - an easy-to-use web application for sonifying data and equations. In: Proceedings of the 3rd Web Audio Conference, London, UK (2017). http://eecs.qmul.ac.uk/~keno/24.pdf
15. Leporini, B., Buzzi, M.C., Buzzi, M.: Interacting with mobile devices via VoiceOver: usability and accessibility issues, pp. 339–348 (2012). https://doi.org/10.1145/2414536.2414591
16. National Federation of the Blind: Statistical facts about blindness in the United States
17. https://nfb.org/blindnes-sstatistics (2014)
18. Neuhoff, J.G., Knight, R., Wayand, J.: Pitch change, sonification, and musical expertise: which way is up? July 2002. http://hdl.handle.net/1853/51370
19. Clark, R.E., Feldon, D.F., van Merriënboer, J., Yates, K.A., Early, S.: Cognitive task analysis. In: Handbook of Research on Educational Communications and Technology, Routledge (2007)
20. Thinking Aloud: The #1 Usability Tool. Nielsen Norman Group. www.nngroup.com/articles/thinking-aloud-the-1-usability-tool/

Man-Machine-Synchrony

Johan de Heer(✉)

Thales Research and Technology, Gebouw N,
Haaksbergerstraat 67, 7554 NB Hengelo, The Netherlands
Johan.deHeer@nl.thalesgroup.com

Abstract. The focus of this (provocative) position paper is on how humans and 'learning' machines team up. Specifically, we look into the concept of synchrony. Systems 'in sync' seem to perform better. Using hyperscanning methods from social neuroscience one may analyse if humans are 'in sync'. We suggest that this methodology might be applicable to study man-machine teaming as well. We hypothesize that various implementations of artificial neural nets lead to different levels of synchronizations with humans.

Keywords: Hyperscanning · Man-machine cooperation · Human behavior analytics

1 Introduction

We are at the beginning of a new technical (r)evolution towards systems with autonomous functions. Based on AI, machine learning techniques and deep learning frameworks the technical and operational potential is considerable [1]. The roadmap towards full autonomy faces many challenges. A step-wise implementation expects to see changes in human-machine interactions that evolve with increasing autonomous functions at the machine side. From human-in-the-loop to human-on-the-loop, and finally human-out-of-the-loop across a variety of human tasks. Man-machine teaming and harmonization in relation with human-machine performance is becoming a challenge in itself.

From both a system and human factors perspective concepts such as mutual trust, cooperation, coordination and even leadership between man and machines will become more important than ever. Do human 'operators' trust systems that learn and evolve, and make decisions on their own, do we allocate specific tasks to systems because they may do a more efficient job, who leads, follows, coordinates subsequent activities and tasks? And vice versa, do these evolving learning systems trust humans regarding their (moral)judgment and decision-making capabilities, which may be characterized by various perceptual and cognitive biases [2]?

In this work in progress paper we like to make the following contributions. First, we introduce the concept of synchronization, borrowed from [3]. Second, we will focus on human – human synchronization based on social neuroscience insights. In particular, we will look into the so-called hyperscanning methodology that allows for the simultaneously recording and analysis of brain activities and relating those to behavioral outcomes (and vice versa). We are intrigued by preliminary results from social neuroscience that indicate that teams 'in sync' perform better, and that we are able to

T. Ahram et al. (Eds.): IHIET 2019, AISC 1018, pp. 460–464, 2020.
https://doi.org/10.1007/978-3-030-25629-6_71

classify if people are in a collaborative mode, trust one another, coordinate their actions, et cetera based on their neural activities. Third, we briefly touch upon the debate if we may consider AI to be 'alive', since it evolves and learns over time. Deep learning techniques and frameworks are to a great extend inspired by biological solutions and aim to find a representative artificial solution. Fourth, if we assume that these artificial systems could be considered 'alive' and we may capture its artificial brain state next to its behavioral outcomes than we examine how these neural nets synchronize with our brains. We (simply) have to look for a kind of 'synchronization' measure. We therefore suggest that hyperscanning provides an interesting methodology to study man-machine synchronization. One may hypothesize, for example, that variations of deep learning implementations may lead to different levels of synchronization, and classifications of trust, collaboration, coordination and leadership. Finally, if man and machines are not 'in sync' but mutually depending on one another, we might even entrain them as such so they will synchronize.

2 Synchronization

The concept of synchronization as a universal concept in nonlinear sciences is well described by [3]. This paragraph is borrowed, copied, paraphrased from and inspired by these authors. Bits and pieces of texts are selected from their book and glued together to form this section. As they argue, synchronization refers to a variety of phenomena in almost all branches of natural sciences, engineering and social life. The phenomena appears to be rather diverse, however, obeys universal laws. Synchronization in biological systems is found from synchronous firing of neurons to different forms of cooperative behavior of insects, animals and humans. In essence, systems adjusts their rhythms to the rhythms of other systems. *The adjustments of rhythms due to an interaction is the essence of synchronization*. In general, the interaction between two systems is nonsymmetrical: one oscillator is more powerful than the other, and the frequency of the driven system is pulled towards the frequency of the drive. Synchronization can also be observed if more than two oscillators interact. Synchronization depends on the number of oscillators as well as on the strength and the type of interaction between each pair. As a consequence, different synchronous states are possible. As the authors mention, non-identical oscillators are like human beings each having their own personality. The driving inputs that come to an oscillator come from all others by one input from the whole ensemble. Indeed, we can say that each oscillator is driven by a force that is proportional to the sum of outputs of all oscillators in the ensemble. This force can entrain many oscillators if their frequencies are close. This force determines whether the systems synchronize, but it itself depends on their oscillation - it is a typical example of self-organization. As they note: to call a phenomenon synchronization, we must ensure that:

- We analyze the behavior of two (or more) self-sustained oscillators, i.e., systems capable of generating their own rhythms;
- The systems adjust their rhythms due to weak interactions;
- If the frequency of one oscillator is slowly varied, other systems follows this variation.

3 Hyperscanning

Hyperscanning technology from social neuroscience permits the study of the brain that underlie social interactions [4]. Hyperscanning is a method by which multiple individuals can interact with one another while their brains are simultaneously scanned. Several hyperscanning architectures have been employed using EEG, fMRI and fNIRS brain activity recordings. In Fig. 1 [taken from 5] a simplified schematic representation of the two main steps for – in this case - fNIRS-based hyperscanning applications is visualized. Data is recorded via a simultaneous measurement of optical imaging data from multiple participants in an experimental hyperscanning study. During the first step information on individual hemodynamic activities for each participant is obtained. Waveforms and activation maps are often used to represent brain data. In the second step of the analysis interpersonal synchronization and inter-brain coupling in hyperscanning is explored with e.g., correlation analysis, coherence analyses, Granger causality modelling.

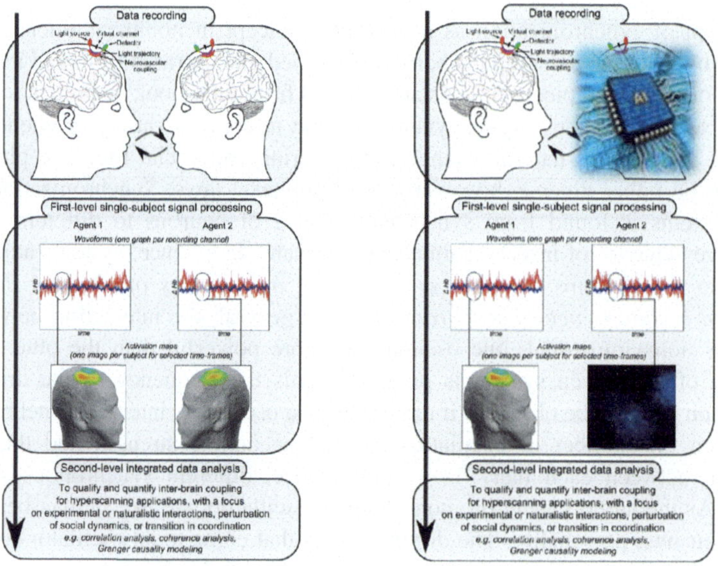

Fig. 1. Left: Framework of the study design from [5]. Right: see paragraph 5.

In addition, as proposed by [6] a network analysis could be the next step in the pipeline. Note that each step of the pipeline requires consideration to the selection of the best fitting method given theoretical and practical constraints, including the research hypothesis. First, brain activities from the number of participants (n) is simultaneously collected using, for example, fNIRS (step 1). In step 2 the oxygenated hemoglobin (HbO) signals from several region of interests (ROI) is averaged. In step 3 the network edge weights are obtained by calculating the correlation coefficients between the ROI-averaged time courses forming a n x n connection matrix. In step 4 the connection matrix is transformed into a binary network. Finally, the graph is visualized, and graph metrics can be used for further statistical analysis.

It has been found in hyperscanning studies that classification of human trust [7], cooperation, coordination and leadership is possible, in some cases even under high threat situations. For example, inter-brain activity coherence was found between participants that indicated better cooperation performance. [8]. Looking at interpersonal neural synchronization (INS) of gamma band oscillations it was that found that INS was enhanced when people are under high threat; increased gamma interbrain synchrony is associated with higher coordination [9]. It has been shown that INS is significantly higher between leaders and followers than between followers and followers, suggesting that leaders emerge by synchronizing their brain activity with that of the followers [10]. And it has been found that entities 'in sync' perform better [11].

4 Man-Machine Synchrony

Let's assume that AI could be considered a self-sustained oscillator and not a passive system that is just controlled by an electrical signal; meaning that it does not function if the signal disappears [3]. If that's the case then we could think of elucidating a metric to examine if human brain activity synchronizes with artificial neural net activities (see Fig. 1 – right). Although, we have no clue yet of what this metric could be. Recent work on visualizing the hidden activity of artificial neural networks may be a good start to look for such a metric [12]. Or, a synchrony based neural network architecture as put forward by [13] as a synchrony based approach for human-robot interaction might be an interesting option to examine. In any case, we hypothesize that various implementations of neural nets -, e.g., Perceptron, Feed Forward, Radial Basis Network, Deep Feed Forward, Recurrent Neural Network, Long/Short term memory, Gated Recurrent Unit, Auto Encoder (AE), Variational AE, Denoising AE, Sparse AE, Markov Chain, Hopfield Network, Boltzman Machine, Restricted BM, Deep Belief Network, Deep Convolutional Network, Deconvolutional Network, Deep Convolutional Inverse Graphics Network (see [13]) – may lead to various levels of correlations with human brain networks. Consequently, changes in human-machine-teaming performances. It would be of interest to start a series of empirical studies to study human-machine teaming ensembles' performances under various conditions of (entrained) neural net variations.

5 Conclusions

Over the last decade the hyperscanning methodology showed to be a valuable paradigm to study social neuroscience. The concept of synchronization is intriguing and we suggest that hyperscanning might be applied to study human brain – artificial network synchronizations. We hypothesized that variations of AI implementations may lead to different levels of synchronization, and classifications of trust, collaboration, coordination and leadership between humans and machines.

References

1. European Defence Agency: remote defence: unmanned and autonomous systems take hold in military toolboxes. EDM European Defence Matters, Issue #16 (2018)
2. Kahneman, D.: Thinking, Fast and Slow. Macmillan (2011). ISBN 978-1-4299-6935-2
3. Pikovsky, A., Rosenblum, M., Kurths, J.: Synchronization: A Universal Concept in Nonlinear Sciences. Cambridge University Press, Cambridge (2001)
4. Hirsch, J.: The grand challenge to understand the brain: neuroimaging by functional near-infrared spectroscopy. Shimadzu J. **5**(1) (2017). https://www.ssi.shimadzu.com/sites/ssi.shimadzu.com/files/Products/literature/Life_science/fnirs-article.pdf
5. Crivelli, D., Balconi, M.: Near-infrared spectroscopy applied to complex systems and human hyperscanning networking. Appl. Sci. **7**, 922 (2017). https://doi.org/10.3390/app7090922
6. Duan, L., Dai, R., Xiao, X., Sun, P., Li, Z., Zhu, C.: Cluster imaging of multi-brain networks (CIMBN): a general framework for hyperscanning and modeling a group of interacting brains. Front. Neurosci. (2015). https://doi.org/10.3389/fnins.2015.00267
7. Akash, K., Hu, W., Jain, N., Reid, T.: A classification model for sensing human trust in machines using EEG and GSR. ACM Trans. Interact. Intell. Syst. **8**(4) (2018). Article No. 27
8. Cui, X., Bryant, D.M., Reiss, A.L.: NIRS-based hyperscanning reveals increased interpersonal coherence in superior frontal cortex during cooperation. Neuroimage **59**(3), 2430–2437 (2012)
9. Mu, Y., Han, S., Gelfand, M.J.: The role of gamma interbrain synchrony in social coordination when humans face territorial threats. Soc. Cogn. Affect. Neurosci. **2017**, 1614–1623 (2017)
10. Jiang, J., Chen, C., Dai, B., Shi, G., Ding, G., Liu, L., Lu, C.: Leader emergence through interpersonal neural synchronization. In: Proceedings of the National Academy of Sciences, vol. 112, no. 14, pp. 4274–4279 (2015)
11. Szymanski, C., Pesquita, A., Brennan, A., Perdikis, D., Enns, J., Brick, T., Muller, V., Lindenberger, U.: Teams on the same wavelength perform better: inter-brain phase synchronization constitutes a neural substrate for social facilitation. Neuroimage **152**, 425–436 (2017)
12. Rauber, P.E., Fadl, S.G., Falcao, A.X., Telea, A.C.: Visualizing the hidden activity of artificial neural networks. IEEE Trans. Vis. Comput. Graph. **23**(1), 101–110 (2017)
13. Van Veen, F.: A mostly complete chart of neural networks (2016). https://towardsdatascience.com/the-mostly-complete-chart-of-neural-networks-explained-3fb6f2367464?gi=56bfca856969

User Experience Study of Live Streaming News with a Second Screen on a Mobile Device

Chien-Hsiung Chen(✉) and Liang-Yuan Che

Department of Design, National Taiwan University of Science and Technology, 10607 Taipei, Taiwan
cchen@mail.ntust.edu.tw, a3n7156@gmail.com

Abstract. With the increasing use of mobile devices, users in recent years tend to use their smart mobile phones or tablets to obtain instant information. While staying at home, users may also like to watch live streaming news on TV and utilize their mobile devices as a second screen to interact with the news in order to share feedbacks to friends or obtain more detailed information pertinent to that particular news. The purpose of this study is to investigate the user experience (UX) when users watch live streaming news on TV and use their smart mobile devices as a second screen for various social interaction requirements. It is hoped users will have more opportunities to share their viewpoints and search for more information regarding that particular news to the public, and their voices can easily be heard.

Keywords: User experience · Live streaming news · Interaction design · Second screen

1 Introduction

A TV is a popular entertainment device often used in a common household. Modern TVs are designed with smart functions that are able to receive news information from various channels, such as air broadcasting news, cable news, and on-line news via the Internet. In addition, a smart mobile device can also provide an important channel to help modern users obtain news information. As the rapid development of digital economy, many TV programs are considering using a second screen from a smart mobile device (i.e., mobile phones or tablets) to extend user interaction with the program, such as when users are watching live streaming news. This study is to explore an innovative user interface design regarding an interactive on-line TV as a social platform. That is, what kind of interaction style a user may adopt when they watch on-line TV? What type of information and value can be provided and added by using the applications in a smart mobile device? These interesting interaction design issues are investigated in this study.

Most of the users are used to watching daily news on TV together with other multimedia information. Nonetheless, users in the modern era also like to obtain instant information via Internet. The way of watching live stream news on the Internet was formed. Users like to watch TV news programs and at the same time browse through the Internet to obtain more detailed information pertinent to that particular news. Their

T. Ahram et al. (Eds.): IHIET 2019, AISC 1018, pp. 465–470, 2020.
https://doi.org/10.1007/978-3-030-25629-6_72

user experiences pertinent to this type of interaction style are worth of further investigation. In addition, many TV programs encourage their viewers to call in or send text comments to share their viewpoints on the program. Therefore, it has become the trend that providing a second screen by using a smart mobile device can help users obtain more relevant information and interact with the TV program to address their personal opinions to other on-line TV viewers.

2 Review of Literature

The term "user experience (UX)" often refers to a user's emotions and perceptions regarding the use of a particular product or a service. Forlizzi and Battarbee (2004) point out the importance of incorporating user experience in designing interactive systems. The user experience regarding how a user watches and interacts with a live streaming news program is important in facilitating the design of an easy-to-use user interface. In this study, the techniques of "persona" and "discount usability engineering" were adopted to facilitate the research process. The term "persona" was introduced by Cooper (2004) to be used as a practical interaction design tool to help define primary user groups. In fact, persona is a type of user profile descriptions created for each represented type of users. In addition, the technique of "discount usability engineering" proposed by Nielsen (1989, 1990) was also adopted in this study. It focuses on cheap, fast, and easy-to-use testing methods, such as user and task observations, scenarios, simplified thinking aloud, and heuristic evaluation. A brief discussion of these methods is provided as follows:

User and Task Observation: To an interaction designer, the purpose of user and task observation is to conduct a non-participant observation by watching users performing a particular task, i.e., the way to watch a live streaming news. Diaper (1989) argues that observation is not an easy technique, especially in the area of interaction design. It is difficult to record the user's behavior in sequence as well. Therefore, in this study, a series of live streaming news-watching tasks were defined in advance to help users perform the experiment.

Scenarios: Scenarios are personalized, fictional stories with characters, events, products and environments (Preece et al. 1994). They can be adopted to help explore design ideas and facilitate the usability testing of a proposed design. Because the scenario can be created in a small scale, an interaction designer can quickly modify it and test each design concepts in order to obtain quick and frequent feedback from users. In this study, the scenarios of watching a live streaming news were created based on the users' requirements generated from persona.

Simplified Thinking Aloud: The simplified thinking aloud method is performed by asking one user at one time to conduct a specific task while "thinking out loud." The interaction designer may find out not only how the user is interacting with the live streaming news interface, but also why s/he is doing it. This method provides the interaction designer with insights into the user's thinking process. These insights can help the interaction designer point out potential interaction problems and make appropriate design modifications. The simplified thinking aloud method was conducted during the users' live streaming news-watching experiment.

Heuristic Evaluation: The heuristic evaluation technique is used to find out obvious interaction problems that a user may encounter during the usability testing process. It requires expert users to perform the test because they have more user experience and can pinpoint potential problems better than novice users. It is also highly recommended to ask several expert users with different expertise to perform the heuristic evaluation because they may locate different types of interaction problems.

3 The Experiment

The way how a user holds and interacts with a smart mobile device are investigated in this study. That is, users use the mobile device as a second screen in horizontal or vertical styles are important regarding how the user interface is designed. A series of news-watching scenarios were created for the participants to conduct experimental tasks while interacting with the live streaming news on TV. At the same time, the users were required to use a smart mobile device as a second screen in horizontal or vertical styles (see Figs. 1 and 2).

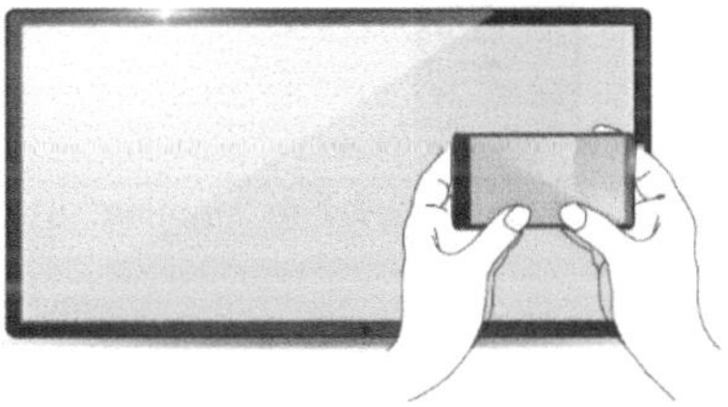

Fig. 1. Users use the mobile device as a second screen in horizontal style

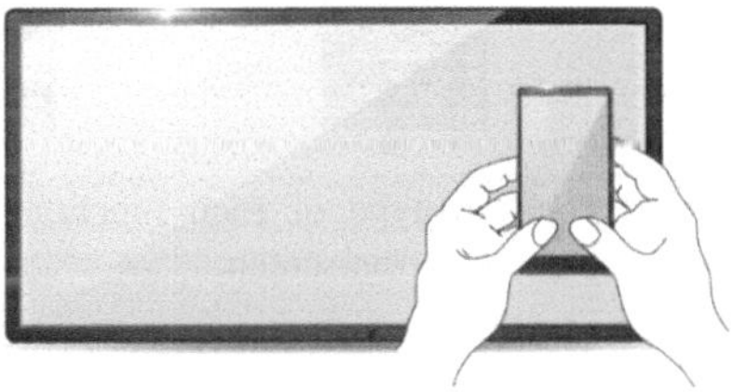

Fig. 2. Users use the mobile device as a second screen in vertical style

The design prototype was created using the Proto.io simulation application for the experimental purpose. The user interface framework was designed with initial screen, screen with function list, and chatroom in both interaction styles illustrated in Fig. 3.

The prototype designed based on the user interface framework was then incorporated with local news to simulate live streaming news (see Fig. 4). Participants were invited to take part in the experiment and perform the assigned tasks.

Before the experiment, a persona was conducted to help generate potential user profiles and evaluate the functions, interaction styles, and user interface designs of the second screen. Six primary users were invited to participate in the news-watching experiment to help obtain information regarding their user needs and requirements by the purposeful sampling method. The design prototypes were created using the Proto.io simulation application emphasizing different user interface designs for the experimental purposes. The simplified thinking aloud technique was used to help acquire users' thinking process and interaction steps when they conducted the assigned tasks.

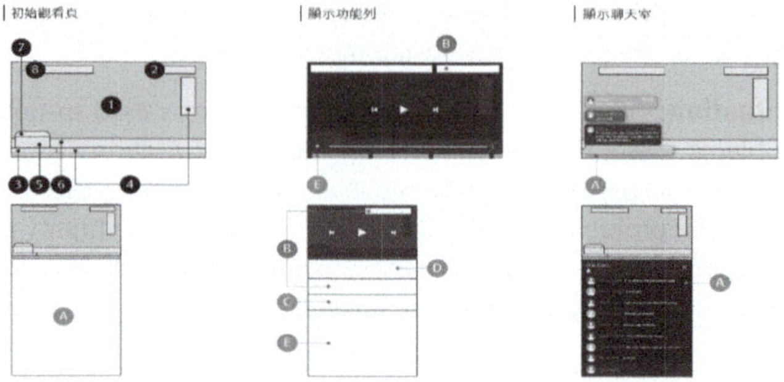

Fig. 3. The user interface framework of initial screen, screen with function list, and chatroom was designed in both horizontal and vertical styles

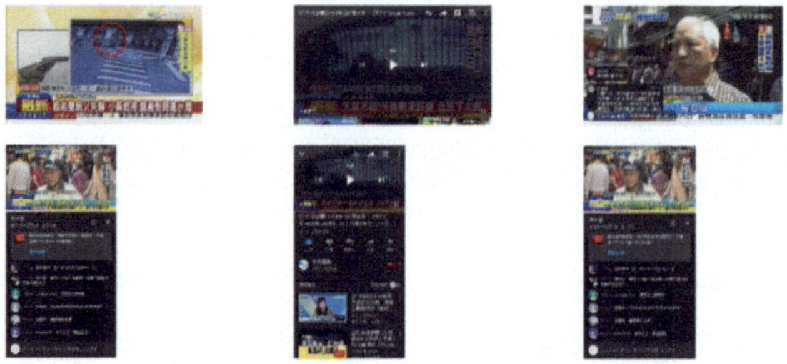

Fig. 4. The prototype of each function was incorporated with local news to simulate live streaming news on the screen

The collected data were analyzed and summarized to help create an innovative user interface for the second screen in the mobile device. After that, three expert users were invited to conduct heuristic evaluation to help find out potential interaction problems. Both observation and interview techniques were adopted for the expert users to help generate more usability testing information for further revision.

4 Results and Discussions

The six primary users were asked to conduct tasks regarding typical activities in watching a live streaming news, such as open the news channel, switch to different channels, and share the channel with a friend. The simplified thinking aloud method was used to help collect users' opinions. The findings were summarized. Among six primary users, five of them had successfully open the live streaming news channel. One user reported that by using keyword searching, it allowed him to obtain the needed news information more quickly than other search techniques. Another user reported that the screen design on the user interface tended to be too complicated to understand. It might take him to spend more time to search for some specific channels.

To those users who liked to hold their smart mobile devices in a vertical style, there existed few problems in leaving a message on the screen. Nonetheless, they might had problems in distinguishing the screen from comment-making area and chatting area. They also felt that the messages left by news readers were moving too fast. It is difficult for them to provide feedbacks or responses to those messages. In addition, to those who liked to hold their smart mobile devices in a horizontal style, the screen position of chatting area might block the live streaming news screen. This might affect their internal feelings. All of them agreed that when interacting with the live streaming news in a horizontal style, the chatting function should be disabled to avoid the news-blocking problem. Moreover, when the users were watching a news with a video clip in the horizontal style, the disabled chatroom function would allow them to concentrate more on the video. By so doing would increase their user experience as well.

In terms of sharing news to a friend, two of the users reported that this task was easy to achieve. One of them liked to click on the located top-right sharing button to share the news to a friend. This is because this button can be noticed easily when a user is watching a video clip.

The results generated from three expert users' heuristic evaluations reported that all of them could open the live streaming news without any problem. Among them, one expert user suggested that the functions of sharing a news, leaving a message, and offering a comment could be incorporated into the same structure level to help catch users' attention. In addition, one expert users reported that the user experience of long-pressing a button just like the function used in other chatroom could be adopted to increase interface usability. Making a comment directly to a particular user in the chatroom is important and the task should be conducted quickly without any problem. Two of the expert users suggested that the message-leaving function could be designed with a popup style. Users were able to turn on or turn off the function and define the degree of transparency to help increase its readability. It is very likely that a user might receive phone calls or other instant messages while watching a live streaming news. It is highly suggested that the live streaming news can be left in the background when a user is required to interact with other applications in the same mobile device. Once the additional task is completed, the user can go back to the live streaming news immediately without opening the application again.

5 Conclusions

After the experiment was completed and the data were analyzed, the generated results revealed that: (1) The messages left by news readers on the screen should be displayed with a certain speed so that users are able to provide feedbacks or responses to those messages. (2) When the user interface is designed to be used in a horizontal style, it is important that the screen position of chatting area should not block the live streaming news area to help increase the news readability. By so doing would increase their user experience as well. (3) It is important to provide an obvious button (often located on the top-right screen) to help users share the news with a friend. This is because this button can be noticed easily when a user is watching a video clip. (4) The functions of sharing a news, leaving a message, and offering a comment can be incorporated into the same structure level to help catch users' attention. (5) Providing a way of long-pressing a button just like the function used in other chatroom is important to help increase interface usability. (6) It is important that the live streaming news can be left in the background when a user is required to interact with other applications in the same mobile device. Once the additional task is completed, the user can go back to the live streaming news immediately without opening the application again.

It is hoped that the proposed interface design suggestions for the second screen of a smart mobile device can meet with users' mental models and offer them a good interface usability to satisfy their interaction needs and requirements. Users will have more opportunities to share their viewpoints and search for more information regarding that particular live stream news to the public so that their voices can easily be heard.

Acknowledgments. Financial support of this study is provided by the Ministry of Science and Technology under the grant number of MOST 105-2410-H-011-012-MY3.

References

Cooper, A.: The Inmates Are Running the Asylum: Why High-Tech Products Drive Us Crazy and How to Restore the Sanit. SAMS Publishing, Indianapolis (2004)

Diaper, D.: Task Analysis for Human-Computer Interaction. Ellis Horwood, Chichester (1989)

Forlizzi, J., Battarbee, K.: Understanding experience in interactive systems. In: Proceedings of the 5th Conference on Designing Interactive Systems: Processes, Practices, Methods, and Techniques, pp. 261–268. ACM, Cambridge (2004)

Nielsen, J.: Usability engineering at a discount. In: Salvendy, G., Smith, M.J. (eds.) Designing and Using Human-Computer Interface and Knowledge Based Systems. Elsevier, Amsterdam (1989)

Nielsen, J.: Big paybacks from 'discount' usability engineering. IEEE Softw. **7**(3), 107–108 (1990)

Preece, J., Rogers, Y., Sharp, H., Benyon, D., Holland, S., Carey, T.: Human-Computer Interaction. Addison-Wesley, Harlow (1994)

Barcode Representation of Face Image Combining LGFA and Windowing Technique

Sanjoy Ghatak[1(✉)] and Debotosh Bhattacharjee[2]

[1] Department of CSE, Sikkim Manipal Institute of Technology, Majitar, Sikkim, India
sanjoylcs@yahoo.co.in

[2] Department of CSE, Jadavpur University, Kolkata, West Bengal, India
debotoshb@hotmail.com

Abstract. This paper represents a novel work for standard type rectilinear barcode from illumination invariant confront pictures. This method finds out the qualification in slopes of picture sparkle utilizing LGFA and Windowing technique, at that point, it requires discovering normal of the angles into a limited number of interims utilizing standardization. After this, the aftereffect of quantization is changed over into the breaking points of decimal digits from zero to nine and the chart is converted into an extreme straight standardized identification. Surely, the present strategy creates the quality sort direct EAN-8 standardized tag of the best piece of face picture. In any case, in the present work, a system which is proposed to extract edge-based information utilizing LGFA and window method. LGFA helps us to generate gradient information from illumination invariant face image and by using the windowing technique; we scan the input image horizontally and take the upper 75% and 70% of the gradients. The barcode for these two cases are extracted from face images of five datasets, and it is found that the present technique is useful to account, discovery, acknowledgment and look for people in a group.

Keywords: LGFA · Facial picture · EAN-8 barcode · Image angle · Real-time framework · Illumination invariant face image

1 Introduction

Scanner tag innovation is an essential innovation in our regular day-to-day existence for recognizable proof of different item, merchandise, fund records, installments, promoting materials and administrations. The method, which described standardized tags mark on the individual body, does exclude any biometrical highlights of individual [1]. If a scanner tag brings some biometric characteristics, it will be taken up as a "popular token," as well as the reasonable arrangement of human acknowledgment. Some techniques [4, 5] already exist for tagging human face information as a bar code, but those suffering from the constraint of illumination variation aspect of human face images. To overcome this problem, a new approach is introduced in this paper. The name of this approach is "Bar code representation of face image combining LGFA and windowing technique. In [11], it is noticed that LG-Faces are more effective for light

T. Ahram et al. (Eds.): IHIET 2019, AISC 1018, pp. 471–475, 2020.
https://doi.org/10.1007/978-3-030-25629-6_73

invariant and heterogeneous face acknowledgment. This approach also performs consistently within sight of muddled variety, i.e. involvement of noise and disguise. Different illumination conditions create a key barrier to face recognition and quality bar code generation because they can greatly affect the looks of the facial image, therefore strongly increasing the inter-class variation. It has been observed that the execution of the face acknowledgment framework is significantly degraded if the illumination of face images is changed. So, in this method, for generating linear barcode, both windowing technique and LGFA have been considered.

This paper is organized as Sect. 1 for Introduction; Sect. 2 describes the proposed approach: Sect. 3 contains experimental results, and the paper is concluded in Sect. 4.

2 Proposed Approach

The technique, proposed in this paper and shown in Fig. 1, consists of the following four steps: (a) Image preliminary processing (b) Feature Extraction using LGFA and window technique (c) Feature coding (d) Barcode maker.

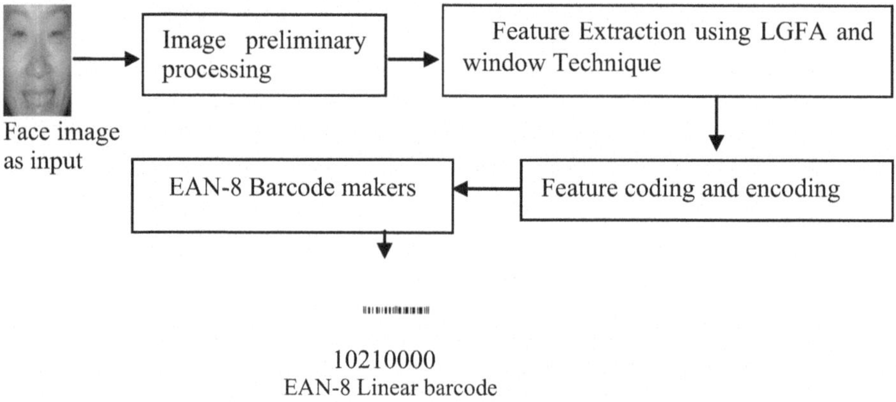

Fig. 1. Ventures of EAN-8 scanner tag generation

Image Preliminary Processing: Facial area is cropped from the background, and median filtering is applied to remove noise.

Feature Extraction Using LGFA and Window Technique: For features extraction, LGFA is used. LGFA is based on illumination Reflectance model, which is described in the paper [12]. To take out the light part from the image, Division Method Applied to sets of connecting pixels. LGFA is the combination of the law of universal gravitation which is described in the paper [11, 14] and Local Gravity face (LG-face) which is explained in the paper [11, 13]. The formulas, which are used for calculating local gravity faced, are discussed in the paper [11]. Following formula are used for local gravity face angle:

$$\alpha = \arctan\left(\frac{-\frac{R_2}{2\sqrt{2}} - R_3 - \frac{R_4}{2\sqrt{2}} + \frac{R_6}{2\sqrt{2}} + R_7 + \frac{R_8}{2\sqrt{2}}}{-R_1 - \frac{R_2}{2\sqrt{2}} + \frac{R_4}{2\sqrt{2}} + R_5 + \frac{R_6}{2\sqrt{2}} - \frac{R_8}{2\sqrt{2}}}\right) \tag{1}$$

Applying this formula, gradients are computed, and an image formed by gradients; thus computed is shown in Fig. 2(b).

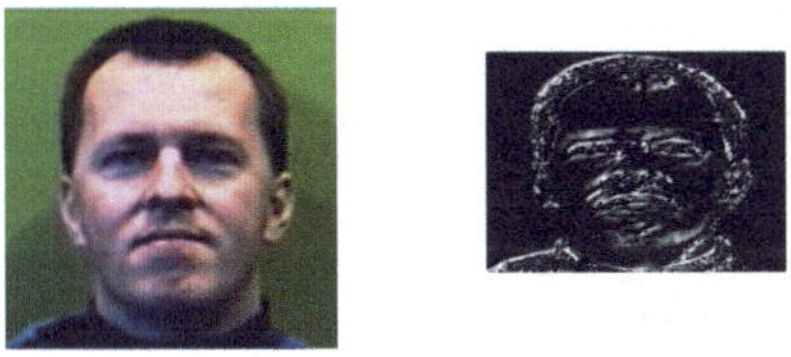

(a) (b)

Fig. 2. (a) Actual face image; (b) Gradient of actual face image after applying LGFA

After getting the image gradient by using LGFA, window technique is applied in image gradient, which is discussed in the paper [2, 3, 10]. For generating a stable bar code, the windowing technique has been used.In window technique; sliding window is applied for scan the image gradient of face image. It start scanning at the "hair/sanctuaries" obliges and concluded at the nether uttermost spans of the nose. Human face scanning start from the forehead and end below the nose using the window. Window is one unit square mask. It scans the face horizontally because most of the information of human face is kept in horizontally. Details of window technique are discussed in paper [2, 3].

Feature Coding and Encoding: Encoding is performing by a vital number of decimal digits. For feature code, succeeding errands are conducted which is discussed in paper [10]. Components of the angle (vectors) are standardized to an extreme estimation of inclination (max_gradient).

EAN-8 Barcode Marker: At this stage, the last eight digits EAN-8 standardized tag is created. Figure 3 demonstrates the last yield of info picture, which is spoken to as an EAN-8 direct standardized identification. Add up to quantities of digits are 8 in this scanner tag. Yield of eight digits, the eighth digit is contemplated as checksum digit for the initial seven digits. A detail of EAN-8 barcode and checksum digit is described in the paper [10]. In Fig. 3 checksum digit is 2. The checksum digit is used for error correction.

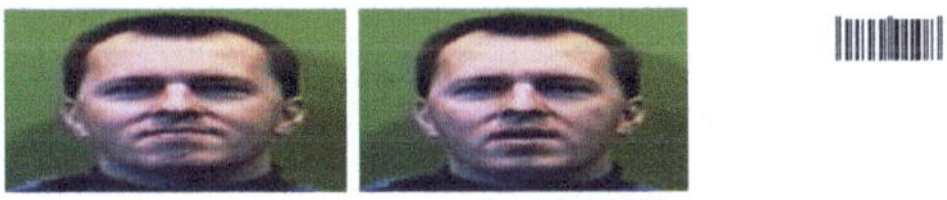

11001102
EAN-8 linear Barcode

Fig. 3. EAN-8 straight barcode

3 Experimental Results

Experiments are carried out to evaluate the durability of made systematized tag of the face picture in various face affirmation conditions. In this procedure, experiments are conducted on a few datasets: “Face94” [6], “Face Dataset YaleB” [8], “FERET face dataset” [7], “FG-NET creating face dataset” [9], “NIR-VIS edited dataset” [15], “LWF Dataset” [16] and “a composite appearances face dataset at changed ages”. The systematized tag is made in light of 70%, and 75% of the top bit of the facial image except for the part hack down the purpose of the assembly of the nose/mouth for check the idea of scanner label utilizing the LGFA and Windowing Technique. The comparative result of windowing technique and combining LGFA and window technique is shown in Tables 1 and 2. From these tables, it is clear that more stable barcode can be generated from illumination invariant face image using the proposed method i.e. combination of LGFA and windowing technique.

Table 1. Accuracy rate of creating institutionalized labels for different datasets.

Name of dataset	Windowing technique		Combining LGFA and windowing technique	
	75% of upper face image	70% of upper face image	75% of upper face image	70% of upper face image
FACE94 dataset	78	80	80	85
FERET database	65	70	75	80
Face dataset YaleB	10	15	70	75
NIR-VIS cropped dataset	15	20	70	73
IFW dataset	20	25	70	72

Table 2. Examine the rate of life of the made scanner labels to developing of looks.

Name of dataset	Window technique		Combining LGFA and windowing technique	
	75% of upper face image	70% of Upper face image	75% of upper face image	70% of upper face image
Aging dataset FG-NET	75	80	80	85
Aging dataset of composite faces	80	83	81	85

4 Conclusions

The paper demonstrates a novel calculation for face acknowledgment utilizing straight EAN-8 scanner tags. This proposed system of making straight EAN-8 standardized tags from face pictures is expanded on the utilization of the window procedure, inclinations computation, angle bearings, standardization, and quantization. At last, input faces are converted to tags with the assistance of EAN-8 straight standardized identifications. Dataset Face94, Face dataset YaleB, dataset FERET, Aging dataset FG-NET, composite face database (total No. 20), NIR-VIS cropped dataset and LWF dataset are used for performing the test. The test works out as expected had shown that the calculation which is depicted confirmation the idea of the made standardized names by uprightness of slight reflecting of the main image, when the plane, point, and apparent looks became different. This standardized identification can be used for an account, recognizing confirmation, affirmation and search for individual

References

1. Barcode/Tattoos. http://www.barcodeart.com/store/wearable/tattoos/. Accessed 15 Mar 2014
2. Matveev, Y., Kukharev, G., Shchegoleva, N.: A simple method for generating facial barcodes. In: Conference on Computer Graphics, Visualization and Computer Vision in Co-operation with EUROGRAPHICS Association Exchange Anisotropy, WSCG 2014, Academic, Czech Republic, pp. 213–220 (2014)
3. Kukharev, G., Matveev, Y., Shchegoleva, N.: Barcode generation for face images. Data Analysis and Intellectual System, Business Information No 3(29) (2014)
4. Forczmanski, P., Kukharev, G., Shchegoleva, N.: An algorithm of face recognition under difficult lighting conditions. Electr. Rev. **88**(10), 201–204 (2012)
5. Matveev, Y.N.: Technologies of biometric identification of a person by voice and other modalities. Vestnik MGTU, Priborostroenie, Special Issue "Biometric Technologies", pp. 46–61 (2012). (in Russian)
6. Face94 database. http://cswww.essex.ac.uk/mvallfaces/face94.html
7. CHUK face Sketch FERET database. http://mmlab.ie.cuhk.edu.hk/cufsf
8. http://cvc.yale.edu/projects/yalefacesB/yalefacesB.html
9. FG-NET Aging database (2010). http://www.fgnet.rsunit.com
10. Ghatak, S.: Facial representation using linear barcode. In: Bhattacharyya, S., Chaki, N., Konar, D., Chakraborty, U., Singh, C. (eds.) Advanced Computational and Communication Paradigms, vol. 2, pp. 791–801. Springer, Singapore (2018)
11. Roy, H., Bhattacharjee, D.: Local-Gravity-Face (LG-face) for illumination invariant and heterogeneous face recognition. IEEE Trans. Inf. Forensics Secur. **11**(7), 1412–1424 (2016)
12. Horn, B.K.P.: Robot-Vision. MIT Press, Cambridge (2011)
13. Kundu, S.: Gravitational clustering: a new approach based on the spatial distribution of the points. Pattern Recogn. **32**(7), 1149–1160 (1999)
14. Olenick, R.P., Apostol, T.M., Goodstein, D.L.: The Mechanical Universe: Mechanics and Heat. Cambridge University Press, New York (1985)
15. Li, S.Z., Yi, D., Lei, Z., Liao, S.: The Casia NIR-VIS 2.0 face database. In: IEEE Conference on Computer Vision and Pattern Recognition Workshops, pp. 348–353 (2013)
16. Kawulok, M., Emre Celebi, M., Smolka, B. (eds.): Advances in Face Detection and Facial Image Analysis, pp. 189–248 (2016)

A Pilot Study on Interactive Information Visualization of Multi-dimensional Data

Ting Tan(✉) and Zhanxun Dong

School of Design, Shanghai Jiao Tong University, No. 800 Dongchuan Road, Minhang District, Shanghai, China
{tanting, dongzx}@sjtu.edu.cn

Abstract. In recent years, with the popularity of electronic products, interactive information visualization has been widely used in various fields. In this paper, we describe a solution of interactive information visualization applied in displaying the bird habitat information and discussed what level of optimizations is achieved and what remains to be done. The experimental results show an increase in the efficiency of users collecting information and user satisfaction when the Zijingang Birdwatching Guide is used. This pilot study provides opportunities for further improvement on bird protection and interactive information visualization.

Keywords: Information design · Interaction · Multi-dimensional data

1 Introduction

Interactive information visualization is an information display method that adds interactive experience to information visualization. Compared with traditional information visualization, it can express more information and be more vivid. In recent years, with the popularity of electronic products, interactive information visualization has been widely used in medical, educational, and industrial fields.

In this paper, we introduce the Zijingang Birdwatching Guide, an application using interactive information visualization as the core to display multi-dimensional information about bird protection in the Zijingang Habitat in Hangzhou, Zhejiang Province, China. The Zijingang Birdwatching Guide is taken as a case to study how interactive information visualization can improve the efficiency of information expression when dealing with multi-dimensional information and discuss the application prospect of interactive information visualization.

Two experiments were done among 40 students from Shanghai Jiao Tong University, China. These students were divided into experimental group and control group. In the first experiment, in order to compare the efficiency of two methods, the Zijingang Birdwatching Guide and the traditional charting application, two groups were asked to use two methods respectively to get the same amount of information. In the second experiment, two groups were asked to use two different versions of the Zijingang Birdwatching Guide, one with interactive prompts, such as prompt bubbles, and one without, to evaluate the impact of two versions on user satisfaction.

T. Ahram et al. (Eds.): IHIET 2019, AISC 1018, pp. 476–481, 2020.
https://doi.org/10.1007/978-3-030-25629-6_74

2 Relate Work

Currently, interactive information visualization has applied research in many areas, In 2015, the American Medical Informatics Association (AMIA) officially established a Visual Analysis Working Group to study the development of information visualization in the medical field [1]. In education, Guolong Quan and Xiaoqing Gu have determined how students use visualization tools to distinguish the behavior features of learners [2]. Jeffrey Heer, Stuart K. Card et al. have created prefuse, a software framework for creating dynamic visualizations [3].

In the aspect of multi-dimensional information analysis, David HS Chung, Philip A Legg et al. present a glyph-based conceptual framework as part of a visualization process for interactive sorting of multivariate data. They focused on glyph-based sorting framework design, giving analysts new insights [4]. At the same time, many people have made efforts in the collection and sharing of raw data, Chia-Yuan Lin implement an automatic bird data capture system from social network websites and stores them in the database [5].

3 Zijinggang Birdwatching Guide

Zijingang Birdwatching Guide is the application to display the information of birds in Zijingang habitat, in Hangzhou, Zhejiang province, China. Zijinggang Birdwatching Guide uses interactive information visualization to display multi-dimensional information of local birds. The paper takes the design procedure of Zijinggang Birdwatching Guide as the example to discusses the relationship between using interactive information visualization to display multidimensional information and the efficiency of users getting information.

There are three steps to design the Zijingang Birdwatching Guide, namely, (1) selecting a bird habitat, and collecting the data of local birds; (2) determining the dimension of information; (3) formulating a reasonable display method and creating an interactive information display carrier. Here, the Zijingang Birdwatching Guide is taken as a case to study how interactive information visualization can improve the efficiency of information expression when dealing with multi-dimensional information and discuss the application prospect of interactive information visualization. Figure 1 shows the steps to design the Zijingang Birdwatching Guide.

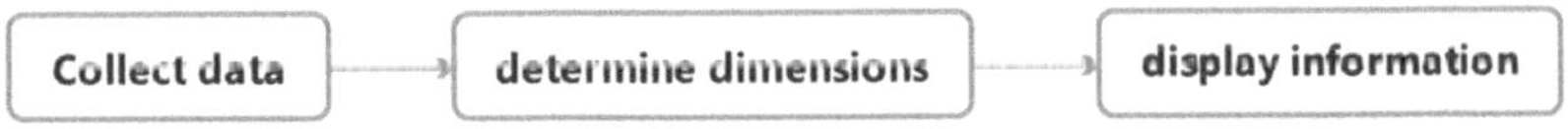

Fig. 1. Steps to design the Zijingang Birdwatching Guide.

3.1 Data Sources

Zijinggang habitat is located around Xixi-Wetland, Hangzhou, Zhejiang Province, China. The habitat has a rich diversity of birds. Not only there are many kinds of birds permanently inhabiting here, but also a variety of birds stay here temporarily during migration.

The data of this application are obtained from many sources, including logs from local bird watchers, Chinese bird-watching websites, China Weather, and so on. The information includes the occurrence of each bird at each location of the day in a year, weather and temperature of each day, air quality index (AQI), and introductions of each kind of bird, etc.

3.2 Data Dimension

The collected data can be classified into three dimensions, namely Location Dimension, Time Dimension, and Bird Information Dimension, which are represented respectively by "where", "when", and "what" in the frame of bird information in Fig. 2.

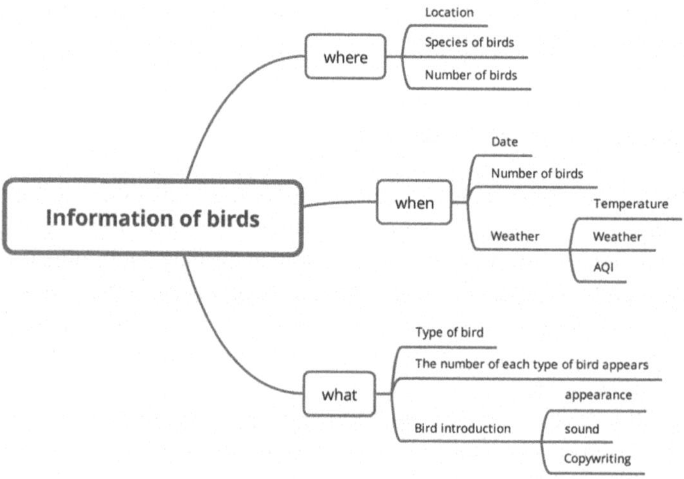

Fig. 2. The frame of bird information.

Location Dimension consists of the number of bird species and the occurrence rates in each position. Weather and temperature of each day and the number of birds is classified to Time Dimension. Bird Information Dimension includes the appearances, voices and text introduction of each bird species.

3.3 Display Mode

Figure 3 is the main interface of Zijingang Birdwatching Guide. There are relations between three dimensions of bird information. Location Dimension is displayed by the electronic map, which can show the distribution of birds in the habitat, as shown in Fig. 3(a). When users click at one position in the electronic map, Time Dimension information of this position will appear.

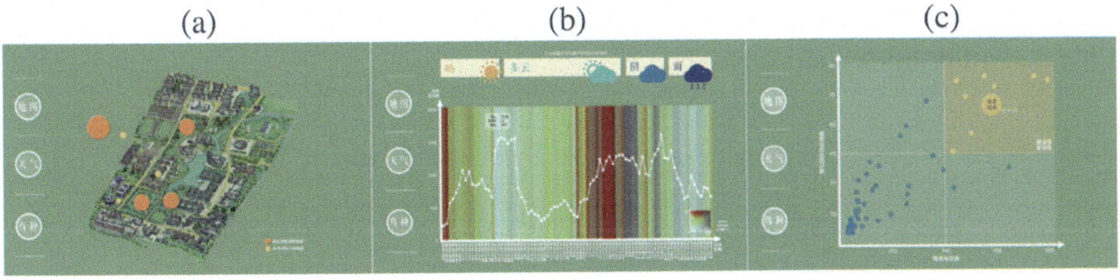

Fig. 3. The main interface of Zijingang Birdwatching Guide.

Figure 3(b) is the chart of Time Dimension. The background color temperature indicates the temperature of the day, color saturation represents AQI, the line indicates the bird number of the day. The detailed information of the day will appear, when the cursor stays at the corresponding position. The user interface will show weather and temperature information individually, when the users click on the Weather Button above.

Figure 3(c) is the chart of Bird Information Dimension. The horizontal axis is the total number of one kind of bird appearing in one year, and the vertical axis is the total days of this kind of bird appearing in one year. The migratory bird and native bird can be distinguished, and the most normal bird species can be concluded by this chart. The popup window of detailed introduction of the bird will appear, including photograph, sound button, and text introduction, when the users click on the points in the chart.

4 Experiment and Discussion

Two experiments were done among 40 students. These students were divided into two groups equally, that is, experimental group and control group. In the first experiment, in order to compare the efficiency of two methods, the Zijingang Birdwatching guide and the traditional charting application, two groups were asked to use two methods respectively to get the same amount of information. In the second experiment, two groups were asked to use two different versions of the Zijingang Birdwatching Guide, one with interactive prompts, such as prompt bubbles, and one without, to evaluate the impact of two versions on user satisfaction.

4.1 Experimental Design

The first group is asked to finish the Experiment I. 20 students are required to search one specific information by the traditional charting application realized by Microsoft Excel and Zijingang Birdwatching Guide respectively. The time that the students spend in getting the same amount of information by two different methods are recorded and compared.

The second group is asked to finish the Experiment II. The other 20 students are required to search the specific information by two different versions of Zijingang Birdwatching Guide. The consumed time are recorded respectively and compared.

Figure 4 is the interfaces of two versions. The first version doesn't have prompt bubbles, while the second one has.

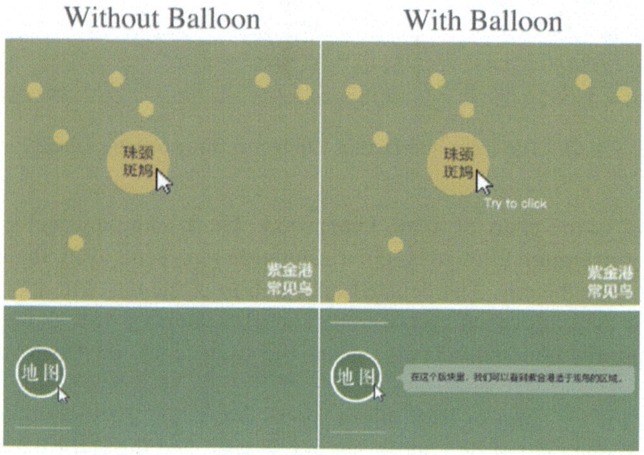

Fig. 4. The interfaces of two versions of Zijingang Birdwatching Guide.

4.2 Results and Analysis

The results of the first experiment are displayed in Table 1. In term of efficiency, the results show an increase in the efficiency of users collecting information and user satisfaction when the Zijingang Birdwatching Guide is used. The average consumed time is reduced by 2.35 min, and the efficiency of 85% of students collecting information is well improved.

Table 1. Number of people in each time period in experiment one.

Time	Traditional chart	Zijingang Birdwatching Guide
<1 min	0	2
1–2 min	1	5
2–3 min	4	9
3–4 min	8	3
4–5 min	5	1
>5 min	2	0

The results of the second experiment are displayed in Table 2. The second version with hint messages in prompt bubbles has better user experience, because the users can find the way to the next interface more easily under the guidance of prompt bubbles. The experiment also indicates that users will lose their patience if the Zijingang Birdwatching Guide doesn't response their requests in 5 s.

Table 2. Number of people in each time period in experiment one.

Time	Zijingang Birdwatching Guide without balloon	Zijingang Birdwatching Guide with balloon
<1 min	0	4
1–2 min	1	9
2–3 min	1	5
3–4 min	7	2
4–5 min	7	0
>5 min	4	0

5 Conclusion and Future Work

In this paper, we describe a solution of interactive information visualization applied in displaying the bird habitat information. The first experiment proves the efficiency of collecting information by the interactive information visualization can be improved. The second experiment indicates interactive prompts, such as prompt bubbles, in interactive information visualization can improve user satisfaction.

In the future work, we will continue to optimize the user experience of Zijingang Birdwatching Guide by interactive information visualization, such as further improving the efficiency of collecting information and displaying the information by VR/AR.

References

1. Gotz, D., Borland, D.: Data-driven healthcare: challenges and opportunities for interactive visualization. IEEE Comput. Graphics Appl. **36**(3), 90–96 (2016)
2. Quan, G., Xiaoqing, G.: Visualization forms in the cross-cultural collaborative activities of design and development of a digital resource for education. J. Educ. Comput. Res. **56**(3), 439–463 (2018)
3. Heer, J., Card, S.K., Landay, J.A.: Prefuse: a toolkit for interactive in-formation visualization. In: Proceedings of the SIGCHI Conference on Human Factors in Computing Systems. ACM (2005)
4. Chung, D.H.S., et al.: Glyph sorting: interactive visualization for multi-dimensional data. Inf. Vis. **14**(1), 76–90 (2015)
5. Lin, C.-Y., et al.: The design of automatic bird data capture systems. In: 2018 IEEE International Conference on Consumer Electronics-Taiwan (ICCE-TW). IEEE (2018)

Smart Learning Environments: A Blend of ICT Achievements and Smart Pedagogy for the World Sustainable Development

Vasiliki Karampa(✉) and Foteini Paraskeva

Department of Digital Systems, University of Piraeus, Karaoli Dimitriou Street 80, 185 34 Piraeus, Greece
{bkarampa, fparaske}@unipi.gr

Abstract. In the context of a sustainable development the mitigation of the energy consumption could be achieved by the incorporation of Information and Communication Technology (ICT) as well as the exploitation of smart computing in every day sectors, formulating a smart society constituted by energy conscious citizens. According to this assumption a smart society is necessary to be built on foundations of a smart education which aims to orchestrate best practices and methods based on smart pedagogies, in order to accomplish optimized learning through the development of Smart Learning Environments (SLEs). This paper presents the emergency of developing SLEs as a robust solution for the humans' well-being. It classifies the fundamental features of SLEs highlighted by the international literature the past decade, into affordances arising from services that come from both accelerating technological achievements and pedagogical issues regarding energy. It also provides conclusions that foster research to this direction.

Keywords: Smart Learning Environments (SLEs) · Smart pedagogy sustainable · Development

1 Introduction

Faced with the phenomenon of climate change, energy over-consumption as well as the emergency for green planet, international organizations [1–3] and large electronics and telecommunications companies e.g. Ericsson [4], collectively formulate energy saving policies in line with the UNESCO's sustainable development goals [5]. These policies lead to the development of smart ecosystems [6], which in turn compose a "smart society", that is, an environmentally friendly, safe and comfortable and where citizens share high quality goods, products and services.

However, a smart society is established on the foundations of a smart education that not only incorporates the rapidly advancing information and communication technological (ICT) achievements, but above all, orchestrates best practices and methods to provide optimized learning. Therefore, the development of that kind of learning environments, also called "smart learning environments" SLEs [7], sets all the conditions for the emergence of "smart" learners who will dispose digital competences and high order thinking skills, and will be capable of solving the major problems of the

T. Ahram et al. (Eds.): IHIET 2019, AISC 1018, pp. 482–488, 2020.
https://doi.org/10.1007/978-3-030-25629-6_75

humanity. Beyond the incorporation of modern technological achievements and the diffusion of intelligent computing into all areas of life, including educational institutions (schools, universities and campuses), the goal of sustainable development is achieved through education and learning.

The international literature highlights the need for rethinking and evolving pedagogy in our century [8], as to better support the acquisition of skills and competences. According to this point of view, the present article highlights the paving way to sustainable development and citizens' well-being. It indicates basic features of smart learning environments, in order to provide opportunities for efficient learning and eventually transform learners into future operators of the energy field. Therefore, the authors attempt to classify these features into affordances arising from both technological advances and pedagogical and learning aspects over the energy sector and provide conclusions in order to foster research in this direction.

2 Smart Learning Environments

Over the past few years researchers are been striving to illuminate the vast and prominent area of Smart Learning Environments, by articulating definitions and conceptual frameworks [9–15]. They mainly focus on the aspects of the three basic disciplines: (a) education, (b) computer science and (c) organization & management. Considering that a learning environment is determined by giving precise answers to the dimensions of space, time, technology, control and interaction [16], most researchers argue that the potential of SLEs is enhanced by a series of words that in turn imply smart services. Therefore, international research is predominantly dominated by the words: fast, flexible, comfortable, efficient, effective, scalable, engaging, motivating, adaptive, reflective, collaborative, that can in total be replaced by a single word, that of "optimized". From the authors' viewpoint, the following sections give a clear picture of the words mentioned before, translated into affordances and distributed to the two key components of the SLE blend referring to the energy perspective: ICT and Pedagogy.

2.1 The "ICT" Component: Digitization for Energy Saving and Energy Efficiency

Nowadays, global warming and climate change are crucial issues for all the citizens of the world. The reduction in greenhouse gas emissions mainly from the industrial sector, the rising cost of fossil fuels (coal, oil, natural gas) and the lack of such resources lead to policy-making towards sustainable development. A positive direction is maximizing energy savings with international initiatives to increase energy efficiency [17] in industry [18], transport, buildings [19, 20], housing and appliances, as well as drafting laws and regulations to establish efficiency standards, financial incentives, tax credits and funding of research programs. In this context, the European Commission in specific, announces policies regarding three key factors known as 3D: decarbonization, decentralization and digitization.

With respect to the digitization, these policies underline the growing importance of ICT [21] for energy efficiency. The guidelines for safe, clean and efficient energy include the capabilities of smart controls, sensors and network actuators, smart components and systems and advanced programming algorithms [22]. Lighting, robotics, nanoelectronics, flexible and portable electronics are important digitalized technologies in the industry. In addition, IoT digital technologies, Big Data and cloud computing technologies allow a wide range of competitive solutions in the energy sector, including renewable energy, smart grids and energy storage and conservation as well. In other words, Europe's dominant trend is "Smart Everything Everywhere". However, while the rate of digitization is accelerating and covering more and more key areas of the European data infrastructure, there are still significant shortcomings in areas such as education. From this perspective, digitization in the educational sector could be represented by the development of smart learning environments mainly laid on two layers: (a) the core layer, encompassing the hardware, namely smart technological infrastructure for pervasive computing, networking and storage, electronic devices connected to others or networks for collecting data mainly through sensors or sensing technologies (e.g. RFID, GPS and QR codes) as well as computers and mobile devices, interactive whiteboards, smart tables, e-bags, smartphones, wearable devices, etc. [9] (b) the software layer of smart applications such as learning analytics, big data analytics and augmented reality (AR) [9, 15]. Hence, smart services arise from the innovative technological incorporation, providing the following affordances:

Mobility, Portability and Affordability. The emergence of mobile devices has transformed learners to nomadic users, who carry small, eco-friendly and portable devices and use computing resources anywhere, at any time. Innovative techniques like wireless charging, improve functionality and efficiency, providing opportunities for energy replenishment at low cost [23].

Awareness. In the context of ambient intelligence, awareness consists of learners' location, situation and context. The exploitation of more energy-efficient 5G technology provides extremely fast, very stable and highly versatile data transportation between devices and learning systems [4, 9].

Interoperability. It implies operation between different standards of learning resources, services, and platforms [11]. Standardization, in turn implies energy performance improvements and energy optimized products [4, 15].

2.2 The "Pedagogy" Component: Energy Culture and Lifelong Learning

According to UNESCO, every individual is entitled to a good quality education. The quality stems indirectly from the education and culture of people and the empowerment of collective thinking about a sustainable future. Conversely, sustainable development leads to high-level services and gifted humans with augmented skills and thus maintain, even strengthen the quality of the education. Through this perpetual cycle two significant educational issues emerge referring to the smart learning environments. The first refers to the instructional design considering social and affective factors of learning. It is widely accepted that culture is determined by inherited ideas, beliefs, values, attitudes, feelings, behaviors and knowledge as well. Similarly, energy culture consists of the cultivation of energy consciousness, changes in perceptions or attitudes to environmental protection through individual or social action. On the other hand, the second issue refers to the cognitive learning content. The enhancement of high-order thinking skills and digital competences is achieved by activities oriented to STEM and IoT which in turn provide deeper knowledge about energy management and expertise.

Research has shown barriers to the lack of energy awareness raising among consumers and insufficient knowledge, training or expertise [24, 25]. Smart pedagogy paves the way to the instrumentation of holistic type solutions by incorporating methodologies that focus on self-determination of the individual through self-regulated and self-directed learning choices as well as STEM epistemology [26]. Internationally STEM is the target of primary and secondary education. At the same time, adult specialization or retraining is equally important. Energy innovation creates a huge need for new talents that have skills and expertise. Across this line and because of the rapidly created job opportunities, many workers must be trained, up-skilled or re-skilled. Considering the above-mentioned and primarily highlighting the smart pedagogical perspective, the smart learning environments provide smart services referring to the following affordances:

Motivation and Engagement. Research has shown that the learning process is enhanced by the incorporation of strategies and techniques based on affective and psychological factors of learning. For example, Self Regulating Learning Theory, Self-Determination Theory as well as the ARCS motivational model and the Technology Acceptance Model (TAM), in combination with methodologies related to games (gamification/game-based learning), provide great opportunities for high engagement and motivation and consequently positive learning outcomes.

Sociality and Collaboration. SLEs provide automatic matched communities and communities of practice, where learners share ideas through dialogue, enrich their learning experience and cultivate their social skills. At the same time, while new methods of interaction appear, CSCL scripts are enriched, changing their traditional form and fostering communication and collaboration.

Individualization and Personalization. SLEs are developed on a learner-centric consideration and therefore they cultivate self-teaching, self-direction and learning autonomy. In addition, considering the different needs and preferences of every individual, by incorporating learning methods like BYOD (bring your own device) which implies technological features such as mobility, portability and adaptivity, the learning environment is augmented by personal independency.

Authenticity. It refers to authentic frameworks based on real world activities. Similarly, authentic assessment is bolstered by self or peer to peer interaction providing opportunities for system's self-organization [15] and learners' better cognitive performance.

Situated Learning. Considering that learning workspaces are partially real and virtual/digital (the recent years are also described by the term "phygital" [6]), formal and informal, new pedagogies based on situated learning framework and learning spaces theories [27] emerge.

Inquiry and Action. Since the design follows reusable instructional models with positive research outcomes, such as Problem Based Learning, Project Based Learning, even Challenge Based Learning, enhanced by strategies and techniques that foster inquiry and action, as well as pedagogies based on robotics and practical application, high order thinking skills (problem solving, critical thinking, creativity, innovation etc.) are developed or improved.

Intercontextuality and Content Enrichment. When learners enrich transferred content by linking new information to old, they cultivate meaningful knowledge and metacognitive abilities [9].

Reflectiveness and Pervasiveness. SLEs track learning status and evaluate learning progress. Through learning analytics, they predict and suggest solutions [9, 11] to future potential problems. This encourage new learning strategies to be implemented.

3 Conclusions

In this paper, the authors ventured to present Smart Learning Environments as a blend of smart technology and pedagogy, aiming to boost the research focus on the urgent and crucial issue of energy management. With the appropriate orchestration, both technology and pedagogy provide smart services which mainly are based on fundamental features of SLEs, investigated the recent years. However, while technology rapidly accelerates and new innovative and intelligent ICT achievements mitigate the energy consumption, the gravity should be given on education, especially on learning and pedagogy. There is no point of being innovative in technology without being conscious of using it effectively for the benefit of the humanity. Main task should be this generation's learners to become the next generation's smart citizens and consumers, cultivated with wisdom [10], who will dispose stronger conduct ability and will use their knowledge and experience to make good decisions and judgments for energy management. Since SLEs are innovative learning environments, pedagogy should be explored in detail, clearly implemented and evolved. As such, optimum techniques and methods of teaching and learning will emerge and will contribute to the fulfillment of the goals of sustainable development.

Acknowledgment. This work has been partly supported by the Research Center of the University of Piraeus.

References

1. European Energy Research Alliance – EERA. A sustainable energy future at the center of Horizon Europe. https://www.eera-set.eu/
2. International Energy Agency –IEA. https://www.iea.org
3. Organization for Economic Co-operation and Development – OECD Green growth and energy efficiency. http://www.oecd.org/greengrowth/greening-energy/greengrowthand-energyefficiency.htm

4. Ericsson Sustainability and Corporate Responsibility Report. https://www.ericsson.com/assets/local/about-ericsson/sustainability-and-corporate-responsibility/documents/scr-reports/ericsson-sustainability-and-corporate-responsibility-report-2017.pdf
5. United Nations Educational, Scientific and Cultural Organization – UNESCO. Sustainable Development Goals. https://en.unesco.org/sdgs
6. Giovannella, C.: Smart learning eco-systems: "fashion" or "beef"? J. e-Learning Knowl. Soc. **10**(3) (2014)
7. International Association of Smart Learning Environments – IASLE. http://iasle.net/
8. Luna Scott, C.: The futures of learning 3: what kind of pedagogies for the 21st century? (2015)
9. Zhu, Z.T., Yu, M.H., Riezebos, P.: A research framework of smart education. Smart Learn. Environ. **3**(1), 4 (2016)
10. Hwang, G.J.: Definition, framework and research issues of smart learning environments-a context-aware ubiquitous learning perspective. Smart Learn. Environ. **1**(1), 4 (2014)
11. Mikulecký, P.: Smart environments for smart learning. In: Proceedings of DIVAI 2012—9th International Scientific Conference on Distance Learning in Applied Informatics, pp. 213–222 (2012)
12. Tikhomirov, V., Dneprovskaya, N., Yankovskaya, E.: Three dimensions of smart education. In: Smart Education and Smart e-Learning, pp. 47–56. Springer, Cham (2015)
13. Spector, J.M.: Conceptualizing the emerging field of smart learning environments. Smart Learn. Environ. **1**(1), 2 (2014)
14. Singh, A.D., Hassan, M.: In pursuit of smart learning environments for the 21st century (Current and critical issues in curriculum series, No. 12, IBE/2017/WP/CD/12). UNESCO, Geneva (2017)
15. Hoel, T., Mason, J.: Standards for smart education–towards a development framework. Smart Learn. Environ. **5**(1), 3 (2018)
16. Piccoli, G., Ahmad, R., Ives, B.: Web-based virtual learning environments: a research framework and a preliminary assessment of effectiveness in basic IT skills training. MIS Q. **25**, 401–426 (2001)
17. Ang, B.W.: Monitoring changes in economy-wide energy efficiency: from energy–GDP ratio to composite efficiency index. Energy Policy **34**(5), 574–582 (2006)
18. Herrmann, C., Thiede, S.: Process chain simulation to foster energy efficiency in manufacturing. CIRP J. Manufact. Sci. Technol. **1**, 221–229 (2009)
19. Heppell, S., Chapman, C., Millwood, R., Constable, M., Furness, J.: Building learning futures. Building Futures (2004)
20. Taylor, A.: Linking Architecture and Education: Sustainable Design for Learning Environments. UNM Press (2009)
21. Hilty, L.M., Coroama, V., de Eicker, M.O., Ruddy, T., Müller, E.: The role of ICT in energy consumption and energy efficiency. Report to the European Commission, DG INFSO, Project ICT ENSURE: European ICT Sustainability Research, Graz University, vol. 1, pp. 1–60 (2009)
22. Bunse, K., Vodicka, M., Schönsleben, P., Brülhart, M., Ernst, F.O.: Integrating energy efficiency performance in production management–gap analysis between industrial needs and scientific literature. J. Clean. Prod. **19**(6–7), 667–679 (2011)
23. Lu, X., Niyato, D., Wang, P., Kim, D.I., Han, Z.: Wireless charger networking for mobile devices: fundamentals, standards, and applications. IEEE Wirel. Commun. **22**(2), 126–135 (2015)

24. Jennings, P.: New directions in renewable energy education. Renew. Energy **34**(2), 435–439 (2009)
25. Worrell, E., Bernstein, L., Roy, J., Price, L., Harnisch, J.: Industrial energy efficiency and climate change mitigation. Energ. Effi. **2**(2), 109 (2009)
26. Psycharis, S.: STEAM in education: a literature review on the role of computational thinking, engineering epistemology and computational science. Computational STEAM pedagogy (CSP). Sci. Cult. **4**(2), 51–72 (2018)
27. Bligh, B., Crook, C.: Learning spaces. In: Technology Enhanced Learning, pp. 69–87. Springer, Cham (2017)

Understanding Peripheral Audiences: From Subtle to Full Body Gestures

Francisco J. Martínez-Ruiz[1(✉)], Sebastian F. Rauh[2], and Gerrit Meixner[2]

[1] Autonomous University of Zacatecas, Zacatecas, Mexico
javier.martinezruiz@uaz.edu.mx
[2] Usability and Interaction Technology Laboratory (UniTyLab), Heilbronn University, Max-Planck-Straße 39, 74081 Heilbronn, Germany
{sebastian.rauh,gerrit.meixner}@hs-heilbronn.de

Abstract. Full body interaction is used to allow a more immersive and cognitive implication of users in some contexts, for instance, in a museum. However, full body gestures can be stressful for some users in some environments. Specially, if these interactions are performed in the presence of an audience. We have analyzed a spectrum of full body gestures to understand the reaction of the Peripheral audience. Instead of the interactive users, the Peripheral audience is tested against selected gestures.

Keywords: Gesture design · User-defined gestures · Gesture elicitation · Gesture analysis methodology · Gesture annotation · Gesture context-aware · Aesthetics · Interaction design · Human-computer interaction · Performance theory · Experience design

1 Introduction

Interactive public systems (e.g., Smart TVs or public displays) are used in many environments to inform and entertain users (single and group). Today, due to the fast progress of user tracking technologies, allowing the user to employ his/her body to interact with the system becomes feasible. This so-called full body interaction allows a more immersive and cognitive implication of users in some environments, as described e.g. by Roberts [16]. Many studies discuss reactions and preferences of interactive (direct) users [6, 10, 13, 17, 19, 20]. In contrast, in this work we address the effect of these interactive systems on spectators (indirect users) in the surrounding area.

Users are usually alone and control the full experience (e.g., sound volume, colors, and information display) in private contexts. Meanwhile, there is a peripheral audience (PA) of Non-Interactive users in public spaces (e.g., museums, airports, malls). This PA affects the interactive user, because there is social awareness [7]. On the other hand, the PA is also influenced by the user's gestures. However, it is no clear whether the influence is positive or negative, or no influence can be determined at all.

For robots Mori describes the concept of "uncanny valley", which suggests that there is a point where robots too realistic seem creepy or unnatural [12]. Cafaro et al.

T. Ahram et al. (Eds.): IHIET 2019, AISC 1018, pp. 489–495, 2020.
https://doi.org/10.1007/978-3-030-25629-6_76

used this concept in full body gestures of interactive systems [1] and concluded that more realism could derivate in this effect.

In this paper, we argue that there is an uncanny valley of full body interactions affecting the PA, since some of these gestures could be unpleasant, disturbing, or even aggressive for the PA. We analyze the reaction of PA in the surroundings of the interaction space. Besides that, we propose an ad hoc taxonomy to expose the PA to some selected gestures, looking for the effect of uncanny valley in the spectrum of full body gestures.

2 Related Work

There are numerous Human Gesture Classifications [3–6, 9, 10]. Instead of trying to build a new one, this work proposes categories or dimensions to be included in current taxonomies with the purpose of helping and guiding designers in the construction of new applications in specific contexts. For instance, the gesture taxonomy in [6] included nine dimensions divided in multiple features (cultural, meaning, workspace among others). Nevertheless, interesting features are missing (e.g., Sound as result of the gesture production). Note: In [21] the sound was used as feedback for different tasks. Here, it is included as a side effect.

Also, the role of users is examined in this study. According to Dalsgaard and Hansen [2], there are three roles that users take during interaction: Performer, Spectator, and Operator. They stated that some of those spectators are looking to become next users. Reeves et al. considered that experience designers should contemplate spectators [15]. Gestures, in the context of games, were better studied than other kinds [18]. Most gestures are regarded as acceptable in the context of games. Also, the role of spectator (PA) is underestimated in most of the settings.

3 Methods and Results

In this paper, the PA and the impact of different types of gestures is examined. That's why, the spectrum of full body gestures is introduced, considering three scopes (see Fig. 1). We consider that full body gestures require a more refined hierarchy to study better, different groups of gestures. First, hand gestures are incorporated in the subtle category as part of gestures related to fine motor skills and the head (cf. Fig. 1a). Second, Medium range includes torso as a unit (with hands, arms, shoulders, and chest, cf. Fig. 1b). And third, Full body gestures include and process the whole body (the previous categories plus, hips and legs, cf. Fig. 1c) as tools to interact with public displays in the context studied in this paper. In addition, we included three types of users. The performer (Fig. 1d), PA interested in participating (Fig. 1e), and PA unable or unwilling to participate. Nevertheless, they are aware of the interaction (Fig. 1f). It is an important remark that PA is not defined in terms of location, i.e., a PA member wishing to participate, could be far away from the performer while another member of the PA unwilling to participate could be next to the performer.

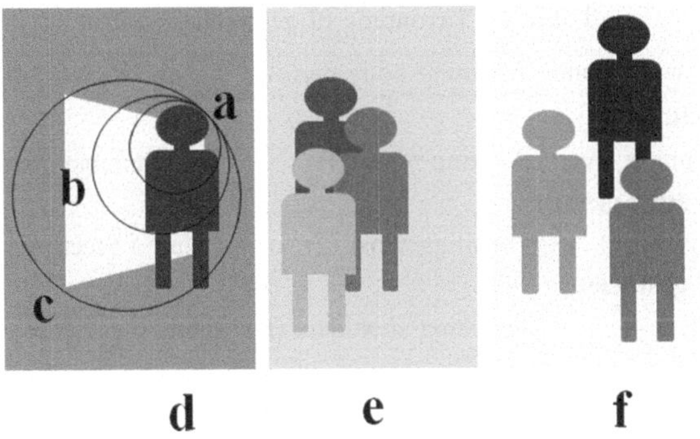

Fig. 1. Defining gesture scope (Subtle *a*, Medium *b* and Full body *c*) and User roles (Performer *d*, PA interested in participating *e*, and PA unable to participate *f*).

Two groups of participants have been defined (performers and PA). All of them, students of the Computer Science Faculty at the University of Zacatecas. Each experience included an interacting user and a PA. The PA group was composed by 26 users. Two tasks were proposed: moving from left to right (and vice versa) using the gestures. For instance, Finger snapping (a Subtle Gesture) is done with the left hand to move to the left and the same gesture with the right hand, a movement to the right in a Photo gallery mockup. Each gesture was repeated ten times by 3 different performers to produce 270 repetitions.

After the study, users completed an online survey [8] in order to rate the following concepts in a semantic differential scale: (1) enjoyable, (2) understandable, (3) exciting, (4) predictable, (5) bad, (6) easy, (7) not secure, (8) practical, (9) unfriendly, (10) disagreement to perform the gesture, (11) comfortable, and (12) encouraging.

A set of 9 gestures was proposed. This set was based on the taxonomies of Grijincu et al. [6], Maricchiolo et al. [9], Taralle et al. [17], besides the concept of social acceptance of new gestures [11], sound as result of the gesture with no feedback purpose [21] and the taboo of touching (Chapter 7) [14]. It is worth mentioning that these gestures were selected to test conditions that could be considered not socially accepted. In Montero et al. [11], they have stablished that a meaningful action is socially acceptable. Hence, we have proposed gestures with no meaning prior interaction (see Table 1). The main idea was to test the emergence of the uncanny valley effect in the PA while using gestures related to the taboo of touching, acceptance of producing sound, and using unknown objects in public spaces.

We collected the following results: 29 students have collaborated in the experiment. (7 females, 22 males; age: 18–21 = 51.72%, 22–25 = 37.93%, 26–30: 6.90%, >31 = 3.45%). This was a group with experience in the use of technology. Most of the users are aware of gestures from touch screen devices and game environments. 44.83% of users used an application in a public display (big screen in public). 79.31% of users

Table 1. Taxonomy of gestures tested.

Combined with sound	Touching body parts	Using tangible objects
Subtle gestures		
Finger snapping (A)	Pointing nose (B)	Using a small box (C)
Medium range gestures		
Hand clapping (1)	Touching wrist (2)	Using a Steering wheel (3)
Full body gestures		
Jumping (I)	Touching shoulders (II)	Using a cylinder (III)

were familiar performing gestures in a touch screen and 34.48% were aware of mid-air ones. 65.52% of users executed gestures on computers, Smartphones 86.21%, Tablets 27.59%, game consoles 37.93% and 6.90% do not use gestures with any device. All the gestures were considered easy (Note: Semantic Differential value 6). Subtle gestures were interpreted as more secure (7) than Medium and Full body ones. Also, a general discomfort (10) was observed with gestures associated with touching body parts in all the gesture range. Although, sounds were interpreted as understandable (2). The attitude or qualification of users to them was not significative. More studies are required to deal with this important feature. Finally, the use of tangible accessories was more comfortable for PA than other categories (11) (Figs. 2, 3 and 4).

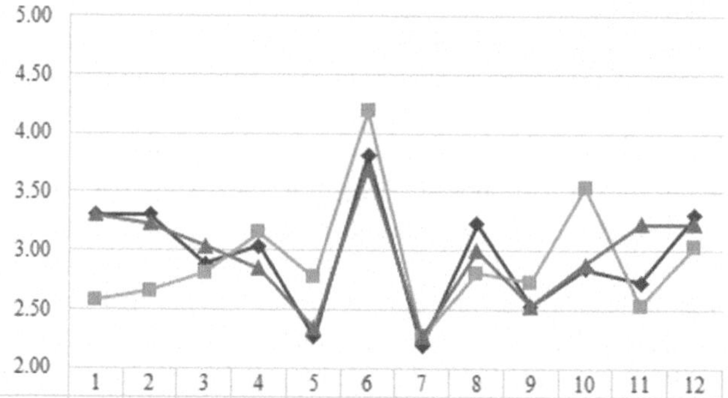

	1	2	3	4	5	6	7	8	9	10	11	12
A AVG	3.31	3.31	2.88	3.04	2.27	3.81	2.19	3.23	2.54	2.85	2.73	3.31
B AVG	2.58	2.65	2.81	3.15	2.77	4.19	2.27	2.81	2.73	3.54	2.54	3.04
C AVG	3.31	3.23	3.04	2.85	2.35	3.69	2.27	3.00	2.54	2.88	3.23	3.23

Fig. 2. Results of subtle gestures A, B and C.

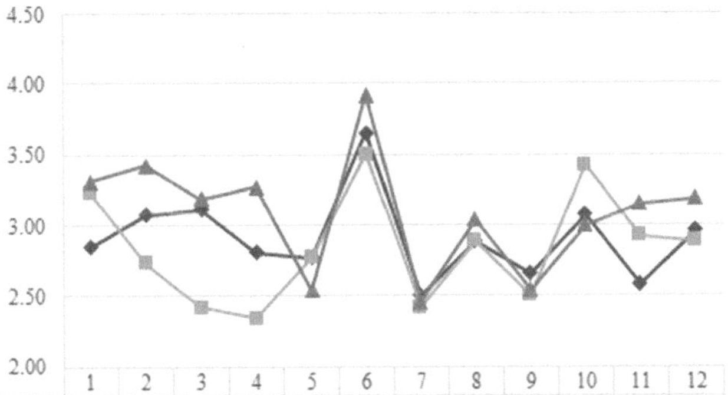

	1	2	3	4	5	6	7	8	9	10	11	12
1 AVG	2.85	3.08	3.12	2.81	2.77	3.65	2.50	2.88	2.65	3.08	2.58	2.96
2 AVG	3.23	2.73	2.42	2.35	2.77	3.50	2.42	2.88	2.50	3.42	2.92	2.88
3 AVG	3.31	3.42	3.19	3.27	2.54	3.92	2.46	3.04	2.54	3.00	3.15	3.19

Fig. 3. Results of medium gestures 1, 2 and 3.

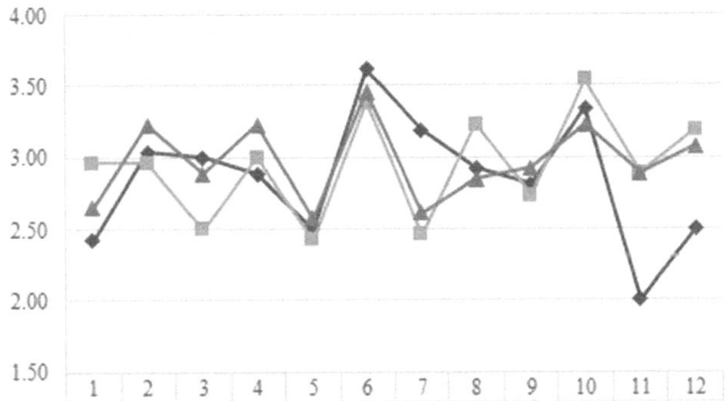

	1	2	3	4	5	6	7	8	9	10	11	12
I AVG	2.42	3.04	3.00	2.88	2.50	3.62	3.19	2.92	2.81	3.35	2.00	2.50
II AVG	2.96	2.96	2.50	3.00	2.42	3.38	2.46	3.23	2.73	3.54	2.88	3.19
III AVG	2.65	3.23	2.88	3.23	2.58	3.46	2.62	2.85	2.92	3.23	2.88	3.08

Fig. 4. Results of full body gestures I, II and III.

4 Conclusions and Future Work

Our proposal is a first approach to understand PA in the spectrum of full body gestures besides adding new categories. These categories were selected to test the taboo of touching [14], acceptance of producing sound with no feedback purpose, and using unknown objects in public spaces. A total of 9 gestures are proposed. This set is based, partially, on the taxonomies of Grijincu et al. [6], Maricchiolo et al. [9], Taralle et al. [17] and the concept of social acceptance of new gestures [11]. In this study subtle gestures were described by users as more secure while "touching body parts" gestures were perceived as not acceptable to perform. Gestures including sounds were interpreted as understandable. Furthermore, the use of tangible accessories was comfortable for PA.

The uncanny valley effect was not clear. Nevertheless, medium, and Full body gestures scored higher in "disagreement to perform the gesture" than subtle gestures. Finally, a more exhaustive and systematic procedure is needed to select and validate the proposed taxonomy. Also, more categories (for instance, gender and cultural ones) and natural spaces (e.g., a mall) can be added in the future studies.

References

1. Cafaro, F., et al.: The uncanny valley of embodied interaction design. In: Proceedings of the 2014 Conference on Designing interactive systems - DIS 2014, pp. 1075–1078. ACM Press, Vancouver (2014). https://doi.org/10.1145/2598510.2598593
2. Dalsgaard, P., Hansen, L.K.: Performing perception—staging aesthetics of interaction. ACM Trans. Comp. Hum. Interact. **15**(3), 13:1–13:33 (2008)
3. Efron, D.: Gesture and Environment. King'S Crown Press, Oxford (1941)
4. Eisenstein, J., Davis, R.: Visual and linguistic information in gesture classification. In: Proceedings of the 6th International Conference on Multimodal Interfaces, pp. 113–120. ACM, New York (2004). https://doi.org/10.1145/1027933.1027954
5. Ekman, P., Friesen, W.V.: The repertoire of nonverbal behavior: categories, origins, usage, and coding. Semiotica **1**(1), 49–98 (2009). https://doi.org/10.1515/semi.1969.1.1.49
6. Grijincu, D., et al.: User-defined interface gestures: dataset and analysis. In: Proceedings of the Ninth ACM International Conference on Interactive Tabletops and Surfaces, pp. 25–34. ACM, New York (2014). https://doi.org/10.1145/2669485.2669511
7. Jacob, R.J.K., et al.: Reality-based interaction: a framework for post-WIMP interfaces. In: Proceeding of the Twenty-Sixth Annual CHI Conference on Human Factors in Computing Systems, CHI 2008, p. 201. ACM Press, Florence (2008). https://doi.org/10.1145/1357054.1357089
8. Limesurvey GmbH: LimeSurvey: the online survey tool. https://www.limesurvey.org/
9. Maricchiolo, F., et al.: Coding hand gestures: a reliable taxonomy and a multi-media support. In: Esposito, A., et al. (eds.) Cognitive Behavioural Systems, pp. 405–416. Springer, Heidelberg (2012)
10. McNeill, D.: Hand and Mind: What Gestures Reveal about Thought. University of Chicago Press, Chicago, London (1996)
11. Montero, C.S., et al.: Would you do that? Understanding social acceptance of gestural interfaces. In: Proceedings of the 12th International Conference on Human Computer Interaction with Mobile Devices and Services - MobileHCI 2010, p. 275. ACM Press, Lisbon (2010). https://doi.org/10.1145/1851600.1851647
12. Mori, M.: The Uncanny Valley: The Original Essay by Masahiro Mori. https://spectrum.ieee.org/automaton/robotics/humanoids/the-uncanny-valley
13. Obaid, M., et al.: A framework for user-defined body gestures to control a humanoid robot. Int. J. Soc. Rob. **6**(3), 383–396 (2014)
14. Payne, H. (ed.): Essentials of Dance Movement Psychotherapy. Routledge, London, New York (2017)
15. Reeves, S., et al.: Designing the spectator experience. In: Proceedings of the SIGCHI Conference on Human Factors in Computing Systems, pp. 741–750. ACM, New York (2005). https://doi.org/10.1145/1054972.1055074

16. Roberts, J.: Exploring effects of full-body control in perspective-based learning in an interactive museum data display. Presented at the Proceedings of the Ninth International Conference on Tangible, Embedded, and Embodied Interaction, 15 January 2015
17. Taralle, F., et al.: A consensual and non-ambiguous set of gestures to interact with UAV in infantrymen. In: Proceedings of the 33rd Annual ACM Conference Extended Abstracts on Human Factors in Computing Systems, pp. 797–803. ACM, New York (2015). https://doi.org/10.1145/2702613.2702971
18. Tomitsch, M., et al.: Who cares about the content? An analysis of playful behaviour at a public display. In: Proceedings of the International Symposium on Pervasive Displays, pp. 160:160–160:165. ACM, New York (2014)
19. Williamson, J.R., et al.: Understanding performative interactions in public settings. Pers. Ubiquit. Comput. **18**(7), 1545–1549 (2014). https://doi.org/10.1007/s00779-014-0819-7
20. Wobbrock, J.O., et al.: User-defined gestures for surface computing. In: Proceedings of the 27th International Conference on Human Factors in Computing Systems - CHI 09, p. 1083. ACM Press, Boston (2009). https://doi.org/10.1145/1518701.1518866
21. Wolf, K., et al.: Touching the void: gestures for auditory interfaces. In: Proceedings of the Fifth International Conference on Tangible, Embedded, and Embodied Interaction, pp. 305–308. ACM, New York (2011). https://doi.org/10.1145/1935701.1935772

Programming Assistant System Using Improved Flowchart for the Visually Impaired

Ryo Hirakawa(✉), Rin Hirakawa, Hideaki Kawano, Kenichi Nakashi, and Yoshihisa Nakatoh

Electrical and Electronic, Kyushu Institute of Technology, 1-1 Sensuicho, Tobata Ward, Kitakyushu, Fukuoka Prefecture, Japan
{hirakawa.ryo844,hirakawa.rin151}@mail.kyutech.jp, {kawano,nakashi,nakatoh}@ecs.kyutech.jp

Abstract. The purpose of this study is to assist the visually impaired to develop applications. There is a method for the visually impaired to develop applications by reading program codes with screen reader. In this method, the visually impaired can read code on line by line and select a line by knocking the up and down arrow key on the keyboard. After that, they can read the processing and describe an instruction before and after the processing. However, such an operation takes them a long time. Therefore, we suggested the system which let develop applications by editing flowcharts. This system converts program code into flowchart and read blocks in the flowchart. In this system, they can select blocks by knocking the left, right, up and down arrow key. We compared the time for rewriting programs between approach and the proposed system. As a result, the time reduced in all programs.

Keywords: Programming · The visually impaired · Visual programming · Flowchart · Audio guide

1 Introduction

One of challenges of modern society is employment status of the visually impaired [1]. They can get little information with their sight. Therefore, they have limited opportunities to make use of their skills than the sighted. As a result, it is difficult for them to get jobs. However, the information from eyes is not necessary in software development with audio guides [2]. In addition, the number of software engineers is insufficient for the needs of the world. For these reasons, we thought that the visually impaired may be able to work as software engineers by supporting to their programming. Currently, there is a method for the visually impaired to develop applications by reading program codes with screen reader. In this method, the visually impaired can read code on line by line and select a line by knocking the up and down arrow key on the keyboard. After that, they can read the processing and describe an instruction before and after the processing. However, such an operation takes them a long time. Therefore, we decided to build new development environment with reading mechanism specialized for developing the software so that the visually impaired can read efficiently about the

T. Ahram et al. (Eds.): IHIET 2019, AISC 1018, pp. 496–501, 2020.
https://doi.org/10.1007/978-3-030-25629-6_77

software. In this paper, we describe the operation of the proposed system and the result of the experiment for confirming the usability of this system.

2 Paper Preparation

We proposed this system referring to visual programming. This system converts source code to flowchart and users can develop the software by editing flowchart during listening to audio guides with this system. The behavior of this system is shown in Fig. 1. First, this system waits for commands. Then, this system classifies commands and operate in accordance with commands. Commands are roughly divided into three classes.

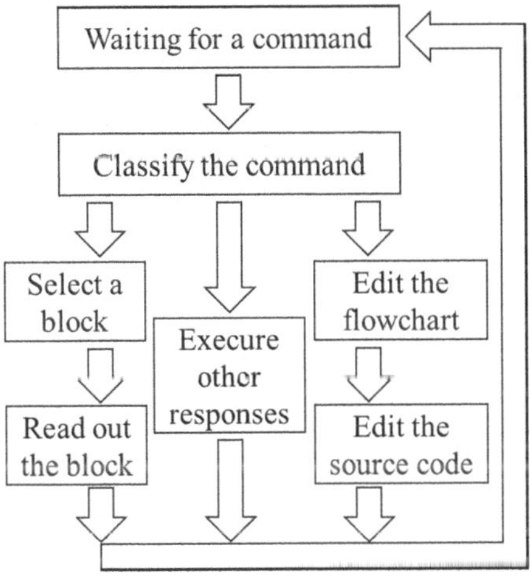

Fig. 1. Behavior of the proposed system

1. Commands for reading flowcharts
2. Commands for editing flowcharts
3. Other commands

Commands of 1 are for reading the specific processing in the flowchart. The visually impaired can grasp the flowchart by associating the processing read by the system with the contents inputted by themselves. When these commands are inputted, the system selects the block of the processing. Then, the system reads out the block. Commands of 2 are for creating the software by making and editing the flowchart. When these commands are inputted, the system edits the flowchart. Then, the system edits the source codes of the software to comply with editing the flowchart. Commands of 3 are for the processing of the system. Example of these commands are shown in Table 1.

We describe the method of reading flowcharts in Sect. 2.1 and the method of editing flowcharts in Sect. 2.2.

Table 1. Relationship of inputted commands and response.

Command	Type	Response
↑, ↓, ←, →	Reading commands	Selecting the block in the inputted direction and reading it
z		Shifting from the integrated block to the flowchart which is subdivided the block integrated
r		Shifting from the flowchart which is subdivided the block integrated to the integrated block
Enter	Editing commands	Adding a new block next the selected block
Delete		Deleting the selected block
Backspace		Editing the processing of the selected block
Escape	Other commands	Converting flowchart to source code and saving it

2.1 Flowchart Reading Method

This system reads the process of the block when users select the block in the flowchart by inputting commands. The flowchart used in this system has 3 features.

First, ends of conditional statements are converted into blocks. It is difficult to guide ends of conditional statements by the voice because the merging of arrows means it. This system converts ends of conditional statements into blocks in order to solve this problem.

Second, some blocks repeated by loop statement is integrated into "loop block". When "loop block" has selected, users can select any block repeated by loop statement with this system if they input "z key" with keyboard.

Third, this system converts a comment into "comment block" and makes "comment flowchart" with only "comment block". Users can select blocks easily with "comment flowchart". We describe the convenience of "comment flowchart" with Fig. 2. With conventional flowchart, users have to input "down arrow key" for 5 times in order to select "printf" when the system selects "Start". However, users can select "printf" by inputting "down arrow key" for 2 times and "z key" for 1 time.

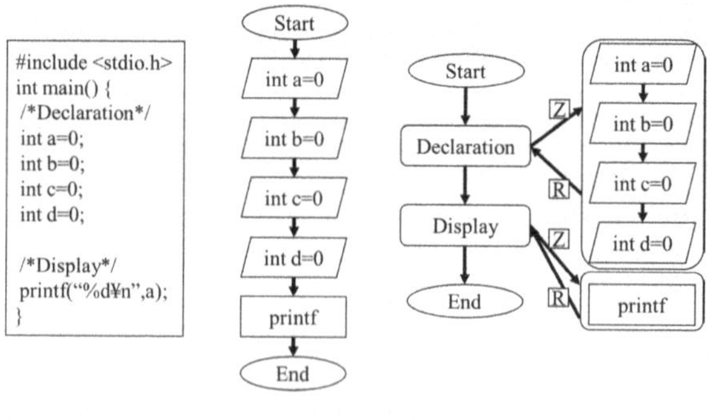

Fig. 2. Example of the comment flowchart

2.2 Flowchart Editing Method

The method of editing flowcharts is incomplete. So, we described the current specifications of this system.

There are three types of editing mechanisms for flowcharts.

First, I describe "add". Users can add a new block under the selected block by inputting "Enter" key in this system. The block added in the flowchart at that time isn't set the processing.

Second, I describe "edit". Users can set the processing for the selected block by inputting "BackSpace" key. In addition, users can reset the processing for the block which is set the processing before.

Third, I describe "Delete". Users can delete the selected block by inputting "Delete" key. Users can edit the flowchart with these keys.

We describe the behavior of this system with Fig. 3. Initially, the shape of the flowchart is like (a). This systems "int a = 0;" at that time. Then, the shape of the flowchart is like (b) when users input "Enter" key. In short, a block which isn't set the processing is added under the selected block. Then, the selected block is set the processing like (c) by inputting "BackSpace" key. This system finishes to set the processing for the block when users input "Enter" key. Also, the shape of the flowchart changes from(c) to (a) when users input "Delete" key at "int x = 0;" in the flowchart like (c). In short, "int x = 0;" is deleted in the flowchart.

3 Verification of Improvement of Understanding by Proposed System

In order to confirm the validity of this system, we made 10 subjects rewrite programs with screen reader or the proposed system. We describe the method of the experiment in Sect. 3.1 and the result of the experiment in Sect. 3.2.

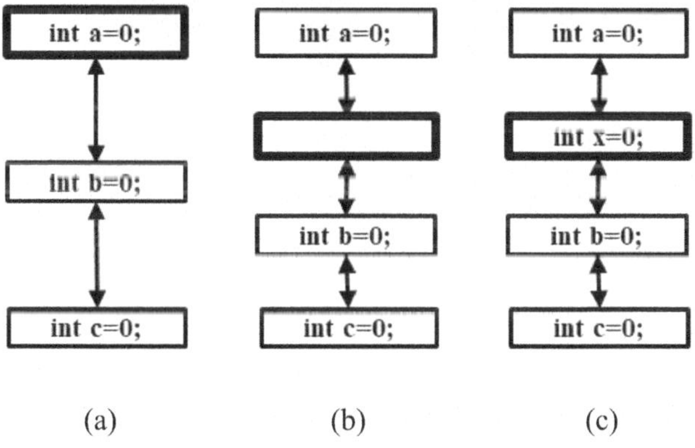

Fig. 3. Example of editing the flowchart

3.1 Experiment Method

We used 5 programs which have about 100 lines of source code in this experiment. In addition, we set the difficulty of the experiment by the position of the process to rewrite. (Level 1: less than 33 lines, Level 2: less than 66 lines, Level 3: within 100 lines)

Subjects rewrote programs 10 times for each difficulty level. In short, they rewrote programs 30 times. In addition, they rewrote programs without the display.

In this experiment, we assessed the proposed system with the time rewriting the programs. In addition, we killed the experiment 3 min after the start of rewriting programs.

3.2 Results and Discussion

Figure 4 shows average for each difficulty level to rewrite programs.

First, we describe about the result of level 1. It took 42.29 s to rewrite the program with conventional screen reader. On the other hand, it took 40.24 s to rewrite the program with proposed system. In short, there was almost no gap between each the result of method. However, the gap widened as increasing difficulty level. In the experiment of level 2, it took 73.58 s with conventional screen reader and 41.01 s with proposed system. In the experiment of level 3, it took 82.60 s with conventional screen reader and 38.48 s with proposed system.

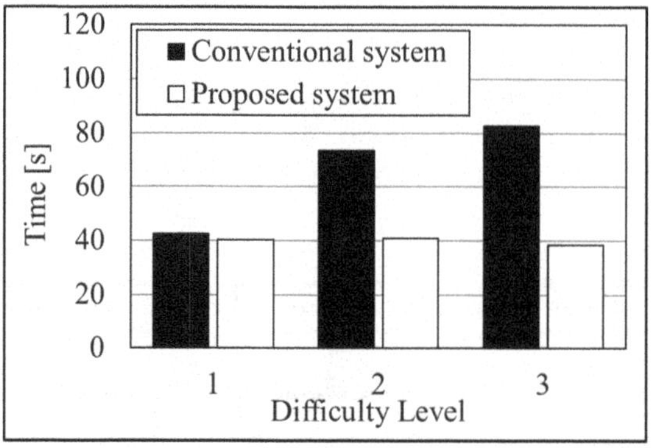

Fig. 4. Result of the experiment

In short, with proposed system, the wider the program to be read, the shorter the time for rewriting the program.

Also, in 300 experiments, subjects made 11 mistakes about the rewriting position with the conventional system and made 4 mistakes about the rewriting position with the proposed system. In addition, subjects exceeded the time of the experiment 3 times with the conventional system and exceeded the experiment 2 times with the proposed system.

A factor from which these results were obtained is the proposed system makes subjects easily to image the structure of the program. Based on the above, it can be said that the proposed system is useful in programming without visual information.

4 The References Section

In this paper, we confirmed that proposed system is more useful than conventional method in programming without visually information because the time of rewriting programs reduced. In particular, the proposed system is useful for developing large softwares.

In the future, we will improve usability in operating the system so that the visually impaired can operate easily and the system for reading and editing flowcharts. In addition, we would like to test that the visually impaired is able to use this system.

References

1. Ministry of Health, Labor and Welfare: Fiscal year 2016 - Employment introduction situation of person with disabilities etc., May 2017. https://www.mhlw.go.jp/file/04-Houdouhappyou-11704000-Shokugyouanteikyokukoureishougaikoyoutaisakubu-shougaishakoyoutaisakuka/0000166291.pdf
2. Nagaoka, H.: Vocational usefulness of software development skills of the blind. Vocat. Rehabil. **16**, 43–51 (2003)

Evaluating Green Light Optimum Speed Advisory (GLOSA) System in Traffic Flow with Information Distance Variations

Hironori Suzuki[1(✉)] and Yoshitaka Marumo[2]

[1] Department of Robotics, Nippon Institute of Technology, 4-1 Gakuendai, Miyashiro, Saitama 3458501, Japan
viola@nit.ac.jp

[2] Department of Mechanical Engineering, Nihon University, 1-2-1 Izumicho, Narashino, Chiba 2758575, Japan
marumo.yoshitaka@nihon-u.ac.jp

Abstract. The use of green light optimal speed advisory (GLOSA) systems is seen as a key application for achieving more environmentally friendly, time efficient and safer traffic flows at signalized intersections. However, while previous GLOSA systems provide optimum speed advice to drivers, we have proposed a GLOSA system concept that informs drivers of the appropriate *position* of their vehicle instead of their optimal *speed*. This paper reports on a performance evaluation of our proposed GLOSA system using information distance variations. Information distance is defined as the distance between the subject vehicle and the closest traffic signal where the GLOSA system first becomes active. Traffic simulator experiments showed that the earlier activation of the GLOSA system is particularly effective when the approach traffic demand is relatively lower. In other situations, the partial assistance (PA) mode, in which the GLOSA system is activated only when the signal is red, performed well.

Keywords: GLOSA · ADAS · Travel time · Traffic simulation · Fuel consumption · CO_2 emissions

1 Introduction

The use of green light optimal speed advisory (GLOSA) systems is expected to play a key role in achieving more environmentally friendly, time efficient and safer traffic flows at signalized intersections. The GLOSA system concept was originally designed to advise drivers on their optimum speeds when approaching signalized intersections in order to avoid the need for complete stops [1–7]. However, another GLOSA concept, which we proposed previously, calls for providing advice to drivers on the most appropriate position for their vehicle instead of the optimal speed in order to achieve timely, energy efficient, and safe intersection transits [8, 9].

In use, our GLOSA system is designed to project a combination of green and red-colored planar rectangle shapes placed adjacent each other onto the road surface ahead of the vehicle. If the vehicle is on the green portion, the GLOSA system is advising the driver to maintain his/her current speed in order to cross the intersection without

T. Ahram et al. (Eds.): IHIET 2019, AISC 1018, pp. 502–508, 2020.
https://doi.org/10.1007/978-3-030-25629-6_78

making a complete stop. However, if the vehicle is on the red rectangle, the driver is advised to decelerate until the vehicle enters the green portion.

In our previous studies, we confirmed that our proposed GLOSA system was effective when traffic demands are relatively low, but that it significantly worsened traffic efficiency under high traffic volume scenarios [8, 9]. In such cases, significant traffic congestion developed because the assisted vehicles traveling on red rectangles were advised to slow down even though the upcoming signal was green. Accordingly, in order to make the use of this GLOSA system more effective, it may sometimes be necessary to delay system activation under high approach demand conditions.

In this paper, we introduce the concept of "information distance", which is defined as the distance between the assisted vehicle and the traffic light where the GLOSA system first becomes active. We then conduct traffic simulation experiments using information distance variations in order to evaluate the performance of our updated GLOSA system.

2 Methodology

2.1 GLOSA System Outline

Our proposed GLOSA system assumes that connections exist between the vehicles and traffic lights via a vehicle-to-infrastructure (V2I) communication system and uses the system data to calculate the distance required to cross the intersection without making a complete stop. Refer to [9] for more details about our GLOSA system.

As shown in Fig. 1, the GLOSA system consists of a combination of green and red rectangles placed adjacent to each other on the road surface.

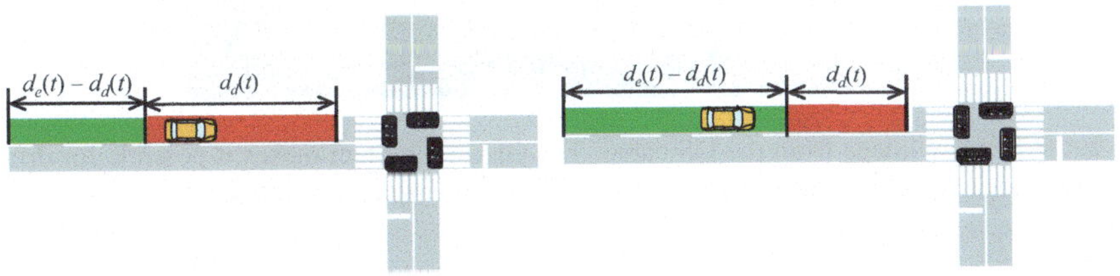

Fig. 1. The green and red rectangles are placed adjacent to each other. The driver is advised to maintain his/her current speed when the vehicle is travelling on the green rectangle in order to pass through the signalized intersection without stopping (right). In contrast, if the vehicle is on the red portion, the driver is advised to decelerate until the vehicle enters the green portion (left).

The length of both rectangles are computed as:

$$d_e(t) = v(t) \times \text{TTR and } d_d(t) = v(t) \times \text{TTG}. \tag{1}$$

Here, $d_e(t)$ and $d_e(t)$ are the length of green and red rectangle shapes, TTR and TTG are the times to red and green that are equivalent to the remaining green and red times, respectively. $v(t)$ is the current vehicle speed at time step t.

As long as the assisted vehicle is traveling on the green rectangle, the driver will not need to make a complete stop or accelerate in order to meet the onset of a green signal. In contrast, the driver of a vehicle travelling on the red rectangle is advised to decelerate at 1 m/s^2 until the vehicle enters the green portion, after which he or she should maintain a constant speed to ensure that the vehicle will be able to pass through the intersection without stopping when the traffic light changes to green. Our proposed system design calls for these rectangle shapes to be projected on the road surface ahead of the assisted vehicle through a head-up display (HUD).

In our earlier study, we equipped a driving simulator with our proposed GLOSA system and carried out DS experiments to investigate its performance [10]. A front-view image from the DS cabin is shown in Fig. 2. This system setup makes it possible for a driver to easily control the vehicle so that he/or she will keep traveling on the green rectangle.

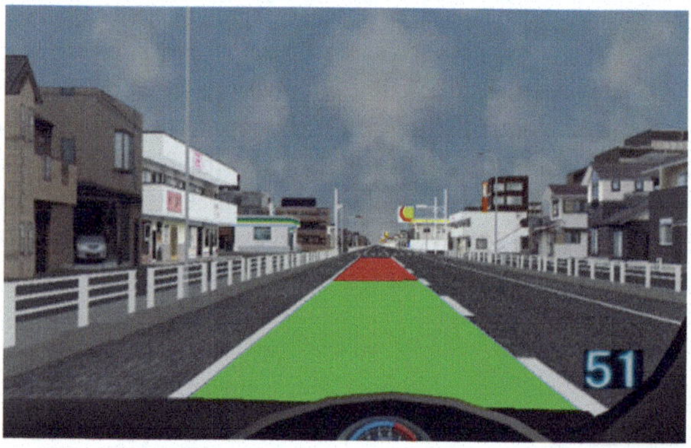

Fig. 2. Front view image from the DS cabin. The GLOSA system makes it possible for drivers to easily recognize if they are traveling on either the red or green rectangles.

2.2 Traffic Simulator

Our DS experiment showed that GLOSA system use resulted in higher fuel economy, less driver distraction, increased driver comfort, and less stop-and-go behavior in a limited environment [10]. To extend this experiment by inserting an isolated vehicle into the traffic flow, a time-scanning traffic simulator (TS) was developed and validated by one of the authors of this paper, after which it was integrated into the GLOSA system. The vehicle acceleration is calculated using Eq. (2):

$$\ddot{x}(t) = a\left(\frac{\Delta v}{d}\cdot v^{\alpha}\right) + b\left(\sqrt[\delta]{\beta\cdot v^{\gamma}} - \frac{v}{d}\right) + c\left(\frac{R}{1+m\exp(n\cdot d)} - v\right) + \Phi. \qquad (2)$$

where, a, b, c, Φ, α, β, γ, δ, R, m, and n are the parameters, d is a headway distance from the preceding car (m), and v is the velocity (m/s).

3 Numerical Analysis by Traffic Simulation

3.1 Test Setup

With the exception of the signal phase, the simulation test field used in this study was identical to the one that appeared in our previous study [8].

Geometry: A corridor consisting of four 500 m straight links was prepared as a scenario. Traffic lights are installed at the end of each link. The speed limit was set to 16.7 m/s for all links.

Simulation Parameters: The simulation duration was set at 2400 s and the time interval was set at 0.1 s. Vehicles were generated at the entrance of the first link but only injected into the road within the first 600 s.

Measurements: Traffic detectors for all four links were installed at locations 50 m in front of the traffic lights in order to measure the distributions of time headway, accelerations, spot speed, and link traffic count.

Signal Phase: A pre-timed control in which the green, amber, and red phases were set to 62, 3, and 35 s, respectively, was assumed for all signals.

3.2 Test Conditions and Scenarios

Information Distance: The information distances at which the GLOSA system first became active were set to 500, 333, and 167 m upstream the intersection. They are referred to as 500 ID, 333 ID, and 167 ID, respectively.

Traffic Demand: Traffic demands were assumed 100, 200, 400, 800, and 1200 vehicles per hour (VPH).

Penetration Rate: The penetration rate of the GLOSA-assisted vehicle was assumed to be 100%. In addition, we prepared a partial assistance (PA) mode in which the GLOSA system only activates during red signals, thus avoiding the extremely low driving speeds that result at green signals at times of heavy traffic [9].

Measures of Effectiveness (MOE): The traffic flow characteristics were evaluated in terms of travel time, fuel consumption rate, and CO2 emissions. The travel time is defined as the elapsed period from the vehicle generation until it exits the last link. The test conditions are summarized in Fig. 3.

3.3 Simulation

Figure 4 shows the travel time reductions (upper left), fuel economy improvements (upper right), and CO2 emission reductions (lower). If the data are allocated in the

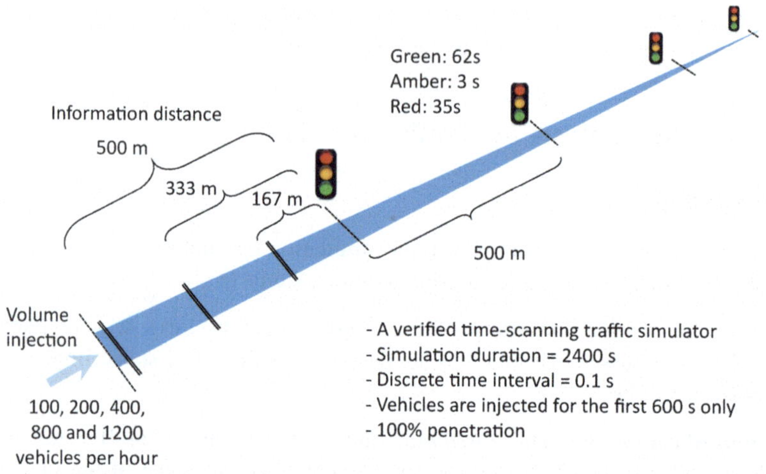

Fig. 3. Traffic simulation experimental conditions. A vehicle is travelling along a 2000 m long straight corridor equipped with four traffic lights. The GLOSA systems is activated 167, 333, and 500 m upstream from the traffic lights.

positive side, it indicates that the GLOSA system imparts a positive impact on the MOE. In any traffic demands, the system performance improved as the information distance lengthened. In fact, the 500 ID showed more than a 7% improvement in terms of fuel efficiency and a 10% reduction in CO2 emissions. However, 167 ID worsened

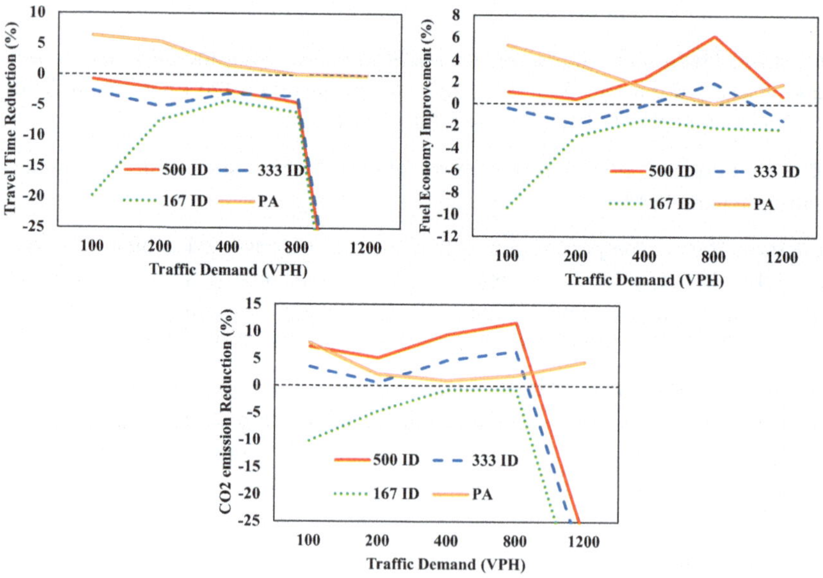

Fig. 4. Travel time reductions (upper left), fuel economy improvements (upper right), and CO2 emission reductions (lower). It can be seen that performance improvements increased as information distances lengthened, except for the 1200 VPH demand.

the traffic flow quite significantly. These results indicate that the GLOSA system should be activated as early as possible.

However, under high traffic demand conditions such as 1200 VPH, the information distance variations had no effect and even worsened the efficiency and environmental factors. This is because the assisted vehicles had to slow down on the red portion even though the signal was green. Although this problem cannot be eliminated by early system activation, can be alleviated by use of the PA mode, in which the GLOSA system is only activated when the signal is red. Our results show the PA mode did not increase travel time, improved fuel economy by 2%, and reduced CO2 emissions by 5% even when traffic demands were extremely high.

4 Conclusion

In this work, we tested the performance of our proposed GLOSA system in scenarios where the system activation time was varied. It can be concluded that an earlier activation of the system was particularly effective when the approach demand was less than 800 VPH. In other situations, the PA mode, in which the GLOSA system is activated only when the signal is red, performed well.

Except for extremely congested situations, such as morning or evening peak periods, the GLOSA system can be expected to have a positive effect on the efficiency and environmental factors related to traffic flow.

Acknowledgments. Research supported by the Japan Society for the Promotion of Science (JSPS) KAKENHI Grant-in-Aid for Scientific Research (B) JP17H02055.

References

1. Eckhoff, D., Halmos, B., German, R.: Potentials and limitations of green light optimal speed advisory systems. In: 2013 IEEE Vehicular Networking Conference, pp. 103–110 (2013)
2. Katsaros, K., Kernchen, R., Dianati, M., Rieck, D.: Performance study of a green light optimized speed advisory (GLOSA) application using an integrated cooperative ITS simulation platform. In: 2011 7th International Wireless Communications and Mobile Computing Conference, pp. 918–923 (2011)
3. Nguyen, V., Kim, O.T.T., Dang, T.N., Moon, S.I., Hong, C.S.: An efficient and reliable green light optimal speed advisory system for autonomous cars. In: 2016 18th Asia-Pacific Network Operations and Management Symposium (APNOMS) (2016)
4. Seredynski, M., Dorronsoro, B., Khadraoui, D.: Comparison of green light optimal speed advisory approaches. In: Proceedings of the 16th International IEEE Annual Conference on Intelligent Transportation Systems (ITSC 2013), pp. 2187–2192 (2013)
5. Seredynski, M., Mazurczyk, W., Khadraoui, D.: Multi-segment green light optimal speed advisory. In: 2013 IEEE 27th International Symposium on Parallel & Distributed Processing Workshops and PhD Forum, pp. 459–465 (2013)
6. Bodenheimer, R., Brauer, A., Eckhoff, D., German, R.: Enabling GLOSA for adaptive traffic lights. In: 2014 IEEE Vehicular Networking Conference (VNC), pp. 167–174 (2014)

7. Bodenheimer, R., Eckhoff, D., German, R.: GLOSA for adaptive traffic lights: methods and evaluation. In: 2015 7th International Workshop on Reliable Networks Design and Modeling (RNDM), pp. 320–328 (2015)
8. Suzuki, H., Marumo, Y.: A new approach to green light optimal speed advisory (GLOSA) systems and its limitations in traffic flows. In: Proceedings of the 1st International Conference on Human Systems Engineering and Design (IHSED 2018), pp. 776–782 (2018)
9. Suzuki, H., Marumo, Y.: A new approach to green light optimal speed advisory (GLOSA) systems for high-density traffic flow. In: Proceedings of the 21st IEEE International Conference on Intelligent Transportation Systems, pp. 362–367 (2018)
10. Nakanishi, T., Yamazaki, K., Marumo, Y., Suzuki, H.: Driver assistance system to pre-vent unnecessary deceleration at signalized intersection using signal information. In: 4th International Symposium on Future Active Safety Technology Toward Zero Traffic Accidents Fast-Zero (2017)

A Data-Driven Methodology to Assess Text Complexity Based on Syntactic and Semantic Measurements

Diego Palma[1(✉)], Christian Soto[1], Mónica Veliz[1], Bernardo Riffo[1], and Antonio Gutiérrez[2]

[1] University of Concepción, Concepción, Chile
{dipalma, christiansoto, mveliz, bernardo}@udec.cl
[2] Georgia Southern University, Statesboro, USA
agutierrez@georgiasouthern.edu

Abstract. In this paper we propose a data driven methodology to assess text complexity of Spanish school texts. We model the problem as a classification task, that can be solved in a data-driven fashion using machine learning techniques. We show empirically that the discriminative power of the classifier depends on school grade level. Our proposal includes multiple predictors that capture different dimensions of text complexity such as coherence and cohesion. We provide an importance analysis of predictors across several complexity levels. Finally, we assess the model performance using accuracy and correlation measurements. The proposed model achieves accuracies of 0.7.

Keywords: Text difficulty assessment · Natural language processing · Artificial intelligence · Machine learning · Educational systems

1 Introduction

In education, for reading comprehension assessment it is important that the texts that are presented to learners fit a certain level, so learners can be challenged and learn better about text content. To achieve this, it is critical that the texts are not too difficult or too easy for that particular level. In this manner, the ideas from the text can be processed more efficiently.

In this paper we introduce a new methodology to assess text difficulty levels based on coherence and cohesion predictors in the Spanish language. We prove that text difficulty level assessment can be modeled as a classification problem, and that the degree to that predictors have discriminative power depends on school grade level. Our proposal includes multiple predictors that capture different dimensions of the text complexity. Such dimensions are classified in three groups: lexical-semantic, syntactic and content.

For the semantic dimension of our proposal, we use predictors based on word embeddings, such as word2vec [1] model and latent semantic analysis (LSA) [2]. We try to capture different properties of text coherence in such predictors. For example, we approximate local coherence as the average meaning between adjacent sentences. To

T. Ahram et al. (Eds.): IHIET 2019, AISC 1018, pp. 509–515, 2020.
https://doi.org/10.1007/978-3-030-25629-6_79

achieve this, we use vector representation of word embeddings to encode sentences as mathematical vectors, and then we use cosine similarity to extract a measurement of coherence in the text. We also extended these measurements and tried to capture givenness which is defined as the amount of new information of the text that is added through sentences. To measure this, we form a hyperplane of previous sentences and compute the orthogonal component of the new sentence to all other sentences. This gives us a measure of what amount of new information is the sentence adding to the text [3].

For the syntactic dimension we use several ratios involving pronouns, adjectives, functional words and average measurements per sentences. In this manner, we try to capture cohesion properties of the text [4]. We also are using syntactic modelling from computational linguistics, such as entity grids [5] and entity graphs [6] to assess local coherence of a text. On the other hand, we use information from lexical-semantic norms (e.g. concreteness, imageability) to capture how easy/difficult is for the reader understanding a text based on the words that composes it. We also use lexical diversity measurements such as type token ratios (TTR), because the literature has shown correlations between TTR and text difficulty. On top of this, we also use the Kullback-Leibler divergence as a measurement of lexical complexity of a text [7].

We also assess content of texts using a bag of words modelling, because school curricula are also dependent on content, and there are different topics that are assessed through different school grade levels.

Finally, we use all the predictors and artificial intelligence techniques to end up with a classifier that can assess texts based on different predictors [8]. We show that important predictors for different school grade levels vary (e.g. for higher grade levels semantic relationships are more important than TTRs). We obtain classification accuracies of 0.7.

2 Related Work

Readability and text complexity assessment was computed using shallow features from texts in the early days. Features such as sentence length and number of syllables in a word were considered in measurements such as the Flesch-Kincaid formula [9]. Nevertheless, such measurements of text complexity over-generalize what makes a text complex, for instance they are not considering cohesion or coherence properties of a text, which can differ between texts composing the same word structure, but different grammar or linguistics resources used. On the other hand, these approaches are not considering semantic properties of the text, which might impact readers' perception of the text complexity.

In the literature, there have been several approaches to assess text complexity, but they have drifted to assess intrinsic text properties such as cohesion and coherence, and tools have been developed in order to assist research in this field [10]. This has been done considering syntactic properties of the text. In the mentioned approaches, cohesion and coherence are tried to be captured indirectly, and research has shown good levels of correlations between measurements and text complexity.

For the semantic view of the text complexity problem, research has focused on bag of word modelling. Latent semantic analysis (LSA) have been widely used for analyzing text complexity, and even to create automatic tools that assess texts based on content and semantic relationships between sentences and paragraph [11]. The problem is that this approach is not considering sentence ordering or syntactic complexity.

To address drawbacks from syntactic modelling and semantic modelling, research have focused in combining approaches for text assessment [8]. Nevertheless, text difficulty might depend on different predictors depending on target readers (e.g. school students). Such issues provide an opportunity to explore and research a data-driven methodology for text complexity assessment.

3 A Data-Driven Architecture for Text Complexity

In this paper, a data-driven methodology for text complexity assessment is proposed. The approach is capable of assessing text complexity based on textual coherence and cohesion by merging semantic measurements and syntactic patterns. Unlike the state-of-the-art text complexity assessment methodologies, the contribution of this research is twofold:

- The approach sets up a methodology for text complexity assessment and measurements selection.
- A text's complexity is measured by using corpus-based semantics and discourse patterns extraction (i.e. entity grids).

In order to evaluate the effectiveness of our proposed approach for text complexity assessment, a computational prototype was built using SPACY [12] and sci-kit learn libraries available for Python language. Several experiments were conducted, to check that the proposed method has predictive power (i.e. comparing to a dummy baseline) and to study which of the predictors are more important in several scenarios.

3.1 Data Collection

Texts from Chilean school system were collected from Chilean school textbooks. The corpus consisted on several texts for different grade levels and three different disciplines: social science, humanities and literature, and natural sciences. We had linguistics experts and school teachers gathering the data and carrying out the data digitalization for further processing. We also considered texts between 100–500 words. Corpus description is detailed on Tables 1 and 2. In total, we collected 1395 texts.

For generating word embeddings (word2vec) for Spanish, we used the Spanish billion-word Corpus [13].

3.2 Data-Driven Text Complexity Assessor Performance

In these experiments, the proposed method DDTCA (Data-Driven Text Complexity Assessor) was compared against a baseline which consisted on predicting always the most frequent grade level. The rationale for this comparison is that, if the method is not

Table 1. Text CORPUS used for experiments first 8 levels.

Grade	# of texts	School level
1	64	Elementary
2	101	Elementary
3	119	Elementary
4	121	Elementary
5	92	Middle
6	129	Middle
7	137	Middle
8	134	Middle

Table 2. Text CORPUS used for experiments for high school.

Grade	# of texts	School level
9	121	High-school
10	127	High-school
11	129	High-school
12	121	High-school

better than a dummy approach, then there is no gain on using a data driven approach. The performance was measured by using accuracy metric and the standard *Quadratic Weighted Kappa (QWK)*, which estimates the agreement between two raters, being 1 perfect agreement, and close to zero or even negative if there is no agreement. In order to perform the experiments, the following tasks were needed:

- Feature extraction: Each text was analyzed to extract shallow features such as average word per sentences, and TTR indices. To compute the Kullback-Leibler divergence we considered comparing the token distribution against a uniform distribution. For grammar-based features, texts were tagged using SPACY Python package. For content analysis using bag of word modelling, punctuation, numerals and stopwords were removed, and to reduce variability of texts, a *stemmer* was applied, respectively. For semantic coherence measurements, we used word embeddings from a word2vec representation. For the semantic givenness measurement, we used Gram-Schmidt orthogonalization to compute the vector space of the hyperplane composed by previous sentences word vectors. Then, we computed the orthogonal component of the sentence vector to the vector space and the givenness measurement is given by the cosine between the sentence and the orthogonal projection.
- Feature selection: We used Boruta algorithm [14]. As it will be discussed on results, many of the proposed features are relevant for this classification task.
- Generating the predictive model: We tried several machine learning models, but the best results were obtained using Random Forests classifier. This model ensembles multiple decision trees in the training phase, and prediction is produced by a voting scheme using predictions from each decision tree. Unlike other classification

methods, random forests classifier avoids overfitting and it is robust to noise in data. To assess the model performance, we split the dataset into two set, training (80%) and test (20%) sets.

We considered four classification tasks: elementary/middle school vs high school, only high school level, only elementary/middle school levels, and all. Results on Table 3 show the top five predictors on each classification task. Performance results are shown in Table 4. The decrease in performance while increasing granularity is the effect of having more classes defined in the problem. It is worth noting that QWK for baseline is always zero because it is equivalent than predicting at random.

Table 3. Top five features for different classification tasks.

Elementary/Middle vs High School	High-School levels	Elementary/Middle levels	All levels
Lemma TTR	Lemma TTR	Lemma TTR	Lemma TTR
Adjective incidence	Adjective incidence	Auxiliary verb incidence	NP-density
KL divergence	Noun-phrase density	Letters per word	Givenness
Entity graph coherence	Syllables per word	Closed class words	Funct. TTR
Average concreteness	Average imageability	Lexical overlap	Clause len

Table 4. Performance (accuracy|QWK) comparison between baseline and proposed approach

Method	Elementary/Middle vs High School	High School levels	Elementary/Middle levels	All levels
Baseline	(0.64|0.0)	(0.45|0.0)	(0.30|0.0)	(0.17|0.0)
DDTCA	**(0.71|0.35)**	**(0.62|0.26)**	**(0.52|0.66)**	**(0.39|0.64)**

From results, we can see that our proposed approach outperforms the baseline in all the scenarios. This means that, empirically the approach has a predictive power, and that AI techniques can make use of the approach to generate accurate predictions. We also observe that QWK is relatively high in high granularity scenarios, and this means that predictions are closer to what a human rater would predict. On the other hand, best predictors changed depending on the classification scenario. Additionally, we observe that at least for the dataset, the lemma TTR was always present as one of the best predictors. This is expected, since this is a measurement of vocabulary usage, which can help in distinguishing texts from different complexity levels.

4 Conclusions

In this paper, a novel methodology that takes into account semantic and syntactic information is proposed for text complexity assessment. The approach combines several predictors from linguistics research and discourse patterns in order to predict complexity of texts by using a random forest classifier. Unlike state-of-the-art approaches, our methodology relies on data, and thus, it can be adapted for different scenarios and different types of texts.

Experiments showed that the proposed predictors are closely related to the text complexity, and that their predictive power depends on context and the type of texts considered.

As future work, we consider enhancing the methodology by adding multiple layers for the model learning (model stacking and meta-learners). On the other hand, there are other features to consider such as the text narrativity, which might be correlated with a specific aspect of text complexity.

Acknowledgments. This research was supported by FONDEF (Chile) under Grant IT17I0051 *"Desarrollo de una herramienta computacional para la evaluación automática de textos en el sistema escolar chileno." ("Development of a computational tool for automatic assessment of Chilean school texts").*

References

1. Mikolov, T., Sutskever, I., Chen, K., Corrado, G.S., Dean, J.: Distributed representations of words and phrases and their compositionality. In: Advances in Neural Information Processing Systems, pp. 3111–3119 (2013)
2. Deerwester, S., Dumais, S.T., Furnas, G.W., Landauer, T.K., Harshman, R.: Indexing by latent semantic analysis. J. Am. Soc. Inf. Sci. **41**(6), 391–407 (1990)
3. Hempelmann, C.F., Dufty, D., McCarthy, P.M., Graesser, A.C., Cai, Z., McNamara, D.S.: Using LSA to automatically identify givenness and newness of noun phrases in written discourse. In: Proceedings of the 27th Annual Conference of the Cognitive Science Society, pp. 941–946. Erlbaum, Mahwah (2005)
4. Crossley, S.A., Kyle, K., McNamara, D.S.: The tool for the automatic analysis of text cohesion (TAACO): automatic assessment of local, global, and text cohesion. Behav. Res. Methods **48**(4), 1227–1237 (2016)
5. Barzilay, R., Lapata, M.: Modeling local coherence: an entity-based approach. Comput. Linguist. **34**(1), 1–34 (2008)
6. Guinaudeau, C., Strube, M.: Graph-based local coherence modeling. In: Proceedings of the 51st Annual Meeting of the Association for Computational Linguistics (Volume 1: Long Papers), vol. 1, pp. 93–103 (2013)
7. Salesky, E., Shen, W.: Exploiting morphological, grammatical, and semantic correlates for improved text difficulty assessment. In: Proceedings of the Ninth Workshop on Innovative Use of NLP for Building Educational Applications, pp. 155–162 (2014)
8. Palma, D., Atkinson, J.: Coherence-based automatic essay assessment. IEEE Intell. Syst. **33**(5), 26–36 (2018)

9. Kincaid, J.P., Fishburne Jr., R.P., Rogers, R.L., Chissom, B.S.: Derivation of new readability formulas (automated readability index, fog count and flesch reading ease formula) for navy enlisted personnel (1975)
10. Graesser, A.C., McNamara, D.S., Louwerse, M.M., Cai, Z.: Coh-Metrix: analysis of text on cohesion and language. Behav. Res. Methods Instrum. Comput. **36**(2), 193–202 (2004)
11. Wade-Stein, D., Kintsch, E.: Summary Street: interactive computer support for writing. Cogn. Instr. **22**(3), 333–362 (2004)
12. Honnibal, M., Montani, I.: spacy 2: natural language understanding with bloom embeddings, convolutional neural networks and incremental parsing (2017, to appear)
13. Cristian Cardellino: Spanish Billion Words Corpus and Embeddings, March 2016. https://crscardellino.github.io/SBWCE/
14. Kursa, M.B., Jankowski, A., Rudnicki, W.R.: Boruta–a system for feature selection. Fundamenta Informaticae **101**(4), 271–285 (2010)

Study on User Experience Design of Mobile Application Interfaces

Taian Xu(✉)

Zaozhuang University, Zaozhuang 277160, Shandong, China
tyanxu@163.com

Abstract. With the development of big data technology, the smartphone has become essential tool of people's life and work. APP interface, the core of smartphone application program and the APP interface to construct the user experience mode, is an important means to improve APP product performance and satisfy users' demand. This paper studies the interface design of smartphone APP so as to construct the interface design of user experience oriented smartphone APP from the three levels of feeling, cognition and sense.

Keywords: User experience · Smartphone · Interface

1 Introduction

With the development of big data technology, smartphone has been widely applied in people's life and work. The application of various intelligent devices largely depends on the control of mobile application programs. The users' demand is also being satisfied by the convenience of mobile operation systems. However, with the continuous development of Internet technology, traditional mobile interfaces has no longer met the growing need of users. Therefore, people have put forward higher requirements for the form and contents of mobile interface design. In other words, users should get better service level in the aspect of user experience, and accurate info-transformation between providers and target users, thus implement the application quickly and effectively.

2 Smartphone APP User Experience Layer Model

2.1 Analysis on User Experience of Smartphone APP Interface Design

User experience includes instinct layer, behavior layer and reflection layer. Instinct layer means that the product is leaving the most direct experience on users by stimulating people's sensory system. Instinct layer, the foundation of all experience, stimulates people's sensory system for a very short time and does not last for long, which will quickly disappear if it cannot be converted into higher layer experience. Behavior layer is users' experience through the use of various parts of the body and operation of products. We can carry out the innovation of user experience design from three aspects in the behavior layer [1]. First, the new operation of product can bring new user experience to users. Second, the new operation of products through body

T. Ahram et al. (Eds.): IHIET 2019, AISC 1018, pp. 516–521, 2020.
https://doi.org/10.1007/978-3-030-25629-6_80

parts can bring new user experience to users. Third, users can gain new user experience by actively participating in product design.

The reflection layer is users' emotional response in product using. The significance of emotional components in the interaction design has not been widely recognized. Emotional experience in the interaction design may be more important than sensory experience and behavior experience. The user experience of reflection layer usually depends on user' general impression on a kind of interface.

Based on the analysis on the user experience of instinct layer, behavior layer and reflection layer in interface design and characteristics of smartphone APP interface design, the user experience layers of smartphone APP interface design can be divided into sensory perception experience layer, emotional experience layer, and cognitive evaluation experience layer.

2.2 Study on Experience Layer of Smartphone APP Interface Design

2.2.1 Sensory Perception Experience Layer of Smartphone APP Interface Design

Sensory perception experience layer is users' visual, auditory and tactile sensations brought by various elements in the smartphone APP interface design. The information in the brain constitutes the formation of activities, which is closely related to various exterior information received by the sense organ. There are many factors affecting the sensory perception experience layer. Sensory experience of interface design constitution and color enables users to produce visual perception for text and picture when users use the same APP interface [2]. Users will have tactile perception when operating on the touch screen and have auditory experience through the feedback of voice interaction in the design interface. The most direct sensory stimulation by users is of great significance for the interface design. Good sensory experience can enhance the experience of the final interface. Interface design is based on the orientation of sensory experience and information display should be clear and easy to understand for users before operation. The design space of text and text should be allocated rationally and the zoom images should conform to users' operation habit so as to avoid the touch barrier. We should carry out module interface design and reasonable interface interaction so as to eliminate users' anxiety in using. The visualization effect of element in any smartphone APP interface design will bring users a strong visual sensory experience. However, be different sensory perception experience layers focus on different aspects in different types of APP interface design. For example, a notepad app may focus on the clearness of the recording content, humanized input mode and convenience in its sensory perception experience layer [3]. The a MEITUAN group-buying app may emphasize the fluency of the interface in its sensory perception experience layer so as to facilitate users to search the coverage of the products they need and pay conveniently.

2.2.2 Emotional Experience Layer of Smartphone APP Interface Design

Emotional experience layer is users' feeling in the operation of products. The emotional experience of smartphone APP enables users to have an expecting, comfortable, interesting and warming feeling in use, which emphasizes the emotional exchange service full of sense of design, story, interaction, entertainment and humanization between user and interface as well as the attractive, interesting and unforgettable product or service to users. In terms of smartphone APP interface design, the nerve centre of users' brain will have the ability to handle and judge the transmission information more quickly and accurately when users are operating the interface in positive emotional status so that they will have more pleasant and relaxing for feedback. Positive emotional status is easy to arouse users' curiosity, stimulate users' creativity, and easy to accept and understand interference stimulus information in the outside world. The positive or negative results of emotional experience play an important role in the success of APP interface design. Emotional experience has become the main trend to judge whether human-computer interaction products can succeed in the information era so as to make human-computer interaction process become natural, appropriate, aesthetic and anticipating [4]. Therefore, based on users' feeling, it is necessary to make the APP interface design in line with users' emotional style, understand users' inner demand and preferences and design the desired product characteristics for users, thus enhancing users' final experience for products and increasing the market share of products.

2.2.3 Cognitive Evaluation Experience Layer of Smartphone APP Interface Design

Cognitive evaluation experience layer is able to bring more practical and reflective experience for users while satisfying their fundamental demands, thus enabling users to have unexpected surprise in operation. APP product in cognitive evaluation experience layer will bring innovative and unforgettable memory as well as unexpected shock to users so that the products can have good user viscosity and market competitive advantage. In the process of smartphone APP interface design, apart from the fundamental function of user emotional experience layer, the pursuit for cognitive evaluation experience layer can bring innovative, peculiar and imaginative effect to users. It is an important method for the designers to carry out product differentiation in the cognitive evaluation experience layer.

3 User Experience Layer Model Oriented Smartphone APP Interface Design

3.1 Direction of Smartphone APP Interface Design

First, we need to construct the user experience based APP interface design according to users investigation. Specifically, we need to refine and divide the user groups. For example, we need to determine the specific user group according to smartphone APP property and function.

Second, APP interface design should be concise but not simple. The leading mode of recognition and emotion should be determined to ensure that the APP interface design should meet users' demand. All elements of all APPs have their mission. If a certain element is visually prominent, it has the most important function.

Third, APP function and interaction are customized. With clear priority of user demands, we should focus on users' key demands.

Fourth, it is necessary to create a warm and interesting mobile APP experience atmosphere from the perspective of design. The design of APP is similar to film photography. We need to seize people in the performance. Game app is particularly important to guide users into a certain situation. It trends to have this consciousness in the tool APP, which is inclined to design a process that constantly affect users' emotion. Therefore, many APPs will display the inquisitive pictures or videos at the homepage.

Fifth, we have enjoyment in the APP playing. Different contents will be displayed in different or interactive ways, thus bring different pleasures. Good apps can make full use of characteristics of mobile equipment, such as geographical location positioning, gyroscope, sound, camera, etc., which actually provide pleasures for users by using interaction channels.

3.2 Flow of Smartphone APP Interface Design

3.2.1 List of Users' Demand Customization

In the process of product development, the user centered design activates the participation of different user group and enables users to have a strong purchase desire because of security, comfort and high efficiency. In the design process, user demand should be fully taken into account because the intensity of user demand is able to improve product viscosity. At the same time, users should be invited to participate in the design process. Users not only put forward demand in the early stage of design but actively give their feedback opinion in the interface test process, which provides experience basis for final evaluation [5].

We should determine the target user group according to the use and interaction experience of the existing products. Users with interaction experience of the product and system can provide more effective information for the design compared with users with no interaction experience [6]. Therefore, we should first take into account of the users of the designed products or users with use experience of similar products for the collection of user experience information. Under the most perfect circumstance, designers can obtain users' sensory impression through a certain technique or research method and grasp their emotional experience in users interaction experience of products. However, these subjective experience information are difficult to be collected through laboratory method and conveyed by scientific description. Therefore, we can only seek a practical user experience method close to users, i.e., in-depth interviews and on-site observation.

3.2.2 Architecture Design of Interface

Architecture design is mainly for the construction of product information, including navigation design and information layout design of the user interface, aiming to enable users to get the information they need at the cost of least cognition, which is characterized by high efficiency, low recognition cost, etc. Users can easily understand the main function of the products and the organization relation among each functional module. Due to the restrictions of mobile equipment screen, user use method and other conditions on the mobile Internet app, its architecture structure is generally carried out on the basic layer structure. The information architecture of mobile Internet app can be divided into 4 basic types (as shown in Fig. 1), superficial and wide, narrow and superficial, wide and deep, narrow and deep information architectures [7].

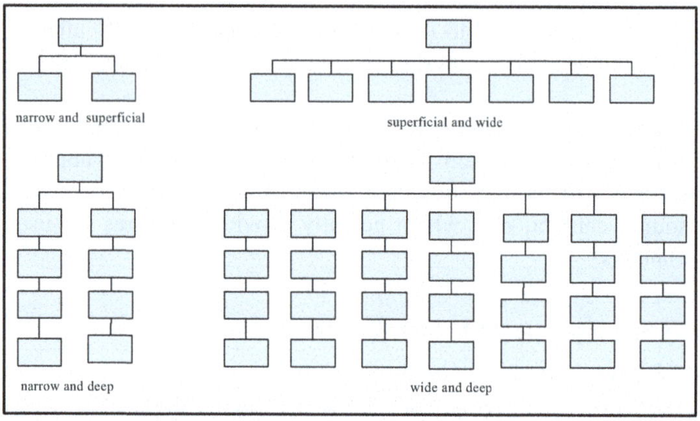

Fig. 1. Types of information architecture

3.2.3 Interface Process Design and Wireframe Design

Interface design flow chart is the basic process to vivid construct the user interface design in graphical form, which can be regarded as the guiding drawing of design process. This drawing can help designers with the design according to routine, high efficient communication among different design departments and good logical guidance of new users and complex flow. Wireframe design is the APP function realization targeted and centered design graphic display, which expounds the basic constitution and basic relation of pages. The wireframe diagram gives a good description of information logical relation according to priority information, thus providing design blue print for interface design [8].

3.2.4 Visualized Design of Interface

There are some differences of apps in serviceability due to different appearances similar to the interface design mode. Furthermore, the visual style of the interface may greatly affect users' evaluation on the app when users use the service for the first time. Good visual style enables users to leave good impression on its service and use it for a long time.

At present, the prominent style of smartphone is the basic style of iOS application, Android application and Windows application. Among them, iOS application and Android application have their own default style. In addition, people are familiar with two visual styles, i.e. quasi-physical design and flat design.

Quasi-physical design is a simulation of real design through a certain material. Its interface shows the real objects, which give prompt to users about its function. Users who use this kind of design style for the first time can quickly understand the usage of various interfaces. This kind of design not only improves the operability but also get the distance with users closer. However, it still have some shortcomings. Overprecise prototype texture reduces the usability on the contrary.

The whole interface is in flat style in the flat design. The buttons and other parts for users' operation are all in flat design with no indication for user click. The interface of flat design is of simple structure, even tone and unified style. Among them, Windows8 application gives full play to the plat style. Its style has no redundant elements, suitable for frequently daily use application, which is able to reduce users' disgust due to daily contact. It is also the mainstream interface style currently.

Visual design is the part that has most direct contact with users. Reasonable visual design conforms to the interaction process in the interaction design and the interface is full of sense of layer, which is able to accurately convey the brand image and pass on the most important information to users.

4 Conclusion

The integration of user experience in APP design is an important way to gain more user groups. Particularly, as the 5G era is coming, it provides wider opportunity platform for the development of APP. Based on the development status of APP currently, we need to correctly understand the necessity of user experience integration and improve in the interface design and content design, thus promoting the improvement of comprehensive competitive strength.

References

1. Yang, L., Wei, Y.: Visual thinking based user interface design. Design **4**, 109–111 (2015)
2. Jiao, J.: Mobile User Interface Design (UI) and Development Trend. Northwest University, Xi'an (2013)
3. Chaofan, S.: Visual aesthetics principle in mobile terminal interaction design. Art Lit. Masses **06**, 118 (2014)
4. Sida, L.: Introduction to Interaction Design, p. 162. Tsinghua University Press, Beijing (2011)
5. Huijuan, W.: Study on the Interaction Design in Mobile Context. Zhejiang University of Technology (2016)
6. Libin, H.: Study on the Interaction Effect of Mobile Application. Zhejiang University (2015)
7. Zhen, C.: Impact of Interaction Design on Mobile User Experience. Fudan University (2003)
8. Xiaolu, Z.: Study on the User Experience Based APP Interaction Design. SouthWest JiaoTong University (2015)

Studmap 3.0 – An Interoperable Web-Based Platform for Geospatial Data Offers in Academic Life

Ștefana Cioban[1(✉)], Vitor Santos[1], and Torsten Prinz[2]

[1] NOVA IMS – Universidade Nova de Lisboa, Campus de Campolide, 1070-312 Lisbon, Portugal
stefanacioban@yahoo.com, vsantos@novaims.unl.pt
[2] WWU – Institut für Geoinformatik, Universität Münster, Heisenbergstraße 2, 48149 Münster, Germany
prinz@uni-muenster.de

Abstract. Geographic Information Systems has now entered the realm of web and yields for feasible solutions to balance the technology offers with the users' needs to share, access and explore the massive amounts of geodata available. Challenges occur when moving forward from old 2D platforms towards innovative and integrated webGIS systems that align functionality with the necessity to grant a complete understanding of the surrounding reality. 3D space responds to this necessity but, however, stands only at the beginning of its era and cannot yet reach the development of 2D web integration. Research is now aiming at possible webGIS solutions to adapt to the special structure imposed by 3D data. In this context, this paper focuses on designing an architecture for 2D and 3D geospatial data integration on a student-oriented web platform. This concept was further delivered and validated through a real case scenario – Studmap 3.0, a webGIS platform to serve the students of the University of Muenster in their academical life. The portal currently grants availability of geospatial data and web services of regional interest in a smart GIS environment that allows access and comparison of official services with own data. The implementation of Studmap 3.0 aided in the continuous improvement of the proposed architecture model and hence, developed under a design science research methodology. The cycle reached its end once the final approval of its users was attained via a mixed usability evaluation. Final strengths and drawbacks of the proposed architecture were ultimately identified in terms of data, system functionality, ease of implementation and usability. The usability for academical use was evaluated via a customized expert inspection, followed by a standardized student usability test of the resulting portal interface. The results fall under the acceptable range with an 83.75 score for the System Usability Scale standardized questions when addressed to experts and a score of 83.87 when addressed to students. A summary of future participants' opinion on the benefits, drawbacks and proposed improvements was also delivered according to the answers to the final open-ended questions. Peers interested in similar concepts can use both this model and its final remarks as a reference for their work.

Keywords: WebGIS · Geodata · 3D · Web portal

T. Ahram et al. (Eds.): IHIET 2019, AISC 1018, pp. 522–527, 2020.
https://doi.org/10.1007/978-3-030-25629-6_81

1 Introduction

New tendencies of GIS integration with Internet technologies or simply, webGIS, enable geospatial data to move towards a new accessibility and interoperability culmination [1]. Due to the flood of geodata available, an increasing number of users and a limited number of resources to cope with them, the technological advances are pushing the geospatial sciences to rethink the way data are understood, stored, handled and delivered [2].

WebGIS allows the efficiently sharing of the geospatial data among its users around the world [1]. To synchronize with the current tendencies in GIS and geodata offers across the web, students crosscutting with this realm now require a smart, 3D-friendly web environment to respond to their practical needs: to allow the access of public and official data and to upload and share own data with the others. In this scenario, this paper is motivated by the lack of scientific solutions to balance both 2D and 3D functionality in a webGIS system dedicated to the student's academic needs. Therefore, we aim to offer a new architecture for an integrated web platform intended to allow the download, exploit and upload of the datasets of regional interest in a webGIS environment.

Researchers in the GIS field are delivering innovative ideas to promote progress usually in written forms which are not always applied to real-world practices [3]. The present research responds to this call as the validation of the proposed architecture was done via a practical implementation of Studmap 3.0 [4], a webGIS platform designed to support the students of WWU University of Muenster in real life altogether with a design science framework that can always be adapted according to specific needs and improved upon feedback. The implemented architecture wishes to serve as a reference tool for all peers interested.

2 Methodology

The aim of the research is to integrate complex geospatial data and web-based services on an interoperable web platform by proposing and evaluating a GIS client-server architecture. Hence, design science research framework [5] is adopted as the intention is to build knowledge through the creation of reality (Fig. 1).

The awareness of the problem phase is introduced by the objectives of the research: the proposal and implementation of a client-server architecture for complex GIS data and web services integration. The suggestion phase reflects in the solutions proposed by the existing GIS integration research and the empirical experience gained through the operation and goal knowledge discovery. The development phase is the construction of the artefact based on the suggestion phase. The artefact is represented by the proposal and design of a client-server architecture to serve for the integration of the motivated data and services. The evaluation consists of the practical implementation of the proposed architecture and validation of its functionality throughout the student dedicated platform: Studmap 3.0 [4]. The outcome of this phase is feed back to the previous one and hence, the artefact is reshaped accordingly. The process iterates as experience is accumulated and new theories emerge. The conclusion is drawn from the

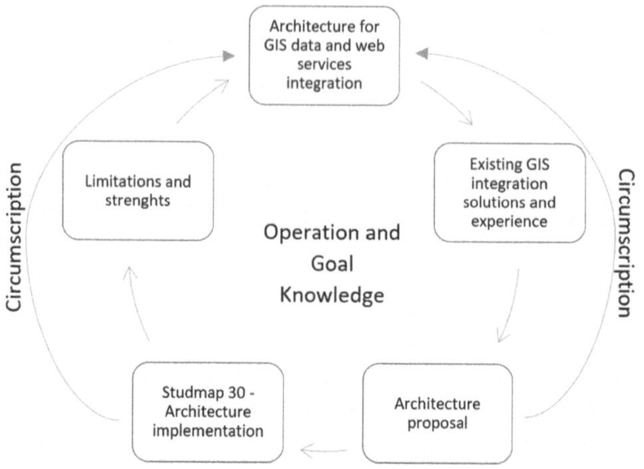

Fig. 1. Design-science research framework implementation

evaluation of the artefact. As a measure for the ultimate approval of the end-user to terminate the process, a customized usability evaluation is designed.

Among the software solutions available, ArcGIS Server was chosen for its powerful geoprocessing functions. The ArcGIS Server Site is federated with the Portal for ArcGIS and configured as a hosted server using registered ArcGIS Data Stores to allow the publication of cached maps, feature and scene layers as hosted services [6]. An enterprise database was chosen to work with the ArcGIS Data Stores to allow the real-time updates and the fully administrator management of the GIS services in parallel with the ArcGIS managed ones. The database was created using the PostgreSQL open source database management system because of its extended spatial functionality, ease of administration and compatibility with the ESRI software. For an intuitive web applications configuration on top of the GIS server, WAB SDK [7] was used. The aimed webGIS services compatible with the software choice, are OGC compliant web map services that reduce the need to store the data locally and to take the workload off the GIS server to give fast responses to the users' requests.

A three-tier client-server architecture was chosen [8] to divide the workload between different machines and enhance the overall functionality. The presentation tier is represented by the web browsers that allow the users and administrators to interact with the GIS server and portal. The application tier consists of the web servers and the GIS server holding the logic of the system. The GIS server provides the core GIS functionality of the system and supports the derived web maps [1]. The database tier is represented by two relational databases -a PostgreSQL enterprise database and an ArcGIS managed data store- and a non-relational database -the ArcGIS tile cache data store. While the relational databases hold the GIS function of handling 2D and basic 3D features, the tile cache the manages hosted scene layers which allow storage and manipulation of the complex 3D data. To secure the communication between the components of this architecture, all communications are restricted to HTTPS-only. The administration of the requests is done via the REST API and is handled by two web applications, the ArcGIS Server Administrator Directory or the ArcGIS Server Manager [9].

3 Results

To validate the artefact, the client-server architecture was implemented and evaluated using the Studmap 3.0 portal (Fig. 2). The data was generated from three different sources: an old portal, Studmap 1.4 [10][1], the students' UAS2018 projects and some relevant third-party providers. The data coming from the old portal and the recent projects are stored in a common PostgreSQL geospatial database. The complex 3D data, in this case the point cloud layer generated from the UAS2018 project, are stored locally in a converted format, SLPK [11] as this type of data structure doesn't allow storage in a database. The data coming from the third-party servers are represented by the web map and feature services provided by the official geodata servers of the German state of North Rhine-Westphalia [12] and by the cloud-based platform of the Institute for Geoinformatics of the WWU University of Muenster [13].

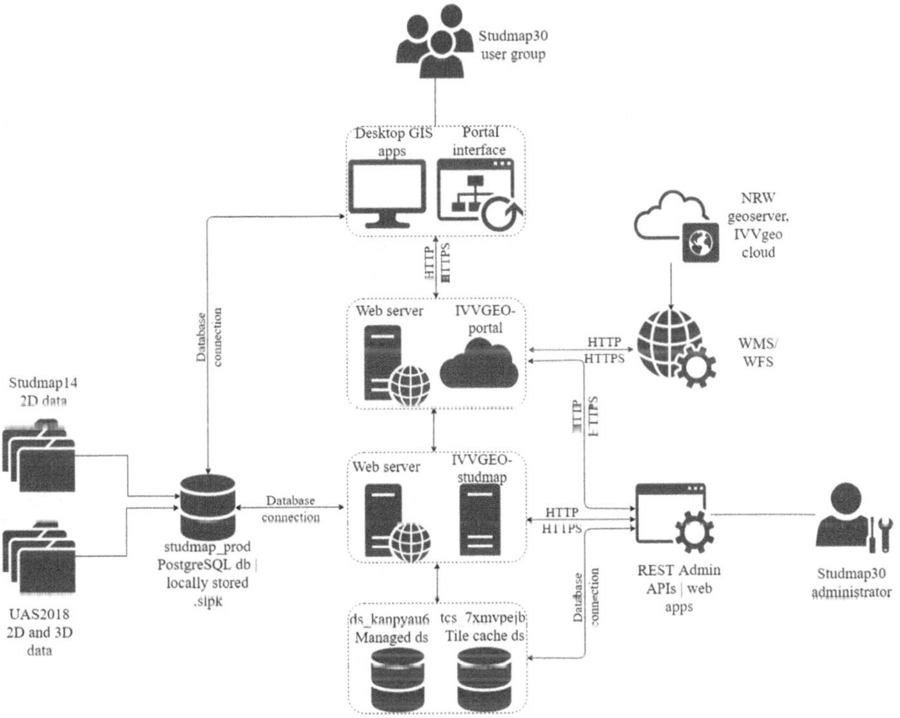

Fig. 2. General diagram of the architecture implementation for Studmap 3.0

The implemented web portal has a hybrid system architecture at all three component levels. The presentation tier consists of desktop GIS applications (ArcGIS Map and ArcGIS Pro) and web applications (Portal for ArcGIS, ArcGIS Server Manager) or

[1] Source derived from the intranet (not publicly available) of WWU Muenster.

REST Admin APIs (ArcGIS Portal Directory, Portal Administrator Directory, ArcGIS Server Administrator Directory) that allow the users and administrators to interact with the IVVGEO portal and server. As for the application layer, it consists of the two web servers holding the logic for both the portal and the server and the IVVGEO Server itself. The database tier consists of two relational data stores (a PostgreSQL enterprise geodatabase and the Managed ArcGIS Data Store) and one non-relational data store (the Tile Cache ArcGIS Data Store).

4 Discussion and Conclusion

A comparison between the concept and implementation of the proposed architecture was done in terms of data, system functionality, system usability and ease of implementation. The first three criteria were specified according to nowadays' mapping trends [14] and focus on the technical objectives of this study, while the latter focuses on the overall implementation of the system. The proposed and evaluated architecture is limited by a series of non-functional requirements depending on the context of the implementation of the Studmap 3.0 portal. The first dependency is given by the resources available in terms of both hardware and software and influences the overall performance of the system. System security comes as the second dependency as the communications of the implemented systems are done via both HTTP and HTTPS protocols which gives a less secure alternative compared to the conceptual model. Last, the cost of equipment comes as a restriction for the designed architecture as the chosen software to offer the main GIS function is provided by ESRI.

The output of this study is Studmap 3.0 [4], an integrated webGIS platform to grant relevant services and geospatial data to students. To evaluate the users' appreciation of the platform and to reach the end of the design science cycle, a mixed usability evaluation was developed. First, the study was done by two experts that were asked to inspect the interface of the portal and answer questions formulated according to its intended functionalities and audience. Second, the interface was evaluated by 20 students that were given a set of tasks designed corresponding to the intended functionality of the platform. The tasks were generally well received, with a completion rate of 100% for all students whose graphics were compatible with the products' requirements. All participants responded to a standardized SUS questionnaire [15] which delivered a score of 83.75% for the experts and 83.87% for the students. The benefits, drawbacks, future improvements and overall opinion were summarized for both categories of participants and should contribute to further improve the platform.

Two main strengths were identified: the platform provides students with an effective tool to interact with available official data and previous projects via an interactive web mapping portal interface and it integrates both 2D and 3D features in a smart webGIS environment. One essential compromise was necessary to fit with the chosen schema: the storage of the SLPK datasets is done separately from the databases, in a local folder.

An additional usability study is recommended to further improve of the platform and to provide comparative results. Moreover, an extension of the machines hosting the main components should be considered to increase the overall performance. For an improved quality of the storage system, a solution to organize the complex 3D data files needed to be saved locally is required. Nonetheless, this work can be perceived as a reference for any peers interested in similar problems.

References

1. Agrawal, S., Gupta, R.D.: Web GIS and its architecture: a review. Arab. J. Geosci. **10**, 518 (2017)
2. Yang, C., Huang, Q., Li, Z., Liu, K., Hu, F.: Big Data and cloud computing: innovation opportunities and challenges. Int. J. Digital Earth. **10**, 13–53 (2016)
3. Gahegan, M.: Our GIS is too small. Canadian Geographer/Le Géographe canadien. **62**, 15–26 (2017)
4. Digitale Karten - Universität Münster. https://www.uni-muenster.de/ZDMgeo/angebot/digitalekarten.html. Accessed 15 Apr 2019
5. Kanellis, P., Papadopoulos, T.: Conducting research in information systems. In: Information Systems Research Methods, Epistemology, and Applications, pp. 1–34. IGI Global (2009)
6. Portal for ArcGIS - Apps and functionality that require ArcGIS Data Store. http://enterprise.arcgis.com/en/portal/latest/administer/windows/what-requires-arcgis-data-store.htm. Accessed 11 Jan 2019
7. Web AppBuilder for ArcGIS (Developer Edition). https://developers.arcgis.com/web-appbuilder/guide/xt-welcome.htm. Accessed 05 Jan 2019
8. Shekhar, S., Xiong, H., Zhou, X. (eds): Encyclopedia of GIS (2017). http://dx.doi.org/10.1007/978-3-319-17885-1
9. ArcGIS Server. http://enterprise.arcgis.com/en/server/latest/get-started/windows/what-is-arcgis-for-server-.htm. Accessed 06 June 2018
10. StudMap14 Dokumentationen. https://ivv6-wiki.uni-muenster.de/neu/dokuwiki/doku.php?id=dev_studmap14:old:inhalt:dokumentation. Accessed 16 Dec 2018
11. OGC Indexed 3d Scene Layer (I3S) and Scene Layer Package Format Specification. http://docs.opengeospatial.org/cs/17-014r5/17-014r5.html. Accessed 16 Apr 2019
12. OpenNRW - Open Data. https://open.nrw/suche. Accessed 08 Jan 2019
13. IVVgeo - Gallery for Geo Münster. http://ivv6.maps.arcgis.com/home/index.html. Accessed 09 Jan 2019
14. Veenendaal, B., Brovelli, M.A., Li, S.: Review of web mapping: eras, trends and directions. ISPRS Int. J. Geo-Inform. **6**, 317 (2017)
15. Sauro, J., Lewis, J.R.: Standardized usability questionnaires. In: Quantifying the User Experience, pp. 185–248. Elsevier (2016)

Medicine, Biomechanics, Sports and Healthcare

A Serious Game for Thrombosis Prophylaxis – Only for the Healthy?

Daniel Steffen[1(✉)], Juliane Pietschmann[2], Thomas Jöllenbeck[2], and Gabriele Bleser[1]

[1] AG wearHEALTH, Technische Universität Kaiserslautern, Gottlieb-Daimler-Straße, 67663 Kaiserslautern, Germany
{steffen, bleser}@cs.uni-kl.de
[2] Institute for Biomechanics, Klinik Lindenplatz, Weslarner Straße 29, 59505 Bad Sassendorf, Germany
{juliane.pietschmann, thomas.joellenbeck}@klinik-lindenplatz.de

Abstract. The rates of thrombosis without any prophylaxis range from 40% to 50% after orthopedic surgery like hip or knee replacement. Besides pharmacological measures, the muscle-vein-pump (MVP) is a typical exercise that is recommended for thrombosis prophylaxis. However, this exercise can be mundane and boring, which will compromise adherence to the rehabilitation program. Serious Games for Health have been suggested to motivate exercise training in rehabilitation and prevention. This paper describes a serious game for thrombosis prophylaxis. 41 participants volunteered in our user study and tested either an application counting the repetitions or a serious game controlled through MVP repetitions. All participants were patients after a hip or knee replacement surgery of a rehabilitation hospital. We evaluated the effect of application type on usage, i.e., duration, repetitions, and repetitions per minute. Additionally, we applied different questionnaires, e.g., System Usability Scale, Technology Acceptance Model, Intrinsic Motivation Inventory among others.

Keywords: Serious game for health · Thrombosis prophylaxis · Hip and knee replacement · Rehabilitation hospital · User study

1 Introduction

The number of hip and knee replacements has increased rapidly since 2000 in most OECD countries. While the rate of hip replacement increased by 30% between 2000 and 2015, the rate of knee replacement nearly doubled [1]. The risk of a deep vein thrombosis after a hip or a knee replacement is between 40% and 50% without any prophylaxis [2]. Pharmacological prophylaxis is recommended for patients after hip or knee replacement. Additionally, mechanical measures (e.g. compression stocking) as well as basic measures including early mobilization, movement exercises and instructions for self-exercises should be applied [3]. The muscle-vein-pump (MVP) is a typical physical exercise that is frequently recommended for thrombosis prophylaxis. It belongs to the category of repetitive movement exercises. To activate the MVP users flex their feet downward the sole and afterwards towards their knee.

T. Ahram et al. (Eds.): IHIET 2019, AISC 1018, pp. 531–537, 2020.
https://doi.org/10.1007/978-3-030-25629-6_82

Simple movement exercises like the MVP, however, can be mundane and boring due to their repetitive nature, which will compromise adherence to the rehabilitation program [4]. Serious games for Health have been suggested as one way to motivate regular training in prevention and rehabilitation, which include such monotonous and mundane exercises. However, researchers support as well as reject the hypotheses that serious games support and motivate regular exercise training [5–7].

2 User Study

2.1 Design

To address the above mentioned problems within the context of thrombosis prophylaxis we used a between-subject design with the independent variable *Application* (with two levels: *Counter* and *Game*). While the control group (CG) used the *Counter* application the treatment group (TG) used the *Game* application. The dependent variables were the *number of repetitions* a participant performed the MVP, the *duration* he used the application, and the *repetitions per minute*. Additionally, we used the following questionnaires: Borg's Rating of Perceived Exertion (RPE) [8], System Usability Scale (SUS) [9], Intrinsic Motivation Inventory (IMI) [10], AttrakDiff2 [11], Technology Acceptance Model (TAM) [12, 13], Technology Affinity – Electronic Devices (TA-EG) [14]. Ethical approval was obtained from the University of Paderborn Ethics Committee.

2.2 Participants

All participants were patients in a rehabilitation hospital after hip or knee replacement. Due to a technical issue one participant canceled the user study and was excluded. 41 participants (27 female), aged 49 to 78 (M = 60.6, SD = 7.3), volunteered in the user study. 21 participants (11 treatment group) had undergone a hip replacement and 20 participants (9 treatment group) had a knee replacement.

From the total sample, 17 participants (9 control group) had already used a game console supporting movement-based interaction, e.g. Nintendo's Wii. We asked the participants how many hours per week they had spent playing computer games. 24 participants (11 control group) had never played computer games. Nearly all participants (98%) owned a mobile device, i. e. either a smart phone or a tablet PC or both.

The results of the TA-EG questionnaire show no significant difference between control and treatment group for the constructs *enthusiasm* ($M_{CG} = 2.81$, $SD_{CG} = 0.93$; $M_{TG} = 2.98$, $SD_{TG} = 1.24$; $t(35.28) = -0.48$, $p = 0.63$), *competence* ($M_{CG} = 3.02$, $SD_{CG} = 0.99$; $M_{TG} = 3.03$, $SD_{TG} = 1.09$; $t(38.189) = -0.00$, $p = 0.99$), *positive attitude* ($M_{CG} = 3.62$, $SD_{CG} = 0.41$; $M_{TG} = 3.54$, $SD_{TG} = 0.39$; $t(38.98) = -0.19$, $p = 0.60$) and *negative attitude* ($M_{CG} = 3.89$, $SD_{CG} = 0.79$; $M_{TG} = 4.02$, $SD_{TG} = 0.54$; $t(35.27) = -0.62$, $p = 0.54$) with electronic devices.

2.3 Apparatus

A portable system has been developed using a an Apple iPad2 and two inertial measurement units fastened to the participants 'feet to measure the flexion angle during the MVP. The user controls the application by stretching and bending his left and right ankle joint. The *Counter* application only counts and displays the number of MVP repetitions. The *Game* is a movement-based side-scroller game (see Fig. 1).

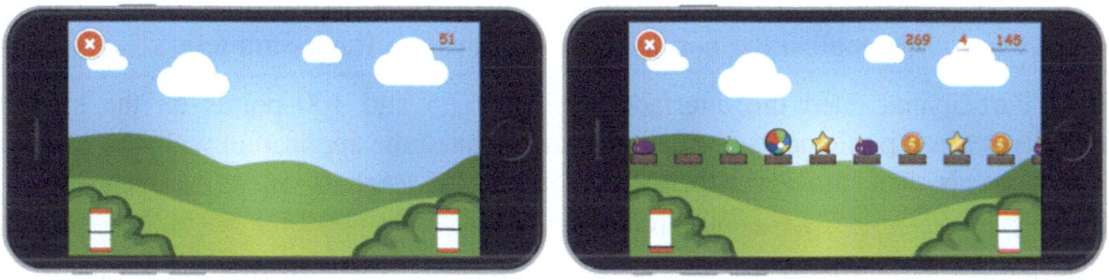

Fig. 1. Participants of the control group used the *Counter* application (left). The *Game* application (right) was used by participants of the treatment group.

2.4 Procedure

The experiment was conducted in the laboratory of the Institute for Biomechanics, Klinik Lindenplatz, Bad Sassendorf, Germany. Participants were randomly assigned to the two application conditions. They were recruited through notices in their mailbox or by telephone call. At the beginning of the experiment, the participants signed an informed consent. Furthermore, we gave some general information about thrombosis prophylaxis and the MVP exercise. We then asked them to fill in the 11-point Numeric Rating Scale for Pain (NRS). Participants were asked twice to comment on any pain: (1) before (NRS_{before}) starting the application and (2) immediately after (NRS_{after}) they finished the application.

To ensure a good fastening, participants had to take off their shoes. Next, the participants laid down on a medical couch in a comfortable posture. To prevent early dislocation by limiting the flexion of the hip (less than 90°) after a hip replacement we fastened the sensors on the participants' feet. For hygienic reasons the sensors were wrapped in a plastic bag and fastened using self–adherent bandages, which were thrown away afterwards.

Before starting the application, the participants calibrated the system. We explained the participants how to perform the MVP exercise correctly and set the task: "Please use the exercise application as long as you like". The application stopped in the following cases: (1) the participant pressed the exit button, (2) he completed the application, or (3) he played longer than 30 min. Participants were not aware about the latter two exit conditions. To validate and extend the data collected during the application different constructs were measured subsequently. Starting with the NRS_{after} we used the questionnaires mentioned above. Besides their gaming habits, participants commented on the usability of the wireless IMUs and reported on the demographic variables (e. g. year of birth, gender, etc.). As a surprise, participants received a voucher for the local cafeteria after they finished the user study.

3 Results

The experimental user study took approximately one hour (M = 52.32, SD = 15.65). We will describe the objective and subjective measurements. Where applicable we used the parametric independent t-test to analyze the data. If the assumptions to use the t-test were violated, we applied the non-parametric Wilcoxon Rank-Sum test.

SUS: Participants rated the interface between 62.5 and 100 points on the system usability scale. 7 participants (5 treatment group) rated the application with a maximum of 100 points. The difference between *Counter* (M = 89.40, SD = 7.47) and *Game* (M = 91.75, SD = 9.78) was not significant, $W = 153$, $p = 0.14$, $r = -0.23$.

Sensor Usability: The usability of the wearable IMUs was evaluated using 3-items on a 7-point Likert scale. Overall, the treatment group (M = 6.98, SD = 0.07) as well as the control group (M = 6.80, SD = 0.31) found the application very usable. The difference between the *Game* and the *Counter* application was significant, $W = 149$, $p < 0.05$, $r = -0.36$.

TAM: The average value for *perceived usefulness* was significantly different between treatment group (M = 6.78, SD = 0.35) and control group (M = 6.02, SD = 1.07), $W = 126.5$, $p < 0.05$, $r = -0.36$. The *perceived enjoyment* using the *Game* application was significantly larger (M = 6.38, SD = 0.90) than using the *Counter* application (M = 5.52, SD = 1.18), $W = 115$, $p < 0.05$, $r = -0.40$. No difference was found for the construct *perceived ease of use* between the two applications ($M_{CG} = 6.46$, $SD_{CG} = 0.62$; $M_{TG} = 6.81$, $SD_{TG} = 0.40$; $W = 152$, $p = 0.08$, $r = -0.27$).

IMI: A 20–item version (each item on a 7-point Likert scale) of the IMI was used to evaluate the four categories *enjoyment*, *perceived competence*, *usefulness*, and *pressure*. The participants rated the construct *enjoyment* significantly higher using the *Game* (M = 6.00, SD = 1.45) than using the *Counter* application (M = 5.19, SD = 1.47), $W = 135.5$, $p < 0.05$, $r = -0.31$. No significant difference was found for the categories *usefulness* ($M_{CG} = 5.67$, $SD_{CG} = 1.52$; $M_{TG} = 5.85$, $SD_{TG} = 1.49$; $W = 199.5$, $p = 0.78$, $r = -0.04$), *perceived competence* ($M_{CG} = 5.14$, $SD_{CG} = 1.36$; $M_{TG} = 5.55$, $SD_{TG} = 1.20$; $W = 174.5$, $p = 0.35$, $r = -0.17$), and *pressure* ($M_{CG} = 1.81$, $SD_{CG} = 1.62$; $M_{TG} = 1.85$, $SD_{TG} = 1.65$; $W = 219.5$, $p = 0.77$, $r = -0.05$).

AttrakDiff2: This AttrakDiff2 questionnaire uses semantic differentials to assess the user experience of a product. No significant differences were found between the *Counter* and the *Game* application for the categories: *attractivity* ($M_{CG} = 5.95$, $SD_{CG} = 0.90$; $M_{TG} = 6.00$, $SD_{TG} = 1.22$; $W = 187.5$, $p = 0.55$, $r = -0.09$), *pragmatic quality* ($M_{CG} = 2.81$, $SD_{CG} = 1.59$; $M_{TG} = 3.5$, $SD_{TG} = 1.53$; $W = 150$, $p = 0.11$, $r = -0.25$), and *hedonic quality* ($M_{CG} = 4.86$, $SD_{CG} = 1.35$; $M_{TG} = 5.13$, $SD_{TG} = 0.96$; $W = 169$, $p = 0.41$, $r = -0.13$).

Increased Pain Intensity: In total, 11 out of 41 participants rated the pain intensity on the NRS_{after} higher than on the NRS_{before}. When asked about the type and location, nearly all of them mentioned a sense of pain in the lower legs that had stopped, when they stopped the exercise.

RPE: Although participants of the control group rated their perceived exertion slightly higher ($M = 11.42$, $SD = 2.48$) than the treatment group ($M = 10.65$, $SD = 2.83$), the difference was not significant, $t(37.73) = 0.91$, $p = 0.37$, $r = 0.15$.

Figure 2 presents the results for the dependent variables duration, number of repetitions and repetitions per minute for the two application conditions.

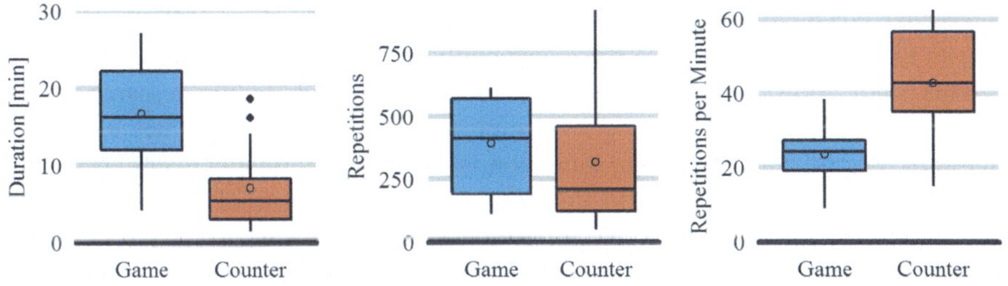

Fig. 2. Participants of the treatment group used the *Game* application significantly longer than the control group the *Counter* application. No significant difference was found between the conditions for *the number of repetitions*. In contrast, participants in the control group performed the MVP significantly faster than the treatment group.

Duration: Participants of the treatment group used the *Game* application significantly longer ($M = 16.6$ min, $SD = 6.47$) than the control group the *Counter* application ($M = 6.99$, $SD = 4.72$), $W = 49$, $p < 0.001$, $r = 0.70$.

Number of Repetitions: However, the difference in number of repetitions for the treatment group ($M = 391.45$, $SD = 182.31$) was not significantly different from the control group ($M = 314.95$, $SD = 258.35$), $W = 146$, $p = 0.10$, $r = -0.26$.

Repetitions per Minute: In contrast, the number of repetitions per minute of the control group ($M = 42.59$, $SD = 13.67$) was twice as big as for the treatment group ($M = 23.48$, $SD = 6.70$). The difference was significant, $W = 364$, $p < 0.001$, $r = -0.67$.

4 Discussion and Conclusion

The presented user study evaluated the effects of a serious game for thrombosis prophylaxis with patients after knee or hip replacement in a rehabilitation hospital. No significant difference was found for the *number of repetitions*. Since past studies showed a significant effect when used by healthy participants [5], the usage environment might have an effect on the *number of repetitions*. The dependent variables *duration* and *repetitions per minute* of the MVP exercise were significantly different.

Participants using the *Game* application played 2.4 times longer than participants of the control group. The frequency of repetitions was significantly higher for the control group. On average, participants of the control group performed a MVP repetition every 1.4 s. Participants of the treatment group completed a MVP repetition only after 2.56 s. This result might be due to the additional cognitive load while playing. The lower frequency of MVP repetitions while playing might be more effective, since longer exercise intervals show a tendency to increase the amount of blood flow velocity [15].

The high ratings of the SUS indicate an excellent usability of both the *Counter* and the *Game* application. These findings are strengthened by the high scores for the constructs *perceived ease of use, perceived usefulness,* and *perceived enjoyment* of TAM. A significant difference between the application conditions for *perceived usefulness, perceived enjoyment* and for the construct *enjoyment* of the IMI questionnaire indicate that the intention to use the *Game* application in future is higher.

This study, however, focused on the first-time contact. Future research has to analyze how these effects develop over time and has to conduct studies evaluating long-term use and adherence. One limitation is with respect to participants' perceived pain. Although, they were told to quit the application in case of pain, participants continued to use the application. No difference was found for increased pain intensity between the applications. Future work will have to find the reasons for the increased pain intensity and will have to answer the question "Why didn't participants cancel the application?". Moreover, the applications have to introduce exercise breaks depending on the users' individual characteristics and/or performance to avoid overexertion.

Acknowledgments. We would like to thank all our participants volunteering in the user study. The research group wearHEALTH is funded by the German Federal Ministry of Education and Research (16SV7115).

References

1. OECD: Health at a Glance 2017. OECD Publishing, Paris (2017)
2. Rabe, E., Bauersachs, R.M., Pannier, F., List, S.M.: Venenerkrankungen der Beine, Gesundheitsberichterstattung des Bundes, Heft 44 (2009)
3. Encke, A., Haas, S., Kopp, I.: The Prophylaxis of Venous Thromboembolism. Deutsches Aerzteblatt International **113**(31–32), 532–538 (2016)
4. Kato, P.M.: Video games in health care: closing the gap. Rev. Gen. Psychol. **14**(2), 113 (2010)
5. Steffen, D., Christmann, C.A., Bleser, G.: jumpBALL - Ein mobiles Exergame für die Thromboseprophylaxe. In: 'Mensch und Computer 2017 - Tagungsband', Gesellschaft für Informatik e.V., Regensburg, pp. 27–36 (2017)
6. Peng, W., Crouse, J.C., Lin, J.-H.: Using active video games for physical activity promotion. Health Educ. Behav. **40**(2), 171–192 (2012)
7. Kari, T.: Can exergaming promote physical fitness and physical activity?: a systematic review of systematic reviews. Int. J. Gaming Commun. Mediat. Simul. **6**(4), 59–77 (2014)
8. Borg, G.: Borg's Perceived Exertion and Pain Scales, Human Kinetics (1998)
9. Brooke, J.: SUS - A Quick and Dirty Usability Scale. CRC Press, Boca Raton (1996)

10. Deci, E.L., Ryan, R.M.: Intrinsic Motivation and Self-Determination in Human Behavior (Perspectives in Social Psychology). Springer, New York (2013)
11. Hassenzahl, M., Koller, F., Burmester, M.: Der user experience (UX) auf der Spur: Zum Einsatz von. In: Brau, H., Diefenbach, S., Hassenzahl, M., Koller, F., Peissner, M., Röse, K. (ed.) 'Tagungsband UP08', Fraunhofer Verlag, Stuttgart, pp. 78–82 (2008). www.attrakdiff.de
12. Davis, F.D.: Perceived usefulness, perceived ease of use, and user acceptance of information technology. MIS Q. **13**(3), 319–340 (1989)
13. Venkatesh, V., Davis, F.D.: A theoretical extension of the technology acceptance model: four longitudinal field studies. Manage. Sci. **46**(2), 186–204 (2000)
14. Karrer, K., Glaser, C., Clemens, C., Bruder, C.: Technikaffinität erfassen–der Fragebogen TA-EG. Der Mensch im Mittelpunkt technischer Systeme **8**, 196–201 (2009)
15. Toya, K., Sasano, K., Takasoh, T., Nishimoto, T., Fujimoto, Y., Kusumoto, Y., Yoshimatsu, T., Kusaka, S., Takahashi, T.: Ankle positions and exercise intervals effect on the blood flow velocity in the common femoral vein during ankle pumping exercises. J. Phys. Ther. Sci. **28** (2), 685–688 (2016)

Ergonomic Analysis of Community Health Agents During Homecare Visits

Ana Cristina Forain Bartz[1], Adalgiza Mafra Moreno[2], Redha Taiar[3], Christiano Bittencourt Machado[4](✉), and Luis Guilherme Barbosa[4]

[1] National Cancer Institute (INCA), Rua Marquês de Pombal, 125, 12th floor, Rio de Janeiro, Brazil
[2] University of Nova Iguaçu, Av. Abílio Augusto Távora, Nova Iguaçu 2134, Brazil
[3] Université de Reims Champagne-Ardenne, Chemin des Rouliers, BP1036, 51687 Reims, France
[4] Graduate Program on Family Health, Estácio de Sá University, Av. Presidente Vargas, 642, Rio de Janeiro, Brazil
cbmfisio@gmail.com

Abstract. This work aimed at analyzing ergonomic conditions of community health agents (CHAs) in homecare visiting, mapping the performed activities, observing daily routine and describing the working process of CHA during visits. A descriptive study was carried out by a systematic observation of the reality. Eleven CHA's from a public health unity at Rio de Janeiro, Brazil, were accompanied during their home visits. About 54.5% of the CHAs were well trained, with undergraduate certification and more than five years of work experience. A predominance of dynamic positions (less harmful) over static was noted. Despite the common presence of hot temperatures during home visits, the ergonomic risk was considered low. According to the Body Mapping Tool, the location of affected body areas can be related to the professional profile of the CHA. There was no evidence of mental disorders, as well as ergonomic inadequacies or work-related disorders during CHA's daily work routine.

Keywords: Community health agents · Brazilian Unified Health System · Family Health Strategy · Ergonomics · Work-related health

1 Introduction

The Brazilian Health Unified System (*Sistema Único de Saúde* – SUS) was implemented in the 1990's, leading to an increase in health care access across the country. One of SUS's strategies is the Family Health Programme (*Programa de saúde da Família* - PSF), consisting in family health-care teams: one doctor, one nurse, one auxiliary nurse, and four to six community health workers. These PSF teams are located at PSF clinics and they are assigned to specific geographical areas inside the municipality. The aim is to offer a first reference for local health attendance and at the

T. Ahram et al. (Eds.): IHIET 2019, AISC 1018, pp. 538–542, 2020.
https://doi.org/10.1007/978-3-030-25629-6_83

same time is integrated to other health facilities for diagnostic exams and hospital care, for example [1].

Community health agents (CHAs) are professionals who should live in the community itself. Some of their roles are working with families within a well-defined geographical area. CHAs must collect data using interviews, home visits, family registers, community mapping and community meetings, in order to analyze community needs, and to foster health promotion and disease prevention [2].

The PSF team usually has to work in underserved areas with severe social vulnerability (which is common in Brazil). Some of the great challenges are precarious sanitation, housing, and transportation, an increase in unemployment and violence associated with the drug traffic [3]. Therefore, ergonomics (or human factors) is of great importance since its main goal is to reduce human error, increasing productivity and enhancing safety and comfort of the work process [4].

In this context, the aim of this work was to analyze ergonomic conditions of community health agents (CHAs) in homecare visiting, mapping the performed activities, observing daily routine and describing the working process of CHA during visits. A descriptive study was carried out by a systematic observation of the reality.

2 Materials and Methods

2.1 Subjects

A total of eleven CHA's from a public health unity at the downtown neighborhood of Lapa, Rio de Janeiro, Brazil (all women, mean age 42 ± 12 years old, range 21 to 65 years old) were accompanied during their home visits, and information was collected about environment conditions, dressing and work tools, complaints and perceptions. They signed an informed consent for participation in the study and publication of data. This work was approved by Estácio de Sá University's Ethics Committee (CAAE n° 76465617.3.0000.5284) and follows the guidelines of the Declaration of Helsinki.

2.2 Study Protocol

First of all, a questionnaire was applied to collect self-referenced personal data (sociodemographic, socioeconomic and occupational information). Weight and height were also measured for the calculation of the body mass index (BMI = kg/cm^2), consequently classifying the nutritional status. Then, the Body Maping Tool (BMT) [5] was used to assess for painful symptoms with temporal evolution and its location. The Couto's Questionnaire (or check list) [6] with 25 questions was also applied in order to evaluate the biomechanical factors in the risk for upper limbs work-related musculoskeletal disorders (scored from 0 to 25, i.e., no risk to high risk, respectively), and finally the Self-Reporting Questionnaire (SRQ-20) [7] was used for screening of psycho-emotional factors of community health agents, scoring from 0 (unlikely) to 20 (extreme likely to present mental disorders).

After this initial assessment, the CHAs were accompanied in different days during their home care visits by one of the researchers. Qualitative data were then collected about relevant ergonomic aspects, such as environmental conditions, clothing, materials, tasks performed, time working at the PSF, complaints and reported perceptions, as well as the ergonomic demands. Before the visits, all the materials transported by the CHA in that day was weighted (in kg) using a scale.

Descriptive statistics was used to present the results, and the Spearman's correlation coefficient ($p < 0.05$) was applied to verify if there are correlations among some variables collected in this study.

3 Results

Sociodemographic data showed that 72.7% of the CHAs self-referred as brown color, and 27.3% as white; the average individual income is R$ 1,110.36 (approximately 298 American dollars); the average family income is R$ 2,152.72 (approximately 560 American dollars); 45.5% are single; all of them have completed a high school degree; 54.5% were classified as presenting "overweight" (it was identified one CHA with obesity); 72.7% have at least one child. The average weight transported by the CHA during the visits was 2.2 ± 0.7 kg.

After a qualitative and systematic ergonomic assessment, it was observed that all the CHAs visited houses in the community by walking, with solar exposure. Travelled distances ranged from 190 to 710 m, with an average duration of 21 min. Eight CHAs (72.7%) reported a strong sensation of heat (three of them during a sunny day and five with an overcast sun).

Ten CHAs were using a cotton sweater with short sleeves, an ACS with a sweater under the uniform vest. Four CHAs were using vests. Two of them reported that the vests are very uncomfortable because the heat up. Six CHAs wore jeans pants, and other five choose to use fabric or knit pants by judging them more comfortable. Nine CHAs (81.8%) used sneakers (although they apparently did not present the adequate cushioning for long walks). The other two CHAs wore inappropriate shoes for the activity: apparently leather shoes, with no cushion for walking and sneaker moccasin, with a flat sole, without any elevation in the region of the heel.

The agents informed us that sunscreen was not recently available. There are hats (caps) for protection; nevertheless the CHAs were not using them at the time of the visit.

It was observed that all eleven CHAs remained in orthostatic position at the entrance of the house to be visited, waiting for the authorization to come in during one to ten minutes (average waiting time of three minutes). Four CHAs carried a plastic folder with papers and backpack; three CHAs carried a bag; two CHAs carried a clipboard with papers and bag, and the other two CHAs carried only one item: a backpack or a plastic folder with papers.

It could not be disregarded the influence of structural aspects of the visited houses which may affect the work process of CHAs. Five CHAs were able to sit down shortly after arrival at the site; three agents remained in orthostasis throughout the entire visit; other three agents were in orthostasis for up to ten minutes, and after that period, they could sit, alternating between the orthostatic and sitting position. It was noticed that there was a predominance of dynamic tasks, which can be justified by the need of performing multiple health care interventions.

Figure 1 shows the results from the three questionnaires applied for all the eleven subjects. All correlation coefficients were estimated with $p > 0.05$, and for that reason they will not be presented here.

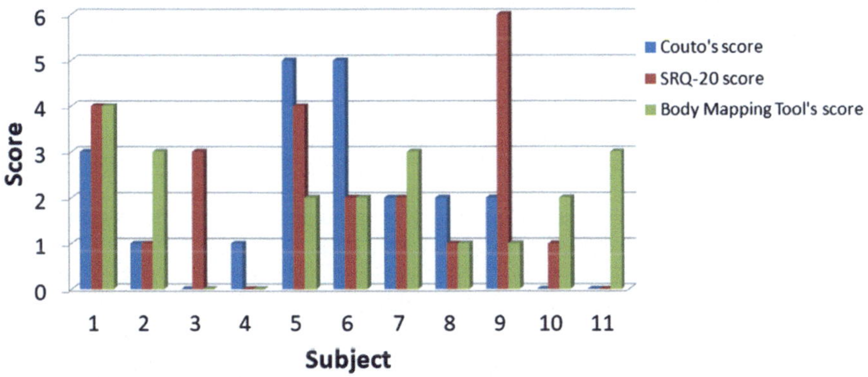

Fig. 1. Scores from the three questionnaires applied: Couto's questionnaire, the SRQ-20 and the Body Mapping Tool, for each subject.

4 Discussion and Conclusions

It is well known that CHAs are the link between health professionals and the community. Several challenges have to be overcome by these agents, for example, the resistance to orientation, areas of difficult access, the crescent violence due to drug trafficking etc. [2]. This study presented some other additional and important aspects about CHAs: (1) low income levels for a reasonable living condition, especially in Rio de Janeiro; (2) temperature at uncomfortable levels; (3) long-distance walks to visit houses in the community; (4) inappropriate wearing during work.

As shown in Fig. 1, there were no high scores in all three questionnaires, for all the eleven subjects. However, the health unit could create individual strategies for risk assessment and health intervention using the present results. Healthier CHAs may lead to a better community service, since they are the key for the success of primary care policy in Brazil.

There is a concern about the aggravation of the existing underfinancing of the SUS. Brazil has passed for several budget cuts for health since 2015. In 2016, the Brazilian Congress approved a 20-year freeze on the federal budget for health and education, which may heavily affect the SUS in the next years [3]. The consequences on CHAs work process due to these cuts are unknown.

One may suggest that PSF teams should increase the mentality of safety during labor. The update on ergonomics trends, guidelines for prevention of musculoskeletal disorders and a periodic assessment by a specialist would help on health prevention.

The present work assessed only one health unit in Rio de Janeiro (Lapa), with eleven CHAs. It is evident that the results obtained here cannot extrapolate for all the country, even for the city of Rio de Janeiro, considering the differences among the territories. Nevertheless, it brings up questions to be answered: do the conditions qualitatively observed here have the potential to aggravate health conditions on CHAs? How do the financial cuts by the government affect the work process for them? May the creation of policies be beneficial for individual approaches on CHA's health care? Further investigations could answer these questions with longitudinal studies (cohort), larger samples, and a variety of health units in the entire country.

References

1. Paim, J., Travassos, C., Almeida, C., Bahia, L., Macinko, J.: The Brazilian health system: history, advances, and challenges. The Lancet **377**, 1778–1797 (2011)
2. Kluthcovsky, A.C.G.C., Takayanagui, A.M.M.: Community health agent: a literature review. Rev. Latino-Am Enfermagem **14**, 957–963 (1996)
3. Coelho Neto, G.C., Antunes, V.H., Oliveira, A.: The practice of Family and Community Medicine in Brazil: context and perspectives. Cad Saúde Pública **35**, 1–4 (2010)
4. Soares, M.M., Rebelo, F.: Ergonomics in Design: Methods & Techniques. CRC Press, New York (2017)
5. Messing, K., Vézina, N., Ève, M., Ouellet, S., Tissot, F., Couture, V., Riel, J.: Body maps: an indicator of physical pain for worker-oriented ergonomic interventions. Policy. Pract. Health Saf. **6**, 31–49 (2016)
6. Souza, N.L.S.A., Oliveira, L.S.N., Araújo, C.L.O.: Check List de Couto: simplified evaluation of the biomechanical factor in a hospital institution located in Vale do Paraíba. IOSR J. Nurs. Health Sci. **6**, 60–65 (2017)
7. Santos, K.O., Carvalho, F.M., Araújo, T.M.: Internal consistency of the self-reporting questionnaire-20 in occupational groups. Rev. Saude Publica **50**, 1–10 (2016)

Coupling of Integral and Differential Numerical Models Applied in the Evaluation of Integral Thermal Comfort, Air Quality and Draught Risk

Eusébio Conceição[1,2(✉)], João Gomes[2], Maria Lúcio[1], Maria Conceição[3], and Hazim Awbi[4]

[1] FCT-Universidade do Algarve, Campus de Gambelas, 8005-139 Faro, Portugal
econcei@ualg.pt

[2] CINTAL, Campus de Gambelas, 8005-139 Faro, Portugal

[3] Instituto Superior Técnico, Av. Rovisco Pais, 1049-001 Lisbon, Portugal

[4] School of Built Environment, University of Reading, Reading RG6 6AW, UK

Abstract. In this work is used the coupling of integral and differential numerical models applied in the evaluation of integral thermal comfort, indoor air quality (IAQ), Draught Risk (DR) and Air Distribution Index (ADI). In this study, a confined space, using a new Heating, Ventilation and Air-Conditioning (HVAC) system, based in confluent jets ventilation systems (CJVS) is used. This system is built with four vertical ducts, located in the corner of the wall surfaces, with horizontal nozzles turned to the two vertical walls. This study, done in summer conditions, evaluates the thermal comfort, the air quality, the DR around the occupants and the ADI for two possible arrangement of the nozzles: 0.5 m or 1.5 m. The results show that DR is acceptable for both cases but the ADI is better for the 0.5 m than the 1.5 m nozzles arrangement.

Keywords: ADI · Air quality · Confluent jets · Draught Risk · HVAC system · Numerical simulations · Thermal comfort

1 Introduction

The main objectives of a ventilation system installed in a building are to improve the IAQ and simultaneously ensure the thermal comfort of a significant percentage of occupants. However, the operation of a ventilation system will have an effect on air movement, which will affect the perception that people have on thermal comfort inside a building [1]. According to [2], the two most common airflow distribution systems in indoor spaces are based on mixed ventilation (MV) and displacement ventilation (DV). The performance of MV ventilation systems is poor, requiring high airflow rates to remove contaminants, and having low values of energy efficiency [3]. On the other hand, MV systems are easily designed [1]. The advantages of DV systems are its high air-exchange efficiency (usually above 50%) and ventilation effectiveness [4]. The weaknesses of DV systems are, for example, that they cannot be used for heating loads,

T. Ahram et al. (Eds.): IHIET 2019, AISC 1018, pp. 543–548, 2020.
https://doi.org/10.1007/978-3-030-25629-6_84

the large vertical temperature gradient, the existence of DR at ankle level, and poor efficiency in removing contaminants at floor level [4, 5]. In order to overcome these disadvantages, new types of hybrid ventilation systems have been developed. Among them, the CJVS have the potential to simultaneously reduce energy consumption and improve thermal comfort [3]. CVJS can also be used both for cooling and heating and are able to create a well distributed airflow [1].

A confluent jet can be described as multiple circular free jets, coming from nozzles that are in the same plane, flowing in parallel directions in which, at a certain distance downstream, they start to coalesce and behave as unique jet [2]. Several studies have been conducted on the area of CJVS. These studies show, for example, that the total airflow rate directly influences the flow and velocity patterns in each nozzle [6], CVJS can guarantee good levels of thermal comfort and IAQ in the conditioned space [7], and CVJS can produce enough momentum to spread and cover almost the entire space and reach the opposite wall [8].

The aim of this work is to analyze the performance of a CJVS constituted by four vertical ducts, with round nozzles equally distributed along the axis of each duct, for two possible arrangements of the nozzles: 0.5 m or 1.5 m. In this work, the numerical simulation is done considering a coupling between the Computational Fluid Dynamics (CFD) and the Human Thermal Response (HTR) numerical models.

2 Numerical Models

In this work, the HTR numerical model is used to establish, simultaneously, the level of thermal comfort of each occupant [9]. It operates in steady-state or transient regimes for non-isothermal conditions and its details are presented in [9].

The used CFD model simulates the tri-dimensional turbulent airflow in steady-state non-isothermal conditions within an occupied room. This CFD is described in detail for isothermal conditions in [10] and for non-isothermal conditions in [11].

In order to evaluate the influence of this CJVS in the human thermal behavior, the surrounding environmental variables are numerically calculated. To evaluate simultaneously each occupant thermal comfort level, each occupant air quality level and the ventilation system efficiency, the Air Distribution Index (ADI) is used.

The building thermal behavior numerical model used in this work estimates the floor, ceiling, walls and windows surrounding surfaces temperatures, the indoor surfaces temperatures and the indoor air temperatures [12].

In the evaluation of the thermal comfort level, the Predicted Percentage of Dissatisfied people (PPD) index, developed by Fanger [13], is used. The percentage of people dissatisfied with DR index is used to evaluate the DR [14].

The ADI is an index that allows an integral evaluation of the thermal comfort, IAQ and energy efficiency of a ventilation system (please, see details in [2, 15]). ADI depends on the thermal comfort number (TCN) and the air quality number (AQN). In turn, the TCN is function of the effectiveness for heat removal and the PPD, and the AQN is function of the effectiveness for contaminant removal in the breathing area and the percentage of dissatisfied (PD) with IAQ.

3 Numerical Methodology

Numerical simulations are performed in a virtual chamber equipped with a square table and with 4 virtual manikins located on each side of the table. The virtual manikins used in the HTR and CFD are presented in Fig. 1. The virtual chamber is equipped with this new CJVS, which consists of 4 vertical ducts, located in each corner, and equipped with two sets of round nozzles equally distributed, each set directed parallel to adjacent walls, and one extractor located at the middle area of the chamber ceiling. In this study, two arrangements of the nozzles are considered: Case A, vertical duct with 0.5 m of nozzles (Fig. 2, left side); Case B, vertical duct with 1.5 m of nozzles (Fig. 2, right side).

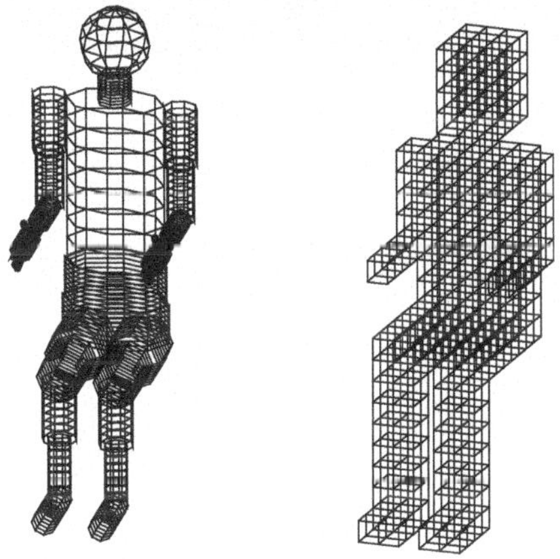

Fig. 1. Virtual manikins used in the HTR (left side) and CFD (right side).

The numerical simulations were made for a typical summer day conditions with an inlet air temperature of 25 °C and an indoor air relative humidity of 50%. It was considered a typical clothing level of 0.5 clo and a typical activity level of 1.2 met. The inlet air velocity is 2.8 m/s for the case A and 1 m/s for the case B.

4 Results and Discussion

The effectiveness for heat removal, PPD, TCN, CO_2 concentration in the breathing area, effectiveness for contaminant removal, PD, AQN and ADI results are presented for summer conditions, for cases A and B, respectively, in Tables 1 and 2.

The obtained results show that the effectiveness for heat removal is slightly higher in case A than in case B but the PPD is better for case B, though in both cases PPD values are inside category B of ISO 7730 [14]. The TCN values are similar for both cases. The effectiveness for contaminant removal and CO_2 concentration in the breathing area results are much better in Case A than in Case B. However, for both Cases, the CO_2 concentration values are below the standard value of 1800 mg/m^3 [16]. The AQN is much better for Case A than Case B. Finally, the ADI is much better for

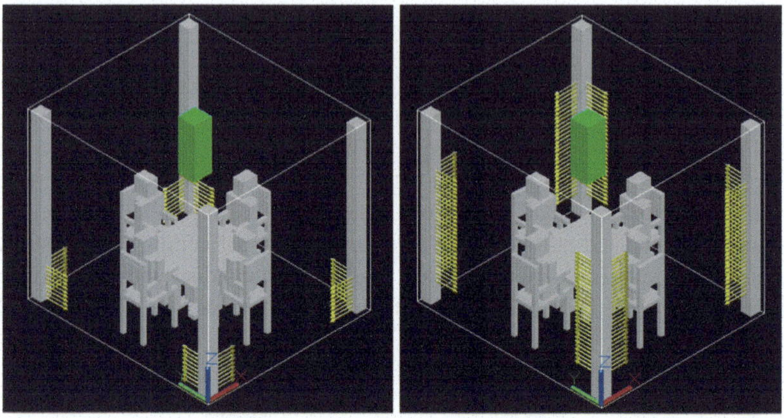

Fig. 2. Virtual chamber equipped with a CJVS and an *extractor system* (*green*). Case A (left side): set of 0.5 m of *nozzles* (*yellow*). Case B (right side): set of 1.5 m of *nozzles* (*yellow*).

Table 1. ADI that each occupant is subjected, in summer conditions, for Case A.

Occupant	1	2	3	4	Average
Effectiveness for heat removal (%)	91.85	91.80	88.73	94.52	**91.72**
PPD (%)	11.69	12.66	8.67	8.00	**10.25**
TCN	7.86	7.25	10.23	11.82	**9.29**
CO_2 concentration in the breathing area (mg/m^3)	1321.8	695.3	982.1	963.6	**990.7**
Effectiveness for contaminant removal (%)	7.76	32.64	13.23	13.75	**16.85**
PD (%)	0.76	0.76	0.76	0.76	**0.76**
AQN	10.27	43.21	17.51	18.20	**22.30**
ADI	**8.98**	**17.70**	**13.38**	**14.67**	**13.69**

Table 2. ADI that each occupant is subjected, in summer conditions, for Case B.

Occupant	1	2	3	4	Average
Effectiveness for heat removal (%)	86.70	92.92	90.89	88.38	**89.72**
PPD (%)	8.42	10.43	7.87	12.09	**9.70**
TCN	10.29	8.91	11.55	7.31	**9.51**
CO_2 concentration in the breathing area (mg/m^3)	1944.6	890.5	1274.1	2004.4	**1528.4**
Effectiveness for contaminant removal (%)	3.25	12.02	6.06	3.12	**6.11**
PD (%)	0.57	0.57	0.57	0.57	**0.57**
AQN	5.68	21.03	10.61	5.46	**10.70**
ADI	**7.65**	**13.69**	**11.07**	**6.32**	**9.68**

case A than case B. As conclusion, the thermal comfort level is similar for both cases, but Case A presents much better IAQ and ventilation efficiency.

In Fig. 3(a) and (b), the DR distribution around the occupants, in summer conditions, for Cases A and B, respectively, are presented. For both cases, the obtained results show that the DR distribution around the occupants is generally uniform and it is acceptable for all occupants according to category B of ISO 7730 [14]. However, the DR is slightly lower for Case B than Case A.

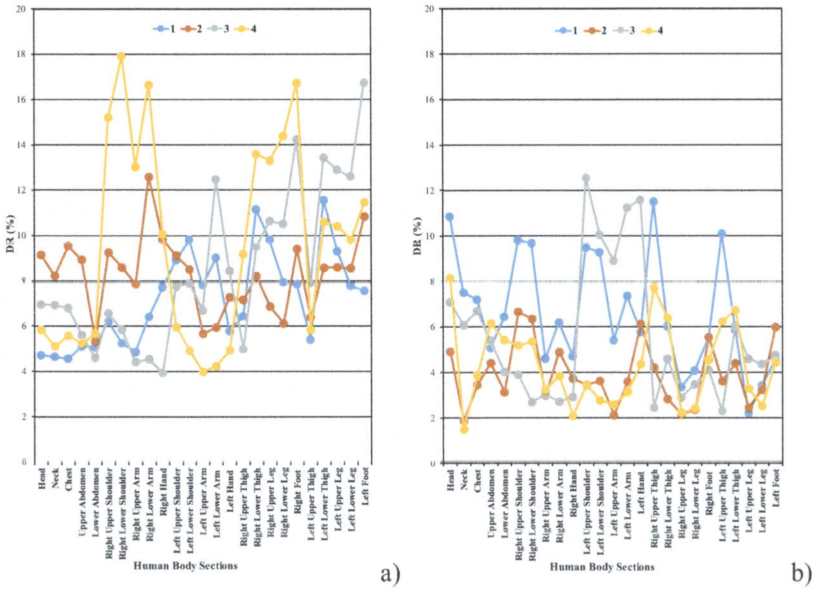

Fig. 3. Draught Risk (DR) distribution around the occupants, in summer conditions, for (a) Case A and (b) Case B.

5 Conclusions

In this numerical work, it is used a virtual confined space with four virtual manikins and equipped with a CJVS. Two configurations of this ventilation system were considered: the nozzles are distributed within 0.5 m (Case A) or 1.5 m (Case B) of the vertical duct.

For both cases, the PPD results show that thermal comfort is acceptable within category B of ISO 7730 [14], and the DR is also acceptable for all occupants within category B of ISO 7730 [14]. The IAQ is better for Case A than Case B. The ADI index results are highest for Case A. Therefore, the configuration with the nozzles distributed along the 0.5 m of the duct shows the best performance, mainly due to its greater efficiency in extracting the contaminants from the breathing zone.

Acknowledgments. The authors would like to acknowledge the support of the project supported by Algarve Regional Operational Program (CRESC Algarve 2020), under the PORTUGAL 2020 Partnership Agreement, through the European Regional Development Fund (ERDF) and the National Science and Technology Foundation (FCT).

References

1. Larsson, U., Moshfegh, B.: Comparison of ventilation performance of three different air supply devices: a measurement study. Int. J. Vent. **16**(3), 144–154 (2017)
2. Awbi, H.: Ventilation of Buildings. Taylor & Francis, London (2003)
3. Yin, H., Li, A., Liu, Z., Chen, T.: Experimental study on airflow characteristics of a square column attached ventilation mode. Build. Environ. **109**, 112–120 (2016)
4. Janbakhsh, S., Moshfegh, B.: Experimental study of a ventilation system based on wall confluent jets. Build. Environ. **80**, 18–31 (2014)
5. Shan, X., Zhou, J., Chang, W., Yang, E.: Comparing mixing and displacement ventilation in tutorial rooms: students' thermal comfort, sick building syndromes, and short-term performance. Build. Environ. **102**, 128–137 (2016)
6. Andersson, H., Cehlin, M., Moshfegh, B.: Experimental and numerical investigations of a new ventilation supply device based on confluent jets. Build. Environ. **137**, 18–33 (2018)
7. Arghand, T., Karimipanah, T., Awbi, H., Cehlin, M., Larsson, U., Linden, E.: An experimental investigation of the flow and comfort parameters for under-floor, confluent jets and mixing ventilation systems in an open-plan office. Build. Environ. **92**, 48–60 (2015)
8. Janbakhsh, S., Moshfegh, B.: Numerical study of a ventilation system based on wall confluent jets. HVAC&R Res. **20**, 846–861 (2014)
9. Conceição, E.: Evaluation of thermal comfort and local discomfort conditions using the numerical body of the human and clothing thermal system. In: Proceedings of the 7th International Conference on Air Distribution in Rooms – RoomVent'2000, Reading, UK, 9–12 July 2000
10. Conceição, E., Vicente, V., Lúcio, M.: Airflow inside school buildings office compartments with moderate environment. HVAC&R Res. **14**, 195–207 (2008)
11. Conceição, E., Lúcio, M., Rosa, S., Custódio, A., Andrade, R., Meira, M.: Evaluation of comfort level in desks equipped with two personalized ventilation systems in slightly warm environments. Build. Environ. **45**, 601–609 (2010)
12. Conceição, E., Lúcio, M.: Numerical simulation of the application of solar radiant systems, internal airflow and occupants' presence in the improvement of comfort in winter conditions. Buildings **38**, 1–20 (2016)
13. Fanger, P.: Thermal Comfort. Danish Technical Press, Copenhagen (1970)
14. ISO 7730: Ergonomics of the thermal environments – analytical determination and interpretation of thermal comfort using calculation of the PMV and PPD indices and local thermal comfort criteria. International Standard, Switzerland (2005)
15. Conceição, E., Lúcio, M., Awbi, H.: Comfort and airflow evaluation in spaces equipped with mixing ventilation and cold radiant floor. Build. Simul. **6**, 51–67 (2013)
16. ASHRAE Standard 62.1: Ventilation for acceptable indoor air quality. American Society of Heating, Refrigerating and Air-Conditioning Engineers, Atlanta, GA, USA (2010)

Energy Consumption Assessment of College Tennis Players Based on Actigraph GT9X Accelerometer

Tianyu He[1(✉)] and Qi Luo[2]

[1] Graduate School, Wuhan Sports University, Wuhan 430079, China
499132717@qq.com
[2] College of Sports Engineering and Information Technology, Wuhan Sports University, Wuhan 430079, China

Abstract. With the continuous development of tennis in China, tennis has been accepted by the masses. At the same time, tennis in colleges and universities is a very popular elective course among college students. Therefore, the accurate and simple monitoring and intervention of tennis sports is of great significance to the cultivation of college students' physical activities and physical quality. In this paper, ActigraphGT9X is used to collect the data of sports energy consumption of college tennis beginners and skilled players, and to explore the influence of energy consumption in different body parts of tennis on the technical level of tennis.

Keywords: Acceleration sensor · Sports energy consumption · Tennis · College students

1 Introduction

As one of the most popular and widely developed sports in the world, tennis can not only meet the sports needs of different ages and technical levels, but also achieve fitness goals [1]. In recent years, with the international success of Chinese tennis players, especially Chinese women's tennis player Li Na won two Grand Slam titles, tennis has gradually become more and more popular and concerned [2]. Therefore, with the increase of beginner tennis players, understanding the energy consumption of different parts of tennis is of great significance for scientifically guiding sports and enhancing sports levels. In order to study the influence of energy consumption of different parts on the energy consumption of tennis sports, the energy consumption data of different parts of professional athletes and non-professional athletes are collected by three-dimensional accelerometer method, and the data is tested and analyzed for beginners or tennis fitness. And theoretical support for sports training and the rational use of acceleration sensors [3].

T. Ahram et al. (Eds.): IHIET 2019, AISC 1018, pp. 549–555, 2020.
https://doi.org/10.1007/978-3-030-25629-6_85

2 Research Objects and Research Methods

2.1 Research Object

In this study, 20 college tennis players with basic tennis training (professional tennis training or one year or more of study) were selected as the professional group. In addition, 20 college students who had preliminary study or less than one year of tennis were required to be non-professional group. The two group were compared. Table 1 is a basic information table for professional and non-professional groups.

Table 1. Basic information of the subjects

Anthropometric features	Professional group (n = 20)		Non-professional (n = 20)	
	Male (n = 10)	Female (n = 10)	Male (n = 10)	Female (n = 10)
Age	20.08 ± 0.51	19.7 ± 0.48	22 ± 1.22	22 ± 1.22
Height (cm)	175.92 ± 4.94	167 ± 6.77	165 ± 6.82	165 ± 6.82
Weight (kg)	67.83 ± 7.74	56.4 ± 5.93	54.6 ± 5.03	54.6 ± 5.03
BMI (kg/m^2)	21.94 ± 2.63	20.21 ± 1.72	20.06 ± 1.63	20.06 ± 1.63

2.2 Test Plan

In this study, the basic physical characteristics of the subjects were collected before the formal test. In the formal test, the subjects held a GT9X accelerometer on the wrist, waist and ankle for collecting the acceleration signal per second. In the movement, the right forehand shot, the left backhand shot, the right front forehand shot, and the left front backhand shot are monitored for energy consumption monitoring. Each test time is 2 min, and each test interval is 1 min.

2.3 Data Processing

Daily activities during the experiment collected relevant data using an ActiGraph GT9X accelerometer device, which was sampled at 80 Hz, respectively [4]. After the test is finished, the data is imported into the computer, the body energy index such as the EE (Energy Expenditure) energy consumption, the MET (Metabolic Equivalent of Energy) and so on are obtained by the self-contained data analysis software Actilife 6. After the data is collected, Statistics were analyzed by SPSS20 statistical software, where the data were expressed as mean ± standard deviation ($x \pm s$). Descriptive statistical analysis was performed for each variable, and t-test was used to compare changes in energy consumption between different genders and different parts [5]. Among them, the GT9X has improved the energy consumption algorithm worn on the wrist compared with the GT3X, enabling it to measure relevant data more accurately.

3 Research Results

3.1 Comparison of EE Values Between GT9X Professional Group and Non-professional Group in Different Wearing Parts

The EE values of professional and non-professional groups are measured by ActiGraph6's own algorithm freedson VM, as shown below.

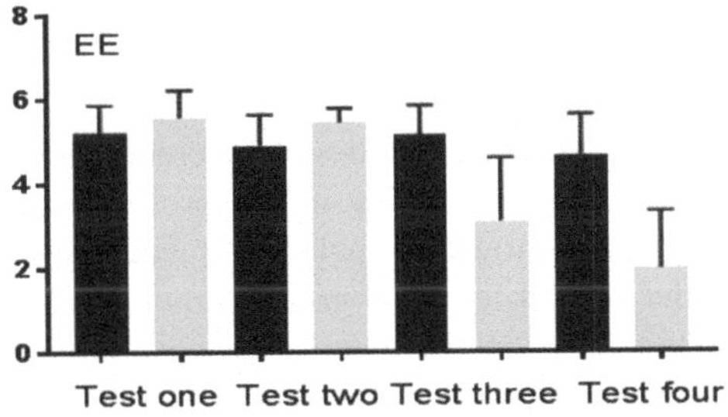

Fig. 1. Male wrist EE values in professional and non-professional groups (left)

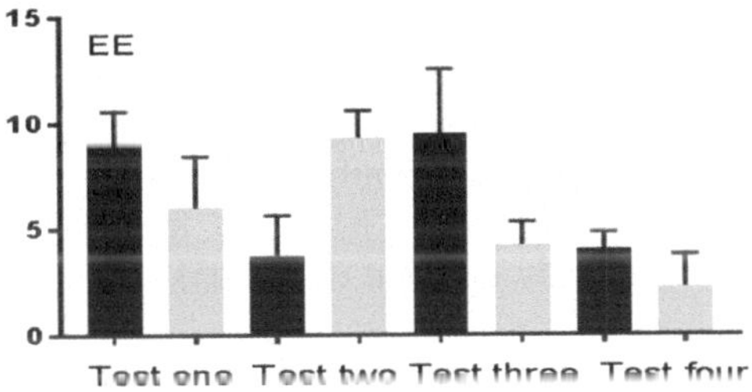

Fig. 2. Male waist EE values in professional and non-professional groups (right)

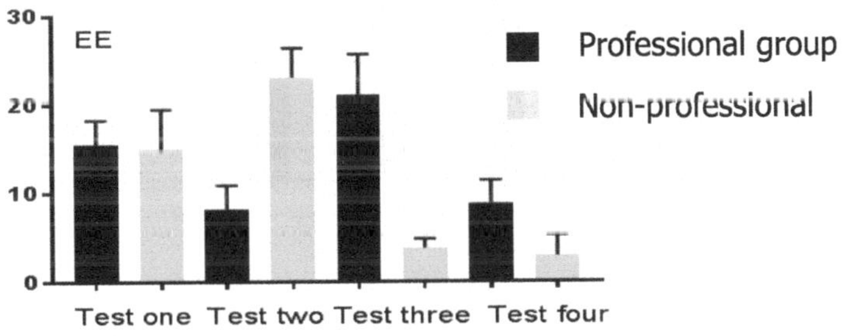

Fig. 3. Male foot EE values in professional and non-professional groups

The first experiment is the right forehand shot, the second is the left backhand, the third is the right front forehand, and the fourth is the left front backhand.

Table 2. F-test and T-test analysis results of male EE values in professional and non-professional groups

Wearing part	Right forehand				Left backhand				Right front forehand				Left front backhand			
	F test		T test		F test		T test		F test		T test		F test		T test	
	F	P(F <=f)	T	P(T <=t)	F	P(F <=f)	T	P(T <=t)	F	P(F <=f)	T	P(T <=t)	F	P(F <=f)	T	P(T <=t)
Waist	0.48	0.12	4.73	0.00	0.75	0.32	–4.76	0.00	3.08	0.04	5.31	0.00	0.25	0.03	2.72	0.03
Wrist	0.36	0.05	–1.07	0.30	2.47	0.20	–1.72	0.10	0.68	0.23	5.28	0.00	0.49	0.15	4.91	0.00
Ankle	0.39	0.09	1.49	0.15	0.23	0.01	–9.55	0.00	21.12	0.01	9.00	0.04	3.66	0.03	3.75	0.00

P < 0.05 means significant difference

There is a difference between the EE values of different parts of GT9X. Figures 1, 2 and 3 show the male EE measured values in the professional group and the non-professional group, and Table 2 shows the male F-test and T-test analysis results in the professional group and the non-professional group. Among them, the average value of the waist in the professional and non-professional groups in the right forehand test was 8.91 and 6.01, which were significantly different (P < 0.01). The average values of the wrist and ankle were 5.2, 5.55, 15.51, and 15.05, respectively. There was no significant difference between the two (P > 0.05). In the lumbar energy consumption monitoring, the apparent non-professional group has less energy consumption than the professional group. In the left backhand test, the measured values of EE in the lumbar and ankle were 3.74, 9.27, 8.21, and 23.08, respectively, (P < 0.05), but there was no significant difference in the measured value of wrist EE (P > 0.05). In the right front forehand and left front backhand test, there was no significant difference between the right front forehand wrist and the EE in the waist, hand and foot (P > 0.05), and other EE measured values were significantly different (P < 0.05).

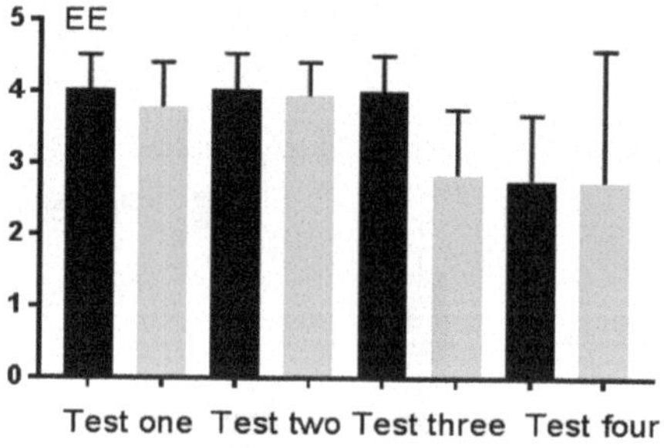

Fig. 4. Female wrist EE values in professional and non-professional groups (left)

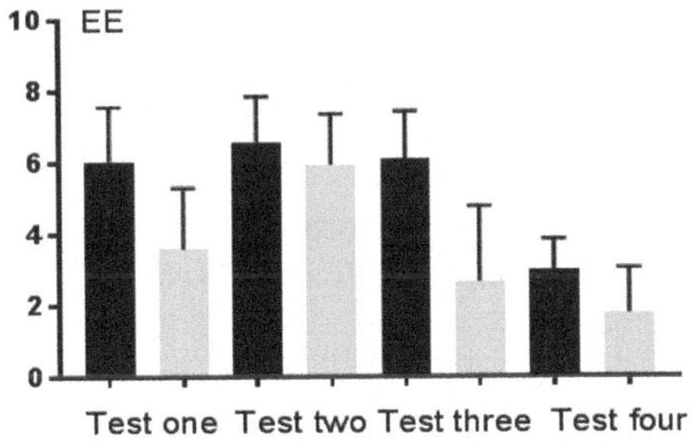

Fig. 5. Female waist and EE values in professional and non-professional groups (right)

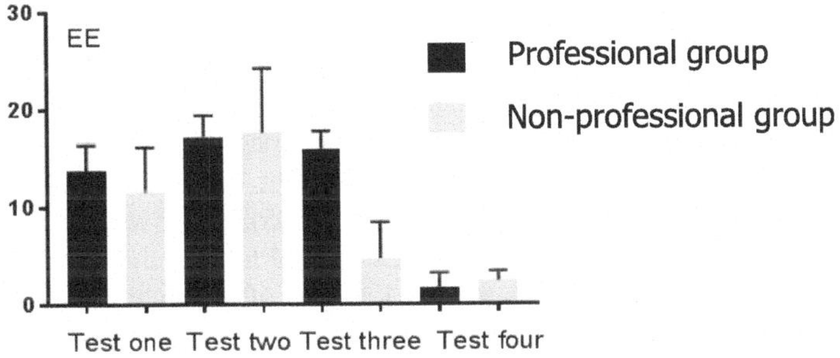

Fig. 6. Female foot EE values in professional and non-professional groups

Table 3. F-test and T-test analysis results of female EE values in professional and non-professional groups

Wearing part	Right forehand				Left backhand				Right front forehand				Left front backhand			
	F test		T test		F test		T test		F test		T test		F test		T test	
	F	P(F <=f)	T	P(T <=t)	F	P(F <=f)	T	P(T <=t)	F	P(F <=f)	T	P(T <=t)	F	P(F <=f)	T	P(T <=t)
Waist	2.52	0.17	– 0.76	0.47	0.79	0.35	0.89	0.39	0.40	0.12	3.87	0.00	0.47	0.16	2.16	0.05
Wrist	0.60	0.24	4.57	0.00	0.57	0.30	0.35	0.73	0.29	0.06	3.28	0.01	0.24	0.04	0.18	0.37
Ankle	0.32	0.07	1.22	0.25	0.11	0.00	– 0.14	0.89	0.23	0.03	6.40	0.00	2.21	0.23	– 0.91	0.38

P < 0.05 means significant difference

Figures 4, 5 and 6 show the measured values of female EE in the professional and non-professional groups. Table 3 shows the results of female F-test and T-test analysis in the professional and non-professional groups. Among them, the average EE of the professional group and the non-professional group in the right forehand test were 4.03 and 3.79 respectively, and the female group in the professional group was significantly larger than the non-professional group, there was a significant difference (P < 0.05), while the difference in the waist and ankle was not obvious. (P > 0.05). In the backhand shot test on the left side, there was no significant difference in the three parts (P > 0.05), indicating that the degree of body movement of the left backhand shots tends to be the same level. In the right front forehand shot test, the three data had very significant differences ($P < 0.01$) indicating female athletes. In the left front backhand shot test, the waist EE measurements were 0.27 and 1.66, respectively, and there was a significant difference ($P < 0.05$).

3.2 Comparison of MET Values Between GT9X Professional Group and Non-professional Group in Different Wearing Parts

The male MET measured in the professional group was 4.38 ± 0.67 in the right forehand test, compared with 4.79 ± 0.96 in the non-professional group ($P < 0.05$). The data on the wrists of the wrists are not much different. There was a significant difference in the measured values of MET between the wrist and ankle in the left-hand backhand test ($P < 0.05$), and the waist difference was not obvious ($P > 0.05$). The mean MET values of the wrist and ankle in the right front forehand and the left front backhand test were 3.58, 3.34, and 5.64, and 4.02, respectively, which were significantly higher than those of the non-professional group of 3.05, 2.91, and 3.03, and 3.02, respectively < 0.05).

Among the females in the professional group and the non-professional women, the waist test was the most obvious difference in the four tests, and there was only no significant difference in the left backhand test ($P > 0.05$). There was only a significant difference in the hand test for the right front forehand test. In the comparison of the measured values of the ankle MET, the MET values of the right front hand and the right front forehand professional group and non-professional group have similar characteristics, the difference is not obvious, and there is a big difference in the left backhand and the left front backhand test ($P < 0.05$).

4 Conclusion

This study measured their energy expenditure and metabolic equivalent of energy in the energy experiment of tennis beginners and skilled players. By comparing the energy expenditure of the two group in tennis and the metabolic equivalent of energy, it is found that the energy consumption of different parts has a certain influence on the level of tennis. Professional athletes usually consume more energy in the ankle area, while non-professional athletes consume less energy at the waist, indicating that non-professional athletes have not fully mastered the correct tennis posture. In the wrist area, there is no significant difference between the two. This shows that in the process of learning tennis, the beginners have practice of gripping and hitting the ball at the beginning, so the difference with the skilled players is not obvious. However, the energy consumption of tennis hit is not only determined by the wrist, but also related to the arm, shoulder, etc., and these parts will continue to be tested in subsequent studies.

Acknowledgments. Fund Project Support: China Postdoctoral Science Foundation (2015M580 655), Hubei Natural Science Fund Project (2017CFB560), 2018 Wuhan Institute of Physical Education Graduate Education Innovation Program

References

1. Zhu, L., Chen, P.: Three-axis motion accelerometer (GT3X) measures the establishment and test of the energy consumption prediction equation for adolescents (11 ~ 14 years old). China Sport Sci. Technol. **50**(03), 73–77 (2014)
2. Liu, D.: Construction of college students' physical fitness and energy consumption model of daily physical activity. Wuhan Institute of Physical Education (2014)
3. Yuan, C., Chen, Q.-G.: Study on monitoring energy consumption of tennis sports based on ActiGraph GT3X. J. Hebei Inst. Phys. Educ. **31**(04), 83–91 (2017)
4. Hoppe, M.W., Baumgart, C., Freiwald, J.: Do running activities of adolescent and adult tennis players differ during play? Int. J. Sports Physiol. Perform. **11**(6), 793–801 (2016)
5. Ondrak, K.S., Mcmurray, R.G.: Comparison of energy expenditure of youth playing tennis during practice and match settings. J. Phys. Act. Health **13**, S21–S23 (2016)

A Study on Transparent Access to Medical Information by Implementing Automatic Authentication in Emergency Situations

Su-Chong Joo(✉) and Gyu-Sung Ham

Department of Computer Software Engineering,
Wonkwang University, 460 Iksandaero, Iksan, South Korea
{scjoo, haml231}@wku.ac.kr

Abstract. In this paper, we designed and implemented an automatic authentication for accessing medical information and IoTs based biometric information through user-owned mobile terminals. The medical information server determines whether patient's healthcare situation is a normal status or an emergency status by using IoTs based biometric information, according to a given disease-specific emergency status condition defined by hospital policies. As soon as the emergency status for a patient is determined, the medical staff (user) receives an emergency notification message service notification with an emergency code from the medical information server. The authentication procedures of user and user's mobile terminal is automatically performed by sending to the authentication server with a text message composed only of the user password including the defaulted ID, emergency code and mobile terminal's current location. Finally, if a patient is in a normal state after a successful first-aid with the authentication confirmation of the medical staff, the authorized access of the authorized medical staff also returns to a normal state.

Keywords: Automatic authentication · Biometric and medical information · Normal and emergency status · User and User-owned mobile terminal authentication

1 Introduction

With the advent IoTs based ICT technologies recently, the medical information systems are being constructed in an integrated u-health environment through cloud services, IoT technologies, and mobile applications [1]. These medical information systems should provide medical staff with authorities to access patients' medical information for emergency status' treatments or general therapeutic purposes.

In this paper, we propose and develop an automatic authentication mechanism using IoTs based biometric information obtained real-timely from medical IoTs biosensor and medical devices, installed in hospital wards and patient's body, so that according to the patient's health situations, medical staff can access and manage the patient's medical information through a prompt authentication [2]. In this paper, user and medical staff use the same meaning in a point of view of authentication after this.

T. Ahram et al. (Eds.): IHIET 2019, AISC 1018, pp. 556–562, 2020.
https://doi.org/10.1007/978-3-030-25629-6_86

As a core of this paper, the authentication for user and user-owned mobile terminal is to identify an emergency status of the patient using IoTs based biometric information, and then, according to a normal status or an emergency status of a patient, manual or automatic authentication procedures can be performed. Also, the authenticated user has transparent access rights to patient's medical information through his or her owned authenticated mobile terminals. With the authentication attributes we used, in user authentication, ID & PWD and emergency code attributes are used. In the mobile terminal authentication, attributes such as a role of an owner of the mobile terminal, the working time, the working location, like ward-room, and the current position of the mobile terminal are used. Finally, if a patient is in a normal status after medical staff' successful emergency aids with authentication confirmation, the authenticated medical staff's access rights also return to a previous normal status.

This paper is organized as follows. Section 2 describes the medical information system environment for showing automatic authentication. Section 3 explains the design and implementation of medical DB information and authentication DB information for supporting medical information service and authentication. In final Sect. 4, we summarized our research contents, and suggested the improvements of our researched results by reflecting the practical considerations in hospital fields to the hospital information system.

2 Medical Information System Environment for Automatic Authentication

Our medical information system environment for executing the automatic authentication consisted of 3 units are shown in Fig. 1 [3, 7]. The authentication procedures divided into of user authentication and user-owned mobile terminal authentication.

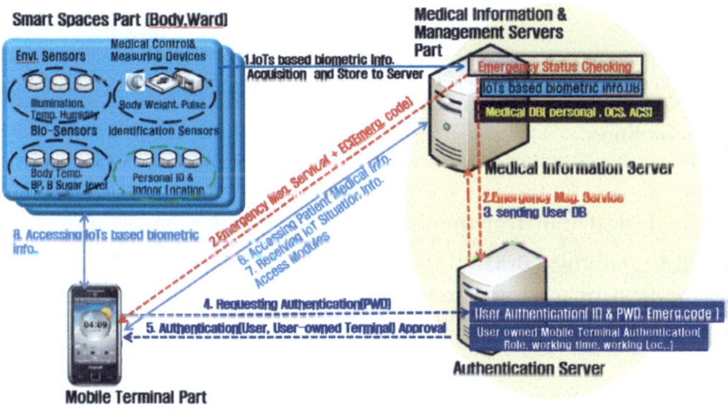

Fig. 1. Automatic authentication procedures in medical information system environment

The Smart Space Part consists of hospital ward-rooms installed or attached biosensors and medical devices for obtaining IoTs based biometric information. The Medical Information Server Part contains the medical information server and the authentication server. The medical information server stores and manages IoTs based biometric information and patient medical information and checks patient's emergency situations real-timely. The authentication server executes authentication procedures of user and user-owned mobile terminal using user-related information and mobile terminal-related information. The Mobile Terminal Part requests the authentications to authentication server and receives the confirmation of authentications of user and user-owned mobile terminal [4]. And then users can access not only IoTs based biometric information generated real-timely from the Smart Space Part but also patient's medical information constructed in the medical information server.

A patient's emergency condition is checked using IoTs based biometric information that real-timely stored to patient's medical information DB scheme in medical information server. If a patient's healthcare condition is in a range of a given emergency status, the emergency notification message including an emergency code is sent to Authentication Server and the mobile terminal of medical staff in charge through message service.

After the completion of procedures of automatic authentication, the authenticated user, medical staff, will receive the access rights. And then authenticated users can access medical in-formation and IoTs based biometric information using authenticated user-owned mobile terminal.

We assume that the patient's medical information is categorized into the 3 groups (level 1, level 2, level 3) by a given disease-specific emergency status condition according to the hospital's privacy policies as shown in Fig. 2.

Graded Medi. Info.
Level 1
Level 2
Level 3

Role	Normal	Emergency
Nurses	Level 1	Level 1,2
Doctors	Level 1, 2	Level 1, 2, 3

Fig. 2. An example of the 3 level-grouped medical information by a given disease-specific emergency status condition

Hence, medical staff can transparently access the 3 level-grouped medical information according to patients' normal or emergency status. The ETD of the whole of the detailed authentication procedures mentioned above is shown as Fig. 3.

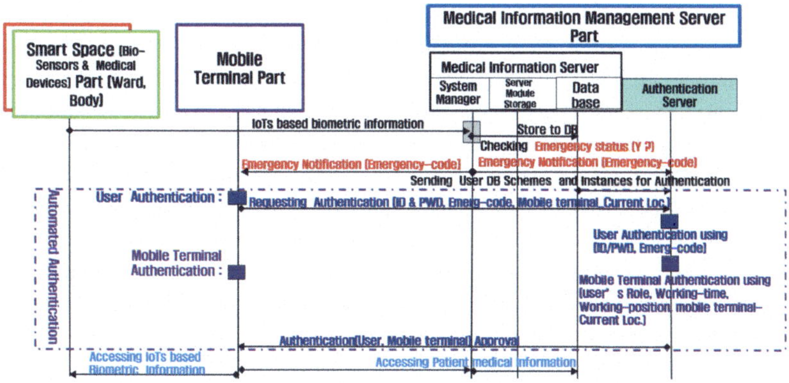

Fig. 3. The event tracing diagram showing of user and user-owned mobile terminal's authentications in medical information system environment

3 Design and Implementation of Medical Information and Authentication Information

We designed and implemented the medical DB information and authentication DB information for supporting medical information service and authentication service. The Fig. 4 is showed the Entity Relationship Model to design the medical information schemes and authentication information schemes.

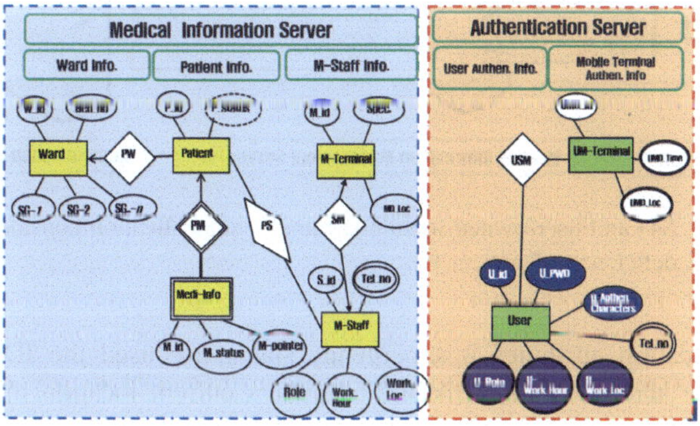

Fig. 4. The entity-relationship diagram for designing medical DB information and authentication DB information schemes.

The detailed description of this model's entities and relationships are skipped with page limits. Based on the implemented medical DB and authentication DB [5], we added the condition box for reflecting a given disease-specific emergency status condition to the ER Diagram showed in Fig. 4. As soon as an emergency status for a patient is satisfied by referring IoTs biometric information, medical staff receives an emergency notification message service included an emergency code from the medical information server system. The authentication procedures of user and user-owned mobile terminal are performed automatically together with that user forwards the emergency text message itself to the authentication server. In order to support automatic authentication, the DB of medical information is constructed with IoTs based biometric information of the patient, patient-medical staff medical information for user authentication, medical staff-mobile terminal medical information for user-owned mobile terminal authentication. The Fig. 5 is showing to the procedures of user authentication and user-owned authentication using patient medical information in the medical information server and authentication information in the authentication server, after occurring the patient's emergency status.

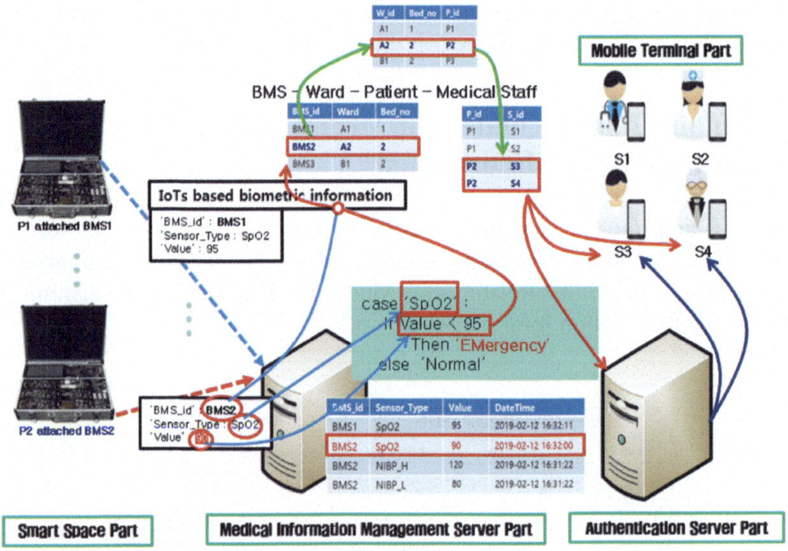

Fig. 5. User (S3, S4) and user-owned mobile terminal's authentication considering emergency situation of SpO2 deficiency of patient P2.

As authentication attributes in emergency status, we used the ID & PWD, the emergency code and user-owned mobile terminal's current location in user authentication. In the user-owned mobile terminal authentication after user authentication phase, we used the attributes such as a role of an owner of the mobile terminal, the working time, the working location sent from medical information server and information sent from the phase of user authentication are used. These authentication phases are automatically executed using only authentication attributes enumerated above inside the authentication server without any external interactions with user's mobile terminals and the medical information server.

After two phases of authentication are confirmed, users have the access permissions to access selectively the 3 level-grouped medical information by a given disease-specific emergency status situation as shown in Fig. 2. For a proving example, let P2 are a patient and medical staff in charge of P2 are nurse S3 and doctor S4 as referring Fig. 5. In our experiment, the biometric information of each patient is obtained through the BMS board installed biosensors and medical devices' interfaces.

In an emergency status, S3 and S4 had the confirmation of user authentication and user-owned mobile terminal. According user's role, users access the 3 level-grouped medical information of patient P2. A nurse S3 access the level 1 in normal status, and the level 1, 2 in emergency status. Also, a doctor S4 access the level 1, 2 in normal status and all the level 1, 2, 3 in emergency status. The Fig. 6 is showing the leveled parts of medical information grouped on screen of user-owned mobile terminal according to the access rights of users such as Nurse S3, Doctor S4.

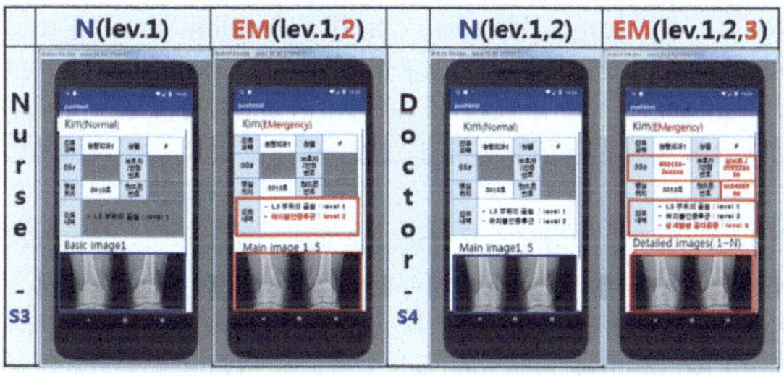

Fig. 6. An example of medical information accessing by mobile terminals of medical staff in patient's emergency and/or normal status

4 Conclusion

In this paper, we designed and implemented an automatic authentication mechanism accessing whole of medical information in emergency status, and authentication DB for user and user-owned mobile terminals authentication. The medical information designed to the 3 level-grouped medical information accessing in accordance with medical staff's roles (Nurse, Doctor) and patient's healthcare situations (emergency status, normal status). Authentication DB in the authentication server is constructed to User relation for user authentication and UM-Terminal relation for mobile terminal authentication. The phases of User and user-owned mobile terminal's authentications are used the attributes as user ID/PWD, emergency code, medical staff's role, working time, working location and user owned mobile terminal's location extracted from DB stored in medical information server.

After authentication confirmation, the authenticated user can access medical information via M-pointer attribute in Patient-related Medi-Info relation, and real-time IoTs based biometric information using authenticated their mobile terminals. Finally, if the patient is in the normal status after medical staff' successful emergency aids, the authenticated medical staff's access rights also return to a previous normal status.

In future, we are to study for mining the anterior symptoms of emergency using IoTs based biometric information of patient situation. And we will improve authentication and access mechanisms of the medical information system with our researched results by reflecting practical considerations in hospital fields.

Acknowledgement. This work was supported by Basic Science Research Program through the Ministry of Education of R.O.K and National Research Foundation in 2019 (NRF-2017-R1D1A1B03029210).

References

1. Kim, S.K., Hwang, H.J.: Security requirements of personal health service. J. Inst. Korean Electr. Electron. Eng. **19**(4), 548–556 (2015)
2. Park, J.H.: Technology and market trends of health care wearable device. Mag. IEEE **45**(3), 48–56 (2018)
3. Ham, G.-S., Seo, O.-J., Jung, H., Joo, S.-C.: Implementation of dynamic situation authentication system for accessing medical information. J. KISS **19**(12), 31–40 (2018)
4. Woo, S., Li, Z., Mirkovic, J.: Good automatic authentication question generation. In: Proceedings of the 9th INLG Conference, Edinburgh, UK, pp. 203–206, 5–8 September (2016)
5. Abdelkader, G., Naima, H.S., Adda, A.P.: Secure authentication approach based new mobility management schemes for mobile communication. J. Inf. Process Syst. **13**(1), 152–173 (2017)
6. Aslam, M.U., Derhab, A., Saleem, K., Abbas, H.: A survey of authentication schemes in telecare medicine information systems. J. Med. Syst. **41**, 14 (2017). https://doi.org/10.1007/s10916-016-0658-3
7. Joo, S.-C.: Automatic Authentication method Based on Dynamic Context for Transparent Access for Medical Information, Patent application in R.O.K.(10-2018-0029551), 14 March 2018

Digital Support in Logistics of Home-Care Nurses for Disabled and Elderly People

Karin Reinhold[1](✉), Piia Tint[1], Ada Traumann[2], Piret Tamme[3], Viiu Tuulik[3], and Silja-Riin Voolma[4]

[1] Faculty of Economics, Department of Business Administration, Tallinn University of Technology, Ehitajate 5, 19086 Tallinn, Estonia
{karin.reinhold,piia.tint}@taltech.ee

[2] TTK University of Applied Sciences, Pärnu 62, 10135 Tallinn, Estonia
ada.traumann@tktk.ee

[3] Lifelong-Learning Centre, Tallinn Health Care College, Kännu 67, 13418 Tallinn, Estonia
piret.tamme@ttk.ee, viiu@gmail.com

[4] Cognitive Psychology Department, National University of Singapore, 21 Lower Kent Ridge Rd, Singapore 119077, Singapore
siljariinvoolma@gmail.com

Abstract. The paper gives results of possibilities to use information technology organizing the work of health care nurses while working at patients' homes. Information technology helps to improve care-quality of patients and has positive an economic impact. This paper analyses the results of three studies investigating Estonian healthcare nurses in the workplace. This study was conducted in 2007–2019. Significant changes have taken place in this timeframe. New improvements are possible if the latest information technology is utilized: tablets, mobile phones, wearables, etc. In the countryside, services are more patient-centric, but nurses in rural areas must commute further than care professionals who live in towns. Some Estonian retired people do not have enough resources to live in nursing homes. Instead, the elderly and their families make the economic decision to live at home.

Keywords: Healthcare · Home-nurses · Disabled patients · Ageing people

1 Introduction

Homecare is long-term support for people who need ongoing support in everyday life. Ageing and disabled people who require personal homecare may also need nursing and additional health services. The analysis shows that in Estonia, long-term is underfunded and disorganized. The lack of resources and community-based services in Estonia decreases the number of years that elderly populations can successfully live at home.

This issue is compounded by the fact that the Estonian population is ageing. It is recognized that there is a need to develop a user-centric, comprehensive, and integrated long-term care system where services are equally accessible to all members of society. Based on the experience of other countries, the use of ICT is facilitated by greater and

T. Ahram et al. (Eds.): IHIET 2019, AISC 1018, pp. 563–568, 2020.
https://doi.org/10.1007/978-3-030-25629-6_87

more efficient use of ICT opportunities by long-term system [1]. The Estonian healthcare system is in the process of adopting digital health. Digital patient data is available to doctors and home nurses. The Estonian second-generation e-prescription system is widely used by citizens, healthcare providers and administrators. However, there are gaps in measuring the impact of the service, especially with respect to timesaving and improved healthcare quality. To ameliorate this issue, future nationwide e-health services should be more rigorously evaluated during the design and implementation stages [2, 3]. The current care burden in Estonia is approximately 30,000 women and 17,000 men. The burden on caregivers is high both in providing care and paying for care services. People are left out of the labour market due to the burden of care (according to the Labor Force Survey, 8,000 people in Estonia cannot work because the burden of caregiving is too high. Another 5,000 are working part-time) or are being cared for by family members who also work full-time.

People with chronic illnesses and those in need of home care are commonly diagnosed with cardiovascular diseases, lung diseases, diabetes, cancer, stroke, or spinal cord damage. ICT homecare solutions for people with chronic illnesses most commonly take advantage of video technologies, text messaging and health monitoring, or combinations thereof. Video technologies use video telephones, videoconferencing, health monitoring, as well as home-based care and counselling based on the data obtained. Using these technologies improves communication with homecare professionals, enables experts to get involved more efficiently, and provides emotional support to the patient. Text messaging helps patients cope with the symptoms of disease in everyday life by increasing their quality of life. ICT health status monitoring allows for the collection of real-time data on the functional state of all organ systems. Alerts can be created to help caretakers respond to changes in health status.

2 The Experience of Other Countries in Home Nursing

The Finnish home care model [4] focuses on cooperation and partnership between national and private medical institutions, nursing companies and ICT companies. When Finland introduced technological solutions, it was important to save on maintenance costs, decrease time spent on professional home visits and to speed up the flow of health information between hospitals and home care, including doctors and nurses.

In Canada's home care work [5], the main outcomes of ICT adoption are improved communication between home care team members. The use of ICT enables the patient and the care team to be adequately advised on a real-time basis, based on health monitoring data of the person in need. However, the need for the development and refinement of standards for the delivery of digital information, including the clinical terminology and technologies used, has been emphasized. On the positive side, the use of tele monitoring in telemarketing makes it possible to improve the effectiveness of treatment and care while reducing the cost of treatment.

In the home care of England [6], the personality of care work and the achievement of individualized care are considered important. Different strategies are drawn up before the care, caregivers and specialists of everything, and then the ideology of using the technologies. At the same time, the use of ICT enables public and private companies to become more transparent in the maintenance system. England also emphasizes the need to develop a system of standards that ensures the availability of necessary information and adequate decision-making by care workers and patients.

In Ireland, the EU is developing a ProACT [7] project for a home care model for elderly people with chronic diseases. Partners in home care, industry (IBM, Philips, etc.) and academic institutions are involved in the project. The aim of the project is to enable elderly people with chronic illnesses (diabetes, chronic cardiovascular diseases, etc.) to live at home as long as possible using different assistive technologies. The project will develop interfaces to integrate new technology solutions (sensors, new aids, etc.) introduced into home care with integrated systems in healthcare. New home care model has highlighted the need to develop patient-centred solutions.

New Zealand [8] invests heavily in ICT and technological innovation in order to shape individual patient support. Developing ICT systems (such as IBMs Watson) ensure interaction between health data and people, enabling it to be continuously applied (reprogrammed). By using telemedicine and transmitting information by telecommunication means, a person can get a better view of his health. At the same time, attention is paid to the safe storage and transmission of data on health status and confidentiality.

The rapid development of technologies has made it possible to significantly improve the quality of home care in Japan [9]. In addition to the state, academic and private companies, including high-tech companies, contribute to the use of ICT in home care. The use of ICT in home care is the classification of needs, the collection of data on the use of assistive devices (including robotics), the conduct of market research, the monitoring of high-tech health care at home and the response to changes. The importance of using ICT in developing a telemedicine model, focusing on the needs of the patient, their awareness and accurate and adequate documentation of care and treatment, has been emphasized separately. Home nursing enables continuous monitoring of the patient's health status in chronic diseases, as well as the possibility to advise the elderly and those with disabilities.

Worldwide, older adults are in many cases the fastest growing computer and Internet user group. Internet use and access drop off significantly after age 75. Internet usage is much less prevalent in the older group than among younger groups, reaching only 47% among 75–79 year olds, while home access was 34%, an increase from earlier years, but still low [10]. Social capital also affects Internet use by the elderly. Elderly people approach the Internet and health information technology differently than younger people, but have growing rates of adoption. Assistive technology, such as sensors or home monitors, may help "aging in place", but these have not been thoroughly evaluated. Elders face many barriers to using technology for healthcare decision-making, including issues with familiarity, willingness to ask for help, trust of the technology, privacy, and design barriers to acceptance and use.

3 Materials and Methods

Three investigations have been conducted as the basis in the current study: the first was carried out in 2007 in Pärnu county with 272 questionnaire answers. In this satisfaction study with social care, the patients graded the care service from of home-nurses positively: the mean score given by patient was 2.88 (in 3-point system) [11]. By that time, the e-health system was not in practice, yet. The second investigation was carried out by Viljandi hospital in 2016 [12]. It studied patients' satisfaction with the home-nurses work as well. Sixty two questionnaires were sent out; the response rate was 75.8. The mean age of the patients was 82 and the ICT use from the side of the patients was negligible. To the question "how do you assess the service of the home-nurse?", in 5-point scale, the answer 5 was given by 77% of the patients. The communication means with the home-nurse were not studied. Usually, the patient first visits the family doctor and afterwards, the communication with home-care nurse takes place by the phone. The e-health system is used only in the hospital, but not by the home-nurse. The third and very recent investigation "E-client file for home care and home nursing - pre-analysis and initial task preparation" lasted from June 2018 to January 2019 [13] and describes the computer-system for better service of ageing people at home by the home-nurses. The aim of the project is to conduct a preliminary analysis of the need for social care and home nursing information system and to propose an optimal and modern technical solution. The task is accurate enough to prepare the information system procurement documents, and the needs and expected benefits (paperless, fast, timesaving) of different service providers and beneficiaries are outlined in the pre-analysis document. The total cost of the project is EUR 30,657.6, of which the self-financing is EUR 4598.64 and the European Regional Development Fund support 26, 058.96 EUR.

4 The Model for Logistics of Home Care Nurses

The centre for the care is hospital or home-care nurses unit. The nurses are equipped with the small cars, smart-phones and computers. The patients are equipped with phones and tablets. There are many patients who are disabled contemporarily and the retirement is long away. They have to go back to work and their knowledge in ICT is rather advanced. In addition, the ICT capabilities are improving very quickly for ageing people. The scheme for improvement the care is presented in the Fig. 1.

5 Discussion and Conclusions

A literature review [14] shows that patients with possibilities of being cared for and using telecare at home preferred a combination of telecare and traditional healthcare delivery. Therefore, ICT applications must be used as an adjunct and not as replacements for standard care; otherwise, the positive results might be not be replicated [15]. Many patients prefer being involved and participate in decision making regarding the care they will receive. Despite this, caring programs will be developed without caregiver's participation [16].

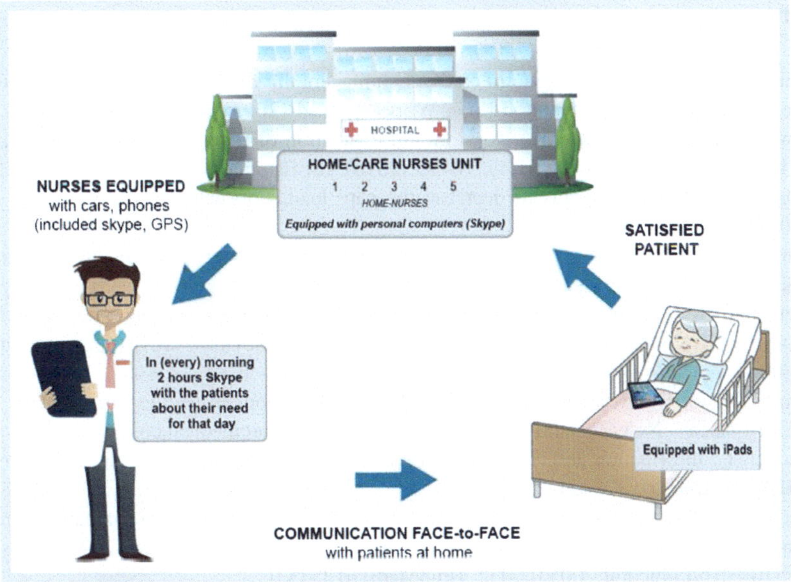

Fig. 1. The use of digital tools in the care of old and disabled people (original painting by authors).

In many countries, older adult population is increasing at a dramatic rate due to better health care, technology, and improved living conditions. However, as individuals 65 years and older begin to live longer and experience multiple life changes, there is a larger incidence of social isolation leading to loneliness, depression, and a general decline in health.

The most important issues that have to be considered while caring the ageing people at home are the following:

- The possibility to carry out continuous monitoring of the patient's health status in chronic diseases,
- Advice possibilities for the people with disabilities.

The methods more suitable to older people can be advised as:

1. Timely and regular consultations by Skype on IPad.
2. Coordinated work by the hospital unit with co-operation of home-nurses.
3. Application of the 'smart home' - an innovative living environment (continuously ready to respond to a request for environmental assistance).

References

1. Lai, A.: The situation of long-term care in Estonia and the challenges of the state in reducing the burden of carers. Sotsiaaltöö (Soc. Work) **4**, 9–14 (2017). (in Estonian)
2. Parv, L., Kruus, P., Mõtte, K., Ross, P.: An evaluation of e-prescribing at a national level. J. Inform. Health Soc. Care **41**(1), 78–95 (2016). (in Estonian)
3. Tarum, H.: The first means to decrease the care load. Sotsiaaltöö (Soc. Work) **4**, 15–17 (2017). (in Estonian)
4. Sami, P.: Technology on elderly care Finland. EPTEC (2012). https://www.epliitto.fi/images/EHealth_in_Finland_Per%C3%A4l%C3%A4.pdf
5. Canadian Home Care Association on the issues- ICT (2015). www.cdnhomecare.ca
6. Homecare UK-Homecare Reviews & Nursing Agencies Reviews (2016). https://homecare.co.uk
7. ProAct-Major EU Research Project (2016). http://www.homeinstead.ie
8. ICT Homecare New Zeeland (2017). https://www.homecaremedical.co.nz/
9. Kamei, T.: Information and communication technology for homecare in future. J. Nurs. Sci. **2013**(10), 154–161 (2013)
10. Rice, R.E.: Influences, usage, and outcomes of Internet health information searching: multivariate results from the pew surveys. Int. J. Med. Inf. **75**(1), 8–28 (2006). https://doi.org/10.1016/j.ijmedinf.2005.07.032. [PubMed:16125453]
11. Kõre, J.: Satisfaction with patient service in Pärnu city (2007). https://parnu.ee/failid/uuringud/Rahulolu_sotsiaalteenustega_Parnu_linnas.pdf. (in Estonian)
12. Tammesalu, S.: Pre-analysis of the E-client file of the information system. HEISIT OÜ. Tallinn, Bureau Veritas (2018). https://www.tallinn.ee/est/E-klienditoimik-koduhooldusele-ja-koduoendusele. (in Estonian)
13. Ülesoo, G.: Patient Satisfaction Survey Survey Viljandi Hospital (2016). http://www.vmh.ee/public/Kodu6endus_2016.pdf. (in Estonian)
14. Williams, T.L., May, C.R., Esmail, A.: Limitations of patient satisfaction studies in telehealth care: a systematic review of the literature. Telemed. J. e-Health **7**(4), 293–316 (2001)
15. Ducharme, F., Baudet, L., Legault, A., Kergoat, M.-J., Levesque, L., Caron, C.: Development of an intervention program for Alzheimer's family care givers diagnostic disclosure. Clin. Nurs. Res. **8**, 44–67 (2001)
16. Vahdat, S., Hamzehgardeshi, L., Hessam, S., Hamzehgardeshi, Z.: Patient involvement in health care decision making: a review. Iranian Red Crescent Med. J. **16**(1) (2014)

Literature Review of the Application of Wearable Device GT3X in Monitoring Physical Activity

Tong Wan[1(✉)] and Qi Luo[2]

[1] Graduate School, Wuhan Sports University, Wuhan 430079, China
760009436@qq.com
[2] College of Sports Engineering and Information Technology, Wuhan Sports University, Wuhan 430079, China

Abstract. After years of development, ActiGraph GT3X has been used in many fields, and the health effects of physical activity are also very obvious, and people are paying more and more attention to it. This paper systematically explains the basic principles of GT3X and the research status of GT3X in monitoring daily physical activities. By reviewing the two databases of CNKI and Clarivate Analytics Web of Science, the papers have been compared and summarized in a simple way. It is found that the research on monitoring physical activity through GT3X at home and abroad has been widely applied, but compared with foreign research fields and research results, there is still a lot of room for improvement in China. It is necessary to increase the research on the daily physical activity of wearable devices represented by GT3X in China, so as to make scientific and in-depth research on the physical activity of different periods of time and research and develop a guide for healthy physical activity that is most suitable for the Chinese population.

Keywords: ActiGraph GT3X · Physical activity · Energy consumption · Monitor

1 Concept of Physical Activity

There are many concepts about physical activity. Zhu et al. [1] mentioned that the early definition of physical activity is any body movement caused by skeletal muscle contraction that can lead to energy expenditure. Later, there is a new definition, that is, at the metabolic level, any activity that has skeletal muscles that move the body and can cause an increase in energy consumption in the body. In 2001, scholars gave a new definition that physical activity is the movement of the body caused by skeletal muscle contraction, including daily energy consumption. It concludes physical activity, competitive sports and leisure sports, although there is a deeper explanation of physical activity, but I think the most acceptable is the activity of skeletal muscle contraction at the level of basal metabolism (BMR), which causes the increase of body energy consumption. According to daily activities, it includes occupational physical activity, physical exercise and so on.

T. Ahram et al. (Eds.): IHIET 2019, AISC 1018, pp. 569–575, 2020.
https://doi.org/10.1007/978-3-030-25629-6_88

2 Principles and Functions of GT3X

The GT3X series of accelerometers are manufactured by Actigraph Inc. of the United States to measure the amount of physical activity in the human body's daily life. 2 Not only can the daily physical activity, intensity, and activity patterns be monitored, but also the energy expenditure of human activities. It has been used by more than 1,500 institutions and research institutions in more than 60 countries around the world. The GT3X device is the size of a watch and is easy to wear. Subjects can wear it 24 h a day, and can be recorded in a variety of environments without being affected by space. The GT3X sensor device mainly consists of a piezoelectric element and a vibrating body. When the external body receives the induction, the vibration body is deformed, and the piezoelectric element changes when it is connected. The deformation of the piezoelectric element forms an electrical signal and an electrical signal. The intensity is the magnitude of the acceleration. After numerical simulation and conversion, the electrical signal is converted into a digital signal, and the digital signal is converted into the final acceleration count (counts) by mathematical conversion. We can analyze the intensity and time of daily physical activity through counts. The recorded data can be analyzed by the matching software Aritilife (Figs. 1 and 2).

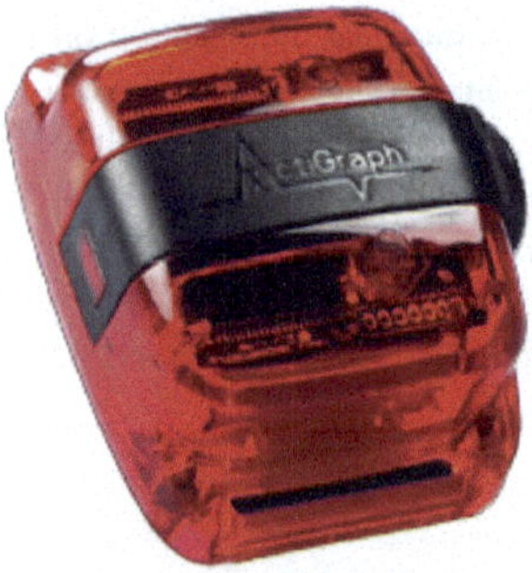

Fig. 1. GT3X appearance

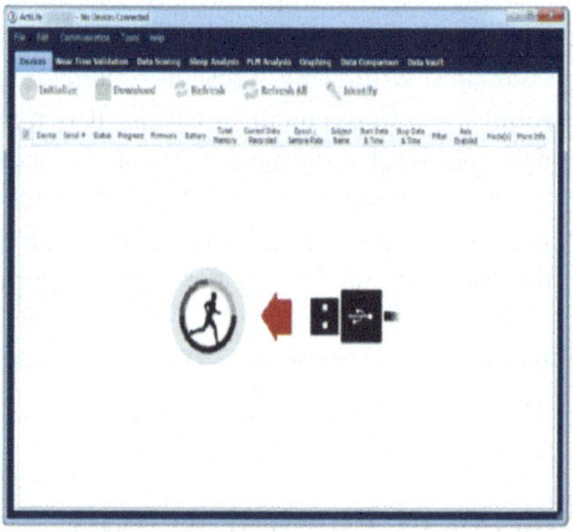

Fig. 2. Artilife work interface

3 GT3X Research in Monitoring Physical Activity

There are many types of wearable devices on the market, and the GT3X wearable device has made great contributions in many fields such as preventing physical illness, enhancing physical fitness, and rehabilitation. The following is the application of GT3X in physical activities of people of different ages.

3.1 GT3X in Monitoring the Physical Activity of Young Children (0–3 Years Old)

As a special period, infants and young children aged 0–3 have just learned to walk and start using tools, language and thinking begin to occur, early self-awarenessappears. It is difficult to have an experiment and test. However, because of its simple equipment, the GT3X does not have any effect on the child's daily physical activity during the experiment. Table 1 is a list of literature on GT3X monitoring physical activity in young children.

Table 1. List of literature on GT3X in monitoring physical activity in young children

Literature	Research purposes
Elin Johansson	Exploring the differences in physical activity of children of this age
Sanne L.C. Veldman	Exploring the relationship between infant muscle and physical exercise
Sílvia Costa	Exploring the predictive validity of GT3X at different cut points between sedentary and mid-high-intensity exercise

Elin et al. [2] collected physical activity and sedentary time of 2-year-old children through GT3X, assessed average activity, low-intensity and high-intensity physical activity, sedentary time, and found that children of this age are a kind of Intermittent exercise patterns, with no link to gender, body mass index, motor skills or parents; Veldman et al. [3] measured the physical activity of Australian 11–29 month old children through GT3X, through multi-level linear regression Analysis to assess the link between motor skills and physical activity, and found that the large muscle motor skills in the sample have nothing to do with physical activity, which confirms the existence of a potential age for improving large muscle motor skills; Costa et al. [4] through GT3X, NHANES, Trost and Pate measure sedentary behavior and physical activity in children aged 2–2 years, and compare the predictive validity of GT3X with a cut-point of 5-s to the 15-s predictive validity of NHANES, Trost and Pate. The high accuracy of 5-s indicates that this critical point is useful for studies of sedentary and physical activity in children aged 2–3 years [4].

3.2 GT3X in Monitoring the Physical Activity of Young Children (3–12 Years Old)

Younger children (3–12 years old) is a key period of growth and development. Many scholars have studied children in this period and made great contributions to the healthy growth of children. Table 2 is a study of GT3X monitoring physical activity of young children. List of documents.

Lin et al. [5] collected data on 24-h behavioral activities of children aged 9–11 through GT3X, and analyzed data by multi-layer linear model to verify there is a two-way connection in children's sleep time, daytime PA (physical activity) and SED (sedentary time); JP Chaput et al. collect energy consumption during daily physical activity of Canadian children aged 9–12 through GT3X, and evaluate the independent and joint associations with physical activity, sedentary time, sleep time and obesity of Canadian children through cross-sectional studies [6]; Cohen et al. [7] performed 26 specific exercises on children in low-income communities through GT3X, and conducted randomized controlled trials to obtain a linear mixed model of the data obtained. This will improve the overall ability of basic motor skills (FMS) and improve the cardio-pulmonary health of children in low-income communities.

Table 2. List of literature on GT3X's research on monitoring physical activity in young children

Literature	Research purposes
Yingyi Lin	Verify two-way contact between sleep time and daytime physical activity and sedentary time
J-P Chaput	Explore children's sedentary, sleep time, MVPA and obesity
Kristen E. Cohen	Improve the cardiorespiratory health of children in low-income communities
Cheryl A. Howe	Assess children's MVPA levels
Kristen E Cohen	Improve children's basic motor skills and MVPA levels

3.3 GT3X Monitors Physical Activity Among Adolescents (12–17 Years Old)

Adolescence is a period of psychological and physical maturity. The physical development and physical fitness of adolescents (12–17) has always been the focus of social attention. How to improve the fitness and health of adolescents has become the focus of attention now. Table 3 is a list of literature on GT3X's research on monitoring physical activity in adolescents.

Table 3. List of literature on GT3X's research on monitoring physical activity of adolescents

Literature	Research purposes
WangYi Bo	Improve physical education curriculum and improve teaching level
HongJun Rui	Enhance the physique of young people
Viciana, Jesús	Increase moderate to strong physical activity among young people in Latin America
Rosenkranz, Richard R.	Improve the PA level of Australian youth
Danilo R. Silva	Reduce the sedentary time of teenagers and increase MVPA

Wang et al. [8] collected the sports load data of junior high school physical education students through GT3X, and conducted comparative research, successfully improving the scientific basis for digital physical education; Junrui et al. [9] collected through GT3X 10- Energy consumption data of 17-year-old students in pre-puberty, middle and late physical activity, analysis of Chinese youth physique, improvement of appropriate training recommendations, and enhancement of youth physique; Silva [10] using GT3X for sixth graders'daily physical activity was collected and recorded, and a controlled trial was set up. Successfully found that standing desks can increase students' MVPA levels.

3.4 GT3X in Monitoring Adult Physical Activity

Adults are a large group and the most extensive. By examining this population, we can examine the characteristics of normal human movements. Table 4 is a list of literature on GT3X's research on monitoring physical activity in adults.

Table 4. List of literature on GT3X's research on monitoring physical activity in adults

Literature	Research purposes
Wang Li Jun	Better predicting body energy consumption
Pedro B. Júdice	Verify that sedentary effects affect many diseases
Faisal A. Barwais	Verify that increasing standing time can prevent obesity
YuanChuan	Prediction of the energy consumption of tennis
A.V. Rowlands	Validating wristband monitors is a viable option for future bone research

Wang Lijun et al. [11] collected the energy consumption of running sports for 19–29 year olds through GT3X, and analyzed with GT3X's own analysis software Actilife to find a more suitable sports energy prediction equation for young people in China; Júdice et al. [12] collected the sedentary time and energy expenditure of obese adults in daily life through GT3X. Through randomized controlled trials, it is found that people may now be underestimated that "sedation may affect many diseases". Barwais et al. [13] through GT3X for standing, lying, sitting time, daily physical activity of 22–30 year old adults, through questionnaires and data analysis, successful discovery can increase the standing time Good prevention of obesity.

3.5 GT3X in Monitoring the Physical Activity of the Elderly

Nowadays, the aging is serious, and the health of the elderly is also a point that cannot be ignored. Table 5 is a list of literature on GT3X's research on monitoring physical activity in the elderly.

Aguilar Farias et al. [14] used GT3X to collect sedentary time and energy expenditure in the free life of the elderly. The optimal threshold for determining the sedentary time of the elderly by ROC curve analysis is 200/min; Ortlieb et al. [15] collecting and recording the daily physical activities of 65–89 year olds through GT3X, and using the multivariate regression linear model to predict the functional exercise ability (FEC), and explore a physical activity pattern of the elderly. To help healthy exercise for the elderly; Andrea Z. LaCroix et al. [9] collect and record the daily

Table 5. List of literature on GT3X's research on monitoring physical activity in the elderly

Literature	Research purposes
N. Aguilar Farias	Find the best threshold for sedentary elderly people
Sandra Ortlieb	Exploring the physical activity patterns of the elderly
Andrea Z. LaCroix	Exploring the relationship between exercise and cardiovascular disease in older women
Kim, Miji	Verifying the relationship between sleep patterns and body composition in older women
Holmquist, Sofie	Exploring the high-risk characteristics of depression in the elderly

physical activity of 63–99 year old women through GT3X, and combine the bedtime and questionnaire to assess the direct connection with cardiovascular disease with body movements of the elderly.

4 Summary

After decades of development, GT3X has been applied in many fields. This article gives an overview of GT3X and its application in different age groups, mainly from children, children, adolescents, adults, and the elderly. A systematic review, analysis of existing research success can lead to the following inference:

(1) According to the existing research situation, the monitoring of daily physical activity of GT3X is very accurate, and the reliability and validity of the prediction of body strength and energy consumption are very high. With the development of GT3X, it is believed that the device will be more widely used in the world in the future, which will be the future development trend.

(2) The success of the research collected in this paper is mainly in the field of daily physical activity of people of different ages. Learning from children and young people's physical activities, we can improve the school education methods and promote growth; learn from the technical movements of tennis, we can promote the research results to golf, table tennis and other balls; learn from the movements of patients waiting for lumbar surgery Methods and drawbacks can be applied to other types of surgical patients or rehabilitation exercises. Drawing on the study of sedentary and disease in adults and the elderly, research can be applied to the construction of fitness, exercise and fitness equipment. There are differences in the body of people of different ages. By referring to the physical activity models of people of different ages, the physical activity model can be extended to many educational institutions or scientific research institutions and many other fields to increase the physical fitness of the whole people.

Acknowledgments. This work was supported by Hubei Natural Science Foundation Project (2017CFB560).

References

1. Zhu, F., Xu, K.: Research status of GT3X measurement of physical activity. Sports Res. Educ. **30**(S1), 104–107 (2015)
2. Elin, J., Maria, H., Viktoria, S., Anna, E., Michaela, F.: Objectively measured physical activity in two-year-old children – levels, patterns and correlates. Int. J. Behav. Nutr. Phys. Act. **12**, 3 (2015)
3. Veldman, S.L.C., Jones, R.A., Santos, R., Sousa-Sá, E., Pereira, J.R., Zhang, Z.: Associations between gross motor skills and physical activity in Australian toddlers. J. Sci. Med. Sport **21**, 817–821 (2018)
4. Costa, S., Barber, S.E., Clemes, S.A.: Calibration and validation of the ActiGraph GT3X+ in 2–3 year olds. J. Sci. Med. Sport **17**, 617–622 (2014)
5. Lin, Y., Tremblay, M., Katzmarzyk, P., Fogelholm, M.: Temporal and bi-directional associations between sleep duration and physical activity/sedentary time in children: an international comparison. Prev. Med. **111**, 436–441 (2018)
6. Chaput, J.P., Leduc, G., Boyer, C., Bélanger, P., LeBlanc, A.G., Borghese, M.M., Tremblay, M.S.: Objectively measured physical activity, sedentary time and sleep duration: independent and combined associations with adiposity in canadian children. Nutr. Diabetes **4**, e117 (2014)
7. Cohen, K.E., Morgan, P.J., Plotnikoff, R.C., Callister, R., Lubans, D.R.: Physical activity and skills intervention: SCORES
8. Wang, Y.: Application of "accelerometer" to assess the sports load of junior high school physical education class. Shanxi Normal University (2017)
9. LaCroix, A.Z., Rillamas-Sun, E., Buchner, D., Evenson, K.R., Di, C., Marshall, S., LaMonte, M.J., Hunt, J.: The objective physical activity and cardiovascular disease health in older women (OPACH) study. BMC Public Health **17**, 192 (2017)
10. Silva, D.R., Minderico, C.S., Pinto, F., Collings, P.J., Cyrino, E.S., Sardinha, L.B.: Impact of a classroom standing desk intervention on daily objectively measured sedentary behavior and physical activity in youth. J. Sci. Med. Sport **21**, 919–924 (2018)
11. Wang, J., Zhang, B., Jia, L., Sun, Z., Zheng, Z.: The validity of actigraph (GT3X) accelerometer in measuring the energy activity of physical activity of Chinese people aged 19–29 years. Sports Sci. 32(12), 71–77+92 (2012)
12. Júdice, P.B., Santos, D.A., Hamilton, M.T., Sardinha, L.B., Silva, A.M.: Validity of GT3X and Actiheart to estimate sedentary time and breaks using ActivPAL as the reference in free-living conditions. Gait Posture **41**, 917–922 (2015)
13. Barwais, F.A., Cuddihy, T.F., Rachele, J.N., Washington, T.L.: ActiGraph T3X determined variations in "free-living" standing, lying, and sitting duration among sedentary adults. J. Sport Health Sci. **2**, 249–256 (2013)
14. Aguilar Farias, N., Peeters, G., Brown, W.: ActiGraph GT3X + threshold for classifying sitting/lying activityin older adults in free-living environments. Friday 2 November Papers/J. Sci. Med. Sport **15**, S188 S264 (2012). S34 S126 (2013)
15. Ortlieb, S., Dias, A., Gorzelniak, L., Nowak, D., Karrasch, S., Peters, A., Kuhn, K.A., Horsch, A., Schulz, H.: Exploring patterns of accelerometry-assessed physical activity in elderly people. Behav. Nutr. Phys. Act. **11**, 28 (2014)

Application of Computational Fluid Dynamics in Biofluids Simulation to Solve Actual Surgery Tasks

Alex G. Kuchumov(✉) and Aleksander Selyaninov

Department of Computational Mathematics,
Mechanics and Biomechanics, Perm National Research Polytechnic University,
Komsomolsky Prospekt 29, 614990 Perm, Russia
kychymov@inbox.ru

Abstract. Computational fluid dynamics (CFD) is a dynamically developing tool in mechanical engineering and interdisciplinary research. Medicine is one of the areas, where the application of current computational methods is extremely necessary. This study presents the results of using computational fluid dynamics methods to solve actual problems of surgery (modeling of blood flow in the patient-specific aorta of a child with congenital heart disease during bypass surgery; modeling of the flow of bile in the biliary system to predict cholecystectomy outcome; modeling of the chyme flow in the colon). *Simulation of blood flow in the aorta during shunting*. Cardiovascular diseases are most common in the population and cause the prevailing part of premature mortality and disability in both adults and children. Blalock – Taussig shunting is mainly used to eliminate pathological changes in children. However, this procedure is carried out empirically: surgeons use their own experience. CFD enabled to numerically evaluate the shunt parameters and its location for proper lung development in children with congenital heart disease after shunt installation. *Biomechanical analysis of the bile flow in healthy state, pathology, and after cholecystectomy.* Cholecystectomy (removal of the surgical gallbladder) is usually taken to treat patients suffering from gallbladder disease and gallbladder pain. However, it should be noted that the results of the operation are not always successful. The biomechanical patient-specific model was created to assess the cholecystectomy outcome. *Study of the chyme flow features in the colon.* The large intestine is a long hollow muscle tube of complex shape, which digests and absorbs nutrients and water from food (which is commonly called chyme in medicine). The goal is to create a patient-specific model of the chyme and feces flow in the colon in the healthy state and pathology. Clinical applications of this model can be expressed in the description and understanding of the causes of the disorders as well as drug efficiency assessment to reduce the number of patients.

Keywords: CFD · Shunt · Cholecystectomy · Chyme

T. Ahram et al. (Eds.): IHIET 2019, AISC 1018, pp. 576–580, 2020.
https://doi.org/10.1007/978-3-030-25629-6_89

1 Introduction

Computational fluid dynamics (CFD) is a dynamically developing tool in mechanical engineering and interdisciplinary research. Medicine is one of the areas, where the application of current computational methods is extremely necessary.

This study presents the results of using computational fluid dynamics methods to solve actual problems of surgery (modeling of blood flow in the patient-specific aorta of a child with congenital heart disease during bypass surgery; modeling of the flow of bile in the biliary system to predict cholecystectomy outcome; modeling of the chyme flow in the colon).

Simulation of Blood Flow in the Aorta During Shunting. About 25–30% of all congenital heart anomalies are related to aorta coarctation [1]. It is necessary to use systemic-pulmonary anastomoses for radical correction [2, 3]. The first Blalock-Taussig operation was performed in 1945 [4]. In 1975 de Leval modified this technique by using a polytetrafluoroethylene shunt known as the modified Blalock Taussig shunt (MBTS) [5]. This method has become a standard intermediate palliative operation for the cyanotic heart diseases to provide a dosed pulmonary blood flow.

It is noteworthy that literature data indicate MBTS as a relatively high-risk procedure with a total mortality of 7.2% [6, 7]. It competes with the risk of mortality in the range of many neonatal open-heart procedures with artificial circulation [8]. Potential disadvantages of these shunts include excessive volumetric load, acute thrombosis and low diastolic blood pressure, which leads to coronary insufficiency [9–11].

Biomechanical Analysis of the Bile Flow in Healthy State, Pathology, and After Cholecystectomy. Gallstones affect 10 to 15% of the adult population in the World at average. Cholecystectomy is the most commonly performed abdominal operation for the treatment of patients suffering from gallbladder disease in Western countries [12, 13]. Nevertheless, the operation outcome is not always positive. To predict outcomes of cholecystectomy, the computational simulations are good tool for providing more realistic choledynamic factors (bile flow velocities, pressures, WSS). A thorough review of current publications in this field reveals that bile flow has been mostly investigated in separate ducts of the biliary system. Some attempts to make patient-specific models of cystic ducts [14] and biliary tree [15] have been made. So far, however, there has been no attempt to create a patient-specific model of bile flow. The aim of work is to study bile flow to predict outcomes of surgical operations using patient-specific approach and created the entire biliary system model.

Study of the Chyme Flow Features in the Colon. The diseases of the intestine, as a rule, include inflammatory forms of the disease (most often it is Crohn's disease or ulcerative colitis), benign or malignant neoplasms, and functional disorders [16]. According to statistics, about 5 million people in the world suffer from various kinds of inflammatory bowel diseases, in Europe - about 0.3% of the population. In 2018, colon and rectal cancer was diagnosed in 1.8 million people.

Treatment of bowel disease may be conservative or operative. In the case of surgery, the percentage of complications reaches up to 60%. When functional disorders of the intestine are applied, as a rule, conservative methods of treatment [17].

The causes of intestinal diseases are hereditary factors or external - sedentary lifestyle, bad habits, unhealthy diet, stress. To understand the processes occurring in the intestine in normal and pathological conditions, as well as to assess the effectiveness of treatment, it is necessary to consider a number of factors: the movement of chyme, mixing, absorption of nutrients. Methods of mathematical modeling allow us to describe the transport of chyme in the intestine, taking into account peristalsis, to take into account changes in the properties of the intestinal wall due to various diseases.

2 Materials and Methods

Simulation of Blood Flow in the Aorta During Shunting. Based on MRI, we constructed a patient-specific models of system "aorta–pulmonary artery–shunt" to analyze hemodynamics in 10 children with congenital heart pathology.

Blood was considered as a Newtonian fluid. The boundary conditions for children were obtained using ultra-sound measurement techniques. The aim was to get the main hemodynamical parameters (velocity, pressure, flow rate, Qs/Qp, OSI, WSS, TAWSS, e.t.c.) at different shunt configurations to evaluate the surgery effectiveness.

Biomechanical Analysis of the Bile Flow in Healthy State, Pathology, and After Cholecystectomy. Different models (for example, Windkessel model, peristaltic fluid motion, FSI algorithm) can describe fluid motion in the elastic and compliant ducts. Our approach is decomposition of the biliary system into three compartments (extra-hepatic biliary tree, gallbladder, major duodenal papilla). Bile flow in the extra-hepatic ducts is simulated using FSI algorithm. Bile flow in the gallbladder can be described as flow in the reservoir with compliant ducts using Windkessel model. Bile flow in the major duodenal papilla is considered as peristaltic fluid motion, because the wall contraction is really important factor of fluid motion in that segment. The coupling of these compartments is performed by boundary conditions. The biliary system geometry was obtained using MRI patient-specific data. It was confirmed that normal bile can be modeled as Newtonian fluid and lithogenic bile can be modeled as non-Newtonian fluid (Carreau fluid). Bile ducts were modeled as hyperelastic material. Bile flow analysis was performed for several patients.

Study of the Chyme Flow Features in the Colon. MRIs of colon were used. Chyme was considered as a non-Newtonian power-law fluid. Navier–Stokes equations and the continuity equation were used for CFD computations

$$\rho\left(\frac{\partial \mathbf{v}}{\partial t} + (\mathbf{v} \cdot \nabla)\mathbf{v}\right) = -\nabla \cdot \boldsymbol{\sigma} + f,$$

$$\nabla \cdot \mathbf{v} = 0,$$

where $\mathbf{v}$ is chyme velocity, ρ – density, $\boldsymbol{\sigma}$ – the stress tensor, f – mass forces.

Rendering and segmentation of MRI was performed by open source software ITK-Snap to create patient-specific 3D colon model. OpenFOAM software was adopted to permorm CFD simulations.

3 Results and Conclusions

Simulation of Blood Flow in the Aorta During Shunting. Velocity, pressure and WSS distributions were numerically obtained. It was shown that blood flow in the pulmonary arteries is asymmetric. Wall shear stress, which is a biomechanical assessment of thrombosis formation, has maximal values in the shunt region. Biomechanical modelling enables to predict an effectiveness of shunt functioning at its different modifications.

Biomechanical Analysis of the Bile Flow in Healthy State, Pathology, and After Cholecystectomy. The effect of bile pathology on the velocity and pressure distributions in the patient-specific extrahepatic biliary tree was investigated using a one-way FSI approach. Several patients were analyzed. Comparisons were made for healthy and lithogenic bile in terms of fluid flow, WSS and pressure. Lower values of pressure in the extrahepatic biliary tree in the case of the healthy bile were related to the difference in the rheological properties (the lithogenic bile was more viscous than the healthy bile). It was shown that bile rheology and geometry changes played an important role in the changes of the velocities, pressures and stresses, which could lead to gallbladder disease progression. Moreover, cholecystectomy changes in the bile flow and stress distributions were found. Therefore, the proposed model could be applied to medical practice to evaluate the circumstances of surgical interventions.

Study of the Chyme Flow Features in the Colon. As a result of the implementation, a model of the flow of chyme and feces in the three-dimensional geometry of the intestine, obtained by processing MRI images of a particular patient, was obtained. The resulting model will open up broad prospects in medicine and pharmacology:

- assessment of the effect of drugs on the transport of chyme and feces;
- analysis of the current state of the patient on the basis of a numerical assessment of the hydrodynamic parameters of the chyme in this segment of the digestive system, as well as a comparison with normal values for a particular patient;
  strength analysis of colorectal anastomoses to reduce a high mortality;
- evaluation of the effectiveness of the treatment of inflammatory bowel disease for a particular patient.

Acknowledgments. The research is performed under financial support of Perm Region Government. The work was partially supported by Russian Government Assignment (Project No. 19.7286.2017/8.9).

References

1. Zinkovskiy, M.: Congenital Heart Diseases. Nauka, Russia (2010). (in Russian)
2. McKenzie, E.D., Khan, M.S., Samayoa, A.X.: The Blalock-Taussig shunt revisited: a contemporary experience. J. Am. Coll. Surg. **216**, 699–704 (2013)
3. Williams, J.A., Bansal, A.K., Kim, B.J.: Two thousand Blalock-Taussig shunts: a six-decade experience. Ann. Thorac. Surg. **84**, 2070–2075 (2007)
4. Moulton, A.L., Brenner, J.I., Ringel, R.: Classic versus modified Blalock-Taussig shunts in neonates and infants. Circulation **72**, 1135–1144 (2007)
5. de Leval, M.R., McKay, R., Jones, M., Stark, J., Macartney, F.J.: Modified Blalock-Taussig shunt. J. Thorac. Cardiovasc. Surg. **81**, 112–119 (1981)
6. Gold, J.P., Violaris, K., Engle, M.A.: A five-year clinical experience with 112 Blalock-Taussig shunts. J. Card. Surg. **8**, 9–17 (1993)
7. Curzon, C.L., Milford-Beland, S., Li, J.S.: Cardiac surgery in infants with low birth weight is associated with increased mortality: analysis of the society of thoracic surgeons congenital heart database. J. Thorac. Cardiovasc. Surg. **135**, 546–555 (2008)
8. Petrucci, O., O'Brien, S., Jacobs, M., Jacobs, J., Manning, P., Eghtesady, P.: Risk factors for mortality and morbidity after the neonatal Blalock-Taussig shunt procedure. Ann. Thorac. Surg. **92**, 642–651 (2011)
9. Myers, J.W., Ghanayem, N.S., Cao, Y.: Outcomes of systemic to pulmonary artery shunts in patients weighing less than 3 kg: analysis of shunt type, size, and surgical approach. J. Thorac. Cardiovasc. Surg. **147**, 672–677 (2017)
10. Li, J.S., Yow, E., Berezny, K.Y.: Clinical outcomes of palliative surgery including a systemic-to-pulmonary artery shunt in infants with cyanotic congenital heart disease: does aspirin make a difference? Circulation **116**, 293–307 (2007)
11. Ahmad, U., Fatimi, S.H., Naqvi, I.: Modified Blalock-Taussig shunt: immediate and short-term follow-up results in neonates. Heart Lung Circ. **17**, 54–58 (2008)
12. Luo, X., Li, W., Bird, N., Chin, S.B., Hill, N.A., Johnson, A.G.: On the mechanical behavior of the human biliary system. World J. Gastroenterol. **13**, 1384–1392 (2007)
13. Portincasa, P., Moschetta, A., Palasciano, G.: Cholesterol gallstone disease. Lancet **368**, 230–239 (2006)
14. Al-Atabi, M., Ooi, R.C., Luo, X.Y., Chin, S.B., Bird, N.C.: Computational analysis of the flow of bile in human cystic duct. Med. Eng. Phys. **34**, 1177–1183 (2012)
15. Lo, R.C., Huang, W.L., Fan, Y.M.: Evaluation of bile reflux in HIDA images based on fluid mechanics. Comput. Biol. Med. **60**, 51–65 (2015)
16. Dumic, I., Nordin, T., Jecmenica, M., Stojkovic, M., Milosavljevic, T., Milovanovic, T.: Gastrointestinal tract disorders in older age. Can. J. Gastroenterol. Hepatol. **2019**, 1–19 (2019)
17. Yamamoto, T., Watanabe, T.: Surgery for luminal Crohn's disease. World J. Gastroenterol. **20**, 78–90 (2014)

Numerical Evaluation of Sport Mouthguard Application

Anna Kamenskih[1], Tatyana Ustugova[1], Alex G. Kuchumov[1(✉)], and Redha Taiar[2]

[1] Department of Computational Mathematics, Mechanics and Biomechanics, Perm National Research Polytechnic University, Komsomolsky Prospekt 29, 614990 Perm, Russia
anna_kamenskih@mail.ru, kychymov@inbox.ru
[2] Groupe de Recherche en Sciences Pour l'Ingénieur (GRESPI/MAN), Université de Reims Champagne-Ardenne (URCA), 9 Villa Douce, 51097 Reims Cedex, France
redha.taiar@univ-reims.fr

Abstract. Dental system pathology has a negative impact on the quality of life. Abrasion, chipping, and loss of teeth are the main consequences of non-carious damage to the dental system elements. These factors are often associated with different levels of physical and emotional stress. One of the ways to reduce the physical loads on the dental system elements is the use of protective mouthguards during a sports activity. Therefore, studying the deformation behavior of the prosthetic structure and elements of an individual's dental system and analyzing contact parameters are necessary for examining the structure's operation and optimization. In this study, stress distribution in the teeth was obtained during a contact interaction without considering prosthetic structures and a single-layer prosthetic structure with a biting force of 200 N. Stress intensity distribution (max σ_i) in hard tooth tissues was obtained. Results showed that sports mouthguards reduced the maximum stress intensity in hard tooth tissues by 1.5 times on the tooth surface and 3.7 times near the zone of occlusion.

Keywords: Contact · Dentofacial system · Mouthguard · Polymer · Numerical simulation

1 Introduction

A number of socially significant diseases of the human dental system significantly affect the quality of life of a patient [1]. During powerlifting and working with a psycho-emotional overload, functional loads can significantly exceed normal values. The muscle force overload causes the gradual abrasion and dyeing of the teeth [1–3]. The worst consequence is a partial or complete loss of teeth. One of the most optimal ways to reduce the stress of the dental system is using mouthguards [1, 3].

A number of works [3–6] have analyzed the effect of protective prosthetic structures with different designs on the state of the elements of the human dental system. In the last five years, there has been an increase in patents related to a change in the

T. Ahram et al. (Eds.): IHIET 2019, AISC 1018, pp. 581–585, 2020.
https://doi.org/10.1007/978-3-030-25629-6_90

geometric configuration of protective mouthguards. However, there has been no wide-scale biomechanical modeling aimed at assessing the influence of the geometric features of mouthguards on the stress-strain state in the dental system.

This work aims to biomechanically analyze the deformation behavior of a pair of teeth in contact with and without a single-layer mouthguard.

2 Problem Statement

A biomechanical analysis of the deformation behavior of a pair of teeth was performed in contact with and without a single-layer mouthguard made of ethylene-vinyl acetate (EVA) polymer material (Fig. 1). The geometrical configuration of the dentition elements was obtained using computed tomography in the framework of clinical studies by the research team of Perm State Medical University (Professor N. Astashina and Dr. E. Sergeeva).

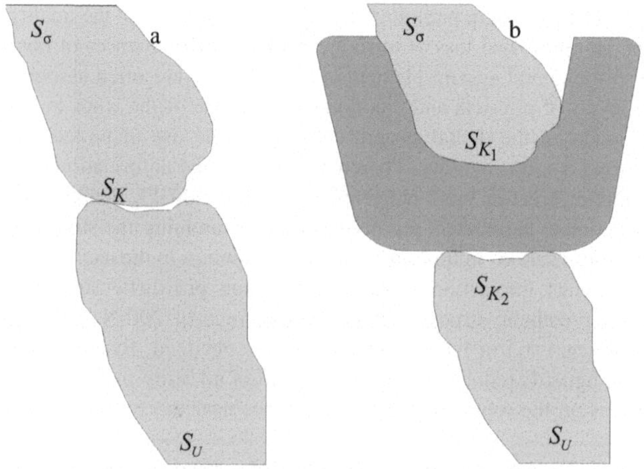

Fig. 1. Contact between teeth without a mouthguard (a) and with a single-layer mouthguard (b)

Earlier, the experiments to determine the mechanical properties of EVA were performed in the framework of interdisciplinary studies [5]. The Young's modulus and the Poisson's ratio were found as $E = 17.3$ MPa and $\nu = 0.46$, respectively.

3 Results and Conclusions

A numerical assessment was performed to evaluate the effect of a single-layer mouthguard on the deformation behavior of the patient's dental system elements. Figures 2, 3 show the stress intensity distributions in the upper and lower teeth at an indentation force of 200 N. In case of mouthguard usage, the stress intensity distribution changes: the maximum value observed near the roots of the teeth is 1.5 times less and 5 times less in the zone of teeth closing compared with the case of contact without a mouthguard. The level of max σ_I in the tooth from the lower dentition with the strength of indentation of 200 N is less than 2 times in the main volume of the tooth and less than 3.8 times in the zone of teeth closing in the case of mouthguard application. The dependence of the maximum stress intensity on the indentation force is close to linear. A significant decrease in the level occurs when a pair of teeth contact through an individually adapted single-layer mouthguard: the stress intensity in the tooth of the upper dentition is, on average, 1.5 times less than when contacting without considering the mouthguard, in the area of teeth closing, on average, more than 5.5 times less (Fig. 4).

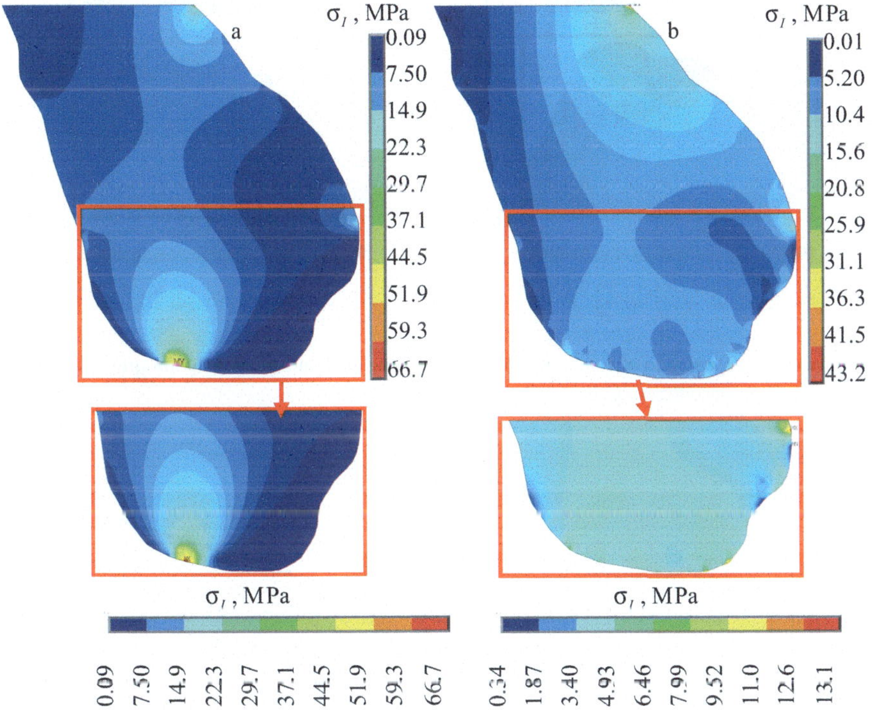

Fig. 2. Stress intensity in the upper tooth at F = 200 N: contact without mouthguard (a) and with single-layer mouthguard (b)

In case of mouthguard application, the stress in the lower tooth is 2.1 times less than that in the case of the contact without this protective construction. The stress in the area of teeth occlusion is approximately 3.7 times more than that in the case of mouthguard application

Thus, within the framework of the study, a numerical model of the problem of contact interaction of two teeth of the upper and lower dentition was developed with and without considering an individually adapted single-layer mouthguard.

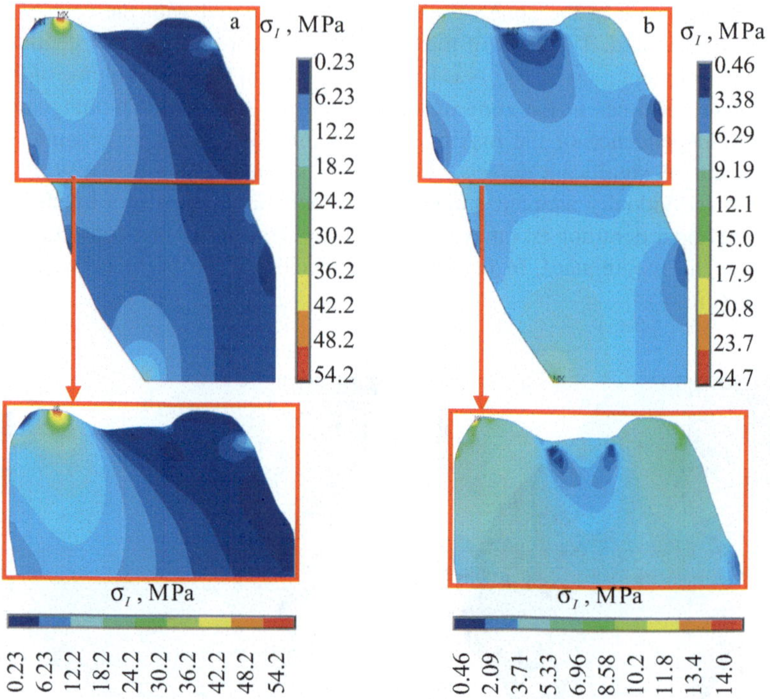

Fig. 3. Stress intensity in the lower tooth at $F = 200$ N: contact without mouthguard (a) and with single-layer mouthguard (b)

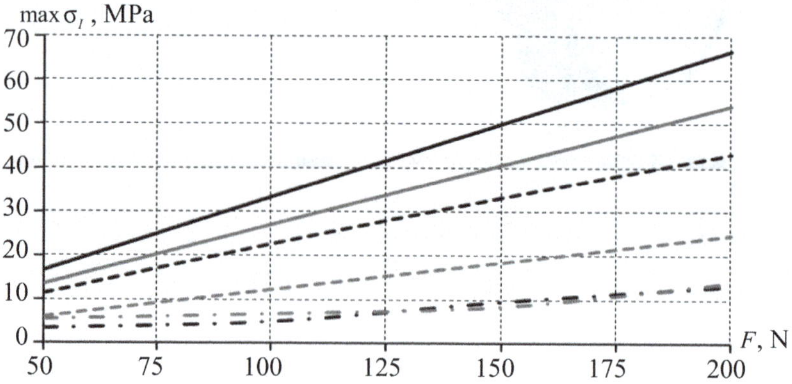

Fig. 4. Dependence of max σ_I on F: 1, 3, 5 – upper tooth; 1, 2 – contact without mouthguard; 3, 4 – max σ_I at contact through a single-layer mouthguard; 5, 6 – max σ_I in the occlusion area during the contact through a mouthguard

The de-formation behavior of the biomechanical contact assembly under different functional loads was analyzed. Within the framework of a series of numerical experiments, the dependence of the nature and magnitude of the parameters of the contact zone on the level of physiological load was established. Contact pressure and contact shear stress for models with and without a protective mouthguard were compared. The effect of the prosthetic structure on the deformation of hard dental tissues for one clinical case was analyzed. The results showed that the use of a single-layer mouthguard led to a significant decrease in maximum stress intensity.

Acknowledgments. The research is performed under financial support of Perm Region Government. Anna Kamenskih and Alex G. Kuchumov also acknowledge financial support of Russian Foundation for Basic Research (Project No. 17-48-590411 r_a).

References

1. Roettger, M.: Modern Sports Dentistry. Springer, Switzerland (2018)
2. Hernandez, F., Wu, L.C., Yip, M.C., Laksari, K., Hoffman, A.R., Lopez, J.R., Grant, G.A., Kleiven, S., Camarillo, D.B.: Six degree-of-freedom measurements of human mild traumatic brain injury. Ann. Biomed. Eng. **8**, 1918–1934 (2014)
3. Kamenskih, A., Astashina, N.B., Lesnikova, Y., Sergeeva, E., Kuchumov, A.G.: Numerical and experimental study of the functional loads distribution in the dental system to evaluate the new design of the sports dental splint. Ser. Biomech. **1**, 3–15 (2018)
4. Demidov, D.A., Zakiev, V.N., Borisov, V.V., Shakaryants, A.A.: Comparative characteristics of thermoplastic and individually made protective mouthguards fit on polyurethane models. Dent. Forum **4**, 21–22 (2016)
5. Tiwar, V., Saxena, V., Tiwari, U., Singh, A., Jain, M., Goud, S.: Dental trauma and mouthguard awareness and use among contact and noncontact athletes in central India. J. Oral Sci. **56**(4), 239–243 (2014)
6. Lokhov, V.A., Kuchumov, A.G., Merzlykov, A.F., Astashina, N.B., Ozhgikhina, E.S., Tropin, V.A.: Experimental investigation of materials of novel sport mouthguard design. Russ. J. Biomech. **4**, 409–420 (2015)

Preliminary Results on the Assessment of Temperature Distribution on Hands After Typing on Ergonomic and Non-ergonomic Postures

Bruno Erthal de Souza Vianna[1(✉)], Pedro Kaíque Rodrigues Leite[1], Emma Butterworth[2], Redha Taiar[3], and Christiano Bittencourt Machado[1]

[1] Biomedical Ultrasound Laboratory, Estácio de Sá University, Rua Eduardo Luiz Gomes, 134, Niterói 24020-340, Brazil
cbmfisio@gmail.com
[2] Northumbria University, Newcastle-upon-Tyne NE18ST, UK
[3] Université de Reims Champagne-Ardenne, Chemin des Rouliers, BP1036, 51687 Reims, France

Abstract. The objective of this work was to assess temperature distribution on hands after typing on ergonomic and non-ergonomic postures, using infrared camera. Three volunteers performed four activities: control, ergonomic typing (10-min typing in an ergonomic posture), non-ergonomic typing 1 (wrist extension) and non-ergonomic typing 2 (wrist flexion). There was no significant trend seen in temperature between the different days as they fluctuate across all the different subjects. There was an increase in temperature in the difference between metacarpophalangeal and finger extremities and the dorsal temperature and finger extremities after typing. There was a slight increase in temperature because small muscles were used as the typing task required a minimal amount of work intensity, therefore less heat was produced. The temperature increase could also be due to increased blood flow to the working muscles, suggesting the elevated temperature is secondary to increased blood flow.

Keywords: Infrared thermography · Ergonomy · Temperature · Image processing

1 Introduction

It is known that changes in the production process have taken place in recent decades. Activities are more monotonous and repetitive, and workdays are excessively prolonged, as well as night jobs. Efficiency was increased during production, thus generating serious consequences for physical and mental health [1].

In this context, work-related musculoskeletal disorders (WMSDs) are represented by a group of diseases and by the occurrence of symptoms such as paresthesia (i.e. numbness, tingling or decreased sensation), pain in various parts of the body, sensation of muscle weight and/or fatigue, especially affecting the upper limbs [2].

T. Ahram et al. (Eds.): IHIET 2019, AISC 1018, pp. 586–591, 2020.
https://doi.org/10.1007/978-3-030-25629-6_91

Currently, infrared thermography has been used for health assessment. A thermographic camera is capable of measuring the infrared radiation emitted by a body that has thermal energy. The aim of this application is to correlate skin temperature with the subcutaneous perfusion level, and its diagnostic potential has been widely explored [3]. There has been many large correlations reported between musculoskeletal disorders and jobs involving extensive keyboard use [4, 5].

Some works can be highlighted in this area. Gold et al. [6] were able to discriminate individuals with cold extremities with the probable cause of a reduced blood flow. They demonstrated that reduced skin temperature could be a sign of sympathetic nervous system disturbance. In another study, they found that a typing speed over 50 words per minute affected blood temperature and volume, and that skin temperature could reflect muscle perfusion in the hand [7].

Thus, the objective of this work was to present preliminary results on the effect of non-ergonomic positions on the wrists during typing task in the distribution of temperature of the hands and fingers, measured by infrared thermography.

2 Materials and Methods

2.1 Subjects

Three volunteers were recruited to this study: a man (M1, 21 years old) and two women (W1 and W2, with 23 and 24 years old, respectively). They signed an informed consent for participation in the study and publication of data. This work was approved by Estácio de Sá University's Ethics Committee (CAAE nº 32015514.6.0000.5284) and follows the guidelines of the Declaration of Helsinki.

Exclusion criteria were: presence of Raynaud's phenomenon, presence of carpal tunnel syndrome, recent surgery or cervical spine pathology, diabetes, acute upper limb injury, osteoarthritis, or use of beta blockers or calcium channel blockers for disorders cardiac disorders. To avoid temperature increases not associated with intervention sessions, volunteers were instructed not to engage in intense exercise or to use a computer keyboard, not to consume coffee or cigarettes (at least 60 min before the sessions).

2.2 Experimental Setup

The intervention occurred on four distinct days, one week interval. Before each intervention, the patient was in an air-conditioned environment (between 22.5 °C and 23.5 °C), sitting for 20 min. Magazines were offered to them as a pastime. After this period, the volunteer went to a simulation of an ideal office, with the chair and monitor adjusted according to each individual, following the guidelines of Dul and Weerdmeester [8].

On the first day, the individual only performed a thermographic evaluation of the hands before and after 10 min sitting at the work place, without performing any task. On the second day, the subject entered a text for 10 min, with the highest speed he could achieve the task, with the wrists aligned with the forearm and hands, as described in [8] as a recommended ergonomic position. On the third and fourth day, the individual performed the same task, but with a 10° wrist extension and flexion, respectively, which was accomplished by placing the keyboard above the level of the forearm using a wooden block (extension) or a supporting object below the distal forearms (flexion). Thermographic evaluations were performed before and after these tasks.

A thermographic camera (i7, Flir® Systems Inc., USA, image resolution: 140 × 140 pixels, thermal sensitivity: 0.1 °C, spectrum: 7.5 to 13 μm, accuracy: ± 2 °C, emissivity: 0.95) was used to capture temperature distribution on the dorsal aspect of hands and fingers. The camera was positioned 63 cm above the table of the simulated workstation, in parallel with the ground. The volunteer placed his hands under the camera, inside a rectangular marking of 30 × 26 cm, with the thumbs of both hands in contact. The images were collected and saved on memory cards for later processing, using an intensity-based algorithm, implemented in Matlab (MathWorks Inc., USA), for the extraction of several parameters.

2.3 Algorithm for Image Processing

The user enters the name of the desired file (.csv worksheet). The thermographic image appears on the screen (Fig. 1) and he/she is asked to draw a square with the mouse in the dorsal region of the right and left hands, defining the region of interest (ROI). Then the user is asked to click on each location of the metacarpophalangeal joints (right and left, always starting at the first joint). Finally, the location of the tip of each finger is requested (right hand first, first to fifth finger). This procedure will be used to calculate the parameters: average temperature at the dorsal region of the hand ("Dorso"), the temperature difference between the metacarpophalangeal joint and the distal phalanx (DMFFD) and between "Dorso" and the distal phalanx (DDFD).

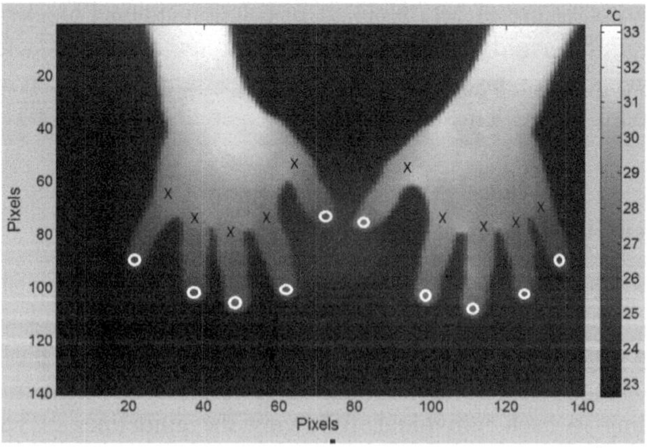

Fig. 1. Example of an infrared image. Metacarpophalangeal joints are marked with a mouse (black "X") as well as finger extremities (white circles).

3 Results

Figure 2 depicts an example of a infrared images from the 2nd day, for subject W2, before (left) and after (right) typing in ergonomic posture. Differences in temperature distribution can be observed mainly in finger extremities.

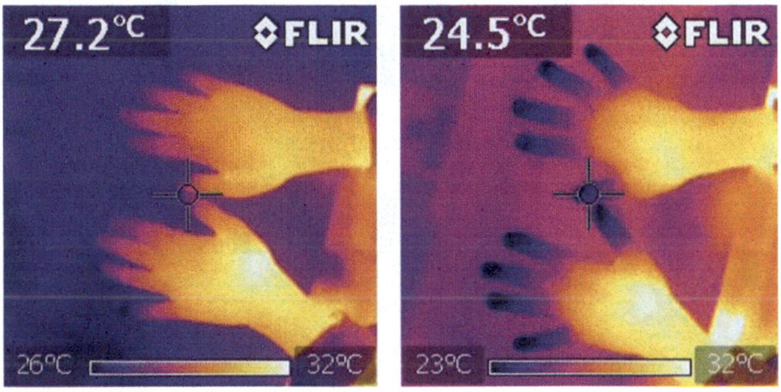

Fig. 2. Infrared images from the 2nd day, subject W2, before (left) and after (right) typing in ergonomic posture. It is possible to observe differences in temperature distribution (markedly in finger extremities).

Figures 3, 4 and 5 show the results for subjects M1, W1 and W2, respectively. The two first bar charts are results for the right and left hands, respectively (pre- and post-intervention). The third bar chart depicts the difference between post- and pre-intervention for both hands. The number after each parameter at the x-axis represents the intervention day (1 to 4).

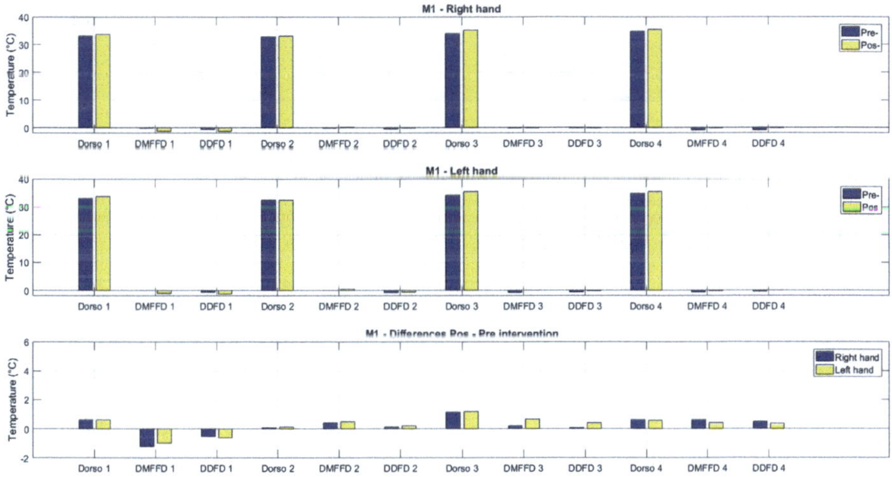

Fig. 3. Results for subject M1.

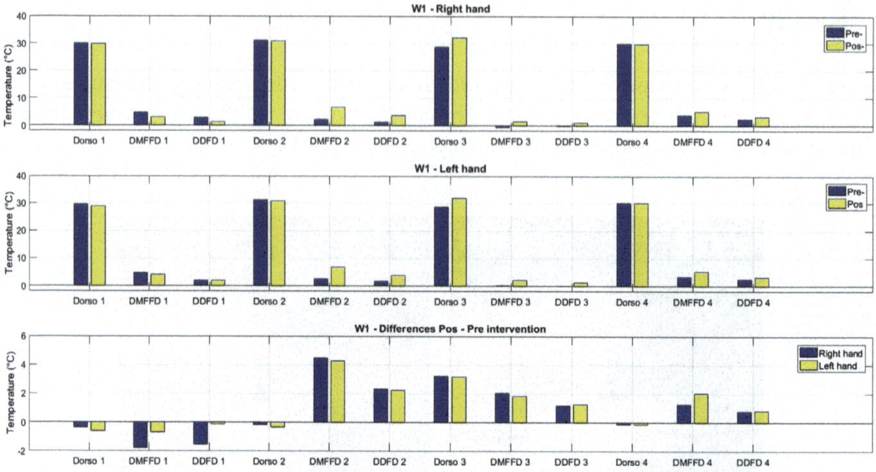

Fig. 4. Results for subject W1.

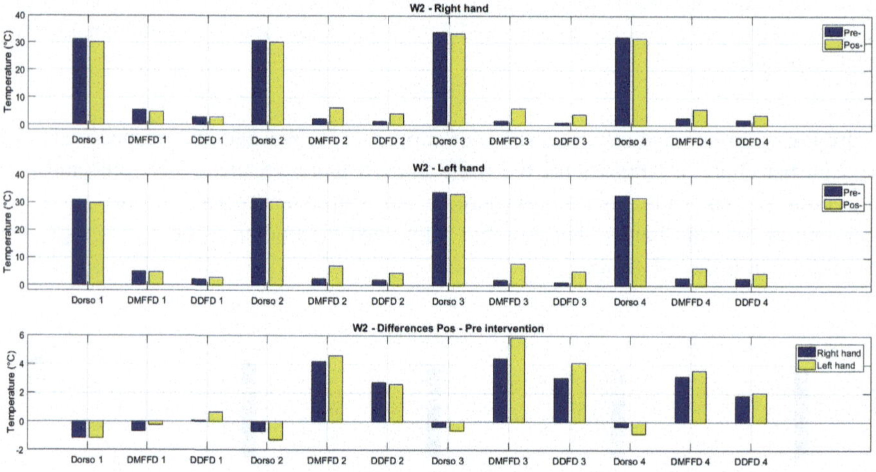

Fig. 5. Results for subject W2.

4 Discussion and Conclusions

Distinct patterns were recognized from the infrared images, in the comparison of the temperatures of the hands before and after typing for 10 min, in ergonomic and non-ergonomic positions. From the results, it can be observed that there was an increase in the difference between metacarpophalangeal and finger extremities and the dorsal temperature and finger extremities, after the subject has typed (2nd, 3rd and 4th day). This may be accounted for by the decrease in finger extremity temperature during typing (Fig. 2), which increases the overall difference. However, there was no observable trend in the temperature of the dorsal region alone.

When examining how the different positions affect the temperature and therefore blood flow, there was no observable trend between the different days as they fluctuate across all the different subjects. As there was a very small sample size (N = 3), it limits statistical power, making it hard to draw definite conclusions. However, our findings may corroborate papers showing that the temperature of the hands after typing can increase or decrease, depending on the subject [6, 7]. Further research and more subject recruitment would solidify this conclusion.

It is still not known how reliable infrared imaging actually is. Skin temperature can change throughout the day due to many things, such as certain medical conditions or the menstrual cycle [9]. These factors were not taken into account in this investigation.

Each subject typed at different speeds, using typing different styles. This is unique to each individual and cannot be standardized. Moreover, the subjects only typed for 10 min, and this might not be long enough as office workers work for long periods of time. A longer typing period is needed for a more accurate representation of the office workers everyday life and would increase the reliability of these results.

To conclude, there is a visible trend that there was an increase in the difference between metacarpophalangeal and finger extremities and the dorsal temperature and finger extremities, after the subject has typed for 10 min, no matter the posture is (ergonomic or non-ergonomic). Further investigation is needed to make any conclusion on if the position in which a person is typing affects the blood flow. This should be done using a larger sample size and using an extended typing period.

References

1. Soares, M.M., Rebelo, F.: Ergonomics in Design: Methods & Techniques. CRC Press, New York (2017)
2. Simoneau, S., St-Vincent, M., Chicoine, D.: Work-Related Musculoskeletal Disorders (WMSDs): A Better Understanding for More Effective Prevention. IRSST, Québec (1996)
3. Vollmer, M., Möllmann, K.P.: Infrared Thermal Imaging. Wiley-VCH, Wineheim (2010)
4. Gerr, F., Monteilh, C., Marcus, M.: Keyboard use and musculoskeletal outcomes among computer users. J. Occup. Rehabil. **16**, 259–271 (2006)
5. Juul-Kristensen, B., Kadefors, R., Hansen, K., Byström, P., Sandsjö, L., Sjøgaard, G.: Clinical signs and physical function in neck and upper extremities among elderly female computer users: the NEW study. Eur. J. App. Physiol. **96**, 136–145 (2004)
6. Gold, J.E., Cherniack, M., Hanlon, A., Dennerlein, J.T., Dropkin, J.: Skin temperature in the dorsal hand of office workers and severity of upper extremity musculoskeletal disorders. Int. Arch. Occup. Environ. Health **82**, 1281–1292 (2009)
7. Gold, J.E., Cherniack, M., Hanlon, A., Soller, B.: Skin temperature and muscle blood volume changes in the hand after typing. Int. J. Ind. Ergon. **40**, 161–164 (2010)
8. Dul, J., Weerdmeester, B.: Ergonomics for Beginners: A Quick Reference Guide. CRC Press, New York (2008)
9. Kräuchi, K., Konieczka, K., Roescheisen-Weich, C., Gompper, B., Hauenstein, D., Schoetzau, A., Fraenkl, S., Flammer, J.: Diurnal and menstrual cycles in body temperature are regulated differently: a 28-day ambulatory study in healthy women with thermal discomfort of cold extremities and controls. Chronob. Int. **31**, 102–113 (2013)

Ergonomic Interventional Study of Lighting Atmospheres in Textile Company

Amira Omrane(✉), Asma Dimassi, Chayma Harrathi, and Lamia Bouzgarrou

Department of Occupational Medicine and Ergonomics, Faculty of Medicine, University of Monastir, Monastir, Tunisia
omraneamira@yahoo.fr

Abstract. An ergonomic intervention in a textile company was conducted after an initial request focusing on the recrudescence of workers' visual complaints, and the defects of articles at the end of the chain. This intervention included three stages: an initial evaluation of the lighting atmosphere of the 6 workshops, an improvement of the compliance with industrial lighting standards and a re-evaluation of the lighting atmosphere. The total study population was composed of 718 workers, spread in six workshops. The evaluation concluded of non-compliance with the lighting standards of 60% of the workstations studied.

Keywords: Ergonomic interventional study · Lighting atmospheres · Textile industry integration

1 Introduction

The Safety and well-being of workers are conditioned by the work environment. Particularly, in industrial settings, adapted workplace lighting ensures optimum comfort and safety, reduces visual fatigue and accidents at work, and maximizes productivity and efficiency. An ergonomic intervention in a textile company was conducted following an initial request which focused on the recrudescence of workers' visual complaints, and of the errors and defects of articles at the end of the chain reported by the supervisors.

2 Presentation of the Company

Our study was conducted in a company located in the governorate of Monastir in the center of Tunisia, created since 1984 and specialized in the manufacture and washing of articles "sportswear", including jeans. It is a limited liability, fully bonded, fully exporting company with a monthly capacity of 120,000 items.

T. Ahram et al. (Eds.): IHIET 2019, AISC 1018, pp. 592–598, 2020.
https://doi.org/10.1007/978-3-030-25629-6_92

3 Patients and Methods

3.1 Patients

The number of employees of the company was 2412. The administration and the maintenance department were excluded from this survey. Thus, this study concerned 718 workers, spread into six workshops: cutting; preparation, washing, development, brushing, ironing. The majority of workers (80%) in the clothing workshop were female. Stratified random sampling was conducted using the Epi info 6 program. The criteria for non-inclusion were tenure in the workstation of less than two years.

3.2 Methods

This study was conducted in three stages:

- **1st stage:** initial evaluation of lighting in the six workshops using a luxmeter and referring to standard NF 35-103.
- **2scd stage:** a lighting intervention conducted based on the recommendations from the first assessment.
- **3thrd stage:** a reassessment of the lighting associated with an assessment of visual disturbances and worker satisfaction. These data were collected using a 50-item semi-open questionnaire on socio-occupational characteristics, ophthalmological history, history of eye injuries, ocular and musculoskeletal manifestations, and a subjective assessment of worker satisfaction.

4 Results

4.1 Initial Evaluation of the Lighting

The results of the measurements of the lighting are shown in Table 1. The lowest level of illumination was 90 lx and was measured at the storeman's workstation in the cutting workshop. The highest level of illumination was 1320 lx and was measured at a checkpoint in the brush shop. No workshop had a normative lighting in all of workstations. In the cutting workshop, the embroidery station which concerned 51.78% of the workers of this workshop, was concerned by a gap from the standard with levels of 210 lx for recommended standards of 500 lx. In the garment shop, the machine sewing stations had lighting below the recommendations, i.e. 84.7% of the workers in the workshop were working in non-normative lighting environments.

4.2 Intervention in the Lighting Environments

An action plan adapted to each workshop was presented, according to the tasks carried out in workstations, referring to the results of the initial evaluation and according to the available means.

In the cutting workshop a cleaning of the fixtures of the entire cutting workshop was done and coupled with a quarterly periodic cleaning. For the embroidery sector,

Table 1. Measurements of the lighting los of the first and third stages of the study in the different workshops

Workshops	Recommended lighting (lux)	Initial measurement of lighting (step 1)	Measurement of lighting after intervention (step 3)
Cutting *(n = 162)*	300	320	320–580
	300	90	200
	500	210	250
Confection *(n = 245)*	700–1000	700–1000	700–1000
	300	330	340
	500	350	690–740
Washout *(n = 113)*	700–1000	780	780
	300	205	150
	300	160	132
Development *(n = 12)*	300	380	390
	1000–1500	1230	1300
	300	200	180
Brushing*:* *(n = 107)*	500	800	900
	300	410	500
	700–100	840–1320	1300
	500	250	250
Ironing *(n = 79)*	700–1000	270	720
	150	226	350
	300	480	520

requiring a lot of precision, an increase in the number of luminaries with the installation of additional lighting; has been programmed. A matt coating of the floor and walls was planned in a 2nd intervention. A replacement of defective fluorescent tubes, with cleaning of the luminaries was carried out in the store room.

In the clothing workshop, the lighting distribution was not harmonious; the cladding of the walls is done by a bright dark gray hue. Transparent covers have been installed in the luminaries. In addition, a implantation of the production lines respecting the light sources has been proposed coupled with light scrolling grids, auxiliary lamps for all machine workstations and a matt floor covering, and walls of any kind of workshop. An arrangement of the premises of this workshop aiming to a compromise between natural and artificial lighting was planned at a later stage.

In the fading workshop the single fluorescent lamps were replaced by lamps with scrolling grilles installed. At the control stations, the luminaries were equipped with transparent covers to reduce glare, and devices for height adjustment, coupled with wall cladding and worktops.

4.3 Reassessment of Lighting

The results of the illumination measurements made after the intervention phase are shown in Table 1. The lowest level of lighting was 132 lx and was measured at the dryer station in the washroom. The highest level of illumination was 1300 lx, measured respectively at the checkpoint in the brushing and color control workshop in the development workshop. The garment and ironing workshops had normative lighting in all the workstations, for a total of the 324 workers. In these 2 workshops, we noted the most notable increases in lighting levels compared to the initial assessment. In the other workshops (cutting, developing, washing and brushing), the overall rate of workers occupying positions with lighting levels below the recommended standards was 22.4%. The largest and most persistent standard deviations from the re-evaluation of lighting were noted at the branding station of the horizontal dummy brushing and cutting shop in the brush shop (with a measured level of 132 lx for a recommended minimum level of 300 lx).

4.4 Study of Visual Symptoms and Satisfaction of Light Environment

This sample was composed of 250 workers with a sex ratio of 0.66, an average age of 30 years [22–55 years]. This sample is essentially composed of blue-collar workers (80%). The average job tenure was 4.5 years ± 6 months [2–10 years]. The average tenure in the garment and clothing sector was 7 years ± 2 years [4–17 years].

Among the workers surveyed, 243 had no history of chronic disease. A refractive disorder was noted in 59 subjects (23.6%). A musculoskeletal disorder was reported by 25% of subjects. The most commonly reported ocular symptoms are headache, itchy eyes and eye burns.

After the intervention, a decrease in ophthalmological symptoms was noted in 176 workers (70.04%) and in headaches in 40 workers (16%).

The overall percentage of satisfaction was 58%. The highest satisfaction rates were in the workshops of washing (100%), ironing (74.07%) and cutting (71.42%).

5 Discussion

The current study was carried out following a request aroused by both a large number of complaints related to visual fatigue, and high error rate of articles at the end of the chain. This study aimed to preliminary analyze the lighting conditions in six workshops of the company, intervene on these conditions in order to improve the visual comfort of workers and to reduce the rate of non-compliant articles at the end of the chain. The initial and secondary evaluation of the lighting conditions were made by a luxmeter enabling the integration and measurement of all the light rays regardless their angle of incidence. In addition, working conditions could be cofactors of certain visual symptoms noted such as; dust, heat, the relative humidity level of the air… The comparison of the measurements made during these two evaluations must take into account the fact that they were carried out in different conditions of sunshine (according to the period of the year). Moreover, the intervention on the lighting conditions was largely limited by the financial conditions. The evaluation of the impact of the lighting conditions on health workers and their satisfaction was limited by the absence of a screening of visual disturbances by visiotests or specialized examinations. In the literature, the theme of the eye at work has been approached through different index, including exposures and traumatologie [1–9]. Few articles concerned the issue of vision at work outside these particular issues and more rarely the precision and industrial work. Yet, the quality of visual perception at work, largely conditioned by the lighting, ensure safety and comfort for workers.

In this study, the prevalence of visual fatigue was 48% (which corresponds to the association of 3 or more symptoms). Most frequent reported symptoms were: eye burns (90, 4% of cases); the feeling of blurred vision (54% of cases) and tingling eyes (40% of cases). These results are comparable to those of others Tunisian study [10, 11]. Indeed, a study conducted among 361 workers spread over 3 Tunisians confection companies, noted a frequency of visual disturbance of 24.3%. The increase of visual complaints associated to lighting failure, was significantly related to the seniority, and control and sewing highest rates of visual disturbances [11]. In a study conducted in a garment factory in the central region of Tunisia, covering 400 employees, N. Bayoudh reported visual disturbances in 52.25% of the population studied. The control workshop was the most exposed to fatigue. This workstation requires a lot of precision and vigilance to detect defects [10]. This rate was comparable to those reported in periodic plant worker surveys carried out by the Work and environment Office; 38–56% [12]. The inadequate lighting conditions contribute to an increase of the workload, and may cause discomfort or visual fatigue [11, 13, 14]. The term visual fatigue, or asthenopia refers to a subjective psycho physiological and objective, behavioral and phenomena that reflect a weakening of visual sensory and/or motor functions. These phenomena, generally generated by a predominantly visual work, are reversible after rest [13]. Glare is one of the main factors of visual discomfort. According to the International Commission on Illumination (CIE), this term refers to the visual conditions in which the subject experiences either discomfort or a reduction in the ability to distinguish between objects and/or an excessive contrast in space and time as a result of improper distribution of luminance in the visual field [14, 15]. In the context of industrial work, and more specifically in the case of working inside; the most common cause of glare is the inadequate distribution of lighting, is an inadequate location of the light sources in relation to the workers, or the insufficient protection of these sources of artificial light (lamps and lights) or natural light sources. Their high luminance causes glare directly or indirectly, by reflection [14, 16–18].

A study was conducted in the jewelery and electronics industry in Thailand, involving 472 workers assigned to various positions, aiming to the assessment of work-related visual fatigue [19]. The authors used questionnaires, a binocular vision test [19]. The prevalence of visual fatigue was equal to 52.1% and explained by the high level of precision of the tasks performed and the inappropriate lighting conditions founded [19]. This survey was completed by an intervention focusing on the improving the lighting conditions especially cleaning and replacement of defective luminaries and increasing their number. Moreover, authors insured the introduction of intermittent breaks of 10 min every 2 working hours. This intervention reduced the visual complains to 48.3%, with persistence of an inadequate level of illumination in 24.3% of cases [12]. Furthermore, some others studies focusing on visual fatigue among workers with visualization terminals, noted the importance of the contribution of interventions to the levels of illumination. Indeed, beneficial effect of brief breaks on the whole visual symptoms mainly fatigue were particularly imminent among workers over 40 years of age with uncorrected presbyopia [2, 12, 20].

In this sample, after the intervention, visual symptoms was noted among 176 workers (70.04%) and in headaches in 40 workers (16%). The global prevalence of satisfaction was 58%. The term visual satisfaction is used to describe the acceptability of the real light environment by the user [14]. Concerning activities involving working in closed enterprise, the visual satisfaction of the operator depends on the lighting condition. This latter enables him to work easily. Besides, the pleasant nature of the luminous environment is important both when focusing on the task, and when looking elsewhere to relax. Specifically, visual satisfaction is influenced by the level of illumination of the surfaces, especially the work plan, the composition of the colors, the contrasts, the reflections and the other factors which diminish the visual comfort (such as glare…) [12, 14].

6 Conclusion

Lighting atmospheres are an important component in the working environment in the textile sector. Prevention advisor - in particular the occupational physician and ergonomist- should emphasize when developing strategies of the prevention and improvement of safety and well-being at work.

References

1. Cole, B.L.: The handicap of abnormal colour vision. Clin. Exp. Optom. **87**, 258–275 (2004)
2. Darker, I.T., Gerret, D., Filik, R., Purdy, K.J., Gale, A.G.: The influence of 'Tall Man' lettering on errors of visual perception in the recognition of written drug names. Ergonomics **54**, 21–33 (2011)
3. Gehin, D.: Endotoxines en milieu de travail [Thesis]. University of René Descartes, Faculty of Medecine Cochin Port-Royal, Paris V (2009)
4. INRS. Eclairage des locaux de travail. TJ 13 Aide mémoire juridique (2000). http://www.inrs.fr/inrs-pub/inrs01.nsf/inrs01_rechavancee_view/CDE7DE53A6A67137C1256CC60045BEC0/$File/tj13.pdf
5. INRS. Fiche pratique de sécurité ED82: L'éclairage naturel (2008). http://www.inrs.fr/inrs-pub/inrs01.nsf/inrs01_ts_fps_view/318BF50FC08ECB8EC1256E2E003885BA/$File/ed82.pdf
6. Muller, G.: Œil et travail surveillance et prévention dans un service médical interentreprises. University of René Descartes, Faculty of Medecine Cochin Port-Royal, Paris V (2005)
7. Owsley, C., McGwin Jr., G., Lee, P.P., Wasserman, N., Searcey, K.: Characteristics of low vision rehabilitation services in the United States. Arch. Ophthalmol. **127**, 681–689 (2009)
8. Portail Santé.lu.Poste informatique: Variables ergonomiques à considérer. http://www.sante.public.lu/publications/impacts-milieu-vie/sante-travail/ergonomie-poste-informatique/ergonomie-poste-informatique-fr.pdf
9. Reidy, A., Minassian, D.C., Joseph, J., Wu, J., Desai, P., Connolly, A.: Prevalence of serious eye disease and visual impairment in a north London population: population based, cross sectional study. Br. Med. **316**, 1643–1646 (1998)

10. Blehm C, Vishnu S, Khattak A, Mitra S, Yee RW. Computer vision syndrome: a review. Surv Ophthalmol;50:253-62 (2005)
11. Lemercier, C.: Dépistage des troubles visuels en médecine du travail. Revue Francophone Orthoptie **2**, 84–87 (2009)
12. Zimmermann, G., Quartier, V., Bernard, M., Salamin, V., Maggiori, C.: Qualités psychométriques de la version française de la TAS-20 et prévalence de l'alexithymie chez 264 adolescents tout-venant. Encéphale **33**, 941–946 (2007)
13. Cavalleri, A., Gobba, F.: Reversible color vision loss in occupational exposure to metallic mercury. Environ. Res. **77**, 173–177 (1998)
14. INRS, Conception des lieu et situation de travail (2000). www.inrs.fr/dms/inrs/CataloguePapier/ED/TI-ED-950/ed950.pdf
15. Benavides, F., Benach, J.: Types of employment and health: analysis of the second European survey on working conditions. Gac. Sanit. **13**, 425–430 (1999)
16. INRS. Fiche pratique de sécurité ED85: Eclairage artificiel au poste de travail (2018). http://www.inrs.fr/inrs-pub/inrs01.nsf/inrs01_ts_fps_view/A187DF901244952DC1256CD900504C87/$File/ed85.pdf
17. Janabi-Sharifi, F., Vakanski, A.: Analysis of visual acuity and motion resolvability as measures for optimal visual perception of the workspace. Appl. Ergon. **42**, 473–486 (2011)
18. Lam, B.L., Lee, D.J., Zheng, D.D., Davila, E.P., Christ, S.L., Arheart, K.L.: Disparity in prevalence of self-reported visual impairment in older adults among U.S. race-ethnic subgroups. Ophthalmic Epidemiol. **16**, 144–150 (2009)
19. Untimanon, O., Pacharatrakul, W., Boonmeepong, K., Thammagarun, L., Laemun, N., Taptagaporn, S., et al.: Visual problems among electronic and jewelry workers in Thailand. J. Occup. Health **48**, 407–412 (2006)
20. de Jonge, J., Bosma, H., Peter, R., Siegrist, J.: Job strain, effort-reward imbalance and employee well-being: a large-scale cross-sectional study. Soc. Sci. Med. **50**, 1317–1327 (2000)

Health-Related Quality of Life in Male Steel Industry Workers in Tunisia

Amira Omrane(✉), Chayma Harrathi, Taoufik Khalfallah, and Lamia Bouzgarrou

Department of Occupational Medicine and Ergonomics, Faculty of Medicine, University of Monastir, Monastir, Tunisia
omraneamira@yahoo.fr

Abstract. The current exhaustive cross-sectional study aims to assess the Health-related quality of life (HRQoL) and capacity of work among steel industry workers in Tunisia. Two validated questionnaires were used to assess the work ability (the «WAI») and the HRQoL (the «SF12»). Among young, productive workers good preserved work ability was conflicting to altered HRQoL. Indeed, work ability was felt excellent or moderate by 30.8% of workers and poor HRQoL was noted in 49.23% of cases for physical dimension and in 50.77% of them for mental dimension. Steel workers need more concern about determinants of physical and mental components of HRQoL.

Keywords: Health related quality of life · Ability of work · Steel industry · Tunisia

1 Introduction

The perceived health, health-related quality of life (HRQoL) and work ability are associated with the future health status and even mortality [1]. Historically, the painful occupation described has been physically heavy activities such as work in the mines, iron and steel or construction. In recent decades, hard work have been topical issues, widely debated by researchers in the field of occupational health but also policy makers and union forces [2, 3].

Moreover, the evidence literature suggests that high job stressors could alter the health related quality of life (HRQoL) and are related to serious health problems such as cardiovascular diseases, musculoskeletal disorders, gastrointestinal illness, psychiatric diseases, occupational injuries, absence from work, sleep problems, depression, and anxiety [4]. These conditions could alter the capacity of work and then generate an early retirement. In Tunisia, the active population occupies the majority of the sectors with physical load [5]. The steel sector, despite the economic difficulties it faces, remains an important sector [5]. This study aims to assess the HRQoL and the capacity of work in steel industry workers in Tunisia.

T. Ahram et al. (Eds.): IHIET 2019, AISC 1018, pp. 599–605, 2020.
https://doi.org/10.1007/978-3-030-25629-6_93

2 Material and Method

A cross-sectional study was conducted in a steel company, located in the central Tunisian governorate of Monastir, specialized in the manufacture of truck springs. The list of personnel with their age, a work schedule and job assignment was obtained from the Human Resources Management Department. All workers were included in the study population. Before the start of the survey and during an individual interview, each subject was informed of the objectives and the anonymity guarantee, and his right to refuse to participate. The data were collected using a questionnaire comprising 50 items divided into five sections relating to the individual characteristics (age, weight, height, level of study, lifestyle,..), professional (sector of activity, professional seniority, work position,…), HRQoL, work ability and work experience. The HRQoL was assessed using the French version SF-12 containing 12 questions assessing eight dimensions of health (physical activity, life and relationships with others, physical pain, perceived health, vitality, limitations due to physical state, limitations due to psychic state and psychic health) [6, 7]. This self-questionnaire assess the HRQoL in its mental and physical dimensions. The HRQoL score ranges from 0 to 100. Values tending toward 100 indicate a better quality of mental life. The average US benchmark is 50. A recent study in Tunisia established a baseline score for the Tunisian population of 47.96 [8]. According to the usual recommendations of this questionnaire, for each population and in order to optimize the analysis of the results, the median value of the population have to be used to divide it into two groups according to the HRQoL score. Work capacity was assessed using the WAI questionnaire "Work Ability Index". It includes seven questions concerning: current work capacity compared with the best of the past, the ability to work in relation to the demands of work, the number of current diseases diagnosed by the doctor, the assessment of work difficulties due to diseases, sick leave in the last twelve months, personal estimate of work capacity in two years, and mental resources. The score ranging from 7 to 49, enables to define four categories: from low work capacity to excellent work capacity [9, 10].

The work experience was evaluated using a six-ladder likert scale. The worker was asked to answer to the question "How do you judge your day's work?", Choosing the most representative figure of his perception and going from "lived very good" to "lived very bad" [11].

3 Results

A total of 65 male workers were included. Table 1 presents the socio-occupational characteristics. Our study population works 40 h a week with the possibility to add 8 h of work per week. The shiftworkers had two shifts (2×8), with rotation between shifts being weekly, but some workers were temporarily and temporarily assigned to the afternoon shift.

- **Health:** Fifty-seven percent of workers rated their health as "good". The average body mass index was 27.3 ± 3.5 kg/m^2 with extremes ranging from 17.8 to 38.7 kg/m^2. More than two-thirds of workers (66.1%) were overweight or obese (BMI > 25 kg/m^2).

Table 1. Study population characteristics

	Number (%)
Socio-demographic characteristics	
*Mean age ± SD (extremes)	37,8 years ± 9,5 years [22 - 54 years]
* Level of education	
Primary	21 (32,3%)
Secondary or higher	44 (67,7 %)
* BMI (kg/m^2)	
<18	1 (1,5%)
Normal [18-25]	10 (15,4%)
Overweight[25-30]	43 (66,1%)
Obesity type I [30-35]	9 (13,8%)
Obesitytype II (>35)	2 (3%)
Professional characteristics	
* Mean Job tenure ± SD (extremes)	12,8 years ± 11,9 years [1- 35 years]
* Workshops	
Oven	19 (29,23%)
Adjustment, Punching, Belting	26 (40%)
Maintenance	14 (21,54%)
Painting	6 (9,23%)
* Workstation requirements	
Prolonged standing	62 (96,9%)
Medium to heavy whole body efforts	42 (64,6%)
Medium-to-heavy Wrist and hands efforts	49 (75,4%)
Uncomfortable postures of the arms	30 (4,6%)
The experience of the working day	
Bad	0
Medium	6 (9,2%)
Good	56 (86,1%)
Excellent	3 (4,6%)

- **Work Experience:** In this study, 85.15% of employees described their work day as average to good. Concerning work equipment and relations with colleagues and the hierarchy, all the workers expressed their satisfaction.
- **HRQoL:** The mean score for physical HRQoL was 51.1 ± 8.8 with extremes ranging from 26.4 to 61.8. Among the workers surveyed, 49.23% said they had a poor physical HRQoL. The mean HRQoL score for those under 45 years group was 54.45 ± 6.14. The mean HRQoL score for those aged over 45 group was 44.82 ± 9.76 with a statistically significant difference (p < 10-3) between these two groups. Nor personnel characteristics (obesity) nor occupational ones (job tenure, workstations) were identified as determinant for the physical HRQoL score.

The mean score of the mental dimension of HRQoL was 44.5 ± 5.3 with extremes equal to 29.36 and 53.2. Among the workers surveyed, 50.77% had a poor mental HRQoL. The mean mental HRQoL score for those aged under 45 group was 45.74 ± 3.46. The mean mental HRQoL score for those aged over-45 groups was 41.81 ± 7.20. The difference was not statistically significant.

- **Work ability:** The average WAI was 39.8 ± 6.1 with extremes equal to 19 and 49. According to this index, 30.8% (n = 20) of the subjects felt that their work ability was excellent and 9.1% (n = 2) rated it as low. The WAI for those under the age of 45 years group was 41.82 ± 4.32. The work ability index for the over-45 age group was 35.71 ± 7.21, with a statistically significant difference (p = 10-3) between these two groups. The ability of work was not correlated to the mental or physical HRQoL. Besides the BMI and job tenure were not statistically correlated to the WAI.

4 Discussion

This survey was based on a questionnaire of the 65 workers in the steel company. The informed consent of these workers was obtained prior to the start of the investigation. This survey identified the main socio-demographic characteristics and invests the work ability, the HRQoL and the experienced day working by the subjects. We adopted the SF12 questionnaire to evaluate the HRQoL and the WAI index for the assessment of work capacity. These two questionnaires have the advantages of being validated in French, widely used in the literature and easy to use, particularly with a limited number of items in each questionnaire. However, since the low educational level of the interviewed workers, this questionnaire was not used as as a self-administered questionnaires. The sheet was filled in by the investigator who attempted, as much as possible, to maintain the same speech and attitude with all subjects.

4.1 Professional Features

The steel and iron sector is one of the five major sectors of metallurgy; the industrial activity of converting ore into metal and manufacturing materials [12, 13]. In Tunisia, this sector has more than thirty years old [12]. According to scientific literature, this sector is known for these heavy physical constraints and is often described as "painful" [13]. This study population worked 40 h a week with the possibility to add 8 h of work per week. The shiftworkers had two shifts (2 × 8), with rotation between shifts being weekly, but some workers were temporarily and temporarily assigned to the afternoon shift. Allen et al. [14] suggested that long working hours can lead to adverse health effects; in particular, work that exceeds 60 h per week is a health problem. In Germany, where hours of work are fixed in each occupational sector by a collective agreement between the social partners (within an average of 48 h per week imposed by law); five branches have a working week of 35 h per week (including metallurgy since 1990) [15].

4.2 The Individual Characteristics of the Operators

Our population was exclusively male. This was also the case for steelworkers in South Africa [16]. However, a Finnish survey of metalworkers showed that there were 813 men and 552 women in the metal industry matched according to sex and sector [17]. Similarly, a study in Australia of steelworkers (n = 469 workers) noted the presence of 33 women [18]. In Tunisia, the steel sector has always employed an exclusively male population since this sector is considered "hard". Yet, some other sectors, reserved to men and considered heavy or very heavy, begin to employ women workers in Tunisia such as the construction sector [19].

Our population was relatively young with an average age of 37.8 ± 9.5 years; 26 workers (40% of the population) were under 35 years of age. The median job tenure was 6 years and the average was 12.8 ± 11.9 years old. The distribution according to the age of the population is comparable to those reported by other studies carried out among workers in the iron and steel sector. Vurren et al. [16] in a study of 366 steel workers showed an average age of 31.8 ± 7.8 years. The average age found by Suadicani [20] among 469 workers in the iron and steel industry was 40 ± 12 years. Toumi [21] in his prospective study of metallurgical workers found a slightly higher average age of 43.9 ± 9.5 years.

Concerning job tenure, Vurren et al. [16], in a survey of 366 steelworkers, noted tenure of 6.7 years ± 5.4 years. The relatively young age of the workers in our series can be partly explained by physical workload of the activity. Indeed, the hardness of work conditions accelerates physiological aging with gradual decline in physical abilities, which may explain early departure of this workplace with the almost continuous recruitment. According to Tunisian legislation, early retirement are allowed in this sector and proposed for 50 years old workers.

4.3 Work Ability (WAI)

The mean WAI index was 39.8 ± 6.1 [19–23]. According to this index, 30.8% (n = 20) of subjects in our population felt that their work capacity was excellent and 9.1% (n = 2) rated it as low. This study revealed a significant difference in terms of better work capacity among younger workers (<45 years) and older workers ($\geq$45 years).

Other authors have also concluded that there is a negative correlation between work ability and age [21–23]. Toumi [21] in his cross-sectional survey of metalworkers initially found a WAI index equal to 42.3 in 1998 and then evaluated at 40.77 in 2000. Makowiec-Dabrowska et al. [22] showed that WAI was inversely proportional to age and workload. In addition, Kang et al. [23], through a study of the VO2max on a bicycle ergometer survey of 507 metal workers in Korea, found a negative correlation between maximum physical capacity and workload in all levels and age groups.

4.4 Health-Related Quality of Life

Regarding the physical HRQol, the mean score of the study population was 51.1 ± 8.8 with extremes of 26.4 and 61.8. Among the workers surveyed, 49.2% had a poor quality of physical life.

The mean score of the mental dimension of the SF-12 questionnaire was 44.5 ± 5.3 with extremes equal to 29.3 and 53.1. Of the workers surveyed, 50.8% had a poor quality of mental life. According to Student's test, the average physical quality of life score for the under-45 age group was 54.45 ± 6.14. The mean quality of life score for the over-45 age group was 44.82 ± 9.76 with a statistically significant difference.

Toumi [21], in a cross-sectional study of 1,389 42-year-old middle-aged employees, investing the mental HRQol through 5 items of the Bradburn Scale of Psychological Wellbeing questionnaire, found a mental well-being score of 3, 3. In this study HRQOL was not correlated to WAI or personnel characteristics (BMI) or job tenure. Sôensena and all found a significant association between the WAI and HRQoL scores (all domains concerned) and concluded that the promotion of work ability may have beneficial effects on quality of life [1].

5 Conclusion

Overall, the mental quality score seems to be decreased in our population. It is diminished further among the population with a high workload. Yet, it seems difficult to decide if the workload alters the mental health score. However a further study of the psychological demand, decision-making autonomy and social support by the Karasek questionnaire among these workers seems justified.

References

1. Sôrensen, L.E., Pekkonen, M.M., Männikkö, K.H., Louhevaara, V.A., Smolander, J., Alén, M.J.: Associations between work ability, health-related quality of life, physical activity and fitness among middle-aged men. Appl. Ergon. **39**, 786–791 (2008)
2. Converso, D., Sottimano, I., Guidetti, G., Loera, B., Cortini, M., Viotti, S.: Aging and work ability: the moderating role of job and personal resources. Front. Psychol. **8**, 2262 (2018). https://doi.org/10.3389/fpsyg.2017.02262
3. Cloostermans, L., Bekkers, M.B., Uiters, E., Proper, K.I.: The effectiveness of interventions for ageing workers on (early) retirement, work ability and productivity: a systematic review. Int. Arch. Occup. Environ. Health. **88**(5), 521–532 (2014). https://doi.org/10.1007/s00420-014-0969-y
4. Mokarami, H., Stallones, L., Nazifi, M., Taghavi, S.M.: The role of psychosocial and physical work-related factors on the health-related quality of life of Iranian industrial workers. Work **55**, 441–452 (2016). https://doi.org/10.3233/wor-162405
5. Agency for the Promotion of Industry and Innovation, Mechanical and Metallurgical Industries in Tunisia, Year (2014). http://www.tunisieindustrie.nat.tn

6. Montazeri, A., Vahdaninia, M., Mousavi, S.J., Omidvari, S.: The Iranian version of 12-item short form health survey (SF-12): factor structure, internal consistency and construct validity. BMC Public Health **9**, 341 (2009)
7. Kontodimopoulos, N., Pappa, E., Niakas, D., Tountas, Y.: Validity of SF-12 summary scores in a Greek general population. Health Qual. Life Outcomes **5**, 55 (2007)
8. Younsi, M., Chakroun, M.: Measuring health-related quality of life: psychometric evaluation of the Tunisian version of the SF-12 health survey. Qual. Life Res. **23**(7), 2047–2054 (2014). https://doi.org/10.1007/s11136-014-0641-8
9. Coomer, K., Houdmont, J.: Occupational health professionals' knowledge, understanding and use of work ability. Occup. Med. **63**, 405–409 (2013)
10. Mazloumi, A., Rostamabadi, A., NaslSaraji, G., Foroushani, A.R.: Work ability index (WAI) and its association with psychosocial factors in one of the petrochemical industries in Iran. J. Occup. Health **54**, 112–118 (2012)
11. Van den Berg, T., Elders, L., de Zwart, B., Burdorf, A.: The effects of work-related and individual factors on the work Ability Index: a systematic review. Occup. Environ. Med. **66**, 211–220 (2009)
12. Wibail, A.: L'évolution économique de la sidérurgie belge de 1830 à 1913. Bull. Inst. Sci. Écon. **5**, 31–61 (1933)
13. Freyssenet, M.: La sidérurgie française 1945–1979. https://halshs.archives-ouvertes.fr
14. Allen, H.M.J.R., Slavin, T.: Do long work hours impact health, safety, and productivity at a heavy manufacturer? J. Occup. Environ. Med. **49**, 148–171 (2007)
15. Chenu, A.: Les horairesetl'organisation du temps de travail (HAL Id: hal-00521872). https://hal.archives-ouvertes.fr
16. Vuuren, B.J., Becker, P.J., Van Heerden, H.J., Zinzen, E., Meeusen, R.: Lower back problems and occupational risk factors in a South African steel industry. Am. J. Ind. Med. **47**, 451–457 (2005)
17. Vitalis, A., Pournaras, N.D., Jeffrey, G.B., Tsagarakis, G., Monastiriotis, G., Kavvadias, S.: Heart rate strain indices in Greek steelworkers. Ergonomics **37**, 845–850 (1994)
18. Ratnaddep, S., CahndraDey, N., Samanta, A., Biswas, R.: A comparison of cardiac strain among drillers of tow different age groups in underground manuel coal mines in India. J. Occup. Health **50**, 512–520 (2008)
19. Ben Laiba, M.: Profil National de Santé et Sécurité Au Travail En Tunisie, Rev Inst Santé Séc Trav République Tunisienne (2007)
20. Suadicani, P., Hansen, K., Fenger, A.M., Gyntelberg, F.: Low back pain problems among steelworkers. Ugeskr. Laeger **159**, 5240–5243 (1997)
21. Tuomi, K., Vanhala, S., Nykyri, E., Janhonen, M.: Organizational practices, work demands and the well-being of employees: a follow-up study in the metal industry and retail trade. Occup. Med. **54**, 115–121 (2004)
22. Makowiec-Dabrowska, T., Sprusińska, E., Bazylewicz-Walczak, B., Radwan-Włodarczyk, Z., Koszada-Włodarczyk, W.: Ability to work–new approach to evaluation methods. Med. Prev. **51**, 319–333 (2000)
23. Kang, D., Woo, J.H., Shin, Y.C.: Distribution and determinants of maximal physical work capacity of Korean male metalworkers. Ergonomics **50**, 2137–2147 (2007)

Patterns of the Relationship Between the Anatomical Formations of the Chambers of the Heart of Human Fetuses

Galina Spirina(✉)

Ural State Medical University, Yekaterinburg, Russia
profspirina@gmail.com

Abstract. The phenomenon of symmetry in the forms of biological bodies has long served as one of the main points in the ideas about the existence of specific laws of morphogenesis. By analogy with the three-member kinematic blocks of the musculoskeletal system of the human body, the relationships between the three anatomical formations of the heart chambers were determined by the formula for calculating the wurf: the parameters of the right atrium and the length of the distance between the holes of the cava veins; opening area of the vena cava and right atrioventricular opening; the length of the sinus and trabecular parts (in the department of inflow and outflow) of the right ventricle. The material served as 93 hearts of human fetuses preparations of 13–36 weeks of development. It was established that the relationship between the digital values of the three anatomical formations of the chambers of the heart of human fetuses can be expressed as a wurf proportion. The average size of wurfs of three-membered blocks of formations of chambers of the heart of human fetuses is close in magnitude to the "golden wurf" (1.309). This testifies to the action of the laws of conformal transformations in the process of the growth of the heart of human fetuses.

Keywords: Fetus · Hear · Conformal symmetry

1 Introduction

The deepening of biological knowledge is accompanied by the discovery of all new facts of subordination to the principles of symmetry of various biological objects differing in scale and level of organization. Petukhov [1–3], Nigmatullina et al. [4] found that three-membered kinematic blocks dominate in the human body. The criterion for conformal symmetry between blocks of three consecutive straight line segments is a wurf. In the studies of Spirina [5–8], the parameters of the heart and kidneys are presented in the form of three-term blocks connected by conformal symmetry. The study of morphogenesis is one of the fundamental biological problems. The literature provides different approaches to its study. Measurements of the proportions of body parts have traditionally been carried out on the basis of affine (simple) relations between the indices of two anatomical measurements [4]. However, the human body cannot be reduced to the proportions of two-member structures. In a large number of publications, the opinion is expressed that the structure of each organ is determined by

T. Ahram et al. (Eds.): IHIET 2019, AISC 1018, pp. 606–611, 2020.
https://doi.org/10.1007/978-3-030-25629-6_94

adaptation to environmental conditions. At the same time, the authors believe that there are no own laws in morphogenesis or they do not play a significant role. The phenomenon of symmetry in the forms of biological bodies has long served as one of the main points in the ideas about the existence of specific laws of morphogenesis. According to Petukhov [1] in the variety of forms has its own orderliness, independent of the function. The author points to the need to study symmetry in forms, regardless of the function they perform. Petukhov [3] represents the entire musculoskeletal system of the human body as a set of three-term kinematic blocks. From the moment of birth of an individual, body growth occurs with preservation of the wurf value of each three-term kinematic block. All three-member kinematic chains of the human body obey the rule of the "golden wurf" [3]. Further conclusions of Petukhov [1] were confirmed by studies of Nigmatullina et al. [4]. Based on the above theoretical assumptions, we carried out anthropometric studies of the human heart and kidneys [7]. The implementation of the principle of conformal symmetry in the structure of the heart of people of different ages has been noted [5, 6, 8].

1.1 Objective

To identify patterns of communication between the anatomical formations of the heart chambers in human fetuses of different ages. The study material consisted of 93 hearts of human fetuses preparations 13 to 36 weeks of development. The parameters of the heart and its shape were determined. Anthropometric studies of the anatomical formations of the heart chambers were carried out in order to identify and describe the harmonious proportions between them. To calculate wurf indices, we used the determination of the area of the openings of the upper and lower cava veins, the area of the right atrioventricular opening, the width and height of the right atrium. The length of the distance between the holes of the cava veins at the confluence, the length of the sinus and trabecular (in the inflow and outflow) parts of the right ventricle was determined. By analogy with the three-membered kinematic blocks of the musculoskeletal system of the human body, three values of the measured anatomical structures were used, taking into account the age of the fetus and the shape of the heart, to calculate conformal symmetries of the formations inside the heart chambers. The magnitude of the wurf between the three formations of the heart chambers was determined by the formula [3]:

$$W = \frac{(C - A) * (D - B)}{(C - B) * (D - A)}$$

Three values of the measured anatomical structures were used according to the formula for calculating the wurf: (a) the width and height of the right atrium, the length of the distance between the holes of the cava veins; (b) the area of the holes of the cava veins and the right atrioventricular opening; (c) the length of the sinus and trabecular parts of the right ventricle (in the department of inflow and outflow).

2 Research Results

According to the results of the study, three forms of the heart were found in the human fetuses of the same age: narrow and long (with an index less than 0.80), transitional (with an index from 0.80 to 0.95), wide short (with an index more than 0.95). In all age groups, the predominance of the transitional form was found. The hearts of the extreme forms have a harmonious ratio of overall dimensions (length, width, thickness), sizes of parts of the interventricular septum, a triad of sizes: the length of the distance between

Table 1. Values of wurfs (W) of a three-member block consisting of the width of the right atrium, its height and the length of the distance between the holes of the cava veins in a human fetus with a narrow long heart shape (a):

Fetal age (weeks)	The width of the right atrium (mm)	The height of the right atrium (mm)	The length of the distance between the holes of the cava veins (mm)	Wurf values (arbitrary unit)
13 - 16	6,22 ± 0,43	5,96 ±0,84	5,36 ± 0,36	1,29
17 - 20	7,45 ± 0,47	6,50 ± 0,87	7,35 ± 0,58	1,30
21 - 24	7,50 ± 0,34	7,55 ± 1,24	7,50 ± 0,89	1,33
25 - 28	10,2 ± 0,92	9,47 ± 0,63	9,78 ± 0,85	1,30
29 - 32	12,95± 0,82	11,26 ±0,46	11,65 ± 0,72	1,28
33 - 36	13,58 ±1,02	15,03 ±1,54	13,02 ± 1,38	1,34

M=1.31

transition (b):

Fetal age (weeks)	The width of the right atrium (mm)	The height of the right atrium (mm)	The length of the distance between the holes of the cava veins (mm)	Wurf values (arbitrary unit)
13 - 16	6,89±0,58	6,02±0,57	6,02 ± 0,36	1,28
17 - 20	8,57 ± 0,64	7,57 ± 0,79	8,10 ± 0,75	1,30
21 - 24	9,25 ± 0,57	9,25 ± 0,98	8,76 ± 0,63	1,31
25 - 28	12,54± 0,85	10,82± 1,58	11,54 ±0,85	1,28
29 - 32	12,69± 0,94	13,02 ± 1,61	11,84±1,31	1,32
33 - 36	15,25 ±0,76	15,93 ± 1,52	15,62±1,09	1,34

M=1.31

wide short (c):

Fetal age (weeks)	The width of the right atrium (mm)	The height of the right atrium (mm)	The length of the distance between the holes of the cava veins (mm)	Wurf values (arbitrary unit)
13 - 16	7,02 ±0,49	6,82±0,71	6,35±0,51	1,23
17 - 20	8,60 ± 0,73	8,25±1,20	8,26±0,57	1,31
21 - 24	8,56 ± 0,48	8,44±0,91	8,75±0,48	1,40
25 - 28	13,68±0,87	11,61±0,82	11,73±0,47	1,27
29 - 32	14,68±1,05	14,58±2,00	13,04±1,25	1,40
33 - 36	15,02±0,75	17,28±0,74	16,37±1,50	1,28

M=1.315

the openings of the cava veins, departments of inflow and outflow of the right ventricle. An analysis of the height, width of the right atrium, the length of the distance between the holes of the cava veins near the heart of the human fetuses with its different shape. The numerical values of these parameters can be represented as a wurf (wurf ratio).

Table 2. Values of wurfs of a three-member block consisting of the area of the openings of the upper and lower cava veins and the right atrioventricular opening in human fetuses with different heart shapes: narrow long (a):

Fetal age (weeks)	Hole size of the inferior vena cava (mm²)	Hole area of the superior vena cava (mm²)	The area of the right atrioventricular opening (mm²)	Wurf values (W), rel. units
13-16	5,26 ± 0,42	3,10 ± 0,23	10,38 ± 0,94	1,32
17 - 20	6,22 ± 0,64	3,66 ± 0,37	16,74 ± 0,65	1,34
21 - 24	6,74 ± 0,37	4,52 ± 0,27	22,61 ± 1,85	1,40
25- 28	15,28± 0,91	6,82 ± 0,56	43,22 ± 2,14	1,30
29 - 32	33,68 ±1,59	13,81±1,22	61,39 ± 1,82	1,23
33 - 36	41,97 ±2,63	20,67±1,59	68,37 ± 2,47	1,26

M=1.308

transitional (b):

Fetal age (weeks)	Hole size of the inferior vena cava (mm²)	Hole area of the superior vena cava (mm²)	The area of the right atrioventricular opening (mm²)	Wurf values (W), rel. units
13-16	6,59± 0,27	3,21 ± 0,27	10,62 ± 0,49	1,26
17 - 20	9,59± 0,49	4,49 ± 0,73	23,33 ± 0,86	1, 28
21 - 24	10,96± 0,52	5 ,58± 0,49	32,37 ± 1,74	1,33
25- 28	16,95 ±0,69	7,12 ± 0,34	44,39 ± 1,68	1,27
29 - 32	36,08± 1,76	14,06±0,58	67,23 ± 1,67	1,23
33 - 36	44,67± 2,56	23,07±0,86	80,82± 2,58	1,28

M=1.27

wide short (c):

Fetal age (weeks)	Hole size of the inferior vena cava (mm²)	Hole area of the superior vena cava (mm²)	The area of the right atrioventricular opening (mm²)	Wurf values (W), rel. units
13-16	8,32 ± 0,46	3,72 ± 0,43	12,87 ± 0,65	1,23
17 - 20	10,32±0,68	5,29± 0,45	25,73± 0,79	1,32
21 - 24	10,94± 0,87	7,41± 0,57	29,31± 0,87	1,41
25- 28	18,27± 0,76	7,45± 0,61	49,34± 2,58	1,27
29 - 32	39,91± 1,85	15,33±0,85	67,72± 2,41	1,40
33 - 36	47,25± 2,34	25,64±0,79	75,25± 2,85	1,28

M=1.318

Regardless of age and heart shape, wurf values are grouped around a value of 1.3 (Tables 1 and 2). The average value of the wurf ratio of the area of the openings of the upper and lower cava veins and the right atrioventricular opening in fetuses with a narrow long heart was 1.308; the hearts of the transitional form 1,270; for wide short hearts 1,318. The size of the wurf of the length of the sinus part, the trabecular part (in the inflow and outflow section) of the right ventricle in the heart of the transitional form varied from 1.23 to 1.29.

3 Discussion of the Data

Thus, the area of the holes of the cava veins, right atrioventricular opening, by analogy with the three-member kinematic blocks of the musculoskeletal system [1] can be represented as a three-member block. The width and height of the right atrium and the distance between the openings of the cava veins, the length of the sinus and trabecular parts of the right ventricle (in the inflow and outflow section) are similarly related to each other. The calculations showed that the digital values of the wurf of the area of the holes of the cava veins, the right atrioventricular hole in fetuses 13–36 weeks, regardless of the age and shape of the heart, approach 1.309 (the "golden wurf"). The ratio between the size of the area of the holes of the cava veins and the right atrioventricular opening form a harmonic wurf proportion close to the value of 1.31. The magnitude of the wurf between the parameters of the right atrium and the length of the distance between the holes of the cava veins is also close to 1.31. In human fetuses of different ages, the growth of the heart occurs with the preservation of the value of the wurf of each specified three-member block. Anthropometric studies based on measurements of the proportions of the three anatomical structures offer great opportunities. Petukhov [1–3] indicated that all three-term kinematic chains of the human body obey the rule of the "golden wurf". Subordination to the laws of conformal symmetry is manifested not only in the interplay between the parameters of the heart itself at all ages, but also in the interrelations of anatomical structures inside the heart chambers. The digital values of the wurf of the human heart can serve as an objective indicator of the harmony of its proportions. The Golden Wurf is a three-member canon of not only the human body as a whole, its musculoskeletal system, but also the heart at all stages of individual development.

4 Conclusions

1. The relationship between the digital values of the three anatomical structures of the heart chambers can be expressed as a wurf proportion during the prenatal period of ontogenesis.

2. The values of wurfs for each three-member block (the area of the openings of the cava veins and the right atrioventricular opening; the parameters of the right atrium and the length of the distance between the openings of the cava veins; the length of the sinus and trabecular parts in the right ventricular outflow and outflow) 36 weeks of development, which indicates the action of the laws of conformal transformations in the process of growth of the heart of the human fetuses.
3. The average size of wurfs of three-membered kinematic blocks of the heart of human fetuses is close in magnitude to the "golden wurf".

References

1. Petukhov, S.V.: Biomechanics, bionics and symmetry. Science, p. 240 (1981)
2. Petukhov, S.V.: Geometry of living nature and algorithms of self-organization,vol. 6, p. 46 (1988)
3. Petukhov, S.V.: Symmetries in biology. The appendix to the book: Shubnikov, A.B., Coptik, V.A. "Symmetry in Science and Art", 3rd edn., pp. 489–546 (2004)
4. Nigmatullin, R.T., Gafarov, V.G., Salikhov, A.Y.: Soft core of a person ' s face. Aspects of surgical and functional anatomy. Ufa, p. 99–119 (2003)
5. Spirina, G.: Comparative analysis of the quantitative parameters of the different shapes of the heart in human fetuses. In: Intelligent Human Systems Integration. Proceeding of the 1st International Conference on Intelligent Human Systems Integration (IHSI 2018): Integrating People and Intelligent Systems, Dubai, United Arab Emirates, 7–9 January, 6 p. Springer (2018)
6. Spirina, G.A.: Realization of the principle of conformal symmetry in the structure of the heart. In: Advances in Human Factors in Simulation and Modeling. Proceeding of the AHFE International Conference of Human Factors in Simulation and Modeling, Los Angeles, California, USA, 17–21 July 2017, vol. 26, pp. 175–183. Springer (2017)
7. Spirina, G., Yalunin, N.V.: Phenomenon of conformal growth of the human heart in ontogenesis. Book of Abstracts of XXVI International Symposium of Morphological Sciences (2018). Praha.- P., pp. 69–70
8. Spirina, G.A.: Application of the principle of conformal symmetry in the structure of human internal organs. In: Materials of 1st International Conference on Human Systems Engineering and Design: Future Trends and Application, Reims, France, 25–27 October, pp. 585–588. Springer (2018)

Modeling of Contact Interaction of an Endoprosthetic Knee Joint

Roman Pryazhevskiy[1], Ildar Akhtyamov[2], Anna Morgunova[1], Helo Mohammad Jihad[2], Andrey Nevzorov[3], and Oskar Sachenkov[4,5](✉)

[1] Moscow Aviation Institute, Moscow, Russia
pryazhevskiyrd@tdhc.ru, iv.morgunov@yandex.ru
[2] Kazan State Medical University, Kazan, Russia
gidropress3.01@mail.ru, yalta60@mail.ru
[3] DONA-M, Moscow, Russia
dona-m@mail.ru
[4] Kazan Federal University, Kazan, Russia
4works@bk.ru
[5] Kazan National Research Technical University, Kazan, Russia

Abstract. Problems of the endoprosthetic knee joint are an actual problem of modern clinics. It is important to increase the terms of work resource of the endoprosthesis. For this purpose, it is important to get an equation of contact pressure in joint. Nowadays for simulation of contact interaction in joint a finite element method is used, but results of such simulations are sensitive to mesh quality and options for numerical contact model. An analytic model of contact in the knee joint is presented in the paper. The Hertz solution was used as a basic solution. The medial and lateral condyles are described with good accuracy by a sphere in each cross section. Then the pressure distribution obtained is transmitted to the elastic half-space. According to analytical solutions diagrams connecting maximum stress in an endoprosthetic knee joint and patient's weight was built. Results allow using analytic solution in clinical practice.

Keywords: Contact interaction · Endoprosthesis · Knee joint

1 Introduction

Problems of the endoprosthesis joint are an actual problem of modern clinics [1–6], especially in the case of the endoprosthetic knee [7–9]. It is important to increase the terms of work resource of the endoprosthesis. Many anatomic parameters influence the work resource [9–13], more than, the endoprosthesis can influence the knee biomechanics and bone quality [14, 15]. For this purpose, it is important to get an equation of contact pressure in joint. Nowadays for simulation of contact interaction in joint a finite element method [16–19] and others [20] are used, but results of such simulations are sensitive to mesh quality and options for numerical contact model. An analytic model of contact in the knee joint is presented in the paper. The idea of solution based on splitting the equation of contact interaction and influence of contact pressure on the

T. Ahram et al. (Eds.): IHIET 2019, AISC 1018, pp. 612–617, 2020.
https://doi.org/10.1007/978-3-030-25629-6_95

media [21, 22]. For this purpose the Hertz solution was used as a basic solution. The medial and lateral condyles were described with good accuracy by a sphere in each cross section. Liner was described by elastic half-space.

2 Materials and Methods

The pressure in the contact area is expressed as follows:

$$p(x_1, x_2) = \frac{3P}{2\pi a^3}\sqrt{a^2 - x_1^2 - x_2^2}. \quad (1)$$

The and radius of the contact area and mutual penetration we obtain the following approximation expression-hypotheses:

$$a = \sqrt[3]{\frac{3}{4}CPR}, \quad (2)$$

$$\alpha = \sqrt[3]{\frac{1}{R}\left(\frac{3}{4}CP\right)^2}, \quad (3)$$

where C – stiffness parameter taking into account Young's modulus and Poisson's ratios of both bodies, R-radius of indentor, P-external load.

The parameters of the joint for which this distribution is obtained are given at the end. Next, we consider the influence of the pressure obtained in the contact area on the elastic half-space.

We will consider the problem of the pressure of a stamp on an elastic body occupying a half-space in the case when there is no frictional force between the elastic body and the stamp. We assume that a given load P acts on the boundary of the half-space at $x_3 = 0$. To find the stress state and displacements in the body it is convenient to use the functions introduced to solve the three-dimensional problem of P.F. Papkovich [23]. Then the displacements u_j are expressed by harmonic functions Φ_0, Φ_1, Φ_2, Φ_3.

$$u_j = \Phi_j - \frac{1}{4(1-\nu)}\frac{\partial}{\partial x_j}\left(\Phi_0 + \sum_{i=1}^{3} x_i\Phi_i\right), \quad (4)$$

where ν - Poisson's ratio.

The following boundary conditions are set at the boundary of the elastic half-space:

$$\tau_{31} = \tau_{32} = 0, \; x_3 = 0 \quad (5)$$

Expressing these boundary conditions through the functions entered earlier (4, 5) we arrive at the following result:

$$\begin{aligned}
&\frac{\partial\Phi_3}{\partial x_1}+\frac{2(1-\nu)}{(1-\nu)}\frac{\partial\Phi_1}{\partial x_3}-\frac{1}{1-2\nu}\frac{\partial}{\partial x_1}(x_1\frac{\partial\Phi_1}{\partial x_3}+x_2\frac{\partial\Phi_2}{\partial x_3}+\frac{\partial\Phi_0}{\partial x_3})=0\\
&\frac{\partial\Phi_3}{\partial x_2}+\frac{2(1-\nu)}{(1-\nu)}\frac{\partial\Phi_2}{\partial x_3}-\frac{1}{1-2\nu}\frac{\partial}{\partial x_2}(x_1\frac{\partial\Phi_1}{\partial x_3}+x_2\frac{\partial\Phi_2}{\partial x_3}+\frac{\partial\Phi_0}{\partial x_3})=0
\end{aligned} \tag{6}$$

However, if two harmonic functions that disappear at infinity coincide on the boundary of a region, then they are equal to each other everywhere in the region. For the harmonic functions [20, 21], we obtain the following boundary value problems:

$$\begin{aligned}
&\frac{\partial\Phi_1}{\partial x_3}=-\frac{1-2v}{2(1-\nu)}\frac{\partial\Phi_3}{\partial x_1};\\
&\frac{\partial\Phi_2}{\partial x_3}=-\frac{1-2v}{2(1-\nu)}\frac{\partial\Phi_3}{\partial x_2};\\
&\frac{\partial\Phi_0}{\partial x_3}=-\frac{1-2v}{2(1-\nu)}(x_1\frac{\partial\Phi_3}{\partial x_1}+x_2\frac{\partial\Phi_3}{\partial x_2}+\frac{\partial\Phi_3}{\partial x_3}).
\end{aligned} \tag{7}$$

Further, we will assume that the normal pressure $-p(x_1,x_2)$ is distributed over a certain region Ω located at the boundary of the half-space, is expressed as follows:

$$\sigma_{33}=\begin{cases}-p(x_1,x_2), & (x_1,x_2)\in\Omega\\ 0, & (x_1,x_2)\notin\Omega\end{cases} \tag{8}$$

From the physical relations, it follows that the stress at $x_3 = 0$ can be expressed in terms of the derivative of the harmonic function introduced earlier (7). We obtain the Neumann problem for determining the function φ_1:

$$\left(\frac{\partial\varphi_1}{\partial x_3}\right)_{x_3\to+0}=\begin{cases}-\frac{1+\nu}{E}p(x_1,x_2), & (x_1,x_2)\in\Omega\\ 0, & (x_1,x_2)\notin\Omega\end{cases} \tag{9}$$

As is known, such a function can be represented as a potential of a simple layer [20]:

$$\varphi_1(x_1,x_2,x_3)=-\frac{1+\nu}{2\pi E}\iint\limits_{\Omega}\frac{p(\xi,\eta)d\xi d\eta}{\sqrt{(x_1-\xi)^2+(x_2-\eta)^2+x_3^2}} \tag{10}$$

Considering the connection between w and φ_1 above we get the following expression:

$$w(x_1,x_2)=-\frac{1-\nu^2}{\pi E}\iint\limits_{\Omega}\frac{p(\xi,\eta)d\xi d\eta}{\sqrt{(x_1-\xi)^2+(x_2-\eta)^2}} \tag{11}$$

From the last expression it follows that if the movement of the stamp in the region is known and there is no friction force, then the harmonic function is known on one side of the region. Due to the parity of the potential of a simple layer this function is also known on the other side with respect to the contact area [23].

Thus, to determine the harmonic function, we obtain a special case of the Direchle problem. The values of the function vanishing at infinity are set on two sides of a flat region located in the $x_3 = 0$ plane.

We present the simplest solution for a spherical indenter that simulates the lateral or medial condyle. The radius of the sphere modeling the condyle is set equal to 15 mm. The force coming to it is set equal to 1400 N. The Poisson coefficient for bone is 0.3, the modulus of elasticity is 6000 MPa. The elastic modulus of the sphere is set to 11200 MPa, the Poisson's ratio is 0.26. Then the value of mutual penetration by Hertz will be 0.342 mm.

3 Results and Discussion

Analyzing the pressure distribution in the elastic half-space it can be concluded that stress decreases rapidly (order of the function is x_3^{-2}). It means that after 20–25% of liner's thickness influences of contact stress is a little. The distribution of displacements in an elastic half-space decreases rapidly too (order of the function is x_3^{-1}). But in this case, only after 40–50% of liner's thickness influences of contact stress is a little. These results mean, that boundary condition influence a little for the static and quasi-static solution of the contact interaction. Generalizing the previous statements it can be concluded, that the maximum stress is in the contact area. The connection between the external load and the maximum contact stress was investigated. For practical usage, the results were recalculated in terms of "patient's weight" and contact stress. It can be shown that the maximum contact stress tends to asymptote (see Fig. 1).

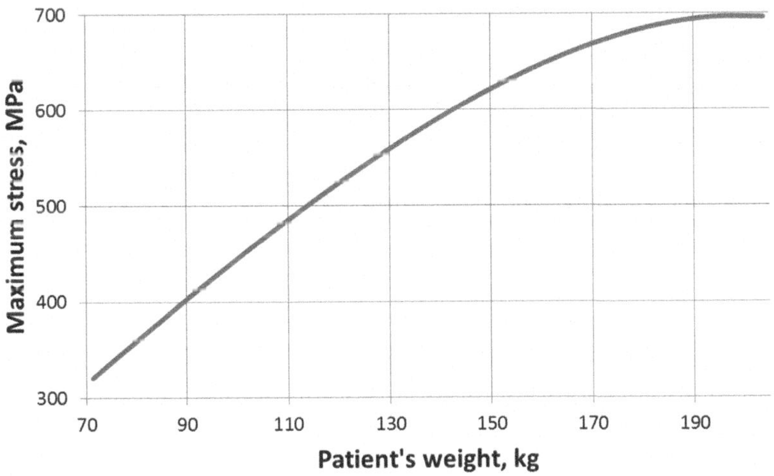

Fig. 1. Distribution of maximum normal stress σ_{zz} (MPa) in the contact area depending on the patient's weight (kg).

4 Conclusion

The result of this work is to obtain analytical solutions for a three-dimensional contact problem. The solutions obtained allow us to verify finite element models for their correctness from the point of view of contact interaction. From the solutions obtained it is clear that displacements in the elastic half-space and contact stresses decay strongly with increasing depth. The solution for maximum normal stress σ_{zz} in the contact area depending on the patient's weight was found.

References

1. Thillemann, T.: Implant survival after primary total hip arthroplasty due to childhood hip disorders: results from the Danish hip arthroplasty registry. Acta Orthop. **79**, 769–776 (2008)
2. Tikhilov, R.M., Shubnyakov, M.I., Boyarov, A.A., Denisov, A.O., Shubnyakov, I.I.: Impact of various factors on the polyethylene wear rate in total hip arthroplasty. Travmatologiya i ortopediya Rossii. **24**(1), 18–28 (2018)
3. Dmitrevich, G.D., Ryzhov, N.G., Al Noumani, S., Tikhilov, R.M., Tsibin, A.B., Vopilovsky, P.N.: Computer-aided design and additive technology engineering of custom acetabular component for revision hip arthroplasty surgery. In: Proceedings of the xix IEEE International Conference on Soft Computing and Measurements, pp. 377–381 (2016)
4. Popov, I., Onuh, S.O.: Reverse engineering of pelvic bone for hip joint replacement. J. Med. Eng. Technol. **33**(6), 454–459 (2009)
5. Saleh, K.J., El Othmani, M.M., Tzeng, T.H., Mihalko, W.M., Chambers, M.C., Grupp, T. M.: Acrylic bone cement in total joint arthroplasty: a review. J. Orthop. Res. **34**, 737–744 (2016)
6. Trepczynski, A., Kutzner, I., Schütz, P., Dymke, J., List, R., von Roth, P., Moewis, P., Bergmann, G., Taylor, W.R., Duda, G.N.: Tibio-femoral contact force distribution is not the only factor governing pivot location after total knee arthroplasty. Sci. Rep. **9**, 182 (2019)
7. Bicanic, G., Delimar, D., Delimar, M., Pecina, M.: Influence of the acetabular cup position on hip load during arthroplasty in hip dysplasia. Int. Orthop. **33**, 397–402 (2009)
8. Aljehani, M., Madara, K., Snyder-Mackler, L., Christiansen, C., Zeni Jr., J.A.: The contralateral knee may not be a valid control for biomechanical outcomes after unilateral total knee arthroplasty. Gait Posture **70**, 179–184 (2019)
9. Nečas, D., Vrbka, M., Galandáková, A., Křupka, I., Hartl, M.: On the observation of lubrication mechanisms within hip joint replacements. Part I: hard-on-soft bearing pairs. J. Mech. Behav. Biomed. Mater. **89**, 237–248 (2019)
10. Yakupov, R.R., Astanin, V.V., Kayumova, E.Z., Minasov, BSh, Minasov, T.B.: Optimization of cementless hip arthroplasty based on acoustic analysis. Russ. J. Biomech. **21**(1), 89–98 (2017)
11. Hettich, G., Schierjott, R.A., Ramm, H., Graichen, H., Jansson, V., Rudert, M., Traina, F., Grupp, T.M.: Method for quantitative assessment of acetabular bone defects. J. Orthop. Res. **37**, 181–189 (2019)
12. Pejhan, S., Khosravipour, I., Gascoyne, T., Bohm, E., Brandt, J.-M., Luo, Y., Wyss, U.: Evaluation of the tibiofemoral contact characteristics of a customized surface-guided knee implant. J. Med. Biol. Eng. **39**, 205–212 (2019)

13. Heyland, M., Checa, S., Kendoff, D., Duda, G.N.: Anatomic grooved stem mitigates strain shielding compared to established total hip arthroplasty stem designs in finite-element models. Sci. Rep. **9**, 482 (2019)
14. Gerasimov, O., Koroleva, E., Sachenkov, O.: Experimental study of evaluation of mechanical parameters of heterogeneous porous structure. In: IOP Conference Series: Materials Science and Engineering, vol. 208, p. 012013 (2017). https://doi.org/10.1088/1757-899x/208/1/012013
15. Gerasimov, O.V., Koroleva, E.V., Sachenkov, O.A., Baltina, T.V., Ahmetov, N.F., Fedyanin, A.O., Baltin, M.E., Lavrov, I.A.: Anisotropic properties of bone tissue changing during unloading hanging. Osteoporos. Int. **29**, 259 (2018)
16. Bolshakov, P.V., Tikhilov, R.M., Mazurenko, A.V., Konoplev, Y.G., Pryazhevskiy, R.D., Sachenkov, O.A.: Numerical study of influence of undercoverage of hip joint. Russ. J. Biomech. **22**(1), 15–24 (2018)
17. Munjal, S., Leopold, S.S., Kornreich, D., Shott, S., Finn, H.A.: CT-generated 3-dimensional models for complex acetabular reconstruction. J. Arthoplasy **15**(5), 644–653 (2000)
18. Sachenkov, O.A., Hasanov, R.F., Andreev, P.S., Konoplev, Y.: Numerical study of stress-strain state of pelvis at the proximal femur rotation osteotomy. Russ. J. Biomech. **20**(3), 220–232 (2016)
19. Konoplev, Y., Fedotenkov, G., Habibullin, A., Pryazhevskiy, R., Sachenkov, O.: Finite element modeling of the contact interaction of the acetabular component and acetabulum. IOP Conf. Ser.: J. Phys. Conf. Ser. **1158**, 032017 (2019). https://doi.org/10.1088/1742-6596/1158/3/032017
20. Berezhnoi, D.V., Gabsalikova, N.F., Miheev, V.V.: Application the particle method in problems of mechanics deformable media. In: IOP Conference Series: Materials Science and Engineering, vol. 158, no. 1, p. 012016 (2016)
21. Tarlakovskii, D.V., Fedotenkov, G.V.: Two-dimensional nonstationary contact of elastic cylindrical or spherical shells. J. Mach. Manuf. Reliab. **43**(2), 145–152 (2014)
22. Tarlakovskiy, D.V., Fedotenkov, G.V.: Analytic investigation of features of stresses in plane nonstationary contact problems with moving boundaries. J. Math. Sci. **162**(2), 246–253 (2009)
23. Papkovich, P.F.: Teoriya uprugosti. Oborongiz, Leningrad (1939). (in Russian)

WAVEX: Physical and Cognitive Research

Acceleration Transmission from an Oscillating Vibration Exercise Platform in Different Postures: A Pilot Study

Renata Marchon[1,3], Christiano Machado[2(✉)], Eloá Moreira-Marconi[3], Patrícia Lopes-Souza[1,3], Anke Bergmann[1], and Mário Bernardo-Filho[3]

[1] Cancer National Institute (INCA), Rio de Janeiro, Brazil
{rmarchon, plopes, abergmann}@inca.gov.br
[2] Estácio de Sá University, Rio de Janeiro, Brazil
cbmfisio@gmail.com
[3] Laboratório de Vibração Mecânica e Práticas Integrativas - LAVIMPI, State University of Rio de Janeiro (UERJ), Rio de Janeiro, Brazil

Abstract. Whole-body vibration exercises (WBVE) are a physical activity modality, promoted by mechanical vibrations generated in oscillating/vibratory platform (OVP). Used in the squatting-posture, but under limiting conditions, an alternative is sitting-posture. The objective was to evaluate acceleration transmission in specific body regions in: (I) squatting-posture; (II) sitting on chair with a free or (III) perpendicular ankle angle to the platform. Four volunteers performed single OVP protocol. An accelerometer was used on knee, lumbar, sternum and head to measure vertical displacement. The root-mean square (RMS) was computed for each signal, as well as the RMS-transmissibility (T_{RMS}). T_{RMS} varied for different parts of body: knees, head and lumbar spine were lowest in seated postures; there was an amplification of the vibration ($T_{RMS} > 100\%$) on the knee in all postures analyzed, a greater attenuation was observed in sternum. Seating positions seem to reduce vibration transmissibility for the upper parts of the body.

Keywords: Whole body vibration exercise · Vibration transmissibility · Accelerometer

1 Introduction

The use of mechanical vibrations (MV) as therapeutic strategies and clinical procedures dates from the mid-nineteenth century, generated by different equipments. Aerospace studies suggested that the vibrations minimized the negative effects of the gravity absence in space, and researches showed that stimulating the gravitational action on the human body allows important biological phenomena [1].

The MV produced in vibratory platform (VP) is a physical agent with wave, sinusoidal and deterministic characteristics [1, 2]. Exercises performed on these platforms generate the so-called whole-body vibration exercises (WBVE). The base of VP

T. Ahram et al. (Eds.): IHIET 2019, AISC 1018, pp. 621–626, 2020.
https://doi.org/10.1007/978-3-030-25629-6_96

may be displayed alternately as a seesaw or vertical (synchronous or triplane) at various frequencies (5–60 Hz) and amplitudes (<1 to 10 mm).

The WBVE is an exercise modality and there are a lot of benefits for the locomotor system [1], muscle activation [2], bone mineralization [2, 3], flexibility [2], balance [2, 4], functional training [4], pain treatment [2], cardiovascular [2, 5], neurophysiologic and hormonal systems [2], osteoarthritis and osteoporosis [1, 3], sarcopenia [4], sequelae of stroke [5], fibromyalgia [1], multiple sclerosis [1, 5], Parkinson [1, 5], cancer (leukemias, peripheral neuropathy) [6] and fatigue resistance [2].

The most used posture over a platform for WBVE is standing with a knee semi-flexion, called the squat posture. It allows the decomposition of the vector forces and muscular damping of the lower limbs, dissipating the vertical transmission of the force aiming at reducing the vibration of the head. In disabling clinical conditions, the sitting position can be adopted; however sitting directly on the VP or positioning the chair on it can generate uncomfortable vibration in the cranial region [7, 8]. It is then suggested that the chair has to be positioned frontally to the VP with the individual's feet leaning on his base [1]. On the other hand, this position provokes different angles of the body segments, causing variations in the force transmission generating different intensities even with identical protocols. For this reason, it is relevant to measure the transmission of MV in different postures, evaluating the energy dissipation through the body in order to produce more effective protocols of WBVE for several clinical scenarios.

The purpose of this study was to evaluate MV transmission during WBVE in four relevant parts of the body – head, sternum, lumbar spine and knee – during three different positions: (I) standing with a knee flexion (squatting position), (II) sitting on a chair with the feet resting on the platform and free ankle angle and (III) ankle perpendicular to the platform.

2 Method

This was a pilot project involving 4 healthy female volunteers recruited at the *Universidade do Estado do Rio de Janeiro* (UERJ), aged between 32 and 58 years old, who signed the Free and Informed Consent Term. The exclusion criteria were clinical manifestations that did not allow to perform exercises or avoid the required positions, the presence of pacemaker, surgeries for less than a year in lower limbs, presence of metal prosthesis or according to the criteria of the evaluator. At the end of the exercise, self-reported discomfort, pain (Numerical Pain - NDT), and effort perception (BORG) were assessed.

The study was developed in the *Laboratório de Vibração Mecânica e Práticas Integrativas* (LAVIMPI). The research is registered at REBEC and it is approved by the Ethical Committee of the institution involved. The following protocol was applied: PV of alternative type (Nova Plate Fitness Evolution), with vibration frequency of 5 Hz with a vibration amplitude of 2.5 mm. The period of intervention was 30 s, with a double resting time to avoid fatigue effect [8], with 3 min of working total time. The subject remained always static, and the protocol was repeated in three different postures as described below (Fig. 1):

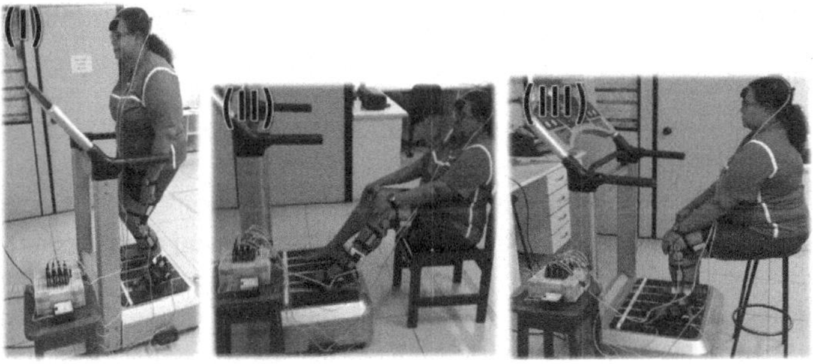

Fig. 1. A volunteer performing WBVE in the squatting posture (*posture I*), sitting with ankle at free angulation (*posture II*), and with ankles perpendicular to VP (*posture III*), with the digital accelerometers and goniometers positioned.

(a) Standing, with 130° knee flexion, arms hanging laterally to the body (posture I);
(b) Sitting in a chair with feet resting on the base of VP with tibia angulation to the surface of 45°, keeping the knee angulation of 130° (posture II);
(c) Sitting in a chair with feet resting on the base of VP with tibia angulation to the surface of the 90° platform, keeping the knee angulation of 130° (posture III);

A height-adjustable seat and a digital goniometer were used at the knee and ankle joints to ensure positioning at the indicated angulation (Model EWF030830/05R, *EMG System do Brasil*). In both sitting postures, hands should be resting on the knees with elbows extended. They were barefoot to avoid influence damping or slippage [9].

In order to measure the magnitude of the effect, the vibration and a_{peak} transmission were analyzed by means of accelerometry with a monoaxial model (Model ACL270303/15, *EMG System do Brasil*), in four distinct points: knee (anterior tuberosity of the tibia), lumbar spine (fourth vertebra lumbar), sternum (manubrium) and head (frontal bone). They were fixed with compressive adhesive tape to prevent displacement of the equipment [8].

Participants were instructed about the procedure, especially for the different positions during the vibration protocol. A short warm-up period was performed in a cycle ergometer and familiarization with VP [7]; each session lasted approximately 25 min, including clarification, data acquisition, period of instruction, heating, adaptation to equipment and acquisition of analysis.

2.1 Data Analysis

Body composition data were provided by the InBody software. The radiofrequency (RF) signal of each accelerometer was analyzed using Matlab® (Mathworks Inc, USA). First, a 9th order Butterworth low-pass filter was designed to filter frequencies higher than 100 Hz. Then, the root mean square (*RMS*) was estimated using the Eq. (1):

$$RMS = \sqrt{1/n \sum_{i=1}^{n} x_i^2} \tag{1}$$

where n is the number of points in the signal, and x_i is the ith point. Finally, the RMS transmissibility (%) for each region was calculated by the Eq. (2) [8]:

$$T_{rms}(\%) = \left(RMS_{body}/RMS_{PV}\right) \times 100 \quad (2)$$

where RMS_{body} is the RMS obtained at the four body regions with an accelerometer, and RMS_{PV} is the RMS obtained with the accelerometer placed directly on the vibrating platform.

A descriptive statistical analysis was carried out by measuring the central tendency and dispersion of data. Non-parametric Wilcoxon tests were run to verify significant differences among the postures (level of significance of 0.05).

3 Results

There were no reports of discomfort or any intercurrence during the execution of the protocol. The collected signals were analyzed for the transmissibility (%) measured at each anatomical point in relation to the vibration emitted by the VP. Descriptive and inferential statistical analysis is depicted in Tables 1 and 2, respectively. There was no significant difference among the postures ($p > 0.05$).

Table 1. T_{rms} central tendency measurements (%) at each anatomical site in the positions studied.

Position_site	Mean	Median	SD	Minimum	Maximum
PE_knee	120.7	126.9	16.1	96.9	132.3
PE_lumbar	45.07	42.69	14.33	31.05	63.84
PE_external	12.69	13.16	4.49	6.85	17.57
PE_head	14.34	14.82	3.28	10.41	17.31
SEN_knee	103.37	103.33	17.32	86.32	120.51
SEN_lumbar	20.66	21.11	2.47	17.24	23.16
SEN_external	8.38	8.33	3.88	3.96	12.91
SEN_head	12.67	11.52	7.47	6.20	21.40
PLA_knee	107.59	100.68	28.64	82.61	146.39
PLA_lumbar	20.12	19.45	3.85	16.66	24.91
PLA_external	11.09	6.69	9.32	5.93	25.04
PLA_head	11.00	10.76	4.69	5.55	16.92

Key: (PE) standing posture in squat; (SEN) sitting posture with free ankle angulation; (PLA) seated posture with ankles perpendicular to VP.

Table 2. Mean differences between paired samples ($p > 0.05$).

Paired samples	Mean difference (%)
PE_knee – SEN_knee	17.42
PE_knee – PLA_knee	13.20
SEN_knee – PLA_knee	–4.21
PE_external – SEN_external	4.30
PE_external – PLA_external	1.59
SEN_external – PLA_external	–2.70
PE_head – SEN_head	1.67
PE_head – PLA_head	3.34
SEN_head – PLA_head	1.67

Key: (PE) standing posture in squat; (SEN) sitting posture with free ankle angulation; (PLA) seated posture with ankles perpendicular to VP.

4 Discussion and Conclusions

The present results were obtained from a pilot study. An ongoing project pretends to obtain a minimum quantitative of 30 women, in order to obtain a greater statistical expression. It was possible to observe that data are in agreement with the findings in literature regarding the effect of the semi-knee position [7], which causes a higher concentration of vibration in the knee joint, as well as a lower vibrational transmissibility in sitting postures.

Although the sample was small, there are some interesting points to note. The knee joint receives a higher vibrational transmissibility ($T_{rms} > 100\%$) in all postures analyzed, which can be justified by the phenomenon of resonance [2, 8]. Seated postures presented lower transmissibility at all regions in comparison to standing posture (Table 1). The non-significant p-value obtained may be due to the small sample ($p > 0.05$). Nevertheless, it was possible to notice a trend of greater variation in knee joint in the posture I in relation to the other postures, and a greater transmission of the force in knee and sternum regions in the posture III compared to the ankles with free angulation (posture II). In relation to the head, the posture of lower vibration was seen in the posture III.

In conclusion, the posture adopted on VP may exert an effect on vibrational transmissibility in different body regions. Further research must be developed to obtain data that are more reliable. In this way, health professionals will be able to develop safe, well-tolerated and effective protocols for individuals with disabilities in performing physical activities. Information obtained from this work can also be used to elaborate protocols, which may be incorporated into research projects involving individuals with different physical limitations.

References

1. Paiva, D.N., Cabezuelo, P.J.M., Bernardo-Filho, M.: Plataforma Oscilante/ Vibratória: Fundamentos e a Prática Clínica. Livraria e Editora Andreoli, São Paulo (2014)
2. Rittweger, J.: Vibration as an exercise modality: how it may work, and what its potential might be. Eur. J. Appl. Physiol. **108**, 877–904 (2010). https://doi.org/10.1007/s00421-009-1303-3
3. Moreira-Marconi, E., Dionello, C.F., Morel, D.S., Sá-Caputo, D.C., Souza-Gonçalves, C.R., Paineiras-Domingos, L.L., Guedes-Aguiar, E.O., Marin, P.J., Cruz, B.D.P., Bernardo-Filho, M.: Could whole body vibration exercises influence the risk factors for fractures in women with osteoporosis? Osteoporos. Sarcopenia. **2**, 214–220 (2016). https://doi.org/10.1016/j.afos.2016.09.003
4. Rogan, S., Taeymans, J., Radlinger, L., Naepflin, S., Ruppen, S., Bruelhart, Y., Hilfiker, R.: Effects of whole-body vibration on postural control in elderly: an update of a systematic review and meta-analysis. Arch. Gerontol. Geriatr. **73**, 95–112 (2017). https://doi.org/10.1016/j.archger.2017.07.022
5. Cochrane, D.J.: Vibration exercise: the potential benefits. Int. J. Sports Med. **32**, 75–99 (2011). https://doi.org/10.1055/s-0030-1268010
6. Streckmann, F., Balke, M., Lehmann, H.C., Rustler, V., Koliamitra, C., Elter, T., Hallek, M., Leitzmann, M., Steinmetz, T., Heinen, P., Baumann, F.T., Bloch, W.: The preventive effect of sensorimotor- and vibration exercises on the onset of Oxaliplatin- or vinca-alkaloid induced peripheral neuropathies - STOP. BMC Cancer **18**, 1–10 (2018). https://doi.org/10.1186/s12885-017-3866-4
7. Vasconcellos, R.P., Schütz, G.R., dos Santos, S.G., Vasconcellos, R.P., Schütz, G.R., dos Santos, S.G.: A interferência da posição corporal na transmissibilidade vibratória durante o treinamento com plataforma vibratória. Rev. Bras. Cineantropometria e Desempenho Hum. **16**, 597 (2014). https://doi.org/10.5007/1980-0037.2014v16n6p597
8. Caryn, R.C., Dickey, J.P.: Transmission of acceleration from a synchronous vibration exercise platform to the head during dynamic squats. Dose-Response **17**, 1–7 (2019). https://doi.org/10.1177/1559325819827467
9. Rauch, F., Sievanen, H., Boonen, S., Cardinale, M., Degens, H., Felsenberg, D., Roth, J., Schoenau, E., Verschueren, S., Rittweger, J.: Reporting whole-body vibration intervention studies: recommendations of the international society of musculoskeletal and neuronal interactions. J. Musculoskelet. Neuronal Interact. **10**, 193–198 (2010)

WBV'S Physiological Effects and Clinical Correlations

Alessandro S. Pin[1,2](✉), Thaísa O. Paiva[1], Fernanda Lima[1], Lucas L. Borges[2], and Victor P. Graciano[2]

[1] Physiotherapy Department, Goiatuba University Center – UNICERRADO, Goiatuba, GO, Brazil
alessandropin@unicerrado.edu.br
[2] Medicine Department, Mineiros University Center – UNIFIMES, Trindade, GO, Brazil

Abstract. WBV is gaining adepts in clinical application on account of the countless benefits arising from its application. The physiological effects that justify its clinical use are diverse. Our purpose was to review the physiological effects of WBV, correlating them with the clinical use of this resource. An analytic literature review of manuscripts was made. Data collection was carried out on data bases using articles published between 2004 and 2019 that addressed the physiological effects and/or the clinical applications of the use of WBV. During low frequency WBV (maximum of 30 Hz) there is an increase in blood flow, Consequently the ventilatory patterns accompany this. It was noted better blood reperfusion in cardiac tissues that had undergone anterior ischemic injury. Biochemical analyzes showed a significant increase in growth hormone (GH) immediately after the end of WBV use, the high levels lasted for 1 h. There was also an improvement in the glycemic status. The mechanical stress offered by the WBV seems to prevent osteoporosis. Vibration training also improved isometric and dynamic muscle strength. WBV acts mainly in the cardiovascular, respiratory and musculoskeletal systems, under neurological and endocrine influence, enhancing organic functioning and cellular activity with many good effects in body.

Keywords: WBV · Physiology · Clinical effects · Vibrating platform

1 Introduction

The use of vibration on the human body was first used in the 1970s in Soviet astronauts, with the intent of making them stay longer in space without causing many changes to their body (such as reduction of bone and muscle mass) due to the low gravity. With the use of the vibration machine on the limbs, there was an increase of 3.5 times in the period that they could stay in space without harmful musculoskeletal alterations [1].

At first, because of the few features offered by the equipment, cable systems were placed in parts over the skin, causing only local vibration. The technological advance resulted in the vibratory platform, that distributed the vibration on to the body in a global way, the Whole-body-vibration (WBV), which is a form of stimulation capable

T. Ahram et al. (Eds.): IHIET 2019, AISC 1018, pp. 627–631, 2020.
https://doi.org/10.1007/978-3-030-25629-6_97

of producing responses equivalent to muscular endurance exercise (2). The physiological responses will form a relation with different organic systems, causing stimulus to the cutaneous receptors and muscle spindles, presenting vibratory tonic reflex responses [1].

The sinusoidal vibration the vibrating platform uses in various frequencies and amplitudes offers the body stimuli for the muscle spindles, which are activated producing vibratory reflex, that activates the α-motoneurons. The greater the number of active motoneurons, the greater will be the production of force and power. The lower the frequency (between 20 or 30 Hz), more intense the muscle activity will be. This fact may be related to the muscular adjustment mechanism, meaning that the low frequency would be closer to the natural resonance frequency of the muscles (between 15 and 20 Hz) [3–5].

Nowadays much is being investigated about the vibratory platform and the physiological changes it causes in the human body. Considering the benefits derived from the use of this resource and the its recent popularization, the authors aimed to compile the physiological changes caused by the application of WBV correlating these changes to their clinical effects.

2 Methodology

An analytical review was carried out in literature, the search for manuscripts was done in electronic bases and libraries: PubMed, Lilacs, Scielo and Google Scholar. The search strategy was advanced search, using combinations of terms connected by the Boolean "and" operator. The search terms used were: "whole body vibration", "WBV", "vibratory platform", "physiology", "clinical effects", combined as follows: "whole body vibration and clinical effects", "WBV and clinical effects", "vibratory platform and clinical effects", "WBV and physiology", "vibratory platform and physiology", "whole body vibration and physiology", "WBV and physiology and clinical effects", "whole body vibration and physiology and clinical effects", "vibratory platform and physiology and clinical effects".

We considered for this research the materials that met the following inclusion criteria: clinical trials, field surveys and systematic reviews that approached the vibratory platform and its organic effects; studies published preferably from 2014, although studies considered relevant with publication date of up to 15 years could be accepted; languages were English, Portuguese and Spanish. We summarily excluded studies that did not meet the requirements previously outlined or of limited electronic availability.

The manuscripts elected were compiled in the following text.

3 Results and Discussion

The analysis of the carried out studies points out a relation between the physiological effects of whole body vibration (WBV) and the improvement of clinical conditions that have increased in modern days, such as diabetes. It is well known that exercise prevents and/ or improve the situation of these diseases. However, physical activities tend to be tiring and time consuming, reducing exercise compliance in young and older people with little time and/or little physical vigor (6). It is important to emphasize that due to the intense effect on the head, the use of the vibrating platform should not be done with the body in full extension position [7].

Regarding the physiological effects, an increase in bone mineral density was observed in women aged 15–20 years that used the WBV for 12 months, for 10 min a day, 5 days a week (5). This finding can be corroborated by a research made in postmenopausal women where WBV was applied for 6 months in 60 individuals. The total bone mineral density (BMD) of the hip increased, as well as the trunk balance and isometric and isokinetic muscle strength [8]. These findings show that WBV training is beneficial for the prevention of osteopenia and osteoporosis.

In strength training associated with WBV (whole body vibration), the physiological alterations that promote its increase are the result of the reduction of the time of depolarization for conduction of the stimulus and the greater activation of muscle fibers of fast contraction [9].

Improvement in oxygenation muscle and peripheral blood flow were also noted after the use of WBV. Vertical vibrations and lateral alternating vibrations, in amplitudes of 2 to 6 mm applied for 30 to 300 s showed an increase in the level of muscular oxygenation at a vibration frequency of 25 Hz and 30 Hz; seen through Near Infrared Spectroscopy - NIRS. The explanation for the increase in blood flow comes from the rate of muscle contraction, lower frequencies enable more time between contractions, allowing greater perfusion and oxygenation [10, 11].

This set of changes results in a better efficiency of the musculoskeletal system, offering greater strength of contraction and resistance. In addition to better kinetic dynamics, the static balance will also be favored by post-use gains derived from the vibratory platform.

The use of WBV in animal models also showed a significant increase in tolerance of injuries caused b myocardial ischemia and reperfusion (IK). This effect comes from increased regulation of heart rate, reduction of infarct size and facilitation of involuntary cardioversion [12].

Hormonal changes can also occur by applying whole body vibrations. The GH levels measured immediately after the end of the application rose significantly, remaining high up to 1 h later, it is important to point out that the increase was directly related to the intensity of the vibration. There was also an increase in testosterone concentration, although the increase was not related to exercise intensity. Inflammatory markers also underwent positive change after the activity [13].

In patients diagnosed with chronic fibromyalgia WBV provided satisfactory results in the inflammatory state and metabolic balance, in addition it demonstrated improved responsiveness to the stress received due to the neuroendocrine mechanism adapted by the therapy [14].

A clinical study on the effects of WBV in chronic obstructive pulmonary disease (COPD) detailed better the latter effect. In COPD patients, the body, especially the pulmonary region, is in a constant inflammatory state, with high levels of interleukin- 8 (IL-8), responsible for maintaining the inflammation; and low levels of Interleukin- 10 (IL-10), this anti-inflammatory. WBV increased IL-10 levels in COPD patients [15].

There is also an improvement in muscle tone through the simultaneity of fiber contraction and synergistic and antagonistic muscle adjustments [16]. This results in better quality of life and respiratory efficiency in a population that normally has serious difficulties in aerial use.

4 Final Considerations

WBV acts mainly in the cardiovascular, respiratory and musculoskeletal systems, under neurological and endocrine influence, enhancing the organic functioning and cellular activity. The most cited clinical effects are: improvement of cardiovascular and respiratory conditioning, increase in bone density and muscle dynamics and possible improvement in the reception of cellular substrates mediated by hormones - case of insulin receptors in patients with DM2. It was also observed the predominant use of low frequency (up to 30 Hz) and different time patterns of vibration application in these cases.

References

1. Pardo, E.M., Páez, L.C., Ramón, P.E.A., Gómez, A.B., Soler, C.N.: Efectos agudos de las vibraciones mecánicas sobre el salto vertical. Ed Fís y Depor. **87**, 81–85 (2007)
2. Bogaerts, A., Delecluse, C., Claessens, A.L., Coudyzer, W., Boonen, S., Verschueren, S.M.: Impact of whole-body vibration training versus fitness training on muscle strength and muscle mass in older men: a 1-year randomized controlled trial. J. Gerontol. Biol. Sci. Med. Sci. **62**(6), 630–635 (2007)
3. Da Silva, R.G., Andreotti, R., Gehring, P.G., de Nunes, M.E., Wallerstein, L., da Fonseca, C. O.M., et al.: Efeito do treinamento vibratório na força muscular e em testes funcionais em idosos fisicamente ativos. Rev Bras Cineantropom Desempenho Hum. **11**(2), 168–175 (2009)
4. Ruymbeke, V.B., Boone, J., Coorevits, P., Vanderstraeten, G., Bougois, J.: Whole-body vibration in breast cancer survivors: a pilot study exploring its effects on muscle activity and subjectively perceived exertion. Int. J. Rehabil. Res. **37**(4), 371–374 (2014)
5. Edionwe, J., Hess, C., Fernandez-Rio, J., Herndon, D.N., Andersen, C.R., Klein, G.L., et al.: Effects of whole-body vibration exercise on bone mineral content and density in thermally. Burns **42**(3), 605–613 (2016)
6. Yin, H., Berdel, H.O., Moore, D., Davis, F., Liu, J., Mozaffari, M., et al.: Whole body vibration therapy: a novel potential treatment for type 2 diabetes mellitus. Springerplus **4**, 578–585 (2015)
7. Vasconcellos, R.P., Schütz, G.R., Santos, S.G.: The interference of body position with vibration transmission during training on a vibrating platform. Rev. Bras. Cineantropom. Desempenho Hum. **16**(6), 597–607 (2014)
8. Verschueren, S., Roelants, M., Delecluse, C., Swinnen, S., Vanderschueren, D., Boonen, S.: Effect of 6-month whole body vibration training on hip density, muscle strength, and postural control in postmenopausal women: a randomized controlled pilot study. J. Bone Min. Res. **19**(3), 352–359 (2003)
9. Licurci, M.G.B., Fagundes, A.A., Arisawa, E.A.S.: Whole body vibration and blood glucose levels in elderly perple: a pilot study. Sci. Med. **27**(4), 3 (2017). ID27604

10. Urso, R.P., Okuno, N.M., Batista, M.A.B., Tricoli, V., Kiss, M.A.P.D., Bertuzzi, R.: O treinamento de força com e sem o uso da plataforma vibratória é capaz de modular a variabilidade da frequência cardíaca em repouso? Motriz: Rev. Educ. Fis. **18**(3), 526–532 (2012)
11. Games, K.E., Sefton, J.M., Wilson, A.E.: Whole body vibration and blood flow and muscle oxygenation: a meta-analysis. J. Athl. Train. **50**(5), 542–549 (2015)
12. Shekarforoush, S., Naghii, M.R.: Whole-body vibration training increases myocardial salvage against acute ischemia in adult male rats. Arq. Bras. Cardiol. **112**(1), 32–37 (2019)
13. Giminiani, R.D., Fabiani, L., Baldini, G., Cardelli, G., Giovannelli, A., Tihanyi, J.: Hormonal and neuromuscular responses to mechanical vibration applied to upper extremity muscles. PLosOne **9**(11), e111521 (2014)
14. Ribeiro, V.G.C., Mendonça, V.A., Souza, A.L.C., Fonseca, S.F., Camargos, A.C.R., Lage, V.K.S., et al.: Inflammatory biomarkers responses after acute whole body vibration in fibromyalgia. Braz. J. Med. Biol. Res. **51**(4), e6775 (2018)
15. Lage, V.K.S., Lacerda, A.C.R., Neves, C.D.C., Chaves, M.G.A., Soares, A.A., Lima, L.P., et al.: Acute effects of whole body vibration on inflammatory markers in people with chronic obstructive pulmonary disease: a pilot study. Rehabil. Res. Pract. **2018**, 7 (2018). 5480214
16. Cardoso, M.C.S., Sayão, L.B., Souza, R.M.P., Marinho, P.E.M.: Pulmonary rehabilitation and whole-body vibration in chronic obstructive pulmonary disease. Motriz: Rev. Educ. Fis. **22**(2), 44–50 (2016)

Short-Term Effect of Whole-Body Vibration in Static Posture: A Randomized Controlled Trial

Mayara Sampaio[1], Thays Ingrid Ribeiro[1], Larissa Fialho[1], Susana Vidal[1], Antônio Marcos Lopes[1], Christiana Valois[3], Danúbia Sá-Caputo[2], Mário Bernardo-Filho[2(✉)], Redha Taiar[4], and Christiano Machado[1]

[1] Physical Therapy Department, Estácio de Sá University, Niterói, Brazil
cbmfisio@gmail.com
[2] IBRAG, State University of Rio de Janeiro, Rio de Janeiro, Brazil
[3] Globus, Codogné, Italy
[4] Université de Reims Champagne-Ardenne, Reims, France

Abstract. The present study aimed at evaluating the short-term effect of one whole-body body vibration (WBV) session in the static posture of apparently healthy young adults, by means of a randomized controlled trial. Twenty-one volunteers were recruited and randomly assigned to one of three blinded interventions: (1) vibration group - VG; (2) placebo group – PG; and (3) control group - CG. Static posture of all volunteers was blind assessed before and right after interventions using computerized biophotogrammetry. Significant differences were observed in CG (tibial tuberosity horizontal alignment: $p = 0.04$) and in VG (pelvic horizontal alignment: $p = 0.04$). The intergroup analysis showed no significant differences ($p > 0.05$). The initial hypothesis was that if WBV provides strong reflex muscle contractions, posture alterations could be detected after a session. It was not possible to observe a short-term effect of a WBVE session on static posture as assessed by biophotogrammetry.

Keywords: Whole-body vibration · Posture · Rehabilitation · Biophotogrammetry

1 Introduction

An exercise modality involving mechanical vibration generated in an oscillating/vibratory platform (OVP) is known as whole-body vibration (WBV). Several studies have been demonstrating the effects of this modality on the musculoskeletal system. WBV stimulates muscle spindle and produces muscular contractions similar to tonic reflexes, which may lead to muscular strengthening [1].

WBV exercises have been proposed for several purposes [1]. Recent studies indicate benefits in patients, for example with metabolic syndrome [2], respiratory diseases [3], among others. Muscle strengthening and flexibility has been also influenced by vibration [4].

T. Ahram et al. (Eds.): IHIET 2019, AISC 1018, pp. 632–637, 2020.
https://doi.org/10.1007/978-3-030-25629-6_98

A question that may arise is that WBV could influence postural control. Some evidence can be found in the literature. Chow et al. [5] determined the effects of WBV applied in standing and seated postures, on spinal proprioception. They verified that it could improve body posture, lumbar repositioning ability, maximum reaching distance and lumbopelvic coordination. Liang et al. [6] analyzed the center-of-mass movement of children and young adults before, during, immediately after, and 5 min after WBV in quiet standing. Volunteers could adapt their postural control system to WBV and maintain balance during and after vibration. Dickin and Heath [7] studied the effect of whole body vibration on postural stability in young adults, and they concluded that vibration might impair postural control with low level of sensorial challenge, and improve stability with high-level challenge. Moreover, it has been shown that 5-consecutive daily WBV sessions can improve the time of response to recover the uprightness after sudden disturbances [8].

Therefore, the present study aimed at evaluating the short-term effect of a whole-body body vibration (WBV) session in the static posture of apparently healthy young adults, by means of a randomized controlled trial.

2 Materials and Methods

2.1 Subjects

Twenty-one university students were recruited (6 men and 15 women, mean age = 23.76 ± 3.86 years old; mean weight = 61.85 + 13.45 kg; mean height = 1.64 + 0.09 m) and randomly assigned to one of three blind interventions: (1) vibration group - VG; (2) placebo group – PG; and (3) control group – CG, each of them with seven volunteers. They signed an informed consent for participation in the study and publication of data. This work was approved by Estácio de Sá University's Ethics Committee (CAAE nº 28761314.9.0000.5284) and follows the guidelines of the Declaration of Helsinki.

Inclusion criteria were apparent healthy students between 18 and 30 years old, both genders, who never were submitted to a WBV session. The exclusion criteria were subjects with neurological and orthopedic diseases, which could prevent locomotion or balance, and subjects who have already been submitted to WBV exercises.

2.2 Interventional Protocol

All the interventional protocol was blind applied. For the vibration group (VG), subjects underwent a WBV session using a vertical vibration platform (G-Vibe 800, Globus®, Italy), frequency of 30 Hz, peak-to-peak amplitude of 4 mm, during five minutes (or until muscle fatigue reported by the volunteer). A knee flexion of 60° was always maintained.

For the placebo group (PG), subjects were asked to maintain for five minutes the same knee flexion on the platform, but no vibration was produced. Finally, subjects from control group (CG) stood still during the same period.

2.3 Postural Assessment

Static posture of all volunteers was blind assessed before and right after interventions using computerized biophotogrammetry, in a separate room. Pictures were taken in anterior, lateral and posterior view using a digital camera (Sony®, model DSC-W110, 7.2 megapixels) and a tripod, adjusted to be perpendicular to the anatomical planes at a distance of 1.67 m from the subject and a height of 0.92 cm from the floor. The subjects were in standing position, and dressed to allow the visualization of the anatomic landmarks considered for this study. Vertical calibration of the images was done using a plumb line.

The landmarks were bilaterally marked using styrofoam balls and double-faced adhesive tapes, as described by literature [9], to estimate parameters using the software Corel Draw®, as described in Table 1.

Table 1. Parameters for postural analysis and landmarks bilaterally marked in the body.

View	Parameter (in degrees)	Landmarks
Anterior	Head horizontal alignment (HHA)	Ear tragus
	Acromial horizontal alignment (AHA)	Acromial process of scapula
	Anterior superior iliac spine alignment (ASISHA)	Anterior superior iliac spine (iliac bone)
	Tibial tuberosity horizontal alignment (TTHA)	Tibial tuberosity
Lateral	Head vertical alignment (HVA)	Ear tragus
	Pelvic horizontal alignment (PHA)	Anterior superior and posterior superior iliac spines (iliac bone)
Posterior	Ankle angle	Calcaneus tendon (between malleolus) and calcaneum (posterior)
	Scapular horizontal alignment (SHA)	Inferior angle of scapula
	Posterior superior iliac spine horizontal alignment (PSISHA)	Posterior superior iliac spine (iliac bone)

2.4 Statistical Analysis

Wilcoxon tests were run to test the null hypothesis that there is no difference between "before" and "after" interventions, and the Kruskal-Wallis test were used to verify whether there are significant differences among groups. All statistical analysis were made in SPSS® (IBM, EUA) with a significance level of 0.05.

3 Results

Table 2 shows descriptive statistics (minimum, maximum, average and standard deviation) of the postural parameters before intervention, for all volunteers.

Table 2. Descriptive statistics of postural parameters before interventions (SD = standard deviation). Negative and positive values refer to the orientation of the alignment (left or right side down).

Parameter	Minimum (degrees)	Maximum (degrees)	Average (degrees)	SD (degrees)
Head horizontal alignment (HHA)	–5.87	9.69	0.81	3.50
Acromial horizontal alignment (AHA)	–3.08	2.40	0.03	1.23
Anterior superior iliac spine alignment (ASISHA)	–1.92	2.02	0.13	0.95
Tibial tuberosity horizontal alignment (TTHA)	–1.97	2.70	–0.19	1.20
Head vertical alignment (HVA)	–5.91	4.59	–0.61	2.67
Pelvic horizontal alignment (PHA)	–1.92	3.58	0.62	1.56
Ankle angle	–3.74	2.73	–0.36	1.55
Scapular horizontal alignment (SHA)	–2.89	3.44	–0.26	1.74
Posterior superior iliac spine horizontal alignment (PSISHA)	–1.78	3.54	0.62	1.43

Statistical analysis have shown that significant intragroup differences were obtained only for two parameters: TTHA (for the CG) and PHA (for the VG), both with $p = 0.04$. All other intra- and intergroup analysis have provided $p > 0.05$. Figure 1 presents two boxplots of two of these variables: HHA and PHA.

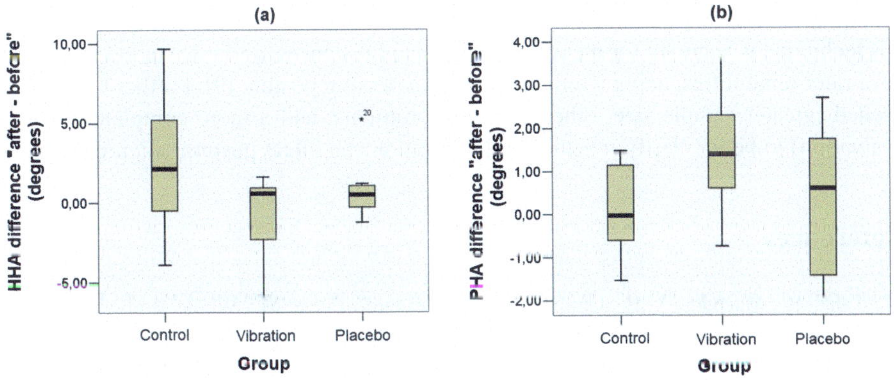

Fig. 1. Boxplots of "after – before" intervention differences for parameters (a) HHA and (b) PHA (CG, VG and PG) ($p > 0.05$).

4 Discussion and Conclusions

To our knowledge, the present work was the first approach to study the effect of WBV on static posture by means of a postural analysis with biophotogrammetry. Initially, the hypothesis raised was that WBV could affect posture since evidence shows that motor units can be activated under the influence of vibration [1]. Reflex contractions in muscle fibers could lead to a change in the pattern of muscle activation responsible for maintaining the upright posture, among others.

However, muscle activation is not the only necessary element to maintain body posture. Other elements involved are proprioceptors in muscles, tendons, joints, ligaments, capsules and in the labyrinth of the inner ear. These receptors (Golgi tendon organs, muscle spindles, Ruffini endings, Pacini and Meissner corpuscles, free terminations) receive the impulses produced from body positions and movements and transmit them to the central nervous system [10].

Overall, the results have shown that the proposed vibration protocol did not lead to significant changes in posture ($p > 0.05$) as compared with control and placebo groups. The frequency used was 30 Hz, as seen in the work of Cardinale and Lim [11], who analyzed the responses of the vastus lateralis muscle to different frequencies through electromyography (EMG). They found a higher EMG activity at 30 Hz, caused by the greater reflex response in the muscle.

Several limitations can be pointed out here. First, the postural analysis took into account some of the anatomical landmarks regularly used in clinical practice, but several other postural parameters were not considered, mainly because the styrofoam balls were not correctly placed during the assessment and it was preferred to neglect them. Moreover, the sample size was considered small ($N = 21$ divided in three groups).

In conclusion, a 5-min bout of WBV at 30 Hz did not lead to short-term alterations in posture as assessed by a protocol of computerized biophotogrammetry. One may say that this technique is accurate for measuring angles and distances, and it has good inter- and intra-rater reliabilities, being a reliable tool for assessing posture [9]. Further research is needed (greater sample size, other vibration protocols, and a more complete postural evaluation) to better clarify whether body vibration can affect postural alignment.

References

1. Taiar, R., Machado, C.B., Chiementin, X., Bernardo-Filho, M.: Whole Body Vibrations: Physical and Biological Effects on the Human Body. CRC Press, Boca Raton (2018)
2. Sá-Caputo, D., Paineiras-Domingos, L.L., Francisca-Santos, A., Anjos, E.M., Reis, A.S., Neves, M.F.T., Oigman, W., Oliveira, R., Brandão, A., Machado, C.B., Chiementin, X., Taiar, R., Sartório, R., Bernardo-Filho, M.: Whole-body vibration improves the functional parameters of individuals with metabolic syndrome: an exploratory study. BMC Endocr. Disord. **19**, 1–10 (2019)
3. Zhou, J., Pang, L., Chen, N., Wang, Z., Wang, C., Hai, Y., Lyu, M., Lai, H., Lin, F.: Whole-body vibration training – better care for COPD patients: a systematic review and meta-analysis. Int. J. COPD **13**, 3243–3254 (2018)

4. Di Giminiani, R., Manno, R., Scrimaglio, R., Sementilli, G., Tihanyi, J.: Effects of individualized whole-body vibration on muscle flexibility and mechanical power. J. Sports Med. Phys. Fitness **50**, 139–151 (2010)
5. Chow, D.H.K., Lee, T.Y., Pope, M.H.: Effects of whole body vibration on spinal proprioception in healthy individuals. Work **61**, 403–411 (2018)
6. Liang, H., Beerse, M., Ke, X., Wu, J.: Effect of whole-body vibration on center-of-mass movement during standing in children and young adults. Gait Posture **54**, 148–153 (2017)
7. Dickin, D.C., Heath, J.E.: Additive effect of repeated bouts of individualized frequency whole body vibration on postural stability in young adults. J. Appl. Biomech. **30**, 529–533 (2014)
8. Diego, I.M.A., Hernández, C.P., Rueda, F.M., Cuerda, R.C.: Effects of vibrotherapy on postural control, functionality and fatigue in multiple sclerosis patients. a randomised clinical trial. Neurología **27**, 143–153 (2012)
9. Ferreira, E.A.G., Duarte, M., Maldonado, E.P., Burke, T.N., Marques, A.P.: Postural assessment software (PAS/SAPO): validation and reliability. Clinics **65**, 675–681 (2010)
10. Hall, J.E.: Guyton and Hall Textbook of Medical Physiology. Elsevier, New York (2015)
11. Cardinale, M., Lim, J.: Electromyography activity of vastus lateralis muscle during whole-body vibrations of different frequencies. J. Strength Condit. Res. **17**, 621–624 (2003)

Whole-Body Vibration Exercises Associated with Pressure Threshold Device for Inspiratory Muscular Training

Leiner Costa[1], Viviane Souza[1], Vinícius Maldonado[1], Redha Taiar[2], Christiano Machado[1](✉), Sandra Helena Mayworm[1], and Antônio Marcos Lopes[1]

[1] Physical Therapy Department, Estácio de Sá University, Niterói, Brazil
cbmfisio@gmail.com
[2] Université de Reims Champagne-Ardenne, Reims, France

Abstract. This work aimed at evaluating the effect of whole-body vibration exercises (WBVE) associated with a pressure threshold device for inspiratory muscular training (IMT). A blind randomized design was carried out with 15 women, divided into two groups: G1 (WBVE and threshold IMT) and G2 (threshold IMT). There was no significant difference ($p > 0.05$) between maximal inspiratory pressure (MIP) before and after interventions for day 1 (G1: -1 ± 13 cmH_2O; G2: $+1 \pm 8$ cmH_2O) and day 8 (G1: -1 ± 9 cmH_2O; G2: -2 ± 5 cmH_2O). However, when comparing measurements before intervention between day 1 and 8, it was found a significant p-value (G1: $+30 \pm 11$ cmH_2O; G2: $+14 \pm 11$ cmH_2O; $p = 0.02$). The association of WBVE and pressure threshold IMT led to a significant increase in MIP after 8 sessions, suggesting a benefit in combining these two techniques in clinical practice.

Keywords: Whole-body vibration exercises · Threshold IMT · Diaphragm · Pulmonary rehabilitation · Maximal inspiratory pressure

1 Introduction

An exercise modality involving mechanical vibration generated in an oscillating/vibratory platform (OVP) is known as whole-body vibration (WBV). Several studies have been demonstrating the effects of this modality on the musculoskeletal system. WBVE stimulates muscle spindle and produces muscular contractions similar to tonic reflexes, which may lead to muscular strengthening [1].

Evidence suggests that WBVE can improve respiratory function. A recent meta-analysis [2] showed that patients with chronic obstructive pulmonary disease (COPD) presenting a significant reduction in muscle force and resistance may benefit from WBVE because it improves neuromuscular activation and blood circulation, as well as alleviating clinical symptoms. WBVE also significantly increased maximal inspiratory (MIP) and expiratory (MEP) pressures, chest wall total volume, and quality of life in elders [3]. The combination of WBVE with conventional endurance and strength training for patients after lung transplantation led to improvement in six-minute walk test with no adverse effects [4].

T. Ahram et al. (Eds.): IHIET 2019, AISC 1018, pp. 638–643, 2020.
https://doi.org/10.1007/978-3-030-25629-6_99

On the other hand, evidence suggests that inspiratory muscular training (IMT) using a pressure threshold device increases respiratory muscle strength, exercise capacity and quality of life. When a person inhales through a threshold IMT, a spring-loaded valve provides a resistance for respiratory muscles training [5, 6]. Up to the present moment, the association of these two techniques was never addressed. Therefore, this work aimed at evaluating the effect of WBVE associated with a pressure threshold device for inspiratory muscular training (IMT).

2 Materials and Methods

2.1 Subjects

Fifteen female volunteers were recruited to this study, and randomly assigned to one of two groups: G1 (WBVE + Threshold IMT) with 7 subjects (mean age = 23 ± 2 years old) and G2 (Threshold IMT) with 8 subjects (age = 26 ± 5 years old). They signed an informed consent for participation in the study and publication of data. This work was approved by Estácio de Sá University's Ethics Committee (CAAE nº 09635418.4.0000.5284) and follows the guidelines of the Declaration of Helsinki.

Inclusion criteria were: being female, sedentary, aging from 20 to 35 years old, without any musculoskeletal disorder and with no recent history of regular physical activity. Subjects who did not attended these criteria were not included, as well as presenting respiratory or cardiac diseases, abdominal effusion, blood hypertension, recent surgery or trauma, abdominal hernia, acute middle ear disease, glaucoma or retinal detachment, neurological disorders, swallowing disorders, or mental illness.

2.2 Inspiratory Pressure Assessment

The maximal inspiratory pressure (MIP) was blinded assessed before and after each intervention (to be explained in Sect. 2.3). An analogic manovacuometer (model NAM, Muremas®, operating range = ±120 cmH_2O) was used. All measurements were made in the same room at 25 °C by the same researcher. Volunteers remained at sitting posture, with feet flat on floor, knees at 90º flexion and a nose clip. They were then asked to keep their lips tightly closed over the mouth in order to perform the forced inspiration maneuver from residual volume during 3 s. The procedure was repeated three times with a one-minute interval, and the greater MIP value was considered for analysis [7]. After the first evaluation, the predicted threshold IMT load for each subject was obtained as 30% of the greater MIP measured.

2.3 Interventional Protocol

Volunteers from G1 were submitted to an 8-sessions intervention with WBVE and threshold IMT, simultaneously, twice a week. The WBVE protocol was applied as follows: a vibration platform GLOBUS® (G 800 VIBE, Italy) was used during one minute (standardized amplitude of 2.0, frequency of 35 Hz), and at the same time the subject inhaled in a Threshold IMT (Philips® Respironics) with the load predicted during initial assessment. Volunteers from G2 were submitted only to threshold IMT in a sitting posture (Fig. 1).

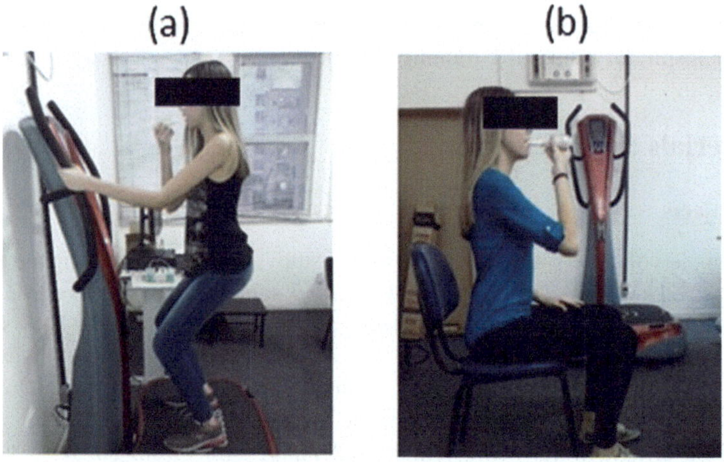

Fig. 1. Intervention protocol. In (a), the simultaneous application of WBVE and threshold IMT (G1); in (b), only threshold IMT (G2).

2.4 Statistical Analysis

Descriptive statistics provided average, confidence intervals, standard deviation, median, minimum and maximum values. The Wilcoxon signed rank and Mann-Whitney U-test were applied to verify intragroup and intergroup significant differences, respectively, assuming a significance level of 0.05. All statistical computations were performed using SPSS® software (IBM).

3 Results

Table 1 shows statistics (average, confidence interval, standard deviation, minimum and maximum) obtained from MIP values of sessions 1 and 8 (before and after intervention, difference between after and before, and difference between the 8th and 1st session). Figure 2 depicts boxplots with the difference in MIP values for the two groups in the following cases: (a) difference "after – before" in the first day ($p = 0.87$), (b) difference "after – before" in the eighth day ($p = 0.26$) and (c) difference in the "before" measurement between days 8 and 1 ($p = 0.02$).

Table 1. Descriptive statistics of the MIP measurements (1st and 8th sessions).

MIP measurement	Group	Average ± SD (cmH_2O)	CI 95% (cmH_2O)	Minimum (cmH_2O)	Maximum (cmH_2O)
1st session (before)	G1	73 ± 16	55 to 88	50	100
	G2	87 ± 28	64 to 111	50	120
1st session (after)	G1	71 ± 9	63 to 79	60	80
	G2	88 ± 34	60 to 116	40	120
1st session (after - before)	G1	−1 ± 13	−13 to 11	20	0
	G2	1 ± 8	-5 to 7	−10	10
8th session (before)	G1	103 ± 9	94 to 111	90	120
	G2	101 ± 22	82 to 120	70	120
8th session (after)	G1	101 ± 15	88 to 115	80	120
	G2	99 ± 22	80 to 117	70	120
8th session (after - before)	G1	−1 ± 9	−10 to 7	−20	10
	G2	−2 ± 5	−6 to 1	−10	0
Differ. 8th – 1st session	G1	30 ± 11	19 to 41	10	40
	G2	14 ± 11	5 to 23	0	30

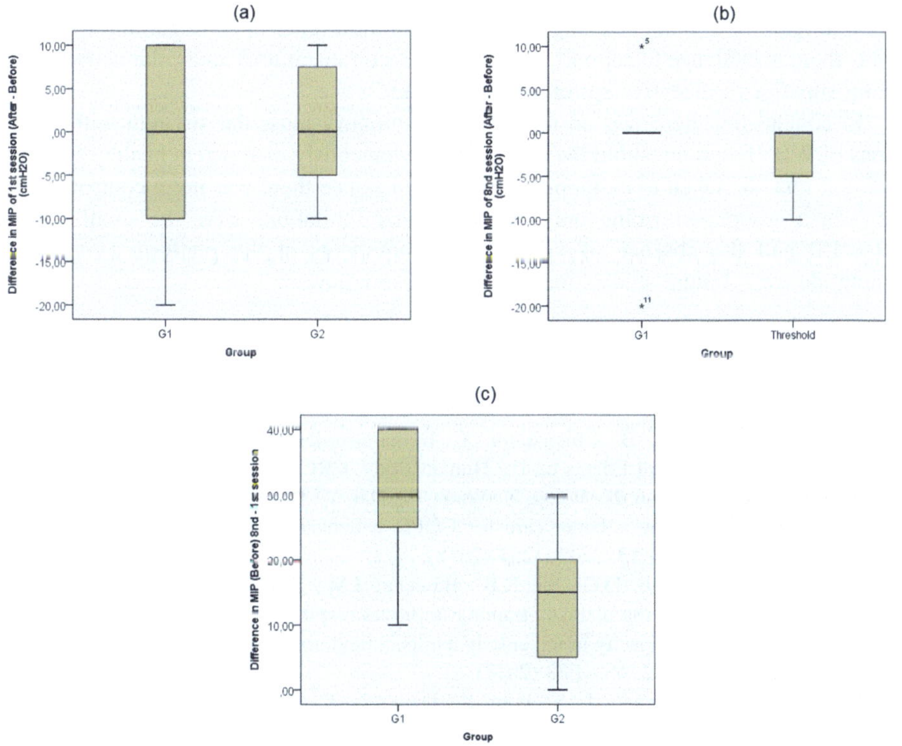

Fig. 2. Boxplots comparing G1 and G2: (a) the difference in MIP values (after – before) in the 1st session (p = 0.87); (b) the difference in MIP values (after – before) in the 8st session (p = 0.26); (c) the difference in MIP values (before) between sessions 8 and 1 (p = 0.02).

4 Discussion and Conclusions

There was no significant differences ($p > 0.05$) when comparing before and after intervention measurements in 1st and 8th sessions. One may say that the techniques did not lead to changes in muscular strength (mainly the diaphragm muscle) right after the intervention. For example, in the boxplot of G1 in Fig. 2(b) it is possible to observe that several subjects presented MIP differences of zero in the 8th session (no change in muscular strength) except for some outliers. However, when analyzing the baseline MIP values at the 1st and 8th sessions (see Table 1), a significant difference was observed (average value for G1 = 30 ± 11 cmH_2O; for G2 = 14 ± 11 cmH_2O; $p = 0.02$), suggesting that somehow both methods applied together may lead to an addictive effect.

WBVE are seen as an alternative or complementary training method in the last decades by several researchers and health professionals. It is becoming more popular each day, mainly by physical therapists, physical educators and trainers because of its effects on the neuromuscular system [8]. To our knowledge, this is the first study to propose the simultaneous application of WBVE and threshold inspiratory training.

The increase in muscular strength by mechanical vibration can be explained by the neurophysiologic mechanisms generated from vibration stimuli that drive neuromuscular spindles (mainly alpha), which leads to muscle contraction and increases muscle strength (similar to that occurring with tonic vibration reflex) [9]. Regarding threshold IMT, there is evidence to support its effectiveness on inspiratory muscular activity [10] being superior to incentive spirometry (Voldyne).

In conclusion, there was an increase in inspiratory muscular strength with 8 sessions of WBVE and threshold IMT applied simultaneously in apparent healthy females. Caution must be taken to extrapolate these results since there was not a control group, or even a group performing only WBVE. Other limitations were the small sample (N = 15) and the absence of vibration measurements at the platform (frequency, amplitude etc.). Future studies may address these issues.

References

1. Taiar, R., Machado, C.B., Chiementin, X., Bernardo-Filho, M.: Whole Body Vibrations: Physical and Biological Effects on the Human Body. CRC Press, Boca Raton (2018)
2. Zhou, J., Pang, L., Chen, N., Wang, Z., Wang, C., Hai, Y., Lyu, M., Lai, H., Lin, F.: Whole-body vibration training – better care for COPD patients: a systematic review and meta-analysis. Int. J. COPD **13**, 3243–3254 (2018)
3. Pessoa, M.F., Brandão, D.C., Sá, R.B., Barcelar, J.M., Rocha, T.D.S., Souza, H.C.M., Andrade, A.D.: Vibrating platform training improves respiratory muscle strength, quality of life, and inspiratory capacity in the elderly adults: a randomized controlled trial. J. Gerontol. Biol. Sci. Med. Sci. **72**, 683–688 (2017)
4. Gloeckl, R., Heinzelmann, I., Seeberg, S., Damisch, T., Hitzl, W., Kenn, K.: Effects of complementary whole-body vibration training in patients after lung transplantation: a randomized, controlled trial. J. Heart Lung Transplant. **34**, 1455–1461 (2015)

5. Wenninger, S., Greckl, E., Babačić, H., Stahl, K., Schoser, B.: Safety and efficacy of short- and long-term inspiratory muscle training in late-onset Pompe disease (LOPD): a pilot study. J. Neurol. **266**, 133–147 (2019)
6. Hartz, C.S., Sindorf, M.A.G., Lopes, C.R., Batista, J., Moreno, M.A.: Effect of inspiratory muscle training on performance of handball athletes. J. Hum. Kinet. **63**, 43–51 (2018)
7. Costa, T.R., Lima, T.P., Gontijo, P.L., Carvalho, H.A., Cardoso, F.P.F., Faria, O.P., Cavalcanti Neto, F.F.C.: Correlation of respiratory muscle strength with anthropometric variables of normal-weight and obese women. Rev. Assoc. Med. Bras. **56**, 403–408 (2010)
8. Marín, P.J., Múnera, M., García-Gutierrez, M.T., Rhea, M.R.: Effect of mechanical vibration on performance. In: Taiar, R., Machado, C.B., Chiementin, X., Bernardo-Filho, M.: Whole Body Vibrations: Physical and Biological Effects on the Human Body, p. 91. CRC Press, Boca Raton (2018)
9. Pessoa, M.F., Souza, H.C.M., Fuzari, H.K.B., Marinho, P.E.M., Andrade, A.D.: Effects of whole body vibration on the elderly. In: Taiar, R., Machado, C.B., Chiementin, X., Bernardo-Filho, M.: Whole Body Vibrations: Physical and Biological Effects on the Human Body, p. 102. CRC Press, Boca Raton (2018)
10. Paiva, D.N., Assmann, L.B., Bordin, D.F., Gass, R., Jost, R.T., Bernardo-Filho, M., França, R.A., Cardoso, D.M.: Inspiratory muscle training with threshold or incentive spirometry: which is the most effective? Port J. Pneumology **21**, 76–81 (2015)

Acute Responses of the Passive Whole-Body Vibration on Clinical Parameters of the COPD Individuals: Preliminary Outcomes

Laisa Liane Paineiras-Domingos[1,2,3(✉)], Eliane de Oliveira Guedes-Aguiar[1,3], Maria Eduarda S. Melo-Oliveira[1], Adriana Lírio[1], Tiago Eduardo-Santos[1], Diego Eduardo-Santos[1], Danúbia da Cunha Sá-Caputo[1,2,3], Arlete Francisca-Santos[1,3], Aline Reis-Silva[1,4], Redha Taiar[5], and Mario Bernardo-Filho[1]

[1] Laboratório de Vibrações Mecânicas e Práticas Integrativas, Departamento de Biofísica e Biometria, Instituto de Biologia Roberto Alcântara Gomes e Policlínica Américo Piquet Carneiro, Universidade do Estado do Rio de Janeiro, Rio de Janeiro, RJ, Brazil
laisanit@gmail.com

[2] Programa de Pós-Graduação em Ciências Médicas, Faculdade de Ciências Médicas, Universidade do Estado do Rio de Janeiro, Rio de Janeiro, RJ, Brazil

[3] Faculdade Bezerra de Araújo, Rio de Janeiro, RJ, Brazil

[4] Mestrado Profissional em Saúde, Medicina Laboratorial e Tecnologia Forense, Universidade do Estado do Rio de Janeiro, Rio de Janeiro, RJ, Brazil

[5] GRESPI, Research Group in Engineering Sciences, University of Reims Champagne-Ardenne, Reims, France

Abstract. COPD is characterized by persistent limitation in air flow, major chronic inflammation, associated with various local and systemic complications and high frequency of exacerbations, besides the skeletal muscle dysfunction. The passive whole-body vibration (pWBV) is perform when the individuals are exposed to WBV in the sitting position on an auxiliary chair placed in front of the vibrating platform (VP), with the foot position on the base of the VP. This prospective study aimed to show preliminary acute responses of the clinical parameters of the COPD individuals exposed to pWBV. 15 individuals were randomized and allocated into 2 groups: control group and group exposed to pWBV on alternating VP. The individuals were barefoot, 2.5 mm of the peak-to-peak displacement, 25 Hz of the frequency, 5 bouts, working time of 1 min interpased with a rest time of 1 min. Clinical parameters were assessment in the begin and after a single session. The GraphPad Prism 6.0 program was used and appropriate tests were applied ($p \leq 0.05$). Clinical parameters did not change after pWBV. The pWBV seem to benefit COPD individuals maintained clinical parameters, without exacerbation of the symptoms.

Keywords: Chronic obstructive pulmonary disease · Clinical parameters · Exacerbation · Mechanical vibration

T. Ahram et al. (Eds.): IHIET 2019, AISC 1018, pp. 644–649, 2020.
https://doi.org/10.1007/978-3-030-25629-6_100

1 Introduction

Chronic obstructive pulmonary disease is the variable combination of chronic bronchitis and emphysema, which share a common cause (cigarette smoking) and physiologic outcome (expiratory airflow obstruction). Various complications including dyspnea, malnutrition, dysfunction of skeletal muscles impairing functional capacity, impacting the quality of life and recurrent exacerbations are involving with the chronic nature and prevalence of the COPD leading to hospitalization and increased mortality [1].

For Goldestein *et al.* [2] there is a high level of evidence for the clinical relevant benefits of pulmonary rehabilitation (PR) in patients with COPD. Authors [3, 4] affirmed that he physical activity represents a major component of PR programs.

Whole-body vibration (WBV) exercises have been recommended as a modality of physical activity for many populations, included individuals with COPD [5]. For Gloeckl *et al.* [6], PR and WBV exercises may have enhanced exercise tolerance, and did not elicit exacerbations of the disease. WBV exercises are performed when individuals are exposed to mechanical vibration generated on a vibrating platform (VP) in operation, in contact with the base of this VP, standing with flexed joints [7] or in different positions [8, 9]. However for individuals with significant functional limitation and clinical compromise, WBV has been recommended passively (pWBV). The pWBV is defined as the action of mechanical vibration in individuals who are in contact with the VP in operation, in a seated posture with a chair positioned in front of the VP and the feet supported on the base. It is also recommended that these individuals place their hands on the knees, allowing a better propagation of the mechanical vibration [10].

Both WBV, performed actively on VP and pWBV can be considered as a therapeutic intervention strategy for individuals with COPD. This study aimed to evaluate acute effects of pMV on clinical parameters of this population.

2 Methods

2.1 Design

This prospective, randomized controlled and crossover trial was approved by an Ethics Committee (CAAE: 49219115.3.0000.5259). This study is in accordance with the principles expressed in the Declaration of Helsinki and all individuals must sign a consent form before any procedure.

Twenty-four COPD individuals, over 40 years, randomized and allocated into 2 groups: (1) control group (CG) with their normal daily routine, without exposure to WBV exercises; (2) group exposed to pWBV in the sitting position once a week (pWBVG) on side alternating VP. In the pWBVG, individuals were positioned seated in a chair placed in front of the VP with their hands resting on the knees and the feet on the base of the VP.

As inclusion criteria, individuals of (i) both sexes and (ii) outpatient at the *HUPE*, diagnosed with COPD based on criteria established by the GOLD with stable disease with Expiratory Volume Forced in the 1st Second (FEV1) < 50% and independents were considered. As exclusion criteria, individuals with exacerbation of the disease for less than 3 months; some diseases like labyrinthitis, osteoporosis, decompensated cardiovascular disease or other respiratory diseases; malnutrition; "fear" to the movements on the VP or serious or incapacitating clinical illness, at the decision of the investigator, were considered.

2.2 Intervention

The individuals were barefoot, the peak-to-peak displacement was 2.5 mm, frequency was 25 Hz, 5 bouts, with working time (WT) of 1 min interpased with a rest time (TR) of 1 min. The VP used was a Novaplate fitness evolution, *DAF Produtos Hospitalares Ltda*, from Estek As, *São Paulo,* Brazil.

The protocol was performed in three days: (1) in the first day, the individuals performed an evaluation with personal data reporting, (2) in the second day (acute session), only the pWBVG performed the VP. Before and after this single session, clinical parameters were evaluated and; (3) in the third day, the reassessment of the individuals was performed; the analysis and the tests of the first day were repeated.

2.3 Assessments of Clinical Parameters

For evaluate the clinical conditions were assessment: (1) the systolic blood pressure (SBP) and the diastolic blood pressure (DBP) (mmHg); (2) the heart rate (HR) (beats per min – bpm) and (3) the respiratory rate (RR). To determine the SBP, DBP and HR, in the begin and in the final of the session, an automated device was utilized (OMRON, model HEM-7113, China) [11]. The measurement was performed on the left arm of the individuals after a 5 min rest seated and with 1 min of rest was done in each measurement, for three times. The RR was evaluated during the intervals (rest) of the measurement of the SBP, DBP and HR. During this time (1 min), the evaluator observes the movement of the costal beds of individuals with COPD, sitting in a chair, facing the evaluator.

2.4 Sample Size and Data Analysis

For a statistical power of 95%, sample size of 13 subjects was calculated. The software used was the Graph Pad Prism 6.0. Normality data distribution was evaluated using the Shapiro-Wilk test. Wilcoxon test, for paried analysis and Mann–Whitney test, for unpaired analysis were applied later. The results were described as mean ± standard deviation (SD). The $p \leq 0.05$ was used for significance level.

3 Results

Twenty-four subjects were selected to participate in this study. However, after the baseline analysis, 09 subjects gave up participating in the study and were withdrawn. 15 were randomly allocated to CG (n = 8) and pWBVG (n = 7), as presented in the flowchart (Fig. 1).

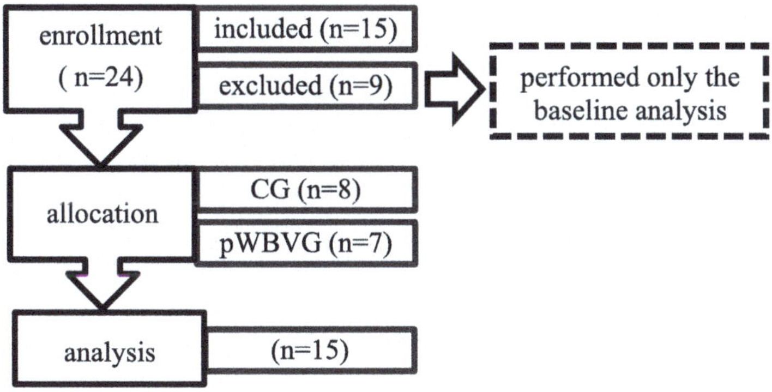

Fig. 1. Flowchart of this current study

Anthropometric data and clinical parameters: O2 saturation (SpO2), maximal inspiratory pressure (PImax), maximal expiratory pressure (PEmax), SBP, DBP, HR, RR) were assessment in the baseline and are presented in Table 1. There was no significant difference of any of these data, when compared the CG with the pWBVG individuals, confirming the homogeneity of the sample.

Table 1. Anthropometric data and baseline clinical parameter.

Baseline	CG (n = 8)	pMV G (n = 7)	*p* value
Age (years)	67.63 ± 11.49	69.29 ± 6.99	0.69
Mass (kg)	80.23 ± 16.83	82.06 ± 19.10	0.71
Height (cm)	1.62 ± 0.06	1.63 ± 0.06	0.70
Sp02 (%)	95.25 ± 2.12	93.14 ± 1.77	0.08
PImax (cmH2O)	−54.75 ± 26.68	−50.00 ± 36.97	0.67
PEmax (cmH2O)	78.13 ± 23.44	63.57 ± 24.28	0.19
SBP(mmHg)	115.3 ± 13.35	113 ± 9.89	0.92
DBP (mmHg)	64.87 ± 4.22	64.81 ± 4.48	0.99
HR (bpm)	84.71 ± 11.41	89.33 ± 10.10	0.39
RR (irpm)	21.29 ± 3.12	21.52 ± 3.31	0.59

CG - control group, pWBVG - passive WBV group, SpO2 - O2 saturation, PImax - maximal inspiratory pressure, PEmax - maximal expiratory pressure, SBP - systolic blood pressure, DBP - diastolic blood pressure, HR - heart rate, RR - respiratory rate, SD - standard deviation. Data express in mean ± SD. $p \leq 0.05$

3.1 Clinical Parameters

Table 2 shows the clinical parameters of the individuals in this study. There was no difference in the values ($p > 0.05$), comparing the values before and after the protocol.

Table 2. Analysis of the clinical parameters of the CG and pWBVG, before and after the single session.

	CG before	CG after	p#	pWBVG before	pWBVG after	p#	p
SBP (mmHg)	119.30 ± 13.08	126.60 ± 23.03	0.14	113.40 ± 12.26	123.10 ± 12.92	0.17	0.39
DBP (mmHg)	67.63 ± 5.90	72.71 ± 11.80	0.46	65.57 ± 5.39	67.29 ± 5.99	0.34	0.21
HR (bpm)	87.75 ± 10.65	87.43 ± 14.89	0.67	88.14 ± 9.40	86 ± 8.18	0.14	0.87
RR (irpm)	21.88 ± 3.09	22.57 ± 1.27	0.87	22.43 ± 4.35	23.43 ± 4.57	0.18	0.77

CG - control group, pWBVG - passive WBV group, SBP - systolic blood pressure, DBP - diastolic blood pressure, HR - heart rate, RR - respiratory rate, SD - standard deviation. P - p value. p# - intragroup. Data express in mean ± SD. $p \leq 0.05$

4 Discussion

This present study evaluated the acute effects on the clinical parameters of individuals with COPD undergoing pWBV. During the protocol no exacerbation of the symptoms was reported by the individuals. The clinical parameters did not altered after the protocol and a maintained of RR, can suggest the viability of this kind of exercise for individuals with COPD.

Furness *et al.* 2014, showed that WBV did not exacerbate symptoms of COPD that can be associated with physical inactivity. Comparing the combining squat exercises with WBV in patients with severe COPD, with the squat training without WBV, Gloeckl *et al.* [12], found that it did not affect ventilatory requirements, concluding that the WBV could be an effective, safe and feasible exercise modality in patients with stable severe COPD. Lage *et al.* [13], in an acute session, showed that the WBV can increase the cardiorespiratory responses in patients with COPD, no significant difference in cardiorespiratory parameters, reaching values similar to that of the control group.

5 Limitations

There are limitations of this study that should be considered. First, the sample size of COPD patients analyzed in this study is small (15), in contrast to the high number of dropouts (9). Second, there are additional situations to the diagnosis of COPD that may interfere with the results presented, and which were not adjusted as: gender, level of physical capacity and medications administered.

6 Conclusion

This research presented favorable results for the inclusion of pWBV in PR. The maintenance of clinical parameters suggests that this intervention is adequate and can be performed safely in COPD population. However, there is still no consensus on the most adequate protocol, considering biomechanical parameters, sample size, placements on the VP and the periodicity of the intervention.

References

1. Barnes, P.J., Celli, B.R.: Systemic manifestations and comorbidities of COPD. Eur. Respir. J. **33**, 1165–1185 (2009)
2. Goldstein, J., Plioplys, S., Zelko, F., Mass, S., Corns, C., Blaufuss, R., Nordli, D.: Multidisciplinary approach to childhood epilepsy: exploring the scientific rationale and practical aspects of implementation. J. Child Neurol. **19**(5), 362–378 (2004)
3. Ries, A.L., Bauldoff, G.S., Carlin, B.W., Casaburi, R., Emery, C.F., Mahler, D.A., Make, B., et al.: Pulmonary Rehabilitation: Joint ACCP/AACVPR Evidence-Based Clinical Practice Guidelines. Chest **131**(5 Suppl), 4S–42S (2007)
4. Spruit, M.A., Singh, S.J., Garvey, C., et al.: ATS/ERS task force on pulmonary rehabilitation, an official american thoracic society/european respiratory society statement: key concepts and advances in pulmonary rehabilitation. Am. J. Respir. Crit. Care Med. **189**(12), 1570 (2014)
5. Furness, T., Joseph, C., Naughton, G., Welsh, L., Lorenzen, C.: Benefits of whole-body vibration to people with COPD: a community-based efficacy trial. BMC Pulm. Med. **14**, 38 (2014). https://doi.org/10.1186/1471-2466-14-38
6. Gloeckl, R., Heinzelmann, I., Baeuerle, S., Damm, E., Schwedhelm, A., Diril, M., Buhrow, D., Jerrentrup, A., Kenn, K.: Effects of whole body vibration in patients with chronic obstructive pulmonary disease – a randomized controlled trial. Respir. Med. **106**(1), 75–83 (2012)
7. Paineiras-Domingos, L.L., da Cunha Sá-Caputo, D., Reis, A.S., Francisca Santos, A., Sousa-Gonçalves, C.R., Dos Anjos, E.M., Dos Santos Pereira, M.J., Sartorio, A., Bernardo-Filho, M.: Assessment through the short physical performance battery of the functionality in individuals with metabolic syndrome exposed to whole-body vibration exercises. Dose Response **16**(3), 1559325818794530 (2018). https://doi.org/10.1177/1559325818794530
8. Boeselt, T., Nell, C., Kehr, K., et al.: Whole-body vibration therapy in intensive care patients: a feasibility and safety study. J. Rehabil. Med. **48**, 316–321 (2016)
9. Chaves, J.R., Borges, D.L., Fortes, J.V.S., Vale, T.F.S., Borges, M.G.B., Silva, L.M., Sá-Caputo, D.C., Bernardo-Filho, M.: Study of the effect of whole body vibration exercise in cardiac surgery postoperative care: a protocol proposition. Braz. J. Health Biomed. Sci. **17**(1), 7–11 (2018). https://doi.org/10.12957/rhupe.2018.39167
10. Neto, S.B.S., Marconi, E.M., Kutter, C.R., Frederico, E.H.F., de Paiva, P.D.C., Meyer, P.F., Chang, S., Sá-Caputo, D., Bernardo-Filho, M.: Beneficial effects of whole body mechanical vibration alone or combined with auriculotherapy in the pain and in flexion of knee of individuals with knee osteoarthritis. Acupunct. Electrother. Res. **3**(4), 185–201 (2017)
11. Sá-Caputo, D.C., Paineiras-Domingos, L.L., Oliveira, R., Neves, M.F.T., Brandão, A., Marin, P.J., Sañudo, B., Furness, T., Taiar, R., Bernardo-Filho, M.: Acute effects of whole-body vibration on the pain level, flexibility, and cardiovascular responses in individuals with metabolic syndrome. Dose Response **16**(4), 1559325818802139 (2018). https://doi.org/10.1177/1559325818802139
12. Gloeckl, R., Richter, P., Winterkamp, S., Pfeifer, M., Nell, C., Christle, J.W., Kenn, K.: Cardiopulmonary response during whole-body vibration training in patients with severe COPD. ERJ Open Res. **3**(1), 00101–2016 (2017). https://doi.org/10.1183/23120541.00101-2016
13. Lage, V.K.S., Lacerda, A.C.R., Neves, C.D.C., Chaves, M.G.A., Soares, A.A., Lima, L.P., Matos, M.A., Leite, H.R., Fernandes, J.S.C., Oliveira, V.C., Mendonça, V.A.: Cardiorespiratory responses in different types of squats and frequencies of whole body vibration in patients with chronic obstructive pulmonary disease. J. Appl. Physiol. **126**(1), 23–29 (1985). https://doi.org/10.1152/japplphysiol.00406.2018

Effect of Vibration Exercise in the Modified Push-Up Position on Hand Neural Efficiency in Rheumatoid Arthritis: Preliminary Results

Ana Cristina Lacerda[1,2,3](✉), Ana Carolina Oliveira[1,2,3], Vanessa Mendonça[1,2,3], Luciana Martins Santos[1,3], Sueli F. Fonseca[1,3], Jousielle Marcia Santos[1,3], Vanessa G. Ribeiro[1,3], Angelica de Fatima Silva[1,2], Hercules R. Leite[1,2,3], Pedro Henrique Figueiredo[1,2,3], Fabio Martins[1,2], and Mario Bernardo-Filho[4]

[1] Universidade Federal dos Vales do Jequitinhonha e Mucuri (UFVJM), Diamantina, MG, Brazil
lacerdaacr@gmail.com

[2] Programa de Pós-Graduação em Reabilitação e Desempenho Funcional (PPGReab), Diamantina, MG, Brazil

[3] Centro Integrado de Pós-Graduação e Pesquisa em Saúde (CIPq-Saúde), Diamantina, MG, Brazil

[4] Universidade Estadual do Rio de Janeiro (UERJ), Rio de Janeiro, RJ, Brazil

Abstract. The aim of this study was to investigate a single session of whole-body vibration (WBV) exercise in the modified push-up position on hand neural efficiency (NE) in women with rheumatoid arthritis (RA). Twenty-one women with RA (diagnosis of disease: +8 years, erythrocyte sedimentation rate: +24.8, age: 54 $\pm$ 11 years, BMI: 28 $\pm$ 4 kg.m^{-2}) received three experimental tests for the upper limbs in a randomized cross-over clinical trial: Control, Placebo, and Vibration. Participants remained five minutes in each test. Before and immediately after the three experimental tests, the handgrip strength (HS) and electromyographic activity (EMG) of the flexor digitorum superficialis muscle of the dominant hand were measured for determination of the ratio between EMG and HS. Thus, the lower neuronal ratio represents the greater NE. This study suggests the WBV applied directly under the hands improves the hand NE in women with AR.

Keywords: Vibration · Neuronal ratio · Chronic disease

1 Introduction

Rheumatoid Arthritis (RA) causes progressive changes in the musculoskeletal system, compromising neuromuscular control, especially of the hands. In Brazil, the prevalence is 1–2%, and of two to three times higher in women, predominantly between the ages of 20 and 65 years [1]. Therapeutic strategies that enhance hand neural efficiency (NE) are important in the context of rehabilitation [2].

T. Ahram et al. (Eds.): IHIET 2019, AISC 1018, pp. 650–652, 2020.
https://doi.org/10.1007/978-3-030-25629-6_101

Whole-body vibration (WBV) exercise is a neuromuscular stimulus method that has recently received popularity in the health sector, local gyms, fitness and rehabilitation centers, as an additional or substitute method to conventional training and therapy [3], representing an alternative strategy for the treatment of patients diagnosed with chronic inflammatory diseases [4].

Few studies have investigated the effects of WBV in rheumatoid arthritis [5, 6], and only one study used the static modified push-up position to assess the effects of WBV on healthy subjects [7]. Therefore, the present study aimed to investigate a single session of whole-body vibration in the modified push-up position on hand NE in women with RA.

2 Methods

Ethics Committee of the Universidade Federal dos Vales do Jequitinhonha e Mucuri (N° 2.544.850). Clinical trial registry number (ReBEC: RBR-2n932c).

Twenty-one women with RA (diagnosis of disease: +8 years, erythrocyte sedimentation rate: +24.8, age: 54 ± 11 years, body mass index: 28 ± 4 $kg.m^{-2}$) received three experimental tests in a randomized cross-over clinical trial: (A) Control- Seated with feet on the floor and hands supine in the lower limbs without vibratory stimulus; (B) Placebo- Push-up with hands on the vibratory platform that remained disconnected, but with sound stimulus mimicking vibration; (C) Vibration- push-up with hands-on vibratory platform turned on (45 Hz/2 mm/159.73 $m.s^{-2}$). Participants remained five minutes in each test.

Before and immediately after the three experimental tests, the handgrip strength (HS) and electromyographic activity (EMG) of the flexor digitorum superficialis muscle (FSD) of the dominant hand were measured for determination of the ratio between EMG and HS. Thus, the lower ratio represents the greater hand NE.

Statistical analysis was performed by ANOVA two-way design mixed test, with Bonferroni post hoc. The level of significance was set at $p < 0.05$.

3 Results

Hand neuronal ratio was similar at baseline between experimental tests. Only the vibration decreased around 25% the neuronal ratio between-tests, indicating greater neural efficiency (Table 1).

Table 1. Effect of experimental tests on hand neuronal ratio (NR).

Variables	Control	Placebo	Vibration 45 Hz/2 mm	*Between-tests*			*Within-tests*			*Interaction*		
				p1	F	η^2	p2	F	η^2	p3	F	η^2
NR Baseline (%rms. Kg^{-1})	3.88(2.13)	3.68(2.21)	3.42(2.21)	0.008	5.520	0.79	0.067	3.739	0.56	0.022	4.208	0.15
NR After (%rms. Kg^{-1})	3.71(2.13)	3.63(2.28)	2.74(2.08)*#									

Whole-body vibration 45 Hz, 2 mm. Measures performed in the baseline and after the experimental tests. Data are presented as Mean (Standard Deviation). p1: Between-tests; p2: Within-tests; p3: Interaction. F values. Eta partial η2. N = 21 participants in each experimental test. *p < 0.05 to baseline; #p < 0.05 to experimental tests.

4 Conclusion

Whole body vibration applied directly under the hands improves the neural efficiency of the hands in women with Rheumatoid Arthritis.

Acknowledgments. CAPES, CNPq, FAPEMIG, UFVJM.

References

1. Sangha, O.: Epidemiology of rheumatic diseases. Rheumatology **39**, 3–12 (2000)
2. Bosco, C., Cardinale, M., Tsarpela, O.: Influence of vibration on mechanical power and electromyogram activity in human arm flexor muscles. Eur. J. Appl. Physiol. Occup. Physiol. **79**, 306–311 (1999)
3. Alam, M.M., Khan, A.A., Farooq, M.: Effect of whole-body vibration on neuromuscular performance: a literature review. Work **59**, 571–583 (2018)
4. Chanou, K., Gerodimos, V., Karatrantou, K., Jamurtas, A.: Whole-body vibration and rehabilitation of chronic diseases: a review of the literature. J. Sports Sci. Med. **11**, 187–200 (2012)
5. Prioreschi, A., Makd, M.A., Tikly, M., Mcveigh, J.A.: In patients with established RA, positive effects of a randomised three month WBV therapy intervention on functional ability, bone mineral density and fatigue are sustained for up to six months. PLoS ONE **11**, e0153470 (2016)
6. Prioreschi, A., Tikly, M., Mcveigh, J.A.: A three month controlled intervention of intermittent whole body vibration designed to improve functional ability and attenuate bone loss in patients with rheumatoid arthritis. BMC Musculoskelet. Disord. **15**, 403 (2014)
7. Ashnagar, Z., Shadmehr, A., Hadian, M., Talebian, S., Jalaei, S.: The effects of whole body vibration on EMG activity of the upper extremity muscles in static modified push up position. J. Back Musculoskelet. Rehabil. **29**, 557–563 (2016)

Effects of Whole-Body Vibration in Cardiorespiratory and Hormonal Parameters in Elderly People: Preliminary Results

Fabiana Angelica de Paula[1(✉)], Vanessa K. Lage[1], Guilherme P. Silva[1], Hellen C. Almeida[1], Liliana P. Lima[1], Joyce N. Santos[1], Anna Gabrielle Pinto[1], Daniela P. Castro[1], Camila F. Paixão[1], Ana Luiza Rodrigues[1], Hercules Ribeiro Leite[1], Ana Cristina Lacerda[1], Mario Bernardo-Filho[2], and Vanessa Mendonça[1]

[1] Universidade Federal dos Vales do Jequitinhonha e Mucuri – UFVJM, Diamantina, MG, Brazil
vaafisio@hotmail.com
[2] Universidade Estadual do Rio de Janeiro – UERJ, Rio de Janeiro, RJ, Brazil

Abstract. The aging process is accompanied by reduced muscle mass, referred to as sarcopenia, which contributes to fragility, loss of functional mobility, independence and mortality in the elderly. Although resistance exercises are preferred, whole body vibration exercise (WBV) has recently been introduced as an alternative training modality. Recent studies have demonstrated that the application of WBV in sarcopenic elderly improves bone mineral density, hormonal status, mobility, balance, reduction an prevention of falls and fractures. Thus, the present study aims to evaluate the cardiorespiratory and hormonal responses during the exercise of a dynamic squat with and WBV in the elderly population. The individuals who underwent both intervention protocols: squats with and without WBV. The exercise protocol was 40 Hz and 4 mm, with eight sets of the 40 s of exercise and rest. This study suggests that cardiorespiratory and hormonal responses after different types of exercise were similar in both groups.

Keywords: Whole-body vibration · Sarcopenia · Elderly

1 Introduction

Aging is accompanied by reduced muscle mass, referred to as sarcopenia [1] a complex, multifactorial, progressive, syndrome involving muscle, neural and hormonal changes. In Brazil, the overall prevalence of sarcopenia in the elderly was 17.0%, 20.0% in women and 12.0% in men [2].

Although resistance training is preferred, full-body vibration exercise (WBV) has recently been introduced as an alternative training modality capable of promoting gains in strength and lower limb power in young [3, 4] as well as in the elderly [5].

T. Ahram et al. (Eds.): IHIET 2019, AISC 1018, pp. 653–657, 2020.
https://doi.org/10.1007/978-3-030-25629-6_102

The whole-body vibration (WBV) training has been shown to be effective in producing neuromuscular adaptations, increased bone mineral density, improved postural control, changes in hormonal status, improved mobility and balance, as well as benefits related to physical function, reduction of falls and fractures in the elderly [6].

Thus, the present study aims to compare dynamic squat with and without WBV in sarcopenic elderly variables: heart rate (HR), cortisol and oxygen saturation (SPO_2).

2 Methods

Ethics Committee of the Universidade Federal dos Vales do Jequitinhonha e Mucuri with the number 2.282.653, the register in the Registro Brasileiro de Ensaios Clínicos (ReBEC).

This was a randomized crossover trial involving non-sarcopenic (n = 7) and sarcopenic (n = 11) individuals who underwent both intervention protocols: squats with and without WBV. The exercise protocol was 40 Hz and 4 mm, with eight sets of 40 s of exercise and rest. The participants were evaluated by Dual Energy Radiological Absormetry and performed physical strength tests of upper and lower limbs, respiratory and functional assessments.

Immediately before and after the test, systemic arterial pressure, heart rate (HR), oxygen saturation (SpO2), level of dyspnea and fatigue of the lower limbs (Borg Scale). Peripheral blood samples were collected before and after the situations (with and without vibration).

Data were analyzed for mean, standard deviation and delta. In the statistical analysis were used independent T-test or Mann-Whitney and the interaction by ANOVA two away for repeated measures and Person or Spearman correlation. The significance considered was $p \leq 0.05$.

3 Results

The characteristics of the participants at the beginning of the study are shown in Table 1 and the results of the analysis of the effects of the WBV exercise on the variables evaluated are presented in Table 2 and correlations hormonal parameters and functionality Fig. 1.

Table 1. Clinical, demographic and functional characteristics of participants.

Variable	Non-sarcopenic (n = 07)	Sarcopenic (n = 11)	*p*-value
Age (years)	75.3 ± 7.1	72.3 ± 8.3	0.4411
BMI (kg/m^2)	26.7 ± 2.7	20.7 ± 2.3	0.0001*
WC (cm)	94.1 ± 9.0	75.9 ± 8.0	0.0003*
BF (%)	32.1 ± 6.7	30.9 ± 9.6	0.7825
FFM (kg)	42.7 ± 5.8	32.2 ± 5.5	0.0013*
BMD (g/cm^2)	1.107 ± 0.16	0.926 ± 0.12	0.0170*
RSMI (g/m^2)	7.5 ± 0.6	5.6 ± 0.4	0.0001*
6MWT (m)	501.7 ± 67.8	433.7 ± 82.6	0.0880
SPPB	10.5 ± 1.1	9.5 ± 1.5	0.1435
5STS (sec)	8.5 ± 1.9	11.7 ± 2.4	0.0041*
GS (m/s^2)	1.801 ± 0.3	1.377 ± 0.4	0.0224*
MIP$^{(\#)}$ (cmH_2O)	84.3 ± 32.0	40.0 ± 12.2	0.0006*
HGS (Kg)	34.1 ± 7.9	26.0 ± 7.9	0.0536
MMSE	26.4 ± 1.7	22.0 ± 5.3	0.0502

Abbreviations: BMI (Body mass index), WC (waist circumference), BF (Body fat), FFM (Fat free mas), BMD (bone mineral density), RSMI (relative skeletal muscle index), 6MWT (6-minute walk test), SPPB (Short Physical Performance Battery), 5STS (Sit and stand up), GS (Gait speed), MIP (Maximal inspiratory pressure), MMSE (Mini-Mental State Examination), HGS (Handgrip strength). Values are means ±SD or number. Independent Test- t. Statistical significance P < 0,05. $^{\#}$ n = 8

Table 2. Variation of hormonals and cardiorespiratory parameters before and after exercise of (WBV) or squat in groups sarcopenic (n = 11) and non-sarcopenic (n = 07)

Variable	Non-sarcopenic WBV	Sarcopenic WBV	Non-sarcopenic Squat	Sarcopenic Squat	P
Δ HR	10.3 ± 2.3	9.3 ± 6.6	1.4 ± 4.0	5.0 ± 4.4	0.18
Δ SPO_2	1.3 ± 1.1	−0.09 ± 0.8	−0.5 ± 2.0	−0.6 ± 1.8	0.21
ΔTestosterone Male$^{\#a}$	11.2 ± 34.9	−1.6 ± 38.5	0.8 ± 41.4	−16.6 ± 67.1	0.92
ΔTestosterone Female$^{\#b}$	2.0 ± 2.8	−4.1 ± 4.9	−3.5 ± 4.9	−7.7 ± 12.6	0.86
Δ Cortisol	0.5 ± 3.5	−1.9 ± 2.3	−1.3 ± 1.5	−0.3 ± 7.3	0.27

Abbreviations: HR (Heart Rate), SPO_2 (Oxygen saturation). Mean ± SD. Independent t test. ANOVA two-way. *Statistical significance (P < 0.05). $^{\#a}$ non-sarcopenic = 5 and sarcopenic = 3; $^{\#b}$ non-sarcopenic = 2 and sarcopenic = 8

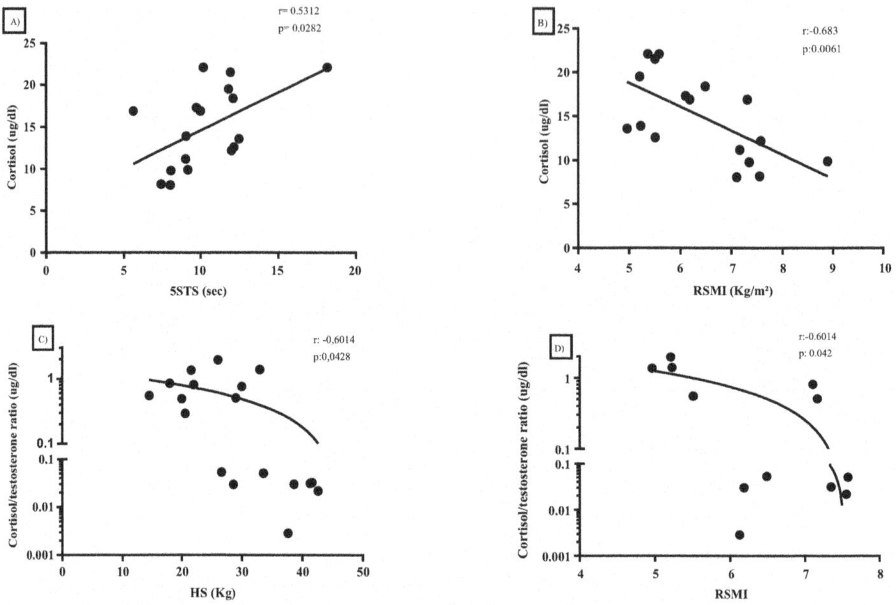

Fig. 1. Correlation between cortisol and 5STS (p = 0.0282) (A) and RMSI, (p = 0.0061) (B). Correlation between cortisol/testosterone ratio with handgrip strength (p = 0.0191) (C) and RSMI (p = 0.042) (D).

4 Conclusion

The results of this study are still preliminary, and we observed that elderly patients with sarcopenia presented worse body composition and functional performance however, cardiorespiratory and hormonal responses after different types of exercise were similar in the groups.

Acknowledgements. CNPq, FAPEMIG (APQ- 01328-18), CAPES, UFVJM.

References

1. Almeida Fechine, B.R. Trompieri, N.: O processo de envelhecimento: as principais alterações que acontecem com o idoso com o passar dos anos. InterSciencePlace (2012)
2. Diz, J.B.M., Leopoldino, A.P.O., Moreira, B.S., Henschke, N., Dias, R.C., Pereira, L.S.M., Oliveira, V.C.: Prevalence of sarcopenia in older Brazilians: a systematic review and meta-analysis. Geriatr. Gerontol. Int. **17**, 5–16 (2017)
3. Sehl, M.E., Yates, F.E.: Kinetics of human aging: I. Rates of senescence between ages 30 and 70 years in healthy people. J Gerontol. A Biol. Sci. Med. Sci. **56**, 198–208 (2001)
4. Delecluse, C., Roelants, M., Verschueren, S.: Strength increase after whole-body vibration compared with resistance training. Med. Sci. Sports Exerc. **35**(6), 1033–1041 (2003)

5. Petit, P.D., PensinI, M., Tessaro, J., Desnuelle, C., Legros, P., Colson, S.S.: Optimal whole-body vibration settings for muscle strength and power enhancement in human knee extensors. J. Electromyogr. Kinesiol. Off. J. Int. Soc. Electrophysiol. Kinesiol. **20**, 1186–1195 (2010)
6. Machado, A., García-López, D., González-Gallego, J., Garatachea, N.: Whole-body vibration training increases muscle strength and mass in older women: a randomized controlled trial. Scand. J. Med. Sci. Sports **20**, 200–207 (2010)

Effects of Whole-Body Vibration Exercises on the Body Fat Distribution of the Metabolic Syndrome Individuals: Preliminary Outcomes

Aline Reis-Silva[1,2,3], Eliane de Oliveira Guedes-Aguiar[1,2], Laisa Liane Paineiras-Domingos[1,4,5], Arlete Francisca-Santos[1,4], Adriana Lírio[1], Cristiano Bittencourt Machado[6], Ana Cristina Lacerda[7], Vanessa Amaral Mendonça[8(✉)], Anelise Sonza[9], Adérito Seixas[10], Redha Taiar[11], Mario Bernardo-Filho[1], and Danúbia da Cunha Sá-Caputo[1,4,5]

[1] Laboratório de Vibrações Mecânicas e Práticas Integrativas, Departamento de Biofísica e Biometria, Instituto de Biologia Roberto Alcântara Gomes e Policlínica Américo Piquet Carneiro, Universidade do Estado do Rio de Janeiro, Rio de Janeiro, RJ, Brazil

[2] Mestrado Profissional em Saúde, Medicina Laboratorial e Tecnologia Forense, Instituto de Biologia Roberto Alcantara Gomes, Universidade do Estado do Rio de Janeiro, Rio de Janeiro, RJ, Brazil

[3] Hospital de Força Aérea do Galeão (HFAG), Rio de Janeiro, Brazil

[4] Faculdade Bezerra de Araújo, Rio de Janeiro, RJ, Brazil

[5] Programa de Pós-Graduação em Ciências Médicas, Faculdade de Ciências Médicas, Universidade do Estado do Rio de Janeiro, Rio de Janeiro, RJ, Brazil

[6] Universidade Estácio de Sá University, Niterói, Brazil

[7] Centro Integrado de Pós-graduação e Pesquisa em Saúde (CIPq-Saúde), Universidade Federal dos Vales do Jequitinhonha e Mucuri, Diamantina, MG, Brazil

[8] Laboratório de Inflamação e Metabolismo (LIM), Universidade Federal dos Vales do Jequitinhonha e Mucuri, Diamantina MG, Brazil

vaafisio@hotmail.com

[9] Departamento de Fisioterapia, Universidade do Estado de Santa Catarina, UDESC, Florianópolis, Brazil

[10] Escola Superior de Saúde, Universidade Fernando Pessoa, Porto, Portugal

[11] GRESPI, Moulin de la Housse, Université de Reims Champagne Ardenne, 51687 Reims Cedex 2, France

Abstract. Metabolic syndrome (MetS) is a public health problem that including risk factors, such as central obesity, hypertension, insulin resistance and dyslipidemia. Inadequate reserve of fat promotes a redistribution of free fatty acids to other tissues such as muscle and viscera, increasing metabolic risks. Studies have shown the association of subcutaneous and visceral fat with cardiovascular risk factors, oxidative stress and atherosclerosis. This population has a resistant profile both to start and to maintain an exercise routine. Whole-body vibration exercises (WBVE) can be considered as physical exercise. The aim of the present study was to analyze the effect of WBVE on body composition in MetS individuals. WBVE participants trained 2 times per week for 6 weeks at the vibratory platform (alternating) with frequency from 5 Hz up to 16 Hz

T. Ahram et al. (Eds.): IHIET 2019, AISC 1018, pp. 658–664, 2020.
https://doi.org/10.1007/978-3-030-25629-6_103

which peak to peak displacement of 2.5/5.0/7.5 mm. This study suggest that WBVE can improve percentage segmental body fat in MetS individuals.

Keywords: Whole body vibration · Metabolic syndrome · Body composition

1 Introduction

Metabolic syndrome (MetS) is a public health problem that including risk factors, such as central obesity, hypertension, insulin resistance and dyslipidemia. According to International Diabetes Federation (IDF), obesity seems to be fundamental to the development of MetS. The diagnosis is made through by increasing abdominal circumference plus two other conditions as: hypertension, high triglycerides, hyperglycemia or low cholesterol high density [1]. The MetS is associated with increased of cardiovascular risk, different types of cancers including breast, pancreatic, colon and mortality [2].

The accumulation of adipose tissue in abdominal region has been associated with metabolic disturbances [3]. Excess of subcutaneous and visceral adipose tissue can contribute to abdominal obesity, but they differ in metabolic activity and structural composition. Positive caloric balance in individuals with impaired adipogenesis can result in adipocyte hypertrophy, energy storage impairment and adipose tissue dysfunction subcutaneous [4]. This inadequate reserve of fat promotes a redistribution of free fatty acids to other tissues such as muscle and viscera, increasing metabolic risks [5].

The increased of total fat mass has been significantly associated with glucose intolerance, insulin resistance, risks to diabetes mellitus type II and cardiovascular disease (CVD) [6]. This inflammatory changes in adiposity tissue can promote a chronic inflammation strongly associated with systemic metabolic disorder [7].

The treatment of MetS individuals consists in lifestyle modifications, including calorie restriction diet and exercises. Changes in lifestyle can favor a positively effect on the prevalence of cardiovascular risk factors in these individuals. The benefits of regular exercises are well established for prevention and treatment of many non-communicable chronic diseases as obesity (that is strongly related to MetS). [8].

These positives effects may modify single metabolic risk factors i.e. Insulin resistance, hypertension, hyperlipidaemia and improve the body composition [9].

However, this population has a sedentary habits and resistant profile both to start and to maintain an exercise routine [10].

Whole-body vibration exercise (WBVE) is considered as a type of exercise that can be considered as easy, feasible and safe [11]. WBVE promotes rapid stimuli that modify the length of the tendon muscle complex, generating an eccentric-concentric continuous muscle work and reflexive muscle contractions [12].

WBVE is produced when the individual is in direct contact with the base of vibratory platform (VP) in working. To establish a WBVE protocol, it is necessary to adjust some biomechanical parameters, as: frequency, expressed in hertz (Hz), peak-to-peak displacement, expressed in millimeter (mm) and peak acceleration, expressed as a multiple of standard gravity (g). In addition to the biomechanical parameters, it is necessary to establish the positioning, type of exercise (static or dynamic), number of bouts, working time and rest [13].

Studies have reported that WBVE could reduce accumulation of fat mass and adipogenesis in rats [14]. In humans, Nam *et al.* 2016 reported that WBVE was effective as aerobic exercises in reduction of fat mass when associated with hypocaloric diet [15]. Milanese *et al.* 2012, founded a significant decrease in body fat mass without changes in body weight after 8 weeks of WBVE [16]. However, Tapp *et al.* 2014, no founded changes in the body composition after 8 weeks of WBVE [17].

Authors have been demonstrated effects in the WBVE in MetS individuals. Sá-Caputo *et al.* 2018, founded significant changes on the flexibility, gait speed, lower limb and handgrip strength after 5 weeks of WBVE [18]. Carvalho-Lima *et al.* 2017, observed that a WBVE protocol (one or two times per weeks) can improves the quality of life in MetS individuals [19]. The aim of this study was to evaluate the segmental body fat mass of the MetS individuals performed WBVE.

2 Materials and Methods

This study was performed according to Declaration of Helsinki and was approved by the Research Ethics Committee of the *Hospital Universitário Pedro Ernesto* of the *Universidade do Estado do Rio de Janeiro* (HUPE/UERJ) with the number CAAE 54981315.6.0000.5259, the register in the *Registro Brasileiro de Ensaios Clínicos* (ReBEC) with the number RBR 2bghmh and UTN: U1111–1181-1177.

2.1 Individuals

Six individuals participated of the study. They were recruited from of the *Ambulatório de Clínica Médica*, in the HUPE-UERJ with MetS diagnosis, according IDF criteria. All individuals signed the consent form. The inclusion criteria were females or males older than 18 years of age with diagnostic of MetS according to IDF. The exclusion criteria were individuals with very high blood pressure levels ($\geq 180 \times 110$ mmHg), cardiovascular disease and conditions that not permitted the correct position on the vibratory platform (VP).

Participants were instructed to be continue their lifestyle during the study.

2.2 Study Design

WBVE Protocol

The platform used in the study was an alternating vibratory platform (Novaplate fitness evolution, DAF Produtos Hospitalares Ltda, São Paulo, Brazil). The individuals were positioned barefoot, in a stand position with 130° of knee flexion. Individuals performed squat static and dynamic squat in intercalated sessions. Biomechanical parameters used were: (i) peak-to-peak displacement (D) -2.5, 5 and 7.5 mm, (ii) frequency - 5 Hz in the first session, increasing 1 Hz per session, up to 16 Hz in the last session. The sequence of WBV was performed following: (I) 1 min of work time in the D 2.5 mm, followed by 1 min of rest; (II) 1 min of work time in the D 5 mm, followed by 1 min of rest, (III) 1 min of work time in the D 7.5 mm, followed by 1 min of rest. This sequence was performed 3 times in the (1–4 session), 4 times in the (5–8 session) and 5 times in the (9–2 session). The force g used during the protocol ranged from 0.13 g a 3.86 g. The protocol was performed during 6 weeks, twice a week.

Position of the individuals during the protocol: barefoot, second finger (anatomical point of force distribution) in the direction of established peak-to-peak displacement; knee flexion of 130°; trunk straight; hands lightly supported on the sidebar of the VP; head in neutral position, keeping staring straight ahead; semi static squat (130° knee flexion) and dynamic (1 squat every 3 s).

Clinical Measures
The anthropometric measures: height, waist circumference (WC), neck circumference (NC), and cardiovascular parameters (blood pressure and heart rate) were measured before and after the protocol.

The height was measured with participants standing erect, back straight, heels together, without shoes to the 0.1 cm with a stadiometer (MIC 200 micheletti, São Paulo, Brazil). The WC was measured as the narrowest point between the lower costal border and the iliac crest using a non-elastic tape. The NC was measured using a non-elastic type, with increments down to 0.1 cm, with the individual at erect position and the tape was placed just below the laryngeal prominence.

Blood pressure and heart rate is checked before and at the end of each session.

Multi-frequency bioelectrical impedance analysis (BIA) was assessed using the In Body 370-Korea equipment, in accordance with the previous guidelines regarding the preparation before the first and after the last WBVE session. It was performed to estimate waist-hip ratio, body mass index (BMI), body mass, segmental fat mass (left upper limb, right upper limb, trunk, left lower limb and right lower limb).

2.3 Simple Size

The body mass parameter was used for the sample calculation, with a standard deviation of (1, 9), a maximum error of estimation of 1 and a level of significance of 5% [16]. According to the calculation, the sample size of 14 individuals for each group [20].

2.4 Statistical Analysis

The Prism 6 Software (GraphPad Inc., USA) was used with appropriate statistical tests. The significance considered was $p \leq 0.05$.

3 Results

The characteristics of the participants in the baseline are demonstrated in the Table 1.

Table 1. Characteristics of participants

Variable	WBVE (M ± SD)
Age (years)	57.6 ± 14.15
Height (cm)	1.628 ± 00.14
Body mass (kg)	81.46 ± 15.33
WHR	0.964 ± 00.04

(continued)

Table 1. (*continued*)

BMI (kg/m^2)	30.48 ± 02.21
WC (cm)	104.2 ± 08.46
NC (cm)	38.15 ± 03.06

Abbreviations: BMI (body mass index); WHR (waist to hip ratio); WC (waist circumference); NC (neck circumference); Values expressed with median (M) standard deviation (SD).

The results concerning the effects of WBVE on body composition are presented in Table 2. Following 6 weeks of WBVE, percentage segmental fat mass on left upper limb was reduced ($p \leq 0.05$).

Table 2. Effects of WBVE on body composition

	WBVE		
Variables	Pre	Post	p
Segmental fat (%)	**M ± SD**	**M ± SD**	
LUL	53.60 ± 2.28	52.80 ± 2.73	**0.016***
RUL	52.60 ± 2.42	51.70 ± 2.80	0.063
Trunk	46.10 ± 1.98	46.00 ± 2.87	0.156
LLL	43.40 ± 2.91	42.60 ± 3.96	0.078
RLL	43.50 ± 2.89	42.50 ± 3.99	0.156
Segmental fat (kg)	**M ± SD**	**M ± SD**	
LUL	3.70 ± 1. 1 4	3.70 ± 1.20	0.062
RUL	3.50 ± 0.63	3.30 ± 0.63	0.406
Trunk	19.80 ± 1.80	20.30 ± 2.17	0.844
LLL	5.60 ± 0.75	5.00 ± 0.75	0.156
RLL	5.70 ± 0.80	5.00 ± 0.75	0.125

Abbreviations: LUL (left upper limb), RUL (right upper limb), LLL (left lower limb), and RLL (right lower limb); (M) Median and (SD) Standard Deviation
*p < 0,05

4 Discussion

The aim of the present study was to analyse the effect of WBVE on body composition in MetS individuals. This study demonstrates that 6 weeks of WBVE protocol can reduce fat mass of these individuals. Until the present moment, this is the first study about the effects WBVE on body composition of these population.

Some studies demonstated the effects of WBVE in obese individuals on the profile of body composition. Sang-seok Nam et al. (2016) suggested that long term WBVE combined with hypocaloric diet was effective like the association of diet with aerobic exercises on the improvement of fat mass in obese individuals [15]. Sañudo *et al.* (2018) also verified significant reduction of fat mass only in the vibration group associated with diet and high interval training after the 8 weeks in obese adults [21].

However, other studies did not identify significant changes in fat mass. Stengel *et al.* 2012, observed changes in body fat but there was no difference when comparing the group that performed WBVE and exercises and the group of only exercises for 18 months in postmenopausal women [22]. Roelants *et al.* 2004, did not found significant changes in total body fat mass and subcutaneous after a 24-week WBVE protocol in untrained females [23]. Rubio-Arias *et al.* 2015 investigated the segmental body fat, using 6 weeks of WBVE in healthy individuals and also did not found significant results [24].

There are some limitations in this study. The number of individuals who completed the protocol was small. The caloric intake and balanced caloric intake diet were not verified.

5 Conclusion

The results of this study are still preliminary, but a significant decrease in percentage fat mass in the left upper limb was observed. According to the outcome of the study, WBVE seems to be benefic to lead modifications on the body composition of individuals with MetS.

References

1. Ford, E.S.: Prevalence of the metabolic syndrome defined by the IDF in the U.S. Diabetes Care **28**, 2745–2749 (2005)
2. Shin, J.A., Lee, J.H., et al.: Metabolic syndrome as a predictor of type 2 diabetes, and its clinical interpretations and usefulness. J Diabetes Investig. **4**, 334–343 (2013)
3. Park, J., Lee, E.S., et al.: Waist circumference as a marker of obesity is more predictive of coronary artery calcification than body mass index in apparently healthy Korean adults. Endocrinol. Metab. **31**, 559–566 (2016)
4. Bays, H.E., et al.: Pathogenic potential of adipose tissue and metabolic consequences of adipocyte hypertrophy and increased visceral adiposity. Expert Rev. Cardiovasc. **6**, 343–368 (2008)
5. Tan, C.Y., Vidal-Puig, A.: Adipose tissue expandability: the metabolic problems of obesity may arise from the inability to become more obese. Biochem. Soc. Trans. **36**, 935–940 (2008)
6. Neeland, I.J., Turer, A.T., et al.: Dysfunctional adiposity and the risk of prediabetes and type 2 diabetes in obese adults. JAMA **308**(11), 1150–1159 (2012)
7. Sell, H., Habich, C., Eckel, J.: Adaptive immunity in obesity and insulin resistance. Nat. Rev. Endocrinol. **8**(12), 709–716 (2012)

8. Bayley, A., de Zoysa, N., et al.: Comparing the effectiveness of an enhanced motivational interviewing intervention (MOVE IT) with usual care for reducing cardiovascular risk in high risk subjects: study protocol for a randomized controlled trial. Trials. **16**, 112 (2015)
9. Pedersen, B.K., Saltin, B.: Exercise as medicine - evidence for prescribing exercise as therapy in 26 different chronic diseases. Scand. J. Med. Sci. Sports **25**, 1–72 (2015)
10. Pedersen, B.K., Saltin, B.: Exercise as medicine - evidence for prescribing exercise as therapy in 26 different chronic diseases. Scand. J. Med. Sci. Sports **20**(25 Suppl 3), 1–72 (2015)
11. Zago, M., Capodaglio, P., et al.: Whole-body vibration training in obese subjects. A systematic review. PLoS ONE **13**(9), e0202866 (2018)
12. Rauch, F., Sievanen, H., et al.: Reporting whole-body vibration intervention studies: recommendations. J. Musculoskelet. Neuronal Interact. **10**, 193–198 (2010)
13. Rittweger, J.: Vibration as an exercise modality: how it may work, and what its potential might be. Eur. J. Appl. Physiol. **108**, 877–904 (2010)
14. Maddalozzo, G.F., Iwaniec, U.T., et al.: Whole-body vibration slows the acquisition of fat in mature female rats. Int. J. Obes. **32**, 1348–1354 (2008)
15. Nam, S.-S., Sunoo, S., et al.: The effects of long-term whole-body vibration an aerobic exercise on body composition and bone mineral density in obese middle-aged women. J. Exerc. Nutr. Biochem. **20**, 19–27 (2016)
16. Milanese, C., Piscitelli, F., et al.: Ten-week whole-body vibration training improves body composition and muscle strength in obese women. Int. J. Med. Sci. **10**, 307–311 (2013)
17. Tapp, L.R., Signorile, J.F.: Efficacy of WBV as a modality for inducing changes in body composition, aerobic fitness, and muscular strength. Clin. Interventions Aging **9**, 63–72 (2014)
18. Sá-Caputo, D., et al.: Whole-body vibration improves the functional parameters of individuals with metabolic syndrome: an exploratory study. BMC Endocr. Disord. **19**, 6 (2019)
19. Carvalho-Lima, R.P., Sá-Caputo, D.C., et al.: Quality of life of patients with metabolic syndrome is improved after whole body vibration exercises. Afr. J. Tradit. Complement. Altern. Med. **14**(4 Suppl), 59–65 (2017)
20. Tamanho de amostra – Lee. http://www.lee.dante.br/cgi-bin/uncgi/calculo_amostra
21. Sañudo, B., Munõz, T., et al.: High-intensity interval training combined with vibration and dietary restriction improves body composition and blood lipids in obese adults: a randomized trial. Dose Response **16**, 3 (2018)
22. Von Stengel, S., Kemmler, W., Kalender, W.A., et al.: Effect of whole-body vibration on neuromuscular performance and body composition for females 65 years and older: a randomized controlled trial. Scand. J. Med. Sci. Sports **22**(1), 119–127 (2012)
23. Roelants, M., Delecluse, C., et al.: Effects of 24 weeks of whole-body vibration training on body composition and muscle strength in untrained females. Int. J. Sports Med. **25**, 1–5 (2004)
24. Rubio-Arias, J.A., Esteban, P., et al.: Effect of 6 weeks of whole body vibration training on total and segmental body composition in healthy young adults. Acta Physiol. Hung. **102**(4), 442–450 (2015)

Effects of Passive Whole-Body Vibration and Auriculotherapy on the Surface Electromyographic Pattern of the Vastus Lateralis Right Muscle in Individuals with Knee Osteoarthritis

Eloá Moreira-Marconi[1,2], Adriana Lírio[1(✉)], Marcia Cristina Moura-Fernandes[1,2], Alexandre Meirelles[1,3], Tânia Lemos Santos[1], Luiz Felipe Ferreira de Souza[1], Maria Eduarda S. Melo-Oliveira[1,3], Renata Marchon[1,3], Ygor Teixeira Silva[1,4], Patrícia Lopes-Souza[1,4], Arlete Francisca-Santos[1,5], Aline Reis-Silva[1,3,8], Eliane de Oliveira Guedes-Aguiar[1,5], Laisa Liane Paineiras-Domingos[1,4,5], Danúbia da Cunha Sá-Caputo[1,4,5], Adérito Seixas[6], Borja Sañudo[7], and Mario Bernardo-Filho[1]

[1] Laboratório de Vibrações Mecânicas e Práticas Integrativas, Departamento de Biofísica e Biometria, Instituto de Biologia Roberto Alcântara Gomes e Policlínica Américo Piquet Carneiro, Universidade do Estado do Rio de Janeiro, Rio de Janeiro, RJ, Brazil
eloamarconi@gmail.com, adrianaliriolavimpi@gmail.com

[2] Pós-Graduação em Fisiopatologia Clínica e Experimental, Universidade do Estado do Rio de Janeiro, Rio de Janeiro, Brazil

[3] Mestrado Profissional em Saúde, Medicina Laboratorial e Tecnologia Forense, Instituto de Biologia Roberto Alcantara Gomes, Universidade do Estado do Rio de Janeiro, Rio de Janeiro, RJ, Brazil

[4] Programa de Pós-Graduação em Ciências Médicas, Faculdade de Ciências Médicas, Universidade do Estado do Rio de Janeiro, Rio de Janeiro, RJ, Brazil

[5] Faculdade Bezerra de Araújo, Rio de Janeiro, RJ, Brazil

[6] Escola Superior de Saúde, Universidade Fernando Pessoa, Porto, Portugal

[7] Departamento de Educación Física y Deporte, Universidad de Sevilla, Seville, Spain

[8] Hospital de Força Aérea do Galeão (HFAG), Rio de Janeiro, Brazil

Abstract. Knee osteoarthritis (KOA) is a cause of public disability, mainly in elderly. The management of KOA symptoms requires a combination of conservative interventions for the joint, including both pharmacological and non-pharmacological strategies. The analysis of the surface electromyographic pattern (sEMG) of the Vastus lateralis right(VLR) muscle may increase the understanding of some functions that are impaired by KOA and investigate if passive whole-body vibration (pWBV) or auriculotherapy (AT) increases the neuromuscular activity in these individuals. This study aimed to evaluate the effect (immediate and cumulative effects of a 5-week intervention). The immediate and

T. Ahram et al. (Eds.): IHIET 2019, AISC 1018, pp. 665–671, 2020.
https://doi.org/10.1007/978-3-030-25629-6_104

cumulative effects of the interventions on the sEMG behavior of the VLR muscle were evaluated in all participants. AT, alone or combined with pWBV, significantly increased the recruitment of muscle fibers after 5 weeks of intervention in KOA patients.

Keywords: Knee osteoarthritis · passive Whole Body Vibration · Auriculotherapy · Electromyographic

1 Introduction

Knee osteoarthritis (KOA) is the most prevalent form of arthritis [1]. Cartilage degradation with joint space narrowing, bone remodeling, *formation* of new *bone* at the *joints* margins (*osteophytes*), reduced muscle strength, swelling, stiffness, joint inflammation and loss of normal joint function may be present in patients with KOA [2–6]. Neuromuscular function is highly relevant in the development and/or progression of KOA [7] and as it was reviewed by Mills et al. [8] neuromuscular alterations in muscle amplitude and muscle activity have been reported Therefore, the analysis of the surface electromyography (sEMG) plays an important role to understand changes in neuromuscular function that are impaired in the KOA individuals [9]. Whole body vibration (WBV) [10] or other alternative therapeutic techniques related to the Traditional Chinese Medicine, including acupuncture [11] and auriculotherapy (AT) [12–14], have been used to induce clinical benefits in KOA individuals (i.e., auriculotherapy). Therefore, the aim of this study was to determine the effectiveness (*Vastus lateralis* right muscle activation) of these non-pharmacological interventions (WBV and AT) on different functional tests.

2 Materials and Methods

This study was approved by local Ethics Committee in Research and clinical trial registration (*CAAE* - 19826413.8.0000.5259 and RBR-7dfwct, respectively).

As inclusion criteria the subjects should be 40 years old or more, with clinical diagnosis of KOA according to the criteria established by Ahlback and should sign the declared informed consent [15]. Exclusion criteria included the presence of other musculoskeletal disorders, neurological diseases and uncontrolled hypertension. Participants who declined to sign the were also excluded.

One hundred thirteen participants with KOA diagnosis were allocated in six groups: (a) pWBV group, (b) AT group, (c) WBV + AT and respective control groups, (d) pWBV_CG, (e) AT_CG and pWBV + AT_CG. The individuals performed a protocol 2 days/week during 5 weeks (Fig. 1). To record sEMG activity of the VLR muscle, the individuals were instructed to sit on a chair, back straight, feet approximately shoulder-width apart, and placed on the floor, and the arms crossed over the chest. From the sitting position, participants' were instructed to stand up completely and then back down, the test measures the actual time subjects needed to perform five rises as fast as possible without using the upper limbs (5CST) [16]. The electromyographic activity of the VLR during the 5CST was assessed before and after the first session, and before and after the last session (5 weeks). The RMS values recorded after the first, and before and after the last intervention session were normalized using the RMS values recorded before the first intervention session.

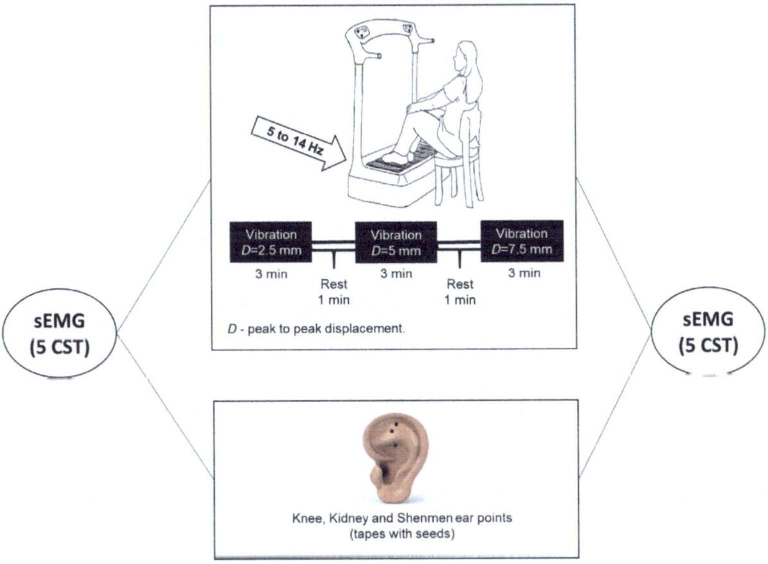

sEMG -surface electromyography, 5 CST – five times-sit-to-stand test

Fig. 1. Protocols of the interventions

3 Statistical Analysis

The statistical analyses were performed using BioEstat for Windows (version 5.3). The Shapiro-Wilk test was used to assess the data distribution of each variable. As it was significant ($p < 0.05$), the nonparametric Wilcoxon test was used to compare RMS values recorded during the intervention period and the Mann-Whitney test was used to compare the RMS between groups.

3.1 Results

Table 1 shows the results of the VLR activation (RMS) after the first session (immediate effect). There were no significant difference in the RMS of the participants subjected to all the interventions, when compared to the participants of the control groups.

Table 2 shows the results of the VLR activation (RMS) after the last session (immediate effect). It was verified that there were no significant differences in the RMS of the participants of the intervention groups, when compared to the participants of the control groups.

Table 1. Immediate effect of the vastus lateralis right electromyography in the first session

	Control (RMS%)	Intervention (RMS%)	*p* value
pWBV	98.95 ± 9.05	102.10 ± 14.35	0.97
AT	92.64 ± 9.25	96.86 ± 11.90	0.74
pWBV + AT	102.00 ± 13.83	95.89 ± 10.06	0.27

pWBV - group submitted to passive whole-body vibration, AT - auriculotherapy group, pWBV + AT - group submitted to combined intervention, RMS - root mean square.

Table 2. Immediate effect of the vastus lateralis right electromyography in the last session

	Control (RMS%)	Intervention (RMS%)	*P* value
pWBV	95.25 ± 27.60	97.08 ± 21.50	0.80
AT	93.66 ± 10.95	103.6 ± 15.86	0.07
pWBV + AT	86.14 ± 20.53	100.40 ± 7.41	0.06

pWBV - group submitted to passive whole-body vibration, AT - auriculotherapy group, pWBV + AT - group submitted to combined intervention, RMS - root mean square.

Table 3 shows the results of the VLR activation (RMS) before and after the protocol (cumulative effect). A significant difference can be observed in the groups submitted to auriculotherapy (AT) and in the group undergoing the associated treatment (pWBV + AT). In the group submitted to pWBV, there was no significant difference in this percentage of RMS in relation to the participants in the control groups.

Table 3. Cumulative effect of the vastus lateralis right electromyography

	Control (RMS%)	Intervention (RMS%)	*P* value
pWBV	91.51 ± 18.71	100.50 ± 28.47	0.67
AT	84.29 ± 16.07	100.40 ± 19.06	0.05*
pWBV + AT	79.15 ± 17.00	97.93 ± 15.27	0.03*

pWBV - group submitted to passive whole-body vibration, AT - auriculotherapy group, pWBV + AT - group submitted to combined intervention, RMS - root mean square.
*$p < 0.05$.

Statistical analysis was considered with the Mann Whitney test.

4 Discussion

The effect of non-pharmacological interventions (AT, pWBV and combined AT and pWBV) on the electromyographic profile (immediate and cumulative effects) of the vastus lateralis muscle (right lower limb) of KOA individuals was assessed. The electromyographic profile of the VLR was not altered due to immediate effect on the first intervention session. However, a significant cumulative effect ($p < 0.05$) was verified to the interventions involving AT alone or combined with pWBV.

Previous research reported that AT would induce this effect by activating the descending pain inhibitory pathways of the brainstem, thereby inhibiting the ascending pain pathway. The effects of AT on the functional capacity of patients with KOA, the clinical responses, seem to be associated with mechanisms related to a close relationship with the autonomic nervous system, the neuroendocrine system, neuroimmunological factors, neuroinflammation, and neural reflex, as well as antioxidation. Previous research has used sEMG as an outcome to quantify the effectiveness of AT. It was reported that the acupressure at a specific point with a somatopic relation to the biceps brachial muscle can modify the electromyographic activity. Furthermore, the response of the acupressure of a sham point has different responses. The maximum voluntary isometric contractions parameters were higher in acupressure treatment than those of control and sham treatments. Moreover, it was also reported significant changes in the pattern of temporal muscle activity after stimulation of the Shenmen, kidney, sympathetic, brain stem and temporomandibular points with mustard seeds.

Although there is no consensus about the mechanisms by which the vibratory stimulus affects the neuromuscular system, it has been suggested that the cause of the increase in motor unit recruitment is an excitatory response of the muscle spindles, due to the stretch reflex mechanism [17–19]. Moreover, It is suggested that neurophysiological factors involved in the response to vibratory stimulus have an important contribution of the oscillation frequency at which body structures are exposed [18, 20].

Considering the cumulative effect (Table 3), a significant improvement on the VLR activation due to the AT alone or combined with pWBV, before the first (with 5 Hz) and after the last session (14 Hz). Trans et al. (2009) [21] have reported that muscle strength and knee-extension range of motion were significantly increased due to the WBV with frequencies from 25 to 30 Hz in individuals with KOA. Fattorini et al. [22], vibration with frequencies pWBV alone has not EMG increased the VLR activation. The improvement of the recruitment of muscular fibers (Table 3) due to the AT alone or combine with pWBV could be associated with analgesic effects of the AT that would be induced by activating the descending pain inhibitory pathway of the brainstem, thereby inhibiting the ascending pain pathway [12, 14]. This would aid patients with KOA to perform tasks that would otherwise increase pain.

5 Conclusion

AT, alone or combined with pWBV, significantly increased the recruitment of muscle fibers after 5 weeks of intervention in KOA patients. However, no immediate effects were observed. Further studies are needed to better understand the effects of WBV and AT in the sEMG of the VL considering also the Vastus Lateralis Left.

References

1. Cross, M., Smith, E., Hoy, D., et al.: The global burden of hip and knee osteoarthritis: estimates from the Global Burden of Disease 2010 study. Ann. Rheum. Dis. **73**(7), 1323–1330 (2014)
2. Holla, J.F.M., van der Leeden, M., Heymans, M.W., et al.: Three trajectories of activity limitations in early symptomatic knee osteoarthritis: a 5-year follow-up study. Ann. Rheum. Dis. **73**, 1369–1375 (2013)
3. Hunter, D.J., Arden, N., Conaghan, P.G., et al.: Definition of osteoarthritis on MRI: results of a Delphi exercise. Osteoarthr. Cartil. **19**(8), 963–969 (2011)
4. Sharma, A.R., Jagga, S., Lee, S.S., Nam, J.S.: Interplay between cartilage and subchondral bone contributing to pathogenesis of osteoarthritis. Int. J. Mol. Sci. **14**(10), 19805–19830 (2013)
5. Vincent, K.R., Vincent, H.K.: Resistance exercise for knee osteoarthritis. PM&R **4**(5 Suppl), S45–52 (2012)
6. Garstang, S.V., Stitik, T.P.: Osteoarthritis: epidemiology, risk factors, and pathophysiology. Am. J. Phys. Med. Rehabil. **85**(11 Suppl), S2–S11 (2006)
7. Sharma, L.: The role of proprioceptive deficits, ligamentous laxity, and malalignment in development and progression of knee osteoarthritis. J. Rheumatol. **70**, 87–92 (2004)
8. Mills, K., Hunt, M.A., Leigh, R., Ferber, R.: A systematic review and meta-analysis of lower limb neuromuscular alterations associated with knee osteoarthritis during level walking. Clin. Biomech. **28**, 713–724 (2013)
9. Bigham, H.J., Flaxman, T.E., Smith, A.J.J., Benoit, D.L.: Neuromuscular adaptations in older males and females with knee osteoarthritis during weight-bearing force control. Knee **25**(1), 40–50 (2018)
10. Bokaeian, H.R., Bakhtiary, A.H., Mirmohammadkhani, M., Moghimi, J.: The effect of adding whole body vibration training to strengthening training in the treatment of knee osteoarthritis: a randomized clinical trial. J. Bodywork. Mov. Ther. **20**(2), 334–340 (2016)
11. Liu, Y.-H., Wei, I.-P., Wang, T.-M., Lu, T.-W., Lin, J.-G.: Immediate effects of acupuncture treatment on intra- and inter-limb contributions to body support during gait in patients with bilateral medial knee osteoarthritis. Am. J. Chin. Med. **45**(01), 23–35 (2017)
12. Hou, P.W., Hsu, H.C., Lin, Y.W., Tang, N.Y., Cheng, C.Y., Hsieh, C.L.: The history, mechanism, and clinical application of auricular therapy in traditional Chinese medicine. Evid. Based Complement Altern. Med. **2015**, 495684 (2015)
13. Suen, L.K.P., Yeh, C.H., Yeung, S.K.W.: Erratum to using auriculotherapy for osteoarthritic knee among elders: a double-blinded randomised feasibility study [BMC Complement AlternMed., 16 (2016), (257)]. BMC Complement Altern. Med. **16**(1), 257 (2016)
14. Round, R., Litscher, G., Bahr, F.: Auricular acupuncture with laser. Evid. Based Complement Altern. Med. **2013**, 22 (2013)
15. Ahlback, S.: Osteoarthrosis of the knee. A radiographic investigation. Acta Radiol. Diagn. **277**(Suppl), 7–72 (1968)
16. Furness, T., Bate, N., Welsh, L., Naughton, G., Lorenzen, C.: Efficacy of a whole-body vibration intervention to effect exercise tolerance and functional performance of the lower limbs of people with chronic obstructive pulmonary disease. BMC Pulm. Med. **12**(1), 71 (2012)
17. Bosco, C., Colli, R., Introini, E., et al.: Adaptive responses of human skeletal muscle to vibration exposure. Clin. Physiol. **19**(2), 183–187 (1999)

18. Cardinale, M., Lim, J.: Electromyography activity of vastus lateralis muscle during whole-body vibrations of different frequencies. J. Strength Conditioning Res. **17**(3), 621–624 (2003)
19. Pollock, R.D., Woledge, R.C., Martin, F.C., Newham, D.J.: Effects of whole body vibration on motor unit recruitment and threshold. J. Appl. Physiol. **112**(3), 388–395 (2012)
20. Bazett-Jones, D.M., Finch, H.W., Dugan, E.L.: Comparing the effects of various whole-body vibration accelerations on counter-movement jump performance. J. Sport Sci. Med. **7**, 144–150 (2008). http://www.jssm.org. Accessed 12 Apr. 2018
21. Trans, T., Aaboe, J., Henriksen, M., Christensen, R., Bliddal, H., Lund, H.: Effect of whole body vibration exercise on muscle strength and proprioception in females with knee osteoarthritis. Knee **16**(4), 256–261 (2009)
22. Fattorini, L., Tirabasso, A., Lunghi, A., Di Giovanni, R., Sacco, F., Marchetti, E.: Muscular forearm activation in hand-grip tasks with superimposition of mechanical vibrations. J. Electromyogr. Kinesiol. **26**, 143–148 (2016)

Human-Technology and Future of Work

Digital Citizenship Behavior in Organization as Indicator for Actors' Co-creative Problem-Solving in Ecosystem-Oriented Work Environments

Thomas Süße[(✉)]

Ruhr-Universität Bochum, Universitätsstr. 150, 44801 Bochum, Germany
thomas.suesse@rub.de

Abstract. Digital technologies foster the fluidity of knowledge and information resources and as such support the emergence of more open and co-creative problem-solving activities. At the same time ecosystem-oriented work environments evolve which are increasingly based on numerous heterogeneous actors' contributions to maintain these work environments' social systems. Thus, this article seeks to shed light on the question how actors' digitally enabled contributions to the social system enable co-creative problem-solving in modern work environments. Based on a quantitative study (N = 187) it shows that actors' digital citizenship behavior fosters co-creative problem-solving while actors' preference for order decreases this positive effect.

Keywords: Digital citizenship · Co-creation · Ecosystem · Modern work

1 Introduction

Digital technologies and smart systems foster the fluidity of knowledge and information resources and as such contribute to human actors' more open and innovative collaboration and interaction processes within ecosystem-oriented work environments [1]. This can expand actors' capacity to co-create products, services or smart solutions in close interactions with customers, users or partners [2]. Thus, smart technologies have the potential to accelerate or support the exploitation and exploration of newly emerging opportunities or stimuli for co creating solutions, e.g. by enabling agile interactions between an increasing number of distributed actors [see e.g. 4]. As such it can be stated that digitalization in general can reshape, open up or recombine existing knowledge structures and information resources for human actors from various domains. This fosters the emergence and the innovative capacity of more interconnected work environments and contributes to actors' ability of co-creating solutions for highly individual (customer) problems [4]. Thus, an accelerated transformation, reconfiguration or recombination of information and knowledge within dynamic, data rich and organic networks of human actors becomes an inherent phenomenon in

Chair for Work, Human Resources and Leadership.

T. Ahram et al. (Eds.): IHIET 2019, AISC 1018, pp. 675–681, 2020.
https://doi.org/10.1007/978-3-030-25629-6_105

modern business environments [5]. At the same time, this may also mean that equivocality and ambiguity of information, knowledge and open collaboration processes are key challenges human actors have to cope with in order to harness the growing amount of various opportunities that emerge in such ecosystem-oriented work environments. Consequently, these developments also reshape the social system within which co-creative problem-solving is organized and performed. However, so far little is known about how human actors maintain such digitally enabled ecosystems of co-creative work. In order to address this gap in research the article seeks to shed light on the question about how human actors' digital citizenship behavior as actors' efforts to maintain the social system may indicate patterns of co-creative problem-solving within ecosystem-oriented work environments. For answering this research question empirical data is gathered in a simulation for ecosystem-oriented work environments with the help of standardized questionnaires. In addition, the psychological concept of human actors preference for order as a sub component of need for cognitive closure which impacts individuals' mode of information processing [6] is taken into account in the model, as well.

2 Theoretical Framing

More innovative solutions can be expected from rather open work contexts organized as collaboration ecosystems [1]. Ecosystems as specific forms of organizing can be defined as digitally enabled integrative problem-solving contexts in which self-organizing heterogeneous actors co-create solutions in mutually beneficial ways [7]. Co-creation as distinct problem-solving pattern of human actors has been discussed as a form of adaptive behavior or response strategy within turbulent environments where the exploitation and exploration of novel stimuli is essential for sustainable success [8]. With the help of digital or smart systems, big data and the emergence of ecosystem-oriented work contexts human actors also gain new opportunities of accessing and utilizing information and knowledge resources or other assets traditionally outside of their direct control [9].

The concept of digital citizenship behavior (DCB) can be regarded as actors' behavioral pattern that plays a crucial role for co-evolution and emergence discussed as prerequisites for adaptive and co-creative interactions [e.g. 10–13]. Major research contributions for DCB are based in the field of education research as well as information technology management and computer science [13–15]. So far, DCB has been defined as actors' ability to actively participate and contribute to digitalized social environments [16] and can be regarded as crucial indicator for co-creation in ecosystem-oriented work contexts conceptualized as institutions of participation [17]. In management research organizational citizenship behavior (OCB) is discussed as human actors' action pattern that contributes indirectly to the organization through the maintenance of the social system [18, with reference to 19]. Thus, both, DCB and OCB share the objective of enhancing or maintaining a social system, e.g. by human actors' participative or engaging behavior. An integrative perspective of DCB and OCB seems to be a fruitful conceptualization with regards to modern digitally enabled work environments. In this article digital citizenship behavior in organizations (DCBO) is regarded as integration of both conceptualizations (DCB & OCB). DCBO is considered to support co-creative problem-solving in ecosystem-oriented work contexts which are determined by a high degree of self-organized actors, co-evolution and emergence [e.g. 10, 17].

However, especially emergence as a reflexive phenomenon can contribute to perceived ambiguity and complexity as "the links between individual agent actions and the long-term systemic outcome are unpredictable" [20]. Weick et al. [21, p. 412] argue that these phenomena of organizing contribute to disorder as evolving phenomena human actors may have to cope with in all work. Research revealed that individual actors showing higher preference for order (PFO) results in their desire to rather avoid ambiguity, uncertainty or disorder [22–24]. Thus, individuals' preference for order may rather hinder co-creative behavior as co-evolution and emergence may not be harnessed, but are rather avoided. This leads to a distinct model where the independent variable X is defined as digital citizenship behavior in organizations (DCBO), the dependent variable Y represents co-creation (CC) and preference for order (PFO) is introduced as moderator variable M influencing the effect of digital citizenship behavior on co-creation. Based on this conceptual outline three hypotheses are deduced. DCBO has a positive effect on CC (H1). PFO has a negative effect on CC (H2). PFO decreases the effect of DCBO on CC (H3). These hypotheses are evaluated within a simulation environment which has been developed as a model of ecosystem-oriented work [25, 26].

3 Research Method

3.1 Sample Structure and Measuring Scales

All data was collected with the help of an online survey in Germany and France from 2016 to 2018. The sample (N = 187) consists of undergraduate and graduate students from engineering and management which all have at least 6 months of work experience. Data was gathered during the participation in the simulation of an ecosystem-oriented work context evaluated in advance [25]. Respondents answered on a seven-step Likert scale, with "1" meaning "I totally disagree" and "7" meaning "I totally agree." DCBO has been measured on a seven-item scale which consists of a combination of scales introduced for DCB [13, 27] and self-rated OCB [28]. The items refer to individual actors' participation, engagement and discursive interaction enabled, supported or fostered by digital tools. For measuring individual actors' PFO a subscale introduced by Webster and Kruglanski [29], reduced by Roets and Van Hiel [30] and translated into German by Collani [31] was applied. The construct CC was measured based on the scale introduced by Voigt [32] which is based on fourteen items referring to individuals' co-creative problem-solving behavior in highly integrative work contexts where success is based on dynamic interactions between customers, partners and solution providers. Reliability of the scales is fully acceptable for PFO (.767), for DCBO (.709) and for CC (.852) [33–35].

3.2 Results

For testing the hypotheses H1, H2 and H3 linear regression analysis has been conducted. Normal distribution of the independent variables (DCBO, PFO) has been checked and both variables have been mean centered in advance. The moderator variable has been calculated based on the mean centered values of both variables. The results (see Table 1) reveal that DCBO has a positive effect on CC ($b_1 = .310$, $p < .001$). PFO has a positive effect on CC ($b_2 = .146$, $p = .035$) as well. The interaction effect of DCBO and PFO represent a negative effect on CC ($b_3 = -.183$, $p = .009$) The whole model is significant ($p < .000$) and shows an R^2 of .143. Multicollinearity among the predictor variables has been tested with the help of variance inflation factor (VIF) which is slightly above the value of 1 for all predicting variables. This means that there might be no multicollinearity between DCBO, PFO as well as the moderating variable in the model [36]. The results show that the positive effect of DCBO on CC is decreased by the moderating variable. In addition, the results also show that a higher PFO also predicts a considerably higher level of CC.

Table 1. Results of the regression analysis and interaction effect

		Coeff ^{s}	*SE*	*t*	*p*
Constant	i_y		.048	112.780	.000
DCBO (X)	b_1	.310	.050	4.533	.000
PFO (M)	b_2	.146	.049	2.124	.035
Interaction effect of X x M	b_3	−.183	.048	−2.656	.009
s: standardized	$R^2 = .143$, MSE = .424 $F(3,183) = 4.31$, $p < .000$				

4 Discussion

This article seeks to reveal further insights about key indicators of human behavior for co-creative problem-solving in digitalized ecosystem-oriented work environments. Based on the theoretical outline three hypotheses have been deduced and tested with the help of linear regression analysis.

The empirical results that are based on a sample of 187 participants in a simulation for ecosystem-oriented work contexts reveal that hypothesis H1 (*Digital citizenship behavior in organization has a positive effect on co-creative problem-solving*) and hypothesis H3 (*Preference for order decreases the effect of digital citizenship on adaptive co-creation*) can be confirmed while hypothesis H2 (*Preference for order has a negative effect on co-creative problem-solving*) has to be rejected. It rather shows that actors' preference for order can predict co-creative problem-solving. One explanation for this result is that even more open and highly dynamic co-creative interactions might be based on a specific set of standards (e.g. rules, roles, norms etc.) that are perceived as helpful by human actors to interact efficiently in ecosystem-oriented work environments or orchestrate other contributing actors. The decreasing effect of preference for order on the contribution of digital citizenship behavior to co-creation reveals, that actors' open-mindedness towards and the capacity of recognizing the growing number of highly novel and digitally enabled opportunities seems to be a critical factor in ecosystem-oriented work environments.

These findings show that higher engagement in digitally enabled cooperation, communication and participation processes can be regarded as contributing elements for open collaboration and co-creation [1].

Finally, it can be concluded that co-creative problem-solving in ecosystem-oriented work environments will more likely be performed by human actors who show a higher tendency to contribute to the evolvability of these work environments' social system with the help of exploring and exploiting digitally enabled opportunities generated by more fluid information and knowledge resources. In further research the effect on collaborative and co-creative problem-solving should be interpreted in context with additional actor-related facets, contextual and technological factors as well as human actors' capabilities of using digital systems efficiently in complex interactions.

References

1. Brunswicker, S., Bertino, E., Matei, S.: Big data for open digital innovation – a research roadmap. Big Data Res. **2**, 53–58 (2015). https://doi.org/10.1016/j.bdr.2015.01.008
2. Barkema, H.G., Baum, J.A.C., Mannix, E.A.: Management challenges in a new time. Acad. Manage. J. **45**, 916–930 (2002). https://doi.org/10.2307/3069322
3. Lerch, C., Gotsch, M.: Digitalized product-service systems in manufacturing firms: a case study analysis. Res.-Technol. Manag. **58**, 45–52 (2015). https://doi.org/10.5437/08956308X5805357
4. Lenka, S., Parida, V., Wincent, J.: Digitalization capabilities as enablers of value co-creation in servitizing firms. Psychol. Mark. **34**, 92–100 (2017). https://doi.org/10.1002/mar.20975
5. Lusch, R.F., Vargo, S.L., Tanniru, M.: Service, value networks and learning. J. Acad. Mark. Sci. **38**, 19–31 (2010). https://doi.org/10.1007/s11747-008-0131-z
6. Kruglanski, A.W., Webster, D.M., Klem, A.: Motivated resistance and openness to persuasion in the presence or absence of prior information. J. Pers. Soc. Psychol. **65**, 861 (1993)
7. Barnett, M.L.: The keystone advantage: what the new dynamics of business ecosystems mean for strategy, innovation, and sustainability. Acad. Manag. Perspect. **20**, 88–90 (2006). https://doi.org/10.5465/AMP.2006.20591015
8. Ramaswamy, V., Ozcan, K.: What is co-creation? an interactional creation framework and its implications for value creation. J. Bus. Res. **84**, 196–205 (2018). https://doi.org/10.1016/j.jbusres.2017.11.027
9. Zahra, S.A., Nambisan, S.: Entrepreneurship and strategic thinking in business ecosystems. Bus. Horiz. **55**, 219–229 (2012). https://doi.org/10.1016/j.bushor.2011.12.004
10. Hearn, G., Pace, C.: Value-creating ecologies: understanding next generation business systems. Foresight. **8**, 55–65 (2006). https://doi.org/10.1108/14636680610647147
11. Moore, J.F.: Predators and prey: a new ecology of competition. Harv. Bus. Rev. **71**, 75–83 (1993)
12. Sussan, F., Acs, Z.J.: The digital entrepreneurial ecosystem. Small Bus. Econ. **49**, 55–73 (2017). https://doi.org/10.1007/s11187-017-9867-5

13. Choi, M., Glassman, M., Cristol, D.: What it means to be a citizen in the internet age: development of a reliable and valid digital citizenship scale. Comput. Educ. **107**, 100–112 (2017). https://doi.org/10.1016/j.compedu.2017.01.002
14. Jonsson, K., Mathiassen, L., Holmström, J.: Representation and mediation in digitalized work: evidence from maintenance of mining machinery. J. Inf. Technol., 1–17 (2018). https://doi.org/10.1057/s41265-017-0050-x
15. Nordin, M.S., Ahmad, T.B.T., Zubairi, A.M., Ismail, N.A.H., Rahman, A.H.A., Trayek, F.A. A., Ibrahim, M.B.: Psychometric properties of a digital citizenship questionnaire. Int. Educ. Stud. **9**, 71 (2016). https://doi.org/10.5539/ies.v9n3p71
16. Mossberger, K., Tolbert, C.J., McNeal, R.S.: Digital Citizenship: The Internet, Society, and Participation. MIt Press, Cambridge (2007)
17. Muegge, S.: Business ecosystems as institutions of participation: a systems perspective on community-developed platforms. Technol. Innov. Manag. Rev. Ott. **1**, 4–13 (2011). https://doi.org/10.22215/timreview/495
18. LePine, J.A., Erez, A., Johnson, D.E.: The nature and dimensionality of organizational citizenship behavior: a critical review and meta-analysis. J. Appl. Psychol. **87**, 52–65 (2002). https://doi.org/10.1037/0021-9010.87.1.52
19. Organ, D.W.: Organizational citizenship behavior: it's construct clean-up time. Hum. Perform. **10**, 85–97 (1997). https://doi.org/10.1207/s15327043hup1002_2
20. Smith, M.Y., Stacey, R.: Governance and cooperative networks: an adaptive systems perspective. Technol. Forecast. Soc. Change. **54**, 79–94 (1997)
21. Weick, K.E., Sutcliffe, K.M., Obstfeld, D.: Organizing and the process of sensemaking. Organ. Sci. **16**, 409–421 (2005). https://doi.org/10.1287/orsc.1050.0133
22. Acar-Burkay, S., Fennis, B.M., Warlop, L.: Trusting others: the polarization effect of need for closure. J. Pers. Soc. Psychol. **107**, 719–735 (2014). https://doi.org/10.1037/a0037022
23. Kossowska, M., Van Hiel, A., Chun, W.Y., Kruglanski, A.W.: The Need for Cognitive Closure scale: structure, cross-cultural invariance, and comparison of mean ratings between European-American and East Asian samples. Psychol. Belg. **42**, 267–286 (2002)
24. Kruglanski, A.W., Webster, D.M.: Motivated closing of the mind: "Seizing" and "freezing". Psychol. Rev. **103**, 263 (1996)
25. Cibat, J., Süße, T., Wilkens, U.: An ecosystem approach as a design principle for a pss-specific business simulation. Procedia CIRP **64**, 223–228 (2017). https://doi.org/10.1016/j.procir.2017.03.035
26. Süße, T.: Improvisation as a prerequisite for the dynamic interplay of production and service in PSS: insights of an organizational design principle and a game-based learning approach. Procedia CIRP **30**, 366–371 (2015). https://doi.org/10.1016/j.procir.2015.02.186
27. Jones, L.M., Mitchell, K.J.: Defining and measuring youth digital citizenship. New Media Soc. **18**, 2063–2079 (2016)
28. Lau, P.Y.Y., McLean, G.N., Lien, B.Y.-H., Hsu, Y.-C.: Self-rated and peer-rated organizational citizenship behavior, affective commitment, and intention to leave in a Malaysian context. Pers. Rev. **45**, 569–592 (2016). https://doi.org/10.1108/PR-04-2014-0083
29. Webster, D.M., Kruglanski, A.W.: Individual differences in need for cognitive closure. J. Pers. Soc. Psychol. **67**, 1049–1062 (1994). https://doi.org/10.1037/0022-3514.67.6.1049
30. Roets, A., Van Hiel, A.: Item selection and validation of a brief, 15-item version of the Need for Closure Scale. Personal. Individ. Differ. **50**, 90–94 (2011). https://doi.org/10.1016/j.paid.2010.09.004

31. Collani, G.: Eine deutsche Skala zum Konstrukt "Bedürfnis nach kognitiver Geschlossenheit (NFCC)/Persönliches Strukturbedürfnis (PNS). In: Danner, D., Glöckner-Rist, A. (eds.) Zusammenstellung sozialwissenschaftlicher Items und Skalen (2014). https://doi.org/10.6102/zis49
32. Voigt, B.-F.: Coping with the challenges of a heterogeneous working context – a configuration of individual competencies for PSS workers. Procedia CIRP. **30**, 402–407 (2015). https://doi.org/10.1016/j.procir.2015.02.097
33. DeVellis, R.F.: Scale Development: Theory and Applications. Sage Publications, Thousand Oaks (2016)
34. Helms, J.E., Henze, K.T., Sass, T.L., Mifsud, V.A.: Treating cronbach's alpha reliability coefficients as data in counseling research. Couns. Psychol. **34**, 630–660 (2006). https://doi.org/10.1177/0011000006288308
35. Nunnally, J.C., Bernstein, I.H.: The theory of measurement error. In: Psychometric Theory, 3rd edn, pp. 209–247 (1994)
36. Belsley, D.A., Kuh, E., Welsch, R.E.: Regression Diagnostics: Identifying Influential Data and Sources of Collinearity. Wiley, New York (2005)

Assessing Trends of Digital Divide Within Digital Services in New York City

Trisha Sharma, Richard Legarda(✉), and Somesh Sharma(✉)

Institute of Housing and Urban Development Studies,
Erasmus University, Rotterdam, The Netherlands
trisha_sharma@yahoo.com, richard.legarda@gmail.com,
sharma@ihs.nl

Abstract. With the ascension of the new digital economy, conventional means of access have found themselves completely reshaped from the ground up and the paradigm of service provision has shifted towards the online space. Daily services have now found themselves intrinsically tied to various online apps as the digital economy aims at increasing the coverage of services and providing equitable access to all users [5]. While the transition of services to the digital realm has certainly acted as a liberating vessel for many individuals, it has not come without its pitfalls. Chief among these is the concept of the digital divide. As a result of this, many individuals who are technically averse in an online sensibility have found themselves at odds with a concept that is in theory marketed as open and inclusive. With an in-depth empirical study of New York City (NYC), this research explains the conditions (and factors) within the digital economy that is causing a digital divide in New York. The focus of this research is specifically on digital media and its subsequent provision of services & accessibility. Among the deficiencies concerning the digital divide is its ambiguous nature. Be it in definition, the multifaceted nature of it, and the accompanying research that is associated with it. Findings of this research highlighted key areas where policy action is urgently needed. It may help policymakers in bringing right regulatory mechanisms in place and prevent the digital divide becoming a potential barrier to the advancements in digitally provided services.

Keywords: Digital divide · New media · Internet access · Digital technologies · Digital services · New York City · Digital economy · Accessibility

1 Introduction

With the advent of digital technologies in the past decade, the digital economy has been a liberating force in connecting a multitude of individuals to various industries they would otherwise be denied access to [10]. However, due to the involvement of digital platforms in the present-day economy, there are certain outcomes that have prevailed & are discussed in this research.

The expeditious advancement of digital technology, also known as information and communications technologies (ICTs), has largely reworked daily lives all around the

T. Ahram et al. (Eds.): IHIET 2019, AISC 1018, pp. 682–687, 2020.
https://doi.org/10.1007/978-3-030-25629-6_106

globe and how individuals access their needs on a daily basis. "Digital media technologies shape our everyday lives, from unprecedented elections to quotidian rhythms of growing older to watching a favorite television show and discussing it with like-minded others via Twitter" [1]. The Internet is now considered as one of the crucial and most significant infrastructures around the world. A 1.2% hike in per capita GDP expansion can be achieved with an added 10% of internet insertion (World Economic Forum, 2014).

The aftermath of the digitalization of various good and services in different world economies has been deep and only going to proliferate in the future. Technology in it and itself is all-encompassing in the daily life of many. Multiple days to day activities have surrendered themselves or been supplanted by various apps and programs. Technology is moving at such a rapid pace and truly shaping the future outlook of our society. The transition has been so fast and seamless that few if any realize how connected society has become to technology as a whole.

The concept of the cell phone in its infancy a literal mobile phone has transformed into an all-encompassing miniature computer the smartphone. Keeping its user connected with various streaming services, the entirety of social media, breaking news and the occasional phone call. The popularity of the smartphone has also transformed or even replaced the wants and needs of the average consumer. Online shopping continues to rise as brick and mortar stores falter, the future of publishing is increasingly digital, and the food we eat is only a click away. Truly digital media and services have established itself as the dominant force to the point that many cannot imagine a life without it [2].

By utilizing multiple types of technological innovations, modern students have found themselves in a radically new learning environment. One where they are not only expected, but required to connect with their colleagues not only within the confines of their respective school, but extending their learning 'network' to their home, working environment and beyond. These trends are often accessed through analyzing how integration between digital means of technology & accessing of daily needs, services, etc., has facilitated human interaction with the digital economy in general [9].

The advancement of the internet and the digital technology it has brought to the public has truly been a transformative force in society. The ease of this technology and its applications broadened our horizons; connected us in work, play, and thought. Unifying people the world over and has been the driving force in creating a variety of new and exciting communities and opportunities that were not thought possible [3].

1.1 Accessibility to Digital Accessibility

Nonetheless, the proliferation of digital technology has become intrinsically tied to concepts of accessibility. Certainly online accessibility differs from user to user, however providing equal access to all from inception is favorable for all users. It is imperative for web creators to identify the fact that their content will in fact be viewed by a diverse audience who in turn do not process content in a uniform fashion. In other words, this concept is defined as digital accessibility. As suggested by [6], digital accessibility refers to the process of providing equitable access to virtually all forms of web content to users, irrespective of their background of individuals who may have disabilities. Traditionally this concept has been tied to physical spaces, yet the internet has transformed this notion so that accessibility now resides in the online or digital arena. The ever changing nature of the internet continues to redefine the concept of accessibility. It has become ever encompassing representing social and digital media, various apps, and websites. As its audience and reach continues to grow and redefine our society as a whole, those who continue to innovate and watch over our online spaces must keep in mind concepts of accessibility for their end users.

Certainly the scope and importance of digitally provided services will continue to grow over time. While in its infancy the negative outcomes of digital services were minute at best, that being digital divide. Yet our research shows that as this sector continues to grow, digital divide continues to expand with it in a symbiotic fashion. As suggested by [4], "The Digital Divide, or the digital split, is a social issue referring to the differing amount of information between those who have access to the internet (peculiarly broadband access) and those who do not have access". The term gained heavy prominence in the late 1990s due to the proliferation of digitalization & involvement of digital means in various economies, among intrigued group of scholars, policy makers, advocacy troops etc.

> *"The power of the Web is in its universality. Access by everyone regardless of disability is an essential aspect."*
>
> ***-- Tim Berners-Lee, W3C Director and inventor of the World Wide Web***

1.2 Findings and Theoretical Framework

In addressing the various literature concerning digital divide in regards to accessibility, there certainly is a fair amount written on the issue. In identifying access to online services for the end user we do not equate this solely to the internet itself. Rather for the purpose of this research access is tied to Information and Communications Technologies (ICT). The internet is not the determinant factor but rather how the internet is accessed (speed of connection, overall quality etc.) and subsequent services that stem from the internet. However, the overwhelming amount of current research centres around access in a rather simplistic way. Either individuals are connected to broadband internet via a hardlined connection through means of an internet service provider and are able to engage online or they do not and are subsequently excluded. In this sense ICT is outright ignored, the research does not go much further if at all past this paradigm of connected or not connected. More so, the measures that quantify access to high speed internet within the household are a bit muddled. As previously mentioned, at the household level, broadband itself is the key measure for charting access to the internet. Using this indicator, we find that just over 27% (730,000) of households in New York City lack broadband access [7]. Further analyzing this figure, a disproportionate amount of these households are in low socioeconomic areas of the city (See Fig. 1).

New York City Digital Divide Fact Sheet

More than 730,000 households in New York City did not have broadband in 2015 according to the United States Census survey of the Percent of Households with a Broadband Internet Subscription. Nearly half of households in New York City without a broadband subscription are in the Bronx and Brooklyn, respectively, nearly one-third (32.5%) and one-quarter (25.6%).

GCT2801-Geography-United States: PERCENT OF HOUSEHOLDS WITH A BROADBAND INTERNET SUBSCRIPTION – United States -- County by State; and for Puerto Rico - Universe: Households							
2015 American Community Survey 1-Year Estimates	Population	Households	% Households with Broadband	Margin of Error	# Households with Broadband	# Households without Broadband	% Households without Broadband
New York State	19,795,791	7,262,279	77.80%	+/-0.2	5,650,053	1,612,226	22.20%
Bronx County	1,455,444	484,902	67.50%	+/-1.0	327,309	157,593	32.50%
Kings County	2,636,735	931,786	74.40%	+/-0.7	693,249	238,537	25.60%
New York County	1,644,518	750,419	80.70%	+/-0.8	605,588	144,831	8.81%
Queens County	2,339,150	780,644	79.70%	+/-0.5	622,173	158,471	6.77%
Richmond County	474,558	165,784	80.90%	+/-1.8	134,119	31,665	6.67%
New York City	8,550,405	3,113,535			2,382,438	731,097	8.55%

Fig. 1. Percentage of access to broadband internet in New York City. Source: [7]

On the contrary, while access within the home may be restricted in the sense of hard line connectivity, we find that access in general is not. For instance, nearly 96% of those living in New York City own a cell phone, and 80% of this group own a smartphone [8]. Zeroing in on low income residents the study shows that 66.5% of New Yorkers who earn no income whatsoever also possess smart phones [8]. This last figure is quite staggering considering that the national rate for smartphone ownership is at 71% [8]. Comparing this figures it is evident to see that network connectivity itself is not the issue for those in New York City.

We therefore argue that it is not necessarily the access itself that is the core issue, but derivative services within the internet that act as gatekeepers. How do individual users perceive the digital economy and the subsequent services that it provides? Recognizing that there is unequal representation as well as understanding of many web users in navigating the internet. What are these barriers that dissuade individuals from participating in the use of digital services? Gaining insight on these issues will requires a study that will properly address more that just the need for internet access. It requires a theoretical framework that can properly address the external factors of would be users of digital media. As shown in Fig. 2, we have identified four variables that proceed access to digital media services.

That being the socioeconomic status of users, age group of users, their familiarity and skills navigating the internet and finally what sort of access they have to the internet itself. Analyzing these factors, we hope to properly quantify the mechanism(s) that generate digital divide as an output of digital media services within New York City.

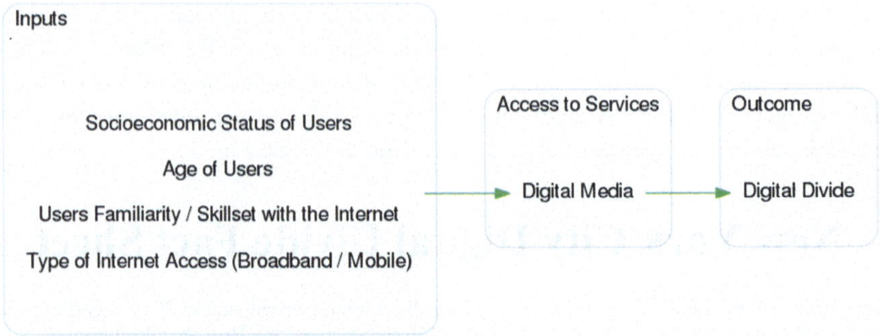

Fig. 2. Framework for comprehension of the linear fashion of digital divide.

2 Conclusion and Recommendations

We believe that the insights that will be gained from such a study will be instrumental in preparing solutions to combat digital divide within New York City. We find that there is both a lack of literature and proper explanation delving into the phenomena of digital divide. As New York City is the leading media market within the United States, what can be learned from such a case study will have the utmost relevance and prove incredibly useful at a national level as well. In addition our proposed theoretical framework, can be extrapolated well beyond the realms of digital media but to other online sectors as well that could be vulnerable to digital divide. Ultimately through engaging policy makers, the tech industry, and appropriate stakeholders, we believe there is an opportunity to flesh out digital divide and further expand equity within digitally provided services.

References

1. Daniels, J., Williams, A., Buggs, S.: Digital media technologies in everyday life. Inf. Commun. Soc. **20**(7), 947–949 (2017)
2. Dixon, I.: The influence of technology on our daily life. The Digital Lifestyle [blog], 02 June 2016. https://thedigitallifestyle.com/w/. Accessed 22 Mar 2019
3. European Commission: Cultural heritage Digitisation, online accessibility and digital preservation: REPORT on the Implementation of Commission Recommendation. 2011/711/EU 2013-2015), European Commission (2016). http://ec.europa.eu/information_society/newsroom/image/document/2016-43/2013-2015_progress_report_18528.pdf. Accessed 14 Apr 2019
4. Internet World Stats: The Digital Divide, ICT, and Broadband Internet: ICT - Information Communications Technologies (2019). https://www.internetworldstats.com/links10.htm. Accessed 2019
5. Kenton, W.: Sharing Economy, 14 December 2017. https://www.investopedia.com/terms/s/sharing-economy.asp. Accessed 01 Mar 2019
6. New York University: What is Digital Accessibility? (2019). https://www.nyu.edu/life/information-technology/help-and-service-status/accessibility.html. Accessed 2019

7. New York City: New York City Digital Divide Fact Sheet [Press release], 16 March 2017. https://benkallos.com/sites/default/files/PressRelease_Spectrum_Internet_Assist_Fact_Sheet_20170316.pdf. Accessed 30 Mar 2019
8. New York City Department of Consumer Affairs: New York City Mobile Services Study: Research Brief. New York: New York City (2015). https://www1.nyc.gov/assets/dca/MobileServicesStudy/Research-Brief.pdf. Accessed 29 Mar 2019
9. Rye, S.A.: Digital communication, transportation and urban structuration in students daily life. Geogr. Ann. Series B Hum. Geogr. **92**(1), 81–96 (2010)
10. Sutherland, W., Jarrahi, M.H.: The sharing economy and digital platforms: a review and research agenda (2018). http://www.sciencedirect.com/science/article/pii/S0268401218301567. Accessed 08 Mar 2019
11. World Economic Forum: Delivering Digital Infrastructure. Advancing the Internet Economy (2014). http://reports.weforum.org/delivering-digital-infrastructure/acknowledgements/)

Deep Water: Predicting Water Meter Failures Through a Human-Machine Intelligence Collaboration

Luca Casini[1], Giovanni Delnevo[1], Marco Roccetti[1(✉)], Nicolò Zagni[2], and Giuseppe Cappiello[2]

[1] Department of Computer Science and Engineering, University of Bologna, Bologna, Italy
{luca.casini7,giovanni.delnevo2, marco.roccetti}@unibo.it

[2] Department of Management, University of Bologna, Bologna, Italy
{nicolo.zagni2,giuseppe.cappiello}@unibo.it

Abstract. Take an AI learning algorithm and a human trainer with an experience in machine intelligence. Take piles of data, in the form of labeled examples. If you think that the task of training a machine that makes accurate decisions is easy as pie, you could not be further from reality. That is what has been missing from this story: getting off on the right foot. For a good start, crucial is the value of data which come large in quantity but low in quality. Beyond how we design our AI, fundamental is making our data valid for learning. We report here our experience in the creation of highly accurate training examples, based on the idea of filtering out all the impurities from a dataset containing 15 million water readings, provided by an Italian water supply company. This was accomplished allowing a human-machine collaboration, down to the implementation of an AI model capable to predict water meter failure.

Keywords: Human-in-the-loop methods · Interactive machine learning · Human machine interaction loop · Water metering

1 Introduction

Modern Artificial Intelligence (AI) can diagnose a medical disease, drive a car and explore an unknown planet. Yet, while impressive capabilities have been demonstrated, many problems are emerging that reveal the possibility that AI systems do not take human concerns as their central mandate. Unpredictable incidents, racism, security and impossibility of explaining why a given decision is taken are just a few remarkable examples of the unintended consequences against which we should protect [1, 2]. The problem becomes evident when we come to the question of how we are instructing our new machines. Either with deep learning or with simpler statistical learning models, we often train our machines to learn patterns from complex piles of data and then claim those intelligences have learned about the world. This fact could not be further from the truth. Only a few systems are capable of a genuine human-like reason, if left alone. Our

T. Ahram et al. (Eds.): IHIET 2019, AISC 1018, pp. 688–694, 2020.
https://doi.org/10.1007/978-3-030-25629-6_107

idea is then that key to create machine learning models whose decisions are accurate and actionable is leveraging both human and machine intelligence [3–5].

We then propose an approach that encompasses the creation of highly accurate training data through an interactive human activity, aimed at filtering out all the incomplete and invalid information, while reinforcing this knowledge with the codification of relevant contextual features [6].

Simply, our model combines the ability of machines at recognizing regularities from vast datasets, with humans that are better at making decisions with less information.

In this paper, we deployed an AI model as an application in the field of water metering, for a water supply company that distributes water over a large area in Northern Italy. Here, the core problem was that of training a machine to predict a failure of water meters, based on a set of meter readings, taken over the past. Another requirement was that of minimizing the number of consecutive readings to be used for such prediction.

In essence, our main result has been to show how an interactive data elaboration can help in managing a complex training process, leading to reliable results, even in the presence of several *impurities* coming from the variety of business processes that have produced those data.

The remainder of this paper is as follows. In Sect. 2 we focus on the problem of filtering out all *impurities* from the initial dataset. Section 3 introduces our approach where learning algorithms were trained with a particular focus on those training examples behind which hidden are those motivations why a given meter fails. Section 4 generalizes to water meters that work properly. Finally, Sect. 5 concludes the paper.

2 Domain Analysis and *Impurities* Filtering

We were provided with an initial dataset comprised of about 15 million water meter readings, corresponding to about 1 million water meters, in the period 2014–2018. Among others, to each reading the following values were associated: (i) time when that reading was taken, (ii) previous reading in time, (iii) time when the previous reading was taken. With respect to the recording of the instant in time when readings are taken, relevant are the following facts: (a) many of these time instants are *incoherent*; (b) a highly variable and unpredictable interval in time may sometimes exist between two *consecutive* readings (even if the Italian regulation recommends two readings per year).

Beyond this specific consideration, the dataset came with other numerous *impurities*, whose causes are to be tracked down to a variety of business processes that contributed to generate those data, including: company policies, specific regulations, as well as human errors in the loop. Other contextual information came with the dataset, for example: date of installation of a given water meter, manufacturer, production date, location of installation, type of use, gauge, and so on …).

To make all these complex piles of data genuinely valid for automatic learning, we designed and developed an interactive procedure that *cleaned* the data.

In particular, a *semantics* was defined, in collaboration with company experts, that ensures that a reading is *valid* for automatic learning, provided that:

- a human operator has confirmed that reading, on site;
- that reading has been correctly transmitted and recorded onto the company ERP;
- that reading has been definitely certified by another human operator on the company ERP; and, finally,
- the instant in time when that reading was taken is *coherent*: i.e., certified as real, by a specific process.

If we take the initial dataset and filter out all those readings that do not comply with the rules of the above semantics, we yield a set of about 8 millions readings on which, now, a safe machine training process can be carried out.

As to the water meters, they:

- were divided over two different classes (those who had failed in the period 2014–2018, and those who did not) and,
- to each of them a set of *valid* consecutive readings was associated, based on the selection that was carried out following the validity semantics above.

Further, to conduct our machine training activities, we finally split the dataset of valid readings into two different portions: (1) all the valid readings from 2014 to early 2018 were used on the training phase; (2) the remaining valid readings (late 2018) were used only for testing.

3 A Focus on Failure

We decided to begin our machine training activity, by concentrating on the water meters that failed, based on the idea to extract, if any, the relationship between failures and history of readings.

To this aim, we employed all the possible water meters that have failed (approx. 15.000) and correspondent valid readings (approx. 80.000). Then, we followed two different directions.

With the first, we took advantage of a variety of machine learning algorithms whose main characteristic is that they **do not** use memory to learn and classify. The second approach went instead towards the direction of using a *deep neural network* (with memory). We review the obtained results in the following two Subsections, in isolation.

3.1 Learning Without Memory

We exploited the following machine learning algorithms: Linear Regression (LR), Lasso (LA), Elastic Net (EN), Classification and Regression Tree (CART), Support Vector Regression (SVR), K-nearest neighbors (KNN), Adaptive Boosting (AB), Gradient Boosting (GB), Random Forest (RF), and Multilayer Perceptron (MLP) with only one hidden layer with 100 neurons.

For all of them, we used the traditional 10-fold cross-validation technique. The area under the receiver operating characteristic curve (AUC-ROC) was our performance metric.

In Fig. 1, a plot with the results obtained with each algorithm is reported, showing that good results can be achieved; for example with the GB and **MLP** algorithms that yield almost an 80% value of accuracy.

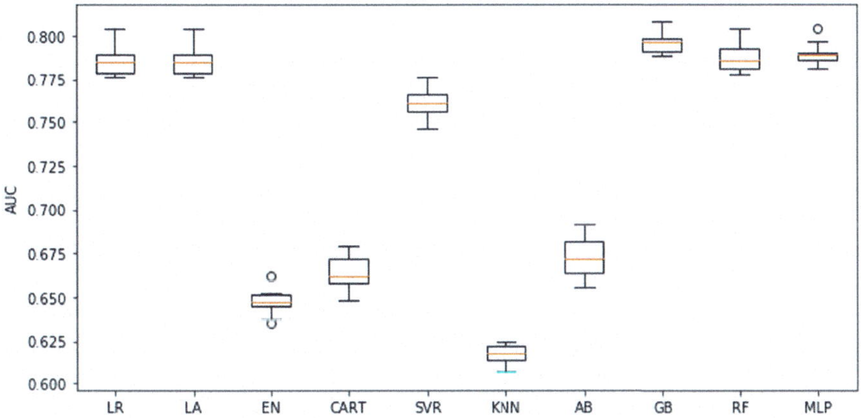

Fig. 1. AUC-ROC – Top to bottom for each represented object, respectively: outliers, maximum, upper adjacent value, third quartile, median, first quartile, lowest adjacent value, outliers

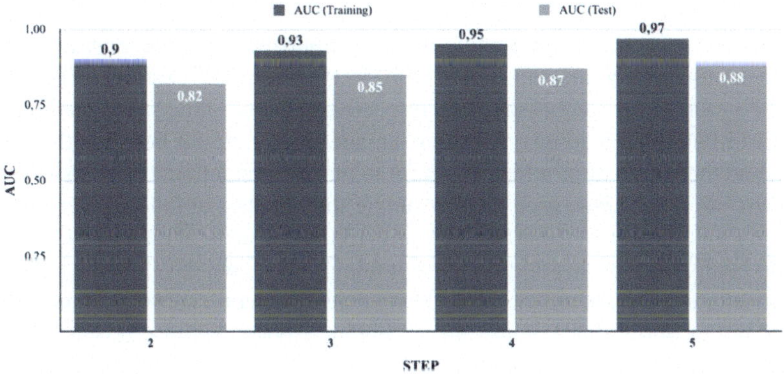

Fig. 2. Deep neural network. Performance with different numbers of readings (2–5)

3.2 Learning with Memory

A deep neural network was used that was able to follow the evolution of water consumption over time. Specifically, such a neural network had two parallel inputs: a feed forward one for the attributes of the water meter and a recurrent one for its reading series. We implemented it using the well-known: *Keras* library. We experimented with series of readings of different lengths, containing from two to five consecutive valid readings. It is easy to notice from Fig. 2 above that the use of memory allows our classifier to predict water meter failures with an increased accuracy, as shown in the grey columns (testing values), ranging from 82% to 88%.

4 Model Generalization

While the preliminary results obtained during the validation phase of our neural network training process were well promising, a crucial factor was left outside.

What about the water meters that never failed? Did our preliminary analysis really take into account all the relevant and various *characteristics* that a *good* water meter can exhibit? Actually not, is the right answer.

For this reason, we developed a further procedure capable to generalize our AI model while taking into account the statistical variety, represented by all the well-functioning water meters.

A confirmation of the importance of this further effort was given by the values of the AUC we got while testing both **MLP** and our deep neural network with those 700.000 valid readings belonging to the portion of data we left out for blind testing (see Sect. 2). Sadly, we yielded only 0.49% and 0.51% accuracy values, respectively.

Nonetheless, this was an expected consequence of the approach we used so far (i.e., our initial focus on faults alone). In essence, one important step still needs to be carried out to finalize the process towards the generalization of our model; it amounts to:

- retraining our **deep neural network** to learn from an adequate variety, in quantity and quality, of positive examples (i.e., well-functioning water meters).

To this aim, we arranged a training dataset comprised of 50.000 positive examples (well-functioning water meters) along with 50.000 negative examples (failed water meters). To each meter were associated, respectively, two or three valid readings, since a number of two/three readings represents an adequate trade-off between the accuracy we need and the length of past history useful to make a prediction. (Needless to say, the *SMOTE-NC* technique was used to oversample the quantity of failed water meters, up to reaching the number of 50.000, with only 15.000 of them actually available).

Upon completion of this additional re-training phase, we developed a final testing experiment for our deep neural network, using that portion of readings that our machines never looked at during the training phase. Figure 3 portrays those results. As clearly demonstrated, there emerges the efficacy of using our AI model, based on a deep neural network; it is able to predict water meter failure with an accuracy of 86–89%.

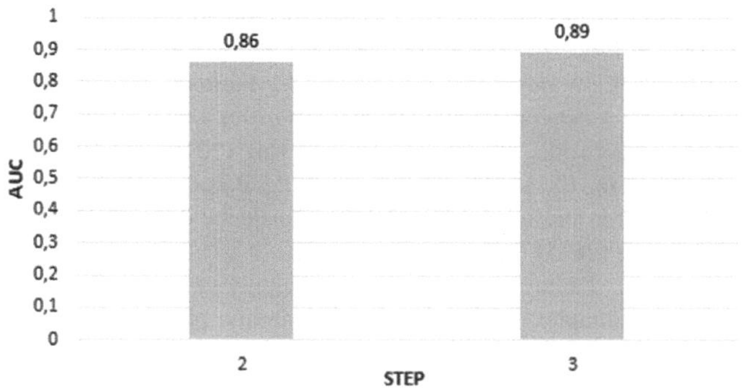

Fig. 3. Re-trained deep neural network: performances

5 Conclusion

The procedures described in this paper have confirmed how still crucial is the role of human intelligence and experience, while training a learning algorithm to the aim of designing a coherent AI model [7–11]. Summarizing, a mix of human attention on the process of cleaning the data to build a correct training dataset and a specialized two-phase machine training procedure has led us to an AI model, based on a deep neural network, capable to predict water meter failures, with an accuracy in the range of 86–89%.

Acknowledgments. We are indebted towards the company that has provided the data. To guarantee its privacy, we keep it here anonymized.

References

1. Garcia, M.: Racist in the machine: the disturbing implications of algorithmic bias. World Policy J. **33**(4), 111–117 (2016). Duke University Press. Project MUSE database. Accessed 20 March 2019
2. Roccetti, M., Marfia, G., Zanichelli, M.: The art and craft of making the tortellino: playing with a digital gesture recognizer for preparing pasta culinary recipes. Comput. Entertainment **8**(4), 1–20 (2010)
3. Nagar, Y.: Combining human and machine intelligence for making predictions. Doctoral dissertation, Massachusetts Institute of Technology (2013)
4. Prandi, C., Roccetti, M., Salomoni, P., Nisi, V., Nunes, N.J.: Fighting exclusion: a multimedia mobile app with zombies and maps as a medium for civic engagement and design. Multimedia Tools Appl. **76**(4), 4951–4979 (2016)
5. Salomoni, P., Prandi, C., Roccetti, M., Nisi, V., Nunes, N.J.: Crowdsourcing urban accessibility: some preliminary experiences with results. In: Proceedings of the 11th Biannual Conference on Italian SIGCHI Chapter - CHItaly 2015. ACM Press (2015)
6. Delnevo, G., Roccetti, M., Mirri, S.: Intelligent and good machines? The role of domain and context codification. Mob. Networks Appl. (2019). https://doi.org/10.1007/s11036-019-01233-7

7. Cabitza, F., Rasoini, R., Gensini, G.F.: Unintended consequences of machine learning in medicine. JAMA **318**(6), 517–518 (2017). https://doi.org/10.1001/jama.2017.7797
8. Walker, D., Creaco, E., Vamvakeridou-Lyroudia, L., Farmani, R., Kapelan, Z., Savic, D.: Forecasting domestic water consumption from smart meter readings using statistical methods and artificial neural networks. In: Procedia Engineering (2015)
9. Mounce, S.R., Pedraza, C., Jackson, T., Linford, P., Boxall, J.B.: Cloud based ma-chine learning approaches for leakage assessment and management in smart water net-works. In: Procedia Engineering (2015)
10. Pietrucha-Urbanik, K.: Failure prediction in water supply system–current issues. In: Theory and Engineering of Complex Systems and Dependability, pp. 351–358. Springer (2015)
11. Haghiabi, A.H., Nasrolahi, A.H., Parsaie, A.: Water quality prediction using machine learning methods. Water Qual. Res. J. **53**(1), 3–13 (2018). https://doi.org/10.2166/wqrj.2018.025

Distributed Connectivity-Preserving Coordination of Multi-agent Systems with Bounded Velocities

Yuan Yang, Daniela Constantinescu(✉), and Yang Shi

Mechanical Engineering, University of Victoria, Victoria, Canada
{yangyaun, danielac, yshi}@uvic.ca

Abstract. This paper presents a distributed control strategy for the coordination with local connectivity maintenance of single-integrator multi-agent systems with bounded velocities. The proposed strategy regards actuator saturation as dynamic scaling of the control. It preserves connectivity by applying gradient-based controls that can monotonically decrease suitably designed local potentials even if saturated. As a result, the controller design is not constrained by the velocity bounds, and can fully exploit the limited velocities for connectivity preserving coordination. Numerical simulations verify the performance of the proposed controller.

Keywords: Multi-agent systems · Connectivity-preserving coordination · Bounded actuation

1 Introduction

Distributed coordination control of multi-agent systems ~ (MAS), whose objective is to drive the multiple agents to a common configuration using only local information exchanges, has been extensively studied [1]. While initial coordination techniques have assumed MAS connectivity [2], more recent strategies have used gradient-based controls to maintain it locally [3–6].

One limitation of gradient-based controls is that they may exceed the actuator bounds or grow unbounded unless the local potentials, which yield the controls, are carefully designed. Local potentials to overcome this limitation have been used in [7–9]. Yet, potentials guaranteeing bounded gradient-based controls are not enough to preserve MAS connectivity. Actuator saturation may still distort the control input and lead to loss of connectivity. The dynamic compensation strategy in [9] has preserved system connectivity by limiting the local controls within actuation bounds, but has increased the order of the system and is conservative when the control signals approach their bounds.

This paper introduces a distributed coordination controller for single-integrator MAS that both maintain the local connectivity and better exploit the bounded velocities. It proposes smooth and bounded local potentials which yield gradient-based controls that behave as Proportional ~ (P) controllers with distance-dependent gains. Innovatively, the new local control laws limit the effect of actuator saturation to a

T. Ahram et al. (Eds.): IHIET 2019, AISC 1018, pp. 695–699, 2020.
https://doi.org/10.1007/978-3-030-25629-6_108

dynamic scaling of the P controls by time-varying positive gains. Hence, the bounded gradient-based controls still implement a distributed P law with time-varying, positive and lower-bounded P gains that decrease the local potentials monotonically while maintaining the sensing links of the MAS. Two sets of numerical simulations verify the performance of the proposed controllers for single-integrator a MAS with bounded velocities.

2 Preliminaries

In a MAS, each agent i, with position $\mathbf{p}_i \in \Re^n$, has limited communication capability. Two agents i and j are adjacent/neighbors if and only if they can, and agree to, exchange information with each other. To be able to exchange information, they must be within their communication distance r. Note that if agent j is within the communication distance of i, $\|\mathbf{p}_{ij}\| = \|\mathbf{p}_j - \mathbf{p}_i\| \le r$, then agent i is also within the communication distance of j, $\|\mathbf{p}_{ji}\| = \|\mathbf{p}_i - \mathbf{p}_j\| \le r$. However, agents within communication distance of each other are neighbors only if they agree to exchange information with each other. Therefore, the set of neighbors of any agent need not change when coordination is achieved and all agents are within communication distance of all other agents.

This paper adopts the following definition of, and assumptions on, of the communication graph of a MAS.

Definition 1. [10] The communication graph of a MAS $G = \{v, E\}$ consists of a set of nodes $v = \{1, \ldots, N\}$, each associated with a different agent in the system, and a set of communication edges $E = \{(i,j) \in v \times v | i \in N_j\}$, each associated with a communication link in the system, where N_j is the set of neighbors of agent j.

Assumption 1. The communication graph is undirected, i.e., $(i,j) \in E$ iff $(j,i) \in E$.

Assumption 2. The undirected communication graph of the MAS is initially connected and each pair of initially adjacent agents (i,j) is strictly within their communication distance, i.e., $\|\mathbf{p}_{ij}(0)\| = \|\mathbf{p}_{ji}(0)\| \le r - \varepsilon$ for some $\varepsilon > 0$.

The paper further adopts the definitions in [10] of the weighted adjacency matrix $\mathbf{A}$, weighted Laplacian matrix $\mathbf{L}$, and incidence matrix $\mathbf{D}$ associated with a graph G. Hence, $\mathbf{A}$ is symmetric, and $\mathbf{L}$ and $\mathbf{D}$ are related via $\mathbf{L} = \mathbf{DWD}^{\mathrm{T}}$[10], where $\mathbf{W}$ is an $M \times M$ diagonal matrix with the diagonal entries equal to the weights of each edge and M the number of edges of graph G.

3 Main Result

Consider an MAS of N single-integrator agents with dynamics:

$$\dot{\mathbf{p}}_i = \mathbf{u}_i \tag{1}$$

where: $i = 1, \ldots, N$ indexes the agents in the system; $\mathbf{p}_i = (p_{i1} \ldots p_{in})^{\mathrm{T}} \in \Re^n$ is the position vector of agent i; and $\mathbf{u}_i = (u_{i1}, \ldots, u_{in})^{\mathrm{T}} \in \Re^n$ is the actual control of agent i.

For each pair of initially adjacent agents $(i,j) \in E$, consider the potential function:

$$\varphi(\|\mathbf{p}_{ij}\|) = \frac{\|\mathbf{p}_{ij}\|^2}{r^2 - \|\mathbf{p}_{ij}\|^2 + \frac{r^2}{Q}} \tag{2}$$

where Q is a positive constant selected to obey $Q > \frac{N(N-1)(r-\varepsilon)^2}{2\left(r^2-(r-\varepsilon)^2+\frac{r^2}{Q}\right)}$. By Assumption 2, all $\varphi(\|\mathbf{p}_{ij}\|)$ are defined on $[0, r]$ at $t = 0$.

The following gradient-based control law serves to coordinate the MAS and preserve its connectivity in this paper:

$$\tilde{\mathbf{u}}_i = -\Sigma_{j \in N_i} \nabla_i \varphi(\|\mathbf{p}_{ij}\|) \tag{3}$$

where N_i is the set of neighbours of agent i at time $t = 0$, and $\nabla_i \varphi(\|\mathbf{p}_{ij}\|)$ is the gradient of $\varphi(\|\mathbf{p}_{ij}\|)$ with respect to $\mathbf{p}_i$. The actual control $\mathbf{u}_i$ on agent i is equal to the designed control $\tilde{\mathbf{u}}_i$ if $\tilde{\mathbf{u}}_i$ is within the agent's actuation bound; otherwise, the agent's actuator saturates and applies only part of $\tilde{\mathbf{u}}_i$:

$$\mathbf{u}_i = \mathrm{Sat}_i(\tilde{\mathbf{u}}_i) = (\mathrm{sat}_{i1}(\tilde{u}_{i1})\ldots\mathrm{sat}_{in}(\tilde{u}_{in}))^{\mathrm{T}} \tag{4}$$

The connectivity preservation and coordination of single-integrator MAS under the bounded gradient-based control law in (4) can be investigated by regarding actuator saturation as scaling of the designed control through time-varying positive gains:

$$\mathbf{u}_i = \mathrm{Sat}(\tilde{\mathbf{u}}_i) = \mathbf{S}_i(t)\tilde{\mathbf{u}}_i \tag{5}$$

where $\mathbf{S}_i = \mathrm{diag}\{s_{i1}(t), \ldots, s_{in}(t)\}, i = 1, \ldots, N$ are diagonal matrices with diagonal elements $s_{ik}(t) > 0$ for all $k = 1, \ldots, n$.

The Lyapunov function that facilitates the proof that the bounded control (5) maintains the initial communication links of the single-integrator MAS (1) is designed as:

$$V = \frac{1}{2}\Sigma_{i=1,\ldots,N}\Sigma_{j \in N_i}\varphi(\|\mathbf{p}_{ij}\|) \tag{6}$$

Algebraic manipulations show that the derivative of this function is non-positive and, thus, that is V monotonically decreasing, i.e., $V(t) \leq V(0)$, for all $t \geq 0$. The same function V, together with the Lasalle Invariance Principle, can be used to deduce coordination. Both proofs are omitted here due to page limits.

4 Simulation Results

This section compares the controller in (3) to that in [9] through simulations of a MAS with $N = 5$ single-integrator agents with: dimension $n = 1$; communication radius $r = 1$ m; actuation bounds 2 m/s, 1 m/s, 1 m/s, 2 m/s and 3 m/s; and initial position

1 m, 1.5 m, 2 m, 2.5 m and 3 m. For the controller in (6), condition (9) is guaranteed by $Q = 40$ after selecting $\varepsilon = 0.1$ m. For the controller in [9], the design parameters are $\alpha_i = 1$, $\varepsilon = 0.1$ and $\beta_i = 11$.

Figures 1 and 2 illustrate that the MAS is coordinated in about 0.7 s by the controller in (6), and in about 10 s by the controller in [9]. The difference in performance arises from a dynamic compensation mechanism in [9] that prevents actuator saturation, as seen in Fig. 2, and thus makes the control conservative and limits the speed of convergence. In contrast, the controller (6) permits simultaneous saturation of several actuators, as shown in Fig. 1, and uses agents' actuation more fully.

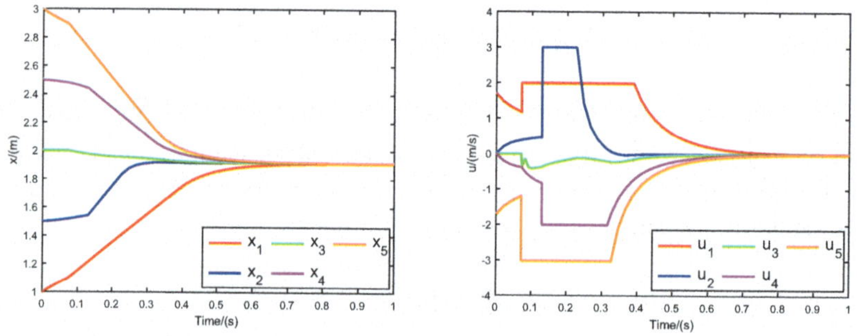

Fig. 1. Coordination of 5 single-integrator agents controlled by (6): positions (*left plot*) and control signals (*right plot*) of all agents.

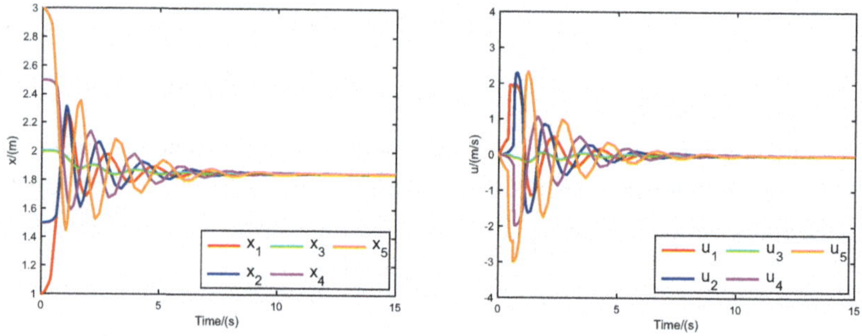

Fig. 2. Coordination of 5 single-integrator agents controlled by the controller in [9]: positions (*left plot*) and control signals (*right plot*) of all agents.

5 Conclusions

This paper has presented a distributed connectivity-preserving coordination controller for single-integrator MAS with bounded actuations. The key steps in the proposed design are: (i) to regard actuator saturation as dynamic scaling of the control; and (ii) to drive the MAS with gradient-based controls derived from local potentials designed to decrease monotonically even when the controls saturate. Then, connectivity preservation results directly from the monotonic decrease of the local potentials. The proposed controller is less conservative than existing distributed connectivity-preserving coordination controllers. With minor modifications, the controller can also guarantee the connectivity-preserving coordination of nonholonomic MAS. Future research will explore sufficient conditions for connectivity-preserving coordination of second-order MAS with bounded actuation.

References

1. Ren, W.: On consensus algorithms for double-integrator dynamics. IEEE Trans. Autom. Control **53**(6), 1503–1509 (2008)
2. Saber, R.O., Murray, R.M.: Consensus protocols for networks of dynamic agents. In: American Control Conference, pp. 951–956. IEEE Press, New York (2003)
3. Ji, M., Egerstedt, M.: Distributed coordination control of multiagent systems while preserving connectedness. IEEE Trans. Autom. Control **23**(4), 693–703 (2007)
4. Zavlanos, M.M., Pappas, G.J.: Potential fields for maintaining connectivity of mobile networks. IEEE Trans. Rob. **23**(4), 812–816 (2007)
5. Dimarogonas, D.V., Kyriakopoulos, K.J.: On the rendezvous problem for multiple nonholonomic agents. IEEE Trans. Autom. Control **52**(5), 916–922 (2007)
6. Feng, Z., Sun, C., Hu, G.: Robust connectivity preserving rendezvous of multi-robot systems under unknown dynamics and disturbances. IEEE Trans. Control Network Syst. **4**(4), 725–735 (2017)
7. Li, X., Sun, D., Yang, J.: A bounded controller for multirobot navigation while maintaining network connectivity in the presence of obstacles. Automatica **49**(1), 285–292 (2013)
8. Ajorlou, A., Aghdam, A.G.: Connectivity preservation in nonholonomic multi-agent systems: a bounded distributed control strategy. IEEE Trans. Autom. Control **59**(9), 2366–2371 (2013)
9. Saboori, I., Nayyeri, H., Khorasani, K.: A distributed control strategy for connectivity preservation of multi agent systems subject to actuator saturation. In: American Control Conference, pp. 4044–4049. IEEE Press, New York (2013)
10. Mesbahi, M., Egerstedt, M.: Graph Theoretic Methods in Multiagent Networks. Princeton University Press, Princeton (2010)

Society 5.0 as a Result of the Technological Evolution: Historical Approach

Andreia G. Pereira[1,2], Tânia M. Lima[1,2(✉)], and Fernando Charrua-Santos[1,2]

[1] Department of Electromechanical Engineering, University of Beira Interior, Calçada Fonte do Lameiro, 6201-001 Covilhã, Portugal
{andreia.gregorio.pereira, tmlima, bigares}@ubi.pt
[2] C-MAST - Centre for Mechanical and Aerospace Science and Technologies, Covilhã, Portugal

Abstract. In the XX century, arises the mass production implemented by Henry Ford to overcome the period of crisis lived in the World. In 1988, the term Lean emerged and this philosophy successfully challenged the mass production implemented in the automotive industry, focused on customers' requirements and satisfaction with the minimum use of resources and waste elimination. A Lean environment can be a promoter in the implementation of the fourth industrial revolution, named Industry 4.0 (I4.0). In the succession of Industry 4.0 emerged the Society 5.0 in Japan, as a strategy to deal with the impact of an ageing population. The focus of this quiet revolution is the humankind and the creation of conditions to promote a happy, motivated and satisfied society with more time for leisure and consequently increase productivity and wealth. This article presents a historical approach to the technological evolution of productive systems, and their influence on societies.

Keywords: Society 5.0 · Industry 4.0 · Lean production · Ageing population · Productivity · Quality of life

1 Introduction

In the twentieth century, Fordism was at the origin of the first industrial revolution, through its philosophy of producing a unique model, thus allowing increasing the production capacity and consequently the reduction of the price of automobiles, which made it possible to acquire them through social classes [1].

After the Second World War, the Lean philosophy has emerged and successfully challenged mass production practices in the automotive industry, with impact in the relation between production and quality as well as production according to customer needs [2]. The production contingency established in Japan allowed the implementation of a production system with a minimum stock of products and services, with tools and practices, which enabled the production of products with more quality, less costs and less production time.

The Industry 4.0 (I4.0) enables the implementation of a dynamic and controlled production autonomously, optimizing the respective supply chains and will be able to

T. Ahram et al. (Eds.): IHIET 2019, AISC 1018, pp. 700–705, 2020.
https://doi.org/10.1007/978-3-030-25629-6_109

join the Lean philosophy with the integration of information and communication technologies [2]. The tools and technological advancements developed by the I4.0 might be used to benefit societies by introducing improvements in their quality of life.

While the world is still adapting to the challenges set by the I4.0, Japan is already moving forward with Society 5.0, with technological development with ambitious goals and the introduction of new methodologies, such as orders delivery made with drones or autonomous trucks [3].

2 From Mass Production to Lean Philosophy

According to Henry Ford's philosophy, the focus was the mass production with the production of standardized products, allowing only a few changes [4].

Fordism featured assembly-line techniques that allowed an improved and more efficient production in standardized and low-cost products. This concept was initially implemented in the automotive sector, although it is also applicable in other manufacturing realities [2].

After the Second World War, Toyota was forced to change its production policy, concerning the limited resources and the necessity to maintain production, that is, to do more with less and emerges the Lean production [4].

According to [5], the industries that apply the Lean production policy are able to produce a wide range of products while maintaining high levels of quality and productivity and this is the first time that the name Lean has appeared. In the Western world, Lean is often referred as Kaizen, which means continuous improvement in Japanese [4].

Concerning the different definitions in the literature, Lean could be defined as an integrated system that produces products and services considering a minimum number of products in stock and low costs [6]. The Lean philosophy enables the implementation of a production system that encourages organizations to adopt continuous improvement practices, through a set of tools and practices that allow them to achieve higher quality, lower costs and shorter execution time [6]. In addition, the Lean philosophy adopts the elimination of all waste, which in Lean terminology is named MUDA [6].

The most common practices commonly associated with Lean production are: bottleneck removal, cellular manufacturing, competitive benchmarking, continuous improvement programs, cross-functional workforce, cycle time reductions, focused factory production, just-in-time/continuous flow production, lot size reductions, maintenance optimization, new process equipment/technologies, planning and scheduling strategies, preventive maintenance, process capability measurements, pull system/ Kanban, quality management programs, quick changeover techniques, reengineered production process, safety improvement programs and total quality management [7].

3 Industry 4.0

In 2011, the German government announced the Industry 4.0 as one of the main initiatives of its high-tech strategy, with an approach that strengthens the competitiveness of the German manufacturing industry [8].

Industry 4.0 is defined as the real-time, intelligent and digital network of people, equipment and objects for industrial management [9] and allows the increasing digitization of all supply chain and the interconnection between people, objects and systems through the exchange of data in real time [10].

The term Smart refers to Industry 4.0 applications including areas such as Smart Factory and Manufacturing, Smart Product and Smart City [11].

The volatile and global market associated with competition enable new challenges for industries concerning the cost, quality and time [9]. The increasing number of competitors and the constant fluctuation of demand/supply in the market allow customers to choose a variety of different products [9]. Due to global competition, it is essential that industries are able to follow innovation and bring products to market very quickly [10]. The interconnection of products, machines and processes with artificial intelligence allows the adaptation to changes independently in the forecast planning [10].

This fourth industrial revolution it is considered the greatest technological revolution with informatization in production, evolution of industrial production systems and consequent reduction of costs, energy, increased safety and quality, improving production processes [12]. It allows the creation of new opportunities for industries, with the challenge of automation and digitalization of production processes [10], a dynamic manufacturing and supply, contemplating the product life cycle [11].

In the future, industries will choose to establish global networks that include machines, storage systems and production facilities from Cyber-Physical Systems (CPS) [8]. CPS is defined as transformational technology for managing systems interconnected between physical resources and the capacities allowed by the computers [9]. In the manufacturing environment, CPS includes intelligent machines, storage systems and production installations with capacity to exchange information autonomously, promote actions and independent control [8].

The applications developed by Industry 4.0 allow the stabilization and support of Lean principles [13]. Although Lean techniques are not in all industrial realities, the intelligent factory that will be promoted by Industry 4.0 will be the reality of the future for industries [13].

4 Society 5.0

Society 5.0 is a quiet revolution starting in Japan to the world, which promises to revolutionize society to improve the humankind life quality, namely focuses on human′ s position in the center of innovation and technological transformation [12]. The main goal of Society 5.0 is to improve the quality of people's lives, using the potentialities acquired by Industry 4.0 [14].

In 2050, it is foreseen that in Japan about 40% of the population will be over 65 years and older, it means that will be the oldest society [15]. The ageing of the Japanese population is a matter of concern and the use of technology such as artificial intelligence, robotics, Big Data, autonomous trucks and drone deliveries will have to be integrated to deal with the dilemma of today's society [12].

In Japan, it is already part of the "growth plan for the future" the training for a super-intelligent society with the capacity to meet the sustainable development goals [3]. Japan will create a Society 5.0 services platform with the purpose to coordinate collaboration between government, academics and industry [3].

This new concept of society aims to promote the idea that industries will be successful if they have happy and fulfilled people at work, by creating all the conditions to improve the day to day of their employees, which will promote a happier, more satisfied and consequently more productive society [12].

Economic growth and social problems can be bridged by the panoply of technologies at the service of humanity and can reduce greenhouse gases, increase production, minimise the loss of food, mitigate costs associated with the ageing of society, sustainable industrialization, redistribution of wealth, correction of regional inequalities, among others [3].

Presently, advances through innovation in science and technology namely in the drastic increase in computing power, contributes to the improvement of business and society [16].

The connection between people and things and between the real and cybernetic worlds will enable the effective and efficient resolution of societal issues to promote a better quality of life for people and to support healthy economic growth [16]. It is expected a change of paradigms of Intelligent Transportation System (ITS) centered on technology for ITS centered on society, with the solution in the CPSS and in the parallel systems methodology [17].

The creation of virtual artificial systems applies a complex analytical approach to the system, which is an ACP approach, which consists of: (A) "Artificial systems"; (C) "Computational experiments"; (P) "Parallel execution" [17].

Society 5.0 is an evolution developed as a continuation of the information society, with the goal of enhancing individual strengths, improving the company's strengths and solving social problems [18].

Technological development allows improving the standard of living of humankind. However, it may have a negative impact on employment and an unequal distribution of wealth and information [19].

The implementation of Society 5.0 has to integrate several dimensions, such as Innovation Policy, Entrepreneurial Spirit and Entrepreneurial Skills, in order for its implementation not to become a purely political-ideological concept [14].

According to Keidanren (2018), digital transformation announced a fifty society. The four precedent societies were marked by Hunting, Agrarian, Industrial, and Information [20]. Figure 1 illustrates the relationship between evolution of Society and Industrial Revolutions.

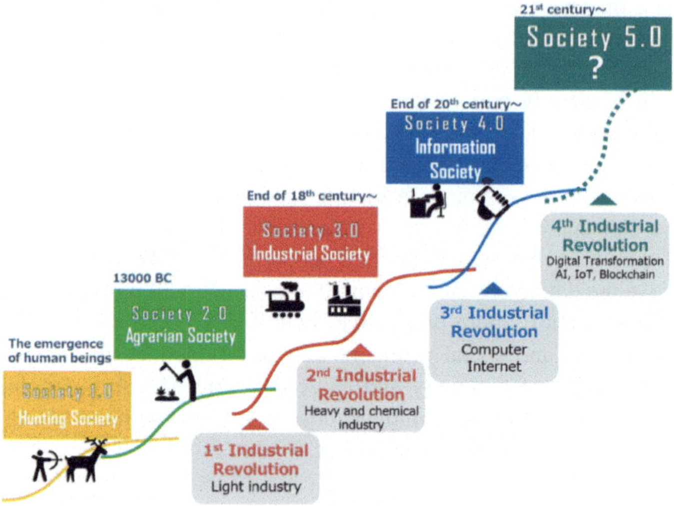

Fig. 1. Relationship between evolution of Society and Industrial Revolutions [20]

5 Conclusion

From the beginning of humankind, the human being sought to find solutions that could improve his working conditions, with this purpose aroused the mechanization of work, electricity and automation, which are part of everyday life today.

The economic crises in the world were an opportunity for industries to promote philosophies that would allow them to produce more with less. At the beginning of the XX century emerged mass production. Later and following another economic crisis, the Lean philosophy emerged with minimal use of resources and the elimination of waste, with a focus on customer satisfaction.

In 2011, Industry it is challenged to follow the technological evolution, with the digitalization of the supply chain and the network interconnection between people, objects and systems, in real time, named fourth industrial revolution or Industry 4.0.

Recently, Japan is concerned with the ageing of the population, and intends to take immediate measures in which the society benefits from the new technologies generated by Industry 4.0 and allows the creation of a system able to improve the quality of life of society, named this new industrial revolution as Society 5.0.

Society 5.0 challenges current societies to use the new technologies of Industry 4.0 to enable them to enjoy a better quality of life by gaining more time for leisure and for personal/family life. However, people may see this as a threat to their jobs and even as a deprivation of interaction with their peers. For this reason, a good part of the success of this new concept of society will depend on the ability of governments to distribute the wealth generated equitably.

Acknowledgments. The authors were funded in part by Fundação para a Ciência e a Tecnologia under project UID/EMS/00151/2019 and C-MAST.

References

1. Smith, C.: Work, Employment & Society, vol. 3, Birmingham (1989)
2. Holweg, M.: The genealogy of lean production. J. Oper. Manage. **25**, 420–437 (2007)
3. Oliveira, H.: A Sociedade 5.0 e a co-criação do futuro, VER – Valores, Ética e Responsabilidade (2019). www.ver.pt/a-sociedade-5-0-e-a-co-criacao-do-futuro
4. Alves, A.C., Kahlen, F.-J., Flumerfelt, S., Siriban-Manalang, A.-B.: The lean production multidisciplinary: from operations to education. In: 7th International Conference on Production Research – Americas, Guimarães (2014)
5. Krafcik, J.F.: Triumph of the Lean Production System, vol. 30 (1988)
6. Naylor, J.B., Naim, M.M., Berry, D.: Leagility: integrating the lean and agile manufacturing paradigms in the total supply chain. Int. J. Prod. Econ. **62**, 107–118 (1999)
7. Shah, R., Ward, P.: Lean manufacturing: context, practice bundles, and performance. J. Oper. Manage. **21**, 129–149 (2003)
8. Hermann, M., Pentek, T., Otto, B.: Design principles for industrie 4.0 scenarios. In: 49th Hawaii International Conference on System Sciences (2016)
9. Dombrowski, U., Richter, T., Krenkel, P.: Interdependencies of industrie 4.0 & lean production systems - a use cases analysis. In: 27th International Conference on Flexible Automation and Intelligent Manufacturing - FAIM2017, Italy, pp. 1061–1068 (2017)
10. Hecklau, F., Galeitzke, M., Flachs, S., Kohl, H.: Holistic approach for human resource management in Industry 4.0. In: 6th CIRP Conference on Learning Factories, Germany, pp. 1–6 (2016)
11. Lu, Y.: Industry 4.0: a survey on technologies, applications and open research issues. J. Ind. Inf. Integr. **6**, 1–10 (2017)
12. Costa, J.M.: Sociedade 5.0, o futuro, pelo presente, Dinheiro Vivo (2018). www.dinheirovivo.pt/opiniao/sociedade-5-0-o-futuro-pelo-presente/
13. Wagner, T., Herrmann, C., Thiede, S.: Industry 4.0 impacts on lean production systems. In: 50th CIRP Conference on Manufacturing Systems, pp. 125–131 (2017)
14. Ferreira, C.M., Serpa, S.: Society 5.0 and Social Development: Contributions to a Discussion, vol. 5 (2018)
15. Granrath, L.: Japan's Society 5.0: Going Beyond Industry 4.0, Japan Industry News (2017). www.japanindustrynews.com/2017/08/japans-society-5-0-going-beyond-industry-4-0
16. Shiroishi, Y., Uchiyama, K., Suzuki, N.: Society 5.0: For human security and well-being. IEEE Comput. Soc. **51**, 91–95 (2018)
17. Wang, F.-Y., Zhang, J.J.: Transportation 5.0 in CPSS: towards ACP-based society-centered intelligent transportation. In: IEEE 20th International Conference on Intelligent Transportation Systems (ITSC): Workshop (2017)
18. Prasetyo, Y. A., Arman, A. A.: Group Management System Design for Supporting Society 5.0 in Smart Society Platform. International Conference on Information Technology Systems and Innovation (2017)
19. Nakanishi, H.: World Economic Forum (2019). www.weforum.org/agenda/2019/01/modern-society-has-reached-its-limits-society-5-0-will-liberate-us
20. Keidanren (2018). www.keidanren.or.jp/en/policy/2018/095_outline.pdf

Using Machine Learning to Optimize Energy Consumption of HVAC Systems in Vehicles

Martin Böhme(✉), Andreas Lauber, Marco Stang, Luyi Pan, and Eric Sax

Karlsruhe Institute of Technology, Institute for Information Processing Technologies (ITIV), Engesserstraße 5, 76131 Karlsruhe, Germany
{martin.boehme, andreas.lauber, marco.stang, eric.sax}@kit.edu

Abstract. The detachment and calculation of functionalities from a vehicle into a cloud creates new chances. By linking different data sources with the in-vehicle data in the cloud, an optimization of these functionalities in terms of energy efficiency can be applied. For example, the Heating, Ventilation and Air Conditioning (HVAC) consumes up to 30% of total energy in a vehicle. Electric vehicles in particular lead to these high values because they are not able to recover the waste heat from combustion engines for interior heating. Therefore, the optimization of energy efficient strategies with respect to the vehicle energy management system becomes more relevant. Forecasts of the interior vehicle temperature are directly related to the HVAC energy consumption. This work focuses on the implementation and accuracy evaluation of Recurrent Neural Networks (RNN) for interior vehicle temperature forecasting.

Keywords: Heating Ventilation and Air Conditioning (HVAC) · Energy efficiency · Internet of Things · Machine learning

1 Introduction

The integration of vehicles with the Internet of Things (IoT) enables a stream of relevant sensor data into a cloud system [1]. The combination of different external data (e.g. weather forecasts, traffic conditions) with in-vehicle data in the cloud allows new strategies for the energy optimization of the HVAC system. Forecasts of the interior vehicle temperature enables the creation of optimized HVAC control (e.g. On/Off schedules). The resulting system predicts future peak loads and preconditions the vehicle according to the created schedules. Such forecasting problems have been an issue of great importance especially for the case of building HVAC systems [2]. Machine learning algorithms allow us to tackle these problems in a novel way as they are able to learn and predict patterns based on different inputs.

T. Ahram et al. (Eds.): IHIET 2019, AISC 1018, pp. 706–712, 2020.
https://doi.org/10.1007/978-3-030-25629-6_110

2 State of the Art of Time Series Forecasting Methods

2.1 Recurrent Neural Networks

In feed-forward neural networks, outputs of one layer is fed as input into the subsequent layers and each unit does relatively simple computations. Outputs are independent of each other i.e., output at time *t* is independent of output at $t - 1$. This idea of independence considered above does not match with sequences such as time-series data which consists of short-long term temporal dependencies that should also be taken into account [3]. For any given sequential data, the output depends upon previous information as well as the current input as shown in the Architecture of RNNs in Fig. 1.

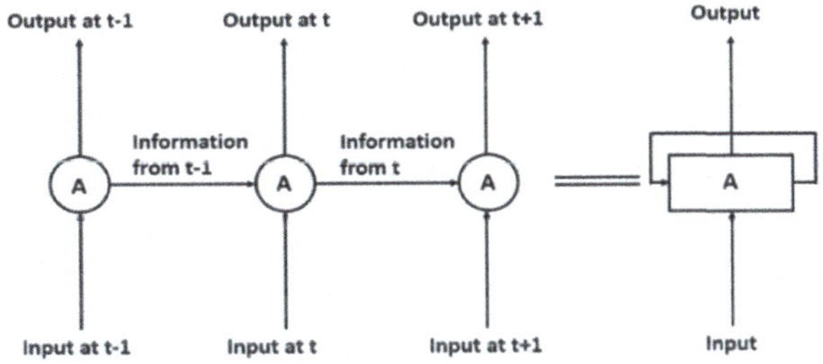

Fig. 1. Architecture of recurrent neural network model [3]

Still RNNs lag in learning as the gap between required previous information and the point of requirement increases to a large extent.

2.2 Long Short Term Memory Networks

LSTM is a special architecture of a recurrent neural network especially used in the field of deep learning. The LSTM contains special units called memory blocks in the recurrent hidden layer. The memory blocks contain memory cells with self-connections storing the temporal state of the network in addition to special multiplicative units called gates to control the flow of information [4].

A schematic of a LSTM block can be seen in Fig. 2. It features three gates (input, forget and output), block input, a single cell (the constant error carousel), and an output activation function. The output of the block is recurrently connected back to the block input and all of the gates [5].

A schematic of a LSTM block can be seen in Fig. 2. It features three gates (input, forget and output), block input, a single cell (the constant error carousel), and an output activation function. The output of the block is recurrently connected back to the block input and all of the gates [5].

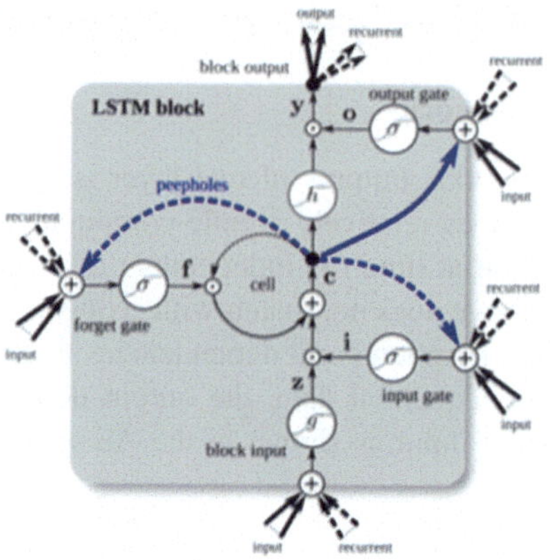

Fig. 2. Detailed schematic of a LSTM block [5]

3 Concept for Vehicle HVAC Optimization

Modern vehicles are equipped with numerous sensors that create huge amount of data transmitted over the vehicle`s bus communication systems [6]. Modern digital communication paves the way to send this data from Controller Area Network (CAN) and other bus systems out of the vehicle into a cloud (V2X). As the cloud is basically a high-performance computer it is able to handle computing-intensive tasks like machine learning. We want to use this data to perform machine learning algorithms in the cloud and return the calculation results back into the vehicle.

In order to optimize the energy consumption of a HVAC system, vehicle sensor data correlated to the operation of the system needs to be streamed into the cloud. The control of HVAC systems is calculated based on different temperature or temperature correlated inputs. The data we used for our machine learning forecasts is described in the following chapter.

4 Datasets and Setup

The Living Lab Bus Project[1] offers development opportunities utilizing the fleet of electric buses running in normal operation on a few of Helsinki Region Transport (HSL) lines. The buses serve as a mobile sensor platform providing extensive selection of real-time and accumulated history data from both existing and third-party devices. We used the data from the sensors that were installed on the bus. The sensor data is measured with a sampling rate of $T = 1\ s$. However, in order to create better forecasting models, each time series is sub-sampled with a period of $T' = 5\ min$.

[1] Living Lab Bus project: http://livinglabbus.fi/.

Three sensor signals were taken into consideration:

- Interior temperature in degrees Celsius. This is the interesting forecasting variable.
- Air pressure measured in kPa.
- Humidity in mass of water vapor mH20.

The data handled needed further preparation as there were missing datapoints and busses didn't have the same operating times each day. The training and testing dataset were created with consecutive days, where each day included the same operating times.

Table 1 displays the training and testing dataset used for further processing.

Table 1. Description of training and testing datasets

Dataset	Number of days	Operating time	Time interval
Training	34	12 h	5 min
Testing	9	12 h	5 min

5 Experimental Results

5.1 Evaluation Measures and Network Architecture

The performance of the described forecasting methods is measured with two different error functions: Mean Average Error (MAE) and Root Mean Square Error (RMSE) [7]. The error is computed comparing target values for the time series $s_{t+1}, s_{t+2}, \ldots, s_{t+z}$ and its corresponding time series prediction $\hat{s}_{t+1}, \hat{s}_{t+2}, \ldots, \hat{s}_{t+z}$.

The network architecture consists of an input shape according to the shape of the training data, followed by 32 LSTM blocks and an output layer that makes a single value prediction.

5.2 Evaluation Results

The following is a summary of the results based on the above-mentioned measures. Two different models were created, one model was trained with all three mentioned features (sensor signals as described in Sect. 4), the other model only used interior temperature as an input. Table 2 shows the results of the multiple features model, whilst Table 3 presents the results of the single feature model. Changing hyperparameters like learning rate ('lr'), dropout ('do') and recurrent dropout ('rdo') had significant impact on MAE and RMSE.

Table 2. Evaluation measures of LSTM model with multiple features and different hyperparameters

Hyperparameter	MAE	RMSE
lr = 0.0001, do = 0.1, rdo = 0.1	0.316055	0.383337
lr = 0.0001, do = 0.2, rdo = 0.3	0.282314	0.349757
lr = 0.05, do = 0.1, rdo = 0.1	0.498570	0.637318

The training and validation loss (MAE) over 20 epochs corresponding to the best model from Table 3 are displayed in Fig. 3. It can be seen that training loss is less than half of validation loss. Training loss seems to improve with the number of epochs while validation loss shows volatility.

Table 3. Evaluation measures of LSTM model with a single feature and different hyperparameters

Hyperparameter	MAE	RMSE
lr = 0.0001, do = 0.1, rdo = 0.1	0.308752	0.378731
lr = 0.001, do = 0.1, rdo = 0.1	0.223504	0.296546
lr = 0.05, do = 0.1, rdo = 0.1	0.498570	0.637318

Figure 4 shows the 12-h prediction of the interior temperature of the best single and multiple feature models presented in Tables 2 and 3. The models are displayed adjoining ground truth. The plot of the single feature model adapts to trends but clearly doesn't show spikes as ground truth. The MAE and RMSE values for the multiple feature model were appropriate but the plot of this model doesn't seem to fit ground truth. The graph doesn't show trends and basically stays within a range of 0.2 °C.

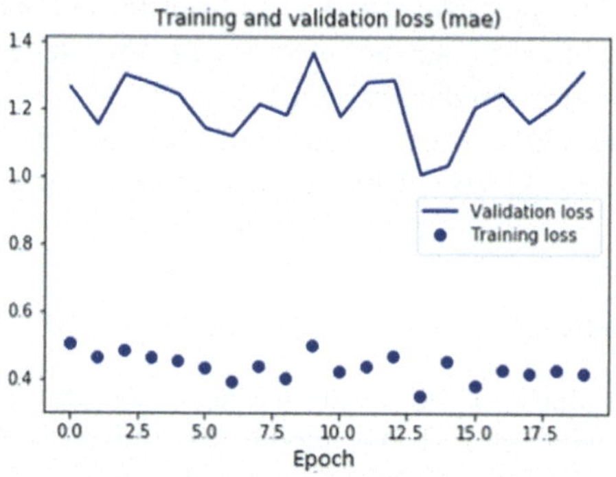

Fig. 3. Training and validation loss (MAE) single feature (LR = 0.001, DO = 0.1, RDO = 0.1)

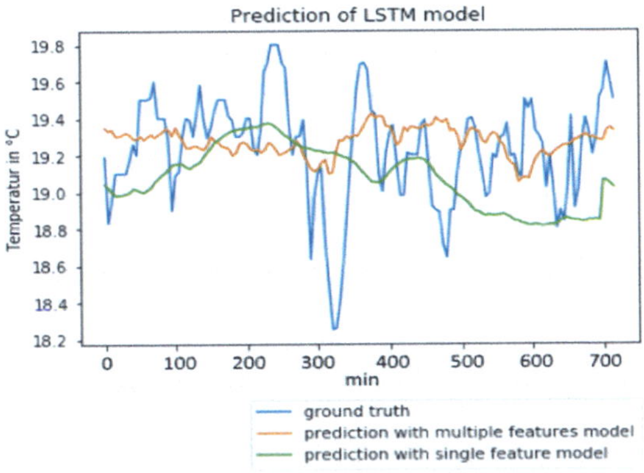

Fig. 4. Prediction of the LSTM model with single and multiple features and ground truth

6 Conclusion

The research in this paper has been focused on how to predict the interior temperature of a vehicle (in this case a city bus), as this is directly related to the HVAC system energy consumption. Both a multiple and a single feature model were followed and their performances were examined with MAE and RMSE. The single feature model (only interior temperature) has shown promising results with a MAE $\approx$ 0.224 °C. The addition of two other features in the multiple feature model didn't show improvements. Air pressure and humidity covariates seem to not add new information to the model in order to improve forecasts.

The results of this work are promising but further research has to be done especially when it comes to the already discussed combination of in-vehicle data with public data. While the overall best result was achieved with only one feature, this is clearly not said for the integration with several other data sources and needs to be examined.

For the purpose of generating HVAC energy optimization, these forecasts have to be used for proactive settings of the HVAC system. Usual set points that can be influenced are temperature set point and fan speed. By calculating an optimized HVAC schedule including the time constants of the HVAC control, the potential energy savings need to be evaluated.

References

1. Traub, M., Vögel, H.J., Sax, E., Streichert, T., Härri, J.: Digitalization in automotive and industrial systems. In: Proceedings of 2018 Design Automation Test in Europe Conference and Exhibition DATE 2018, January 2018, pp. 1203–1204 (2018). https://doi.org/10.23919/DATE.2018.8342198
2. Zamora-Martínez, F., Romeu, P., Botella-Rocamora, P., Pardo, J.: Towards energy efficiency: forecasting indoor temperature via multivariate analysis. Energies **6**, 4639–4659 (2013). https://doi.org/10.3390/en6094639

3. Kurdikeri, R.B., Raju, A.B.: Comparative study of short-term wind speed forecasting techniques using artificial neural networks. In: Proceedings of 2018 International Conference on Current Trends Towards Converging Technologies, ICCTCT 2018, pp. 1–5 (2018). https://doi.org/10.1109/ICCTCT.2018.8550849
4. Sak, H., Senior, A., Beaufays, F.: Long short-term memory recurrent neural network architectures for large scale acoustic modeling. In: INTERSPEECH 2014 (2014). https://doi.org/10.1016/j.edumed.2017.01.001
5. Greff, K., Srivastava, R.K., Koutnik, J., Steunebrink, B.R., Schmidhuber, J.: LSTM: Search Space Odyssey. CoRR. abs/1503.0, pp. 2222–2232 (2015)
6. Massaro, E., Ahn, C., Ratti, C., Santi, P., Stahlmann, R., Lamprecht, A., Roehder, M., Huber, M.: The car as an ambient sensing platform. Proc. IEEE **105**, 3–7 (2017). https://doi.org/10.1109/JPROC.2016.2634938
7. Chai, T., Draxler, R.R.: Root mean square error (RMSE) or mean absolute error (MAE)? - Arguments against avoiding RMSE in the literature. Geosci. Model Dev. **7**, 1247–1250 (2014). https://doi.org/10.5194/gmd-7-1247-2014

An Evolutionary Approach to Hyper-Parameter Optimization of Neural Networks

Marco Stang(✉), Christopher Meier, Vinzenz Rau, and Eric Sax

Institut für Technik der Informationsverarbeitung (ITIV), Engesserstraße 5, 76049 Karlsruhe, Germany
{Marco.Stang, Christopher.Meier, uzdzh, Eric.Sax}@kit.edu

Abstract. The last few years have increasingly been influenced by the emergence of neural networks for classification tasks. Due to the increasing size of the nets, especially concerning deep neural nets, the selection of the optimal topology becomes critical. A set of hyper-parameters determines the topology of a neural network. The selection of suitable hyper-parameters however, is time-consuming or requires expert knowledge. This paper examines the application of an evolutionary algorithm to optimize the hyper-parameters of a neural network. The result of the optimization by evolutionary algorithms can be applied for a variety of use-cases: i.e. detection of anomalies in CAN-bus data, object recognition for autonomous driving or the classification of hydraulic machinery oil.

Keywords: Machine learning · Hyper-parameter optimization · Neural network · Evolutionary algorithm

1 Introduction

Neural Networks can analyze and detect hidden patterns and trends in large amounts of data, far beyond human recognition. An area of application are Intrusion Detection Systems (IDS) in the automotive domain [1]. Furthermore, they are applied for object classification for autonomous driving in a simulated test environment [2] or in this paper for the classification of different oil quality categories. Therefore, they have established themselves as one of the most used concepts in data-mining and machine learning. Their underlying concept, to process input signals with the help of widely connected artificial neurons, mimics the core function of the human brain. The conjunction of these processing units to several stacked layers gives the neural network the ability to learn and predict patterns. One of the key challenges to successfully build and train a new neural network is to find the optimal hyper-parameters (i.e. number of layers, number of neurons, activation functions). Hyper-parameters are model-specific properties set before the start of the learning process. The time-consuming process of configuration, training, and testing with each new set of hyper-parameters enforces the need for an efficient algorithm to identify these values. A strategy to optimize the speed and efficiency of this process is the deployment of an Evolutionary Algorithm. Inspired

T. Ahram et al. (Eds.): IHIET 2019, AISC 1018, pp. 713–718, 2020.
https://doi.org/10.1007/978-3-030-25629-6_111

by the process of biological evolution, this concept encodes parameters in a generic artificial DNA. An integrated validation process ensures that each DNA has only one possible but valid solution to the optimization problem, providing the hyper-parameters for a neural network. The quality of each solution, stored by an individual in a population, is determined by a predefined fitness function. The fitness function is part of an evolutionary method with the target of identifying a global optimum. This evolutionary setup as a hyper-parameter optimization strategy provides a fast, efficient, universal, and simple way to implement and construct optimal neural networks.

2 State of the Art

2.1 Evolutionary Algorithms

Evolutionary algorithms use fundamental concepts of biological evolution to solve complex optimization problems. They are part of population-based optimization techniques and search the given search space using artificial individuals. Each represents a possible solution to the optimization problem. Through the targeted application of genetic operators, generated individuals are modified until the defined termination criterion is reached, and a sufficiently precise solution is found. An artificial population consists of a fixed number of individuals and is responsible for their generation, management, and evaluation. In the course of the optimization process, several successive populations are created [3]. Analogous to biology, these are also called generations. An artificial individual represents exactly one solution of the given optimization problem by its assigned DNA. The quality of this solution is determined by the fitness function and is stored in the individual's fitness value. An individual forms the primary object of the evolutionary algorithm and is subject to the evolutionary process [4]. Each artificial DNA encodes in a list of genes exactly one possible solution to the optimization problem. A gene represents the value of a specific optimization parameter in the number range $0 \leq Gen \leq 1$ [5]. Depending on the given problem, a different number of genes can be used to construct the DNA. An implemented control mechanism ensures that each DNA represents a unique and valid solution in the defined search space. Each individual receives an artificial DNA upon initialization. Recombination is the systematic modification of the genetic material of already evaluated individuals to generate new DNAs with improved genes. The individuals used are determined by the selection method. Subsequently, two individuals (parents) are chosen from this group, depending on their fitness. Their DNA is recombined with the help of genetic operators [6]. The computed DNAs are assigned to new individuals, the so-called children. In this paper, a distinction is made between the following two genetic operators. The single-point crossover operator separates two parent DNA, and alternately combines new children's DNA, [5]. The mutation operator randomly selects genes from a parent DNA and modifies the DNA slightly. The rate of modification is determined randomly and is limited by a maximum tolerated step size [7]. The selection is responsible for picking the parent individuals that should be used to create a new population. The fitness of the particular individuals has a decisive influence since only the best individuals of a population are selected and therefore have a chance of reproduction. The final creation of the new population is determined by the inheritance strategy. This strategy determines the application of the genetic operators and ensures that the defined population size is maintained [6]. The general procedure [4] of the evolutionary algorithm can be described by the following steps:

1. Generating the starting population (Generation 0) with N individuals of random DNA
2. Calculating the fitness of each individual
3. Selection of the best I individuals from the current population (based on the fitness of each individual)
4. Calculation of N new individuals by applying the genetic operators (crossover and mutation) according to a defined inheritance strategy
5. Creating a new population from these resulting individuals
6. Calculating the fitness of each individual of the new population
7. Go back to step 3, if the maximum number of generations is not reached.

2.2 Artificial Neural Networks

The fundamental idea of Artificial Neural Networks (ANN) is to process input signals with the help of widely connected artificial neurons, which mimic the core function of the human brain. The conjunction of these processing units to several stacked layers gives the neural network the ability to learn and predict patterns. The transfer function f_{sum} adds up the calculated products and thereby determines the stimulation of the perceptron. With this excitation and a further threshold value (bias), the activation function f_{act} can calculate the output of the artificial neuron [4].

The Multilayer Perceptron (MLP) is a particular type of artificial neuronal network. A single artificial neuron cannot perform a complicated classification. Thus, several neurons build different layers in order to perform this task. While the neurons of one layer are not connected, successive layers are being connected. Figure 1 (left) shows a sample MLP structure. While each MLP consists of precisely one input layer and one output layer, the number of hidden layers is varying and depends on the complexity of the given classification problem. Given such a problem, MLP seeks to adjust the individual weights and biases of the hidden layers so that the output of the last layer optimally represents a given category. The adjustment of these parameters is repeated several times using an already classified data set and is referred to as "training." After completing the training of a neural network, its performance is evaluated against a previously unknown data set. The accuracy of these predictions allows the evaluation of an MLP's capability to classify. Hyper-parameters are responsible for the definition of the structure of an MLP as well as the definition of essential training parameters. They must be set before constructing an MLP and describe parameters like the number of hidden layers, number of neurons per layer, dropout rate, activation function, and optimization-algorithm. The data set used is generated by synthetically produced oil samples. Various machine oils were examined using infrared spectroscopy and manually subdivided into the categories "Good," "Sufficient," and "Bad" according to their quality (Fig. 1, right).

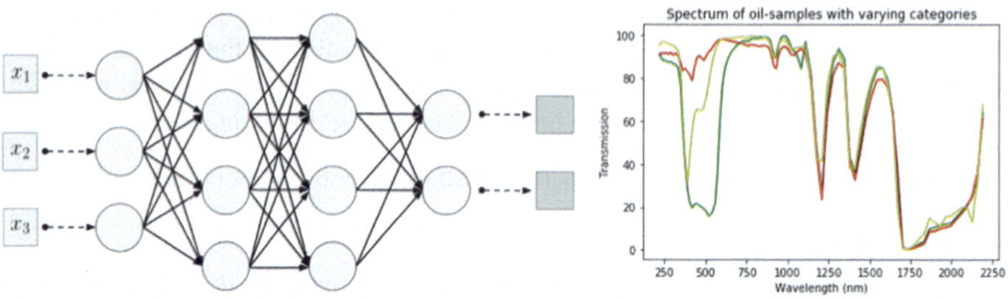

Fig. 1. The basic structure of an MLP (left) [8] and spectrum of oil data samples with three categories (right)

3 Implementation of an Evolutionary Algorithm for Hyper-Parameter Optimization

A learning algorithm optimizes the internal parameters (weights and biases) of an ANN. Since these parameters are responsible for the information flow within the neuronal network and collectively take on the role of a classification function, they are decisive for the achievable accuracy of an MLP. The complexity of this function, in turn, depends on the structure of the MLP and hence on the hyper-parameters. One of the key challenges to successfully build and train a new neural network is to find the best fitting hyper-parameters. The time-consuming process of configuration, training, and testing with each new set of hyper-parameters enforces the need for an efficient algorithm to identify these values. Evolutionary algorithms can efficiently and quickly search, any given search space for global optima. Even minor adjustments in the structure of an MLP can lead to vast improvements in performance, but cannot be reliably foreseen. We have limited ourselves to the optimization of the construction of the MLP. The hyper-parameters, used along with their respective search regions, are displayed in Table 1.

Table 1. Definition and range of used hyper-parameters

Parameter name	Description	Specified range
$num_{hl}(\#n_{hl})$	Defines the number of hidden layers of the MLP	$0 \leq num_{hl} \leq 3$
$num_{neur.}(\#n_{neu})$	Defines the number of neurons of each hidden layer	$1 \leq num_{neur} \leq 200$
$dropout(d)$	Defines the dropout of each hidden layer	$0 \leq dropout \leq 0.4$
activation function (f_{act})	Defines the activation function of each hidden layer	$f_{act} \in \{\text{relu}, \text{sigmoid}, \text{tanh}\}$

Since the hyper-parameters also represent the optimization parameters of the evolutionary algorithm, they must be encoded in genes. For each new layer, the number of neurons, dropout, and activation function must be defined. The parameters are, therefore, not independent of each other. However, in order to achieve a high degree of flexibility in the structure of the individual layers, as many genes are generated as are required for the maximum number of layers. After defining the optimization parameters and the associated structure of the DNA, the initial population can be created. No knowledge about the given search space is available at the beginning, and $N = 10$ individuals are generated with random DNA. In order to be able to calculate the fitness of the different individuals, the MLP encoded in the following steps are performed for each individual:

1. Decoding the DNA of the individual
2. Construction of an MLP using hyper-parameters obtained from the DNA
3. Training the MLP on the training data set and testing the MLP on the test data set
4. Assigning the fitness of the individual according to the performance of the MLP.

The initial population is thoroughly evaluated and provides for the calculation of a new population using the inheritance strategy. The individuals of this population continue to follow the evaluation process described above. This process is carried out for five populations.

4 Results and Discussion

In the course of the optimization process, five populations with ten individuals each were created. Thus a total of 50 MLPs were built, trained, and evaluated. The course of the achieved fitness values of the best and worst individual as well as the average of all individuals of each population are depicted in Fig. 2 (left). The MLP of the best individual found correctly classified 10.544 of the 12.000 test data and consequently achieved a test accuracy of 88.57%. The associated hyper-parameters, as well as the training history of the best MLP, are shown in Fig. 2 (right).

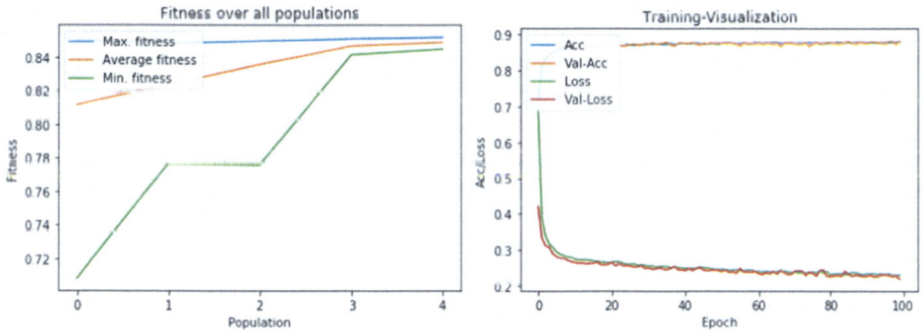

Fig. 2. Fitness overall populations (left), Training history of the best-found individuals (right)

Compared to a manually created MLP, the evolutionary algorithm can increase the performance of an MLP through a better choice of hyper-parameters. It also provides an efficient alternative to traditional algorithms such as random search and grid search through its target-oriented approach. Since each additionally calculated population further examines the search space, better optima can be found with an increasing number of generations and individuals. A further advantage of the evolutionary algorithm lies in the possibility to optimize the structure of ANN to specific characteristics. In addition to the choice of hyper-parameters, the fitness function can also be adapted.

5 Conclusion

Due to their versatile and flexible usage in various fields of technology, ANNs are an essential tool for data processing. The creation of a new neural network is a time-consuming and mostly problem-dependent process. Automated algorithms for optimizing the network structure are becoming increasingly important. In this paper, a promising concept was introduced to how evolutionary algorithms can be applied to optimize the structure of MLPs and further increase their performance. Due to its flexible and universal design, the presented concept can easily be transferred to other types of ANNs and consequently be used in other areas of machine learning.

References

1. Pfeffer, R., Ukas, P., Sax, E.: Potential of virtual test environments for the development of highly automated driving functions using neural networks. Presented at the (2019). https://doi.org/10.1007/978-3-658-23751-6_18
2. Weber, M., Pistorius, F., Sax, E., Maas, J., Zimmer, B.: A hybrid anomaly detection system for electronic control units featuring replicator neural networks. In: Arai, K., Kapoor, S., Bhatia, R. (eds.) Advances in Intelligent Systems and Computing, pp. 43–62. Springer, Cham (2019). https://doi.org/10.1007/978-3-030-03405-4_4
3. Weicker, K.: Anwendung evolutionärer Algorithmen. In: Evolutionäre Algorithmen, pp. 237–291. Springer (2015)
4. Kruse, R., et al.: Computational Intelligence: Eine methodische Einführung in Künstliche Neuronale Netze. Evol. Algorithmen, Fuzzy-Systeme und Bayes-Netze Vieweg + Teubner, Wiesbad (2011)
5. Nissen, V.: Evolutionäre Algorithmen: Darstellung, Beispiele, betriebswirtschaftliche Anwendungsmöglichkeiten, Wiesbaden 1994. Zugl.: Diss., Dt. Univ, (1994)
6. Gerdes, I., Klawonn, F., Kruse, R.: Evolutionäre Algorithmen: Genetische Algorithmen - Strategien und Optimierungsverfahren -Beispielanwendungen. Springer-Verlag (2013)
7. Pohlheim, H.: Evolutionäre Algorithmen: Verfahren. Springer-Verlag, Operatoren und Hinweise für die Praxis (2013)
8. Adam Gibson, J.P.: Major Architectures of Deep Networks. https://www.oreilly.com/library/view/deep-learning/9781491924570/ch04.html#multi-layer-feed-forw

Universal Basic Income: Comparative Analysis of Experiments

Svetlana Tsvirko(✉)

Financial University under the Government of the Russian Federation, Leningradskiy prospekt 49, Moscow, Russian Federation
s_ts@mail.ru

Abstract. The article reveals the features of universal basic income. The objective of the research is to analyze experiments with UBI and to detect advantages and disadvantages of this relatively new, innovative and rather contradictory approach. The method of research is comparative analysis. Several experiments in the sphere of UBI in different types of countries (both developed and developing) are discussed. It is shown that the results of UBI-like experiments are controversial.

Keywords: Universal basic income · Public finance · Social policy · Welfare · Poverty · Inequality

1 Introduction

The study of issues related to the evaluation of results of some experiments in the sphere of universal basic income (UBI) is of current interest.

There is significant amount of publications devoted to the aspects of UBI – both in western economic literature and in Russia. Among them we can name publications by such authors, as Ackerman, Alstott and Van Parij [1], Andersson [2], Coady, Prady and Francese [3, 4], Widerquist [5], researchers from Kela (The Social Insurance Institution of Finland) [6], Istratov, Belyanov [7], Kuznetsov [8]. A number of international organizations have issued their working papers devoted to UBI. For example, OECD is an opponent of UBI in advanced economies as it is revealed in [9]. As for IMF, it does not give direct answer about UBI: in a special announcement the representative of IMF said that IMF is not advocating for or against UBI [10]. There is a specialized website devoted to the concept of UBI [11]. However, it seems that there is no holistic approach to an integrated assessment of opportunities and risks of UBI, which is really necessary to increase efficiency in the relevant sphere.

Experiments in social sphere in different countries have a high degree of uniqueness and specificity, their evaluation is characterized by uncertainty and variety of factors that should be taken into consideration.

In this context the aim of this study is to analyze possibilities and drawbacks of UBI. For achieving the aim of the research, it is necessary to reveal the essence of UBI and the realization of this concept in practice, clarify the problems of evaluation of the results of the experiments with UBI management.

T. Ahram et al. (Eds.): IHIET 2019, AISC 1018, pp. 719–724, 2020.
https://doi.org/10.1007/978-3-030-25629-6_112

2 Essence of Universal Basic Income and Reasons for Popularity of the Ideas of Universal Basic Income

UBI is a periodic payment unconditionally delivered to all on an individual basis, without means-test or work requirement. According to one of the most famous proponents of the idea of UBI Philippe Van Parij, UBI is defined as «income paid by a political community to all its members on an individual basis, without means test or work requirement» [1, page 4].

Relevance of the topic can be explained by the necessity to introduce new approaches to fight with poverty and inequality.

An important reason for the popularity of the idea of UBI was the fear that the labor market would be threatened by automation - smart robotic technologies would force people out of their jobs. There is some evidence that the labor market will face a threat from Artificial Intelligence (AI) in particular and information technology in general. Under the conditions of automation, machines think faster, make more accurate decisions and do their job more carefully than a person. There are industrial robots, unmanned vehicles, systems of collecting and analyzing information, digital assistants - achievements in the field of narrowly focused AI. Although General Artificial Intelligence (comparable in cognitive ability to human, that is, able to solve in completely unforeseen situations, to experiment and invent new scenarios, with self-conscience), according to forecasts, will not appear until 2050, the level of intelligence that robots demonstrate already now disturbs the society. According to the research performed by BCG, when asked about the implications of AI for the economy and society, citizens expressed significant concerns about the availability of work in the future (61% agree) [12]. One of the publications, that caused a wide public response was the publication of Oxford Martin School, where it was stated, that around 47% of total US employment is in the high risk category due to computerization [13]. So, the threat of loss of income makes people turn to the idea of small but guaranteed income.

3 Experiments in the Sphere of Universal Basic Income

Analysis of different countries' experiments in the sphere of social policy, including welfare, can produce relevant data about UBI and provide some understanding of the necessity and possibility to implement UBI as a national or regional policy. Analysis of some UBI-like experiments include cases of the USA, Canada, Finland, Italy, India, Kenya, Uganda (see Table 1).

Our research showed that in practice, there was no full implementation of the concept of UBI in any country of the world. What is given as examples of implementation of UBI can be better defined as different forms of social benefits, which are devoid of either unconditionality, inclusiveness or regularity. The concept of a minimum guaranteed income - a social support system that provides all citizens of the country with enough income for life - is close to the idea of UBI, but is not the same. The minimum guaranteed income is fundamentally different from UBI by the

Table 1. UBI-like social programs

Period	Place of experiment	Number of participants	Payable amount, euro/month	Conditions of inclusion into the program	Comments
1996–nowadays	USA (North Carolina)	8000	862 (in year 2016)	Belonging to the Cherokee tribe	The program budget is formed by gambling revenues
2006–2008	Uganda	12000	329	Age from 15 to 25 years, ultra-low income (less than $ 1 per day)	The program was aimed at increasing employment, reducing poverty and the risk of participation in riots
2010–2012	India (Madhya Pradesh)	6000	21 (per family)	Living in a certain village	The experiment involved 9 villages; performance evaluation was conducted on a wide range of factors: living conditions, nutrition quality, morbidity, etc.
2017–2018	Italy (Livorno)	100 families	460 (per family)	Belonging to the poorest families	In 2018 the experiment was extended to another 100 families
2017–2018	Canada (Ontario)	4000	940	Low income	The project has not been extended
2017–2018	Finland	2000	560	Age 25–58, absence of work	The project has not been extended
2017–nowadays	Kenya	26000	20	Living in a certain village	200 villages were divided into 3 groups with different duration of payments to compare effects of short- and long-term projects

application of some criteria by which the right to receive additional government benefits is assessed. As for minimum guaranteed income, various forms of it now exist in many countries.

It is also necessary to stress difficulties in performing experiments of UBI. The UBI-like programs were performed on a limited scale and cannot be recognized as national scale programs.

Among possible advantages of UBI researchers often name: poverty reduction, the ability to lead a decent life, no matter what happens; insurance against financial disasters in light of the threat of a decline in employment due to the growing automation of processes; possibility for people to spend more time with their families or volunteer activities; reduction of corruption opportunities.

The results of the experiments are contradictory. Some above mentioned advantages were really achieved. For example, in developing countries there were improvements in poverty eradication. In particular in India the following was observed: improvements in health, productivity, and financial stability. In terms of impacts to health, the unconditional cash transfers were associated with better food security and lower rates of malnutrition, especially in female children. Recipient villages had lower rates of illness, more consistent medical treatment, and more consistent medicine intake. As a result they had higher expenditures on schooling and agricultural inputs, promoting better education and higher agricultural yields.

In some experiments the start of payouts led to higher employment and not to its decrease, as some skeptics feared. A number of features were noted: shift from hiring to work based on self-employment (for example, farming), increase in women's business activity, and reduction in the level of migration from the relevant areas.

Finland can be an example of advanced economy with the experiment in the sphere of UBI. In Finland, according to preliminary results, at the end of the experiment the recipients of a basic income perceived their wellbeing as being better than did those in the control group. The recipients of a basic income had less stress symptoms as well as less difficulties to concentrate and less health problems than the control group. They were also more confident in their future and in their ability to influence societal issues. Survey respondents who received a basic income described their financial situation more positively than respondents in the control group. They also experienced less stress and fewer financial worries. The basic income experiment in Finland did not increase the employment level of the participants in the first year of the experiment [6].

One of the controversial issues with UBI is the issue of eliminating of inequality. Proponents argue that UBI can reduce inequality, since income will be the same for all. Opponents claim the opposite, and their arguments are stronger. It is obvious that different people may need different income to maintain the same standard of living for various reasons: different health conditions; different climate and place of residence, etc. Thus, people with problems of any kind will be put in less favorable conditions. This fundamentally undermines the idea of a social state, which supporters of UBI advocate.

The most serious drawbacks of UBI are as follows: burden on public finances, possible tax increases, reduction of other social programs, fraught with public discontent; dismantling of labor and socially useful activities, polarization of society, loss of skills and the inability to return to the labor market. Inflation will lead to a decrease in real income, so an indexing mechanism is required within UBI approach.

Additional complications associated with UBI were found out in the experiment in India and include the fact that within households women's ability to manage income will be limited in favor of men. There is also an argument about the potential overload of the banking system.

We can conclude that given the forms of social relations that have developed in the modern world, the implementation of UBI in the near future seems unlikely. Only from a financial point of view, the UBI concept can be suitable for small countries accumulating income from external sources (for example, offshore and resort countries, gambling territories, etc.). But a change in circumstances in some countries, for instance, the terms of a social contract, may open the way for the implementation of UBI in its ideal form in the long term.

4 Conclusion

In this paper we have revealed the essence of UBI. We have analyzed several experiments with UBI or UBI-like programs and came to the conclusion that, first of all, there are difficulties with proper definition of the concept and evaluation of the results of experiments taking into consideration different factors. Second, it was shown that the results of the experiments in the sphere of UBI are contradictory.

We should look at the UBI from an interdisciplinary perspective with focus on both economic and social factors. It is necessary to combine views of economics, politics, social policy and philosophy into one holistic approach to UBI. An analysis based on survey data that examines the impact of the experiment on the wellbeing of the UBI recipients should be continued. We need to bring together international and national scholars, scientists and activists to have a comparable look at UBI, identify commonalities and differences across countries with UBI and finally learn lessons for more efficient social policies.

References

1. Ackerman, B., Alstott, A., Van Parij, P.: Redesigning distribution: basic income and stakeholder grants as alternative cornerstones for a more egalitarian capitalism (2003). https://www.ssc.wisc.edu/~wright/Redesigning%20Distribution%20v1.pdf
2. Andersson, J.O.: Will Finland be first to introduce a basic income? https://abo.academia.edu/JanOttoAndersson
3. Coady, D., Prady, D.: Universal Basic Income in Developing Countries: Options, and Illustration for India, IMF Working Paper (2018). https://www.imf.org/en/Publications/WP/Issues/2018/07/31/Universal-Basic-Income-in-Developing-Countries-Issues-Options-and-Illustration-for-India-46079?cid=em-COM-123-37543
4. Francese, M., Prady, D.: Univeral Basic Income: Debate and Impact Assessment, IMF Working Paper (2018). https://www.imf.org/en/Publications/WP/Issues/2018/12/10/Universal-Basic-Income-Debate-and-Impact-Assessment-46441
5. Widerquist, K.: A Critical Analysis of Basic Income Experiments for Researchers, Policymakers, and Citizens – 2018. Palgrave Pivot. Springer Nature Switzerland AG, part of Springer Nature (2018)
6. Kela: Experimental Study on a Universal Basic Income (2019). https://www.kela.fi/web/en/basic-income-experiment
7. Istratov, V., Belyanov, A.: Believed in a fairy tale. J. Expert. **35**(1086), 36–39 (2018). (in Russian)

8. Kuznetsov, V.A.: Global challenges in payments industry: “Technological Unemployment” problem and universal basic approach as a possible scenario of its solution. J. Money Credit. **12**, 104–107 (2017). (in Russian)
9. OECD: Basic Income as a Policy Option: Can it Add Up (2017). http://www.oecd.org/employment/emp/Basic-Income-Policy-Option-2017.pdf
10. IMF not Endorsing Universal Basic Income Over PDS in India: Official (2017). https://www.business-standard.com/article/economy-policy/imf-not-endorsing-universal-basic-income-over-pds-in-india-official-117101500053_1.html
11. Basic Income Earth Network. https://basicincome.org
12. Carrasco, M., Mills, S., Whybrew, A., Jura, A.: The Citizen’s Perspective on the Use of AI in Government. BCG Digital Government Benchmarking (2019). https://www.bcg.com/ru-ru/publications/2019/citizen-perspective-use-artificial-intelligence-government-digital-benchmarking.aspx
13. Frey, C., Osborne, M: The Future of Employment: How Susceptible are Jobs to Computerisation? (2013). https://www.oxfordmartin.ox.ac.uk/downloads/academic/The_Future_of_Employment.pdf

User Discrimination of Content Produced by Generative Adversarial Networks

Nicholas Caporusso[1(✉)], Kelei Zhang[1], Gordon Carlson[2], Daniel Jachetta[1], Devon Patchin[1], Spencer Romeiser[1], Noah Vaughn[1], and Angela Walters[1]

[1] Department of Informatics, Fort Hays State University, 600 Park Street, Hays 67601, USA
{n_caporusso, k_zhang4, awalters}@fhsu.edu, {ddjachetta, djpatchin, s_romeiser, nqvaughn}@mail.fhsu.edu

[2] Institute for New Media Studies, Fort Hays State University, 600 Park Street, Hays 67601, USA
gscarlson@fhsu.edu

Abstract. Artificial Intelligence (AI) is increasingly being introduced in several domains for classification and clustering of different types of existing information (e.g., text, images, audio, and video). Recently, improvements to Machine Learning (ML) and new approaches to the design and use of Neural Networks (NNs) enabled the development of algorithms that generate new content that mimics the features of the training dataset. Specifically, Generative Adversarial Networks (GANs) are particularly effective in producing content with unprecedented levels of fidelity. As a result, they can generate realistic images of people, vehicles, and nature. In this paper, we discuss the results of a study that investigated user perception of pictures generated using GANs, with specific regard to portraits featuring faces. Specifically, our experiment involved 551 participants who were asked to classify over 7000 real images and pictures generated by ML algorithms. Our findings show that users show low accuracy in discriminating images and, thus, demonstrate the effectiveness of GANs in producing content that can be perceived as realistic.

Keywords: Artificial Intelligence · Machine Learning · Neural Networks

1 Introduction

In the recent years, Artificial Intelligence (AI) has become increasingly powerful thanks to faster hardware, to the development of new algorithms, and to the availability of open source frameworks and libraries that render AI accessible to larger audiences [1]. As a result, nowadays Machine Learning (ML) is being adopted in different domains (e.g., healthcare [2]) and tasks, such as, image [3], movement [4] and speech recognition, object detection, and autonomous vehicle navigation. In addition to solving traditional problems in the domain of AI, such as, classification and prediction, novel ML techniques aim at overcoming one of the main limitations of AI, that is, the possibility of creating new content.

T. Ahram et al. (Eds.): IHIET 2019, AISC 1018, pp. 725–730, 2020.
https://doi.org/10.1007/978-3-030-25629-6_113

Specifically, Generative Adversarial Networks (GANs) [5] are able to produce original material (e.g., images, speech, and text) with incredible fidelity compared to the training dataset. To this end, their architecture consists of two neural networks competing against one another: a generator NN creates new content based on features and parameters learned from a dataset, whereas a discriminator NN evaluates the output to ensure that its level of realism is consistent with the training set. As a result, GANs can generate high-quality, realistic images featuring non-existing individuals, original artwork that mimics the style of an artist, and text that resembles the rhetoric of a politician. Indeed, empowering machines to develop some degree of creativity and invent new content has incredible potential for applications in several industries. Simultaneously, potential misuse of novel algorithms poses challenges in terms of threats caused by highly realistic and credible profiles and fake news or content. Consequently, there is an emerging need of studying dynamics of human-machine interaction with AI-generated content to study both beneficial and malicious applications of novel Machine Learning systems.

As algorithms will produce more sophisticated and realistic replicas of user-generated content, studying individuals' behavior in the interaction with AI-generated material is crucial for improving the design of ML systems as well as for understanding mechanisms for ensuring users' security and educating them. Previous work focused on analyzing factors, such as, eye blinking, to evaluate whether users are able to distinguish fake faces in real pictures and videos [6].

2 Experimental Study

In this paper, we present a study in which we focused on users' perception of real and AI-generated content. Specifically, we investigated factors involved in the ability to distinguish between authentic and fake images with the objective of evaluating whether users are able to perceive the difference between pictures and discriminate the features that characterize images featuring real humans and AI-generated faces. To this end, we utilized the Generative Adversarial Networks dataset produced using NVIDIA's style-based generator architecture.

Our study consisted of an on-line survey in which participants were presented with random picture from a sample of 20000 images (5000 real and 15000 fake) extracted from the NVIDIA dataset [7]. To this end, we developed a web-based software (publicly available at https://newmedia.fhsu.edu/projects/real-or-ai/) that prompted users with a sequence of 10 randomly-selected non-repeat images from the sample collection. The interface was set to maximize the image width to fit the screen size of users' devices. For each picture, participants were given 5 s to decide between two options, that is, real human or AI-generated, and to click on the appropriate button on the interface of the experimental software.

In addition to recording users' responses, the data collection tool timed each phase of the experiment and acquired the device type (i.e., desktop or mobile) and the display size (i.e., extra-small, small, medium, large, extra-large). Finally, at the end of the session, the data collection tool asked participants for demographic information (i.e., age, ethnicity, gender, and familiarity with computers) and presented a debriefing screen with the results of the experiment, to gamify the experiment and incentivize sharing it (Fig. 1).

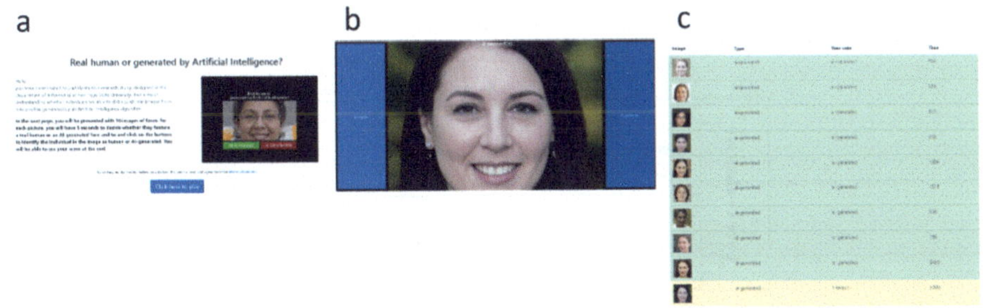

Fig. 1. The experimental software: (a) introduction page showing the instructions and informed consent, (b) trial interface in which users were presented with the image and with buttons (on the left and right sides of the display), and (c) debriefing page. Buttons had the same color to avoid bias.

3 Results and Discussion

551unique subjects participated to the study: among the ones who agreed to share their gender, 216 (39.20%) were females and 220 (39.93%) were males. Their age distribution was the following: 109 (19.78%) were 18-24, 222 (40.29%) aged 25–39, 88 (15.97%) were in the 40–54 bracket, and 34 (6.17%) were in the 55–75 range. Among the ones who agreed to share their nationality, 139 (25.22%) from Europe, 138 (25.04%) were from the US, 89 (16.15%) from China, 43 (7.80%) from other Asian countries, 19 (3.44%) identified as White Caucasian, and 83 (15.06%) were part of other groups. A total of 7137 trials were realized (an average of 12.95 trial per participant), each featuring a different picture (5668 AI-generated and 1469 actual profiles, accounting for 79.41% and 20.58% of the dataset, respectively). There were 742 cases in which the trial timed out due to several factors, including distraction, network performance causing picture rendering delay, and users not being able to identify an image before the 5-s timer expired. Timed-out trials involved 584 AI-generated images and 158 original images, accounting for 10.30% and 10.75% of the datasets, respectively. No statistically significant difference between classes was found. As a result, their values were not considered in our analysis. Consequently, our dataset involved a total of 6395 trials, involving images featuring 5084 AI-generated and 1311 real faces (79.49% and 20.50% respectively).

Figure 2 represents the experimental results as a confusion matrix: as users correctly identified AI-generated images 55.15% of the times, they were basically guessing when discriminating fake profiles, whereas they were slightly more successful (63.92%) in identifying real individuals. Furthermore, we did not find any statistically-significant correlation between accuracy and gender. Also, ethnicity does not seem to be a factor. However, we did not compare the ethnicity of the subject and that of the individual featured in the image, whereas published work on the own-gender and own-race biases [8, 9] suggests that this aspect might need further investigation.

n=6395		Actual		
		AI-generated	*Real*	
User evaluation	*AI-generated*	2804	473	3277
	Real	2280	838	3118
		5084	1311	

Fig. 2. Confusion matrix showing the actual content and participants' evaluation. Users had a total accuracy of 56.95% as they correctly identified images in 3642 trials: 2084 were AI-generated and 838 actual profiles. Users had a higher precision (85.56%) and lower recall (55.15%) in classifying pictures generated with GANs, while they had lower precision (26.87%) and higher recall (63.92%) in identifying images featuring actual humans.

Furthermore, when we analyzed the 3232 trials (50.53%) that contained information about display size, we found no statistical difference across device screens: surprisingly, the 1395 trials (43.16%) that involved desktop displays had an accuracy comparable to the 1837 trials (56.83%) that were executed on mobile devices, demonstrating the difficulty of recognizing distinctive features in images at larger resolutions.

Conversely, our findings show that age is a factor, as detailed in Fig. 3, which might be negatively correlated with accuracy. Although the number of subjects in each age group influences the results, differences in correctly identifying images exist within the groups of users who are younger than 45, which confirms the presence of a trend, though we will address this concern by improving randomization in sampling and data collection.

Also, we found a positive correlation between hours spent per day on PC and accuracy in classifying pictures: longer times spent on the PC are associated with better ability in recognizing real and fake profiles (the correlation coefficient is 0.98). Although we enabled subjects to iterate the experiment multiple times, we were not able to collect enough repeated sessions and, thus, we do not have enough data for analyzing the presence of training effect and for evaluating users' learning curve. Nonetheless, as data collection is ongoing, we aim at addressing this issue in a follow-up paper. The data collected in our experiment is shared in an open repository: a link for downloading the dataset in Comma Separated Values (CSV) format is available on the introduction page of the experimental software.

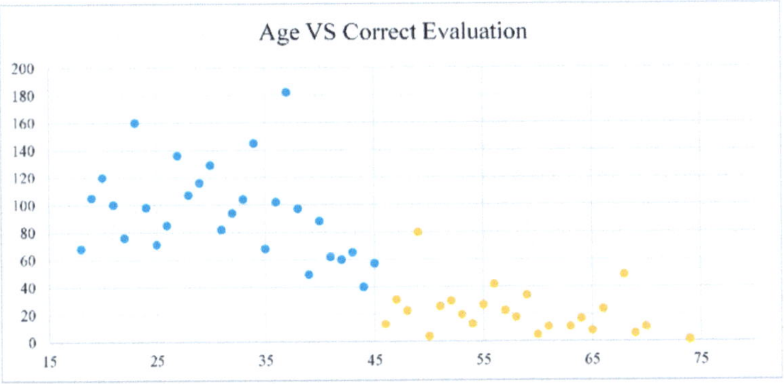

Fig. 3. Age VS correct User Evaluation. Age distribution among subjects partially explains the results, as individuals younger than 40 (331, 60,07%) were more than twice the number of people older than 40 (122–22, 14%). Simultaneously, the 109 participants between 12 and 24 had almost the same number of correct responses of the 222 subjects aged 25–39.

4 Conclusion and Future Work

In the last years, ML algorithms experienced dramatic improvement, especially in the context of image classification and recognition. Furthermore, Generative Adversarial Networks introduce novel ways to leverage AI to produce content. The ultimate objective of our work is to improve content generation Machine Learning systems by taking into account user experience. To this end, in this paper, we detailed the results of the preliminary stage of a focusing on content produced using GANs, with the purpose of our study was to evaluate whether algorithms are mature enough in terms of realism and fidelity. Specifically, the objective of our work was to evaluate whether users can recognize images featuring fake faces generated by AI algorithms and distinguish them from actual humans. To this end, we designed a study that investigated user perception of images created with GANs. Our findings show that participants showed low accuracy in discriminating real from fake profiles. From our results, we can conclude that the level of fidelity of images from the NVIDIA dataset was high enough to succeed in confounding users and triggering them into thinking that they were observing real profiles. Specifically, content produced by AI generated more ambiguity and users were more likely to identify it as authentic, whereas they were more accurate with pictures featuring real humans. Although we investigated images featuring faces, a similar approach can be applied to different types of content and formats.

In our future work, we will realize multiple iterations over the dataset: by collecting several responses for each image, we will be able to rank pictures by realism based on users' perception. Then, we will administer pictures from the ranked dataset to subjects, and we utilized an eye-tracking system to acquire and analyze fixations, in order to identify the key features utilized by individuals to distinguish between real and fake image. Subsequently, we will use the data to identify features that characterize fake images and to help improve both the generator and the discriminator components of the Generative Adversarial Network.

References

1. Caporusso, N., Helms, T., Zhang, P.: A meta-language approach for machine learning, to appear in 2nd international conference on human factors in artificial intelligence and social computing. In: International Conference on Applied Human Factors and Ergonomics. Springer, July 2019, to be published
2. De Pace, A., Galeandro, P., Trotta, G.F., Caporusso, N., Marino, F., Alberotanza, V., Scardapane, A.: Synthesis of a neural network classifier for hepatocellular carcinoma grading based on triphasic CT images. In: Recent Trends in Image Processing and Pattern Recognition: First International Conference, RTIP2R 2016, Bidar, India, 16–17 December 2016, Revised Selected Papers, vol. 709, p. 356. Springer, April 2017 https://doi.org/10.1007/978-3-319-60483-1_13
3. Bevilacqua, V., Uva, A.E., Fiorentino, M., Trotta, G.F., Dimatteo, M., Nasca, E., Nocera, A. N., Cascarano, G.D., Brunetti, A., Caporusso, N., Pellicciari, R.: A comprehensive method for assessing the blepharospasm cases severity. In: International Conference on Recent Trends in Image Processing and Pattern Recognition, pp. 369–381. Springer, Singapore, December 2016. https://doi.org/10.1007/978-981-10-4859-3_33
4. Bevilacqua, V., Trotta, G.F., Loconsole, C., Brunetti, A., Caporusso, N., Bellantuono, G.M., De Feudis, I., Patruno, D., De Marco, D., Venneri, A., Di Vietro, M.G.: A RGB-D sensor based tool for assessment and rating of movement disorders. In: International Conference on Applied Human Factors and Ergonomics, pp. 110–118. Springer, Cham, July 2017. https://doi.org/10.1007/978-3-319-60483-1_12
5. Bevilacqua, V., Trotta, G.F., Brunetti, A., Caporusso, N., Loconsole, C., Cascarano, G.D., Catino, F., Cozzoli, P., Delfine, G., Mastronardi, A., Di Candia, A.: A comprehensive approach for physical rehabilitation assessment in multiple sclerosis patients based on gait analysis. In: International Conference on Applied Human Factors and Ergonomics, pp. 119–128. Springer, Cham, July 2017. https://doi.org/10.1007/978-3-319-60483-1_13
6. Goodfellow, I., Pouget-Abadie, J., Mirza, M., Xu, B., Warde-Farley, D., Ozair, S., Courville, A., Bengio, Y.: Generative adversarial nets. In: Advances in neural information processing systems, pp. 2672–2680 (2014)
7. Li, Y., Chang, M.C., Farid, H., Lyu, S.: In ictu oculi: exposing AI generated fake face videos by detecting eye blinking (2018). arXiv preprint arXiv:1806.02877
8. Karras, T., Laine, S., Aila, T.: A style-based generator architecture for generative adversarial networks (2018). arXiv preprint arXiv:1812.04948
9. Wright, D.B., Sladden, B.: An own gender bias and the importance of hair in face recognition. Acta Physiol. (Oxf) **114**(1), 101–114 (2003)
10. Johnson, K.J., Fredrickson, B.L.: "We all look the same to me" Positive emotions eliminate the own-race bias in face recognition. Psychol. Sci. **16**(11), 875–881 (2005)

Application of a Human Factors-Integrated Information Security Framework to an Oil and Gas Organization

Ahmed I. Al-Darwish and Pilsung Choe(✉)

Department of Mechanical and Industrial Engineering,
Qatar University, 2713 Al Tarfa, Doha, Qatar
aal709549@student.qu.edu.qa, pchoe@qu.edu.qa

Abstract. Information systems support organizations to achieve strategic competitiveness and to improve the decision-making process. In addition, they help timely implementation of projects and effective risk management. A reliable and coherent information system requires a solid security framework that ensures Confidentiality, Integrity, Availability, Authenticity and Auditability of the critical information assets; therefore, managing security is essential for organizations doing a business in a globally networked and competitive environment whilst seeking to achieve their objectives and goals and ensuring the continuity of business. To date, studies have shown that non-technical risks are as important as technical risks in safeguarding. However, little attention has been paid to the role of human factors or organizational factors. This study validates the importance of non-technical factors based on a case study of an incident analysis using the information security framework with a focus of non-technical factors.

Keywords: Security management · Information security culture · Information security · Human factors · Risk Management · Organizational security

1 Introduction

The cyber threat becomes more and more sophisticated and dangerous, and determining the true sources of attacks remains a challenge. Technologies have been a main interest to enhance information security. However, the effect of technologies are limited in practice with many exceptions. Meanwhile, the influence of humans in information security has been somewhat neglected although information security should be everyone's responsibility in an organization. With this practical need for considering humans factors for information security, we proposed an information security framework with a focus of human factors [1, 2, 12–14], and applied this framework to a case to validate if the framework is appropriate to use for real incidents of cyber threats in the organization. We also investigated if this framework is complete and supportive tool to explore relevant actions to prevent or to minimize potential risk in the company. This proposed conceptual framework is based on the information security from four main components: Business, Enterprise Risk Management, Technology, and Human [1]. These four

T. Ahram et al. (Eds.): IHIET 2019, AISC 1018, pp. 731–736, 2020.
https://doi.org/10.1007/978-3-030-25629-6_114

components are essential to achieve a balance between information security and organizational management.

The selected cyber security incident for the case study concerns an International Oil and Gas organization located in Qatar. Cyber security in this organization is a very critical issue because it has a broad range of confidential information shared for work internally, domestically, or internationally by the nature of the oil and gas industry, which often involves complicated exports and imports business relations. In addition, the cyber security incident in the organization is one of the most consequential security breaches that have attracted great attention of all information security professionals. The security breach highlighted the issue of organizational failures in handling very complex issues where people and technology are concerned.

2 Case Study: International Oil and Gas Security Breach

2.1 Incident Overview

On Monday, August 27, 2012, malware was activated within the Company IT System (see Fig. 1) that led to the disruption of Microsoft Windows-based business systems (the "Incident"). The plant DCS (Distributed Control System) was on a separate logical network from the business network and was not compromised, however, there is evidence that the attackers intended to impact the DCS and it is likely that given time they could have accomplished this. SAP and Oracle running on UNIX operating system servers were located on a separate logical network from the Windows-based business network and were similarly not affected [3–7].

Attacker activity is observed as early as April 21, 2012 at The Company, with evidence that the attackers were targeting oil and gas industry in general, resulting in the specific attack on The Company. Logs show that the attacks originated from IP (Internet Protocol) addresses from four different countries, however it is difficult to verify whether these were the attackers' true origins [6, 7].

The initial point of entry for the attackers was on the Company DMZ (Demilitarized Zone) external network recruitment website from the internet on May 2, 2012. The attackers accomplished this by exploiting a vulnerability in a The Company-developed web application by uploading a malware file disguised as a curriculum vitae which gave them complete control of the recruitment server (code injection). This server was then used as a staging ground by the attackers to upload hacker tools to allow them to compromise user ids and passwords and to gain additional control in the DMZ. After using increasingly sophisticated methods, the attackers were finally able to breach the Company internal Windows-based business network from the DMZ via Citrix remote login on 13th August, two weeks prior to the Incident zero date. The attackers then repeated the process of downloading hacker tools to gain additional control in the internal business network [6, 7].

On August 26, The Company IT staff noticed suspicious behavior by a System Administrator account and reset its password. This is believed to have alerted the attackers that they may have been discovered, prompting them to deploy the malware that caused the Incident the following morning August 27, at approximately 3:30 am.

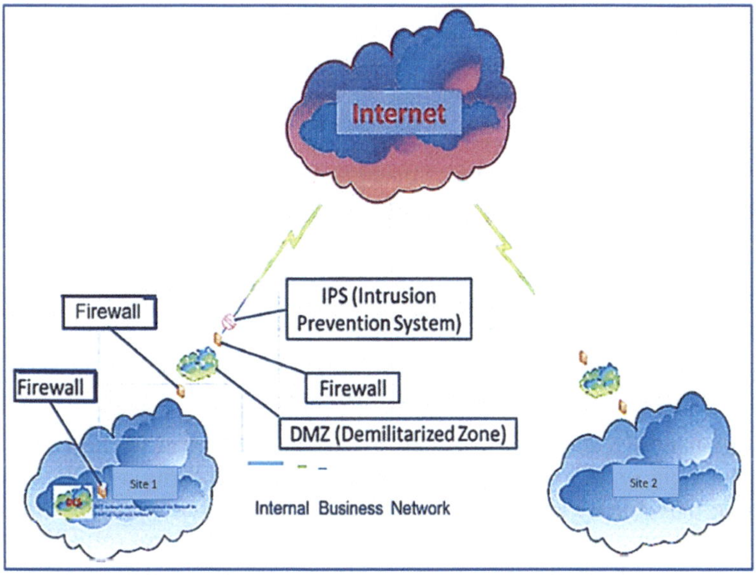

Fig. 1. Internal business network diagram. This shows a brief network structure of the company in relation to information security.

The malware that infected The Company was a new version of the Shamoon/DistTrack worm similar to the one that had previously infected other Oil and Gas company few weeks earlier, and was specifically tailored to "wipe" The Company Windows operating system servers and workstations. The wiping was accomplished by overwriting and thus destroying key data files including documents and critical operating system files rendering the machines inoperable. The malware was able to spread throughout the Windows business network and perform the wiping by utilizing a number of compromised user IDs and passwords that had elevated privileges and were hard-coded into the malware. Of 372 The Company Windows servers, 340 were completely wiped, 26 were partially wiped but could still boot up, and only 6 servers were not infected. All business system Windows servers and approximately 3200 related workstations had to be rebuilt from the ground up, with applications and data restored from clean vendor media and backups, as part of the recovery [8, 9].

Although the initial point of entry was an application on the DMZ recruitment website, there were many vulnerabilities at The Company that were exploited by the attackers or contributed in allowing them to succeed. One of the key contributing root cause factors was a complacent organizational culture which provided a false sense of security and thus a lack of adequate buy-in and urgency regarding the importance of information security [3, 8, 9].

2.2 Analysis and Findings

Incident analysis approach was used for validation study. Two root causes were identified as the source reasons that resulted in the Incident: Culture, and Organization [1].

Organizational Culture. The primary root cause was an organizational culture that provided a false sense of security (not limited, but most relevant in this case, to IT) and thus a lack of adequate buy-in regarding the importance of security. This led to a series of other issues such as inadequate staffing to ensure sufficient security coverage, a heavy organizational focus and priority on maintaining IT operations for the convenience of users, a lack of understanding and awareness of potential security risks, a lack of urgency in dealing with potential security threats, and the development of procedures and guidelines more for the sake of satisfying Audit or Compliance/Controls findings rather than to effectively mitigate risk exposures [1].

Organization (and Governing). Culture is a difficult element to shape, however it starts with strong organizational leadership emphasis on security as demonstrated by clear priorities/policies, organizational roles and responsibilities assigned to sufficient people with the right security skills and experience in effective team structures, and an ongoing interest and follow-up by leadership to provide sufficient governance in order to ensure security remains a top agenda item for continuous improvement of effectiveness in practice [1, 10, 11].

Other key findings include the following Direct and Indirect Human factors:

Ignorance and Negligence. A natural tendency for anyone who has not experienced a particular challenge or difficulty for a significant period of time is to assume that the risk of such an event has spontaneously faded away and is very low. However unless there is good evidence that the environment has changed for the better or that there is some other systemic factor that has resulted in this benefit, it would be a mistake to become complacent and simply assume that this was the case instead of it being the result of simple luck. The lesson is that The Company must remain ever watchful and vigilant, and keep current with the latest information and tools to ensure that it is able to see as sharply as necessary in order to proactively perceive and anticipate change, such as in the cyber-threat landscape, so that it is prepared for it when it does come, for it will.

Audit and Compliance Process. It is not all that difficult to discover risk exposure gaps, or improvement opportunities. Neither is it that difficult to implement some solutions to address these. The trick, however, is that closing a gap improperly can sometimes be worse than not closing it in the first place. By "closing" a gap one can gain a sense of misplaced confidence and security that may in fact be more damaging than recognizing that a gap still exists and needs to be cautiously managed. What's worse is that improperly/inadequately closing gaps uses up resources and introduces additional variation potentially further destabilizing processes. The lesson here is to focus more on the quality of gap closure and improvement, rather than quantity [1, 10, 11].

Individuals' Stress. Resources are almost always limited, in which case effective prioritization, which includes clear communication of expectations, is a critical activity. If after prioritizing there is still a resource shortage that must be filled, then a strong business case should be made and executed for the right resources. This should reduce the incidence of too few resources trying to do too much, including what they may not be adequately skilled for. The IT Manager at the time of the Incident had prepared a proposal for additional resources, and had obtained approval for an IT organization change, however implementation was delayed due to other apparent time demands [1, 3–6].

Employee Engagement. A great deal of technology had been deployed to prevent the type of security breach and Incident experienced by The Company: Intrusion Prevention System, Antivirus, activity logging (ArcSight), email alerts (InTrust), firewall logs, external penetration testing (Acunetix by Comguard), etc. and yet these all failed. People are best positioned to identify anomalous activity which is why empowering them with knowledge combined with explicit policies and procedures is an essential component in the defense against targeted attacks. Without this, technological tools are only partially effective [1, 10, 11].

Management Support. Information security is not only the responsibility of a few people, one section, or one department, it is rather the responsibility of everyone at The Company as security vulnerabilities will always exist to some extent and have the potential to be exploited from many angles. The best defense is a prepared and alert workforce to prevent, or at the very least mitigate damage from future breaches should they occur. Everyone should keep the security of their information top of mind, and adopt appropriate "security hygiene" as a breach for one person can compromise many others [1, 3].

3 Conclusions

Based on the case study, we found that the framework we proposed [1] effectively explained main the main causes of the cyber-attacks and we could be efficiently prepared with appropriate actions focused on each cause to prevent and minimize cyber risk. The factors found in the case study included: Enterprise Risk Management (Social Engineering Attack), human factors (Organizational Culture, Organization & Governing, Ignorance and Negligence, Audit & Compliance Process, Individuals' stress, Employee Engagement, Management Support), Technology (Vulnerabilities, Technology Complexity, Mobility), Economics (the total number of mechanics wiped, restoration/re-build cost, Company reputation) and all causes are appropriately addressed in the framework. We also found that the non technical factors are as important as technical factors for information security. Furthermore, we would conclude that non-technical factors are more carefully managed than technology itself for information security because technology should be properly used by humans that trigger lots of potential cyber risks by physical or cognitive human errors.

We will continue this study to see if this framework will be applied for other industries or cases. We will also continue validating the effect of the framework based on a quantitative analysis.

References

1. Al-Darwish, A., Choe, P.: A framework of information security integrated with human factors. In: HCI International 2019, USA (2019)
2. Audestad, J.: Four reasons why 100% security cannot be achieved. Telektronikk **1**, 38–47 (2005)
3. Internal Company Incident Report, Draft Ver 9.0, Q-CERT, 28 March (2013)
4. Internal Company - Forensics_IR - Technical Report - FINAL - Revision 3, McAfee Strategic Security Foundstone Services, 11 October 2012
5. Internal Company - Forensics_IR - Technical Report - DRAFT vl-3.0.docx, McAfee Strategic Security Foundstone Services, 28 September 2012
6. Internal Company Attack Investigation Executive Review, Symantec, 16 September 2012
7. Internal Company - W32. Disttrack Analysis Report, Symantec, 16 September 2012
8. Microsoft incident Response Report, Microsoft QSTP LLC, 13 September 2012
9. McAfee Labs Threat Advisory-W32-DistTrack b, McAfeeInc., 8 September 2012
10. IT Controls Status Report for Audit Committee Sep 2012 v3, IT Controls Enhancement Team (2012)
11. IT Controls Status Report for Audit Committee Jun 2012 vs, T Controls Enhancement Team (2012)
12. Trustwave 2012 Global Security Report. https://www.trustwave.com/spiderlabs
13. Top Cyber Security Risks Report, Technical Whitepaper, HP DVLabs (2011). http://www.hpenterprisesecurity.com/collateral/report/2011FullYearCyberSecurityRisksReport.Pdf
14. Full Year Top Cyber Security Risks Report, HP DVLabs. http://dvlabs.tippinqpoint.com/imq/Fu11Year2010%20Risk%20Report.Pdf

Development of a Stripper Machine for Al-Mabsili Dates and Evaluation of Human Interactions and Performances

Alaa Al-Waleed Mohammed Al-Hinai and Hemanatha Jayasuriya(✉)

Department of Soils, Water and Agricultural Engineering,
Sultan Qaboos University, Muscat, Oman
s81455@student.squ.edu.om, hemjay@squ.edu.om

Abstract. Al-Mabsili dates are harvested before fully ripen stage and stripped manually. This study aimed to develop a stripper machine for Al-Mabsili dates using different power sources (motor, exercise machine, bicycle) and to compare performances with traditional method. With different power source options, operator's physiological and anthropometric parameters were increased and stabilized after stripping 5 bunches. The calories burnt, energy expenditure were highest in traditional method (2.3 kcal/kg, 14 kJ/kg) while energy expenditure rates were higher in exercise machine and bicycle (24.3 and 25.7 kJ/min). The stripping efficiency of all power sources was above 95%. The Cornell whole-body postural discomfort was lowest in exercise machine and highest in traditional method. Right hand was found more affected in Cornell hands discomfort evaluation. Exercising machine was best in Cornell seat comfort evaluation, traditional method was lowest. The average NIOSH lifting index was satisfactory (0.54). Growers preferred motor as the best power option.

Keywords: Date stripper · Performance evaluation · Ergonomics · Comfort evaluation · Lifting index · Break even analysis · Efficiency · Capacity

1 Introduction

For crop production, postharvest handling is one of the important stages that come before the food processing stages [1]. Improper handling and processing could lead to produce losses and severe reduction of product value and consequently financial losses [2]. In order to obtain good quality and quantity of agricultural products, proper mechanization of sorting, separating and processing should be done that would lead to minimize the low quality products increasing the product market price, and to reduce the time consumption as well as labour needs that required in manual methods [3].

Stripping process is one concept of separating method that required continuous efforts by the designers to improve it up to the modern status [4–7]. There are stripping units in different types of machines which consist of stripping rods like fingers that help to remove the grains, fruits or other agricultural crop products from their bunches, straws or plants [5].

The date palms are one of the most cultivated crops in Oman. Al-Mabsili is one variety out of 200 varieties of date fruits in Oman that are harvested before the fully

T. Ahram et al. (Eds.): IHIET 2019, AISC 1018, pp. 737–742, 2020.
https://doi.org/10.1007/978-3-030-25629-6_115

ripened stage (Al-Besser stage) and then separated manually from the bunches without using any tools or mechanical methods by gathering of all family and neighbors [8, 9]. Al-Tabseel is an important process that begins after harvesting Al-Beser followed by stripping process and then the cleaning, cooking and finally the drying process. [10]. However, not a single study could be found on designing a stripper machine for Al-Mabsili dates.

Al-Mabsili date is source of income for many families and there are 150 Al-Tabseel sites in Al Sharqiyah governorate in Oman. The process of Al-Tabseel requires high effort from the farmers because it takes 12 continuous hours to complete the process. Therefore, in the past, many farmers in Al Mudhaibi area in Al Sharqiyah governorate have faced challenges due to a shortage of local labor because many of them do not wish to participate in this activity. Each year, farmers in the area produce hundreds of tons of Al-Mabsili dates, each small farm producing about 4-8 tones [9]. This prompted many farmers to hire foreign workers, which has caused increase in labor cost [8].

Therefore, the main objective of the study was to conduct the performance and ergonomic evaluation of the developed date stripper prototype. The specific objectives were to design and develop the date stripper prototype with three power sources and to conduct the performance evaluation tests, the break-even analysis, and the questionnaire survey to evaluate the acceptance of the machine.

2 Experimental Method

The developed prototype consisted of main frame to support the feeding tray and stripper drum that contained the stripping blades. All the parts of the machine with the three different power sources (Motor, Exercise machine, Bicycle) were designed and fabricated at the workshop of College of Agricultural and Marine Science, Sultan Qaboos University.

The tests were conducted using dates from two farms. The separation of Al-Mabsili date was done manually by hand without using the date stripper prototype. The stripper machine with bicycle and exercise machine power source were required two operators, one as the feeder and the other as the peddler with three replications whereas in electric motor power source only feeders where each test conducted with three replications. Eighteen operators were used for the experiment (peddlers/feeders) without mixing them during the tests to obtain accurate results.

The machine performance evaluation was done by estimating the stripping efficiency and working capacity. The evaluation of the ergonomic performance was conducted to compare between the traditional and mechanical method with the three power source options. Different discomfort evaluation forms (musculoskeletal, hand and seat) [11, 12] were distributed to the operators after each test run. The NIOSH lifting index is aimed to evaluate whether the load weight is too heavy for the operator. The lifting equation is used for calculating the safe weight recommendations and to prevent any low back injuries from the manual lifting [13]. The NIOSH lifting equation was used to determine each feeder with different power sources and the average was estimated (Fig. 1).

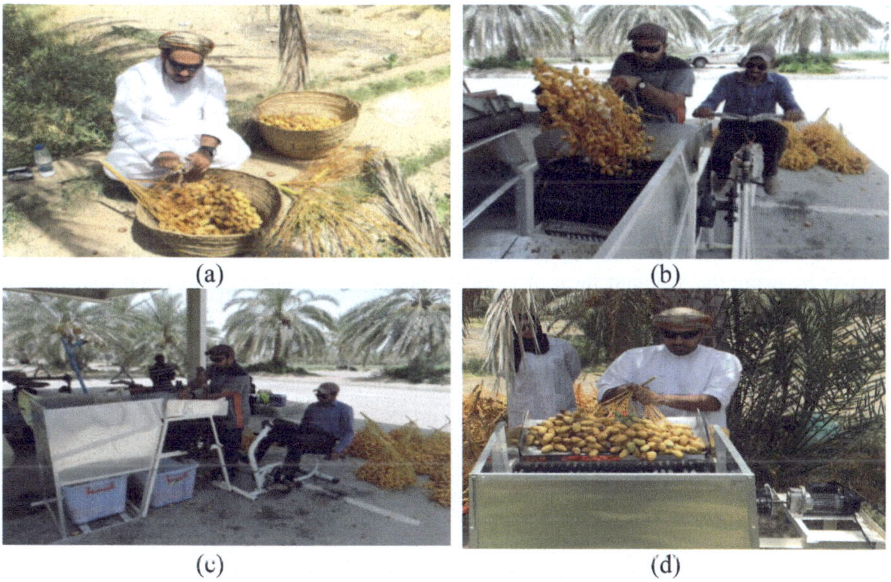

Fig. 1. Testing of the date stripper prototype with three power source options; (a) traditional, (b) bicycle (feeder and peddler), (c) exercise machine (feeder and peddler), (d) electric motor

In Oman, the problems facing agricultural productivity are poor handling at harvest and post-harvest operations, which must be addressed and highlighted [14]. The forms of the questionnaires were distributed among the stakeholders; extension officers, and farm owners and farmers of Al-Mabsili farms in order to obtain the accurate situation of Al-Mabsili potential in the country and the acceptance level of the date stripper machine.

3 Results and Discussion

3.1 Human-Machine Interactions and Performance

The physiological parameters (body temperature, systolic and diastolic pressure, heart-beat) of the operators (feeders and peddlers) were evaluated before and after each test. All the parameters were significantly increased after the test (using the four methods) of all the operators. Traditional method got the highest calories burned (2.3 kcal/kg) and energy expenditure in stripping a kg of dates (13.0 kJ/kg), while at the same time, the energy expenditure rate (10.8 kJ/min) found to be the lowest compared with the mechanical method. However, the bicycle method got the highest expenditure rate (25.7 kJ/min). When evaluating the machine performance, there were no significant differences in stripping efficiency among the three power sources (95.8–97.8%) whereas the bicycle got the highest value in working capacity (804.4 kg/hr). In addition, the evaluation of Cornell postural discomfort [11, 15] showed that, the highest comfort level was observed with the exercise machine option whereas the lowest comfort was observed with the traditional method (Table 1). Moreover, in Cornell hand discomfort [16] test showed that the right hand is more affected than the left hand (Table 2) in all the four methods. Using the Cornell seating comfort [11, 17] evaluation tests, the seating comfort levels of the peddlers were evaluated. The exercise machine was the best (66.7%) followed by the bicycle (51.9%) and the operators with traditional method (9.3%).

Table 1. Comparison of whole-body discomfort between the traditional method and mechanical methods by using the standard form of Cornell musculoskeletal discomfort (modified) method (Summeation of three replications)

The diagram below shows the approximate position of the body parts referred to in the questionnaire.

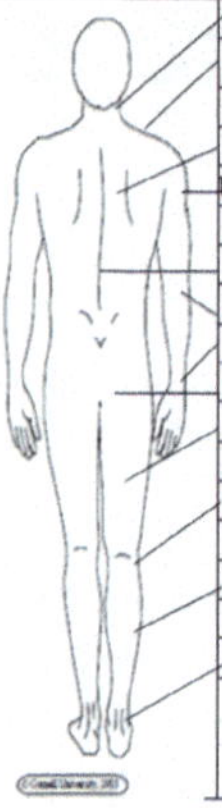

Body Part		Traditional	Bicycle F(a)	Bicycle P(b)	Exercise machine F	Exercise machine P	Electric motor F
Neck			*		*	*	*
Shoulder	(Right)		*		*	*	*
	(Left)					*	
Upper Back		*					
Upper Arm	(Right)						
	(Left)						
Lower Back				*			
Forearm							
Wrist							
Hip/Buttocks		*		*			
Thigh	(Right)			*			
	(Left)			*			
Knee	(Right)			*			
	(Left)			*			
Lower Leg	(Right)						
	(Left)						
Foot	(Right)						
	(Left)						

(b)Peddler

In NIOSH lifting equation, the lifting index was found less than 1 for three feeders of different power sources (average of 0.54) which is a very satisfactory condition.

3.2 Acceptance of Mechanization and Financial Justification

The questionnaires were distributed among the Al-Mabsili farm owners in selected governorates of Oman where Al-Mabsili dates are grown. The number of questionnaires responded was only 8 out of 155 because of the difficulties of finding the farm owners during the Eid holidays, thus the results are not statistically valid. However, the results of the acceptance of the stripper prototype showed that 87.5% of the respondents accepted the date stripper machine in order to solve the problem of labor scarcity and to improve the production as well as the profit and preferred the electric motor power source whereas 12.5% respondents didn't prefer this machine reasoned the problem of possible mixing of Al-Besser date with the fully ripened dates. However, 52.5% of the respondents preferred the bicycle power source as the first option for the farms there is no electricity available.

Table 2. Comparison of the right hand discomfort between the traditional and mechanical methods using Cornell hand discomfort survey (summation of three replications)

The shaded area in the diagrams below show the position of the body parts referred to in the questionnaire							
Four tests / Working during few hours in the day							
(Right Hand)		Traditional	Bicycle		Exercise machine		Electric motor
			Feeder	Peddler	Feeder	Peddler	Feeder
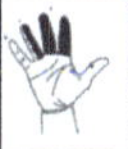	Area A (Shaded area)	*	*	*	*		*
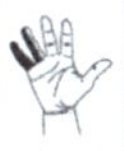	Area B (Shaded area)						
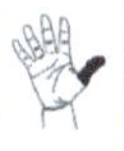	Area C (Shaded area)	*			*		
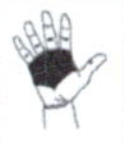	Area D (Shaded area)				*		*
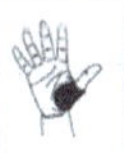	Area E (Shaded area)	*					
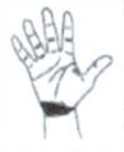	Area F (Shaded area)						

4 Conclusions

The mechanization of date stripping was successfully done and human-machine interactions and performance were evaluated comparing the traditional method with the machine having three power options. The stripping efficiency of the machine with three power sources found to be the same whereas the bicycle power option had the highest working capacity. In ergonomic evaluation part, exercise machine had the highest postural and seat comfort levels, whereas in all power options, more discomfort level found in operator right hand than the left hand. Most of the respondents of questionnaire survey agree about the stripper machine whereas few of them did not accepted because the problem of possible mixing the ripe and unripe dates during the stripping process. Regarding to the respondent ranking, preference scores of power sources in the order of electric motor as a first option and bicycle as a second option followed by exercise machine and finally the traditional method.

References

1. Kader, A.A., Rolle, R.S.: The Role of Post-Harvest Management in Assuring the Quality and Safety Of Horticultural Produce, vol. 152. Food & Agriculture Org. (2004)
2. Madrid, R.M., Philips, H.: Freshwater Prawn Culture: The Farming of Macrobrachium Rosenbergii - Google Books (2008). https://books.google.com.om/books?hl=en&lr=&id=vPQdmZxBGC8C&oi=fnd&pg=PA326&dq=Post-harvest+handling+and+processing&ots=RS8Y77Ghc&sig=fbuAuKMCuJ1i9UXsKEQVeC6MpS0&redir_esc=y#v=onepage&q=Post-harvesthandlingandprocessing&f=false. Accessed 14 Feb 2017
3. Lipinski, B., Hanson, C., Lomax, J., Kitinoja, L., Waite, R., Searchinger, T.: Reducing food loss and waste. World Resources Institute Working Paper (2013)
4. Schafer, A.W.: Machine for pitting fruits such as dates. United State: United State patent (1952). https://docs.google.com/viewer?url=patentimages.storage.googleapis.com/pdfs/US2611403.pdf
5. Troeh, F.R., Hobbs, J.A., Donahue, R.L.: Soil and Water Conservation for Productivity and environmental protection. Soil and Water Conservation for Productivity and Environmental Protection. Prentice-Hall, Inc. (1980)
6. Tado, C.J.M., Wacker, P., Kutzbach, H.D., Suministrado, D.C.: Development of stripper harvesters: a review. J. Agric. Eng. Res. **71**(2), 103–112 (1998)
7. Plants, T.: Palm Fruit Stripper Manufacturer in Rajkot Gujarat India by Tinytech Plants. ID – 139320 (2008). http://www.exportersindia.com/tinytechplants/palm-fruit-stripper-rajkot-india-139320.htm. Accessed 14 Feb 2017
8. Al-Arab Newspaper: Al-Tabseel: Omani Celebration of the date palm (2015). http://alarab.co.uk/?id=58690. Accessed 19 Feb 2017
9. Al-Shueili, A.S.: Tabseel as a source of income for families in Al Mudhaibi - Oman Observer (2014). http://2016.omanobserver.om/tabseel-as-a-source-of-income-for-families-in-al-mudhaibi/. Accessed 14 Feb 2017
10. ONA: Harvest of date palm "Tabseel" a social event in Oman - Times Of Oman (2015). http://timesofoman.com/article/64665/Oman/Heritage/Date-farm-harvesting-relives-an-Omani-tradition. Accessed 14 Feb 2017
11. Hedge, A., Morimoto, S., McCrobie, D.: CUergo: Musculoskeletal Discomfort Questionnaires (1999). http://ergo.human.cornell.edu/ahmsquest.html. Accessed 14 Mar 2017
12. Hedge, A.:. CUErgo: Seating Evaluation Form (2007). http://ergo.human.cornell.edu/ahSEATING.htm. Accessed 14 Mar 2017
13. Waters, T.R., Putz-Anderson, V., Garg, A.: Applications Manual for the Revised NIOSH Lifting Equation. Citeseer, Princeton (1994)
14. Jayasuriya, H.P.W., Al-Ismaili, A.M., Al-Shukaili, T.: Farming systems in Oman and mechanization potentials. Agricult. Mechanization Asia Afr. Latin Am. **48**(2), 66 (2017)
15. CUergo: Cornell Musculoskeletal Discomfort evaluation (2016). http://ergo.human.cornell.edu/ahmsquest.html
16. CUergo: Cornell Hand Discomfort evaluation (2016). http://ergo.human.cornell.edu/ahhandmsquest.html
17. CUergo.: Cornell Seat comfort evaluation (2016). http://ergo.human.cornell.edu/ErgoTools/CHAIREVALUATIONV2.1.htm

Towards Educational Technologies in Language Learning for Children: A Perspective of Linguistic Anthropology

Pingfang Yu, Jiali Du(✉), and Xinguang Li

Guangdong University of Foreign Studies,
Baiyun Avenue North 2, Guangzhou 510420, China
{201310051,201310039,200311088}@oamail.gdufs.edu.cn

Abstract. This paper discussed the language learning from the perspective of educational technologies, e.g. Stanford parser and context free grammar. Language determines our thought, and social context lays an intellectual burden on language learners. Language is the outcome of cultural experience. Sometimes, the existence of ambiguity may delay the further development of language learning and teaching. The effective educational technologies are helpful for disambiguation in language learning and teaching, and stimulate the development of linguistic anthropology.

Keywords: Human factors · Linguistic anthropology · Cross-cultural interaction · Language learning

1 Introduction

Anthropology is not the mindless collection of the exotic, but the use of cultural richness for self-reflection and self-growth. Anthropology whose major concern is human diversity focuses on both culture and thought, e.g. the dependence of meanings on learned schemas, the effect of artifacts on thought and the cross-cultural categorization. It tries to recognize diversity and seek for the ground rules of a viable and humane world society [1–3].

The traditional anthropology comprises four main sub-branches, i.e. biological anthropology, archaeological anthropology, socio-cultural anthropology, and linguistic anthropology (LA). LA, as a cultural resource and practice, is an umbrella term which makes reference to both socio-cultural and linguistic traditions. It studies language in culture and prioritizes social issues, e.g. intercultural misunderstanding, the impact of language contact on speech communities, etc. [4]. It includes discussion of linguistic relativity, the role of language in defining the context of interaction, the focus on performance as opposed to competence, and recent trends such as language socialization, language contact, and language ideology [5]. LA shows the deep relationship between culture and society, and at the same time finds the relevance of cultural and social phenomena for an understanding of language.

Language determines our thought about language [6]. LA examines the role of social interaction in making, mediating and authorizing those contrasts and differences

T. Ahram et al. (Eds.): IHIET 2019, AISC 1018, pp. 743–748, 2020.
https://doi.org/10.1007/978-3-030-25629-6_116

by the semiotic processes on which it relies. Furthermore, language has an existing competence in the alignment which is determined by linguistic diversities, affinity groups, and the politics of educational success [7]. This article will highlight early language learning for young learners to solve a few language-related human problems and to tackle real-life socio-cultural problems.

2 Language Learning and Social Context

Social context lays an intellectual burden on language learners. The modern world is characterized by movements of people, and by exchanges of ideas and things across previously discreet cultural boundaries. Language learners will obviously be affected by the social movement based on the language presentation. The culture concept as the locus of human experience has the special ability to serve its time [8]. Anyone cannot evade for social context and destroy the understanding it is meant to further [9]. It is necessary for an English learner to understand the social contexts of both English and Chinese since the social context exerts the influence on the language acquisition.

Language is the outcome of cultural experience. The process of social movement helps linguistic features to index social groups or activities. Languages can share principles of fine-grained event categorization even though they may differ in how they package the components [10]. Iconic representations depict or display a social group's inherent nature or essence [11]. Cultural factor has developed an impressive distribution to linguistic development.

Bilingual education is helpful for early language learning. In bilingual contexts, schooling for young students is complicated by the social, cultural, and emotional adjustment [12]. Accessing the prior linguistic knowledge in a specific language can activate further languages one knows by using certain skills and strategies for the acquisition. Thus, if bilingual educators are familiar with both English and Chinese social contexts and cultural factors, they can easily lead the young children to the further construction of bilingual language systems. English educators have the responsibility to bring the young learners into both native and alien socio-culture domains by means of the multiplicity of possible interactions between the linguistic systems in the multilingual learner's mind [13].

3 Diversity and Interaction in Early Language Learning

Early English learning is not an easy and simple task for children. The linguistic diversity and inaction, the role of which have a facilitation or inhibition effect on the learner's progress in mastering a new language, make second language learning a complex blend of native and alien cultures. The young learners sometimes follow the imposition of previously learned patterns onto a new learning situation, and as a result they may be positively or negatively transferred. It is controversial whether educators can help children break down the barriers of misunderstanding of languages.

Linguistic diversity exerts an influence on early language learning. The situation of linguistic diversity generally arises from a requirement of cultural diversity. Culture is characterized as human nature, and everyone has the ability to classify experiences and encode classifications symbolically. Different cultures can be developed by different people who live in varied places or circumstances. This provides the real and practical support for linguistic diversity. It seems to accept the existence of universal cognitive processes which seem to be reluctant to accept the impact of culture on these processes [14]. Young learners' social learning can be predicted by the diversity of the communities in which they live [15]. By the contact with other languages, learners' knowledge of language and culture gradually enhances, thus helps the learners understand the way language works and the function language has in society [16]. One man's connection is another man's disconnection, and any object is set in context which is connected by relations to its relevant surroundings [17]. For young learners, it is convenient to enjoy the alien cultures by English. It may be a rational and constructive method for educators to make young learners enjoy both the alien social cultures and diversified languages.

Cultural diversity actively affects early language learning. The diversity of neighborhood environment arouses the children's longing for imitation. Language diversity focuses on the differentiation among linguistic varieties [18]. Linguistic information available outside of the home can greatly affect young learners' social learning. The roles of both English educators and social caretakers are emphasized during the language shift, especially beyond the children's immediate interactions with family members. Young learners can acquire alien culture by means of learning processes of enculturation and socialization. A pure concept of language does not exist outside our ability to comprehend and articulate the nature of that language through language itself.

The connection between language and cultural identity can be strongly felt. Multilingual identities are not an isolated barrier in education which is considered an identity formation process. Educator has the responsibility to show the young children the special characters of national culture. The sentence of (dongtian neng chuan duoshao chuan duoshao, xiatian neng chuan duoshao chuan duoshao) means: "in winter (you should) wear as much as possible; in summer (you should) wear as less as possible." In the Chinese example, a foreigner is very hard to understand the potential meaning of the sentence because no syntactic difference between them except the initial words of dongtian(winter) and xiatian(summer). However, if a qualified educator can teach the students the basic Chinese linguistic characteristics and help them enjoy the pleasure of national culture, young children may improve their lingual ability. The first clause emphasizes "as much as possible" for "neng chuan duoshao chuan duoshao" because of the existence of context of winter since one is expected to wear as much as possible in winter. However, the same phrase of "neng chuan duoshao chuan duoshao" implies the completely opposite meaning because people may be comfortable and relaxed to wear as less as possible in summer. The second phrase of "neng chuan duoshao chuan duoshao" means "as less as possible". The Chinese linguistic character of semantic shift originates from the social and cultural environment. Please see the Chinese sentence Stanford parser parses, and the English sentence context free grammar describes.

Chinese Sentence: dongtian/NT, neng/VV, chuan/VV, duoshao/CD, chuan/VV, duoshao/CD, ./PU

```
Parse
(ROOT
  (IP
    (NP (NT dongtian))
    (VP
      (VP (VV neng)
        (VP (VV chuan)
          (QP (CD duoshao))))
      (VP (VV chuan)
        (QP (CD duoshao))))
    (PU .)))
```

Universal dependencies: nmod:tmod(chuan-3, dongtian-1); aux:modal(chuan-3, neng-2); root(ROOT-0, chuan-3); nmod:range(chuan-3, duoshao-4); conj(chuan-3, chuan-5); nmod:range(chuan-5, duoshao-6); punct(chuan-3, -7).

English Sentence: Until the police arrest the drug dealers control the street.

Until the police arrest the drug dealers control the street.
G={Vn. Vt. S. P}
Vn={S. NP. VP. N. Det. PP. Prep. CP. Conj. IP. V}
Vt={until. the. police. arrest. drug. dealers. control. street}
S=S
P:
a. S→PP NP VP
b. NP→N N
c. NP→Det N
d. NP→Det NP
e. PP→Prep NP
f. CP→Conj IP
g. IP→NP VP
h. VP→V NP
i. Det→{the}
j. Prep→{until}
k. Conj→{until}
l. N→{police. arrest. drug. dealers. street}
m. V→{arrest. control}

Until the police arrest the drug dealers control the street	Rules
Conj the police arrest the drug dealers control the street	k
Conj Det police arrest the drug dealers control the street	i
Conj Det N arrest the drug dealers control the street	l
Conj NP arrest the drug dealers control the street	c
Conj NPV the drug dealers control the street	m
Conj NPV Det drug dealers control the street	i
Conj NPV Det N dealers control the street	l
Conj NPV Det N N control the street	l
Conj NPV Det NP control the street	b
Conj NPV NP control the street	d
Conj NP VP control the street	h
Conj IP control the street	g
CP control the street	f
?	
BREAKDOWN AND BACKTRACKING	

By the analyses above, we can find that, if a foreigner fails to fully understand Chinese sentence's socio-culture, he will not have the ability to distinguish between winter and summer contexts in Chinese example.

And, for a few Chinese children, it is very hard to understand English sentence's social environment and linguistic characters. Firstly, the majority of Chinese children have no experience of drug of abuse, and "drug dealer" has no cognitive psychology concept for young learners. Therefore, educators have to show them something about the drug and the drug control conducted by western governments. Secondly, educators should help the students know the difference between arrest (VT) and arrest (N). If students can know both the verb definition and the nominal definition of arrest, they have the basic ability to understand the sentence. Besides that, the government domain of "until" should be emphasized by the educators. The correct explanation shows (1) "arrest" shifts from VT to N; (2) "until" shifts from conjunction to preposition; (3) "the drug dealers" shifts from object in the clause to subject in the main matrix;

(4) any failure of shifts may lead to garden path effect, namely "to be misled down to the garden path". The correct tree diagram of English sentence is as follows (Fig. 1):

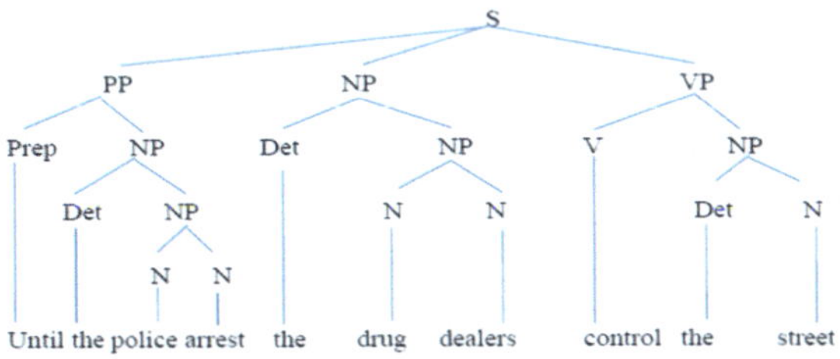

Fig. 1. The tree diagram of English sentence

Second language learning is an active task which needs learners to have access to the alien socio-culture and linguistic systems. As a language learner, he has to understand both culture and linguistic characters. The learning on culture and language promotes the theme of multicultural cognition and development. Multilingual education should be an attempt to integrate the personal multicultural and multilingual background of the students into the school curriculum. In addition, as a language teacher, educator has to help the students to learn more about the language history and culture which are crucial to the success of language learning.

The rich heritage of linguistic and cultural variety should be protected. A complete account of linguistic practice will have to come to terms with the complex interactions between linguistic structure, language usage and language ideologies [19, 20]. Educators bear the responsibility in the transition of culture of complacency into culture of vitality.

4 Conclusion

English language learning in China should be conducted both in a traditional manner and in an alien flavour. Different cultural groups behave and interact in a different way, and systematic instructions from the educators have to be compatible with young learners' cultural characteristics, and meanwhile highlight the cultural flavour of target language. The comparison and contrast between Chinese and English language characters, especially with the help of educational technologies, can stimulate young learners' interest in alien culture, and help them understand native culture from the outside perspective. The diversity of languages and interaction between different cultures can greatly affect the language learning and teaching for young learners in mainland.

Acknowledgments. This article is sponsored by "Thirteen-Five Major Project" for National Science and Technology Terminology Validation Committee (ZD2019001), China Social Science Fund (2018FYY006), China Natural Science Fund (61877013), and Guangdong Science and Technology Department Project (2018A070712032).

References

1. Marcus, G., Fischer, M.M.J.: Anthropology as Cultural Critique: An Experimental Moment in the Human Sciences. Chicago University Press, Chicago (1986)
2. Strauss, C. et al.: Cognitive Anthropology. Encyclopedia of Language & Linguistics, 2nd edn. pp. 529–532 (2006)
3. Hannerz, U.: Anthropology. In: International Encyclopedia of the Social & Behavioral Sciences, pp. 513–519 (2001)
4. Hoye, L.F.: Linguistic anthropology and pragmatics. J. Pragmatics **38**(6), 944–967 (2006)
5. Duranti, A.: Linguistic anthropology. In: International Encyclopedia of the Social & Behavioral Sciences, pp. 8899–8906 (2001)
6. Seargeant, P., et al.: Language ideology, language theory, and the regulation of linguistic behaviour. Lang. Sci. **31**, 345–359 (2009)
7. Souto-Manning, M., et al.: Competence as linguistic alignment: linguistic diversities, affinity groups, and the politics of educational success. Linguist. Educ. **24**, 305–315 (2013)
8. Clifford, J.R.: Travel and Translation in the Late Twentieth Century. Harvard University Press, Cambridge (1997)
9. Scharfstein, B.A.: The Dilemma of Context. New York University Press, New York (1989)
10. Majid, A., et al.: The cross-linguistic categorization of everyday events: a study of cutting and breaking. Cognition **109**, 235–250 (2008)
11. Irvine, J, Gal, S.: Language ideology and linguistic differentiation. In: Kroskrity, P. (ed.), Regimes of Language: Ideologies, Polities, and Identities, pp. 35–83. School of American Research Press (2000)
12. Arbonaa, A.D., Chireaca, S.M.: Language learning methodology for adults: a study of linguistic transfer. Procedia Soc. Behav. Sci. **142**, 318–324 (2014)
13. Hammarberg, B., Williams, S.: A study of third language acquisition. In: Hammarberg, B. (ed.). Processes in Third Language Acquisition. Edinburg University Press Ltd. (2009)
14. Wassmann, J.: Cognitive anthropology. In: International Encyclopedia of the Social & Behavioral Sciences, pp. 2080–2085 (2001)
15. Howard, L.H., et al.: Neighborhood linguistic diversity predicts infants' social learning. Cognition **133**, 474–479 (2014)
16. Cummins, J.: Language. Power and Pedagogy. Bilingual Children in the Crossfire. Multilingual Matters, Clevedon (2000)
17. Dilley, R., et al.: The problem of context in social and cultural anthropology. Lang. Commun. **22**, 437–456 (2002)
18. Ahlers, J.C., et al.: Linguistic variation and time travel: barrier, or border-crossing? Lang. Commun. **38**, 33–43 (2014)
19. Hanks, W.: Language and Communicative Practices. Westview Press, Boulder (1996)
20. Du, J.L., Alexandris, C., et al.: Controlling interaction in multilingual conversation revisited: a perspective for services and interviews in Mandarin Chinese. In: International Conference on Human-Computer Interaction, vol. 10271, pp. 573–583. Springer, Cham (2017)

The Impact of Technology on the Work Process of the Nursing Team Working in Hemodialysis

Saturnina Alves da Silva Martins(✉), Marcia Terra da Silva, and Ivonaldo Vicente da Silva

Paulista University – UNIP, Pindaibal Street 82, São Paulo 08270-060, Brazil
sasmartins@hotmail.com

Abstract. The objective of this study was to identify the impact of technology on the work process of the nursing team who works in hemodialysis services. The methodology used was an integrative review of the literature, whose eligibility criteria of the articles were: be a scientific article, be available in full, corresponding to the publication period from 2008 to 2018. The literature review totaled 1.303 articles, 1.097 were excluded. As results were found 53 articles that had evidence for the proposed study. It was concluded that it was possible to estimate the power that technology represents in the health area. In relation to the nursing team's work process in the hemodialysis, a technological and knowledge advance was identified through the results. Nursing care for patients submitted to hemodialysis evolved positively with the advent of technology.

Keywords: Technology · Nursing · Work process · Hemodialysis

1 Introduction

The evolution of new technological discoveries in the area of health has been evident. The application of new technological discoveries in the area of health is constantly increasing, new machines, equipment, investments in robots for surgical procedures, real-time communication, electronic medical records, among others, are examples of investment and labor market growth for several professionals in this segment [1, 2].

The growth of technology is linked to the advancement of microelectronics, providing a significant improvement in the control of work processes. Studies in the field of health technology become comprehensive and therefore involve a wide range of knowledge [3].

Specific scenarios in the health sector such as Hemodialysis, Intensive Care Units and relating nursing care are described that these professionals are constantly challenged by complex clinical situations in relation to patients, requiring attention and control in real time. Through the correct and safe integration of technology, it is important for the impact on professional work and patient safety to deliver positive results [4]. With this, the guiding question of this study is: How does technology impact on the work process of nursing professionals working on hemodialysis?

T. Ahram et al. (Eds.): IHIET 2019, AISC 1018, pp. 749–755, 2020.
https://doi.org/10.1007/978-3-030-25629-6_117

The objective of this study was to identify the impact of technology on the work process of the nursing team working in hemodialysis services. The methodology used was the review of the integrative literature. It is justified to prepare this review to stimulate and stimulate research on the topic addressed.

2 Theoretical Referential

Chronic Kidney Disease (CKD) is a global public health issue. In Brazil, currently, there are on average 750 units of chronic dialysis according to the census of 2016 of the Brazilian Society of Nephrology (SBN) [5]. Of these 750, 309 units responded to the census indicating 50,807 patients undergoing hemodialysis. Of this total, 83% of the patients performed the procedure through the Unified Health System (SUS) and 17% by health service providers.

For the treatment of Terminal Chronic Renal Disease (CKD), currently the most commonly used conventional therapy of choice is hemodialysis, its operation is performed through a machine with safety sensors, dialyzer filters, arterial, venous and dialytic solutions that replace the function of the patient's kidney. They occur on average three times a week, for a period of three to four hours, depending on the needs of the patient [6].

In recent decades, the development of hemodialysis machines has changed drastically nowadays being more robust and accurate with a series of sophisticated alarms. While in the old machines all the parameters were defined and controlled manually by the health professionals with emphasis to the nursing team that provide direct assistance to the patient, with the new technologies most of the machines became plug and play dealing with most of the problems automatically. This evolution has positive influences on safety and ergonomics, thus reducing labor costs [7].

Continuous monitoring of the patient undergoing hemodialysis procedure becomes important for the effectiveness of the treatment. This monitoring is a potentially useful tool to provide quality assurance in each hemodialysis session, with the intention of reducing the incidence of serious non-physiological events, thus ensuring patient safety, as well as for the professionals involved in the procedure [8, 9].

A specialized nursing team is required to perform the hemodialysis procedure, including the establishment of a therapeutic and interpersonal relationship, treatment of symptoms and attention to the functional limitations that may arise due to intercurrences in the hemodialysis procedure. The role of the Nurse within this team, which besides the leadership aspects of the nursing team, acts directly with the patient, identifying their needs and implementing actions through the elaboration of the Nursing Process [10].

The operation of hemodialysis requires the nursing staff to constantly observe the signs and symptoms presented and referred by the patient during the procedure, monitor the operation of the hemodialysis machine and materials used and the competence to analyze and make assertive decisions to resolve occurrences thus benefiting safety of the patient [11].

To achieve benefits, technology needs to be embedded in the functionality of the system. The technology offers a variety of tangible benefits and is often proposed as a means of increasing the safety of the patient and the nursing staff operating the hemodialysis machines [12].

3 Method

The methodology used was an integrative review of the literature, which is a method whose objective is to gather results obtained in research on a theme or question, in a systematic, orderly and comprehensive way [13].

Scientific papers published in the period 2008 to 2018 followed a six-step protocol [14]: (1) Formulation of the research question; (2) Delimitation of inclusion and exclusion criteria; (3) Readings of articles included; (4) Analysis of selected studies; (5) Interpretation and discussion of results; (6) Synthesis of knowledge. The eligibility criteria of the articles were: to correspond to the descriptors "Technology in Health", "Technology in Hemodialysis" and "Technology and the Work of Nursing in Hemodialysis", to be a scientific article, to be available in the whole. The databases Latin American Literature in Health Sciences - LILACS, International Literature in Health Sciences, MEDLINE and Scientific Electronic Library - SciELO were consulted. The Boolean operators used were "And" and "Or". Regarding the exclusion criteria, publications of the type: editorial, news, commentary, reflection, report of experience, duplicate and incomplete articles, publications with a date lower than 2008 and that did not exhibit some of the mentioned descriptors were discarded. A four-phase flowchart (identification, selection, eligibility and inclusion) of the Preferred Reporting Items for Systematic Reviews and Meta-Analyzes - PRISMA methodology was used to conduct the selection of articles [15].

3.1 Results

The synthesis referring to the data obtained through the search of the studies in the databases listed, considering the descriptors, inclusion/exclusion criteria and methodological variables is described in Table 1.

Table 1. Bibliographic panel, according to the databases and inclusion/exclusion criteria, 2018.

Descriptors	A	B	C	Excluded A – B – C	Included A – B – C	Selected A – B – C
Health technology	08	49	372	07 – 17 – 306	01 – 32 – 66	01 – 23 – 19
Technology hemodialysis	14	216	08	11 – 199 – 06	03 – 17 – 02	01 – 05 – 01
Technology and the work of hemodialysis nursing	50	142	19	35 – 131 – 10	11 – 14 – 09	01 – 01 - 01

Subtitle: (A) Lilacs; (B) Medline; (C) SciELO
Source: Authors, 2018.

The literature review totaled 1.303 articles made available in the three databases through the combinations of the mentioned descriptors as shown in Table 1. Following the exclusion criteria, 1.097 articles were excluded, evidencing the exclusion of 305 articles when using the descriptors Technology in Health on the basis of Scielo data occurred because 53% of the articles the publication were inferior to the year 2008, 41% the texts were published incomplete and 6% were duplicate texts. Regarding the descriptors Technology in Hemodialysis in the Medline database, 199 articles were excluded as a result of 92% being texts with less than 2008 publications, 6% incomplete texts and 2% being biographies.

Related to the descriptors Technology and Nursing Work in Hemodialysis in the Medline database 59% of the articles were excluded due to the publications being inferior to the year 2008, 15% the texts were incomplete and 18% were biographies and editorials. There were 155 articles included that were analyzed in order to qualify them, given the purpose of the review to incorporate them within the scope of this article.

After a careful analysis of the included articles, 53 articles were selected that had evidence on the context of the technologies in the health area, focusing on the work process of the nursing team working on hemodialysis.

In relation to the year of publication of the selected articles for a better understanding is evidenced through Fig. 1.

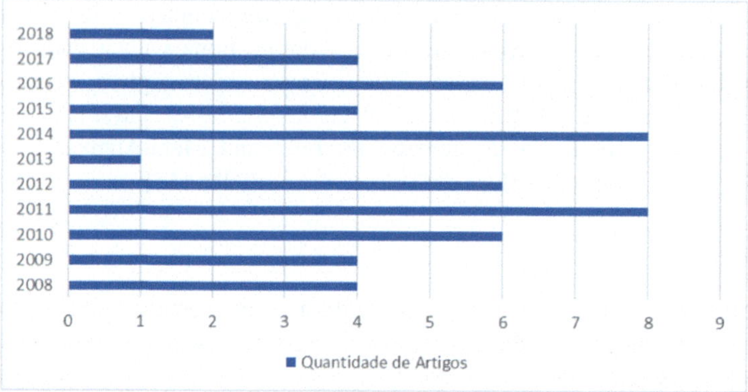

Fig. 1. Illustrates the number of articles selected for the year in which they were published. Source: Authors, 2018.

Continuing the analysis of the articles, for a better organization, a low and exploratory reading of each article was done and in order to systematize the information of the articles, the data extracted from the studies were compiled in a descriptive way, which facilitated the identification and classification of the articles. thematic categorizations as presented in Table 2.

Through the analysis of the selected articles seven topics were considered, thematic 1 Technological innovation and costs in health, it was observed that there is a strong competition of markets among health organizations that is based on the generation of

Table 2. Thematic classification of articles

Main theme	Number of articles	%
1. Technological innovation and health costs	14	26%
2. Technology rationality and work process	24	45%
3. Information technology in the context of health	02	4%
4. Technology management in the Unified Health System - SUS	07	13%
5. Technology and ethical principles	03	6%
6. Technology and knowledge production	02	4%
7. Technology and the environment	01	2%

Source: Authors, 2019.

innovations. So, the pressure of economic interests for the production of new technologies is immense. The capitalist economic logic has been a strong determinant of the directions of technological development in the area of health [16].

Regarding the Thematic 2 Technology Rationality and Work Process reached 45% of the articles. The technologies involved in health services can be classified into: hard technologies (equipment, standards and organizational structures); light-hard technologies (structured knowledge that work in health work); technologies (relations technologies, autonomization, reception and management of the work process). Specifying the issues involving the services of Hemodialysis in Thematic 2, this segment is strongly dominated by technology [17, 18]. Observing the issues involving equipment, machines, needles, medications, skills and knowledge, these are part of the Hemodialysis scenario, and becomes an example of interaction between professionals, patients and technology [19].

Evidencing another thematic of 4 SUS Technology Management, in Brazil the Unified Health System (SUS) is a major technology developer. The Ministry of Health purchases about R$ 8 billion in medicines, equipment and health products per year. At the same time, managers of all instances of the SUS are constantly pressured for new and emerging technologies to be incorporated into the industry [20].

Thematic 3, 5, 6 and 7 no less important reference the questions of Information Technology that applies to the records of the hemodialysis procedure, offering a macro view of the system, also used to plan the supply of services and financial resources [21]. Concerning issues involving ethical principles, production of knowledge and the environment, it is perceived that technology in the context of health should be conducted in order to prioritize the solution of the serious structural and global problems of humanity in a commitment effective way of contributing, in a significant way, to a society that is more dignified, just, solidary and sustainable [1, 22, 23].

4 Conclusion

It was concluded with this research that it was possible to estimate the need and power that technology represents throughout history in the health area. With regard to the work process of the nursing team working in hemodialysis, a significant technological and knowledge advance at the national and international levels was identified through the results. The nursing care provided to patients submitted to hemodialysis evolved positively with the advent of technology. It is worth mentioning that the technology used in the hemodialysis machines and in the equipment for the procedure provide nursing professionals and patients with greater safety, creating perspectives for improvement in the quality of life and patient safety.

References

1. Lorenzetti, J., Trindade, L.L., Pires, D.E.P., Ramos, F.R.S.: Technology, technological innovation and health: a necessary reflection. Texto Contexto Enferm, Florianópolis, Abr-Jun **21**(2), 432–439 (2012)
2. Paim, J.S.: Health surveillance: trends in the reorientation of healthcare models for health promotion. In: Czeresnia, D, Freitas, C.M. (eds.) Health Promotion: Concepts, Reflections, Trends, p. 519–530. Fiocruz, Rio de Janeiro (RJ) (2015)
3. Valentim, R.A.M., et al.: Hospital automation: the state of the art. Braz. J. Technol. Innov. Health **2**(1), 27–38 (2012). ISSN: 2236-1103
4. Bar, D.C.C., Dal Sasso, G.T.M.: Mobile technology at the edge of the bed: computerized nursing process in intensive care from CIPE 1.0®. Text Context Enferm. **19**(1), 54–63 (2010)
5. Brazilian Society of Nephrology. Census (2016). http://www.jbn.org.br/details/1962/en/en/inquerito-brasileiro-de-diali Accessed 19 Apr 2018
6. Oliveira, P.M., Soares, D.A.: Perceptions of people with chronic renal failure on quality of life. Enfermería Global **28** (2012). ISSN: 1695-6141
7. Lameire, N., Biesen, W.V., Vanholder, R.: Did 20 years of technological innovations in hemodialysis contribute to better patient outcomes? Clin. J. Am. Soc. Nephrol. **4**, S30–S40 (2009)
8. Locatelli, F., Buoncristiani, U., Canaud, B., Kohler, H., Petitclerc, T., Zucchelli, P.: Haemodialysis with on-line monitoring equipment: tools or toys? Nephrol. Dial. Transplant. **20**, 22–33 (2005)
9. Lambie, S., Warwick, G.: Intelligent hemodialysis: toys ortools? Hemodial. Int. **11**, 834–838 (2007)
10. Stavropoulou, A., Grammatikopoulou, M.G., Rovithis, M., Kyriakidi, K., Pylarinou, A., Markaki, A.G.: Through the patients' eyes: the experience of end-stage renal disease patients concerning the provided nursing care. In: Healthcare, Multidisciplinary Digital Publishing Institute, Basel, Switzerland (2017)
11. Lima, A.F.C., Fuzii, S.M.O., Pinho, N.A., Melo, C.T., Hashimoto, T.H.F.: Nursing process in the practice of hemodialysis: the experience of nurses at a University Hospital. Revista Referência - II – no. 12 (2010)
12. Perry, S.J., Wears, R.L., Cook, R.I.: The role of automation in complex system failures. J. Patient Saf. **1**(1), 56–61 (2005)
13. Ercole, F.F., Melo, L.S., Alcoforado, C.L.G.C.: Integrative review versus systematic review. REME Rev. Min. Enferm. **18**(1), 1–260 (2014)
14. Mendes, K.D.S., Silveira, R.C.C.P., Galvão, C.M.: Integrative review: research method for the incorporation of evidence in health and nursing. Text Context Nurs. Florianópolis **17**(4), 758–764 (2008)
15. Cervo, A.L., et al.: Scientific Methodology. Pearson Universities, São Paulo (2006)

16. Souza, L.E.P.F.: Health, development and innovation: a contribution of critical theory of technology to the debate. Cad. Public Health, Rio de Janeiro **32**(2), e00029615 (2016)
17. Trindade, E.: The incorporation of new technologies in health services: the challenge of analyzing the factors at play. Cad. Saúde Pública, Rio de Janeiro **24**(5), 951–964 (2008)
18. Santos, W.J., et al.: Evaluation of the technology of care relations in health services: perception of the elderly included in the Family Health Strategy in Bambuí, Brazil. Sci. Collective Health **19**(8), 3441–3450 (2014)
19. Bennett, P.N.: Technological intimacy in haemodialysis nursing. Nurs. Inq. **18**(3), 247–252 (2011)
20. Silva, H.P., et al.: Advances and challenges of the National Policy on Health Technology Management. Rev. Saúde Pública **46**(1), 83–90 (2012)
21. Santos, M.V.R., et al.: Information technology in nephrology. J. Bras Nefrol. **31**(3), 212–219 (2009)
22. Tenório, M., et al.: Policies to foster science, technology and innovation in health in Brazil and the place of clinical research. Sci. Collective Health **22**(5), 1441–1454 (2017)
23. Connor, A., et al.: Clinical transformation: the key to green nephrology. Nephron Clin. Pract. **116**, c200–c206 (2010)

Urban Transport: Comparative Study of Energy Efficiency Between Taxi Drivers in Salvador City, Bahia - Brazil

Euclides Santos Bittencourt(✉), Cristiano Hora de Oliveira Fontes, Jorge Laureano Moya Rodriguez, Salvador Ávila Filho, and Adonias Magdiel Silva Ferreira

Federal University of Bahia, Prof. Arístides Novis 2, Salvador, Bahia, Brazil
euclyd13@gmail.com

Abstract. The objective of this work is to evaluate and quantify the potential of CO2 mitigation in the transportation of passengers, in the use of sub modal urban taxis in the city of Salvador. The complexity and behavior of society influence the behavior of taxi services that are concessions, population increase and consumption. Measures and technologies: (a) the reduction of fuel consumption, as well as (b) the gradual replacement of low-CO2 fuels can contribute to improving the relations of society and the environment. Continued use of fossil fuels is proven to increase the planet's temperature. The methodology used follows the theoretical reference Lee Schipper. The main parameters used to measure emissions relate to the distance traveled, the number of passengers and fuel consumption. Data collection was through a secondary source and primary source, using semi-structured questionnaires at four taxi points through accidental sampling. The hypothesis is that the increase of 0.5 km/l in the energy efficiency of taxis using ethanol instead of CNG could reduce CO2 emissions by about 20%.

Keywords: Measure emissions · Taxi services · Reduce CO2

1 Introduction

Transport logistics is one of the segments of society that bring economic gains and social benefits, from solutions that bring efficiency and good performance in the transfer of material goods. In this sense, estimating the improvement in logistics also estimates reduction in greenhouse gas emissions [1]. The vast majority (94%) of the energy used in transport comes from fossil fuels, which is responsible for emissions of 6,9 Gt of CO2-eq of carbon (CO2) and other greenhouse gases (GHG), whose increase of the concentration in the atmosphere is the dominant factor for climate warming [2].

This paper analyzes experimentally a small sample of the taxi fleet in the city of Salvador/BA/BRAZIL near the Federal University of Bahia (UFBA) Polytechnic School. It was decided to research the taxi fleet in a radius of 3 km in order to construct a comparative study on the consumption of fossil fuels (gasoline, alcohol and gas).

T. Ahram et al. (Eds.): IHIET 2019, AISC 1018, pp. 756–761, 2020.
https://doi.org/10.1007/978-3-030-25629-6_118

The city of Salvador has about 7000 taxis and three different services. The common taxi that voluntarily circulates through the streets of the city, besides having points by all the districts rolled by kilometer (flags 1 and 2, respectively). The cab of cooperatives that operate by radios and the special taxi that make tabulated runs and operate with large cars.

2 Energy Consumption in Urban Transport

The increase in income has historically been translated into a greater demand for faster modes. This justifies an intensive use of transport energy. Transportation accounted for 28% of the total final energy demand in the world in 2012 [3]. Growth in transport energy use has more than doubled since 1970, with a sharp increase in non-OECD growth - Organization for Economic Cooperation and Development [2]. And after 2000 a marked decrease in the OECD countries. Highlight is the transport that, due to the new flight technologies, the sector is experiencing a rapid growth all over the world, in relation to the other molds. On the other hand, non-OECD countries the activity of passenger transport is dominated by the use of the private car.

3 The Urban Population - Transport and Greenhouse Gases

More than half the world's population is now living in urban areas, although urban growth processes vary between OECD and non-OECD [4]. Of course, in populous countries with low intellectual and productive potential, they are against greenhouse gas mitigation because their fleets of vehicles grow year after year, stimulated by credit and consumption policies.

Some cities are experiencing rapid population growth and other [4] population growth has receded. The world population will be concentrated in the urban areas of less developed regions, whose combined populations are projected to increase from 2.7 billion in 2011 to 5.1 billion in 2050.

4 Non-economic Aspects

People's social standards, attitudes, preferences, acceptance, lifestyle, values, and even their attachment to symbolic and affective motives can justify their travel options and behavioral patterns related to transportation. The goal is to achieve voluntary reduction of car use, modal changes, or the promotion of new low-carbon fuels or alternative vehicles.

The use of a taxi requires comparatively a greater amount of 1.65–2.45 MJ/p-km, whereas bicycle transport, although slower, requires 0.1 MJ/p-km [3]. In the city of Salvador due to its topography and cultural issues the use of taxi is frequent and limited to a fleet of 7000 taxis. The other transports, mainly the collective or line bus, operate intermittently, requiring 0.32–0.91 MJ/p-km.

5 Methodology

For emission calculations and estimates of mitigation potential, the baseline and monitoring methodology approved by the United Nations Framework Convention on Climate Change (UNFCCC) was adopted as the reference "AM0090 - Modal shift in transportation from cargo from road transportation to water or rail transportation ". This tool provides procedures for calculating project emissions and/or CO2 leakage.

The sampling was accidental as voluntary taxi drivers set about answering the closed, semi-structured questions, totaling a sample of 10 vehicles (about 7%). The information (data) for the test was collected together with some to the points of taxi, taking with reference the radius of 3 km of the Polytechnic School of the UFBa.

5.1 Formulas Adopted in the Calculation of GHG

5.1.1 Estimation of Baseline Emissions

$$BE_y = T_y \times AD \times EF_{BL} \times 10^{-6} \tag{1}$$

Where:

BEy = Baseline emissions in year y (tCO2);
T,y = Average number of passengers transported per year y (t);
AD,y = Distance traveled (km);
EF_{BL} = Baseline emission factor for passenger transport (g CO2/t.km).

5.1.2 Estimation of the Baseline Emission Factor

$$EF_{BL} = \frac{\sum FC_{BL,i,y} \times NCV_{i,y} \times EF_{CO2,i,y} \times F_{RT,BL}}{T_y \times AD} \tag{2}$$

Where:

EF_{BL} = Baseline emission factor for passenger transport (g CO2/t.km);
$FC_{BL,i,y}$ = Quantity of fuel i consumed by taxis in year y (liters or m^3);
NCVi,y = It is the coefficient of CO2 emission of fuel type i in year y (tCO2/unit of mass or volume).
$EF_{CO2,i,y}$ = CO2 Emission Factor of the fuel i consumed by the trucks in year y;
$F_{RT,BL}$ = Factor for non-empty return trips in the baseline (fraction) scenario.

5.1.3 Factor for Non-empty Return Trips in Baseline Scenario

$$F_{RT,BL} = \frac{T_y \times AD}{T_y \times AD + T_{RT,y} \times RTD_y} \tag{3}$$

Where:
$F_{RT,B}$ = Factor for non-empty return trips in the baseline scenario (fraction);
$T_{RT,y}$ = Number of passengers transported in return taxis in year y (tons);
RTDy = Distance traveled on return trips in year y (km).

5.2 Procedures Performed in Field Research

The data collected in the month of February 2016, concern:

- Average number of passengers carried in the month in the outward itinerary, considering a base year 2015 (ton/year);
- Distance traveled in the year in the basic outward itinerary of 2015 (km);
- Average fuel (gasoline, alcohol or NGV) consumed by the taxi in the year (liters);
- Average number of passengers transported in the year (ton/year); and
- Average distance traveled in the return route in the year (km);

Information on the emission factors of gasoline, alcohol and NGV were obtained from the literature of GHG scenarios up to 2030 of energy efficiency for light vehicles in Brazil, prepared by UFRJ April 2014.

6 Research Results

Daily information on taxi service activity has been deducted for one year. The energy in the form of power of each collective of workers in the taxi points researched deserves further study, but it is worth noting that the energy depends on the amount of car and the cylinder that each car has to design.

For this test we define a power of a car 1.4, since, in general, the cars are bought with this specification to relate the energy gain and average consumption. The power of the setup is by car alcohol (Ethanol - 80 hp (58.8 kW/78.9 HP) @ 6400 rpm).

Research results show that CO2 emissions are a function of the car's moving energy, where tons of fuel are burned without an environmental concern. Usually, taxis pass from one place to another in the city carrying one or a maximum of two people, and eventually at parties, people make round trips to and from their places options.

The CO2 emission values obtained in Fig. 1 reaffirm that without an effectively enlightening energy policy for society we will be helping to accelerate the increase in temperature on the planet. The amount of CO2 emission depends on the amount of heat power of the fuel that releases CO2_equivalent, especially the amount of mileage and the fuel consumption used in the activity.

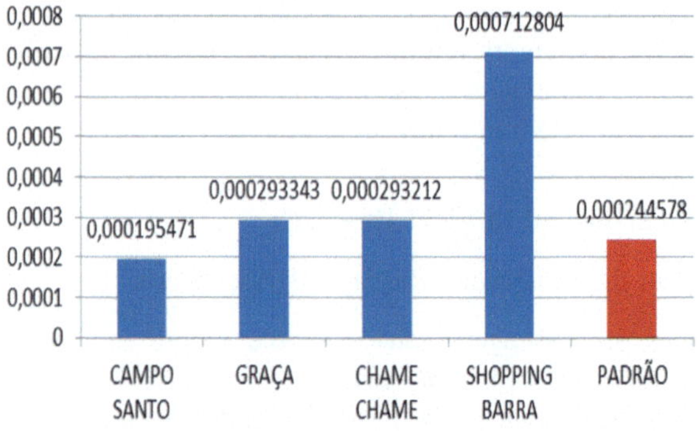

Fig. 1. CO2 emission obtained

7 Discussion

From the model and parameters described in the previous section, the baseline emissions were estimated, i.e. the average emissions observed in the base year of the survey, year 2015. From the data reported by the secondary sources it was possible to define a benchmarket. Second, simulations were performed in order to extrapolate the results from the baseline scenario. This extrapolation sought to estimate the emission mitigation potential resulting from variations in the baseline scenario, due to the adoption of measures that (a) increase the energy efficiency of vehicles, expressed by the increase in the ratio "mileage traveled/liter of fuel" and (b) promote fuel substitution through a progressive increase of the CNG blend for alcohol. With this, it was possible to construct the emission curve, indicating the sensitivity of the mitigation response due to the increase in energy efficiency or in the urban transport segment.

In quantitative terms, a 5% increase in energy efficiency of the taxi fleet studied for inference with the fleet of around 7000 taxis could have an impact on the 5% reduction in CO2 emissions. This means that if measures are adopted that result in a reduction in average fuel consumption of around 0.5 km/l, for example, the resulting GHG emissions are expected to fall by 19.23%.

8 Conclusions

The objective of this study was to compare the CO2 mitigation potential of urban taxis in the city of Salvador and to adopt measures and technologies that (a) reduce fuel consumption, and (b) promote fuel substitution through of a progressive increase of the consumption of Ethanol instead of NGV. The evaluation of these scenarios allowed the construction of a comparative analysis between an emission standard and real emissions. The main parameters used to measure emissions (such as distance traveled, passengers and fuel consumption) were obtained from taxi drivers involved in field research.

References

1. IEA (Int. Energy Agency): Energy Technology Perspectives 2012: Pathways to a Clean Energy System. Inst. Strateg. Energy Anal., Golden, CO (2012)
2. IPCC (Intergov. Panel Clim. Change): Climate Change 2014: Mitigation of Climate Change (2014)
3. Figueroa, M., et al.: Energy for transport. Ann. Rev. Environ. Res. environ.annualreviews.org. https://doi.org/10.1146/annurev-environ-031913-100450
4. Grubler, A., Bai, X., Buettner, T., Dhakal, S., Fisk, D., et al.: Urban energy systems (2012). See Reference 2. http://www.iata.org/whatwedo/cargo/sustainability/Pages/benefits.aspx

Emerging Technologies and Business Applications

Human-in-the-Middle: Increasing Security of Two-Factor Authentication

Kingsley Udenze and Spencer Romeiser(✉)

Department of Informatics, Fort Hays State University,
600 Park Street, Hays 67601, USA
{kzudenze,n_s_romeiser}@mail.fhsu.edu

Abstract. Online security and security of personal information is an important topic in information technology. Due to the recent high-profile security breaches as a result of authentication manipulation, there has been a growing need for enhanced methods of authentication as attackers have become more skilled in defeating existing authentication mechanisms. Attackers have resulted to phishing, social engineering, token interception and other highly sophisticated attackers all to gain access to the accounts of user. These attacks have resulted in serious damages for individuals and organizations. As a result, methods, such as, Two-Factor Authentication (2FA) have been introduced to. Nevertheless, loopholes major vulnerabilities in the existing two-factor authentication implementation. In this paper, This paper analyzes the. The are listed and analyzed, and the methods of manipulation explained. This paper finally suggests a solution of a web platform service which utilizes the mobile phones of users as a form of secure confirmation of the identity of the user through a dedicated mobile application. This solution hopes to eliminate the need for communication of security parameters of the traditional telephone network.

Keywords: Cybersecurity · Two-factor authentication · Human factors

1 Introduction

As attackers develop more sophisticated systems for threatening users and their information [1], individuals are now faced with increasing responsibility concerning the security of their data: malpractices in password generation and management (e.g., reuse of key phrases containing references to personal information) can easily invalidate most prevention measures and facilitate breaches [2, 3]. To this end, novel cybersecurity protocols aim at improving existing services by adopting additional steps in authenticating. Specifically, two-factor authentication (2FA) is a security mechanism that utilizes two types of credentials for verifying the authenticity of a user: in addition to username and password, another piece of information is required from the user to make it harder for unauthorized individuals to gain access to a resource. Typically, this information comes in the form of a code (e.g., pin number) dynamically generated by a hardware token or stored on a chip card. Although two-factor authentication is among the systems at the forefront of the authentication process, several studies demonstrated that its vulnerabilities, especially when 2FA relies on devices, such as, hardware

T. Ahram et al. (Eds.): IHIET 2019, AISC 1018, pp. 765–770, 2020.
https://doi.org/10.1007/978-3-030-25629-6_119

tokens, that can be stolen. Similarly, new solutions based on mobile applications that generate and display the pin number required for authenticating are susceptible to phone theft. Moreover, other types of 2FA systems that deliver the code to the user's phone (e.g., via a text message) or e-mail are vulnerable to techniques, such as, eavesdropping and man-in-the-middle, which can be utilized to listen to communication, hijack transmitted messages, and use the information to successfully breach an authentication system.

In this paper, we describe a system that aims at improving security in 2FA protocols, with specific regard to mobile applications that offer Authentication as a Service (AaaS) for accounts on multiple platforms. The proposed solution consists of additional security measures that are especially designed for preventing man-in-the-middle attacks, as well as the potential risks of breaches related to device theft. To this end, we propose a human-in-the-middle approach, which, in addition to transmitting a dynamically-generated temporary code, leverages information provided by the user to generate or reveal the actual pin to be used for authenticating. By doing this, the proposed solution removes the risks caused by attacks that intercept traffic transmitted to the phone and, simultaneously, introduces a system for securing information stored in 2FA wallets. In addition to describing its architecture, we describe two different implementations based on the human-in-the-middle approach and we demonstrate their interoperability with current solutions. Moreover, we detail the authentication workflow from a user experience perspective and we discuss the implications in terms of usability and convenience.

2 Related Work

The adoption of online services by Internet users has substantially raised the need for better authentication. Most businesses, while trying to make their services available round the clock have resulted to offer cloud-based services which in most cases requires users having accounts on their web platforms. With the increasing number of services which users subscribe to, there is a difficult requirement of remembering various usernames and passwords on the various platforms. The capability of humans to remember large amounts of secrets are still being researched [4]. Today it is common practice for users to select a few passwords that are recycled from service to service [5, 6] Several IT companies have developed applications which are meant to aid the recollection of login credentials and allow for easy access to previously set usernames and passwords. These applications commonly called password managers have been shown by researchers to affect security. Information breaches in the past decades have demonstrated the need for addition layers of security. Judging by the recent happenings, most of the high-profile breaches have come about through unauthorized authentication which occur as a result of the hijacking of the authentication credentials of staffs in an organization. Studies over the years have shown that users could be careless with their login credentials. Users have also been known to share passwords with friends and colleagues, write them down on pieces of paper, stick them on screens of their computers etc. Some users have also been known to repeat the same passwords over several platforms or websites which could also have poor backend security [7].

These recycled passwords may have severe consequences when there is a password leak. These are just some of the ways in which passwords of users can be exposed to attackers. When there are no extra layers of security, and attackers get hold of the login credentials then they have unrestricted access to user information and depending on the role of the user whose information has been compromised, it could lead to huge damages, lawsuits and substantial financial loses. This research identifies the need for extra security of data, the need to make individuals feel a lot more secure about their profiles on various systems and the need to make organizations feel more secure about their organization's data while proposing a solution which implements a more secure form of two-factor authentication.

Two-factor authentication was introduced due to the need for extra security of information and to protect the user's information from unauthorized access. Accessing information for quite a long while was simply by entering a pre-assigned username and a previously set password. The static nature of the parameters needed to gain access to valuable user information made it an easy target for attackers, who only had to get hold of the information once to have unlimited access to the user information. Most individuals were in the habit of repeating passwords across several platforms, so these passwords could easily be remembered, some wrote these passwords down on pieces of papers and stuck them on the monitor screen, some used easy to predict passwords etc. Due to the fact users repeated passwords across various platforms, it meant that if one platform was compromised and the passwords of user collected, they could be applied across other platforms. All these made gaining access to user accounts easy for attackers. Two-factor authentication was introduced to add a dynamic piece into the chain of authentication. A piece which could not easily be predicted by the attacker which in most cases involved a token. Security tokens could either be hardware supplied through a physical token or software supplied through electronic means such as, email and text messages. All these mentioned means of delivery of the token for final authentication can be high jacked by attackers who can take advantage of vulnerabilities and loopholes in the technology behind the token delivery. For example, the man-in-the-middle attack is a common attack used to get or modify the content of communication over Voice Over IP (VOIP), one of the protocols in which users receive the software token for authentication. With the deployment of – and especially the Session Initiation Protocol (SIP) vulnerabilities such as registration hijacking can be used to register the User Agent with a Session Initiation Protocol (SIP) proxy/registrar which allows the proxy to direct inbound calls to the user agent (attacker) [8]. Most organizations have been known to tone down on security because of complaints from customers on the complexity which accompany certain security implementations.

3 System Design

Two-factor authentication is an enhanced authentication mechanism for protecting users that have their password stolen either by leaking a server's password database or through phishing [9]. The increased use of cellphone usage has aided the adoption and implementation of two-factor authentication due to the convenience of delivery of the one-time passwords to the mobile phones of users. Two-factor authentication has been proven to significantly raise the bar for attackers, it is still questioned if the technology can be adopted by majority of the users on the internet as some users complain of the added step included as adding complexity to the authentication process and they would rather operate without it at the expense of having their accounts be vulnerable. It is important to stress that there are so far studies estimating 2FA adoption in a range of 2%–5% [10]. Most authentication mechanisms involve a username and a stored password. These variables can be hijacked by the attackers through various means, and an authentication system without an additional step in the authentication chain would render the account very vulnerable and easy to be hijacked by attackers. We often time think that we have our accounts secure due to the complexity of the passwords which we have set up, but attackers work much harder to find the means to compromise user accounts.

Our A two-factor authentication method is composed of two of the three following authentication verification methods: (1) something the user knows, such a password or a pin code; (2) something the user has, such a token or a smart card; (3) something the user is, such a fingerprint or a retinal scan. Two-factor authentication has found its application in many forms of technology which require utmost safety of personal information and user data. From securing personal emails, online file storage, bank account information and other very critical data. Users generally must confirm that they are indeed the ideal owners of the data being accessed before they can gain access to view, edit or modify the data. They do so by entering the username, password and the final piece of information which confirms their identity.

Current mobile applications can be developed to act as the means of providing the piece of information which the user requires to securely authenticate. The app could synchronize with the web platform of the authentication service and would perform three different functions, depending on the user's choice of authenticating:

- Display a push notification on a login attempt also stating the type of device, operating system and the geographic position of the log in attempt. The user can either click to authorize or deny the authentication.
- The app can generate a timed software token, which would be entered in a text field which would be displayed on the login screen. The login attempt is accepted if the onetime password entered matches the one-time password generated.
- The user can also make use of a random timed QR code option. The authentication service displays a QR code on the login screen which the authorized user must scan using their app. Access is granted if the QR code scanned matches the current QR code enabled for authentication of the account. This method of authentication requires that access be granted to the app to access the user's camera.

A final form of authentication can be implemented which is the hardware token to act as a means of authentication and to accommodate users who do not have smart phones. The hardware token is encrypted and synchronized with the web platform to generated timed secure token to authenticate users.

4 Conclusion

As more and more organizations opt to place their services online to be able to offer round the clock access to customers, it is imperative that only authorized users gain access to accounts. Individuals would also want to feel safe online and not have their personal information harvested from their accounts by attackers. A secure authentication system protects the individual from unauthorized access to the users' personal information and protects organizations from loss of customer data, financial losses and potential law suits as a result of breaches.

Most authentication solutions today implement a less secure model of two factor authentication. Similarities in services exist as AaaS providers like DUO also offer hardware token and push notification. Indeed, users will have to change system in order to be able to use this type of solution. In this regard, previous analysis of switching behavior [12] might be relevant. This service is unique as it implements the highly secure QR code option and most importantly delivers its One-time password only over secure and encrypted internet connection and not through the insecure SS7 telephone network. One of the most used forms of two-factor authentication is the SMS message. Most existing vendors deliver the timed software token over SMS messages or phone call back and this poses a serious security threat to authentication due to the insecurity of the SS7 network over which the text messages are delivered. The SS7 network controls many PTN features, e.g., basic call setup, management, tear down, billing and returning busy signals. Deregulation coupled with PTN convergence with the Internet and wireless networks significantly increase vulnerabilities, enabling attackers to perpetrate fraud, interception and interruption on a potentially massive scale [11]. The proposed service eliminates the need for SMS messages or telephone call back as an option for two-factor authentication.

References

1. Caporusso, N., Chea, S., Abukhaled, R.: A game-theoretical model of ransomware. In: International Conference on Applied Human Factors and Ergonomics, pp. 69–78. Springer, Cham, July 2018. https://doi.org/10.1007/978-3-319-94782-2_7
2. Stainbrook, M., Caporusso, N.: Convenience or strength? Aiding optimal strategies in password generation. In: International Conference on Applied Human Factors and Ergonomics, pp. 23–32. Springer, Cham, July 2018. https://doi.org/10.1007/978-3-319-94782-2_3
3. Fandakly, T., Caporusso, N.: Beyond passwords: enforcing username security as the first line of defense. In: International Conference on Applied Human Factors and Ergonomics. Springer, July 2019, to be published
4. Bonneau, J., Stuart S.: Towards reliable storage of 56-bit secrets in human memory. In: 23rd {USENIX} Security Symposium ({USENIX} Security 14), pp. 607–623 (2014)
5. Florencio, D., Herley, C.: A large-scale study of web password habits. In: Proceedings of the 16th International Conference on World Wide Web, pp. 657–666. ACM, May 2007
6. Caporusso, N., Stainbrook, M.: Comparative evaluation of security and convenience trade-offs in password generation aiding systems. In: International Conference on Applied Human Factors and Ergonomics. Springer, July 2019, to be published

7. Kontaxis, G., Athanasopoulos, E., Portokalidis, G., Keromytis, A.D.: Sauth: protecting user accounts from password database leaks. In: Proceedings of the 2013 ACM SIGSAC Conference on Computer & Communications Security, pp. 187–198. ACM, November 2013
8. Collier, M.: Basic vulnerability issues for SIP security. SecureLogix Corporation (2005)
9. Dhamija, R., Tygar, J.D.: The battle against phishing: dynamic security skins. In: Proceedings of the 2005 Symposium on Usable Privacy and Security, pp. 77–88. ACM, July 2005
10. Petsas, T., Tsirantonakis, G., Athanasopoulos, E., Ioannidis, S.: Two-factor authentication: is the world ready?: quantifying 2FA adoption. In: Proceedings of the Eighth European Workshop on System Security, p. 4. ACM, April 2015
11. Lorenz, G., Moore, T., Manes, G., Hale, J., Shenoi, S.: Securing SS7 telecommunications networks. In: Workshop on Information Assurance and Security, vol. 2, p. 1115, June 2001
12. Xiao, X., Caporusso, N.: Comparative evaluation of cyber migration factors in the current social media landscape. In: 2018 6th International Conference on Future Internet of Things and Cloud Workshops (FiCloudW), pp. 102–107. IEEE, August 2018

Assessment and Design of Employees-Cobot-Interaction

Christoph Mühlemeyer(✉)

Institute of Occupational Health, Safety and Ergonomics (ASER e. V.), Corneliusstraße 31, 42329 Wuppertal, Germany
muehlemeyer@institut-aser.de

Abstract. Prima facie employees-cobot-interaction has the potential to minimize or even eliminate occupational physical and mental health risks. For example when the redesign results in the situation where tasks with high intensity, duration and frequency of physical exposure or monotonous activities are performed by the cobot. But even setting up a modern and inherently safe cobot-workplace does not necessarily mean a prevention of physical and mental health risks and is not automatically ensuring decent working conditions and, at worst, can result in downgraded working conditions. The article - see below - demonstrates this paradoxical situation by a comparison of an employees-cobot-interaction in the sense of industry 4.0 and digitization with its initial situation. For a standardized quantification, the procedural economic, holistic and ergonomic instrument of the BDS-System has been applied practically.

Keywords: Cobots · Holistic approach · BDS-Instrument · Simulation · KPIs · Workplace design · Digital ergonomics · KIM-MHO · Shopfloor transition

1 Introduction

Industrial robots are automatically controlled, freely programmable multipurpose manipulators which are programmable in three or more axes and can be arranged for use in automation either fixed or movable. Furthermore, collaborative operation is considered as a condition where robots are working directly together with employees within a shared space [1]. This kind of collaborating employees-cobot-interaction without safety cages is hereinafter referred as cobot-workplace.

With an inherently safe construction of a cobot, the essential safety and health requirements of machinery directive 2006/42/EC can be met to ensure the free movement of goods in the European Economic Area through product safety which here also includes the holistic product and production related ergonomics [2].

If cobot-workplaces are operated in Germany, the working conditions have to be assessed in accordance with the German act on the implementation of measures of occupational safety and health [3] and the regulations based on it [4] to encourage safety and health protection measures as well as to check their effectiveness. For sure, this applies to both, the 'classic' occupational injury hazards (e.g. mechanical, electrical) as well as health risks which can occur e.g. due to physical and mental exposure and this also includes a verification of special risks for employees with higher

T. Ahram et al. (Eds.): IHIET 2019, AISC 1018, pp. 771–776, 2020.
https://doi.org/10.1007/978-3-030-25629-6_120

protection needs (e.g. disabled, pregnant and breastfeeding women, older employees, newcomers, untrained users).

There is a general assumption that modern and inherently safe cobot-workplaces will easily minimize or even eliminate work-related physical and mental health risks (like manipulators often achieve for lifting tasks). Nevertheless, going live with cobots in the shopfloor does not automatically mean a physical and mental health prevention and is not automatically ensuring decent working conditions for the interacting employees. This is shown by a comparison of a cobot-workplace in the sense of industry 4.0 and digitization with the initial situation (w/o cobot). For a quantified standardization, the procedural economic, holistic and ergonomic instrument of the exposure documentation system (BDS-Instrument) has been applied practically. First, this formed the foundation to evolve the findings to cobot-workplace design proposals and, on the other hand, the article's readers shall also benefit from suggestions and ideas how to improve their own operational processes and being able to also control the shopfloor transition in other fields (e.g. exoskeletons).

2 Methods

2.1 Workplace Description

In the examined cobot-workplace, a female employee performs a sub-task (station) of the packaging process of personal care products by removing tubes (work item) from the delivered boxes (input) to the target packaging (output), here without using any tools [5]. This is performed indoor in an industrial hall (working environment) in individual work within an eight-hour shift [6]. In the same collaborating area, but not working on the packaging product at the same time (synchronous assembly type), the cobot lifts the lid and places it on a conveyor belt [7].

2.2 Holistic Assessment Instrument

Often neglected but very important part of the risk assessment of working conditions process is to determine and implement the required measures to prevent work-related health risks and ensure decent working conditions. Having this in focus, the holistic instrument of the exposure documentation system (Belastungs-Dokumentations-System – BDS) has been developed on the basis of the assessment of the work-related health risks method (Beurteilung arbeitsbedingter Belastungen – BAB) in the 1970s in R&D projects of the German HdA-program [8, 9]. After over 40 years of research, application in practice as well as continuous improvement, today's BDS Production Ergonomics Core Module is subdivided into the main groups physical exposures, mental exposures (work organization), environmental conditions and accident risks. When using the BDS-Instrument, the workplaces' work tasks' intensity and duration are analyzed per exposure type and based on this, shift-related assessment results are aggregated by the underlying methods. This knowledge can be used in the planning phase of workstations as well as in the live phase of workplaces and can also be used to simulate design improvements for checking their effectiveness proactively and afterwards. Table 1 outlines the development and structure of BDS-Instrument [10] as well as the scope of the described practical application for the before/after comparison of the cobot-workplace.

Table 1. BAB-Method and BDS-Instrument - development, structure and practical application for the before/after comparison

BAB/BDS Development	BAB/BDS-Structure	Before/after comparison
1970s: BAB-Development 1980s: Scientific application (steel, metal, glass & ceramics industry) 1990s: Scientific and industrial application (SMEs, Logistics) and development of first digital version 2000s: Development of demographic assessment and network version, application in automotive industry 2010s: Further scientific and international industrial application, national & international awards (e.g. EU-OSHA-Award), KPIS, Inclusion-, reports, tablet-front-end	Core module for production ergonomics & risk assessment incl. shift aggregation & simulation KPI management Gender & demographic filter Inclusion filter & reports Report inclusion Report for ordinance on occupational health care Accidental risks expert-module Mental exposure expert-module Compensation allowances expert-module	Data Gathering Video-Analysis Application of BDS' production ergonomics module Analysis, assessment and simulation of the physical and mental exposures in method detail level: special screening Comparison of eight hour shift aggregation Comparison of KPIs Causal development of design improvements and pre-/post effectiveness-check

2.3 Analysis, Backward Simulation and Comparison

The analysis phase started with data collection for the cobot-workplace. Since the comparison was asked only after the redesign, a backward simulation of the same workplace as a "purely" manual packaging activity (without cobot use) was done with BDS-Instrument to ensure that both production ergonomics scenarios could be compared. Because the 'classic' occupational injury hazards as well as the environmental conditions are very much dependent on every companies' very special conditions (e.g. noise level, climate conditions, lighting level, rules for in-house transport, operating procedures) these are not considered in detail below. Main focus here was to achieve an as informative as possible assessment of the physical and mental health risks by gathering and taking into account the related analysis information (e.g. cycle time, repetition rates, long term assembly line availability, work shift handover regulations, recovery times, personal distribution times, organizational aspects) to be able to aggregate a representative eight-hour shift.

Tasks with high repetitive movements require a valid risk assessment of upper extremity musculoskeletal disorders (UEMSDs). Therefore, BDS provides workplace aggregations [10] based on the key indicator method for manual handling operations (KIM-MHO) [11–13]. After gathering the needed MHO input parameters, finally, the mental exposures for both scenarios were analyzed and compared with BDS' mental exposures group (e.g. repetition of work tasks, connection to the technical process, requirement of concentration, unchallenging work).

3 Results

The result of the eight-hour shift-related workplace bar chart exposure-profile indicates packaging without cobot (backward simulation) as a workplace with various intolerable physical and mental overload. Among physical exposure it is body posture, manual handling operations and distribution of body posture/movement with intolerable overload e.g. due to 7 h of static standing and permanently necessary torsion of the trunk with more than 10° (both, to the right and to the left). Among mental exposures it is the cycle time of 7 s and the unchallenging work (only displacing tasks, no rotation) that lead to intolerable overload (Fig. 1: left-hand side).

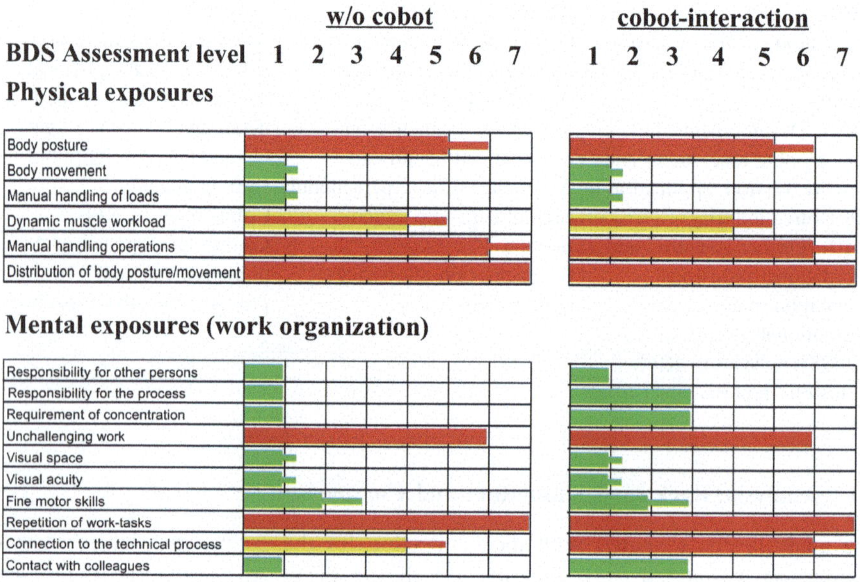

Fig. 1. Comparison of eight-hour shift aggregation with BDS-Instrument (left profile: without cobot, right profile: cobot-interaction)

With implementing the cobot-interaction the ergonomic conditions have deteriorated further. Due to synchronous operation with the cobot, the employees hand movements frequency and total amount per shift increased what now results in a higher UEMSDs risk (KIM-MHO risk score increased from 50,3 to 53,3 points). Due to cycle time reduction from 7 to 5 s (−29%), fewer degrees of freedom and the less contact opportunities to colleagues, the mental exposures deteriorated even more clearly (Fig. 1: right-hand side).

The workplace-variants are associated with multiple intolerable work-related overload in standard (thick bars) and specific (thin bars) assessment and therefore go hand in hand with an increased risk for work-related symptoms and disorders for both, employees with higher protection needs as well as for normally resilient employees. Accordingly, redesign measures need to be implemented to minimize the identified risks. This should be done from a business angle e.g. to increase the own age stability rate as well from the perspective of compliance with the goal to e.g. for Germany meet the AMR 13.2 [14] criteria for MSD risk and the maternity protection criteria [15] for irresponsible Risk (Table 2).

Table 2. BDS - KPIs & reports for packaging w/o cobot vs. cobot-interaction.

Results, KPIs & reports	w/o cobot	Cobot-interaction
KIM-MHO result (risk score)	50,3	53,6
Physical Overload factor/employee (BDS report)	6	6
Cycle time (duration)	7 s	5 s
Repetition of work tasks (BAB level)	7	7
Connection to the technical process (BAB level)	4 (5)	6 (7)
Age stability (BDS KPI)	No	No
MSD risk (AMR 13.2 criteria)	Yes	Yes
Irresponsible Risk (§9 MuSchG criteria)	Yes	Yes
Production Ergonomics Rank	1 of 2	2 of 2
Generally recommended for shopfloor	No	No

4 Discussion

The results demonstrate that operating cobot-workplaces does not automatically ensure healthy working conditions, not even if, with their help exactly this was envisaged. The immense importance of the assessment of product ergonomics in the risk assessment in accordance with Machinery Directive 2006/42/EC and the assessment of production ergonomics according to the respective national health and safety regulations has been pointed out. Essential for valid results is a professionally and correctly consideration of all important method based operating conditions (what also includes e.g. station layout, quantities, space, traffic routes, noise, climate) and conditions of use (e.g. body postures, cycle times, buffers, jumpers). Both, 'classic' workplaces and 'factor 4.0' workplaces need holistic assessment instruments in order to be able to identify the most critical work-related health risks and develop necessary and effective design improvements causally.

For cobot-interaction, it will be very important to transfer especially sub-tasks with high to peak forces, hitting, joint-movements at ranges' limits and sub-tasks where working objects are slippery, soft or sharp edged to the cobot. Especially for the handover sub-task (interface) care should be taken on a neutral (relaxed) joint-position for the employees.

To improve companies' individual operational processes and being able to manage the shopfloor transition professionally it is important to implement a strategy for interdisciplinary analysis, assessment and design. With shorter product lifecycles and increasing workplace complexity, it is getting more important than ever to effectively bringing together the knowledge of diverse operational professionals. This also means to work with KPIs, proactively identify national compliance problems and manage the improvement process to design a competitive, audit-ready safe and healthy shopfloor.

References

1. German Institute for Standardization: Robots and robotic devices - Safety requirements for industrial robots - Part 1: Robots. (ISO 10218-1:2011). German version EN ISO 10218-1:2011. DIN (2011)
2. European Parliament and of the Council: Directive 2006/42/EC of the European Parliament and of the Council of 17 May 2006 on machinery, and amending Directive 95/16/EC (2006)
3. Federal Law Gazette: Act on the Implementation of Measures of Occupational Safety and Health to Encourage Improvements in the Safety and Health Protection of Workers at Work (Deutsches Arbeitsschutzgesetz (ArbSchG)). Bundesgesetzblatt – BGBl. I S. 1246 (2006)
4. Federal Law Gazette: Regulation regarding Safety and Health Protection in Providing Work Equipment and its use in Work. (Betriebssicherheitsverordnung -BetrSichV). Bundesgesetzblatt - BGBl. I S. 49 (2015)
5. German Institute for Standardization: Ergonomics principles in the design of work systems (ISO 6385:2016). German Institute for Standardization. German version EN ISO 6385:2016. DIN (2011)
6. Joint Ministerial Gazette: Gefährdungen an der Schnittstelle Mensch - Arbeitsmittel - Ergonomische und menschliche Faktoren, Arbeitssystem. TRBS 1151. GMBl, no. 17/18, p. 340 (2015)
7. Bauer, W., Bender, M., Braun, M., Rally, P., Scholtz, O.: Leichtbauroboter in der manuellen Montage – einfach einfach anfangen. Fraunhofer IAO (2016)
8. Müller, B.H., Hettinger, Th: Interpretations- und Bewertungsverfahren arbeitswissenschaftlich-ergonomischer Felddaten. Zeitschrift für Arbeitswissenschaft **35**, 82–86 (1981)
9. Peters, H.: Verfahren zur Beurteilung arbeitsbedingter Belastungen BAB. In: Erfassung und Bewertung arbeitswissenschaftlicher Daten. Schriften des IfaA (Hrsg.), no. 62, pp. 64–78, Köln (1986)
10. Klußmann, A., Mühlemeyer, C., Lang, K.-H., Dolfen, P., Wendt, K.-D., Gebhardt, H., Neumann, B., Schäfer, A.: Praxisbewährte Methoden zur Bewertung und Gestaltung physischer Arbeitsbelastungen. Leistung und Lohn – Zeitschrift für Arbeitswirtschaft, BDA – Bundesvereinigung der Deutschen Arbeitgeberverbände (Hrsg.), no. 541–545. Heider-Verlag, Berlin, Bergisch Gladbach (2013)
11. Klußmann, A., Steinberg, U., Liebers, F., Gebhardt, H., Rieger, M.A.: The key indicator method for manual handling operations (KIM-MHO) – evaluation of a new method for the assessment of working conditions within a cross-sectional study. BMC Musculoskelet. Disord. **11**, 272 (2010). https://doi.org/10.1186/1471-2474-11-272. ISSN 1471-2474
12. Steinberg, U., Liebers, F., Klußmann, A., Gebhardt, H., Rieger, M.A., Behrendt, S., Latza, U.: Leitmerkmalmethode Manuelle Arbeitsprozesse 2011. Bericht über die Erprobung, Validierung und Revision. BAuA, Dortmund (2012). ISBN 978-3-88261-722-1
13. Klußmann, A., Liebers, F., Gebhardt, Hj, Rieger, M.A., Latza, U.: Steinberg: Risk assessment of manual handling operations at work with the key indicator method (KIM-MHO) – determination of criterion validity regarding the prevalence of musculoskeletal symptoms and clinical conditions within a cross-sectional study. BMC Musculoskelet. Disord. **18**, 184 (2017). https://doi.org/10.1186/s12891-017-1542-0. ISSN 1471-2474
14. Joint Ministerial Gazette: AMR 13.2 "Tätigkeiten mit wesentlich erhöhten körperlichen Belastungen mit Gesundheitsgefährdungen für das Muskel-Skelett-System". GMBl, 23, no. 76–77, p. 1571 (2014)
15. Federal Law Gazette: Maternity Protection Act. Gesetz zum Schutz von Müttern bei der Arbeit, in der Ausbildung und im Studium (Mutterschutzgesetz - MuSchG). BGBl. I S. 1228 (2017)

Investigating Transparency and Accountability of User Interfaces for Data Visualization: A Case Study on Crowdfunding

Sijia Li and Nicholas Caporusso(✉)

Department of Informatics, Fort Hays State University,
600 Park Street, Hays 67601, USA
s_li93@mail.fhsu.edu, n_caporusso@fhsu.edu

Abstract. Crowdfunding is an innovative form of fund raising that enables individuals and businesses to leverage a large audience of potential supporters for financing their projects: disseminating the message to many potential contributors compensates for the smaller individual commitment. In the recent years, thanks to web-based platforms, crowdfunding received increasing attention and branched into several subtypes, such as, reward-based and equity-based initiatives, which enable supporters to pre-buy products or acquire company shares, respectively. Indeed, crowdfunding platforms have several advantages (e.g., reducing barriers to bottom up initiatives and democratizing access to high-return investments). Simultaneously, as governments are in their early stage of addressing the many risks and grey areas related to the dynamics of crowdfunding, the accountability of platforms has a crucial role. In this paper, we investigate the transparency of the User Interface (UI) of equity crowdfunding platforms and we discuss the implications in enabling users to make better informed decisions about their investments.

Keywords: Crowdfunding · Equity crowdfunding · Reward-based crowdfunding · Data visualization · Visibility · Inferability · Heuristic evaluation

1 Introduction

Crowdfunding is a recent form of fundraising that enables businesses to collect funds for a project by publishing it on an on-line platform and presenting it to an audience of potential supporters and early adopters who are willing to pledge to its future development [1]. Although the initial objective of crowdfunding websites was to help finance small, non-for-profit initiatives, in the last decade it raised a total of 34 billion US dollars worldwide [2], and it evolved into a more sophisticated and structured form of funding for new or established ventures. As a result, nowadays several businesses choose reward- or equity-based campaigns for crowdsourcing funds as alternatives to raising venture capital, and the industry is projected to grow to over 300 billion US dollars by 2025, according to recent statistics [3]. Reward-based crowdfunding typically consists in pre-selling the concept of a variety of initiatives, such as, physical products (e.g., apparel, devices), events and exhibitions, art projects, and services,

T. Ahram et al. (Eds.): IHIET 2019, AISC 1018, pp. 777–782, 2020.
https://doi.org/10.1007/978-3-030-25629-6_121

before they are actually implemented, so that the company can collect the necessary funds to start production. The rules, risks, and best practices of reward-based crowdfunding have been analyzed in several research studies: although most of the projects are successful stories, given the intangible nature of the promise of crowdfunding campaigns, numerous cases resulted in scams or projects that were never realized.

Conversely, in this paper, we focus on the role of User Interfaces (UIs) in crowdfunding platforms, and we detail aspects that have an impact on transparency and, consequently, affect end users. Specifically, we analyze the explicit and implicit dimensions of transparency and their implementation in terms of type of information and data visualization mechanisms currently available on crowdfunding platforms. Moreover, we evaluate the contribution of specific components of the UI in terms of helping users take better informed decisions. We compare the different types of information visualization offered by the most popular websites, and we identify the benefits and potential flaws of the key elements of the UI (e.g., funding goal, fundraising progress, interaction with the audience, investment timeline). Specifically, we consider equity crowdfunding [4], a new form of crowdsourced investment that enables businesses to collect funds by issuing shares of the company. Given its novelty, regulations are still under development and UI is not taken into consideration. Nevertheless, as the audience of equity crowdfunding platforms mainly consists of inexperienced individuals, this type of initiative involves higher risks. From our findings, we demonstrate that information design is a component of governance: User Interfaces have a significant role in providing users with transparent information, increasing their awareness about the risks associated with investments, and improving the effectiveness of crowdfunding platforms in demonstrating their accountability.

2 Accountability and Role of User Interface in Crowdfunding

Many aspects of digital crowdfunding have extensively been explored in the scientific literature [5], despite its introduction is relatively recent. However, the majority of research studies focused on economic aspects [6], factors that contribute to the success of campaigns (e.g., marketing and promotion) [7], and social dynamics, such as herding, that explain the behavior of investors and help understand follow-up investments [8]. Conversely, elements of the user experience that are related to the UI of crowdfunding platforms, such as, the type and quality of information presented to users, data visualization, and the specific components of the GUI, received less attention. This is mainly because most of the work regarded reward-based crowdfunding platforms (e.g., Kickstarter and Indiegogo), in which, similarly to an e-commerce website, information primarily involves a description of the project, a limited number of reward options, and timeline and delivery date. In this case, risks are mainly limited to delayed product receipt or to not receiving the reward at all (e.g., due to production issues or fraudulent campaigns).

On the contrary, as equity crowdfunding platforms (e.g., Seedrs, Companisto, and Mamacrowd) are marketplaces for becoming shareholder of a company in exchange of an investment with potential future returns, there are many more variables and additional pieces of information that need to be disclosed to the user, to make them fully aware of the risks and benefits of the operation. Moreover, currently, most equity crowdfunding platforms have a similar GUI and user journey compared to reward-based websites. However, especially considering the novelty of this form of platforms, there is the risk for non-expert users to assimilate two and, consequently, overlook the inherent risks associated with equity investments. Furthermore, as equity crowdfunding platforms target a diverse audience of stakeholders consisting of investment firms, professional investors and non-experts, it is even more important to make sure all the users have equal access to relevant information and that they can understand it.

Most studies about equity crowdfunding focused on implementation factors pertaining the organization of individual campaigns, such as, financial attractiveness of the business plan, communication and promotion strategy (e.g., updates and responsiveness to comments), and aspects related to founders' ability to use crowdfunding as a digital tool to successfully raise the target amount. Conversely, in this paper, we focus on the design of information, interface, and user experience in crowdfunding platforms, independently from the specific campaign information [9]. Although the design and implementation of user interface are often overlooked, they have a crucial role in increasing transparency and are a fundamental factor of accountability in equity crowdfunding platforms. In the next section, we highlight the best practices and identify areas that need to be improved. As governments recently started studying the complex dynamics of crowdfunding to introduce regulations that address assurance principles and standards, incorporating the concept of transparency in interface design could already contribute to improving the type and quality of information presented to users.

3 Transparency Analysis

In our preliminary analysis, we considered 7 European equity crowdfunding platforms (2 in Germany, 1 in the UK, and 4 in Italy), and we realized a heuristic evaluation of the transparency of their information. Although usability incorporates the concept of transparency, this aspect is inherently elusive and, thus, often overlooked. Therefore, in our study we refer to and adopt the model proposed by [10], which defines the semantic dimensions of transparency, that is, *visibility* and *inferability*, which are necessary and jointly sufficient conditions for there to be transparency. Moreover, [10] details the empirical parameters that can be utilized for measuring the quality of transparency: specifically, visibility represents the degree to which information is complete and findable, whereas inferability describes the extent to which information is disaggregated, verified and simplified. Furthermore, as previously discussed, transparency should be appropriate for the intended audience. To this end, we refer to [11], which differentiated between *indirect* transparency, that is, the level of understanding by experts, and *direct* transparency, which regards the degree to which it is intended to the wider public.

The structure of campaigns on an equity crowdfunding platform typically consists in the following details: (1) project description, which includes video, images and text, that describe the business opportunity, the target market, the proposed solution and its advantages, the team, and the strategy; (2) financials disclose information, such as, amount currently raised, goal of the campaign, equity distribution; (3) updates inform potential investors about accomplishments and milestones achieved during and after the campaign, whereas comments help interested users interact with the team; (4) detailed list of investments promised and secured throughout the campaign. In addition, projects can include additional documentation, such as, investor's deck, business plan, and detailed financial projections, which typically are targeted at a more expert audience. Depending on the specific implementation, elements are arranged over different pages or incorporated in components of the GUI that helps condense and summarize information. Although most platforms include this type of information, they have different criteria in regard to visibility. Furthermore, the systems utilized for visualizing information demonstrate low inferability, which especially decreases indirect transparency.

None of the platforms analyzed in our study included whether the information presented in the project description page is verified and validated by a third-party stakeholder with domain expertise, which would increase direct transparency and, thus, promote trust among non-expert investors. Consequently, although information is visible, its inferability is limited, because it cannot be easily verified. In this regard, reward-based crowdfunding platforms are partnering with companies that analyze whether a project is credible and display a badge on their page, though there are no studies about the effectiveness of this system in terms of amount raised, successful product delivery, or improved trust. Moreover, crowdfunding platforms lack standardization: each campaign utilizes a different system for describing and visualizing data about the market, competition, timeline, funding allocation, and expected growth, which affect the simplification dimension of inferability. Having a single format for presenting similar data would enable users to compare information about different campaigns: although each project is unique, marketplaces should diminish fragmentation to support individuals in deciding about the best investment among the many opportunities advertised. Finally, information about the team is a key factor for determining the likelihood of success of a business. Unfortunately, 4 platforms display only the names of team members, whereas 3 websites provide links to founders' profiles on professional social networks (i.e., LinkedIn), which help infer their expertise.

As for transparency of financial information, several factors render it the most critical aspect among all components. Indeed, this is due to the inherent complexity of investment dynamics. Nevertheless, numerous pieces of information are not visible on most platforms. As an example, only one website shows the difference between promised and committed investment: as raising equity on average involves higher amounts compared to other forms of crowdfunding, users promise a sum that they can commit (i.e., actually pay or transfer) by the end of the campaign. However, as there is no obligation for the investor to fulfil their promise, there often is a discrepancy between the amount promised by users and the funds eventually collected at the end of the fundraising round. While this ambiguity helps demonstrate traction and attract follow-up investments, it might lead to inflating promised amounts and, consequently, affect the success predictability of a campaign based on the amount raised at any given time, and ultimately, decrease the level of trust in the platform. Furthermore, information visibility issues include the relationship between share rights and minimum amount invested: several crowdfunding platforms enable defining different types of shares and assigning them based on the minimum contribution. While direct and indirect transparency are compromised by the lack of visibility of this information, the concern is even greater in terms of inferability, as many non-expert individuals participate in investments. Also, most websites lack transparency in regard to the amount co-invested or raised by founders independently from the platform and assimilate it to the promised or committed amounts, creating further ambiguity in this regard. Many equity crowdfunding campaigns follow the pattern of traditional crowdfunding campaigns, in which the initial commitment is a driver for attracting subsequent investments. As a result, founders typically already secure investment from different sources (e.g., friends and family or professional investors) before or in parallel to launching the campaign. Such investments might involve conditions that are negotiated independently from the platform and might result in different rights compared to users who buy equity on the crowdfunding website. Specifying the amount already secured and the conditions negotiated with the investors would help understand the ratio between founders' ability to raise funds and the effectiveness of the crowdfunding platform, in addition to increasing users' awareness about the convenience of the investment opportunity and the overall structure of the deal. Increasing the visibility and inferability of this type of information is crucial for improving even indirect transparency.

Most platforms include tools for posting updates and comments, which can be utilized to ask for additional information that was not mentioned in the initial package, to clarify specific aspects and, indirectly, to infer the responsiveness and commitment of the team. Also, this component helps dynamically modify and complete the information presented in the other sections based on the feedback received by users.

Finally, platforms lack visibility and inferability of information about investors who contributed to the campaign. In reward-based crowdfunding, who else backs the campaign and the type of reward they choose are not relevant to the supporters and proponents of the campaign: the only concern that matters is that the project is successfully funded. Conversely, as the supporters of an equity crowdfunding campaign will share ownership and responsibilities, their identity should be important to the founders and to other supporters; furthermore, the type and number of shares owned by backers can result in different representation and, thus, have an influential weight in strategic decisions, determine company success and, ultimately, valuation. To this end, 3 of the 7 crowdfunding platforms implement a unique numeric identifier associated with users, so that the investment, equity stake, and portfolio of each investor can be disclosed while preserving their anonymity. Although all platforms examined in our evaluation show the number of supporters, none displays information about the type of shares and their distribution among investors, making it difficult to infer the structure of company shareholders as a result of the campaign.

In addition to the type and quality of information, persistence is relevant for both new users and returning investors. In this regard, platforms have different strategies: 2 websites maintain all the information visible after the end of the campaign, whereas the others remove some or most of the data as soon as the campaign ends, which makes it difficult to compare current investment opportunities with previous campaigns.

4 Conclusion and Future Work

Crowdfunding websites, especially promoting equity-based campaigns, are a novel type of online marketplaces that enables individuals and businesses to raise funds to initiate and develop their projects. Although most campaigns successfully deliver their promise, equity crowdfunding involves several additional risks compared to reward-based campaigns, especially for non-expert investors. Consequently, governments are in the early stages of developing recommendations. Nevertheless, given the current lack of regulations, companies implement what seems to work best in their platforms. In this paper, we highlighted the importance of transparency in User Interfaces, we discussed its implications in terms of risk awareness and information assurance. Specifically, our heuristic evaluation of the main components of the Graphical User Interface focused on transparency, that is, quality and type of information, as well as its visibility and inferability, and did not take into consideration other dimensions of usability. We suggested the implementation of UI elements that should be recommended as mandatory to provide users with information and make them aware of the risks and benefits of investing in a project, so they can make better informed decisions. In our future work, we will expand our study by designing an experiment that will evaluate whether introducing the elements suggested in this paper actually increases transparency and improves awareness of both experts and non-experts.

References

1. Belleflamme, P., Lambert, T., Schwienbacher, A.: Crowdfunding: tapping the right crowd. J. Bus. Ventur. **29**(5), 585–609 (2014)
2. Global Internet Crowdfunding and Wealth Management Market Report 2019. Research Reports World, United States
3. Global Crowdfunding Market Size, Status and Forecast 2025. QYResearch Group, United States
4. Vulkan, N., Åstebro, T., Sierra, M.F.: Equity crowdfunding: a new phenomena. J. Bus. Ventur. Insights **5**, 37–49 (2016)
5. Mollick, E.: The dynamics of crowdfunding: an exploratory study. J. Bus. Ventur. **29**(1), 1–16 (2014)
6. Agrawal, A., Catalini, C., Goldfarb, A.: Some simple economics of crowdfunding. Innov. Policy Econ. **14**(1), 63–97 (2014)
7. Koch, J.-A., Siering, M.: Crowdfunding success factors: the characteristics of successfully funded projects on crowdfunding platforms. In: Proceedings of the 23rd European Conference on Information Systems (ECIS 2015), Muenster, Germany (2015)
8. Astebro, T.B., Fernández Sierra, M., Lovo, S., Vulkan, N.: Herding in equity crowdfunding. (2017). SSRN 3084140
9. Rahmanian, B., Davis, J.G.: User interface design for crowdsourcing systems. In: Proceedings of the 2014 International Working Conference on Advanced Visual Interfaces, pp. 405–408. ACM, May 2014
10. Michener, G., Bersch, K.: Identifying transparency. Inf. Polity **18**(3), 233–242 (2013)
11. Hood, C.: What happens when transparency meets blame-avoidance? Public Manage. Rev. **9**(2), 191–210 (2007)

Designing Systems for the Digital Immortality of Intangible Cultural Heritage

Maurizio Caon(✉)

School of Management, University of Applied Sciences and Arts Western Switzerland (HES-SO), Fribourg, Switzerland
maurizio.caon@hes-so.ch

Abstract. Digital curation of cultural heritage is an urgent and important matter for our society, which is becoming more and more digitized. In particular, preserving intangible cultural heritage requires novel solutions that can enable transmitting all the nuances of values and identity linked to different traditions and communities. The current development of digital copies of human beings, which promises the achievement of digital immortality in the near future, can allow our posterity to experience traditional events or create new artistic performances with deceased people that, otherwise, could not be lived and, therefore, understood.

Keywords: Digital curation · Intangible cultural heritage · Digital immortality

1 Introduction

Our current society is undergoing a tremendous process of digitalization, where everything is being digitized and humanity is generating data at regularly increasing rate. Progressively, this society is building a digital copy of the real world, which is referred to as cyber world and is defined as "a digitized world created on cyberspace inside computers interconnected by networks including the Internet" [1]. This cyber world is becoming a new dimension of human life, as important and impactful as the physical one. The value that this digital world is gaining and generating makes it obvious that it should be built in order to last centuries or, possibly, forever. Although it is obvious that the digitization of information is already happening fast and at a large scale, the management and preservation of digital information are still not mature, and this raises a number of issues. Indeed, the biggest part of the population is exclusively focusing on the creation of new digital content, neglecting the logically consequential phase of conservation of this information; this problematic situation is mainly due to the particular state of elation in our society brought by this new technological revolution. On this matter, Kuny wrote "as we move into the electronic era of digital objects, it is important to know that there are new barbarians at the gate and that we are moving into an era where much of what we know today, much of what is coded and written electronically, will be lost forever. We are, to my mind, living in the midst of digital Dark Ages; consequently, much as monks of times past, it falls to librarians and archivists to hold to the tradition which reveres history and the published heritage of our times" [2].

T. Ahram et al. (Eds.): IHIET 2019, AISC 1018, pp. 783–789, 2020.
https://doi.org/10.1007/978-3-030-25629-6_122

Heritage intended as the preservation of material culture, such as architecture, landscape form, objects of art and of daily use, is a concept formalized in the 20th century and processes, directives and technologies are well established and standardized for the conservation of such tangible artefacts [3]. On the other hand, intangible culture, which comprises performances of dance, music, theater, and ritual, as well as language, human memory and identity, is a concept that was formalized, at least in the Western culture, only recently [3]. For this reason, techniques for their preservation are less explored and standardized. In particular, the process of digitization can still deliver unprecedented opportunities for the conservation of this kind of cultural heritage. In the case of tangible heritage, it is nowadays common to use pictures and interactive 3D models (using also animations) for the digital archiving of monuments and objects, while high-resolution scanners, optical character recognition and semantic technology allow digitizing books, manuscripts and any sort of documents. These techniques fall short in the digitization of intangible heritage and this is even more critical in the case of preservation of digitally native intangible heritage.

The remainder of this paper states the importance of the preservation of intangible cultural heritage, comprising information directly created in the aforementioned cyber world, presenting the future possible perspectives for the digital curation of such information. In particular, the next section describes the ongoing evolution from the digital Dark Ages to the promise of digital immortality. The following section discusses future solutions enabling an augmented digital curation of intangible cultural heritage, with special regard to that intangible heritage directly created in digital form. The last section is dedicated to the conclusion of this paper summarizing the most important points and proposing the future direction of research in this field.

2 Evolving from Digital Dark Ages into Digital Immortality Era

The issue related to neglecting the preservation of digital information is becoming more and more evident as the cyber world is growing in value with reference to the human daily life. This woke up a part of the population, which started searching for solutions involving new technologies, techniques or methodologies in order to create processes and systems able to conserve information for centuries or, hopefully, millennia [4]. The preservation of digital information beyond the human lifespan will create new opportunities, such as the intentional communication with future generations achieving the first type of digital immortality, called by Bell and Gray "one-way immortality" and defined as preserving ideas to communicate with the future [5].

The ongoing process of digital transformation is creating a digital copy of every already existing object and also a huge quantity of original information directly created in this emerging cyber world. The digitalization combined with the advances in artificial intelligence suggests that it will be possible, in the near future, to create also a digital copy of human beings. These digital replicas of people are promised to be able not only to model one's physical characteristics but also to simulate thoughts, ideas and emotions [6]. The final goal of the current research in this domain is to enable the so-called "whole brain emulation", which has been defined as the "one-to-one modeling of the function of the entire human brain" [7]. Ideally, this technology would allow emulating specific brains enabling therefore the creation of back-up copies of people's minds with possible transfer of consciousness [8].

Some call this phenomenon as "digital clones" [9], others as "digital ghosts" [10], while others "digital zombies" [11]. Every definition has a subtle flavor to it: a digital clone is defined as a digital copy of a living being, which is identical to its original individual, and it "can approximate its real counterpart at different levels from external appearance like the vactor, to internal features such as behaviors", where vactor indicates a virtual actor [9]. Digital ghost refers to "a simulation of a specific human life" which "is an intelligent computerized biography that can simulate you at any time of your life" [10]. Digital zombie is defined as "the resurrected dead who remain alive and active in our digital society" [11]. All these definitions describe digital copies that are able to emulate all the information concerning a specific living being and that can survive death since they inhabit the cyber world. All of these definitions refer to the same concept: the two-way immortality, which is defined as "endless experience and learning allowing you, or at least part of you, to communicate with the future in the sense that artifact continues to learn and evolve" [5]. The two-way immortality describes the possibility of creating a digital copy of the self, which can evolve and acquire social agency allowing the extension of one's personhood beyond the boundaries of her body (posthumous personhood) and that can outlive the original individual while keeping to interact with the living [12].

Pragmatically, achieving the digital immortality can be envisioned as feeding all the data generated by a person into an intelligent software that can reconstruct that person's behavior, look, language and logic; this copy has to pass the personalized Turing test: "a close associate (family member, friend, co-worker) of a human is put in a sealed room containing only a teletype. It is linked either to a natural human or the digital copy of that human. The digital copy passes the personalized Turing test if it can convince the associate that it is the natural human" [10]. This intelligent software can also interact with other people in different ways, from the simple written form such as via social media, to more complex as through a multimodal 3D avatar or controlling a humanoid robot. These interactions can happen after the death of the original individual and they can also influence the model of this intelligent software affecting its behavior. One might think that this kind of technology is intended to belong only to the domain of science fiction but, in reality, a number of companies such as *Eterni.me*, *LivesOn* and *Humai*, already proposes some pilot services for the digitization of people and promises to create virtual avatars capable of emulating their behavior in the near future [13].

3 Eternal Preservation of Intangible Cultural Heritage

3.1 Evolution of the "Cultural Heritage" Concept

The definition of cultural heritage shifted its focus from the artistic and historic values as the exclusive parameters to including also the cultural value, the identity and the capacity to interact with memory and, finally, it evolved to include also the capacity of an object to arouse certain values transcending its material aspect. This shift can be tracked through the change UNESCO applied to what it considers as cultural heritage: in 1972 it just included monuments defined as "exceptional universal value from the point of view of history, art or science" [3]. In 2001 UNESCO changed the parameters determining the definition of cultural heritage, which now encompasses cultural goods associated with orality or the immaterial dimension leading to the creation of the lists of intangible cultural heritage [14].

The term intangible heritage refers to "all forms of traditional and popular or folk culture, i.e. collective works originating in the given community and based on tradition" [15]. Nowadays, it goes beyond the preservation of mastery and traditions and it also includes the preservation of living social networks. A new trend claims that now this definition needs to be extended once again to comprehend also the "digital heritage", which is intended as "the accumulation and curation of digital data online, which could form the basis of an inexhaustible resource containing the exact documentation of our digital past" [16]. This perspective enables us to consider living systems of online culture, such as digital social networks and online videogames, as part of our collective intangible heritage [17]. Listing videogames as intangible cultural heritage, as Reinhard pointed out in his paper [18], would be appropriate since also many traditional games are listed in the UNESCO list, for instance the Chogān, which is an Iranian horse-riding game accompanied by music and storytelling. Looking forward to the future, the definition of intangible cultural heritage will one day include digital copies of people.

3.2 Perspectives for Future Digital Curation of Intangible Cultural Heritage

Digital curation is important for the preservation of information in digital format and it should be a priority to digitize the already existing cultural heritage. Some projects are indeed focusing on the digitization of important artefacts, such as manuscripts or buildings, that can be converted into digital information. An outstanding example can be found in the Venice Time Machine, an international scientific program that aims at building a multidimensional model of Venice and its evolution covering a period of more than 1000 years [19]. Researchers and librarians working in this project are digitizing Venetian documents, including books, registries, maps, paintings et cetera. Their aim is to digitize maps and paintings to create a sort of Google Maps with 3D models of the ancient city of Venice, which can be also visualized with reference to a particular period of time in the past, working as a time machine. Moreover, indexing and parsing the content of documents such as birth registrations, death certificates and tax statements will allow reconstructing the social network and simulate how it evolved during the past centuries.

The great effort made for the digital curation of this type of cultural heritage is opportune for monuments, paintings, literature and even the reconstruction of social and economic relationships. However, it falls short when preserving the intangible expressions of human action, which, nonetheless, needs to be protected and preserved. A form of preservation of this kind of cultural heritage can be found in videos, however, this is a limited representation that does not allow for a comprehensive interaction between the user and the content, and it relies on a form of storytelling strictly linked to the view of the person filming and editing the movie. A valid alternative can be found in the adoption of a system such as the ones proposed by the companies mentioned in Sect. 2: a software capable of collecting all the information about a person and then build a model that can replicate that individual's skills, knowledge, behavior and, maybe, personhood. This can, at first, allow the creation of chatbots or social media agents that can interact with other people expressing the values and the identity that a particular performance or tradition can provoke in the original individual. This can, then, evolve in a more sophisticated agent: it would be possible to create 3D virtual models that can show to people in virtual reality the physical aspect of the person, replicate the movements, the sounds and the behavior. The current trend of immersive systems is to also include non-conventional senses in the interaction with digital content, so it is possible to predict that it will also be possible to simulate also touch, smell and taste. The possibilities, introduced by the interaction with such digital copies of people who are the holders of valuable knowledge with reference to a specific tradition or art or craftmanship, can enable the transmission of such intangible cultural heritage preserving also peculiar nuances that would be lost in other formats. This would make a difference similar to what it is possible to understand about an event reading its description, and actually being immerged and living that particular experience. The creation of such digital copies would make possible to improvise Fado music playing with musicians of the past, and that maybe even never met, creating new melodies and songs that were never written before, but which respect the style of this traditional genre. The 3D models can represent the musicians in the virtual space, the immersive audio system will provide the feeling of being surrounded by the music and the haptic feedback will reproduce the vibration created by the instruments and the voice. It would be possible to use robotic system that can allow transmitting the knowledge of these musicians directly guiding the movements of the user through electrical muscle stimulation [20]. Similar concepts can be applied to other examples of intangible cultural heritage: cooking a traditional Neapolitan pizza with Raffaele Esposito (who is considered the inventor of Pizza Margherita) or performing in a Kabuki show (the Japanese traditional theatre form) with actors from the Edo period while other users are attending the spectacle. Possibly, in a few years, also digital artifacts and experiences will be included in the UNESCO lists of intangible cultural heritage and playing or attending a match of StarCraft (an American videogame considered a sport in South Korea [21]) will be valued being a tradition deserving to be safeguarded and transmitted to future generations.

The most important element for the design of such systems generating a digital copy of the holders of this knowledge is providing the possibility to create a narrative with new layers of meaning into the construction of heritage both at the personal and broader cultural level avoiding the homogenization of storytelling and values, as it is happening in the current social media. Designing these systems should encourage the users to critique or to evaluate the significance of digital information because "if people do not begin to set up structures for the future of their data after death, we could be in danger of losing any understandable personal narrative in favor of the vast collection" [17].

4 Conclusion

In this paper, the current trend of digitalization of our society has been analyzed with focus on the promise of a near future where it will be possible generating digital copies of human beings, achieving the so-called digital immortality. This phenomenon can play a crucial role in the preservation of cultural heritage. In particular, it is possible to predict that intangible cultural heritage will benefit from the future development of these digital copies of human beings: first, they will be able to interact with future generations transmitting their knowledge and values beyond the death of their original individuals; second, they will enable the production of personal narratives avoiding the homogenization of language and values in favor of the promotion of cultural identity.

References

1. Kunii, T.L.: The potentials of cyberworlds-an axiomatic approach. In: 2004 International Conference on Cyberworlds, pp. 2–7. IEEE, November 2004
2. Kuny, T.: The digital dark ages? Challenges in the preservation of electronic information. Int. Preserv. News **17**, 8–13 (1998)
3. Vecco, M.: A definition of cultural heritage: from the tangible to the intangible. J. Cult. Heritage **11**(3), 321–324 (2010)
4. Caon, M.: Towards cross-generational system design. In: International Conference on Human-Computer Interaction, pp. 258–267. Springer, Cham, July 2018
5. Bell, G., Gray, J.: Digital immortality (2000). https://www.microsoft.com/en-us/research/publication/digital-immortality. Accessed 18 May 2019
6. Caon, M.: Designing systems in the digital immortality era. In: Proceedings of the 19th International ACM SIGACCESS Conference on Computers and Accessibility, pp. 237–241. ACM, May 2018
7. Sandberg, A.: Feasibility of whole brain emulation. In: Philosophy and Theory of Artificial Intelligence, pp. 251–264. Springer, Heidelberg (2013)
8. Sandberg, A., Bostrom, N.: Whole brain emulation (2008). https://www.fhi.ox.ac.uk/brain-emulation-roadmap-report.pdf. Accessed 18 May 2019
9. Ma, J., Huang, R.: Digital explosions and digital clones. In: 2015 IEEE 12th Intl Conf on Ubiquitous Intelligence and Computing, pp. 1133–1138. IEEE, August 2015
10. Steinhart, E.: Survival as a digital ghost. Minds Mach. **17**(3), 261–271 (2007)
11. Bassett, D.: Who wants to live forever? Living, dying and grieving in our digital society. Soc. Sci. **4**(4), 1127–1139 (2015)
12. Meese, J., Nansen, B., Kohn, T., Arnold, M., Gibbs, M.: Posthumous personhood and the affordances of digital media. Mortality **20**(4), 408–420 (2015)
13. Leaver, T.: Posthumous performance and digital resurrection: from science fiction to startups. In: Kohn, T., Gibbs, M., Nansen, B., van Ryn, L. (eds.) Residues of Death: Disposal Refigured. Routledge, London and New York (2019)
14. UNESCO Intangible Cultural Heritage Lists. https://ich.unesco.org/en/lists. Accessed 18 May 2019
15. Kirshenblatt-Gimblett, B.: Intangible heritage as metacultural production. Museum Int. **56**(1–2), 52–65 (2004)
16. Pitsillides, S., Waller, M., Fairfax, D.: Digital death. In: Digital Identity and Social Media, pp. 75–90. IGI Global (2013)

17. Pitsillides, S., Jeffries, J., Conreen, M.: Museum of the self and digital death. Heritage and social media, pp. 56–68 (2012)
18. Reinhard, A.: Video Games as Archaeological Sites. The Interactive Past: Archaeology, Heritage, and Video Games, pp. 99–106 (2017)
19. Kaplan, F.: The venice time machine. In: Proceedings of the 2015 ACM Symposium on Document Engineering, p. 73. ACM, September 2015
20. Ebisu, A., Hashizume, S., Suzuki, K., Ishii, A., Sakashita, M., Ochiai, Y.: Stimulated percussions. In: Proceedings of the 8th Augmented Human International Conference, p. 33. ACM, March 2017
21. Ok, H.: New media practices in Korea. Int. J. Commun. **5**, 29 (2011)

Let Users Control Their Data – Privacy Policy-Based User Interface Design

Armin Gerl(✉), Bianca Meier, and Stefan Becher

University of Passau, DIMIS, Innstr. 42, 94032 Passau, Germany
{Armin.Gerl,Bianca.Meier,Stefan.Becher}@uni-passau.de

Abstract. Not only are common privacy policies hard to read and understand, but users are usually not experiencing any noticeable reactions of the application to their personal choices, if any are given. The Layered Privacy Language (LPL) is used to present legal privacy policies to the user in a concise way allowing the user fine-grained personalization options. Our contribution consists of the definition and detailing of possible personalization interaction scenarii in the context of web-applications and their validation within our evaluation environment. To simulate a negotiation of a privacy policy, a scenario environment is proposed, simulating several personal privacy preferences and users. Users can hereby perform different privacy policy personalization actions.

Keywords: Consent management · GDPR · Layered Privacy Language · Negotiation · Personal privacy policy

1 Introduction

In the age of digitalization, more and more data is generated, stored, and processed. For example, Google converts 24 petabytes per day, which corresponds to 24 million gigabytes. In order to imagine this figure, Mainzer et al. compares the content with the US Library of Congress, whose data content is generated 6000 times a day by Google [1]. In order to restrict this data collection and strengthen the rights of the data sources, i.e. the users who use these services, the General Data Protection Regulation (GDPR) was introduced on 25th May 2018. The GDPR enforces a data protection declaration that informs about the collection and processing of data. Bitkom Research has conducted a study on 'Privacy in the digital world', which state the users' experience with privacy policies. 90% of the interviewees stated that privacy policies are difficult to read and understand. Another majority, around 80%, state that privacy policies are too long or that they simply agree to the guidelines without really understanding them. Thus the question arises, how the presentation and interaction with privacy policies can be improved. Although GDPR intends to strengthen users' privacy, current implementations of privacy policies seem not to be sufficient to allow truly free and informed consent. To solve these problems the privacy policies must be changed in a way, that (1) they are easier to comprehend, while all required information is still available, and (2) the interaction for giving consent is clearer to allow individual decisions. These aspects are the goal of the machine-readable Layered Privacy Language (LPL), introduced by Gerl et al. [2]. LPL intends to present legal privacy policies to the user in

T. Ahram et al. (Eds.): IHIET 2019, AISC 1018, pp. 790–795, 2020.
https://doi.org/10.1007/978-3-030-25629-6_123

a concise way allowing the user fine-grained personalization options (e.g. consent to purposes). The main contribution of this work is the introduction of user interaction schemes for fine-grained consent management based upon LPL as well as a user interface prototype incorporating such functionality. The remaining of the paper is structured as follows. Section 2 reviews related work. Relevant elements and concepts of LPL are recited in Sect. 3. Section 4 details personalization interaction scenarii for which a prototype implementation is introduced in Sect. 5. Lastly, Sect. 6 concludes and gives an outlook for future work.

2 Related Work

Since privacy languages came up with their most popular representative P3P many solutions for policy visualization and consent simplification were proposed. The Privacy Bird tool [3] takes user preferences as input of a user-interface. In addition to predefined configurations the user can consent or dissent to any given purpose. Then the tool compares P3P policies against this preferences and warns the user, if a mismatch happens giving the user either the possibility to leave the page or continue the process while neglecting the own privacy preferences.

As part of the PrimeLife project [4] an UI was invented that introduces privacy preference changes semi-automatically 'on-the-fly'. When personal data is requested a 'send data' dialog prompts and the user gets information about the privacy policy and can change his preferences as well. Also an abortion of the transaction is possible. Still negotiation of the policies' content is not possible. When a violation of the pre-defined preferences happens the user can either cancel or to allow the mismatch.

A GDPR compliant privacy dashboard was developed for the EU Special project [5]. It offers a time line of given consent for each data item and informs about the privacy policy and third parties. Also there is a graphical representation of data flows to third party processors. Lastly, consent can be withdrawn for any accepted purpose at any time. Therefore, consent to single purposes instead of the whole policy is enabled. This work extends this consent management for even more personalization.

3 Layered Privacy Language (LPL)

LPL and its overarching framework are intended to model privacy policies in both a machine- and human-readable way to enable both free and informed consent as well as an accountable enforcement of privacy policies [2]. Therefore, LPL (see Fig. 1) models a privacy policy as a set of Purpose-elements each denoting the processing of data (set of Data-elements) by specific entities (set of DataRecipient-elements). Furthermore, LPL elements are provided with human-readable headers and descriptions, allowing for a structured presentation of the privacy policy [6].

Each of the Purpose-, Data-, and DataRecipient-elements has the attribute 'required' denoting if the element is required, e.g. due to legal reasons, or is optional and has to be interacted with to be consented to. Based on the structure of LPL, a user would first consent to a purpose and then for data and data recipients. If a purpose is

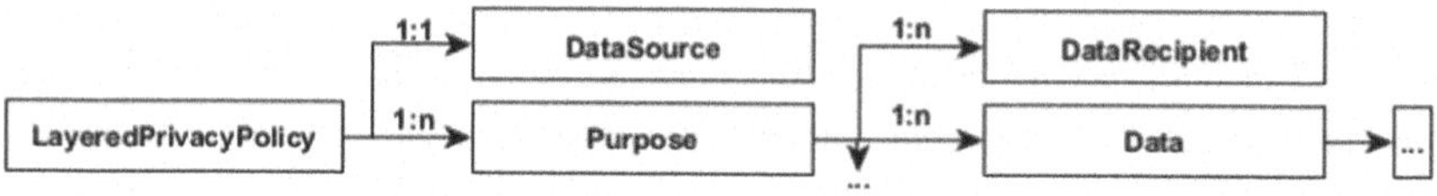

Fig. 1. Structure of core elements of LPL, which are relevant for consent.

consented to, the Purpose-element stores the date and time information in the 'pointOfAcceptance' attribute for compliance. The life-cycle of LPL considers the following scenario. During the Creation step the privacy policy is created by the Data Protection Officer (DPO) and configured within the respective application. Next the privacy policy will be presented to a user, e.g. during the registration process, during which the user can personalize the privacy policy, eventually deciding to consent (or not) to the personalized privacy policy. A policy can only be consented to if all required elements are accepted. After the policy is consented it will be pre-processed and stored alongside the users' data (Sticky Policy concept). The data and policy may be transferred. The personal data can only be processed if the processor is authenticated and authorized [7] and may be de-identified [2, 8].

4 Personalization Interaction Scenario

The previously denoted Negotiation step of LPL is the main focus of this work. During this step the user will get the privacy policy presented by a user interface which is intended to inform the user about the processing of its personal data. The user shall hereby have the free choice on how its personal data is processed and thus personalize the privacy policy.

Usually users only have limited possibilities, often only consent or dissent, regarding the personalization of the usage of their personal data. But with LPL privacy policies more possibilities become available, namely through the Purpose-, Data-, and DataRecipient-elements. Besides the enhanced personalization possibilities, the approach of using a machine- and human-readable privacy language has additional advantages. It allows a structured and unified presentation of the privacy policy, systematic integration approach of privacy in (web-) applications, and actual personalization of the functionality of the application based upon the individuals' decisions.

4.1 Purpose Consent (PC)

The first possible personalization of a privacy policy is to give consent to a specific purpose, which by itself describes in general the processing of the data. We denote Purpose Consent (PC) as opt-in consent for non-required purposes for the application. Opt-in hereby describes that the purpose has to be actively selected and therefore is not pre-selected. Due to the binary 'required' attribute of LPL a purpose is either a mandatory part of the privacy policy, which cannot be dissented to, or the purpose is optional and has to be actively be consented to. For example the purpose 'newsletter', which sends a newsletter to the user, may be non-required. Thus the user can decide to give consent to it. If a purpose is consented to then the attribute 'pointOfAcceptance' will be filled with the current data and time. Not only the consent, but also the dissent to already agreed upon purposes has to be considered, which has to be as easy as the consent to a purpose [9]. A purpose, which is not consented to, will be omitted from the LPL privacy policy and can be added again based upon the original privacy policy provided by the DPO.

4.2 Data Dissent (DD)

Data Dissent (DD) is also one of the actions that can be performed by the data source and denotes an opt-out dissent for optional data in the context of a purpose. For example there is a purpose 'newsletter' for which the required data 'e-mail' and the non-required 'name' exists. The individual can therefore decide to allow the usage of its name for the newsletter, e.g. for personalization of the text. Thus, the fine-grained consent management of data for purposes allows optional functionality for the user. But also the service provider (Controller) may have advantages providing personalization of the services. We assume that users may use service more if they can decide on which personal data is used. Minimal data requirements may be sufficient for basic services but more data may be needed for more advanced services.

4.3 Data Recipient Dissent (DRD)

Similar to PC and DD, the user has one more possibility for personalization with the Data Recipient Dissent (DRD). DRD denotes an opt-out dissent for optional data recipients in the context of a purpose. Therefore, the user can decide which entities may receive its personal data. For example the purpose 'newsletter' defines two data recipients which the user would be registered to. First 'service-newsletter' denoting a newsletter of the service itself, secondly 'third-party-newsletter' denoting a newsletter of cooperating services requiring a transfer of the personal data to other controllers. Both data recipients are not required and therefore the user may choose to only allow a newsletter of the service, but no third party newsletter subscriptions. Therefore, the user has fine-grained control over the processing or transfer of its data by Controllers.

5 Evaluation Environment

To demonstrate and verify the proposed interaction scenarii we propose an evaluation environment for personalized privacy policies. It consists of a database storing both personal data as well as LPL privacy policies. To simulate personal data we used the ADULT data set, from which we use the attributes 'age', 'education', 'marital-status', 'native-country', 'occupation', 'race', 'salary-class', 'sex', and 'workclass'. The frontend consists of login, personal data management, and privacy policy negotiation.

The login site allows a user to authenticate for the web-application with an username and password. The personal data management site allows the user to enter, read, and update its personal data. This view furthermore reacts to the personal privacy preferences of the users, such that it only shows data fields that will eventually be processed according to the privacy policy, thus simulating the restriction of the web-applications' functionality. Finally, the privacy policy negotiation section allows the user to inspect and alter its privacy preferences according to the three introduced interaction scenarii (see Fig. 2).

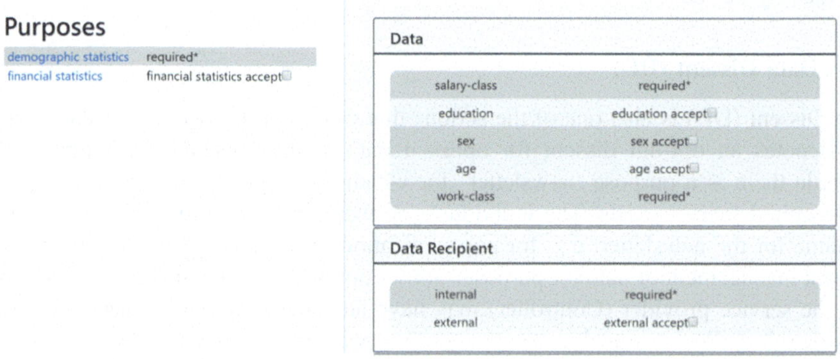

Fig. 2. Negotiation prototype user interface for Purpose Consent (PC), Data Dissent (DD) and Data Recipient Dissent (DRD).

Assuming a scenario in which demographic data is captured via a web-application with the required purpose 'demographic statistics' and the non-required purpose 'financial statistics'. For the required purpose 'demographic statistics' various personal data is collected, but the application offers an additional service to compare ones income to other participants, which requires additional personal information, i.e. 'work-class' and 'salary-class', and optional data for better comparisons, i.e. 'education', 'sex' and 'age'. Furthermore, the functionality allows a comparison to other registered users with the required data recipient 'internal' or with an optional external service provider 'external'. Both 'work-class' and 'salary-class' are unique to the 'financial statistics' purpose. Therefore, the data management site only renders corresponding input fields if the purpose is consented to (see Fig. 3). Thus, the processing (including storage) of data is directly influenced by the users privacy preferences.

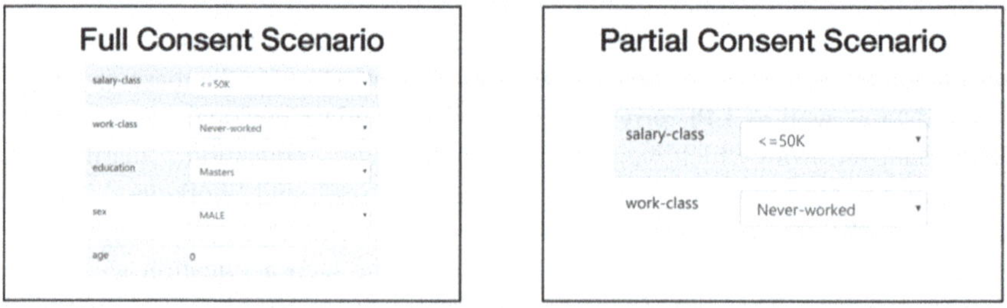

Fig. 3. User Interface adaption to the privacy preferences of the user. The full consent scenario shows all data elements, while the partial consent scenario only shows data elements consented to.

6 Conclusion and Future Works

We introduced a systematic approach on consent management utilizing the machine- and human-readable Layered Privacy Language (LPL). Hereby, LPL serves as the base for personalization of privacy policies by users allowing Purpose Consent (PC), Data Dissent (DD) and Data Recipient Dissent (DRD). Thus, fine-grained consent management is enabled, allowing the user control over the processing of its personal data. Furthermore, we provided a prototype implementation of the consent management user interface based upon LPL.

Investigation of user experiences with the interface will be subject of future research for optimization. Furthermore, the validation of this approach according to real life scenarios and privacy policies is intended. Lastly, variations of the user interface for interaction with children, elderly people or people with disabilities have to be considered in future works.

References

1. Mainzer K.: Big data und die macht der algorithmen. In: Schröder M., Schwanebeck A. (Hrsg.) Big Data - In den Fängen der Datenkraken, pp. 49–70 Die (un-)heimliche Macht der Algorithmen, 1st edn. (2017). ISBN print: 978-3-8487-4147-2
2. Gerl, A., Bennani, N., Kosch, H., Brunie, L.: LPL, towards a GDPR-compliant privacy language: formal definition and usage. In: Springer, Heidelberg, pp. 41–80 (2018)
3. Cranor, L.F., Arjula, M., Guduru, P.: Use of a p 3p user agent by earlyadopters. In: 2002 ACM Workshop on Privacy in the Electronic Society, WPES 2002, pp. 1–10. ACM, New York (2002)
4. Angulo, J., Fischer-Hübner, S., Pulls, T., König, U.: HCI for policy display and administration. In: Springer, Heidelberg, pp. 261–277 (2011)
5. Raschke, P., Küpper, A., Drozd, O., Kirrane, S.: Designing a GDPR compliant and usable privacy dashboard. In: IFIP Advances in Information and Communication Technology (IFIPAICT 2018), Springer. IFIP Summer School 2017, Ispra, Italy, 3–8 September 2017
6. Gerl, A., Prey, F.: LPL Personal privacy policy user interface: design and evaluation. In: Dachselt, R., Weber, G. (Hrsg.) Mensch und Computer 2018 - Workshopband. Bonn: Gesellschaft für Informatik e.V. (2018)
7. Wilhelm, S., Gerl, A.. Policy-based authentication and authorization based on the layered privacy language. In: Meyer, H., et al. (Hrsg.) Datenbanksysteme für Business Technologie und Web (BTW2019) - Workshopband, pp. 245–255. GI, Rostock (2019)
8. Gerl, A., Bölz, F.: Layered Privacy Language (LPL) pseudonymization extension for health care. In: MEDINFO 2019: The 17th World Congress on Medical and Health Informatics Health and Wellbeing E-Networks for All, IMIA MedInfo Proceedings (2019)
9. Council of the European Union: General data protection regulation. Regulation (EU) 2016 of the European Parliament and of the Council of on the protection of natural persons with regard to the processing of personal data and on the free movement of such data, and repealing Directive 95/46/EC, April 2016

BIG IoT - Interconnecting IoT Platforms from Different Domains - Final Results

Thomas Jell[1(✉)], Claudia Baumgartner[2], Arne Bröring[1], and Jelena Mitic[1]

[1] Siemens AG, Munich, Germany
Thomas.jell@siemens.com
[2] VMZ Berlin, Berlin, Germany

Abstract. The Internet of Things (IoT) is today separated by different vertically oriented platforms for integration of all the different devices. Developers who aim to access other platforms and access that data are forced to manually adapt their interfaces to the specific platform API and data models. This paper highlights the work of the BIG IoT project that aims at launching an IoT marketplace and ecosystem as part of the European Platform Initiative (IoT EPI). The project finished end of 2018, so I will be able to present the setup of and the final results of the integration of the use cases that have been implemented in Northern Germany, Italy and Barcelona. Please refer to www.big-iot.eu for further details.

Keywords: BigIoT · Internet of Things · Interconnecting IoT platforms

1 Introduction - The Problem of Missing IoT Interoperability

The idea of the IoT is in widespread use since the last years, collecting sensor data from various application domains. However, so far, these IoT platforms do not form a vibrant ecosystem. There have been lots of research and innovation projects in the context of the IoT. Nonetheless, no broadly used professional ecosystems for the IoT exist today.

One reason for this is the large number of stakeholders who are involved in IoT ecosystems. Among these are providers of platforms and things, as well as application developers, and end users. Another reason for this issue are the high entry barriers for developers of services and applications. This is cased by the heterogeneity of all known IoT platforms. Developers who want to access things and additional data from different platforms need to manually access them by implementing specific adapters. Also, incentives are missing for platform providers to open their systems to third parties.

These different issues all relate to one particular challenge: the missing interoperability on the IoT. Today, various protocols and standards are available on the IoT [2]. This heterogeneity ranges from basic communication protocols such as CoAP [3] and MQTT [4], to focused standard families, such as oneM2 M [5] or OGC SWE [6].

T. Ahram et al. (Eds.): IHIET 2019, AISC 1018, pp. 796–801, 2020.
https://doi.org/10.1007/978-3-030-25629-6_124

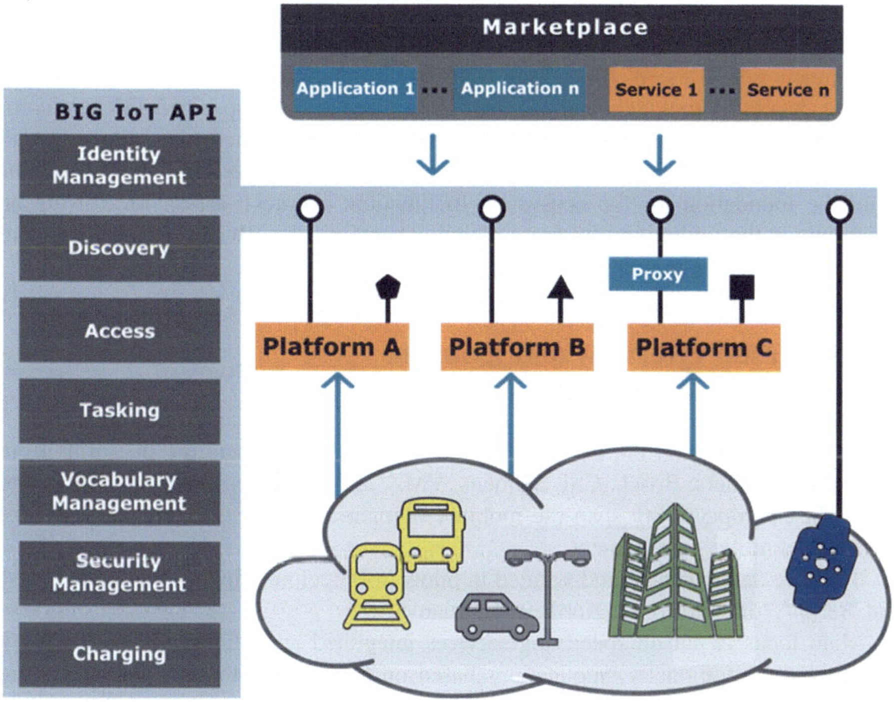

Fig. 1. Overview of the BIG IoT approach (Icons made by Freepik from www.flaticon.com). (Source: [1])

2 The BIG IoT Approach

Bridging the Interoperability Gap of the IoT (BIG IoT) [6] is the project that aims at enabling the access of services and applications from multiple IoT platforms, standards and domains towards building IoT ecosystems.

Previous EC-funded projects that address such enablement of IoT ecosystems are, e.g., IoT-A [http://www.iot-a.eu], by providing a common architecture, FIWARE [http://www.fiware.org] that offers Generic Enablers as building blocks, or projects such as compose [http://www.compose-project.eu] and OpenIoT [http://openiot.eu], which offer dedicated IoT platforms to aggregate other platforms and systems. BIG IoT will not develop yet another platform in order to enable cross-platform IoT applications.

Instead, to reach the above outlined goal, BIG IoT builds up on 3 key pillars for an interoperable IoT ecosystem: (1) a common BIG IoT API, (2) well-defined information models, and (3) a marketplace to monetize access to resources. This approach is illustrated in Fig. 1. Of central importance is the BIG IoT API, which includes functionalities such as ID management and discovery of things, access to things on platforms, tasking of things to send commands, as well as vocabulary management for handling semantics and security management. In order to interact with the marketplace, the API implemented by IoT platforms supports charging for access to things. The generic BIG IoT API as well as the underlying information models have been defined in conjunction with the Web of Things Interest Group at the W3C for standardization.

The details of this technical baseline have already been specified [8] in a comprehensive architectural design. Thereby, particular importance has been given to specific security and privacy requirements [7]. While these technical considerations build the foundation for the ecosystem to function, a crucial aspect to growing an ecosystem is the underlying business model. Therefore, the BIG IoT project has analyzed various business cases and value networks [9].

3 Use Cases: Overview and Example

The BIG IoT project has developed a first prototype of an IoT ecosystem with overall 8 IoT platforms using all the common BIG IoT API. Among them are platforms from most of the partners: Bosch, CSI, Siemens, VMZ, and WorldSensing. The use cases to verify the interoperability span the mobility domain and include smart parking, bike sharing and traffic management.

They are demonstrated and verified in pilots in Barcelona (Spain), Piedmont (Italy) and Berlin/Wolfsburg (NG, Northern-Germany).

Main focus is put on specifying services integrated and offered via the BIG IoT Marketplace. Additionally, applications based on the services that are showcased are specified. The work is executed for all three pilots, taking into account the specific characteristics of the infrastructure as well as pilot-specific requirements.

The Northern Germany Pilot focuses in Berlin on the already installed network of parking sensors (Siemens) in dedicated areas as well as a variety of sensors throughout the city (VMZ).

Additional a semi public parking area at VMZ's premises will be equipped with radar sensors to detect parking vehicles. Provided services and apps will be:

- smart parking,
- smart charging,
- public transport optimization,
- multimodal route optimization,
- parking and charging info and
- reservation of parking spots.

The smart objects are charging stations, parking detectors and Wi-Fi probes as well as location sensors on buses, which deliver their data to availability services for further provision to the BIG IoT ecosystem. The data from those smart objects provided by the availability services are used by other services or by the end user applications directly. The services are:

- Parking spot availability,
- Parking spot WMS,
- Parking reservation,
- People density estimation on bus,

- People density estimation in area,
- Live bus location,
- Charging station availability and
- Charging station WMS.

The services support the different applications with offerings in terms of raw and aggregated data and functionalities.

We will present the first success story showing the integration of parking data from different sources (Berlin, Munich, Barcelona, …) via the already existing Marketplace into integrated end user applications.

4 Northern Germany Pilot

This BIG IoT Pilot makes use of innovative solutions already in place in the mobility innovation labs Berlin and Wolfsburg, the Northern Germany headquarter of automotive industry. The pilot shows how BIG IoT can contribute to mobility innovation in metropolitan areas, middle-sized towns and the connected commuter traffic, addressing the future needs of urban and rural mobility. The pilots' main target is to enable solutions for efficient parking, optimized public transport, better usage of e-mobility infrastructure and multimodal mobility information to support an efficient and sustainable mobility and a better environment. This is done by providing services and apps for:

Smart Parking: Making use of on street Siemens parking radar sensors in Berlin and parking detectors in public car parks in Wolfsburg. BIG IoT provides a Smart Parking App to inform car drivers on location and availability of parking spots. Thus, car drivers find the closest parking spots and parking search traffic - a major cause for urban traffic stress - is reduced. The sensor data are provided by BIG IoT-enabled platforms such as Siemens APM (Advanced Parking Management) platform and BOSCH Bezirk platform. In addition to parking availability, reservation of parking spots will be provided as a service. Being BIG-IoTized enables Siemens Smart Parking App to consume any BIG IoT parking offerings, helps to extend the geographical coverage of parking information and increases business opportunities for service providers. Step one on the way to a European solution has already been done with the integration of WorldSensing parking data of our co-pilot Barcelona – enabled by: BIG IoT.

Public Transport Optimization: Based on wifi-sensors on connected buses Wolfsburg public transport operators get better information on bus occupancy and people waiting at bus stations. Wifi-sensor data is integrated in BIG IoT enabled BOSCH Smart City Platform. This helps to optimize vehicle usage and bus line planning to get more customer demand oriented public transport services.

E-Mobility: Where can I find the next free charging station to charge my e-car, e-scooter, e-van? By providing this crucial information to e-mobility users BIG IoT contributes to the success of e-mobility. E-Mobility in Berlin picked up speed in 2012 with first charging stations on public ground and has been continuously extended to presently more than 350 charging points. Location and status of more than 350 charging stations in Berlin are currently provided via BIG IoT enabled VMZ multimodal mobility platform. With higher numbers of e-vehicles the need to reserve a charging station will increase in the future. Thus BIG IoT reservation service for charging stations is an appreciated Open Call contribution.

Multimodal Commuter App: This App consumes sensor and mobility data coming from various BIG IoT enabled platforms to inform Commuters on the route between Berlin and Wolfsburg. The App provides car and public transport routing functionalities and guides car drivers to available parking spots and charging stations, includes BIG IoT offerings for real time traffic information such as traffic detectors data, incidents and traffic messages for car and public transport. Incorporating diverse data offerings of the BIG IoT Marketplace offering collection the App bridges the interoperability gap of various platforms to provide a multi-modal real-time based information system for mobility end users.

5 Results and Conclusions

BIG IoT provides the common base for enabling different IoT platforms to access their sensors, data and services by a common BIG IoT API and the marketplace behind to orchestrate exchange. The major results achieved have been:

- Subscribe to marketplace is a couple of lines of code, only.
- Connect to data source is a couple of lines of code, as well.
- Effort for integration (as an independent docker container) of data has been reduced from days to minutes.
- More and more Data Sources and Services Providers joined and join allowing to choose in a rich marketplace.
- Marketplace and all other source code is made available open source through an eclipse license.

Acknowledgments. This work is supported by the BIG IoT project that has received funding from the European Commission's Horizon 2020 research and innovation program under grant agreement No 688038. This article presents the current status of work in the project. We thank the consortium partners for their feedback and fruitful discussions. The work will be further evolved as part of the ongoing architecture development in the project.

References

1. Kubler, S., Främling, K., Zaslavsky, A., Doukas, C., Olivares, E., Fortino, G., Palau, C.E., Soursos, S., Podnar Zarko, I., Fang, Y., Krco, S., Heinz, C., Grimm, C., Bröring, A., Mitic, J., Olstedt, K., Vermesan, O.: IoT platforms initiative. In: Vermesan, O., Friess, P. (eds.) Digitising the Industry - Internet of Things Connecting the Physical, Digital and Virtual World, Chapter 9, pp. 265–292. River Publishers (2016). ISBN: 978-87-93379-82-4
2. Bröring, A., Datta, S.K., Bonnet, C.: A categorization of discovery technologies for the Internet of Things. In: 6th International Conference on the Internet of Things (IoT 2016), 7.-9. November 2016, Stuttgart, Germany. ACM (2016). ISBN: 978-1-4503-4814-0. http://dl.acm.org/citation.cfm?doid=2991561.2991570

3. Bormann, C., Castellani, A.P., Shelby, Z.: CoAP: an application protocol for billions of tiny internet nodes. IEEE Internet Comput. **16**(2), 62–67 (2012)
4. IBM and Eurotech: MQTT V3.1 Protocol Specification. http://public.dhe.ibm.com/software/dw/webservices/ws-mqtt/mqtt-v3r1.html. Accessed 24 Apr 2014
5. Swetina, J., Lu, G., Jacobs, P., Ennesser, F., Song, J.: Toward a standardized common M2M service layer platform: introduction to oneM2M. Wirel. Commun. IEEE **21**(3), 20–26 (2014)
6. Bröring, A., Echterhoff, J., Jirka, S., Simonis, I., Everding, T., Stasch, C., Liang, S., Lemmens, R.: New generation sensor web enablement. Sensors **11**(3), 2652–2699 (2011)
7. Hernandez-Serrano, J., Munoz, J.L., Bröring, A., Esparza, O., Mikkelsen, L., Schwarzott, W., Leon, O.: On the road to secure and privacy-preserving IoT Ecosystems. In: Podnar Žarko, I., Broering, A., Soursos, S., Serrano, M. (eds.) 2nd International Workshop on Interoperability & Open Source Solutions for the Internet of Things (InterOSS-IoT 2016) at 6th International Conference on the Internet of Things (IoT 2016), LNCS, pp. 107–122, vol. 10218. Springer, Cham (2017)
8. Schmid, S., Bröring, A., Kramer, D., Kaebisch, S., Zappa, A., Lorenz, M., Wang, Y., Gioppo, L.: An architecture for interoperable IoT ecosystems. In: Podnar Žarko, I., Broering, A., Soursos, S., Serrano, M. (eds.) 2nd International Workshop on Interoperability & Open Source Solutions for the Internet of Things (InterOSS-IoT 2016) at 6th International Conference on the Internet of Things (IoT 2016), LNCS, vol. 10218, pp. 39–55. Springer, Cham (2017)
9. Schladofsky, W., Mitic, J., Metzger, A.P., Simonato, C., Gioppo, L., Leonardos, D., Bröring, A.: An architecture for interoperable IoT ecosystems. In: 2nd International Workshop on Interoperability & Open Source Solutions for the Internet of Things (InterOSS-IoT 2016) at 6th International Conference on the Internet of Things (IoT 2016), LNCS, 7. November 2016, Springer, Stuttgart (2017, forthcoming)
10. Jell, T., Bröring, A., Mitic, J.: BIG IoT – interconnecting IoT platforms from different domains - first success story. In: IEEE, Proceedings of the ITNG (2017)
11. Jell, T., Bröring, A., Mitic, J.: IG IoT – interconnecting IoT platforms from different domains - first success story. In: IEEE, Proceedings of the ICE (2017)
12. Jell, T., Baumgartner, C., Bröring, A., Mitic, J.: BIG IoT – interconnecting IoT platforms from different domains – use case Northern Germany. In: IEEE, Proceedings of the ITNG (2018)

Islamic Interbank Benchmark Rate

Issam Tlemsani(✉)

College of Business Administration,
Prince Mohammad Bin Fahd University, Al Khobar, Saudi Arabia
itlemsani@pmu.edu.sa

Abstract. The aim of this study is to evaluate the Islamic Interbank Benchmark Rate (IIBR) and investigate its relationship to conventional benchmark rates. The methodology in this study relies extensively on multivariate regression, using data culled for IIBR, conventional interest-dependent benchmark rates and oil prices. The study contributes to the understanding of the IIBR's framework principles and its value as a solution to current and future Sharia complaint short term interbank market funding for the Islamic finance industry.

Keywords: Islamic finance · Interbank Benchmark Rate · LIBOR

1 Introduction

The purpose of this study is to evaluate the Islamic Interbank Benchmark Rate (IIBR)'s as a basis for the cost of borrowing between Islamic banks and contrast the sensitivity of IIBR to London Interbank Offered Rate (LIBOR), U.S. Effective federal Funds rate (EFFR), Kuala Lumpur Interbank Offered Rate (KLIBOR), oil prices and conventional interbank rates in the GCC countries. The IIBR indicates average expected return on Sharia compliant short term interbank funding. We aim to demonstrate whether the IIBR is distinct from conventional benchmark rates, and as such whether it can hold its own Islamic identity as an independent finance instrument that is not merely reversely engineered from conventional instruments.

IIBR was introduced by Thomson Reuters on 22nd Nov, 2011 and it is monitored daily. Our data has been provided by Thomson Reuters directly. Seventeen Islamic banks (or fully segregated Islamic banking windows) contribute to the IIBR. When referring to the rate here it is the average expected return on Sharia complaint short term interbank market funding for the Islamic finance industry [1]. This is calculated by removing the highest and the lowest four rates from the 17 Islamic banks. The arithmetic mean (average) is taken to calculate the IIBR. The IIBR is based on conventional cost of debt calculation. Critics could argue that the IIBR is not any different, in terms of methodology and structure from other conventional benchmark rates such as the LIBOR. he IIBR uses the US dollar to have uniformity across contributors as four of the six countries peg their local currencies to the US dollar.

This paper is structured as follows: Sect. 1 is a background to the subject and provides the purpose of this study, why investigating the IIBR is important and its implications. Section 2 provides an overview of the Islamic finance literature. Section 3 outlines the methodology in this study which relies extensively on multivariate

T. Ahram et al. (Eds.): IHIET 2019, AISC 1018, pp. 802–806, 2020.
https://doi.org/10.1007/978-3-030-25629-6_125

regression analysis, using data culled for IIBR, traditional interest-dependent benchmark rates and oil prices which were collected daily over a period spanning from Nov 2011 to June 2015. Section 4 describes analyses and compares the features of the IIBR as a legitimate alternative for Islamic banks looking to operate in accordance with Sharia law. Section 5 presents the result and critically evaluates the findings and the prospects for the findings of this study. Section 6 contains the conclusions.

2 Literature Review

Since Islamic finance has evolved into being part of the mainstream financial service landscape, there is a need to develop an Islamic financial benchmark rate (IIBR) that is Sharia complaint and decoupled from the existing conventional benchmark rates, such as LIBOR [2]. However, current Islamic capital markets literature propose strong correlations between movements of Islamic and conventional financial indices [3–7]. This study contributes to this existing literature.

Iqbal [8] discussed why two different benchmarks are needed when compared to a conventional debt based system where capital is rewarded on the basis of a rate fixed ex-ante, as the Islamic financial system rewards capital on the basis of ex-post return on capital. The Islamic financial system requires all financial products be free from any fixed and predetermined interest rate, instead the system allows and promotes business, equity participation and direct sharing of risk and rewards. By prohibiting interest rates it does not necessarily restrict lawful business nor profits and thus its prohibitions do not imply that the opportunity cost of capital is zero. Iqbal claimed that in an Islamic finance framework the incentive to invest depends on the prospective profitability, where the investor continues to invest until the marginal productivity of capital becomes equal to the marginal cost of capital.

Sukmana and Ibrahim [9] found strong evidence supporting nonlinear reactions of the Islamic investment rates to conventional rates. Their work suggests that Islamic bank rates and pricing do not follow their counterpart conventional rates and have different speed of moving upwards and downwards, which can be considered as an advantage for a consumer based on the consumer reaction hypothesis that is in line with Sharia principles. They thus imply that referring to Islamic banks as interest-based is unfounded.

Azad, Azmat, Chazi, and Ahsan [10] investigated the relationship between IIBR and its conventional counterpart the LIBOR. They concluded that the IIBR and LIBOR are positively correlated in the long and short term. They maintain that the IIBR is not decoupled from LIBOR because they operate in a global financial market where the risk return on Islamic and conventional products are similar and thus Islamic and conventional rates must converge due to arbitrage principles. In our study we have similarly focused on the degree of disjoint between the IIBR and LIBOR, however, we have also considered in our investigation the EFFR, KLIBOR, oil prices and conventional interbank rates in GCC countries. As such, this study provides a more comprehensive evaluation on the IIBR as a benchmark rate.

3 Research Methodology

This study relies on data analysis we extrapolate from trends observed during the period of data collection in order to make educated guesses about the relationship between the observed variables, IIBR and conventional rates, like LIBOR, in the near and long term future. Through regression analysis we are able to analyze how the metrics move in relation to each other during the snapshot in time presented in our data set. The implications of even observing these relationships is that they provide insight on how these variables interacted during our time of record and how they will interact in the future.

Regression analysis is used in our study, the dependent variable is the measure of the IIBR, while the explanatory variables are the conventional benchmark rates. Multiple regression analysis was used to test the sensitivity of the IIBR against oil prices and conventional benchmark interest rates. The same procedure was used to test IIBR's changes relative to fluctuations in the EFFR in order to find the extent to which changes in the EFFR rate resulted in changes in the IIBR.

The implicit hypothesis of this study is that similar changes in conventional benchmark rates have a smaller relative impact on mixed rates, like the KLIBOR, and an even smaller impact on the profit sharing paradigm represented by the IIBR.

4 Results

4.1 Regressions Analysis

Regression Analysis, is a powerful statistical method that allows examination of the relationship between two or more variables of interest. This is useful here to examine if there is an influence of LIBOR and other conventional benchmark rates on IIBR, the dependent variable is the measure of the IIBR, while the explanatory variables are the conventional benchmark rates. Multiple regression analysis was used to test the sensitivity of the IIBR against oil prices and conventional interbank benchmark interest rates. The same procedure was used to test IIBR's changes relative to fluctuations in the EFFR in order to find the extent to which changes in the EFFR rate resulted in changes in the IIBR.

This study relies on data analysis that we extrapolated from trends observed during the period of data collection (Nov 2011 to June 2015) in order to make educated guesses about the relationship between the observed variables, IIBR and conventional rates, like LIBOR, in the near and long term future. Through regression analysis we are able to analyze how the metrics move in relation to each other during the snapshot in time presented in our data set. This observation provides insight on how these variables interacted during our time of record and how they will interact in the future.

We consider different models to capture the variability of the data. Firstly, simple linear regression investigates the relationship between the overnight rates for the IIBR and the LIBOR. We find that although the overnight maturity of the LIBOR is statistically significant $R^2 = 0.123$, nt at the 1% level, this does not explain the variation of the overnight rate of the IIBR.

The explanatory power of the model we consider has an additional independent variable of the EFFR. Adding the EFFR improves the explanatory power of the model slightly as $R^2 = 0.226$. The EFFR is statistically significant at the 1% level and has a bigger effect than the LIBORON on the IIBRON.

Results of all regressions show that all rates are statistically significant either at 1% or 5%. For the Malaysian rate, it has a negative effect on the IIBR. This result is consistent with the correlation coefficient discussed above.

5 Findings

The results of multiple regression analysis confirm most movements of the various LIBOR rates are significantly negatively correlated with the tested IIBR movements. It was noted how LIBOR rates represent more traditional investment prices that depend largely on the world market for loanable funds, and as a key international benchmark rate it helps determine the comparative rates of return on other commercial interest rates and other asset classes.

The findings from regression analysis do not rule out the notion that the IIBR moves independently from traditional interest bearing assets and benchmarks. If the IIBR is independent of conventional interbank rates, this achieves its goal as a Sharia compliant instrument. A further notable feature of the analysis is that the LIBOR (all terms except the overnight rate) is consistently negatively correlated with movements in all terms of the IIBR.

6 Conclusion

One of the major aims of this study was to evaluate the relationship of the IIBR with the conventional benchmark interbank rates such as the LIBOR. As noted in the results section, this study shows that there exists a significant negative correlation between the LIBOR and IIBR at all maturity levels. The only exception is the LIBOR overnight rate, which is positively correlated with the IIBR. This is a significant finding and it has a number of possible implications. As noted above, the IIBR was established to allow for sharia compliant lending practices that avoid riba (usury) and excessive risk taking activities and predatory lending on the part of banks.

A clear result of a riba (usury) free benchmark rate for lending would be that changes in benchmark market oriented interest rates do not directly affect the IIBR. Due to the negative correlation between the LIBOR and IIBR, any potential changes in market rates will affect the IIBR in a way that is consistent with the observed negative correlation. Indeed, market circumstances may dictate that banks using IIBR as a benchmark may experience a flood of liquidity when that rate is below the corresponding LIBOR rate, according to [11].

References

1. Thomson Reuters. http://thomsonreuters.com/content/financial/pdf/cross_asset/iibr_factsheet.pdf. Accessed
2. Khan, F.: How 'Islamic' is Islamic banking? J. Econ. Behav. Organ. **76**(3), 805–820 (2010)
3. Alexakis, C., Pappas, V., Tsikouras, A.: Hidden cointegration reveals hidden values in Islamic investments. J. Int. Financ. Markets Inst. Money **46**, 70–83 (2017)
4. Fakhfekh, M., Hachicha, N., Jawadi, F., Selmi, N., Cheffou, A.I.: Measuring volatility persistence for conventional and Islamic banks: an FI-EGARCH approach. Emerg. Markets Rev. **27**, 84–99 (2016)
5. Aloui, C., Hammoudeh, S., Hamida, H.B.: Co-Movement between Sharia Stocks and Sukuk in the GCC markets: a time-frequency analysis. J. Int. Financ. Markets Inst. Money **34**, 69–79 (2015)
6. Al-Khazali, O., Lean, H.H., Samet, A.: Do Islamic stock indexes outperform conventional stock indexes? a stochastic dominance approach. Pac. Basin Financ. J. **28**, 29–46 (2014)
7. Ajmi, A.N., Hammoudeh, S., Nguyenc, D.K., Sarafraziba, S.: How strong are the causal relationships between Islamic stock markets and conventional financial systems? evidence from linear and nonlinear tests. J. Int. Financ. Markets Inst. Money **28**, 213–227 (2014)
8. Iqbal, Z., Mirakhor, A.: An Introduction to Islamic Finance: Theory and Practice. Wiley Publishers, London (2011)
9. Sukmana, R., Ibrahim, M.H.: How Islamic are Islamic banks? a non-linear assessment of Islamic rate - conventional rate relations. Econ. Model. **64**, 443–448 (2017)
10. Azad, A.S.M.S., Azmat, S., Chazi, C., Ahsan, A.: Can Islamic banks have their own benchmark? Emerg. Markets Rev. **35**, 120–136 (2018). https://www.sciencedirect.com/science/article/pii/S1566014117300845?via%3Dihub
11. Burne, K.: Islamic Banks get A 'LIBOR' of their Own. Wall Street J. (2011)

Analysis of the Mental Workload Applied to the Sorting Activity of Recyclable Materials

Hebert R. Silva(✉)

Industrial Engineering Course,
Federal University of Uberlandia, Ituiutaba, Brazil
hebert@ufu.br

Abstract. In Brazil, the formation of cooperatives that include the involvement of workers excluded from the formal labor market has been promoted for reusing and recycling materials. In this cooperative environment, workers undertaking sorting activities are exposed to various temporal pressures, physical loads, and stress because it is a vital point of the production process. The objective of this research is to ergonomically evaluate the mental workload, tasks, and activities of the sorting activity workers of a material recycling cooperative in the city of Ituiutaba in Brazil. Several observations using filming and interviews were carried out, and the task/activity file and the NASA-TLX method were applied to the sorting activity workers. This research is justified because the level of attention required of the workers is extremely high, and they are required to concentrate on the operation of the machines, materials, their posture, and safety.

Keywords: Solidary economy · Reuse and recycling of solid waste · Mental workload

1 Introduction

In a dynamic work environment, such as in cooperatives, several variables must be taken into consideration, such as lighting, noise, temperature, humidity, and anthropometric standards for high-level work performance [1], as these factors influence the productivity of the workers. Accordingly, ergonomics should be applied judiciously, using Ergonomic Workplace Analysis (EWA), in accordance with the preliminary analysis of demand. Thus, this field study analyzed the material sorting conveyor belt of a recycling cooperative, in order to understand the work of the cooperative, so that improvements can be proposed in the future.

According to Silva [2], the economic sector involving recycling cooperatives has become the target of negative analyses regarding the organization of work, health, ergonomics, and safety, and they have demonstrated low levels of efficiency and productivity. Thus, a critical level of organization in a cooperative directly influences the achievement of its results.

With relation to cognitive analyses, Stanton et al. [3] state that these methods normally provide information about perception, mental processes, and answers. This data can be presented in different forms and aspects, including human failure, human

T. Ahram et al. (Eds.): IHIET 2019, AISC 1018, pp. 807–811, 2020.
https://doi.org/10.1007/978-3-030-25629-6_126

tasks, task time, objectives and subgoals, decisions, workloads, and user preferences. Psychological models of human performance englobe and integrate these data.

In this study, we applied ergonomics techniques and tools to the selection and sorting tasks of a cooperative recycling center, and based on this analysis it was possible to comprehend their tasks and activities and the dynamics of their workplace. This was then used to develop a solution to eliminate the constraints related to their work and improve the quality of life for the employees.

2 Methods

The workplace studied uses a conveyor belt, 12 m long, 1.10 m high, and 1.15 m wide. The sorting of materials is performed on this conveyor belt, as illustrated in Fig. 1.

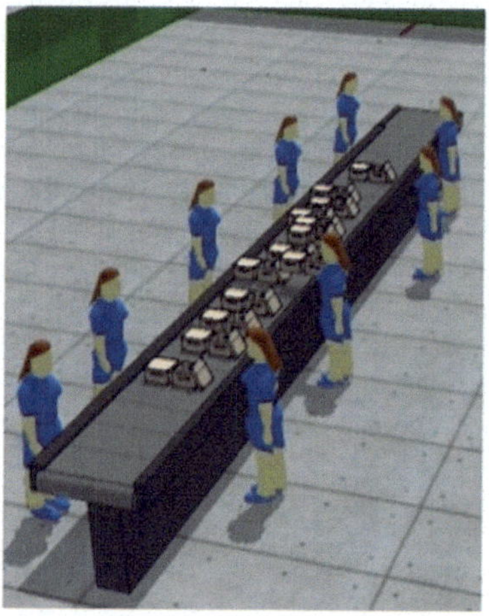

Fig. 1. Conveyor belt for sorting of materials.

The objective of this exploratory research was to understand the activities of the cooperative members allocated to the sorting of materials. Thus, this study involved: (a) bibliographic research, (b) interviews with sorting personnel, (c) observation of the tasks and activities of the sorting personnel, and (d) the application of ergonomic tools, such as the Task/Activity Description Form and NASA Task Load Index (NASA-TLX).

3 Task/Activity Description Form

The Tasks and Activities description form was used along with photos and videos to describe the sorting of the materials and the time used in each cycle. The activities performed by the cooperative are presented in Table 1.

Table 1. Description of tasks/activities during the sorting of materials.

Photograph	Operation name	Operation description	Time
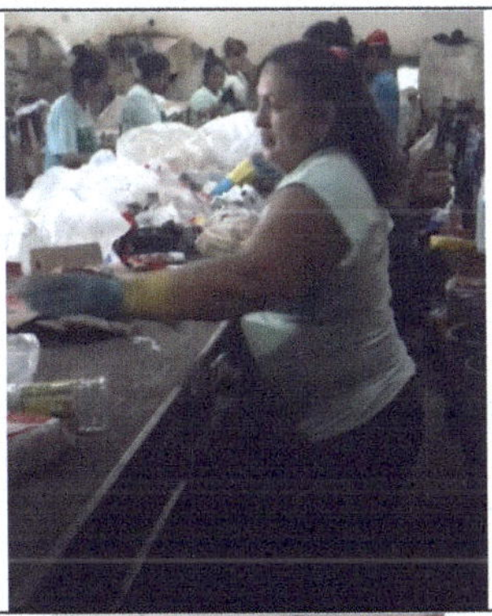	**Sorting of materials**	The member sorts recyclable materials, with slight flexion of the trunk, elevation and abduction of shoulders, slight flexion of the elbows, and fists in the prone position and in a slight extension.	12 seconds
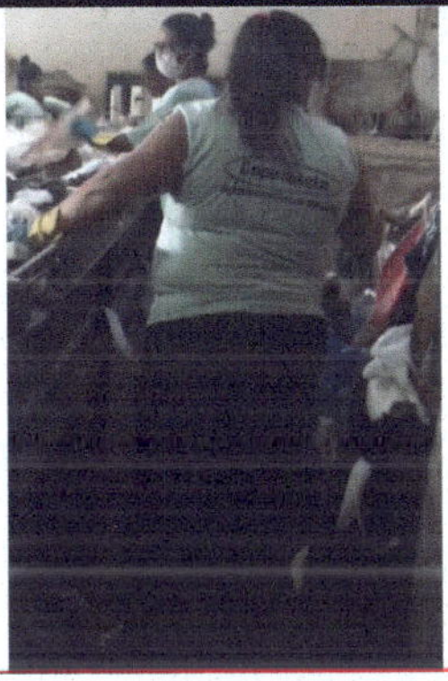	**Sorting of materials**	The member then tosses the materials to containers behind them, performing a rotation of the trunk, lifting with shoulder abduction, flexion and extension of elbows, pronation-supination of wrists, flexed wrists, and palmar flexion of fists.	12 seconds

One of the most critical points regarding inappropriate postures is related to the fixtures in the workplace. These include the lack of planning or adaptation to the sitting position, and how the conveyor belt is not adjustable to the height of the user, does not have a rounded edge, and there are no seats in resting places that can be used during work breaks.

4 Mental Load Evaluation with NASA-TLX

The cognitive assessment used in the NASA-TLX method analyzes the mental load, its dimensions, and its subjective importance (weight). The questionnaire was used to evaluate the mental load activity, given its priorities, generating individual and global results. The data were collected directly from the information sources. The data collection process began with a single natural observation because the observer was included in the work environment. The study proposal was presented to assure the cooperative members that their answers would be used for academic purposes and kept confidential.

This approach is necessary because individual interviews, used for face-to-face assessments of each socioeconomic group, should be performed with caution, as it is necessary to adapt to the environments, customs, and culture, to make the research matter more user-friendly. Table 2 presents the results of the sorting by rates and weight. The NASA-TLX method was applied to three press operators, and the results are presented in Table 2.

Table 2. Representation of the NASA-TLX rates, weight, and indices for press operators.

Factor	Weight	Rate	Weight x rate	Individual loading index
Mental demand	2	60	120	8
Physical demand	5	70	350	23
Temporal demand	4	70	280	19
Performance	0	0	0	0
Effort/Commitment	3	70	210	14
Frustration	1	60	60	4
Perceived workload - global index				68

Among the criteria of the NASA-TLX analysis, Physical Demand had the highest individual load index, which is the amount of physical activity required to perform the work, and it was relatively high (such as push, pull, lift, load, and so on). Temporal Demand, which is the time pressure felt, occupied second place, and the pace of work imposed on the employee, was also relatively high. Effort/Commitment, which refers to the level of physical and mental effort required to reach their level of productivity, was average in relation to the other criteria. Fourth on the individual task load index was Mental Demand (MD), which is related to the amount of mental activity and perspective needed to perform the activity (such as reasoning, calculating, thinking, seeking, deciding, and so on), and this was slightly below average, compared to the other criteria. The fifth criterion that was close to zero is Frustration, where the employee feels irritated, stressed, dissatisfied, and insecure in the performance of their activities. One criterion that did not have an individual load index was Performance, which indicates personal performance, that is, the satisfaction and the performance of the employee given the work performed.

Thus, the dissatisfaction of cooperative members can be noted for their Physical Demand because the physical activity required to accomplish the task is high, and their Temporal Demand, which is the time pressure for the execution of their tasks.

Another observation is that for the values of the NASA-TLX above 61, corrective measures are necessary to reduce the risks and protect the health and quality of life of the members. Therefore, the obtained value of 68 indicates the need for immediate intervention in the workplace.

Accordingly, the NASA-TLX assessment tool confirms the high indices of the physical demands that are perceived in the Tasks and Activities description form, which are constantly present in reuse and recycling cooperatives, as observed in the works of Stanton [3] and Silva [4, 5]. This case study indicates that physical factors and temporal demand stand out more than mental demand.

5 Conclusions

This study indicates that the physical space in which these cooperative members work has several problems. As with the environmental conditions, the physical space is not appropriate to the psychophysiological characteristics of the employees and requires immediate intervention.

The cognitive ergonomics analysis indicates the existence of dissatisfaction in relation to the workplace, expressed as high physical demand, which is related to the amount of physical activity that must be exerted to perform the activity and the time pressure for the execution of their tasks.

Although the mental load is not a significant factor, the results of this study are similar to those obtained by Silva [4], in which several critical postures are adopted in the handling of materials. These results demonstrate the need to use ergonomic solutions to eliminate heavy tasks, flexion of the trunk and neck, and reduce the static posture of the lower limbs. These movements are constantly present in the tasks/activities that are implemented during the selection and recycling of materials.

Therefore, novel human-interaction and engineering approaches, tools, methodologies, techniques, and solutions are need for integrating people, concepts and trends in the Sorting Activity of Recyclable Materials.

References

1. Silva, H.R.: Analysis of the mental workloads applied to press operators during the reuse and recycling of materials. In: Karwowski, W., Ahram, T. (eds.) Advances in Intelligent Systems and Computing, 2nd edn., vol. 903, pp. 673–678. Springer International Publishing, San Diego (2019). https://doi.org/10.1007/978-3-030-11051-2_102
2. Silva, H.R.: Study of the ergonomics applied to the reuse and recycling of materials. In: Karwowski, W., Ahram, T. (eds.) Advances in Intelligent Systems and Computing, 1st edn., vol. 722, pp. 770–775. Springer International Publishing, Dubai (2018). https://doi.org/10.1007/978-3-319-73888-8_119
3. Stanton, N., et al.: Handbook of Human Factors and Ergonomics Methods. 1st edn., p. 760. Phorte, São Paulo (2016)
4. Silva, H.R.: Labor ergonomic analysis applied to a Brazilian solid materials recycling cooperative. In: Advances in Intelligent Systems and Computing, 1st edn., vol. 605, pp. 191–200. Springer International Publishing, Los Angeles (2018). https://doi.org/10.1007/978-3-319-94000-7_13
5. Silva, H.R.: Analysis of ergonomics in the reuse and recycling of solid materials in Brazilian cooperatives. In: Bagnara, S., et al. (eds.) Proceedings of the 20th Congress of the International Ergonomics Association (IEA 2018), vol. VIII, pp. 960–969. Springer International Publishing, Florence (2019). https://doi.org/10.1007/978-3-319-96068-5_104

Complex Predictive Solution for Computerized Processes in Tire Industry

Jan Piesik[1(✉)] and Kazimierz T. Kosmowski[2]

[1] Michelin Polska. S.A., Leonharda 9, 10-454 Olsztyn, Poland
jan.piesik@michelin.com
[2] Gdansk University of Technology,
G. Narutowicza 11/12, 80-233 Gdansk, Poland
kazimierz.kosmowski@pg.edu.pl

Abstract. Following increasing market needs of productivity, cost reduction and safety requirements, computerized industry are faced to finding optimum between economic aspects of business and safety-related risk management. Modern factories equipped with computerized processes and extended diagnostic tools to support operator do not often use of all information's which comes from the equipment. Some of the relations between the events are also omitted or neglected. Authors after analyzing the defects of modern production lines with batch production, noticed a correlation between the defects and the historical information registered by the supervisory system controlling the production process. The problem is that with the multitude of appearing information, they are not analyzed on an ongoing basis. This article presents a new approach to increase machinery reliability, safety and quality increase through predictive data analysis.

Keywords: Reliability · Failure prediction · Data mining · Functional safety

1 Introduction

Until the 40's of the twentieth century, the approach to the failure was based on the reactive approach or principle "broke down, so fix it", this approach began to change during World War II when the reliability of more and more complex technical devices often decided about life or death. This was the beginning of planned repairs and inspections and parts replacement. However, this solution also had some drawbacks, among other things, it brought a high cost of maintenance, as the part which was in very good condition was often exchanged. In particular, the aviation industry, similarly to today, in the 1960s, analyzed the costs of maintaining the fleet of aircraft. With the arrival of Boeing 747 with advanced technology, the Reliability Centered Maintenance (RCM) method was developed [1].

Based largely on a predictive approach analyzing the condition of machines (called Condition Based Maintenance). Due to the rapid development of electronics, it became possible to more and more accurately analyze the parameters of machines and devices. On the other hand, the increasing share of electronics in machines caused that apart from the traditional "bathtub" distribution of damage, several new ones started to

T. Ahram et al. (Eds.): IHIET 2019, AISC 1018, pp. 812–817, 2020.
https://doi.org/10.1007/978-3-030-25629-6_127

appear. Vibroacoustic measurements, oil analyzes and thermographic measurements of machines and electrical cabinets and substations are currently standard in the industry. Various types of real-time measurements are also becoming more and more widely disseminated. Also, thanks to the advances in technology, the sensor market has expanded its offer by testing many physical quantities and at the same time the cost of a single sensor has dropped several dozen times. All this has meant that modern production lines are equipped with hundreds and sometimes thousands of sensors that collect data on an ongoing basis and monitor the state and course of the production process [2].

The problem faced by engineers today is the opposite of that of factories at the beginning of the last century - today it can be seen an excess of information, controllers and through them, Supervisory Control and Data Acquisition (SCADA) systems present hundreds of information to the operator [3]. The most important are filtered and presented in such a way that can be effectively manage the process, but nevertheless a significant part of the data is skipped.

The authors of this article proposed a comprehensive approach to the method of detection of machine defects. The method can be applied and be effective in detecting functional safety anomalies, cyber security threats and can be effective in detecting deviations of quality and energy efficiency analysis, binding together the influence of the parameters of the prescription to increase energy consumption. The last possible profit is the analysis of operator behavior recorded in the machine control systems and then proposing corrective actions.

2 Proposed Prediction Methodology

Every technical device requires human operation and maintenance, the more technically advanced it is, the more trained the operators and maintenance must be, but human behavior remains the same regardless of changes in technology, resulting in the need to implement organisational techniques such as Total Productive Maintenance (TPM) [4] and cost optimization such as RCM. This is the foundation for further work with the advanced solutions proposed in the article.

Authors after analyzing the defects of modern production lines with batch production, noticed a correlation between the defects and the historical information registered by the supervisory system controlling the production process. The problem is that with the multitude of appearing information, they are not analyzed on an ongoing basis. The idea was to create a tool that would generate reports of impending defects with a certain frequency. These reports read by personnel would be verified by inspection. If the predictions of the system were confirmed, actions would be taken to eliminate the anomaly before the occurrence of the defect, or to minimize its impact and the size of the losses [5].

On the market exists the solutions of predictive analytics but their scope is limited to one aspect –maintenance predictive [6, 7]. The proposed solution concerns not only improving the reliability of machines and devices. It also significantly influences the improvement of the safety and quality of manufactured products by reducing anomalies, process disturbances such as defects, a much faster diagnosis of deviations, which reduces the amount of production rework or scrap. The last, however, the most important element improving is the level of cyber security (Fig. 1).

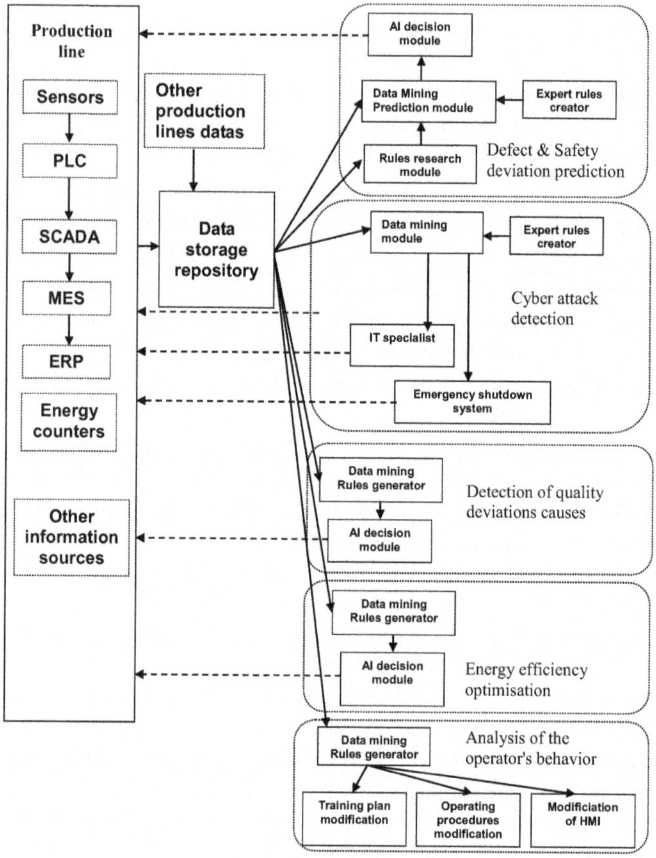

Fig. 1. Integrated concept of factory data mining and prediction supported by artificial intelligence

The main assumptions of each of the above-mentioned functionalities are based on the same tools and mechanism. Therefore, the proposed comprehensive tool will be explained briefly on the example of the section on machine defect & safety deviation prediction module.

The authors propose a prediction tool based on statistical instruments. This tool consists of four modules considered as a comprehensive approach to prediction (Fig. 2). The first element of the system – Data collection - consists of output data from the production line. In modern production lines all data from sensors, inverters, drives, intelligent sensors, networks, programmable logic controllers (PLC), human-machine interfaces (HMI), Supervisory Control and Data Acquisition (SCADA), Manufacturing Execution System (MES) and Enterprise Resource Planning (ERP) are collected in a data storage repository (Fig. 1). These data are, by nature, in different forms.

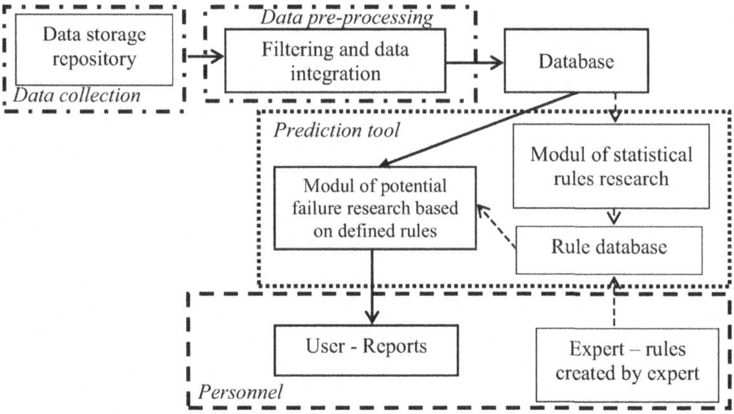

Fig. 2. Functional diagram of proposed solution for defect and safety prediction

The second module - Data pre-processing - is used for data processing by pre-filtering and integrating data into one-dimensional data. The data are then collected in a common database. Next step is that information's has to be classified into two categories – cause or effect. Without this category's algorithm treat every event as a potential cause and effect what leads to a considerable prolongation of time for calculation. The third module - Prediction tool - is the work with the collected and pre-prepared data in order to obtain useful information and conclusions from them. In the first stage, a statistical rule search module is used to analyze historical data. In this case we have to deal with the need to use statistical tools of machine learning and methods of artificial intelligence to discover the relationship between events gathered in the database.

A statistical tool created for this purpose is association analysis [8]. Results of machine learning tool feeds the rules database with ready-made rules. The second stage is to analyze the data gathered on an ongoing basis at specific time intervals. The module filters data through predefined rules using time-frame set for some period defined by the system administrator and searches for potential events.

The last module - Personnel - is the human-system interface module. There is a division into an expert and a user. The role of an expert who also based on knowledge, experience, familiarity with control systems and mechanisms operating in them can supply the database of rules. The second important role is to remove automatically found rules of minimal importance for the goals of the company. The user, on the other hand, is a client of the system who receives ready-made reports with predicted events. Its role is to analyze reports and take preventive steps at the facility.

3 Implementation of Proposed Methodology on the Plant

Two modern production lines equipped with a wide range of sensors monitoring both the process and machine status on-line were selected for pilot implementation. TPM and RCM methods are implemented on these production lines. After collecting and analysing historical data from the period of more than three months, it appeared that on average 11830 messages for operator were generated daily. The test implementation was limited to 6 months and was limited to the defect's prediction module only. The statistical tool created for this purpose was the association analysis. The solution widely used for statistical analyses in recent years, enriched with a package enabling application in industrial plants, was the Statistica software package. Sequential analysis to detect recurring patterns during events resulted in 684 rules with the following indicator levels: minimum support = 0.1, and minimum trust = 0.5. Only simple rules were searched by principle "if the predecessor then a successor". No rules were searched for with a sequence of several preceding events.

Analyzing the results obtained in relation to the predictions, the proportions in which symptoms appear before the occurrence of the defect were proportional. During 8 h before the defect 80% of symptoms appear (Fig. 3).

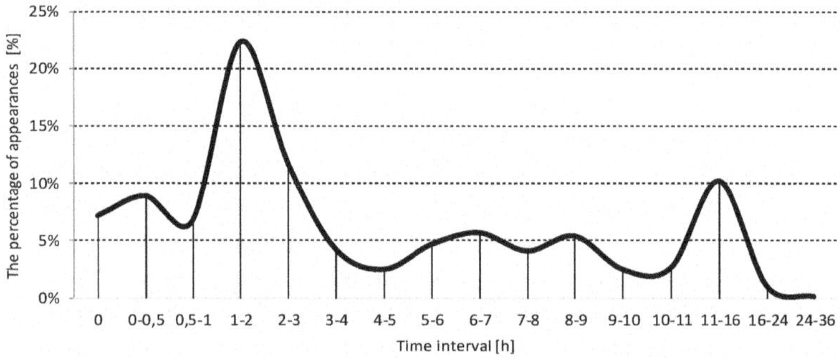

Fig. 3. Chart of time intervals between symptom and effects symptom-effect relationship

It was also puzzling that almost 7% of all relationships appeared in time almost simultaneously with the occurrence of the defect (Fig. 3). The verification of these events showed that some rules should be turned off due to their dull character.

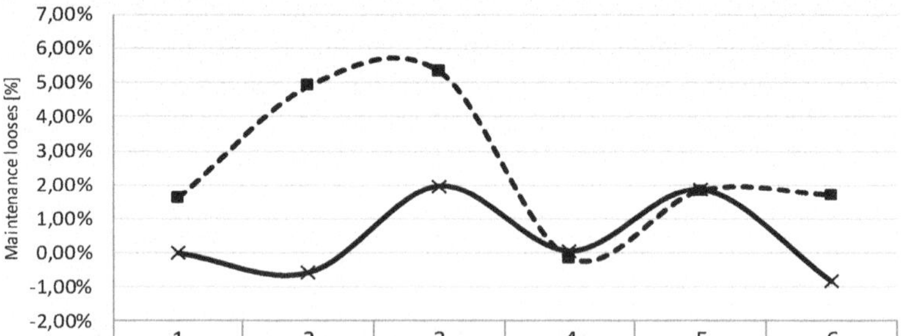

	1	2	3	4	5	6
year n-1	1,60%	4,91%	5,34%	-0,17%	1,84%	1,70%
year n	0,00%	-0,57%	1,96%	0,06%	1,85%	-0,83%

Months

Fig. 4. Losses due to unplanned and planned maintenance activities on line A in the year of tool implementation and previous year.

Analysing the graph of maintenance looses (Fig. 4), where the first month of year *n* (year of tool implementation) was taken as a percentage reference could be seen decrease of 2,13% year to year in maintenance loses indicator. What is also important from the point of view of the maintenance services customer's, compared to the previous year there has been a reduction in the fluctuations in the time load for which the maintenance operations are made. Greater stability results in fewer disturbances, more stable production, which translates into stability of quality results and improvement of production indicators.

4 Conclusion

The results of the test solution showed that it is possible to simultaneously increase machine availability and improve machine safety by predicting faults based on a statistical analysis of the symptoms recorded by the control system. The short test implementation time and limited resources did not allow for the expansion of the system and use of all presented modules, however the results obtained confirmed the effectiveness and usefulness of the tool.

After optimization of the solution, the system can be easily copied and installed on other similar installations in the enterprise. This results in a very fast, cheap and not requiring large human resources increase the reliability and safety and security of machines, which indirectly affects also the improvement of the quality of manufactured products.

References

1. Rausand, M.: Reliability centered maintenance. Reliab. Eng. Syst. Saf. **60**, 121–132 (1998)
2. Kosmowski, K.T. (ed.): Basics of functional safety. Gdańsk University of Technology Publishers, Gdańsk (2016). (in Polish)
3. Piesik, J., Kosmowski, K.T.: Current Reliability and Safety Management issues of production lines. Application of computers in Science and Technology 2016. The Scientific Papers of Faculty of Electrical and Control Engineering Gdansk University of Technology, vol. 51, pp. 155–158 (2016). (in Polish)
4. Suzuki, T.: TPM in Process Industries. Productivity Press, Portland (1994)
5. Piesik, J.: Application of statistical tools to improve the Reliability and Safety of Machinery by predicting failures and improving the diagnostic coverage of machinery (in Polish), Application of Statistics and Data Mining in Scientific research and improvement of production processes with the use of data analysis, Statsoft, Kraków (2015). (in Polish)
6. Google Analytics. https://cloud.google.com/blog/products/data-analytics/
7. IBM Corporation. https://www.ibm.com/us-en/marketplace/ibm-predictive-maintenance-optimization
8. Agraval, R., Srikant, R.: Fast algorithms for Mining Association Rules. In: Proceedings of the 20th International Conference on Very Large Data Bases, pp. 487–499. Morgan Kaufmann Publishers Inc., San Francisco (1994)

Improving Processes Through the Use of the 5S Methodology and Menu Engineering to Reduce Production Costs of a MSE in the Hospitality Sector in the Department of Ancash

Indira Alva[1(✉)], José Rojas[1(✉)], and Carlos Raymundo[2(✉)]

[1] Ingeniería de Gestión Empresarial,
Universidad Peruana de Ciencias Aplicadas (UPC), Lima, Peru
{u201217451, jose.rojas}@upc.edu.pe
[2] Dirección de Investigación,
Universidad Peruana de Ciencias Aplicadas (UPC), Lima, Peru
carlos.raymundo@upc.edu.pe

Abstract. The purpose of this document is to improve inventory management processes and food processing at a restaurant in the region of Ancash by applying the 5S methodology and using specific indicators for the location and type of work. All this was achieved with the implementation of the menu engineering methodology, which consists basically of forecasts, linear programming, long-term orders, and inventory management. The proper operation of the new processes was experimentally validated. First, the main results were that the use of approximately 4.30 m^2 of the work space allocated to unnecessary activities within the work area was optimized, increasing the number of processes that a worker can perform without moving more than 1 m from their work position. Despite the many studies existing on the methodology implemented, there is scarce material that focuses on its application in restaurants, as it is normally developed in industrial areas.

Keywords: 5S · Menu engineering · Forecasts · Restaurant · Hospitality

1 Introduction

The hospitality sector is vital for the country's economy, without which tourism would not be possible. It is impossible to think about traveling without prior planning regarding food and lodging that will be needed in the time away from home. Food is not only a biological need, it is also a part of the country's culture and social development. Perú is going through a complicated period for micro and small enterprises as 90% of them are not able to achieve their desirable sustainability. The most common problems encountered are lack of strategies for quantifying demand, production planning, and continuous process improvement. More specifically, the hospitality sector currently faces a situation of slower economic growth. In addition to this situation, inadequate demand forecasting coupled with poor inventory management can be dangerous for the suitable growth of a company.

T. Ahram et al. (Eds.): IHIET 2019, AISC 1018, pp. 818–824, 2020.
https://doi.org/10.1007/978-3-030-25629-6_128

2 State of the Art

[1] Porter (1996) stated that the strategy is creating a singular and valuable position that entails a distinct set of activities. It is noteworthy since it is an option that will enable an organization to position itself in an unparalleled competitive space. One of the situations that organizations face is achieving market positioning and sustaining it over time. For example, the lean philosophy is a set of methodologies, about which [2] Rodriguez (2014) stated that it is a set of tools aimed at removing everything that does not add value to the product, process or service from production processes. This reduces costs, generates client satisfaction, and improves business profitability, the main objective of all industries that wish to remain in the market. Moreover, [2] Felizzola & Amaya (2014) argued that lean manufacturing is an approach to improve quality and productivity that aims to optimize the way in which a company organizes and manages its relationships with its customers and supply chain, and the development and manufacturing of its products, seeking to generate greater outputs with fewer resources. Lean identifies and differentiates seven types of waste that occur within nearly all companies. In his "Proposal to Improve the Chocolate Sprinkled Bonbon Process," [3] Moreno (2017) defined them as below: Overproduction: Waiting, Overprocessing, Inventory excess, Defects, Motion, Transport.

Among the most used and effective methodologies within everything entailed in the lean philosophy is 5S, which is based on a set of tools to achieve its objective; the elimination of waste. [4] "This tool will result in a substantial improvement in organization, order, cleanliness, standardization, and discipline that will favor resource savings," (Serrano, 2016). A series of steps must be carried out in order to implement 5S.

Once the application of the methodology has been concluded and the work environment is optimal for efficient work without delays that do not depend on employees, the process will proceed to improving organizational levels, such as inventory management and sales forecasting, as part of the menu engineering methodology [5]

To this end, Gracía et al. proposed a matrix that has nine quadrants, with the help of statistical tools to determine the convenience and inconvenience of serving some dishes over others, thus obtaining results and possible strategies to obtain stronger earnings. These forecasts provide important and powerful information to reduce costs. [6] Furthermore, improvements must be implemented in inventory management with respect to the use of inventoried materials. A method called FIFO (first in, first out) essentially aims to get the product that first enters the storage area to be used first. (Viera et al. 2017) stated that inventory management is related to determining record-keeping methods, rotation points, sorting methods, among others, all of which is geared toward actions to help companies manage their inventory. The above is carried out to conclude with a linear programming exercise, to determine the most suitable production with respect to financial efficiency.

3 Method

The study was carried out in an experimental manner. The data obtained was provided by the general manager of the restaurant, who has a record of everything that has occurred since July 2017 to date. Data, such as past sales, profit levels, complaint logs, purchasing records, among others, were obtained to process the information in the best way possible and correctly analyze the problem. The proposed model is built by combining methodologies. First, the well-known 5S was employed to improve each aspect of the work area, for which the processes were defined, each stage of the methodology was implemented which changed, among other aspects, the inventory of instruments within the kitchen, the distribution within the site, and the processes to standardize them. This is all done so that these processes are standardized and become part of each worker's culture. Lastly, the menu engineering methodology was applied, through which processes were implemented that will fulfill the function of maximizing the restaurant's profits and reducing production costs. To this end, the historical demand at the restaurant was analyzed to create a sales forecast. Linear programming was also developed in order to determine the optimal production quantity. This data was used to make purchase orders from approved suppliers, with whom they have long-term contracts. In this manner, inventory management will be carried out successfully. Through the monthly order, it will be known exactly how much of each material has entered the business and how much leaves through sales.

4 Result

4.1 Improvement Proposal

To combat this waste situation, a model was developed that combines two methodologies which, together, seek to establish a long-lasting order in the production area and propose improved purchasing management for the business.

Figure 1 shows that the model was designed in order to address the main problem found in the restaurant studied.

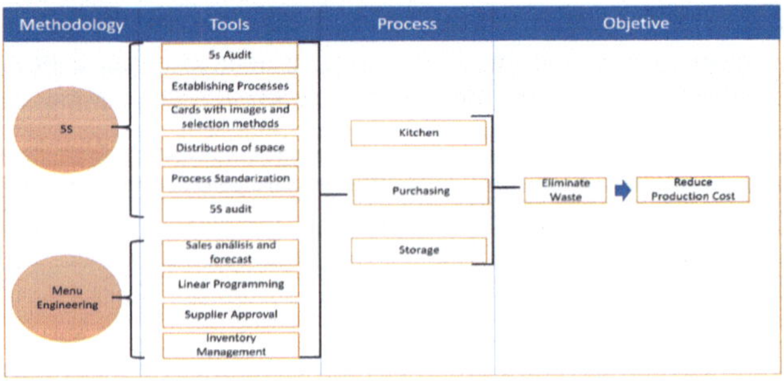

Fig. 1. "Proposed model"

The purpose of applying the 5S methodology is to meet customer requirements and expectations with the least amount of resource use, without generating waste, and eliminating any activity that does not generate value for the consumer.

Moreover, the menu engineering methodology combines several useful tools to manage purchasing and inventory. A 5S audit was carried out as the first step in applying this model, which determined that, in effect, applying the methodology would be very useful in this work area.

- 1S–The first step in implementation entails classifying the need of each element, for which small notebooks are used to define the utensil needs to prepare each dish. These are part of an operations manual that will be created with a complete set of instructions that will be detailed in the process of this proposal. In the first handbooks, the minimum and maximum quantities of utensils that must be near the preparation area will be established.
- 2S–To determine the kitchen's optimum organization, the above procedures are considered. In accordance with the need of each utensil, a place for each element will be established in a specific kitchen area. The procedure will entail identifying the location of each utensil, standardizing containers, and placing the elements in the proper area.
- 3S For cleaning, all the places prone to getting dirty must be identified. The next step is carrying out a detailed account of all the activities and/or incidents that could cause dirtiness. As part of cleaning, freeing up space must also be taken into account. To this end, a list of all the utensils in the kitchen is made, detailing the action to be carried out with them (preserving, storing or discarding), all in accordance with the prior stages' guidelines.
- 4S–As part of the standardization process, management must ensure that not only do these forms exist, but that they are all published in the most appropriate place, according to what is indicated on them. Furthermore, workers will be instructed to report any type of anomaly, such as non-compliance with directions, missing utensils or an excess of the same, among other situations that could cause a return to the prior situation.
- 5S–Lastly, continuous improvement will be achieved by reapplying the 5S audit, in such a manner that first, validates that the work carried out has been efficient and second and seeks ways to continue improving until the audit yields a maximum score.

According to the results from the forecast, the theory of constraints of linear programming will be applied, in order to calculate optimal production to meet future demand, but in a manner that is favorable for the profitability of the business.

At the same time, new policies will be established for negotiating with suppliers, in order to establish longer term contracts with favorable terms for both parties, among other characteristics that were not previously taken into account when purchasing inputs. To this end, food quality standards, price conditions, supplier flexibility, punctuality, among other terms will be established. All of these characteristics will be quantified in order to find the most qualified supplier to enter into long-term contracts with.

4.2 Final Results

One of the main results from all the work carried out was the new arrangement of the kitchen, with visible procedures to be followed by all employees. All stages of the 5S methodology were applied and a favorable result was obtained from its audit.

Table 1 shows the final result of the 5S audit. While there is room to improve the score (maximum score: 50), the change with respect to the initial rating obtained is remarkable (11), for which the following was established:

Table 1. Final results from the 5 s audit

ID	5S	Title	Points
S1	Sort (Seiri)	Separate the necessary from the unnecessary	9
S2	Set in order (Seiton)	A place for everything and everything in its place	8
S3	Shine (Seiso)	Clean the work area and equipment, prevent dirtiness and disorder	9
S4	Standardize (Seiketsu)	Formulate the regulations to consolidated the first three S	7
S5	Sustain (Shitsuke)	Respect the established regulations	7
	Action Plans	5S Score	40
	Conclusion	NEED TO IMPROVE THE SYSTEM	

Operation manuals: Comprised of small forms that indicate what to do, how to do it, what is needed, how a process works, among other specifications that will enable workers to reduce variation in their processes.

Standardized containers: This will help identify maximum and minimum levels for making materials, to prevent waste and avert not being able to prepare certain dishes, by identifying an input replacement point.

Cleaning forms: In order to keep the workplace clean, forms were made. The first identifies sources of grime and the second identifies who cleaned them, when it was performed, if any material was replaced, or if there was anything unusual.

Standardized processes: In order to standardize the kitchen area, a board was installed that displays the procedures for serving food, its preparation, what is needed, among other necessary forms. The cleaning form must be present on this board, so that it is visible to everybody in the kitchen.

Continuous improvement: Applying the 5S audit at least every two months was established as a restaurant policy, and actions must be taken on anything that is not 100% compliant, so that these practices can be implemented for all workers and their culture.

Continuing with the work carried out, a methodology called menu engineering was applied, which includes statistical tools that help forecast changes in demand and consumer preferences, in order to establish reasonable production amounts, taking into account the profitability and popularity that each dish represents for the business.

In addition to these tools, other engineering tools were added in order to detect not only the demand quantity, but also the optimal production quantity for the restaurant according to the profitability of each dish. The following was carried out:

Sales forecasts: Based on information from prior months, a weighted moving average was chosen to forecast the quantities that must be prepared to not waste food and generate waste.

Linear programming: Based on the forecast, a minimum and a maximum production quantity was determined for each dish. The maximum quantity preference will always be given to the dish; pig in a Chinese box, based on the profitability that this dish represents for the restaurant. This is all based on the logic that if the consumer does not find one dish, they will choose another from the menu.

- Advance orders from suppliers: With all the information collected from the linear programming, medium and long-term deals are made with more serious suppliers that are not only reliable, but also offer better contractual terms; among which, the quality and price of the products, supplier flexibility, payment facilities, among other characteristics taken into account when choosing a supplier will be evaluated.
- Inventory management: As the supplier issue and weekly orders will be more standardized, more exhaustive control will be carried out on the materials that enter the restaurant via the FIFO method, that is, that the first inputs to arrive will be the first prepared, through which, it is possible to maintain the freshness of each offered dish.

5 Results Analysis

Below, the results obtained since the implementation of the methodologies will be evaluated with respect to the results obtained in the same period of the previous year. Not only was it possible to increase profit compared to the prior period, it was also possible to reduce expenses incurred by the restaurant to obtain that profit. In other words, more efficient use was made of the money invested.

Moreover, the behavior of the real profit is shown with respect to the proposed objective. The profit target is 25% of total revenue, the profit in the month of November (current month) has reached approximately 20%. It is worth mentioning that this data is from the first three weekends of the month, which means that if the restaurant's profit is projected through the end of the month, it is very likely that the profit target will be reached. This is the result of the production schedule that was made to determine optimal order quantities, so that inputs are not wasted or produced more than can be sold.

References

1. PORTER, Michael: "La ventaja competitiva de las naciones," Cap (1991)
2. Rodríguez: Propuesta de mejora del proceso productivo del vino borgoña semiseco aplicando lean manufacturing, para aumentar la productividad en la empresa bodegas el zarco (Consulta: 25 de mayo) (2014)

3. Moreno Penagos, C.M.: Propuesta de Mejoramiento del Proceso del Bombón Chocolate Grajeas (2017)
4. Serrano, B.: Aplicación de lean management al sector de la restauración: lean restaurant, (Consulta: 01 de mayo) (2016). https://repositorio.comillas.edu/xmlui/bitstream/handle/11531/16776/TFM000612.pdf?sequence=1&isAllowed=y)
5. García Pulido, Y.A., Medina León, A.A., Frías Jiménez, R.A., González Arias, M.: Propuesta de herramienta para la aplicación de la ingeniería de menú en restaurantes de hoteles all-inclusive. Investigaciones Turisticas **12**, 142–162 (2015)
6. Viera, E., Cardona, D., Rodríguez, R., Gutiérrez, B.: Diagnóstico de los modelos de gestión de inventarios de alimentos en empresas hoteleras. Revista Científica ECOCIENCIA, vol. 4(3) (2017)

Implementation of a Compact Wearable Temperature, Pressure, Humidity and Gas Sensing Device

Jordi Palacín, David Martínez(✉), Eduard Clotet, and Marcel Tresanchez

Department of Computer Science and Industrial Engineering, University of Lleida, 25001 Lleida, Spain
{palacin, david.martinez, eclotet, mtresanchez}@diei.udl.cat

Abstract. This paper presents the implementation of a compact wearable sensing device with temperature, pressure, humidity and gas measurement capabilities. The paper focuses on the implementation of an automatic procedure task able to perform periodically readings of the sensor and sending the data through a conventional serial port by the implementation of the USB Communication Device Class (CDC). The wearable sensing device has been tested by gathering measurements of temperature, pressure, humidity and gas sensor resistance when it has moved between two different areas in order to detect data variations and check the correct performance of the automatic procedure task. The objective is to develop a wearable device easy to use, portable and with simple connectivity to any host device in order to measure the ambient environmental conditions. The implemented wearable device is focused to be an easy approach for data measurement of the outdoor and indoor environments that can be used for research, industrial or educational purposes.

Keywords: Wearable device · ARM microcontroller · Ambient environmental measurement

1 Introduction

Recently, intensive efforts have been taken to develop array sensing systems. The advantage of using a sensor array instead of a single sensor is the addition of new dimensions to the observation, helping to estimate more parameters and improve the estimation performance. The array sensing systems has been applied on different scientific fields. On the robotics field, [1] presents the development of a flexible thermal and pressure sensor array to be embedded in mobile robots to perform specific exploratory searching operations [2] or to complement general applications [3]. In the same direction, [4] presents a method to fabricate flexible temperature sensor array that can be used as humanoid artificial skin for sensation system of robots. On the other hand, in [5] presents a flexible wearable sensor array for perspiration analysis. On the chemical field, exist many studies related with the detection of VOCs using an array of gas sensors, an example is described in [6], where is presented a gas sensor array for

T. Ahram et al. (Eds.): IHIET 2019, AISC 1018, pp. 825–830, 2020.
https://doi.org/10.1007/978-3-030-25629-6_129

the simultaneous detection of multiple VOCs. Finally, in [7] presents an ultrasonic array sensor for reliable presence detection in indoor spaces. In this direction, this paper presents the implementation of a compact wearable sensing device using the BME680 sensor. The main idea of this paper is to implement an automatic procedure task that allows periodically readings of the temperature, pressure, humidity and gas of the BME680 sensor, sending the data through a conventional serial port by the implementation of the USB Communication Device Class (CDC). Future work will be focused on improving the wearable sensing device by adding multiple slave sensor devices to develop a wearable array sensing device.

2 Wearable Sensing Device

2.1 Electronic Board Description

The wearable sensing device is based on a small electronic board which includes an ARM microcontroller and a low-cost sensing device (Fig. 1).

The ARM microcontroller is the STM32F070CBT6 from ST Microelectronics. The core is based on 32-bit Cortex-M0 operating at a 48 MHz frequency, 128 Kbytes of Flash memory and 16 Kbytes of SRAM provided in a small surface mount LQFP48 package. The microcontroller offers standard communication interfaces (two I2Cs, two SPIs and four USARTs), one USB Full speed device, one 12-bit ADC with 10 external and 2 internal independent channels, seven general purpose 16-bit timers and an advanced control timer. This microcontroller was selected because it is the smallest low power STM32 microcontroller device able to handle the USB and SPI communication needed to perform the requested task at the same time. The electronic board is powered with 5 V by the USB connector. The 5 V are converted in 3.3 V through a voltage regulator (LD3985M33R) in order to supply the microcontroller and the sensing device. The microcontroller works with an 8 MHz external oscillator. The electronic board also includes a Light Emitting Diode (LED) for status information and a Serial Wire Debug (SWD) pins to program the microcontroller.

The sensor used is the BME680, a low power digital 4-in-1 sensor with temperature, pressure, humidity and gas measurement based on proven sensing principles. The sensor module is encapsulated in a compact metal-lid LGA package. The footprint

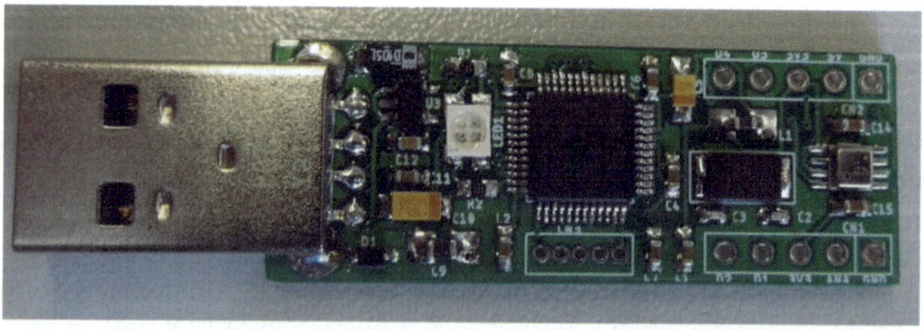

Fig. 1. Image of the wearable sensing device.

measures 3.0 × 3.0 mm^2 with a height of 1.00 mm. The sensor supports the SPI digital interface in order to communicate with external devices. The ARM microcontroller operates as a SPI master and the BME680 sensor operates as a slave device.

2.2 Initialization

The ARM microcontroller configures the basic measurement parameters of the sensor after a power-up sequence. In this case, the versatility of the BME680 sensor enables the measurement of temperature, pressure and humidity with individual oversampling periods, which may increase the resolution of the measurements (16 bits by default). Additionally, the BME680 sensor may be configured to perform gas sensing measurements but this mode is not active by default. The gas sensing contains a heating resistor and a measurement resistor sensitive to gas concentration.

In this sensor, the value of the pressure and temperature (but not humidity and gas sensing result) can be internally filtered by a configurable IIR internal filter in order to remove short-term fluctuations.

Table 1 summarizes the main configuration parameters of the BME680. The microcontroller can disable or skip the measurement of the temperature (T), pressure (P) and humidity (H) by setting the oversampling value. The sensor also enables the configuration of the IIR filter coefficient applied on the temperature and pressure sensor. The configuration of the gas sensor (G) settings can be set by enabling: the heater, the gas conversion, the duration of the heat up stage and the target heater temperature.

Table 1. BME680 main configuration parameters.

Parameters	Values and/or range
Oversampling (T-P-H)	0:Skip - 1:OSx1 - 2:OSx2 - 3:OSx4 - 4: OSx8 - 5:Osx16
IIR filter coefficient (T-P)	0:0 - 1:1 - 2:3 - 3:7 - 4:15 - 5:31 - 6:63 - 7:127
Heat up duration (G)	1–4,032 ms
Target heater temperature (G)	200 °C - 400 °C
Enable heater (G)	1:On - 0:Off
Enable gas conversion (G)	1:On - 0:Off

2.3 Normal Operation

The wearable sensor device operates autonomously by periodically reading the temperature, pressure, humidity and gas of the BME680 sensor. These measurement values are stored internally in order to provide fast data response. The data measured by the microcontroller can be gathered externally through a set of commands using the USB CDC. Figure 2 shows the main non-blocking tasks and the exchange of information between devices of the measurement operation.

The normal operation of the microcontroller includes four main sequential non-blocking tasks. The first task saves the measured data in a buffer by performing all the different SPI communications between the microcontroller and the sensor. The second and third task are aware of the sending and receiving messages between the microcontroller and the host device. Finally, the fourth task can be configured to automatically and periodically send the gathered data without having to send a request command for each data.

The wearable sensing device uses a set of commands in order to configure the operation mode. An example is the time between samples in the automatic mode and the type of measurement that is fully configurable in order to gather temperature, pressure, humidity and gas sensing.

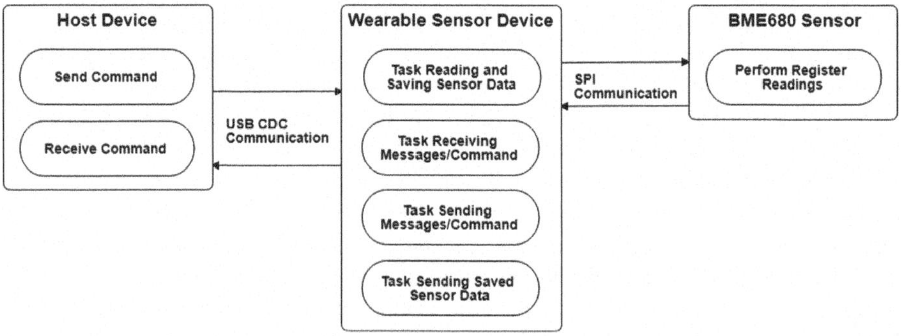

Fig. 2. Diagram of the main non-blocking tasks and exchange of information between devices.

3 Results

This section presents the discussions and the first results obtained with the implementation of the automatic procedure task to perform readings of the temperature, pressure, humidity and gas sensor resistance.

The first aspect to discuss is the challenging task of the manual soldering of the sensor because the small profile of the SMD device packaging (LGA package) which is optimized for automatic soldering, placing the pins under its small metallic package. The second challenging task is the implementation of the USB communication due the complexity of the protocol. After some trials and failures, it has been achieved to develop a full functional USB CDC communication that can be connected to any Host device (computer or mobile) through a conventional serial port.

Focusing on the results, the sensor has been tested carrying out simple measurements of temperature, pressure, humidity and gas sensor resistance. Figure 3 show the evolution of the temperature, pressure, humidity and gas measured by the BME680 sensor during sixty seconds. The wearable sensing device has moved between three different controlled areas to detect changes and verify the correct performance of the measurements. Figure 3(a) shows an initial temperature change from 27.22 °C to 30.30 °C and a final change to 29.55 °C. Figure 3(b) shows an initial pressure of 998.90 hPa that decreased up to 996.30 hPa and then returns slowly to the initial value. Figure 3(c) shows an initial relative humidity of 16.19% that increases suddenly to 23.35% and then decreases to the initial value. Figure 3(d) shows an initial value of gas resistance of 721.30 kΩ that suddenly decreases up to 293.30 kΩ in when forcing a small leakage of methane in the air relative. The value of the gas resistance returns close to the initial value as far as the leakage ends.

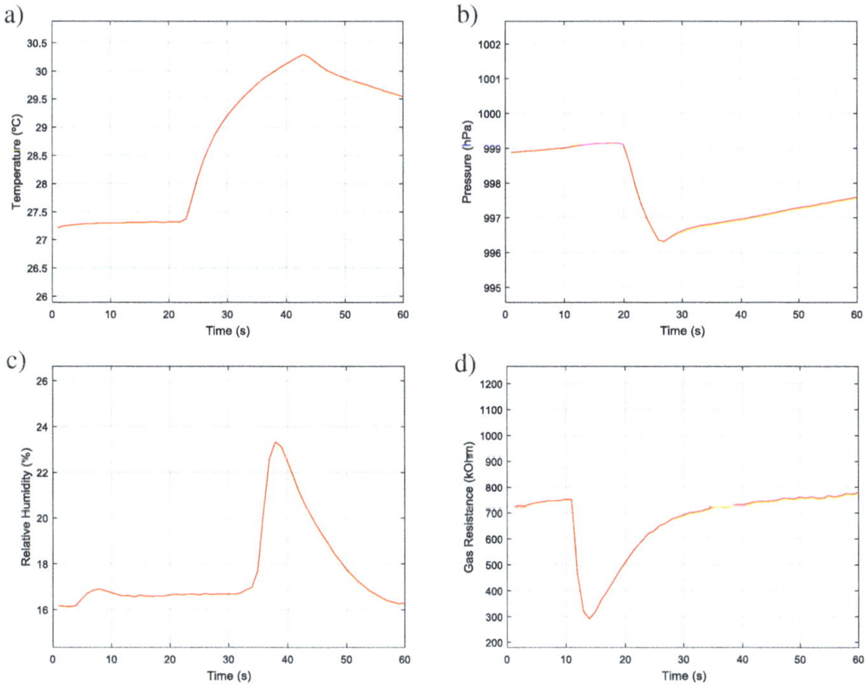

Fig. 3. Example data measurements: (a) Temperature, (b) Pressure, (c) Relative humidity, (d) Gas sensing resistance.

4 Conclusions

This paper presents the implementation of a compact wearable sensing device with temperature, pressure, humidity and gas measurement capabilities. The implementation of the automatic procedure task is able to perform periodically readings of the sensor through a SPI communication. In the other hand, it has also been implemented a USB Communication Device Class (CDC) in order to send and receive messages from the wearable sensing device. The development of these two tasks have allowed fast data readings and easy data management with connection capabilities for any Host device (computer or mobile) through a conventional serial port. Despite the difficulties on the manual soldering process of the sensor and the implementation of the USB communication, the results showed a correct measurement of temperature, pressure, humidity and gas with the BME680 sensor. The next objective will be focused on improving the wearable sensing device by adding multiple slave sensor devices in order to expand the sensing capabilities of the sensor. Then, the sensing device will include an array of BME680 sensors in order to detect and identify the presence of volatile organic compounds in the air.

Acknowledgments. This work is partially founded by the University of Lleida, UdL-Impuls 2017 grant.

References

1. Someya, T., Kato, Y., Sekitani, T., Iba, S., Noguchi, Y., Murase, Y., Kawaguchi, H., Sakurai, T.: Conformable, flexible, large-area networks of pressure and thermal sensors with organic transistor active matrixes. Nat. Acad. Sci. U.S.A. **102**(35), 12321–12325 (2005)
2. Palacín, J., Martínez, D., Clotet, E., Pallejà, T., Burgués, J., Fonollosa, J., Pardo, A., Marco, S.: Application of an array of metal-oxide semiconductor gas sensors in an assistant personal robot for early gas leak detection. Sensors **19**(9), 1957 (2019)
3. Palacín, J., Clotet, E., Martínez, D., Martínez, D., Moreno, J.: Extending the application of an assistant personal robot as a walk-helper tool. Robotics **8**, 27 (2019)
4. Shih, W.-P., Tsao, L.-C., Lee, C.-W., Cheng, M.-Y., Chang, C., Yang, Y.-J., Fan, K.-C.: Flexible temperature sensor array based on a graphite-polydimethylsiloxane composite. Sensors **10**(4), 3597–3610 (2010)
5. Gao, W., Emaminejad, S., Nyein, H.Y.Y., Challa, S., Chen, K., Peck, A., Fahad, H.M., Ota, H., Shiraki, H., Kiriya, D., Lien, D.-H., Brooks, G.A., Davis, R.W., Javey, A.: Fully integrated wearable sensor arrays for multiplexed in situ perspiration analysis. Nature **529**, 509–514 (2016)
6. Zhang, Y., Zhao, J., Du, T., Zhu, Z., Zhang, J., Liu, Q.: A gas sensor array for the simultaneous detection of multiple VOCs. Sci. Rep. **7**, 1960 (2017)
7. Caicedo, D., Pandharipande, A.: Ultrasonic array sensor for indoor presence detection. In: 20th European Signal Processing Conference (EUSIPCO 2012), pp. 175–179 (2012)

Security System Based on S.T.R.I.D.E Using Artificial Intelligence

Sergio Ordoñez(✉), Omar González(✉), Miguel Obregón(✉), Juan Mendoza(✉), and Joaquín Lara(✉)

Pedro de Alba S/N, University City, San Nicolás de los Garza, Nuevo León, Mexico
{sergio.ordonezg, omar.gonzalezest, miguel.obregonvrgs, juan.mendozamldn, joaquin.laramldn}@uanl.edu.mx

Abstract. In the last years hackers have strengthened and have taken advantage of their knowledge and skills, as well as the inappropriate use of technology to search for vulnerabilities in organizations, in order to obtain their own benefit or for third parties. It's imperative to stop this type of attacks, looking for an alternative that allows to know them and learn to classify them, to be prepared for these contingencies. This project seeks to implement a neural network as protection in a computational network. This work will use a multilayer network feedforward that is the type of classifier based on neural networks most widely studied and used. A wide dataset is used for training it and the mean square error (MSE) for the error value measurement. Recently it has been established that neural networks are a promising alternative to several classification methods.

Keywords: Artificial neural network · STRIDE · Computer attack · Multilayer network · Intrusion detection system · NSLKDD

1 Introduction

Each day is more common to hear about new technologies. It's remarkable that everyday companies depend more and more on information, technology and their communications. That's why hackers do what we know as informatic attacks, seeking to serve criminal organizations, the subversion or just for personal economics purposes [1, 2].

One solution to this problem is the use of artificial neural networks, also called multilayer perceptron that are an attractive tool (based on artificial intelligence) to solve classification problems such as pattern recognition, and as in this case, it allows detecting new dangerous packages from previously acquired knowledge [3, 4].

Even so, it is necessary to previously have a classification system for such computer packages. The STRIDE model allows to characterize known threats according to the objectives and purposes of the attacks. This term is the acronym for "Spoofing identity, Tampering with data, Repudiation, Information disclosure, Denial of service, Elevation of privilege" [5].

STRIDE acronym [6]:

(a) Spoofing: Scenario in which an X user pretends to be a user Y by changing their identity and obtains an illegal access to the data resource.

T. Ahram et al. (Eds.): IHIET 2019, AISC 1018, pp. 831–836, 2020.
https://doi.org/10.1007/978-3-030-25629-6_130

(b) Tampering: It refers to the change of data by an illegal person who is not authorized to modify it.
(c) Repudiation: The repudiation is the situation in which any user does not agree to perform an act and cannot identify the one who did it illegally.
(d) Information Disclosure: It helps an attacker or malicious user to achieve confidential information that it is not allowed.
(e) Denial of service. It is an attempt to annoy a resource, network or system in such a way that the intended and valid user cannot use it.
(f) Elevation of Privileges: It is the category of attacks in which the intruder gets the authorization more than what was originally granted.

In this way, this article seeks that the correct use of neural networks is a practical, optimal and reliable alternative for the protection of the different types of more common computer attacks, ensuring the confidentiality of the data of an organization.

2 Objective

Develop a neural network with the capacity to classify data that is not linearly separable, that is, to train the neural network with the best data options allowing it to process a greater quantity of data and results.

The neural network must be prepared to detect any type of attack corresponding to the STRIDE category. It is expected to find the best partially supervised training algorithm, so that by supervising a few data it is possible to be sure that the neural network processed the data correctly in large sets.

3 Justification

Given the information presented previously, it is proposed to use a system that automatically detects possible attacks based on the STRIDE threat model, using the data obtained from the KDD Cup 99 to have information that is already established and in this way to be able to compare the same information with the results obtained with the intrusion detection system (IDS) at the moment of running the tests.

Using an IDS to detect possible threats provides more chances to find them based on learned data during training, thanks to the generalization and learning capacity that have been determined with results obtained in previous investigations of the topic [7, 8].

4 Methodology

4.1 Requirements Analysis

When starting with the procedure of developing the neural network, should consider the following points:

- Generate a security system based on artificial intelligence, specifically using neural networks.

- A dataset should be used that covers the necessary requirements for training, as well as identifying the most appropriate values.
- The training method of the network must be optimal, reliable and effective to detect possible attacks on computer equipment and maximize certainty.
- Conduct tests to identify possible conflicts in the operation.
- The results will be checked, making sure they are the closest to the test results.

4.2 Materials

The knowledge base for the network was taken from the KDD Cup of 1999. The knowledge discovery in databases (KDD) is defined as the non-trivial extraction of implicit, previously unknown and potentially useful information of a dataset [9]. There is an organization called Association for Computing Machinery which has a special interest group in KDD. The SIGKDD annually organizes a competition for data mining and knowledge discovery always with a specific topic. In its third edition it was focused on the detection of intrusion in computer networks. The data is available to the public on the network and divides the attacks into 22 types and one "normal".

For the purposes of this article, the total population of the sample is the NSLKDD Dataset. Even so, the amount of data in this set is higher than what is required for the implementation of the neural network. That is why we selected a sample of this population, which represents it and, of course, it is intended that this sample is a true reflection of the population [10].

The database with the total population of records, has a number greater than 125,000 total records of computer packages of different types. In this case, the sample considered for the implementation of the network will be 1500 registers. Of these, 1050 records will be used for training the neural network; while, the 450 remaining registers will be applied to the trained network, for testing the optimal operation of the neural network. For sampling, a method known as stratified random sampling was used [11].

The selection led to the selection of 1500 records, with an approximate proportional to the original NSLKDD, subdividing the original NSLKDD in the 23 types of computer packages of the record. Having these groups, we proceeded to randomly select some records from each subgroup, to ensure that the 23 types of records were included in the sample. It was decided to use the programming language Python and the Spyder IDE. Both are open source and can be downloaded from their official site.

4.3 System Design

The operation of the neural network was divided into seven stages:

1. Generate random weights for network training.
2. Load the training data.
3. Perform the training.
4. Save training results.
5. Receive the input data of the possible attack to analyze.
6. Identify whether it is a possible attack, if so, identify which type of attack it is.
7. Generate and save results.

4.4 Testing

The first tests were focused on the entry of data through text files which facilitated having to capture each record individually, it was mainly started with CSV (comma-separated values) extension files, but having problems reading this extension it was decided to use the text files maintaining the comma delimited format.

The following tests were then focused on reading and printing the weights generated to document them, testing the collected information and verifying the efficiency of the function and the percentage of the success rate, initializing with values that were far from zero and a minimum number of iterations. Also, the neural network was tested with different quantities of data records (Fig. 1).

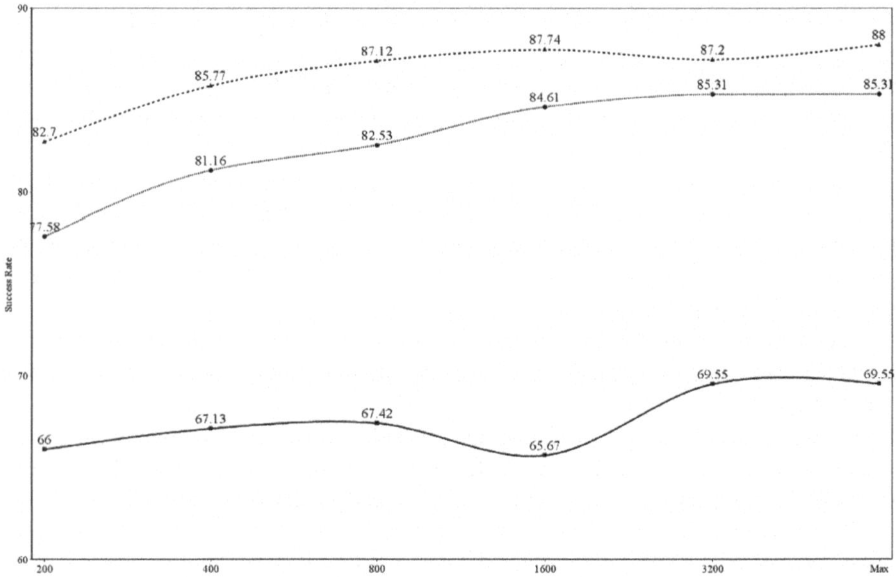

Fig. 1. Success Rate Percentages for the tests with different iterations and quantities of records. *300 records continue line. 900 records dotted line. 1500 records discontinuous line.*

The following values were obtained as success percentage for each case:

Finally, the application was started without a data file to verify that it is necessary to create it from the beginning in order to avoid an error. It checks if the value obtained from the read text file is empty and if the application has data, it could continue the tests without the need to train.

5 Results

During the execution of the program variable results were obtained, it has noticed these changes were due to the random weights generated and the number of iterations that were made for the algorithm to calculate the optimal model. The results are delivered by the system as follows:

```
Optimization terminated successfully.
  Current function value: 0.000218
  Iterations: 3960
  Function evaluations: 3983
  Gradient evaluations: 3983
```

With these values it can be said that the neural network under these training conditions has a success rate of 88%.

This percentage is calculated in this way:

$$\text{Individual Success Rate} = (\text{Result/Expected Result}) * 100. \quad (1)$$

$$\text{Individual Error Rate} = |100 - \text{Individual Success Rate}|. \quad (2)$$

$$\text{Error Rate} = \frac{1}{n}\sum\nolimits_{l=1}^{n} IER_i. \quad (3)$$

$$\text{Success Rate} = 100 - \text{Error Rate}. \quad (4)$$

For the outputs to be closer with a higher success rate, a greater amount of preselected and classified data would have to be used at the time of training, as well as the percentage of attacks should be more equitable since as can be seen in the subject section the amount of attack types varies a lot. This causes that the difference in quantities of training cases generates a possible error in the attack identification tests.

It can be determined then that, although it does not have a success rate of 100%, the network is sufficiently intelligent to identify the attacks.

6 Discussion

It is foreseen that in future tests it will be possible to use more of the data obtained from the dataset in order to prove that the artificial neural network can be more accurate and should promote the use of this type of systems for the identification of possible threats. This could convert the organizational systems in the area of information security in specialized high-tech sectors, eradicating future attacks, since it would look for a possible self-learning of the systems, detecting new attacks and avoiding throwing false positives.

In addition to this, an evolutionary algorithm could be used to evaluate the system, and thus be able to find the dataset that optimizes the network discarding the weakest sets, and therefore yield better results when it comes to identifying the computer information packages.

References

1. Gacharná, F.I.: Hacker ético vs. delincuente informático: Una mirada en el contexto colombiano. INVENTUM **4**(6), 46–49 (2009). https://doi.org/10.26620/uniminuto.inventum.4.6.2009.46-49
2. Mieres, J.: Debilidades de seguridad comúnmente explotadas (2009). By de http://proton.ucting.udg.mx/tutorial/hackers/hacking.pdf
3. Goddard Close, J., Martinez Licona, A.E.: Definición de una red neuronal para clasificación por medio de un programa. Revista Mexicana de Ingeniería Biomédica (1), 4–11 (2001)
4. Benchimol, D.: Hacking desde Cero. RedUsersUsershop, Buenos Aires (2011)
5. Aissa, A.B., Mouna, J., Rabai, L.B.: Classification of security threats in information systems. Procedia Comput. Sci. **32**, 489–496 (2014)
6. Khan, S.: Fuzzy STRIDE model based on werners aggregation operator for computer network threat modelling. Int. J. Comput. Digit. Syst. **6**, 83–88 (2017). https://doi.org/10.12785/IJCDS/060204
7. Britto Montoya, J.A., Isaza Echeverry, G.A., Pérez Rivera, C.A.: Aplicación de Redes Neuronales para la Detección de Intrusos en Redes y Sistemas de Información. Scientia et Technica, X **I**(27), 225–230 (2005)
8. Gupta, R., Paliwal, S.: Denial-of-service, probing & remote to user (R2L) attack detection using genetic algorithm. Int. J. Comput. Appl. **60**(19) (2012). Obtenido de https://pdfs.semanticscholar.org/060d/0c18c3f490720b62e40e7003aa7f75d50941.pdf
9. Frawley, W.J., Matheus, C.J., Piatetsky-Shapiro, G.: Knowledge discovery in databases: an overview. AI Mag. **13**(3), 57–70 (1992)
10. Mata, M.C., Macassi, S.: Cómo elaborar muestras para los sondeos de audiencias, vol. V. ALER, Quito (1997)
11. Casal, J., Mateu, E.: Tipos de muestreo. Barcelona Rev. Epidem. Med. Prev. **1**, 3–7 (2003)

A Method for Audience Extending in Programmatic Advertising by Using Parsimonious Generalization of User Segments

Dmitry Frolov[1(✉)], Zina Taran[2], and Boris Mirkin[1,3]

[1] Department of Data Analysis and Artificial Intelligence, National Research University Higher School of Economics, Moscow, Russian Federation
{dfrolov,bmirkin}@hse.ru
[2] Department of Management, Marketing and Business Admin, Delta State University, Cleveland, MS, USA
ztaran@deltastate.edu
[3] Department of Computer Science, Birkbeck University of London, London, UK

Abstract. We propose a novel method for efficient target audience augmentation in programmatic digital advertising. This method utilizes a novel ParGenFS algorithm for most adequate generalization in taxonomies which was developed by the authors in a joint work. The ParGenFS extends user segments by parsimoniously lifting them off-line as a fuzzy set over IAB content taxonomy into a higher rank 'head subject'. This algorithm was initially intended as an intelligent information retrieval tool. Here it is applied to a very different task of targeted advertisement as an effective tool for augmenting audiences.

Keywords: Programmatic advertising · Targeting · Audience extending · Taxonomy · Generalization

1 Introduction

Programmatic is a novel digital advertisement approach bringing real-time bidding to allow an advertiser to make their purchasing decisions separately for every contact with every user [5, 6, 8]. A real-time bidding system provides an auction for the advertisement impression between multiple advertisers, and each advertiser has a possibility to buy relevant audience only [7, 9, 10]. The audience is classified into segments by user interests, and an advertiser can choose which user segments will be appropriate for them. The segments come from an industrial taxonomy such as IAB (see https://www.iab.com/). Advertising system has to detect users belonging to these segments and provide advertisement impressions for them. Usually, it is done via segment membership weights computed for individual users based on their page visiting behavior [5]. Unfortunately, this approach may fail in providing a sufficient size of the audience because the segments specified for an advertisement campaign appear to be too narrow. Current approaches to augmenting the audience by decreasing the within-segment thresholds or by applying the so-called look-a-like techniques, frequently lead to much

T. Ahram et al. (Eds.): IHIET 2019, AISC 1018, pp. 837–841, 2020.
https://doi.org/10.1007/978-3-030-25629-6_131

diminishing response rates [4]. We propose a novel method for efficient target audience augmentation in programmatic digital advertising. This method utilizes a novel ParGenFS algorithm for most adequate generalization in taxonomies (see, for example, [1]), to extend user segments by parsimoniously lifting them off-line over IAB content taxonomy into a higher rank 'head subject'. This algorithm was proposed as an intelligent information retrieval tool [1]. Here it is applied to a very different task of targeted advertisement. The next Sect. 2 describes our approach, with a background of conventional approaches to targeted advertising. Section 3 describes results of several real-world experiments comparing the conventional approaches and GUS. It appears, our method GUS does increase the number of successful matches between user segments and campaign segments 2.5-3-fold without losing in the targeting quality (click through rate, CTR).

2 Algorithm GUS for Generalization of User Profiles

Our algorithm, Generalization of User Segments (GUS), works over an industrial taxonomy, specifically, the IAB taxonomy [2]. This taxonomy covers all the conventional needs and things as a 4-layer rooted tree whose nodes are labeled by taxonomy topics. Its leaves are referred to as segments further on. A partial fragment of Style and Fashion segment from the IAB taxonomy is presented in Fig. 1.

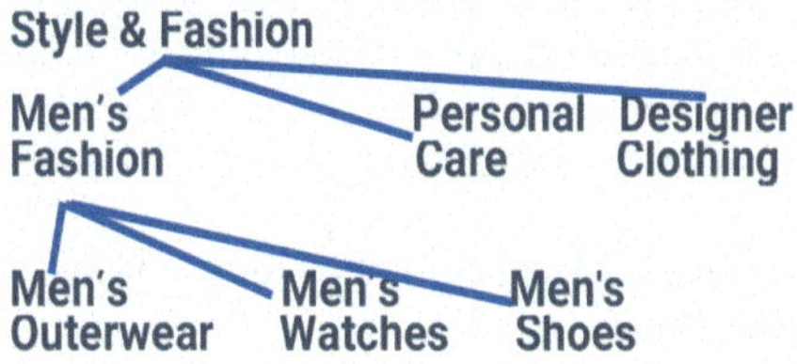

Fig. 1. A partial fragment of the IAB taxonomy

We consider a company, such as start-up Natimatica, Ltd. (see https://natimatica.com) associated with us, that supports a service of native advertising. This service follows millions of individual users visiting popular sites providing news, shopping, specific contents, etc. Information of these users is stored in a special system, Data Management Platform (DMP).

It is assumed that each individual user in the DMP is assigned with a subset of IAB segments relevant to their visits. Each of the segments s is assigned with a real number rs, a fraction of unity, according to the history of the user's visits to the sites under our observation. The history is reflected in texts from the visited pages. These texts are stored and transformed into a numerical format [3], and then classified using a special Random Forest classifier [10] into segments of the IAB taxonomy, thus leading to fuzzy membership values as assigned to them, for each of the users. The totality of the taxonomy segments and membership values assigned to them constitute what can be referred to as the user's profile.

Our next assumption relates to the advertiser. It is assumed that the advertiser can formulate their advert needs as a set of IAB leaves (segments) relevant to the advert. In practice, such a formulation is produced manually by a specially assigned employee, after a detailed discussion of the advert with the advertiser.

Before we formulate our proposed approach to selection of the audience for every specific advertisement, let us formulate a conventional, currently most popular, approach. This approach (CAS) requires to pre-specify a threshold t (usually, t = 0.3 or t = 0.4) and formulate a condition A(t): Given a set S of taxonomy segments and a user's profile, check if the profile has at least one of the S segments with the value rs assigned to them so that rs > t. Then the CAS rule requires to expose the advert involving set S of taxonomy segments, to all those users for whom condition A(t) holds.

An issue with CAS is that the number of users satisfying condition A(t) may be less than the number specified in the advertisement order; say, they want to show their advert to a million users, but only three hundred thousand of those under observation satisfy A(t). In this case, a conventional strategy is to have CAS extended (CASE) by lessening t to t°, t° < t, so that more users satisfy condition A(t°) than A(t). This may increase the number of users exposed to the advert, but it is not warranted that the efficiency remains the same: usually, the added users have a weaker tendency to be impressed by the advert.

Therefore, we propose a different strategy, Generalization of User Segments (GUS) to obtain a set of users to apply condition A(t) to. Specifically, our software preprocesses off-line every user profile by finding one (or, rarely, more) higher-rank taxonomy node generalizing the profile. To this end, we developed a special algorithm, ParGenFS, for finding the most appropriate generalization of fuzzy profile S in the taxonomy [1]. This algorithm "lifts" S to its "head subject", a node in the higher ranks of the taxonomy tree. The head subject is supposed to "tightly" cover the profile S, possibly bringing in some errors, both "gaps" and "offshoots". A gap is a node covered by the head subject but not being in S (1st type error). An offshoot is a node in S, which is not covered by the head subject (2d type error). ParGenFS method globally minimizes a penalty function combining the numbers of head subjects and gaps and offshoots, differently weighted by penalty weights and fuzzy membership values. This method works recursively bottom-up from tree leaves to the root by selecting, at each step, either of two scenarios and corresponding events: (1) the head subject has emerged in the node; or (2) the head subject has not emerged in the node. An example of ParGenFS' results is presented in Fig. 2. Therefore, our strategy GUS for testing condition A(t) is to apply it not to the segment concerned but rather to the head subject derived off-line.

3 Experimental Findings

The follow-up Table 1 presents comparative results of testing our GUS method at real life advertising campaigns in Natimatica, Ltd. Recall three targeting methods under consideration:

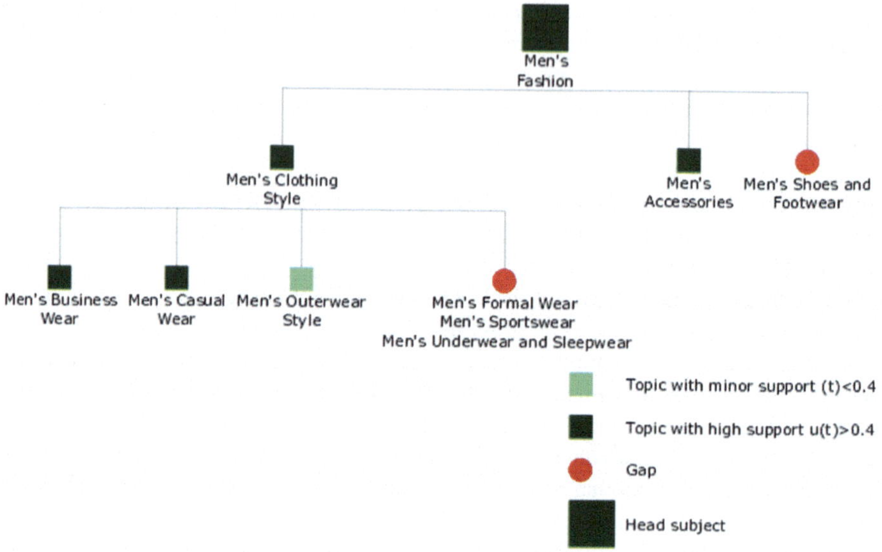

Fig. 2. Illustrative generalization of a profile into "Men's Fashion" head subject.

Table 1. Comparative results of the targeting techniques.

Campaign	Campaign IAB segments	Metric	CAS method	CASE method	GUS method
1. Software for parental control of children. *Duration: 10 days*	{Daycare and Pre-School, Internet Safety, Parenting Children Aged 4–11, Parenting Teens, Antivirus Software}	Impressions	378933	1017598 (+168.5%)	942104 (+148.6%)
		Clicks	1061	1526 (+43.8%)	2544 (+139.8%)
		CTR, %	0.28	0.15 (−46.4%)	0.27 (−3.6%)
2. Frame houses for villages *Duration: 4 days*	{Gardening, Remodeling & Construction, Landscaping, Outdoor Decorating, Houses}	Impressions	87599	160204 (+82.9%)	153032 (+74.7%)
		Clicks	201	288 (+43.3%)	367 (+82.6%)
		CTR, %	0.24	0.18 (−25.0%)	0.24 (+0.0%)
3. Mortgage at a major Russian bank *Duration: 10 days*	{Home Financing, Personal Loans}	Impressions	159342	275035 (+72.6%)	289308 (+81.6%)
		Clicks	749	853 (+13.9%)	1302 (+73.9%)
		CTR, %	0.47	0.31 (−34.0%)	0.45 (−4.3%)

1. Conventional programmatic targeting based on matching segments (CAS);
2. Audience extending by decreasing thresholds (CASE);
3. Audience extending by generalization of user segments (GUS).

Table 1 presents results obtained by application of each of the three targeting methods at three real world advertising campaigns differing by the subject, duration, and the format of "creatives" [5]. In Campaigns 1 and 2, creatives were usual textual graphical blocks. In Campaign 3, the advertiser used more expensive in-read creatives [5], usually leading to higher efficiency due to larger area taken and extended interaction with users.

The comparison criteria are: (a) advertising impressions obtained, (b) numbers of clicks, and (3) click through rates (CTR, (b)/(a)). The last metric is especially meaningful, because it characterizes the quality of the audience impressed by the advertisement. At CASE method, the lessened threshold values were chosen to have audience sizes approximately equal to those emerged at the GUS method.

The results in Table 1 clearly show that our method GUS significantly outperforms the conventional strategies in terms of the targeting quality.

References

1. Frolov, D., Nascimento, S., Fenner, T., Mirkin, B.: Finding an appropriate generalization for a fuzzy thematic set in taxonomy, Working paper WP7/2018/04, Moscow, Higher School of Economics Publ. House, 60 p. (2018). https://wp.hse.ru/data/2019/01/13/1146987922/WP7_2018_04________.pdf
2. IAB Tex Lab Content Taxonomy. https://www.iab.com/guidelines/iab-quality-assurance-guidelines-qag-taxonomy/. Accessed 5 Apr 2019
3. Le, Q., Mikolov, T.: Distributed representations of sentences and documents. In: Proceedings of the 31st International Conference on Machine Learning, ICML 2014, pp. 1188–1196 (2014)
4. Popov, A., Iakovleva, D.: Adaptive look-alike targeting in social networks advertising. Procedia Comput. Sci. **136**, 255–264 (2018)
5. Leung, D.: Digital advertising: theory and research. Shelly Rodgers and Esther Thorson, pp. 457–460 (2017)
6. Li, X., Guan, D.: Programmatic buying bidding strategies with win rate and winning price estimation in real time mobile advertising. In: Pacific-Asia Conference on Knowledge Discovery and Data Mining. Springer, Cham, pp. 447–460 (2014)
7. OpenRTB Protocol. https://www.iab.com/guidelines/real-time-bidding-rtb-project/. Accessed 5 Apr 2019
8. Sayedi, A.: Real-time bidding in online display advertising. Mark. Sci. **37**(4), 553–568 (2018)
9. Wang, J., Yuan, S., Zhang, W.: Real-time bidding based display advertising: mechanisms and algorithms. In: European Conference on Information Retrieval, pp. 897–901. Springer, Cham (2016)
10. Yuan, Y., Wang, F., Li, J., Qin, R.: A survey on real time bidding advertising. In: 2014 IEEE International Conference on Service Operations and Logistics, and Informatics (SOLI), pp. 418–423. IEEE (2014)

Continuous Improvement Model for Inventory Planning Applying MRP II in Small and Medium Sized Enterprises

Hugo Villafuerte[1(✉)], Gino Viacava[1(✉)], and Carlos Raymundo[2(✉)]

[1] Ingeniería Industrial,
Universidad Peruana de Ciencias Aplicadas (UPC), Lima, Peru
{u201111539, pcingvia}@upc.edu.pe
[2] Dirección de Investigación,
Universidad Peruana de Ciencias Aplicadas (UPC), Lima, Peru
carlos.raymundo@upc.edu.pe

Abstract. Planning of resources is a powerful tool in the field of supply chain management and control and in general. Global large-scale companies and enterprises have this implemented in their planning processes. Today, experts in the subject have found issues regarding the implementation of such tools in small- and medium-sized enterprises (SMEs). Therefore, this paper aims to develop an application for the methodology of continual improvement of processes, referred to as the Deming cycle or Plan–Do–Check–Act (PDCA), which adapts to continuous improvements of processes and products in SMEs. The methodology was modeled in a SME dedicated to manufacture and distribution of wine and products (wine and Pisco). The model was simulated through a simulation software, obtaining results of improvement regarding problems like break of stock, taking into account the satisfaction of the client, productivity in the delivery, and shipment time.

Keywords: Supply chain · MRP II · PDCA · Deming cycle · SMEs · Break of stock · Pisquera

1 Introduction

Planning management is a key process of the organization and the supply chain focused on the coordination and effectiveness in the management of materials necessary for a company's various activities [1]. Therefore, past research has studied production planning strategic decisions to enable achieving greater productivity in production areas [2]. In developing a resource planning model for small and medium sized enterprises (SMEs), researchers consider the capacity of the SMEs in question; however, various techniques may not necessarily integrate well in a wine company [3].

This article proposes a manufacturing resource planning (MRP) model for SMEs in the wine industry, based on the use of PDCA as continuous improvement method and manufacturing material requirement. This model aims to respond to issues related to the failure in delivering orders to customers and raw material stock outs [4]. The main product is pisco, a Peruvian wine product [5].

T. Ahram et al. (Eds.): IHIET 2019, AISC 1018, pp. 842–848, 2020.
https://doi.org/10.1007/978-3-030-25629-6_132

2 Literature Review

To propose a viable solution to a company's resource planning, we conducted a literature review [6].

Research Methodology

The wine and pisco companies of Ica were analyzed because they are the most industrialized in pisco production [5]. According to Baeza [7], the collected information was used for the conceptualization of the model (Fig. 1).

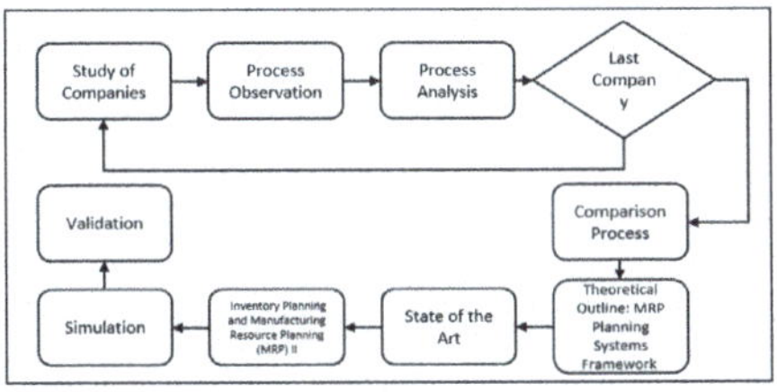

Fig. 1. Research methodology. Based on [7]

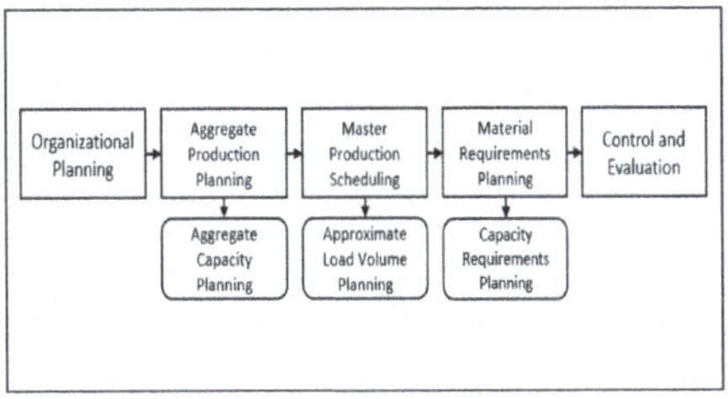

Fig. 2. MRP II implementation system

MRP II

Is a method used for planning the management and use of company's manufacturing resources for production. The Fig. 2 presents the integration of the MRP model with demand planning, master plan control, and other deliverables within the same system manufacturing resource planning [8]. The study has concluded that these tools are limited in the sustainability of their implementation over time [9]. Therefore, the methodology of continuous improvement (Plan–Do–Check–Act: PDCA), or the Deming cycle, will be used for the continuous improvement of these procedures [10].

Supplier Management

The company's supplier and purchasing management is based on the responsiveness of these suppliers and the level of customer service of these intermediaries in supplying the production lines [1].

Inventory Management

Inventory management is defined as the proper management of the input and output flow of products in a company [11].

3 Contribution

The novelty of this contribution is in the implementation of three improvement tools that complement each other in a continuous improvement cycle known as the PDCA or Deming cycle. These tools are MRP II, identification of value chain wastes, and supplier relationship management [1].

We present a case study of a producer and marketer of Peruvian wine products, specifically of wine and pisco [5].

The Fig. 3 below represents the proposed production planning model of this research.

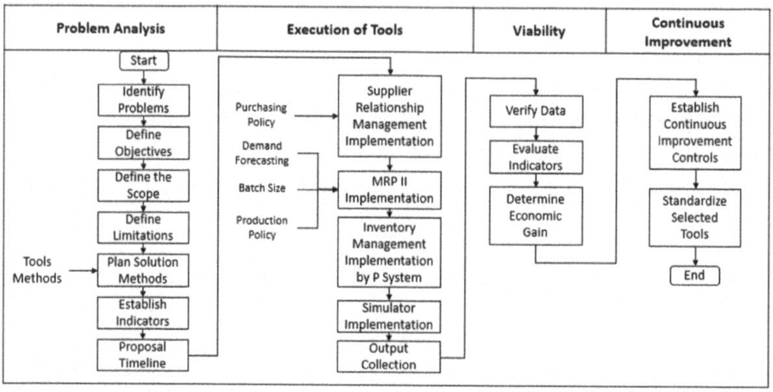

Fig. 3. Procedure of the production planning model

Phase 1: Problem Analysis

In the first phase, the organization establishes the key elements for the methodology implementation [9].

- Objectives: The main objective and specific objectives pursued after implementing the model need to be established, and the problem must be correctly identified [12].
- Defining the scope: The scope of the inventory management model must be treated as the highest point of reference that research can cover.
- Defining limitations: The types of impediments generated throughout the implementation of this model must be specified [12].
- Plan solution methods:
  - MRP II: It is necessary to plan the activity that will be carried out within each MRP II deliverable because it has several outputs that feed the master plan and the total list of materials [13]: Bill of Materials (BOM), Aggregate Production Planning (APP), Inventory Status (INV), Demand Forecasting (DEM), Production Master Scheduling (MPS), and Capacity Requirements Planning (CRP).
  - Supplier Policy: Consists of qualifying different suppliers and objectively analyzing them as per a rating scale [14]. Six aspects need to be evaluated: compliance and delivery, product quality and delivery, documentation and warranties, after-sales service, price, technical support.
  - Inventory Management: The P system will be applied, which is a periodic review system used to review the inventory quantity of a product, if it supplies future orders by means of demand management [15].
- Establishing indicators: It is used to evaluate whether corrections have been successfully implemented, as they measure the improvement or reduction of an aspect of the studied process.
- Proposal Timeline: A proposal timeline must be established, as it is important to determine the implementation duration of the production management model.

Phase 2: Execution of Tools

In this phase, all the activities that have been planned in the first phase are carried out.

- Execution of methods: The three proposed tools will be implemented to improve the model, taking into account an estimated time of MPS timeline.
- Data collection: After the simulation, the most common results will be collected to be analyzed in the next phase.

Phase 3: Viability

This phase aims to examine the simulation results with the data established in the plan, to validate whether the objectives are being achieved as planned [16].

- Verification of the results: The simulation data must corroborate and at least achieve the proposed simulation objectives to be considered a successful implementation.
- Determining the economic gain: The economic gain was calculated with a cash flow tabulation to bring objectivity to the project and ensure a good implementation in an SME.

Phase 4: Continuous Improvement

The last phase consists of rethinking objectives and standardizing what has worked.

- Continuous Improvement Controls: In the case studied, the batch quantity of the MPS of MRP II is changed depending on the type of product and on the product seasonal demand [11].

4 Validation

The applicability of this model proposed in an organization enables verifying its effectiveness and viability.

Manufacturing Resource Planning

The five deliverables already established in the planning phase 1 will be taken into account: Demand forecasting (organizational plan), Aggregate production plan, Master production scheduling, Bill of materials, Evaluation and Control.

Inventory Management

Thus, the analysis of inventories to supply the demand will be maintained and carried out on a weekly basis to cover the entire quantity of products, which are 240 for the pisco product, well monitored through resource planning covering all products. The standard deviation will be used to calculate the maximum inventory of a product and the safety inventory, as shown in Table 2 of the periodic inventory system analysis (Table 1).

This tool was implemented to maintain reduced inventory sizes and obtain a more accurate capacity of safety inventories that protect the company from changes in demand.

Table 1. Inventory result table

Pisco type	SS (units)	Max M (unit)
100A quebranta	4,272	5,014
PG quebranta	87,930	104,646
GP Quebranta	801	1,603
100A acholado	10,589	11,033
PG Acholado	3,895	6,011

Simulation

After the technical implementation of the proposed tools, the proposal stimulation will be implemented. The simulation was carried out in the Arena simulator software, with the aim to provide designers with the service to carry out process modeling works by taking into account all the variables necessary for supply chain management. The variables used and their origin from the tools implemented in phase 2, Execution of Tools, are as follows:

- Inventory → inventory management
- Production → MPS
- Batchsize → Batch size (aggregate capacity plan)
- Target stock → M Max (maximum inventory)
- Demand → Demand management (MRP II)
- OTIF indicators → delivered in full, on time.
- Reorder point → Supplier relationship management and inventory management.
- Order quantity → Sales order to the customer

This information will be used for implementing the simulation, which have two parts of the simulation: order management and bottling. This phase is important for evaluating the changes in improvement after implementation. In total, 25 runs were used to analyze on a varied demand and different data, mainly changing the variables of order quantity and estimated lead time (which should not exceed five days).

Evaluation of Results

After executing the planning model in the simulation, we evaluated the results identified as follows:

- Increase in the lead time from bottling to delivery to the customer.
- Increases in OTIF indicators (service levels).
- Reduction of batch sizes and reduction of associated costs.
- Improved product flow.
- Reduction of orders rejected due to delays.

In addition, there is a monetary saving generated two weeks after implementation, as presented in Table 3.

Table 2. Simulation results

Indicator	Objective	Before	After
IN FULL	>95%	89.24%	96.65%
ON TIME	>91%	82.54%	91.55%
Stock Coverage	>80%	59.12%	77.53%
Supplier Service	<15%	22.66%	14.59%
Supplier Certification	>70%	22.60%	55%

Table 3. Weekly improvement savings

	Before/week	After/week	Savings
Orders Rejected due to Delay	S/17,192,31	S/8,931.23	S/8,261.08
Orders Rejected due to Insufficient Quantity	S/15,695.74	S/4,592.82	S/11,102.92
		Total	S/19,364.00

5 Conclusions

Because there are several proposals for improvement in the literature, this research proposes a model that is more focused on SMEs, as is the wine company studied.

The innovation of this contribution lies in uniting three management tools under a continuous improvement methodology: Manufacturing Resource Planning Tool (MRPII), Supplier Evaluation, and Inventory Management, all of which are based on the PDCA cycle phases. The success of this model consists of improvements in the indicators proposed for analysis, OTIF indicators, ON-TIME service level indicator up to 96% and a 91% improvement for the company's IN FULL service level. Thus, the research objectives have been met.

References

1. Gong, Q., Yang, Y., Wang, S.: Information and decision-making delays in MRP, KANBAN, and CONWIP. Int. J. Prod. Econ. **156**, 208–213 (2014)
2. Benton, W.C., Shin, H.: Manufacturing planning and control: the evolution of MRP and JIT integration. Eur. J. Oper. Res. **110**(3), 411–440 (1998)
3. Koh, S.C.L., Saad, S.M.: Managing uncertainty in ERP-controlled manufacturing environments in SMEs. Int. J. Prod. Econ. **101**, 109–127 (2006)
4. Siddique, P.J., Luong, H.T.: An optimal joint maintenance and spare parts inventory model. Int. J. Ind. Syst. Eng. **29**(2), 177 (2018)
5. Vázquez-Rowe, I., Cáceres, A.L., Torres-García, J.R., Quispe, I., Kahhat, R.: Life cycle assessment of the production of pisco in Peru. J. Clean. Prod. **142**, 4369–4383 (2016)
6. Hidayat, R., Akhmad, S.: Implementation of Enterprise Resource Planning System in Manufacturing Firm in Indonesia **7**(4), 1434–1440 (2017)
7. Baeza Serrato, R.: REDUTEX: a hybrid push-pull production system approach for reliable delivery time in knitting SMEs. Prod. Planning Control **27**(4), 263–279 (2016)

8. Chan, C.K.D., Yung, K.L., Ip, W.H.: The implementation of a model for integration of MRP II and TQM. Integr. Manuf. Syst. **10**(5), 298–305 (1999)
9. Garza-Reyes, J.A., Torres Romero, J., Govindan, K., Cherrafi, A., Ramanathan, U.: A PDCA-based approach to Environmental Value Stream Mapping (EVSM). J. Cleaner Prod. **180**, 335–348 (2018)
10. Lapide, L.: Competitive supply chains: excellence. Supply Chain Manage. Rev. **6**, 4–5 (2015)
11. Singh, D., Verma, A.: Inventory management in supply chain. Mater. Today: Proc. **5**(2), 3867–3872 (2018)
12. Demissie, A., Zhu, W., Kitaw, D., Matebu, A.: Quality assessment and improvement for Ethiopian garment enterprises. J. Ind. Prod. Eng. **34**(6), 450–460 (2017)
13. Miclo, R., Fontanili, F., Lauras, M., Lamothe, J., Milian, B.: An empirical comparison of MRPII and Demand-Driven MRP. IFAC-PapersOnLine **49**(12), 1725–1730 (2016)
14. Yang, F., Zhang, X.: The impact of sustainable supplier management practices on buyer-supplier performance: an empirical study in China. Rev. Int. Bus. Strat. **27**(1), 112–132 (2017)
15. Zare, R., Chavez, P., Raymundo, C., Rojas, J.: Collaborative culture management model to improve the performence in the inventory management of a supply chain. 2018 Congreso Internacional de Innovacion y Tendencias en Ingenieria, CONIITI 2018 (2018)

Project Planning Methodology Based on Lean Philosophy and PMBOK Guidelines for SMEs in the Electricity Sector

Denisse Bazán[1(✉)], Marco Pinedo[1(✉)], José Rojas[1(✉)], and Carlos Raymundo[2(✉)]

[1] Ingeniería de Gestión Empresarial, Universidad Peruana de Ciencias Aplicadas (UPC), Lima, Peru
{u201410153,u201312872,jose.rojas}@upc.edu.pe
[2] Dirección de Investigación, Universidad Peruana de Ciencias Aplicadas (UPC), Lima, Peru
carlos.raymundo@upc.edu.pe

Abstract. Currently, businesses implementing electrical projects lack the theoretical knowledge of ways to correctly develop the projects given that they are based on empirical knowledge. Consequently, a need has developed to implement lean philosophy and project management as distinctive and renowned pillars to ensure high competitiveness in the market of the sector under study. Through case studies, the literature on the subject demonstrated the importance of proper planning based on cost and time pillars. These pillars were analyzed using Ishikawa tools and a problem tree. The following lean tools were chosen: 5S, visual management, and quality circles. These tools and the project management guidelines, specifically the 47 processes published in the 5th edition of the Project Management Body of Knowledge, were applied as a model proposal at a pilot company in which the results of how this combination of solutions reduces delivery times for that organization were compared.

Keywords: Lean project · PMI · Electrical projects · Planning process group

1 Introduction

Small and medium enterprises (SMEs) play an important role in the national economy. They employ 75% of the economically active population (EAP). SMEs represent 96.5% of businesses in Peru, employing more than 8 million Peruvians. This sector contributes to 19.2% of the total production in Peru, 32.1% of which is in metropolitan Lima [1–3]. Due to the concentration of economic activity in the different sectors managed by the country, each company must develop projects for their improvement according to their degree of difficulty and orientation, among other factors.

The electricity sector has experienced remarkable improvements in the last 15 years; accordingly, electrical energy is considered to be a variable that measures regional competitiveness in the country [4]. However, the majority of companies that perform electrification and electrical maintenance do not have access to tools employed by large businesses in their expansion processes. This makes it difficult to commercialize their

T. Ahram et al. (Eds.): IHIET 2019, AISC 1018, pp. 849–855, 2020.
https://doi.org/10.1007/978-3-030-25629-6_133

products and services [5]. Therefore, many projects are not realized due to their improper preparation resulting from material delivery times, unqualified labor, unsuitable workplaces, among other factors.

Accordingly, due to their importance, the national context is demanding rapid responses. Considering strong competition, the time factor becomes a positioning variable in the market. These organizations undertake projects; however, in general, professionals dedicated to project planning possess extensive technical knowledge but limited project management skills [6].

In the current environment, projects have to decrease costs, increase productivity, reduce waste, satisfy even the most demanding clients, improve safety, and be profitable [7]. Using lean philosophy tools and the Project Management Body of Knowledge (PMBOK) guidelines, this study proposes proper project planning to contribute to the economic growth of the electricity sector.

2 State of the Art

2.1 Literature Review

Victor Saravanana et al. [8] revealed that lean tools such as 5S, visual management, and work standardization reduce the time between placing an order and the final product's delivery time by eliminating mudas observed at the beginning of the project during product manufacturing. However, to test new lean techniques, they applied SMED since they considered it to be one of the fastest technique not only in execution but also in implementation in the manufacturing process. This tool was implemented in an injection molding machine because it was identified as a bottleneck in the production process. Consequently, the total time required to perform configuration activities in the selected manufacturing system was reduced by approximately 1623 s. Furthermore, the percentage of reduction in the total configuration time achieved was 67.72%.

2.1.1 Project Management

Several organizations worldwide have published project management guidelines, including the International Organization for Standardization (ISO), Project Management Institute (PMI), Office of Government Commerce (OGC) in the United Kingdom (PRINCE2 guidelines), among others. The set of project management guidelines chosen in this study to evaluate lean manufacturing projects corresponds to the guidelines from the 5th edition of PMBOK. While the PMI is a private organization, their guidelines include all the principals of sound project management. Their selection is justified given that their guidelines are most extensively used in the market [9].

2.1.2 Lean Philosophy

According to Hong, Yang and Dobrzykowski (2014), these practices indicate that lean philosophy focuses on the systematic elimination of an organization's operational waste through a set of synergistic working practices to produce goods and services with the necessary quality within the delivery times required by the client [10, 11].

5S: Agrahari et al. (2015) concurred that 5S is often understood as a simple cleaning and organization strategy. However, this tool can be a powerful application to develop a successful business by implementing a new standard for workplace practices. Many organizations not only apply 5S as the first step to move toward lean but also emphasize eliminating wait times and activities that do not add value [12].

Visual Management: Different definitions of visual management exist in the literature, highlighting different perspectives that have been adopted in its conceptualization. Some authors described the tool as a simple and attractive communication approach made using various devices such as bulletin boards, slogans, indicator lights, cards and display units. Another group of authors emphasized that the tool is part of performance measurement systems. It is manifested as a communication and information center for all employees to understand the strategic directions, performance, and results of organizational improvement initiatives [13].

3 Method

This study focuses on the proper implantation of project planning processes. With increasing competition, responsibility and the relentless need to generate added value and be efficient continue to pressurize organizations. Furthermore, the need for planning and control tools such as project management is constantly increasing. People's desire for competitiveness and the best value in everything pressurizes organizations. However, organization can meet these needs only by effectively using project management in their day-to-day operations. The following figure outlines how the project will unfold.

First, the condition of every activity that is part of planning an electrical project is assessed. For this action, the proposal is based on a flowchart that indicates the correlation of actions to implement a project. This is followed by an analysis of some of the activities' problems using a problem tree to examine the consequences that these generate in the project implementation process.

Second, a formal proposal is made to the company, which is outlined in an act of commitment that formally makes the improvement proposal for the selected SME.

Third, after making model specifications, the project's objectives and those of the company must be correlated to determine the new resources required.

Fourth, once the staff is trained, new forms for purchase orders, sales orders, project closures, and project charters must be created. All these forms must be aligned with the information system, which has a vital role throughout the entire project, as it will serve as a future documentation to implement new projects

Finally, plans are made for the new project. The progress level of the improved activities is evaluated from two perspectives. First, KPIs play a fundamental role in achieving the objectives set out in the first phase. The second perspective considers an empirical context for staff by sending out weekly quality newsletters in which topics of productivity, quality, and new projects are addressed (Fig. 1).

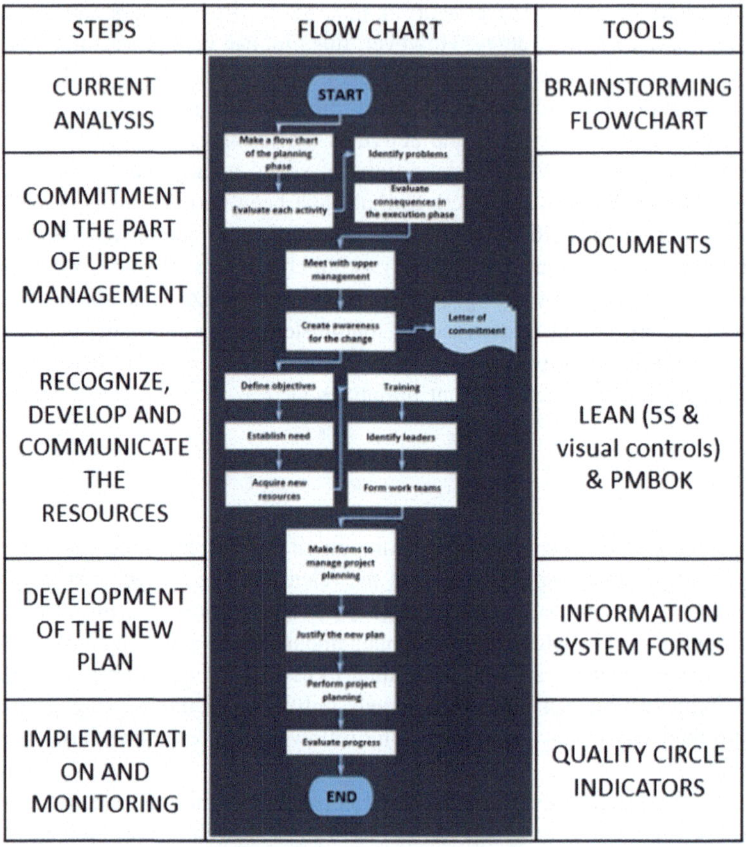

Fig. 1. Methodology flowchart

4 Results

4.1 Contribution

4.1.1 Model Design

A requirement has been observed in the electricity sector in accordance with the research conducted to develop the model and based on studies. Therefore, the development of the archetype must be executed from the client's perspective while understanding that time, cost, and quality are often considered to be the criteria for a project's achievement. These variables determine a project's success. In the majority of cases, it is not possible to maximize or minimize these criteria. A project manager's goal is to reach a satisfactory balance among the three.

Accordingly, this proposed model could represent a balance of time, cost, and performance for a newly planned product, which entails a series of requirements made by the client (Fig. 2).

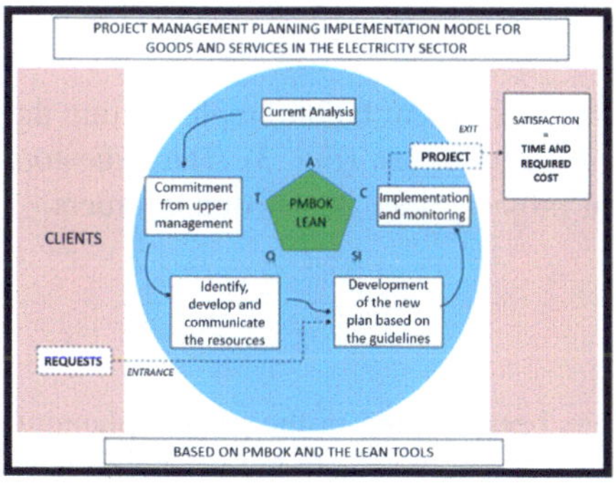

Fig. 2. Proposed model

Indicator	Stoplight			Situation before implementation	Situation from the simulation in Arena	Situation from the pilot test
	DANGER	CAUTION	TARGET			
WOF (Work order fulfillment)	Less than or equal to 50%	Between 51% - 84%	Between 85% - 95%	35%	51%	85%
EVM (Earned Value Management	Less than or equal to 50%	Between 51% - 84%	Between 85% - 95%	37%	55%	87%
Project Knowledge	Less than or equal to 50%	Between 51% - 84%	Between 85% - 95%	31%	60%	86%
% of materials delivered	Less than or equal to 50%	Between 51% - 84%	Between 85% - 95%	28%	66%	88%
% of quantity of materials required in storage	Less than or equal to 50%	Between 51% - 84%	Between 85% - 95%	33%	61%	90%
% of material orders delivered on time	Less than or equal to 50%	Between 51% - 84%	Between 85% - 95%	22%	80%	92%

Fig. 3. Results analysis

The main idea of the proposal is to develop a model that fosters standardization in project planning, as proposed by the PMI in the PMBOK Guide. This would be developed using lean tools to improve service quality provided to the user, thereby increasing their satisfaction, reducing project cost overruns such as extra acquisitions, and not meeting deadlines or penalties. This could generate cost reductions while increasing the financial benefits for the company. The model has five components that include a proposed methodological guide that contributes to project management, in addition to developing a tailor-made format for the proper development of a project in terms of scope, management, time, and cost.

- Current Analysis: The "current analysis" determines the state of the primary activities that constitute the core business of the company.
- Commitment from the upper management: The commitment from the upper management will improve performance and its relation with the organization's profits by strengthening tools known in the business world as organizational environment and culture.
- Recognition, development, and communication of resources: Once the acceptance has been documented and verified by the upper management, short- and long-term objectives must be aligned to the interests of the project team. Objectives represent significant milestones on the path toward the project's final purpose.
- Development of a new plan based on guidelines:
- The development of new project plans will be conducted based on the success criteria of time, cost, and quality. These criteria are selected given that the work must be finished on time, within the established cost, and meet the agreed upon quality standards.
- Implementation and Monitoring: Once the plans have been made, the project manager implements them. As the work progresses, the project manager uses planning and monitoring tools to identify the observed project performance relative to the range of acceptable outcomes.

5 Results Analysis

This point compares the results obtained with the assessment before implementing the proposal, the results in Arena, and the results in the pilot test (Fig. 3). The indicators have been used in electric boards and electrical projects lines in scheduling orders.

6 Conclusion

The methodology used in this research study has been applied in the project planning stage for a goods and services line of an SME. The results conclude that the projects structured by implementing the lean philosophy, following its five principles, indicate a positive trend in their financial evaluation results in terms of the two criterions used: NPV and IRR, which indicate the feasibility of executing the projects to their implementation.

Implementing the lean philosophy in projects provides tools to analyze the feasibility of carrying out a project, eliminating repetitive processes in its implementation, and delivering as per client request.

References

1. Becerra, C.: Pymes emplean 75% de la PEA y destacan en emprendimientos: El Peruano. Recuperado de (2018). https://elperuano.pe/noticia-pymes-emplean-75-de-pea-y-destacan-emprendimientos-67499.aspx
2. Magazine Business: Las Pymes son el 96.5% de las empresas que hay en Perú: Perú Retail Recuperado de (2017). https://www.peru-retail.com/pymes-empresas-peru
3. Flores, C.: Exportadoras: El 82% es micro y pequeña empresa: Diario El Correo. Recuperado de (2018). https://diariocorreo.pe/economia/exportadoras-el-82-es-micro-y-pequena-empresa-833316/
4. Montero, R.: Pyme emplea al 75% de la Población Económicamente Activa del Perú: Andina. Recuperado de (2018). https://andina.pe/agencia/noticia-pyme-emplea-al-75-de-poblacion-economicamente-activa-del-peru-714211.aspx
5. Turkyilma, A., Satir, M., Shoaib, M., Shahbaz, M.: Measuring the performance efficiency of Turkish electrical machinery manufacturing SMEs with frontier method. Benchmarking Int. J. **23**(7), 2004–2026 (2016). https://doi.org/10.1108/bij-09-2015-0089
6. Darlington, J., Francis, M., Found, P., Thomas, A.: Targeting lean process improvement projects for maximum financial impact. Prod. Planning Control **27**(2), 114–132 (2016). https://doi.org/10.1080/09537287.2015.1082665
7. Castillo, G., Alarcón, L.F., Gonzales, V.A.: Implementing lean production in copper mining development projects: case study. J. Constr. Eng. Manage. **141** (2014). https://doi.org/10.1061/(asce)co.1943-7862.0000917
8. Saravanana, V., Nallusamyb, S., Balajic, K.: Lead time reduction through execution of lean tool for productivity enhancement in small scale industries. Int. J. Eng. Res. Africa **34**, 116–127 (2018). https://doi.org/10.4028/www.scientific.net/JERA.34.116
9. Anholon, R., Toshio Sano, A.: Analysis of critical processes in the implementation of lean manufacturing projects using project management guidelines. Int. J. Adv. Manuf. Technol. **84**(9–12), 2247–2256 (2015). https://doi.org/10.1007/s00170-015-7865-9

10. Hong, P., Leffakis, Z.M.: Managing demand variability and operational effectiveness: case of lean improvement programmes and MRP planning integration. Manage. Oper. **28**, 1066–1080 (2017). https://doi.org/10.1080/09537287.2017.1329956
11. Hong, P., Yhan, M., Dobrzykowski, D.: Strategic customer service orientation, lean manufacturing practices and performance outcomes: an empirical study. J. Serv. Manage. **25**, 699–723 (2014). https://doi.org/10.1108/josm-12-2013-0355
12. Agrahari, R., Dangle, P., Chandratre, K.: Implementation of 5S methodology in the small-scale industry: a case study. Int. J. Adv. Res. Innov. **3**, 130–137 (2015)
13. Tezel, A., Koskela, L., Tzortzopoulos, P., Formoso, C.T., Alves, T.: Visual management in Brazilian construction companies: taxonomy and guidelines for implementation. J. Constr. Eng. Manage. **31** (2015). https://doi.org/10.1061/(asce)ME.1943-5479.0000354

Strategic Planning Model to Increase the Profitability of an HR Outsourcing SME Through Digital Transformation

Andrea Bautista[1(✉)], Adriana León[1(✉)], José Rojas[1(✉)], and Carlos Raymundo[2(✉)]

[1] Escuela de Ingeniería de Gestión Empresarial, Universidad Peruana de Ciencias Aplicadas (UPC), Lima, Peru
{u201410643,u201313205,jose.rojas}@upc.edu.pe

[2] Dirección de Investigación, Universidad Peruana de Ciencias Aplicadas (UPC), Lima, Peru
carlos.raymundo@upc.edu.pe

Abstract. The Human Resources (HR) outsourcing market in Peru is growing; however, it is dominated by large companies in this area, which prevents the development of new organizations or small- and medium-sized enterprises (SMEs). The latter, in spite of providing the same services, fail to reach the expected sales volume, thus reporting low profitability. This article analyzes the different factors that impede the growth of SMEs through a fishbone (Ishikawa) diagram and the assessment of initial indicators. It also proposes a model that is based on the three pillars of Digital Transformation and the importance of their alignment in its implementation. A pilot model has been conducted for validation in an SME that provides HR outsourcing services. The research results denote an increase in the company's profitability and capacity.

Keywords: Human factors · Human-systems integration · Systems engineering · Digital Transformation

1 Introduction

In Peru, there are HR service providers, such as TMF Group, Cornerstone International Group, Adecco, and Consulting Advisers, which are widely positioned in the Peruvian market [1]. However, Peru also has SMEs that maintain low profitability when compared with their competitors despite providing the same services and under very similar characteristics. This is due to the fact that these companies have manual and not very agile operating processes in place that do not use technology to bolster their productivity, which results in a low level of sales and under positioning.

This study aims to demonstrate the advantages and increased profitability level of an HR outsourcing SME through the use of Digital Transformation.

T. Ahram et al. (Eds.): IHIET 2019, AISC 1018, pp. 856–862, 2020.
https://doi.org/10.1007/978-3-030-25629-6_134

2 State of the Art

2.1 Digital Marketing

2.1.1 Literature Review

Nowadays, Digital Marketing is used to facilitate sales and communication and improve customer service. Its implementation in industrial companies provides significant competitive advantages and greatly facilitates reaching customers [2, 3].

2.1.2 Tools

Social Media: Social media are considered to be the second most important Digital Marketing tool today, allowing direct and immediate interaction between companies and their customers [4, 5]. Therefore, social media presence is indispensable for positioning the company in the minds of consumers or customers [6–8].

Search Engine Optimization (SEO): Search engine positioning or search engine optimization is the process of improving website visibility in the organic results of different search engines. SEO is necessary to help search engines understand what each page is about and whether it is useful to users [9, 10].

Mailing: Email marketing can be considered to be one of the most important Digital Marketing tools to facilitate communication with customers [11, 12].

2.2 Digital Transformation

2.2.1 Literature Review

Digital transformation is the realignment of technology, business models, and processes. Effective Digital Transformation that is focused on data, information technologies, and people provides a significant competitive advantage to those who have implemented it [13].

2.2.2 Digital Transformation Stages

Analysis: Company analysis prior to the implementation is essential as it allows the identification of key processes and opportunities for improvement.

Execution: The implementation process requires that a digital culture be created and that the incorporated technology be managed. During this process, the company must aim to provide value to its customers in every change made.

Optimization: The optimization process consists of applying corrective action, fostering internal digital talent, and positively sustaining the change momentum [14].

Big Data: Big Data is a set of stored data that helps organizations to identify new opportunities and eliminate problem areas. This, in turn, leads to smarter business moves, more efficient operations, higher profits, and happier customers [15].

2.3 Lean Service

Lean service improves the effectiveness of administrative and support processes in terms of quality, cost, and time. Many SMEs do not appropriately analyze their service quality and the structure of their processes internally. This impedes the obtainment of knowledge regarding the performance and quality levels achieved by the organization. Lean Service provides the following benefits: Standardizes and simplifies activities, Increases speed and reduces service delivery times, Improves productivity and process quality, Increases employee commitment and job satisfaction, Develops employees' skills and versatility.

3 Research Methods

3.1 External Analysis

For the company's external analysis, we used tools such as PESTEL analysis to assess the external factors affecting the business. Also, the BCG matrix was used to analyze the positioning of the company's value proposition in the market.

3.2 Internal Analysis

As part of the company's internal analysis, cross-SWOT tools were used to assess the company's strengths, weaknesses, opportunities, and threats. In addition, we used the issue tree and fishbone diagram to find the main causes of the low profit level. The causes were then subdivided into Manageable and Unmanageable causes so that only manageable causes were considered in our research model. Subsequently, we used the confrontation matrix to evaluate the effectiveness of different tools for the problems encountered, which had been prioritized using Pareto analysis.

3.3 Solution Proposal Model

We formulated this model for our research proposal to increase the profitability of an SME that provides HR outsourcing services specialized in Information Technology personnel. The model is based on three main pillars: Business Process Modeling, Customer Experience, and Technology Optimization, as shown in the following chart (Fig. 1):

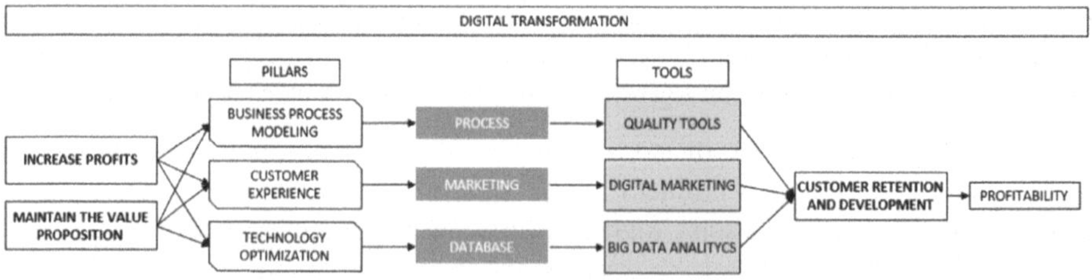

Fig. 1. Solution proposal model

The main objective of the proposal model is to improve the company's sales performance and profitability by sustaining the value proposition—to provide services at low cost and reduced service response time.

The Business Process Modeling pillar focuses on improvement in processes on the basis of quality tools to optimize and increase their productivity. Furthermore, the Customer Experience pillar focuses on the use of Digital Marketing to increase traffic and both customer and candidate attraction. Finally, the Technology Optimization pillar is intended to integrate technology tools into the processes that enhance the company's productivity and efficiency.

In short, the proposal model aims to increase the company's profitability through increased sales and production capacity.

3.3.1 Tool Convergence

Digital Marketing represents a tool for the promotion and sales of the company's services. Also, Big Data analytics allow more effective information management to improve the sales processes.

In addition, the Lean Service, which is aimed at reducing the model wastes selected, will be part of the tools used to maintain the speed of their selection processes and reduce time in the personnel recruitment service, which is part of the company's value proposition.

On the other hand, Digital Transformation will be used as a support tool for the company's process maintenance. The goal will be to implement its use in the general culture in a stable and permanent manner such that the focus is on increasing production and its efficiency to achieve a higher level of productivity that is based on Digital Transformation and Lean Service support tools.

4 Results

4.1 Process

In principle, we conducted the company's internal analysis, starting with its strengths and weaknesses through cross-SWOT analysis. Then, we analyzed the external factors that affect the company using the PESTLE tool. In addition, we analyzed the market sector distributed by delivery time and price of services using the BCG matrix.

On the other hand, to identify the causes of the problem, we used the issue tree and the fishbone diagram tools, in which the following main ones are identified: Financial problems, Under positioning, Unrealized sales, Organizational structure.

On the basis of the analysis performed, we subdivided the factors to be tackled as Manageable and Unmanageable.

Manageable Factors: Organizational Structure, Under Positioning, Unrealized Sales. Unmanageable Factors: Financial Problems.

Our research work is aimed at solving the problems classified as manageable. To achieve a deeper understanding thereof, we performed Pareto analysis with the company's most key causes related to the low sales level, the following were identified, in order of importance: lack of process and procedure documentation, lack of following up with potential clients, lack of after-sales service, lack of competitive strategies, lack of market awareness, well-positioned large companies, lack of organizational and functional structure, demand for new services.

To evaluate the possible tools for problem solving, we used a confrontation matrix with different proposals. On the basis of the analysis performed, we defined the tools to be used in the model.

4.2 Subsequent Results

The effectiveness of our proposal will be validated with three main indicators and independent tests that will finally validate the increase in company profitability.

4.2.1 Company Positioning

Number of IT Talent Facebook followers (04/11/18): 11457.

This result confirms the effectiveness of the Digital Marketing tools used in social media as a means of positioning and increasing the company's exposure.

4.2.2 Productivity and Service Response Time

To validate the decrease in customer service response time and therefore the increase in company service capabilities, we simulated the main processes in an improved context and under the estimated conditions.

According to the results obtained, the new capability is eight processes executed per month, which would give a service time of 49.5 h per process when compared with 70.5 h reported before the improvements.

4.2.3 Sales

We noted an increase in company sales consequent to the increase in sales and service capabilities.

As shown in the Fig. 2, the increase in profit started upon tool implementation (month of July). This validates the model's effectiveness for generating an increase in profit.

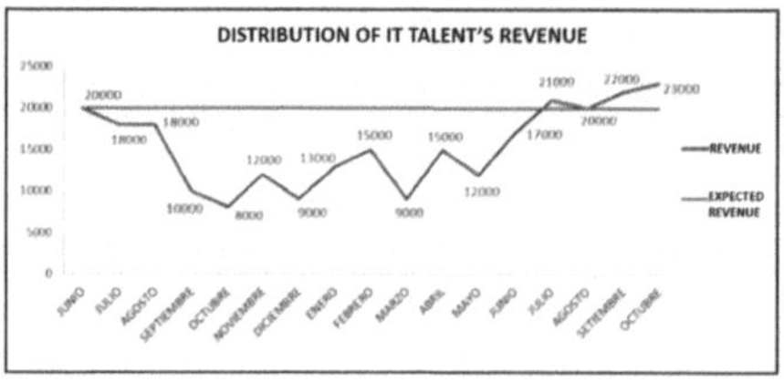

Fig. 2. Distribution of IT Talent's Revenue (2017–2018)

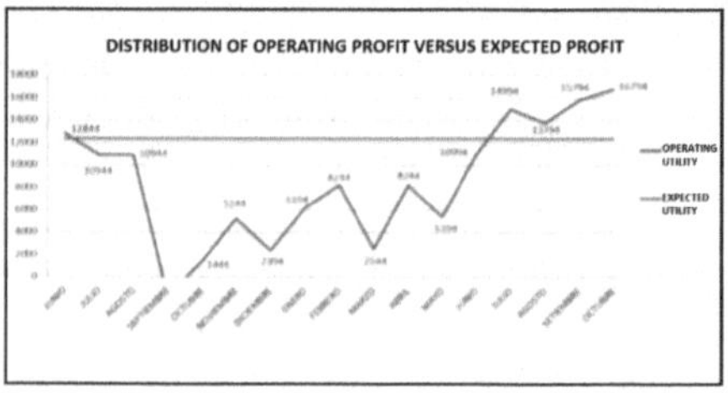

Fig. 3. Distribution of IT Talent's Profits (2017–2018)

5 Comparative Analysis of the Results Obtained

Comparison of Positioning Results
The subsequent results show that the social media placement increased from 2688 to 11417. That is to say, a 425% increase in the year of tool execution. This indicator is considered to be a positioning measurement as it estimates the level of company "followers" and "connoisseurs."

Comparison of Productivity Results
According to the results obtained in the pre (preceding) and post (subsequent) simulations, it was possible to increase production capacity by 60% and reduce the service response time per process by 30%, which would result in a service response time of 49.5 h per process when compared with the 70.5 h obtained before applying the improvements.

Comparison of Sales Results
The company's sales volume increased to a point where it exceeded the expected level, as can be seen in Fig. 2, which denotes revenue behavior from the beginning (April 2017) to the end (October 2018). This was done in a sustainable manner and without raising the expected cost level. This is reflected in the profit level obtained throughout research work and model implementation (Fig. 3). According to the figure, we can conclude that both profits and sales rose above the expected level.

6 Conclusions

As previously discussed, outsourcing SMEs in Peru compete with large companies in the market. However, despite providing the same services, they report much lower sales volumes than large companies. Concerning this problem, our research seeks to increase their revenue and improve the profitability of this sector through the use of the three Digital Transformation pillars, combined with Digital Marketing, Lean Service, and Big Data tools. In the research study, we first analyzed the characteristics of the company and its environment.

Then, we assessed the main causes of the problem so as to determine strategies and the most effective tools for resolving the problem by addressing the causes. The support strategy, together with the Lean Service and Digital Transformation methodologies, helped to eliminate the lack of process and procedure documentation, with this being the cause with the greatest impact on low income. The strategy resulted in the definition of the company's processes, the reduction of time taken, and the elimination of bottlenecks in the personnel selection and recruitment process. The sales strategy, together with the Digital Marketing methodology and the Big Data tool, increased the company's social media placement and the sales volume, exceeding the expected revenue from sales in recent months. Finally, the resale strategy eliminated the lack of customer follow-up by implementing the after-sales service.

Therefore, we can conclude that the methodology used is efficient in increasing the profitability of an SME that provides HR outsourcing services in Peru as it increases the productivity, sales volume, and general indicators of the company.

References

1. NPAworldwide. Obtenido de (2017). http://npaworldwide.com/
2. Taiminen, H.M., Karjaluoto, H.: The usage of Digital Marketing channels in SMEs. J. Small Bus. Enterp. Dev. **22**(4), 633–651 (2015). https://doi.org/10.1108/JSBED-05-2013-0073
3. Karjaluoto, H., Mustonen, N., Ulkuniemi, P.: The role of digital channels in industrial marketing communications. J. Bus. X (2015). https://doi.org/10.1108/JBIM-04-2013-0092
4. Stone, M.D., Woodcock, N.D.: Interactive, direct and digital marketing: a future that depends on better use of business intelligence. J. Res. Interact. Mark. **8**(1), 4–17 (2014). https://doi.org/10.1108/JRIM-07-2013-0046
5. Chahal, H., Rani, A.: How trust moderates social media engagement and brand equity. J. Res. Interact. Mark. **11**(3), 312–335 (2017). https://doi.org/10.1108/JRIM-10-20160104
6. Foroudi, P., Gupta, S., Nazarian, A., Duda, M.: Digital technology and marketing management capability: achieving growth in SMEs. Qual. Market Res. Int. J. **20**(2), 230–246 (2017). https://doi.org/10.1108/QMR-01-2017-0014
7. Bocconcelli, R., Cioppi, M., Pagano, A.: Social media as a resource in SMEs' sales process. J. Bus. Ind. Mark. **32**(5), 693–709 (2017)
8. Kilgour, M., Sasser, S.L., Larke, R.: The social media transformation process: curating content into strategy. Corp. Commun. Int. J. **20**(3), 326343 (2015). https://doi.org/10.1108/CCIJ-07-20140046
9. Park, M.: SEO for an open access scholarly information system to improve user experience. Inf. Discov. Deliv. **46**(2), 77–82 (2018). https://doi.org/10.1108/IDD-082017-0060
10. Luh, C.-J., Yang, S.-A., Huang, T.-L.D.: Estimating Google's search engine ranking function from a search engine optimization perspective. Online Inf. Rev. **40**(2), 239–255 (2016). https://doi.org/10.1108/OIR-042015-0112
11. Lee, S., Jang, W., Lee, E., Oh, S.G.: Search engine optimization: a case study using the bibliofigureies of LG Science Land in Korea. Library Hi Tech. **34**(2), 197–206 (2016). https://doi.org/10.1108/LHT-02-2016-0014
12. Scheinbaum, A.C., Hampel, S., Kang, M.: Future developments in IMC: why e-mail with video trumps text-only e-mails for brands. Eur. J. Mark. **51**(3), 627–645 (2017). https://doi.org/10.1108/EJM-09-20150624
13. Hartemo, M.: Email marketing in the era of the empowered consumer. J. Res. Interact. Mark. **10**(3), 212–230 (2016). https://doi.org/10.1108/JRIM-06-2015-0040
14. Ashwell, M.L.: The digital transformation of intelligence analysis. J. Financ. Crime **24**(3), 393–411 (2017)
15. Shaughnessy, H.: Creating digital transformation: strategies and steps. Strategy Leadersh. **46**(2), 19–25 (2018). https://doi.org/10.1108/SL-12-20170126

Potential Absorptive Capacity, Realized Absorptive Capacity and Innovation Performance

Saad G. Yaseen(✉)

Faculty of Business, Al-Zaytoonah University of Jordan, Amman, Jordan
saad.yaseen@zuj.edu.jo

Abstract. The aim of this research is to investigate the relationship between potential absorptive capacity, realized absorptive capacity, and innovation performance. Drawing on the knowledge- based theory, the current research conceptualizes absorptive capacity as two distinct and separated knowledge dynamic capabilities: potential absorptive capacity and realized absorptive capacity. The research addresses potential ACAP and realized ACAP separately and analyzed their influence on the firm's innovation performance. Using structural equation modeling (SEM) in a sample of 12 firms from Jordanian pharmaceutical industry, the research revealed that potential and realized absorptive capacities have significant and direct relations with firm's innovation performance. The results confirm that potential ACAP along with components (acquisition, assimilation), and realized ACAP (encompassing transformation, exploitation) are antecedents to the firm's innovation performance. The research advances the concept of absorptive capacity by exploring it as two different dynamic capabilities.

Keywords: Potential absorptive capacity · Realized absorptive capacity · Innovation performance

1 Introduction

Knowledge- intensive firms increasingly pursue innovation performance due to heightened level of competition, innovation globalization and accelerated technological development [1, 2, 4, 11]. In this dynamic environment, innovation performance of a firm depends on the knowledge absorptive capacity [1, 5, 7]. From knowledge management perspective, absorptive capacity is crucial in the knowledge economy and society [10, 29]. Cohen & Levinthal [7] initially defined absorptive capacity as the ability of recognizing external knowledge, assimilating and applying it to commercial ends. Therefore, absorptive capacity refers to inter-organizational learning, knowledge transfer and dynamic capability [2, 12]. Absorptive capacity is a complex and multi-dimensional concept that involves ability to value, assimilate and apply knowledge [7, 13]. However, in recent years, researchers have used ACAP across various fields of business entrepreneurship [14], innovation and learning [15], innovation output [16], performance [17], leadership [3], and IT [18]. While there is an extensive literature around the conceptualization of ACAP, the most widely used conceptualization of the

T. Ahram et al. (Eds.): IHIET 2019, AISC 1018, pp. 863–870, 2020.
https://doi.org/10.1007/978-3-030-25629-6_135

construct is that which Zahra and George [21] propose. Following, Zahra and George's reconceptualization spurred a lot of new research in the area and as a result, we now find a rich body of literature on ACAP addressing its antecedents [19, 20], and outcomes [21]. Absorptive Capacity is conceptualized as a dynamic capability composed of potential and realized ACCP, enabling firms to value, acquire, assimilate, transform, and exploit external knowledge [3]. However, in the ACAP literature, a conceptual gap still remains regarding certain ambiguity of the construct's theoretical domain, its antecedents and outcomes [22]. Drawing on the Zahra & George [21] framework, the current research theorizes ACAP as two dynamic capabilities; Namely, PACAP and RACAP but they should be explicitly separated since these two capacities have different knowledge sub processes and activities. The research addresses potential absorptive capacity and realized absorptive capacity separately and analyzes their influence on the innovation performance.

2 Literature Review

2.1 Absorptive Capacity

Cohen and Levinthal [7, 8] introduced the construct absorptive capacity to define the capabilities of the firm to learn innovate and thus, to be dynamic. They argue that the ability of a firm to recognize the value of new external knowledge, assimilate it, and apply it to commercial ends is critical to its innovative capabilities [7]. It depends on the external knowledge resources and prior internal knowledge. Following the original concept, Cohen and Levinthal (1990) conceptualized absorptive capacity as a three-dimensional construct composed of recognizing the value of knowledge, assimilate it, and apply it. However, absorptive capacity has undergone several reconceptualization over the last years [8, 23, 24]. We follow Zahra and George [21] reconceptualization of absorptive capacity. Building upon the dynamic capabilities, Zahra and George [21] suggest that ACAP exists as two subset of potential and realized absorptive capacities with these two subset components, Zahra and George focus on an efficiency view of ACAP; that is efficiency is reducing the gap between PACAP and RACAP [15]. Potential capacity comprises knowledge acquisition and assimilation capabilities and realized capacity contains knowledge transformation and exploitation [21]. According to this view, absorptive capacity is a dynamic capability formed by a set of organizational routines and distinguish between potential and realized ACAP [12].

Potential ACAP has two dimensions: acquisition and assimilation. Knowledge acquisition refers to a firm's capability to identify and acquire externally generated knowledge that is critical to its activities and operations [21]. Assimilation refers to the firm's routines and processes that firm uses to analyze, process, interpret, understand the required knowledge [21]. Realized ACAP comprises transformation and exploitation. The third ability, transformation refers to a firm's ability to build and purify organizational routines that combine existing knowledge with newly acquired assimilated knowledge [19, 28]. The final capability, exploitation is based on the routines that fosters firm's capabilities to leverage competences or to create new ones for commercial application of the new knowledge [7, 17, 21]. Consequently, these four components of absorptive capacity have combined into two subsets; potential ACAP and realized ACAP with different value creating potentials. Thus, the practice raises questions about the multidimensionality of the ACAP and its contribution to innovation performance.

2.2 Absorptive Capacity and Innovation Performance

Cohen and Levinthal [7] argue that the ability of a firm to recognize external knowledge, assimilate it, and apply it is critical to its innovative capacities. Today, the concept of absorptive capacity is used across a wide spectrum of research including but not limited to innovative effort [28], green innovation [14], open innovation [30], innovation and cultural barriers [22], radical innovation [12]. However, little attention has been paid to the question of whether potential ACAP and realized ACAP can independently enhance innovation performance. RACAP is expected to directly improve firm performance. In contrast, PACAP is rather considered an ability to create an organizational memory. Although there is a long history of research on ACAP and innovation outcomes, the evidence of ACAP which highlights the relationship between potential ACAP and realized ACAP with a firm innovation performance is still scare [30]. Nevertheless, firms increasingly pursue innovation strategies that involve an active acquisition and assimilation of newly external knowledge. Influential research papers indicate that the positive effect of potential ACAP on innovation and performance are well established [19, 20]. Thus, it is hypothesized:

H_1: Potential absorptive capacity positively influences innovation performance
Zahra and George [21] suggest that RACAP depends on the existence of well-functioning social integration mechanism. Realized ACAP allow firms to develop, refine organizational routines that facilities combining existing knowledge and newly assimilated knowledge, and incorporating transformed knowledge into its operations [7, 21]. Seen this way, realized ACAP involves transformation and exploitation capacities. The dynamic element of realized ACAP refers to firm's ability to reconfigure its substantive knowledge capabilities for gaining a firm's innovation performance. Thus, it is hypothesized.

H_2: Realized absorptive capacity positively influences innovation performance
The current research posits that potential and realized absorptive capacities have an impact on innovation performance only when newly external knowledge can be acquired, assimilated and transformed, and therefore, exploited. Hence, the distinction between PACAP and RACAP, highlights their different influence on the firm's innovation performance depending on which components are being analyzed.

3 Research Method

3.1 Sampling

Jordanian pharmaceutical industry was chosen as our empirical setting. Pharmaceutical companies in Jordan provide a rich setting for two reasons. First, the Jordanian pharmaceutical industry has accrued good manufacturing practices to extending to more than 60 countries including GCC countries, the US, and the EU, due to its high quality and excellent reputation. This research relies on a cross-sectional data from a survey questionnaire. The basic unit of analysis includes 215 managers, head departments, and knowledge workers was randomly selected from Jordanian Pharmaceutical firms. The participants comprise 44.2% females and 55.8% males. As it is characteristics for pharmaceutical firms, respondent's age range is 20–30 years (21%), 31–40 years (46%), and 41–50 (20.5%), 51 above (12.1%). The respondents are predominantly knowledge workers (62.8%), and (37.2%) of respondents are managers and head departments.

3.2 Measures

The measures for all constructs were operationalized by validated scales, adapted from the extant literature, using 5-points Likert scale. To ensure the face and content validity of the research scales, a qualitative expert assessment with managers regularly engaged in the ACAP activities are conducted. Further, all measurement items and survey questionnaire are validated by ten academic staff for wording, structure and appropriateness of the item. The absorptive capacity is measured via a four dimensions scale of an adapted version of measures developed by Flatten et al. [11], which builds upon the reconceptualization of Zahra and George [21]. The innovation performance captures the capacity of the firm to introduce new products or improve existing products and level of research and development spending.

4 Data Analysis Results

The measurement model included all exogenous and endogenous constructs and their indicators was examined using Smart PLS 2.0. The research's constructs were modeled as reflective. Assessment of convergent and discriminant validity determines the validation of measurement model. All items loading, composite reliability, Cronbach's Alpha and average variance extracted exceeded the commonly accepted thresholds (0.7), implying that all measures consistently represent the same construct. As Table 1 shows, the CR values range from 0.870 to 0.884 and AVE values are more than 50%.

The convergent validity of the scale was verified based on the three criteria suggested; all indicator loading should be significant and exceed 0.7, composite reliabilities should exceed 0.8, and average variance extracted (AVE) by each construct should exceed the variance due to measurement error for that construct [13]. A common measure to establish convergent validity on the construct is the average variance extracted (AVE). AVE value of 0.50 or higher indicates that construct explains more than half other variance of its indicators. The square root of the average variance extracted of each construct should exceed the highest constructs correlation with any other constructs [3, 6, 17]. As shown in Table 2 shows square root of the average variance extracted (AVE) of each latent construct is greater than its highest correlation with other constructs.

Table 1. The measurement model

Construct	Indicators	Loading	Composite reliability	Cronbach Alpha	Average variance extracted
Potential absorptive capacity	ACQ2	0.770	0.884	0.837	0.606
	ACQ3	0.775			
	ASM1	0.827			
	ASM2	0.797			
	ASM4	0.718			
Realized absorptive capacity	EXP1	0.766	0.876	0.811	0.639
	EXP2	0.869			
	EXP3	0.802			
	TRF4	0.757			
Innovation performance	INV1	0.740	0.90	0.870	0.562
	INV2	0.716			
	INV3	0.734			
	INV5	0.796			
	RD1	0.735			
	RD2	0.770			
	RD3	0.754			

Table 2. Latent construct correlations

Construct	Innovation performance	Potential absorptive capacity	Realized absorptive capacity
Innovation performance	0.749		
Potential absorptive capacity	0.489	0.778	
Realized absorptive capacity	0.605	0.467	0.799

4.1 The Structural Model

The key measurements for assessing the structural model are: cross validation (CV) - communality redundancy indices, path coefficients, R2 values and the predictive relevance Q2. Cross validation and communality redundancy indices assess the quality of the structural model. Furthermore, after running the PLS-SEM algorithm, estimates are obtained for the hypothesized relationships among the constructs. The bootstrapping routine delivers a standard error of all relations, the empirical t-value is higher than theoretical t-value of 1.96 for 0.05 probability of error. As a result, one can conclude that all hypothesized relationships are statistically significant. The research results revealed that all path coefficients are significant at P. level of 0.05. The model explains 0.4211 of the variance in a firm's innovation performance. Table 3 provides the structural model results.

Table 3. The structural model results

Construct	Standardized coefficient	Standardized deviation	Standard error	T-statistic	Hypotheses results
Potential absorptive capacity→ innovation performance	0.264	0.267	0.074	3.544	H1 Support
Realized absorptive capacity→ innovation performance	0.482	0.488	0.087	5.493	H2 Support

Overall, the structural model provides confirmation of the direct and positive influence of potential ACAP on the firm's innovation performance. Furthermore, the direct and positive influence of the realized ACAP on innovation performance of the firm was also confirmed.

5 Conclusion, Discussion, and Implications

Research findings revealed that potential ACAP (path coefficient = 0.264; $p < 0.05$) and realized ACAP (path coefficient = 0.481; $p < 0.05$) have significant relations with firm's Innovation performance. The results support research's hypotheses, showing that potential ACAP and realized ACAP positively influence innovation performance. Based on its results, this research provides important evidence in support of the positive and direct impact between potential ACAP, realized ACAP and a firm's overall innovation performance. The current findings are in line with findings from previous studies [7, 12, 21, 27]. The current research has a number of implications to theory and absorptive capacity literature. This research addresses a gap in the literature and, hence, clarifies the direct and positive relationship between potential ACAP, realized ACAP and firm's innovation performance. The excellent fit of the research model and the support for hypothesis H1, H2 are theoretical important findings. However the current research is subject to limitations. The research focuses mainly on three constructs: potential ACAP, realized ACAP and innovation performance. Future research could investigate mediated variables such as cultural values, organizational learning or knowledge sharing.

References

1. Alegre, J., Chiva, R.: Assessing the impact of organizational learning capabilities on product innovation performance: an empirical test. Technovation **28**, 315–326 (2008)
2. Apriliyanti, I.D., Alon, I.: Bibliometric analysis of absorptive capacity. Int. Bus. Rev. **26**, 896–907 (2017)

3. Bagozzi, R., Yi, Y., Phillips, L.: Assessing construct validity in organizational research. Adm. Sci. Q. **36**(3), 421–458 (1991)
4. John, B., Trifilova, A.: Developing absorptive capacity for recombinant innovation. Bus. Process Manage. J. **23**(6), 1094–1107 (2017)
5. Cesar, C., Fores, B.: Knowledge capacity: new insights for its conceptualization measurement. J. Bus. Res. **36**, 707–715 (2010)
6. Chin, W.W., Marcolin, B.L., Newsted, P.R.: A partial least Squares Latent variable modeling approach for measuring interaction effect: results from a Monte Carlo simulation study and an electronic mail emotion, adoption study. Inform. Syst. Res. **14**(2), 189–217 (2003)
7. Cohen, W.M., Levinthal, D.A.: Absorptive capacity: a new perspective on learning and innovation. Adm. Sci. Q. **35**(1), 128–152 (1990)
8. Cohen, W.M., Levinthal, D.D.: Innovation and learning the two faces of R&D. Econ. J. **99**, 569–596 (2017)
9. Cordero, R.: The measurement of innovation performance in the firm: an overview. Res. Policy **19**(2), 185–192 (1990)
10. Drucker, P.F.: Innovation and Entrepreneurship: Practice and Principles. Harper & Row, New York (1985)
11. Flatten, T., Adams, D., Brettle, M.: Fostering absorptive capacity through leadership: a cross-cultural analysis. J. Bus. World **50**, 519–534 (2015)
12. Lusia, F.M., Cooper, S.Y., Oltra, M.J.: External knowledge search, absorptive capacity, and radical innovation in high-technology firms. Europ. Manage., 4–12 (2017)
13. Fornell, C., Larcker, D.: Evaluating structural equation models with unobservable and measurement error. J. Mark. Res. **18**(1), 39–50 (1981)
14. Pernilla, G., Gustafsson, M., Thuvander, L.: An absorptive capacity model for green innovation and performance in the construction industry. Constr. Manage. Econ. **27**(5), 451–464 (2009)
15. Shijia, G., Yeoh, W., Wong, S.F., Scheepers, R.: A literature analysis of the use of absorptive capacity construct in IS research. Int. J. Inform. Manage. **37**, 36–42 (2017)
16. Cui, T., Wu, Y., Tong, Y.: Exploring ideation and implementation openness in open innovation projects. IT-enabled absorptive capacity perspective. Inform. Manage. (2017). https://doi.org/10.1016/j.m.2017,12.002
17. Hair, J.F., Hult, G., Tomas, M., Ringle, C.M., Sarstdt, M.: A Primer on Partial Least Squares Structural Equation Modeling (PLS SEM). Sage Publications Inc, Los Angeles (2014)
18. Jasen, J., Van Den Bosch, F., Volberda, H.: Managing potential and realized absorptive capacity: How do organizational antecedents matter? Acad. Manage. **48**(6), 999–1015 (2015)
19. Lane, P.J., Lubatkin, M.: Relative absorptive capacity and inter-organizational learning. Strateg. Manag. J. **19**(5), 461–477 (1998)
20. Lane, P., Koka, B., Pathak, S.: The reification of absorptive capacity: a critical review and rejuvenation of the construct. Acad. Manag. Rev. **31**(4), 833–863 (2006)
21. Zahra, S.A., George, G.: Absorptive capacity: a review, reconceptualization, and extension. Acad. Manage. Rev. **27**(2), 185–203 (2002)
22. Leal-Rodriguez, A.L., Ariza-Montes, J.A., Jose, L.R., Leal-Millan, A.G.: Absorptive capacity, Innovation, and cultural barriers: a conditional mediation. J. Bus. Res. **67**, 763–768 (2014)
23. Lewin, A., Massini, S., Peeters, C.: Microfoundations of internal and external absorptive capacity routines. Organ. Sci. **22**(1), 81–98 (2011)
24. Ulrich, L., Lichtenthaler, E.: A capability-based framework for open innovation: complementing absorptive capacity. J. Manage. Stud. **48**(8), 1315–1338 (2009)

25. Ulrich, L.: Value of technology and market orientation for external knowledge acquisition. J. Bus. Ind. Mark. **31**, 600–610 (2016)
26. Nika, M., Prodan, I.: Absorptive capacity, its determinants, and influence on innovation output: cross-cultural validation. Technovation **29**, 859–872 (2009)
27. Saeed, N.-T., Sharifi, H., Najafi-Tavani, Z.: Market orientation capability new product performance: the moderating role of absorptive capacity. J. Bus. Res. **69**, 5059–5064 (2016)
28. Nieto, M., Quevedo, P.: Absorptive capacity, technological opportunity, knowledge spillovers, and innovation effort. Technovation **25**, 1141–1157 (2005)
29. Nonaka, I., Takeuchi, H.: The Knowledge-Creating Company: How Japanese Companies Create the Dynamic of Innovation. Oxford University Press, UK (1995)
30. William, P., Ambrosini, V.: Configuration absorptive capacity as a key process for research intensive firms. Technovation **36–37**, 77–89 (2015)

Basic Production Planning and Control Model Based on Process Management to Increase the Productivity of Mango MSEs in Casma

Lizeth Alvarado[1(✉)], Juan Díaz[1(✉)], Juan Quiroz[1(✉)], and Carlos Raymundo[2(✉)]

[1] Ingeniería Industrial, Universidad Peruana de Ciencias Aplicadas (UPC), Lima, Peru
{u201217304,u201415117,pciijqui}@upc.edu.pe
[2] Dirección de Investigación, Universidad Peruana de Ciencias Aplicadas (UPC), Lima, Peru
carlos.raymundo@upc.edu.pe

Abstract. The department with the greatest economic dependence on the fruit is Ancash, and the Province of Casma is most important in production, as it only produces mango; however, at the productivity level, is a marked difference of 8.2 t/ha compared to the highest worldwide producer, Mexico. Taking this data into consideration, an analysis of the MSEs producing mango in Casma was conducted and problems were seen in the management of resources and processes, both at the levels of planning and control. Considering the problems of MSEs from Casma, a basic Production Planning and Control model was designed based on Process Management and agricultural best practices. The model consists of applying process management tools, such as the flow diagram, the SIPOC turtle, data sheet indicators, procedures, and formats for each subprocess, all with the aim of better understanding the proposal's development and increasing the productivity of MSEs.

Keywords: MSEs · Increasing productivity · Process Management · Agricultural best practices

1 Introduction

Currently, the most representative business group in the business distribution are MSEs, as they constitute 99% of the total existing companies in Perú [1]. It is also important to highlight that MSEs generate 70% of employment, and the agricultural sector is the most important sector [2]. When analyzing the Peruvian context, Piura is identified as the largest mango producer. However, the region with the greatest economic dependence on the fruit is Ancash, because 23.5% of the economy consists of agricultural exports [2]. Moreover, 88% of producers are located in the province of Casma, where 99% of the agricultural activity is the production of mango [1]. This shows Casma as a potential province for improvements in the economy and as an attractive area to implement improvements with basic Process Management. Focusing merely on companies from Casma, an analysis was completed. It consisted of

T. Ahram et al. (Eds.): IHIET 2019, AISC 1018, pp. 871–877, 2020.
https://doi.org/10.1007/978-3-030-25629-6_136

conducting an in-depth interview using the snowball method, which is based on interviewing a person, who then provides a contact for the following interview. The biggest problems found were grouped into four areas: Production Planning and Control, Quality, Logistics, and Costs. Considering the study's context and the main characteristics of mango production companies in Casma, a basic model of Production Planning and Control based on Process Management and Agricultural Best Practices applied to mango MSEs in the province of Casma was designed, with the aim of increasing their productivity. The proposal essentially consists of applying process management tools, such as the flow diagram, the SIPOC turtle, data sheet indicators, procedures and forms for each sub-process, all with the aim of better understanding the development of the proposal and increasing the productivity of MSEs.

2 State of the Art

Sterev, Kopeva and Blagoev [3] ensured that economic growth in Bulgaria is based on the use of the right industrial policy, which is based on a dynamic industrial methodology and on an understanding of how companies operate. Decisions (entrepreneurship, innovation, and R&D) at the micro level correspond to the macro level, i.e., GDP growth and innovation policies.

Also, in the Asian context, according to research by Wu, Guo and Marinova [4], Chinese authorities have chosen to make innovation and entrepreneurship the new engines of economic growth in the coming decades. In addition, they explore what can be learned from China's recent experience and how economic growth can be sustained through innovation and improved business productivity.

Considering the importance of business development in a country's economic growth, according to Srivastava [5], it is argued that the micro, small, and medium-sized enterprise sector plays a vital role in the growth of a country's job creation, exports, gross industrial value of production, gross value added, investment in fixed assets, contribution to GDP, manufacturing, services, and infrastructure. Such is the example of the South African context, that according to Masutha and Rogerson's research [6] with the purpose of creating jobs, the political attention is focused on the potential of the environment and microenterprise of the small economy (MYPES).

3 Proposed Model

As detailed above, this article describes the application of Process Management to mango producing MSEs in Casma, Ancash, so as to increase their productivity. So as to obtain representative data from farmers, a sample is taken using the snowball method, which is based on interviewing certain people who, in turn, provide a contact for subsequent interviews, thereby generating a chain of more detailed and higher quality information, as stated by Salganik [7]. The representative sample includes 73 rural farmers out of a total of 1,040, with an error rate of 5%. Two interviews were conducted. The first one aimed to identify processes affecting productivity and the following processes were identified as having a great impact: Quality Management,

Production Planning and Control Management, Cost Management and Logistics Management. The second interview aimed to carry out a specific assessment focused on the area to be improved by group. In this article, a description of the basic Production Planning and Control Model will be carried out.

3.1 Integrated Model Analysis

Four processes with direct impact on the productivity of mango MSEs in Casma were identified, and they have been detailed in a Process Map—a Process Management tool used to model the structure of the Basic Process Management System proposed by the general research group and to demonstrate the importance of the processes in the general system. Below is the Process Map of the general proposal, which is determined by three groups of processes.

3.1.1 Strategic Processes

These are the management processes that General Management is responsible for overseeing. They define the strategies that will guide the development of the MSE, whose main purpose is to produce mangoes that meet quality standards of exports and to supply collecting companies that order high volumes.

3.1.2 Key Processes

These are the processes necessary for mango production, which is the purpose of the MSE.

3.1.3 Supporting Processes

These are the processes necessary for the control, follow-up, improvement, and support of the main activities of mango producing MSEs (Fig. 1).

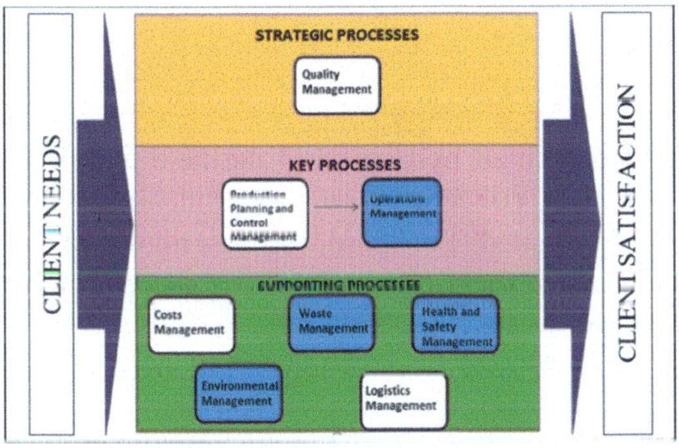

Fig. 1. General processes map

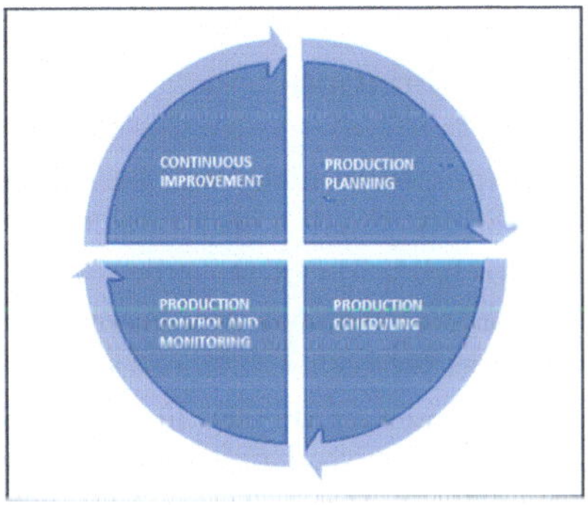

Fig. 2. Sub-processes diagram

Specific Model of Production Planning and Control

After the presentation of the basic model of general management and the description of the interrelations between areas, on which the research group will focus, the creation of a Management Model for the Production Planning and Control of Kent mangoes in

MSEs of Casma, Ancash, is proposed. This model aims to increase productivity and, in turn, the ultimate purpose is to increase the supply of mangoes for export. This Basic Management System for Production Planning and Control is divided into four central sub-processes: Production Planning, Production Scheduling, Production Control and Monitoring, and Continuous Production Improvement (Fig. 2). As can be seen in the diagram, Production Planning develops the production guidelines, and then it goes on to Production Scheduling, in which the time and amount of resources needed for the productive system will be defined. Once the productive process is underway, the results obtained from each stage are compiled, which serve as input for the Production Control and Monitoring sub-process. In this sub-process, what was obtained is compared with what was previously proposed, to identify the variables that have affected the Planning and Scheduling of production. Likewise, Production Improvement will collect the results from the productive system and from Production Control and Monitoring, in order to make improvement decisions and eliminate the variables that influence the initial planning. Finally, Production Planning will use the improvements previously proposed to optimize the mango production process, thus developing a cycle of continuous improvement.

Based on the above, the development of each sub-process is detailed through the use of process management tools. Among the main tools applied to each sub-process are flow diagrams, the SIPOC turtle, indicator sheets, procedures, and documentation forms with indicators, all based on the concept of Process Management. The SIPOC turtle identifies the main activities, inputs, outputs, resources, critical factors, controls, and indicators that allow for measuring and controlling activities. The indicator sheet essentially details the formula and parameters of each indicator. The procedures sheet gives details about the sub-process from the objective, scope, responsible parties, definitions, conditions, and records. The documentation forms specify the plans, follow-up sheets, among other forms that contribute to the deployment of each sub-process.

4 Validation

The proposed model will be validated and verified by experts in the field and users (farmers). Finally, the validation of the data collection and the validation of the characterization of the processes will be presented. For these, the description of the surveys carried out and the identification of the forms, procedures and flows of each process for both validations respectively will be used as evidence.

In order to validate the Production Planning and Control model proposed above, two matrices were prepared. They will allow the validators to give their opinion on the proposed model and to provide a brief evaluation according to the aspects considered important for this research. These matrices are the validation matrix and the impact matrix. The validation matrix takes into account the objectives set by the group and the farmers so that the criteria can assess their main points.

As part of the analysis of results, it has been proposed to identify the degree of general satisfaction of the validators (experts and users) with the proposal and methodology used in the present research study. In both cases (i.e., expert and user validations), the results show high values of satisfaction, as the experts' satisfaction percentage is 89% and the users' satisfaction percentage is 97.5% (Fig. 3).

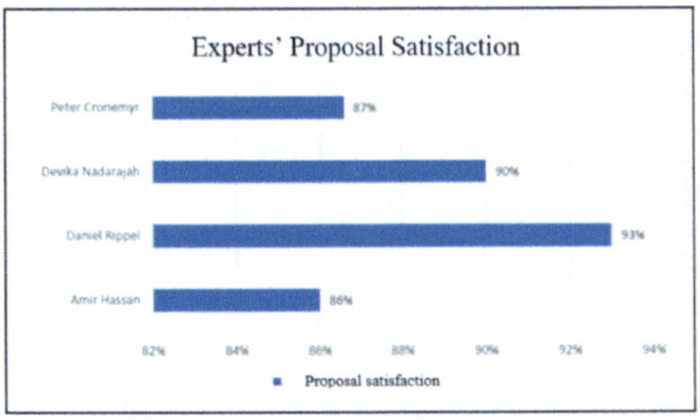

Fig. 3. Experts' satisfaction

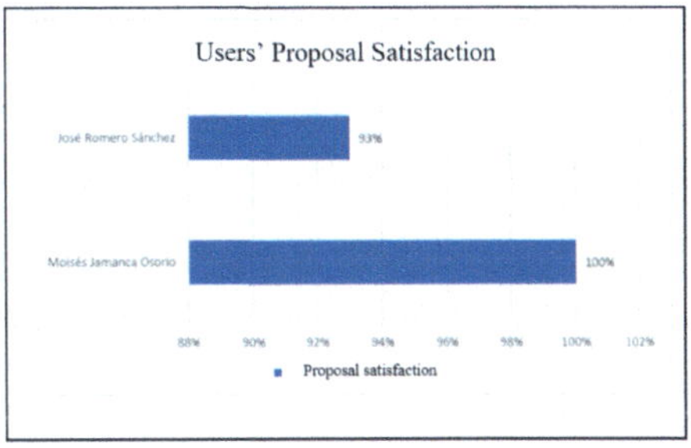

Fig. 4. Farmers' satisfaction

The table below shows the level of satisfaction of users (independent farmers from Casma, Ancash) (Fig. 4).

5 Discussion

- Agriculture in Ancash represents a significant percentage of its economy, specifically, exports represent 23.5% of Ancash's economy, which constitutes a high-impact improvement opportunity. An improvement at the production level can have a significant impact on the final quality of the product and therefore on the economy of each farmer and the farmer's employees.
- The Ancash region is composed of 915 hectares, with an average production of 6,750 tons and an average yield of 7.38 t/ha, a difference of 8.2 t/ha with the main producer, Mexico.
- 88% of farmers are in the province of Casma, which makes it a purely agricultural province that is dependent on this activity. Of these 88%, 97% focus on mango production. As it is a purely agricultural province and it fully depends on mango production as an economic activity, a positive impact on this sector represents an improvement in the economy of families.
- Farmers in the agricultural sector in the province of Casma are divided into two groups: estates and independent farmers. Essentially, the difference lies in the automation of their processes, because estates work with international certifications and a mapping of their processes and the requirements of the certifiers, while independent farmers only handle basic processes and produce at their maximum capacity without monitoring their processes and stages of production.

- 85% have no knowledge of their production capacity. It was found that 86% of farmers have no knowledge of production capacity according to the age of the tree. Farmers provided the data analyzed at the time of asking the question or simply said they did not know and that to calculate final production, they applied an average to all trees in their field without making any distinction of age, density or other variables.
- The farmers notoriously demonstrate an empirical production without optimal referents and deficient production planning, what makes it difficult to project the tons to be produced throughout the productive cycle, thereby managing a deficient production system. According to the interviews, only 5% calculate the resources needed for the production cycle, with respect to materials, labor, and necessary inputs, but this is only a basic calculation in proportion to the hectare of mango.
- 85% do not calculate the production cost and they do not keep track of the costs they incur from the beginning of a new crop to its harvest. Farmers do not use forms that allow them to calculate their production and therefore their profit margin. They work practically at random; the income they obtain will depend on the quality of their production and how much the buyer offers for their fruits. As they do not manage production costs, they do not establish minimum prices for the market. They only decide to sell their product to the highest bidder without knowing for sure if they are making a profit or at least recovering their money. They simply adapt to the price that the market offers. All these facts show poor management of resources and profits.
- 90% do not schedule the processes and do not follow-up on them. The processes follow a pattern according to the independent farmer's experience, leaving aside any updating processes of the sector. They do not consult the Mango and Avocado Production Association—many of them did not know of this association where different conferences are held on the technical improvement of mango seedlings.
- An increased number of professionals are in search of scientific information to improve the sectors affected by poverty, a way to reduce the impact of this social problem on their country.

6 Conclusions

The agricultural sector is a promising market for the application of Process Management with the perspective of meeting export quality standards and solving management level problems.

Process Management and related techniques enable a more efficient production at economic, social, and environmental levels.

References

1. Instituto Nacional de Estadística e Informática - INEI (2016) Evolución de la pobreza monetaria 2009-2015 (2016). Informe técnico, Consultado en: (http://www.inei.gob.pe/media/MenuRecursivo/publicaciones_digitales/Est/Lib1347/libro.pdf)
2. Instituto Nacional de Estadística e Informática - INEI (2014), Evolución de los Indicadores de Empleo e Ingresos por Departamento. Consultado en: (https://www.inei.gob.pe/media/MenuRecursivo/publicaciones_digitales/Est/Lib1200/libro.pdf)
3. Sterev, N., Kopeva, D., Blagoev, D.: Does business cycle have an impact on entrants and exits?. Int. J. Bus. Econ. Sci. Appl. Res. (2017). Consultado en. http://web.b.ebscohost.com/ehost/detail/detail?vid=0&sid=9185cf0e-4251-4efa-bf469843b8392800%40sessionmgr102&bdata=Jmxhbmc9ZXM%3d#AN=122401042&db
4. Wu, Y., Guo, X., Marinova, D.: Productivity, Innovation and China's Economic Growth. ANU Press (2017). Consultado en. http://www.jstor.org.ezproxy.upc.edu.pe:2048/stable/pdf/j.ctt1trkk3v.16.pdf?refreqid=search%3A0400d50e84cace13e87ed255cec9dede
5. Srivastava, J.: The Cordial Link Microfinance sector and Make in India Impact of Make in India on SIDBI. BVIMSR's J. Manage. Res. **9**(1) (2017). Consultado en: http://web.b.ebscohost.com/ehost/detail/detail?vid=0&sid=f5c1b2c8-0603-478d84ef5ccf30adcb2d%40sessionmgr101&bdata=Jmxhbmc9ZXM%3d#AN=123799333&
6. Masutha, M., Rogerson, C.: Small business incubators: An emerging phenomenon in South Africa's SMME economy. Urbanistični inštitut Republike Slovenije. Consultado en: (2014), http://www.jstor.org.ezproxy.upc.edu.pe:2048/stable/pdf/24920931.pdf?refreqid=excelsior%3A1b92568da42708ed70d1fd001ce23973
7. Salganik, M.: Muestreo Bola de Nieve. Obtenido de Muestreo Bola de Nieve (2013). www.ibrarian.net/navon/paper/Muestreo en Bola de Nieve.pdf?paperid=9132610

Integral Model of Maintenance Management Based on TPM and RCM Principles to Increase Machine Availability in a Manufacturing Company

Carlos Moscoso[1(✉)], Alex Fernandez[1(✉)], Gino Viacava[1(✉)], and Carlos Raymundo[2(✉)]

[1] Escuela de Ingeniería Industrial,
Universidad Peruana de Ciencias Aplicadas (UPC), Lima, Peru
{u201420249,u201221066,pcingvia}@upc.edu.pe
[2] Dirección de Investigación,
Universidad Peruana de Ciencias Aplicadas (UPC), Lima, Peru
carlos.raymundo@upc.edu.pe

Abstract. One of the main problems existing in manufacturing companies is the high frequency of machine breakdowns and their high repair time. Therefore, over time, various maintenance strategies seeking to more efficiently manage the scheduled jobs have been presented. However, these are not always as effective as expected, because they are not properly applied, the resources are not available, or the strategy is not aimed at directly solving the problem. Based on the aforementioned, this paper proposes an integral model of maintenance management based on the principles of total productive maintenance and reliability-centered maintenance methodologies in order to increase machine availability in a company in the manufacturing sector. To validate this proposal, a pilot project will be developed to measure the impact that is being sought.

Keywords: Maintenance · TPM · RCM

1 Introduction

The manufacturing sector currently has a dominant presence in Peru, as reflected in its contribution to the national GDP, which is greater than 12% [1]. In Metropolitan Lima, there is a greater concentration of manufacturing companies (approximately 53% of the total), which shows a high level of competition in the sector [2].

One of the main problems in the manufacturing industry is equipment maintenance [3]. The high frequency of production machine breakdowns is a common complication in most companies within the sector.

80% of the unexpected downtime is repetitive and can be resolved by a trained operator, while only 20% requires external assistance [4].

The proposal herein focuses on increasing machine availability in a manufacturing company by applying a model based on total productive maintenance (TPM) and reliability-centered maintenance (RCM) principles. Likewise, through the application

T. Ahram et al. (Eds.): IHIET 2019, AISC 1018, pp. 878–884, 2020.
https://doi.org/10.1007/978-3-030-25629-6_137

of the proposed practices, the average repair times are expected to reduce, just as average times between failures are expected to increase, since these are extremely important indicators when measuring the performance and condition of machines.

2 State of the Art

On one hand, regarding TPM, several authors agree that this is an improvement methodology designed to optimize equipment reliability and availability through the empowerment and active participation of all employees involved in production and maintenance tasks. In addition, it seeks to eliminate the six main equipment losses (equipment failures, machine adjustment, minor breakdowns, reduced operating speed, process defects, and loss of time) [5–8].

TPM is divided into eight pillars: autonomous maintenance, planned maintenance, focused improvements, maintenance prevention, administrative areas, training and coaching, safety and environment, and quality maintenance [9–12].

According to a study carried out in a manufacturing plant, the authors collected data relevant to the research using designed questionnaires, structured interviews, direct observations, and company records. The research results determined that the maintenance department employed 67.6% of its time in repair maintenance, 24.3% in preventive maintenance, and 8.1% in other non-applicable activities. Regarding TPM knowledge, 70.5% of employees were aware of the TPM concepts, while 14.7% indicated that TPM would help improve the current maintenance system and 14.7% were unsure [13].

RCM is a way to capture the possible downtime and underperformance causes by avoiding failures and taking a proactive approach to operations and maintenance [10]. Following are the foundations of this methodology used for the study:

- RCM for specific industries whose processes differ from those already known (specific RCM applicability cases in the mining industry, aviation, and areas of difficult access). Applied at a macro level.
- Application of RCM as an improvement proposal for specific and critical processes and machines and equipment for an organization, requiring special equipment or machine maintenance not commonly provided in the market, and extremely high spare part and repair costs.

Finally, as per some theoretical studies, the results may be enhanced by properly combining the two maintenance strategies. For this reason, we decided to combine several principles from the TPM and RCM methodologies, exploiting the virtues and strengths of each to address the problem posed in this study [7, 8].

3 Contribution

The proposed model associates two methodologies aligned with maintenance in the manufacturing industry, TPM and RCM. Theoretically, TPM comprises eight pillars, and RCM is divided into ten phases. According to the literature reviewed, when implementing these methodologies, it is not recommended to develop them directly and generically, as dictated by the theory. As each organization has different needs and resources, the development of the proposal must be customized for each company. The proposal presented in this paper uses two TPM principles, autonomous maintenance and planned maintenance, and five of the general RCM methodology phases. The merger of these principles is detailed in Fig. 1.

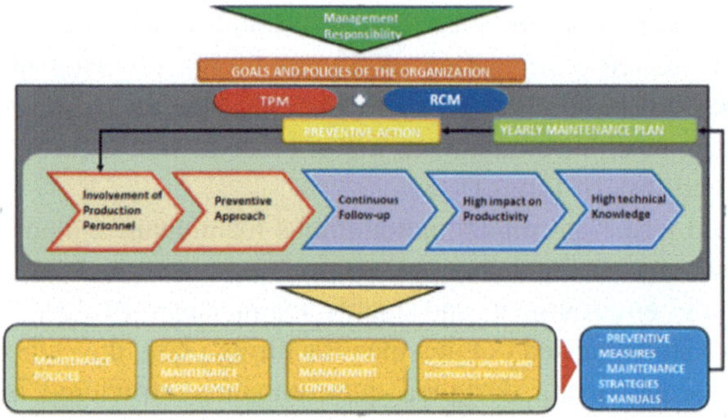

Fig. 1. TPM + RCM

The application of TPM, in particular, focused on simple preventive activities, such as cleaning, lubrication, component adjustment, and verification. With the application of RCM, a new handling and maintenance management system has been established for the machine under study. Improvements were made in safety, environmental impacts, production impacts, reduction of breakdowns caused by excessive maintenance, improvements to the maintenance plan and associated costs, knowledge of the equipment, and reduction of technical dependence on the manufacturers.

3.1 Conceptualization

PM prioritizes the historical information necessary to establish the specific actions required for each equipment piece, so that adequate maintenance times are established, specific prevention activities are defined for equipment with high deterioration, and preventive maintenance tasks are performed based on the criticality and complexity of the equipment.

RCM determines the potential failures of each system through measures such as failure analysis, determination of preventive measures (training plan, modification, procedures), consultation, manuals, and obligations, which will be added to the company's current annual maintenance plan. The levels considered for the corresponding study were identified and determined (Fig. 2).

3.2 Representation

Once the critical machine to which this model will be applied has been defined, it is necessary to identify its composition, i.e., its equipment and components. To define

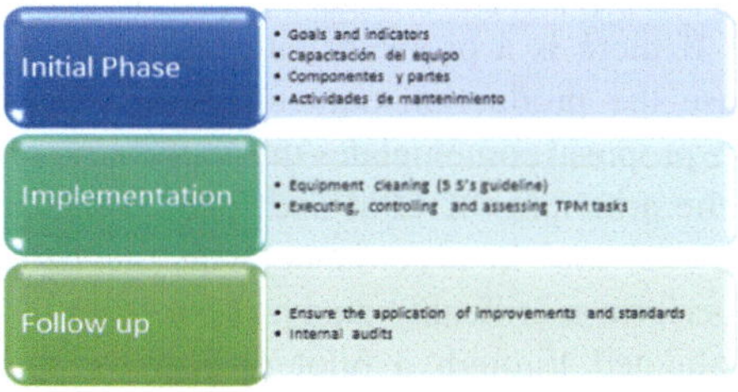

Fig. 2. Stages TPM

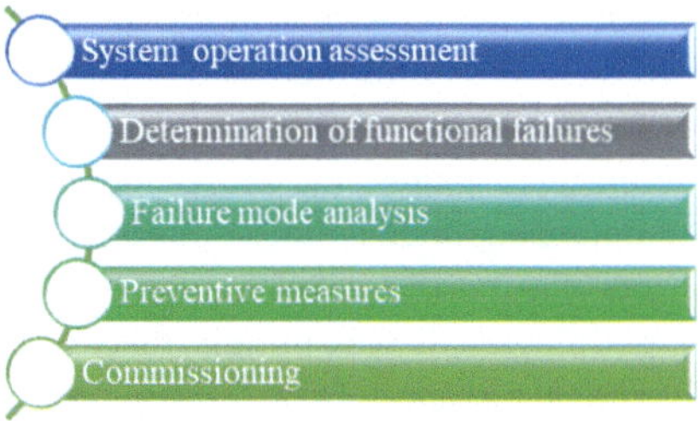

Fig. 3. RCM stages

which components will receive RCM treatment and which will receive TPM treatment, two criteria were considered: cost and criticality. If a component is very expensive and considered very critical, RCM should be applied. Otherwise, this component will be treated with the TPM method. Based on this, both processes were designed so as to maintain the main objective of each methodology. Figure 1 denotes the stages of the TPM section (Fig. 3).

The initial phase presents the initial considerations that must be taken into account before the proposal is implemented. In the implementation phase, the necessary tasks are executed according to the established TPM program. Finally, in the follow-up phase, the observations from internal audits are listed to improve the program.

In the RCM stage, first phase, it is necessary to correctly select the indicators and respective weights for each, in order to know their value before carrying out the study, apply the proposal's conclusions, and measure their effectiveness overall. The second phase refers to sources of information to be consulted and evaluated, such as breakdown history, information provided by maintenance personnel, and production and functional diagrams available in the area. In the third phase, the modes (causes) of the faults found in the previous phase are determined. In the fourth phase, the preventive measures adopted must be related to the importance of the faults to be avoided. Finally, in the last phase, the preventive measures defined in the previous phase must be implemented and their results must be audited.

3.3 Indicators

To achieve a correct follow-up of the proposal, progress-measuring indicators must be established: Mean time to repair (MTTR), Preventive Maintenance Achievement Rate, Corrective Maintenance Task Rate, Reliability, Availability, RCM Efficiency Indicator.

4 Validation

The company where the pilot project was carried out was Bosch,.Worldwide, it is the third best company in the sector. In Peru, it occupies the third position in the market, focusing on manufacturing white goods, such as stoves, refrigerators, and freezers.

Regarding the maintenance area of the company, there is a maintenance coordinator, a maintenance engineer, a maintenance planner, and a TPM assistant. The company considers that three machines are critical for its production areas: a polyurethane injector, a thermoformer, and a paint booth. If there is a problem with any of these machines, the impact caused is great because the production may come to a halt. Therefore, to address the causes mentioned, the proposal contemplates the application of a maintenance management model based on the principles of TPM and RCM.

For the correct implementation of the model and in accordance with the base methodologies, it was initially necessary to perform a criticality analysis per team.

The application of our proposal was validated through a pilot project for the polyurethane injector. First, a series of stages and phases was proposed, which was followed to achieve an adequate TPM implementation. Even when a general sequence has already been established, according to the literature reviewed, it is not always advisable to follow this sequence to the letter as each organization has different resources and needs. Therefore, the implementation sequence was customized with a direct focus on the organization. The stages are presented below:

4.1 TPM Section

4.1.1 Initial Phase

- Forming the work team: First, the work team must be defined. The leading project engineer must be appointed and the number and type of maintenance technicians required to perform the scheduled work must be decided.
- Staff training: Talks and meetings are held to explain the methodology and what the implementation is expected to achieve.
- Defining goals and indicators: These must be clear enough for everyone to understand their ultimate purpose within the application process.
- Determining the machine's equipment and components: After determining the machine on which TPM will be performed, its equipment and components must be defined. This will help to better organize the maintenance activities that will be scheduled, and to perform a more focused follow-up.
- Planning maintenance activities: To better control and follow up on the work, a form will be used to specify who the responsible technicians are, the equipment piece that requires the work done, the specific activities that will be executed, and their frequency of application.

4.1.2 Implementation

- Equipment cleaning: Initial cleaning of the equipment, and of the workstation, before any scheduled activity is performed. This is based on 5S principles.
- Activity execution, control, and assessment: Once the previous step is completed, the actual execution of the maintenance tasks determined in the TPM program begins. Once the tasks are completed, a work completion control, as well as the corresponding evaluation, must be filled out.

4.1.3 Follow-up

- Application of improvements: Improvements in the TPM program should be proposed. This will strengthen the project goals, broaden the scope of the activities in each machine, and verify whether the activities scheduled have been properly completed.
- Internal audits: The program's reports will be checked for completeness and updating, and to make sure that the scheduled activities are being carried out.

5 Conclusion

Through a final assessment of the results, it was verified that the maintenance management improvement proposal presented in this study achieved the expected results, since the objectives of the three main maintenance indicators (availability, reliability, and maintainability) were reached and preventive and corrective maintenance costs were redistributed as required by the company. At the same time, the literature review and the proposal development substantiated and proved that RCM, if developed within the TPM framework, strengthens and facilitates better results, since it focuses on preventive maintenance. The high degree of complementarity between the principles of both methodologies was evident.

As for the final results, a 15% increase was reported in machine availability, yielding an additional availability of 30 h of production. In addition, MTBF increased and MTTR decreased, as expected. In addition, the risk priority number indicated that there was an improvement in the injection head, as the index was reduced from 231 to 210, i.e., a decrease of 10%.

Likewise, it was evidenced that the impact of the implemented proposal turned out to be effective in implementing change in the organization's culture. This involved a series of changes such as implementing several new machines, records, reports, and procedure maintenance activities, which in some complemented the existing activities and covered blank spaces in some processes that required attention.

References

1. MINPRO. Anuario Estadístico Industrial, Mipyme y Comercio Interno2015 (2016). Recuperado de. https://www.produce.gob.pe/documentos/estadisticas/anuarios/anuario-estadistico-mype-2015.pdf (Fecha de consulta: 28 Apr 2018)
2. Cárdenas, G.: ¿Existe aún la industria manufacturera en el Perú? Pensamiento Crítico, **11**, pp. 11–32 (2009). Recuperado de. http://revistasinvestigacion.unmsm.edu.pe/index.php/econo/article/viewFile/9005/7833, https://www.ingenieriaindustrialonline.com/herramientas-para-el-ingeniero-industrial/mantenimiento/eficiencia-general-de-los-equipos-oee/ (Fecha de consulta: 05 May 2018)
3. SPC Consulting Group. 6 Retos que enfrentan las Empresas de Manufactura en la actualidad. México (2014). Recuperado de. https://spcgroup.com.mx/retos-enfrentan-empresas/ (Fecha de consulta: 01 May 2018)

4. Morales, M.J.D., Rodriguez, R.S.: Total productive maintenance (TPM) as a tool for improving productivity: a case study of application in the bottleneck of an auto-parts machining line. Int. J. Adv. Manuf. Technol. **92**(1–4), 1013–1026 (2017). https://doi.org/10.1007/s00170-017-0052-4
5. Kumar, J., Kumar Soni, V., Agnihotri, G.: Impact of TPM implementation on Indian manufacturing industry. Int. J. Prod. Perform. Manage. **63**(1), 44–56 (2014). https://doi.org/10.1108/IJPPM-06-2012-0051
6. Bartz, T., Cezar Mairesse Siluk, J., Paula Barth Bartz, A.: Improvement of industrial performance with TPM implementation. J. Qual. Maintenance Eng. **20**(1), 2–19 (2014). https://doi.org/10.1108/JQME-07-2012-0025
7. Ben-Daya, M.: You may need RCM to enhance TPM implementation. J. Qual. Maintenance Eng. **6**(2), 82–85 (2000). https://doi.org/10.1108/13552510010328086
8. Carrasco, F.J.C.: Characteristics of the systems TPM and RCM in the maintenance engineering. 3C Tecnología **5**(3), 68–75 (2016). https://doi.org/10.17993/3ctecno.2016.v5n3e19.68-75
9. Shen, C.C.: Discussion on key successful factors of TPM in enterprises. J. Appl. Res. Technol. **13**(3), 425–427 (2015). https://doi.org/10.1016/j.jart.2015.05.002
10. Singh, J., Singh, H., Sharma, V.: Success of TPM concept in a manufacturing unit – a case study. Int. J. Prod. Perform. Manage. **67**(3), 536–549 (2018). https://doi.org/10.1108/IJPPM-01-2017-0003
11. Singh, R.K., Gupta, A., Kumar, A., Khan, T.A.: Ranking of barriers for effective maintenance by using TOPSIS approach. J. Qual. Maintenance Eng. **22**(1), 18–34 (2016). https://doi.org/10.1108/JQME-02-2015-0009
12. Ylipää, T., Skoogh, A., Bokrantz, J., Gopalakrishnan, M.: Identification of maintenance improvement potential using OEE assessment. Int. J. Prod. Perform. Manag. **66**(1), 126–143 (2017). https://doi.org/10.1108/IJPPM-01-2016-0028
13. Mwanza, B.G., Mbohwa, C.: Design of a total productive maintenance model for effective implementation: case study of a chemical manufacturing company. Procedia Manufact. **4**, 461–470 (2015). https://doi.org/10.1016/j.promfg.2015.11.063

μσADL: An Architecture Description Language for MicroServices

Tasos Papapostolu(✉)

Faculty of Mathematics and Informatics, Sofia University "St. Kliment Ohridski", 5 James Bourchier Blvd, 1164 Sofia, Bulgaria
papapostol@fmi.uni-sofia.bg

Abstract. In recent years, the MicroServices architectural style has significantly grown in popularity due to its application to large-scale software systems with positive results. In the domain of Software Architecture, textual Architecture Description Languages (ADLs) can be used to describe the architecture of a software intensive system at an abstract level. μσADL is such an ADL, co-created by the author, designed in order to provide to software architects and various stakeholders a practical way for describing software systems that follow the microservices architectural style. In this paper, an example is presented, where a system based upon this style is described using μσADL. The constructs provided by the language concerning the description and dynamic reconfiguration of a microservice architecture are presented.

Keywords: Architecture Description Languages · Microservice architectures · μσADL · Software architecture

1 Introduction

MicroServices [1, 2] architectural style has been applied in building large-scale software applications, with very promising results and has rapidly gained in popularity over the past years. Its aim is to build applications as a collection of independent and as loosely coupled as possible services. Though they present similarities with Service-Oriented Architectures (SOA) and can be viewed as one form of SOA [3], there are differences, e.g. each microservice has its own persistent storage which cannot be modified by other microservices.

Software architecture [4] provides to architects and various stakeholders the conceptual framework in order to be able to abstract over the structure of an application. There is a number of different perspectives, e.g. static or dynamic, each one with different views, which can be used in order to describe in detail and to express the topology and the behaviour of software systems. Focusing on the dynamic perspective, the Component and Connector (C&C) view can be used to express the behaviour of a system during run-time. It consists of components, which express the computational elements, and connectors, which express the communication mechanisms between the components and their environment. A graph with their interconnections can represent the topology of a given system.

T. Ahram et al. (Eds.): IHIET 2019, AISC 1018, pp. 885–889, 2020.
https://doi.org/10.1007/978-3-030-25629-6_138

A formal way to express this in the domain of software architecture is through the use of Architecture Description Languages (ADLs). jADL [5] is a formal ADL, co-created by the author, which follows the C&C paradigm in order to express the architecture of both static and dynamic software systems. μσADL, an extension to jADL, is designed in order to provide to software architects and various stakeholders a practical way for describing MicroService architectures. One of the reasons to create μσADL is to promote the use of ADLs in the industry by hiding too rigorous and unnecessary (from a practitioner's point of view) formalities from the language syntax. The complexity and formalities met in a lot of ADLs constitute one of the main reasons that they are not widely adopted in industrial software development processes, but mostly in academia [6]. Another reason is the fact that the general tendency today for architects is to use architectural languages that describe SOA [7].

In the next section an example is presented, of how a software system, that follows the Microservice architectural style, can be described using μσADL. First, the initial architecture is defined and then the language constructs for handling dynamic reconfiguration are presented. Conclusions and future work are discussed in the final section.

2 μσADL Architecture Description

In the figure below an architecture of a simple eCommerce system is presented in an informal sketch. It comprises of three typical features in such systems; payment, search and review. Each of these processes is modeled as a separate microservice.

Below, the description in μσADL of one of the microservices (*Payment*) of Fig. 1 is presented. The *database* statement allows to simply describe, as a set of attributes, the information about the private database component of each microservice. This way, during the translation, a connector and a component are generated and can be furthermore configured. For the communication between the microservices, a jADL generic implementation of a message bus can be used. It can be directly instantiated and used or a different behaviour can be defined. In order for the attachments between the message bus and the microservices to be successful, a trait (*CommTrait*) needs to be aggregated and a provides port (*p*) needs to be configured.

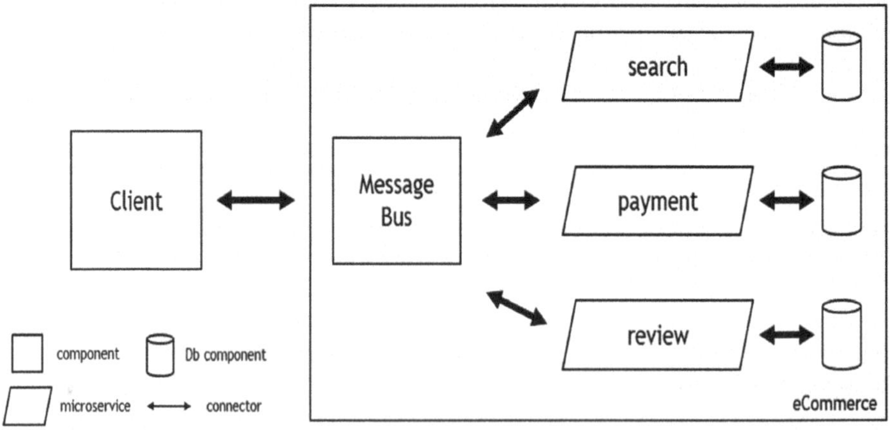

Fig. 1. Architectural sketch of an eCommerce application with microservices.

```
microservice Payment {
  requires port ISubscribe r;

  database {
    location: "localhost";
    connector: "JDBC";
  }

  trait PaymentTrait aggregate CommTrait {
    config p as {
      service void getMsg (Message msg){
        res = rDB.processPayment(msg);
        if (res)
          accept(msg);
        else
          deny(msg);
      }
    }
  }

  instance com1 = new PaymentTrait();

  config pDB as {
    service void getRes (type data){
      com1.r.sendMsg(data);
    }
  }
}
```

The other microservices can be described in a similar way and the instantiation of the initial architecture can be achieved with a script like the one shown in [9], where the description of an analogous system is presented in detail. From here, we focus on the language constructs for reconfiguration presented in the next subsection.

2.1 Dynamic Reconfiguration in μσADL

A common characteristic of microservice architectures is the need for dynamic reconfiguration - i.e. the change (foreseen or unforeseen) of the topology of a software system during run-time. In this example, the payment process can change in the future, hence a new instance of the reconfigured microservice must replace the old one. The language constructs *attach* and *detach* allow to easily describe such a change at the instance level of the given architecture. A script that can handle this reconfiguration is (partly) shown below:

```
component eCommerce {
  //...

  detach(mbus.s, payment.r);
  instance payment2 = new PaymentNew();
  attach(mbus.s, payment2.r);

  //...
}
```

Scalability is another important quality attribute when it comes to microservices. Though it can be challenging, since it can demand the handling of various components, in μσADL one way to address this issue is to use the dynamic load balancer architectural pattern implemented in jADL [8]. In a similar way that the message bus is used in the previous subsection, the architect can use the default implementation or modify the behaviour (a sample implementation is used here for simplicity). Instead of the servers presented in [8], the instances of each microservice can be managed by such a load balancer, after configuring the behaviour concerning the upscaling of each microservice. By applying this to our example, the code concerning the component eCommerce becomes:

```
component eCommerce {
  instance myLB = new DynamicLB();
  instance payment = new Payment();
  instance mbus = new MessageBus();

  attach(mbus.s, myLB.r);
  attach(myLB.p, payment.r);
  myLB.r.subscribe();

  instance myLBs = new DynamicLB();
  instance search = new Search();

  attach(mbus.s, myLBs.r);
  attach(myLBs.p, search.r);
  myLBs.r.subscribe();

  instance myLBr = new DynamicLB();
  instance review = new Review();

  attach(mbus.s, myLBr.r);
  attach(myLBr.p, review.r);
  myLBr.r.subscribe();
}
```

3 Conclusion

The language constructs of μσADL concerning the description and the dynamic reconfiguration of a system have been outlined through an example. μσADL provides an adequate way to simply describe microservice architectures. The majority of the formal definition part of the architecture is handled through the translator, when the script is automatically translated as shown in [9].

Our future work lies in furtherly improving the communication mechanisms provided by μσADL in respect to two important characteristics of microservices; decentralized governance and data management. Additionally, the finalization of the jADL compiler so that software artefacts can be generated from a given architectural description.

Acknowledgments. This work was supported by the project "Information and Communication Technologies for a Single Digital Market in Science, Education and Security" of the Scientific Research Center, NIS-3317.

References

1. Wolff, E.: Microservices: Flexible Software Architectures, 1st edn. Addison-Wesley Professional (2016)
2. Dragoni, N., Giallorenzo, S., Lafuente, A.L., Mazzara, M., Montesi, F., Mustafin, R., Safina, L.: Microservices: yesterday, today, and tomorrow. In: Present and Ulterior Software Engineering. Springer (2017)
3. Fowler, M., Lewis, J.: Microservices: a definition of this new architectural term. http://martinfowler.com/articles/microservices.html. Accessed 05 Apr 2019
4. Clements, P., Bachmann, F., Bass, L., Garlan, D., Ivers, J., Little, R., Merson, P., Nord, R., Stafford, J.: Documenting Software Architecture Views and Beyond, 2nd edn. Addison-Wesley Professional (2011)
5. Papapostolu, A., Birov, D.: Structured component and connector communication. In: Proceedings of Balkan Conference in Informatics 2017, North Macedonia (2017). https://doi.org/10.1145/3136273.3136291
6. Malavolta, I., Lago, P., Muccini, H., Pelliccione, P., Tang, A.: What industry needs from architectural languages: an industrial survey. dipartimento di informatica at the university of L'Aquila, Technical report, TRCS 002/2012 (2012)
7. Francesco, P.: Architecting microservices. In: 2017 IEEE International Conference on Software Architecture Workshops (ICSAW) (2017)
8. Papapostolu, T., Birov, D.: Architectural self-adaptation and dynamic reconfiguration in jADL. In: Proceedings of the Forty-Seventh Spring Conference of the Union of Bulgarian Mathematicians, pp. 168–177 (2018)
9. Papapostolu, T., Birov, D.: Towards a methodology for designing micro-service architectures using μσADL. Lecture Notes in Business Information Processing Book Series (LNBIP), vol. 319, pp. 421–431. Springer (2018)

Waynergy People – Human Interaction with an Emerging Pavement Energy Harvesting Technology

Adelino Ferreira(✉) and Francisco Duarte

Research Center for Territory, Transports and Environment
Department of Civil Engineering, University of Coimbra, Rua Luís Reis Santos, 3030-788 Coimbra, Portugal
adelino@dec.uc.pt, francisco.duarte@uc.pt

Abstract. This paper presents a new pavement energy harvest system that was developed in Portugal by the Waydip Company in collaboration with the Pavement Mechanics Laboratory of the University of Coimbra. After carrying out testing in the laboratory on one Waynergy People prototype module, 25 Waynergy People modules were set up in the entrance to a shopping centre in Lisbon, Portugal. The electrical energy generated by the Waynergy People pilot plant was 15,525.0 J or 4.31 Wh. This energy was harvested from 2,070 people walking over the system, with each person averaging 5 steps, which means that the average energy generated per step was 1.50 J on each module. We recorded a peak value of 4.20 J, which is equal to the energy produced by a person weighing 100 kg jumping. The maximum energy generated during one day was 126,540.0 J, or 35.2 Wh, and the average energy generated per day over the four months of the Waynergy People pilot was 90,417.0 J or 25.1 Wh.

Keywords: Pavement energy harvesting · Prototype · People steps · Electrical energy

1 Introduction

In Portugal, the Waydip Company and the Pavement Mechanics Laboratory of the University of Coimbra have developed Waynergy People, which is a new pavement energy harvesting system [1–3]. A new version of Waynergy People has been released with improvements made to some components and the system has recently been optimized [4–6].

This paper describes the optimized version of the Waynergy People system [7, 8], the laboratory tests that were performed and the implementation of a pilot scheme with 25 modules in a real-world situation at the main entrance of the Colombo shopping centre in Lisbon, Portugal. The main objectives of this study are to evaluate how much energy is generated with this optimized version in comparison to the previous one, and to evaluate the performance of the system in an operational environment, both in terms of the energy it generates and the reliability of the system.

T. Ahram et al. (Eds.): IHIET 2019, AISC 1018, pp. 890–895, 2020.
https://doi.org/10.1007/978-3-030-25629-6_139

2 Waynergy People Pilot Plant Implementation

After the laboratory tests on one Waynergy People prototype, 25 Waynergy People modules were placed in the entrance to a shopping centre in Lisbon, the capital of Portugal. The aim of this project was to measure the energy generated in an operational environment, in which there was no control over the way people stepped on the modules, and guaranteeing a high volume of daily hits.

Each Waynergy People module measures $0.5 \times 0.5 \times 0.16$ m^3, meaning that the pilot plant has a total surface area of 6.25 m^2. Also, each module has an installed power of about 40 W, meaning the pilot plant of 25 modules has a total installed power of 1,000 W.

Energy generated was measured using a carefully calibrated electronic device that measured the voltage and current generated by each module with each hit actuating the system, thus allowing us to calculate the power (W) and energy (J) that was generated. It also counted the total number of actuations.

Figure 1 shows the process installing of the Waynergy People modules. First, the floor was removed to a depth equal to the height of each module (0.16 m) plus the base structure (0.04 m). Then a base structure was built below the floor level to hold the modules in place. Thirdly, the Waynergy modules were mechanically secured to the base, one by one, and connected to each other electrically. Finally, the surface was finished using the same wood material as the surrounding flooring.

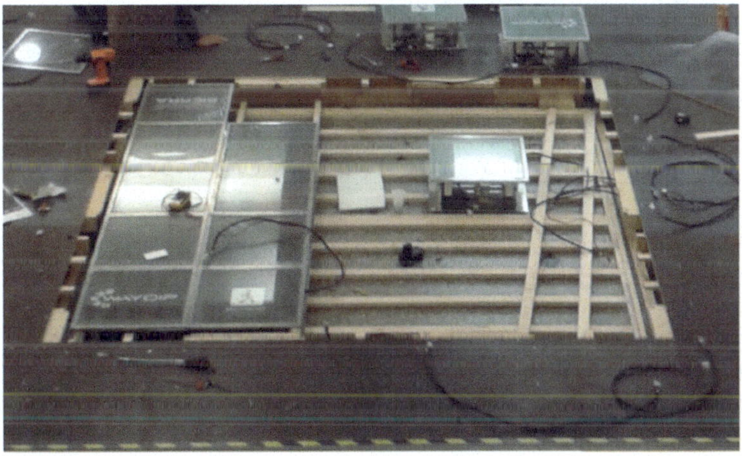

Fig. 1. Installation of the Waynergy People system.

Each Waynergy People module cost 750€ to produce, including the energy harvesting system the finished surface, glass and LED illumination. As well as the Waynergy modules, the pilot plant also included a wooden platform to raise the level of the floor, which cost 750€. Labour costs for the installation were 500€. All included, the total cost of the pilot plant was 20,000€.

3 Waynergy People Pilot Plant Tests and Results

The installation of this Waynergy People pilot plant made it possible to monitor the electrical energy generated by the movement of people in one location (Fig. 2). During peak hour, between 8 a.m. and 9 a.m., 10,350 people steps were measured. Figure 3 shows the electrical energy generated during this peak hour. On analysis, it may be concluded that the electrical energy generated by the Waynergy People pilot plant was 15,525.0 J or 4.31 Wh. This energy was produced by 2,070 people walking over the system, with an average of 5 steps per person, meaning that the average energy generation per step was 1.50 J per module. A peak value of 4.20 J was measured, which is the same energy as would be produced by a person weighing 100 kg jumping.

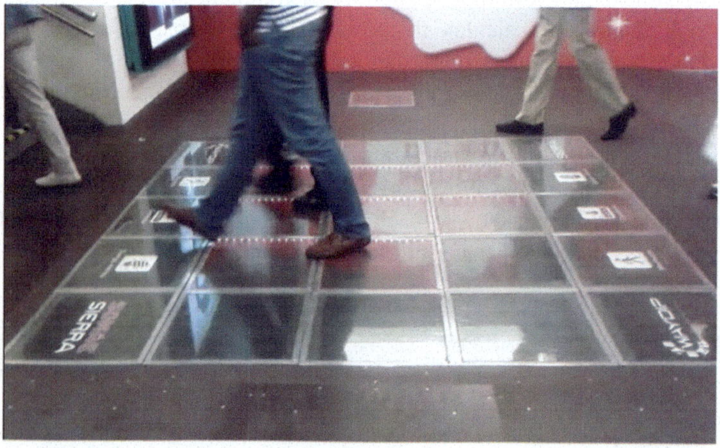

Fig. 2. Waynergy People system in use.

The maximum energy generated in a single day was 126,540.0 J, or 35.2 Wh, while the average daily energy generated, over the four months of the Waynergy People pilot plant, was 90,417.0 J or 25.1 Wh.

The total amount of energy generation was 10,669,223.0 J, or 2,963.70 Wh, for a total number of 7,112,815 measured steps, which is about 1,422,563 people walking on the pilot plant, with an average energy generation of 1.50 J per step. It is important to point out that even after four months, and despite the high number of steps per day, none of modules showed any signs of failure, wear or decreased energy generation, which shows that the system is efficient, reliable and resistant.

Table 1 shows the results for the optimized version of the Waynergy People prototype described in this paper. Analyzing the results presented in this table, it can be seen that, for light steps, 1.1 J and 1.2 J were generated for a person weighing 63 kg and 75 kg, respectively. For normal steps, the energy generated was 1.55 J and 1.70 J, for heavy steps it was 2.46 J and 2.70 J. Jumps generated 3.40 J and 3.80 J, for a person weighing 63 kg and 75 kg, respectively. The conversion efficiency of the

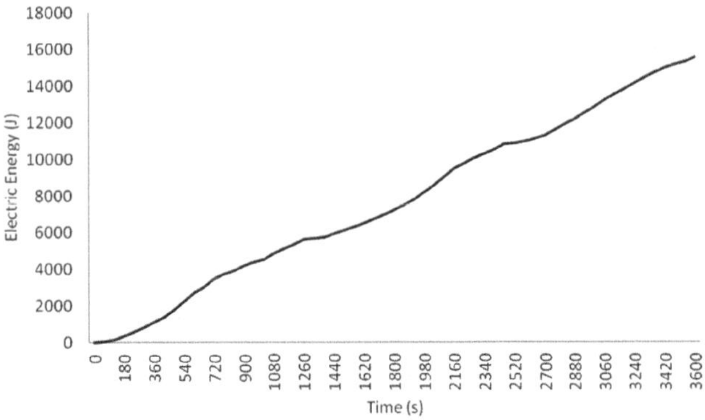

Fig. 3. Electrical energy generated during one hour.

energy harvesting device is defined by the ratio between the generated electrical energy and the energy transmitted by a pedestrian. Table 1 also shows the conversion efficiency for the new version of Waynergy People.

Table 1. Waynergy People prototype results.

Mass of a pedestrian (kg)	Step type	Relative mass (kg)	Energy transmitted (J)	Electric power (W)	Energy generated (J)	Conversion efficiency (%)
63.0	Light	44.1	2.1	17.5	1.1	52.4
	Normal	63.0	3.1	22.9	1.6	51.6
	Heavy	75.6	3.7	30.5	2.5	67.6
	Jump	100.8	4.9	36.0	3.4	69.4
75.0	Soft	52.5	2.6	19.9	1.2	46.2
	Normal	75.0	3.7	25.0	1.7	45.9
	Hard	90.0	4.4	35.0	2.7	61.4
	Jump	120.0	5.9	40.1	3.8	64.4

4 Conclusions

This research describes an optimized version of the Waynergy People system, with a new electromechanical system, including a new electromagnetic generator, a new gear ratio and methodology, and a new electronic controller. After validation in the laboratory, a 25-module pilot plant was installed in the main entrance of a shopping centre. Over a period of four months, the pilot plant was submitted to all kinds of loads and people step types and the energy generated by each module was measured. The results show that, the average energy generated by one step was 1.50 J, and the maximum value measured for one step was 4.20 J. After four months of the pilot plant, the total amount energy generated was 10,669,223.0 J, or 2,963.7 Wh by an estimated number of 1,422,563 people walking over the Waynergy People modules.

With these results, it is clear that the Waynergy People system is ready to be implemented in any indoor or outdoor site with large numbers of people on foot, who will generate electrical energy through their movement. The electrical energy generated can be directly consumed by electrical equipment connected to the modules or can be stored internally and consumed when necessary. The system also presents an additional feature for monitoring people steps, allowing people movement in different places to be counted and monitored, which could be useful for safety purposes, marketing or, in a smart-city, for generating real-time information.

In the near future, our research into energy harvesting will continue in two main directions. First, we will strive to further optimize some components of the Waynergy People system, including the development of new technology to store the electrical energy it generates using. for example, rechargeable batteries. Second, all the knowledge acquired so far will be used to develop a new system for use on road surfaces, in particularly on speed control humps on urban roads, with a view to generating electrical energy from the movement of vehicles. This electrical energy can not only be used for charging batteries, but also for general consumption by injecting it into the electric grid. It can also be used directly by nearby electrical equipment, such as public lighting, traffic lights, or outdoor advertising.

Acknowledgments. The present research work has been carried out in the framework of project PAVENERGY – Pavement Energy Harvest Solutions (PTDC/ECM-TRA/3423/2014), co-financed by the European Regional Development Fund (POCI-01-0145-FEDER-016676) through the Operational Programme for Competitiveness Factors (COMPETE) and by national funds through the Portuguese Foundation for Science and Technology (FCT). The author Francisco Duarte is also grateful to the FCT for the financial support provided to this study through Grant SFRH/BD/95018/2013. The author Adelino Ferreira is also grateful to the ACIV for its financial contribution for the presentation of this paper in the International Conference on Human Interaction and Emerging Technologies.

References

1. Duarte, F., Casimiro, F.: Pavement module for generating electric energy from the movement of people and vehicles. International Patent Application PCT/IB2011/052164, Patent WO2011145057 A2, November 2011
2. Duarte, F., Casimiro, F.: Electromechanical system for electric energy generation and storage using a surface motion. International Patent Application PCT/IB2013/050616, Patent WO2013114253 A1, August 2013
3. Duarte, F., Casimiro, F., Correia, D., Mendes, R., Ferreira, A.: Waynergy people: a new pavement energy harvest system. ICE Proceedings Municipal Engineer **166**(4), 250–256 (2013)
4. Duarte, F., Ferreira, A.: Energy harvesting on road pavements: state of the art. Energy, Institution of Civil Engineers **169**(2), 79–90 (2016)
5. Duarte, F., Champalimaud, J., Ferreira, A.: Waynergy vehicles: an innovative pavement energy harvest system. ICE Proceedings Municipal Engineer **169**(1), 13–18 (2016)

6. Ferreira, A.: Briefing: recent developments in pavement energy harvest systems. ICE Proceedings Municipal Engineer **165**(4), 189–192 (2012)
7. Duarte, F., Ferreira, A., Champalimaud, J.: Waynergy people: application in an operational environment. Energy, Institution of Civil Engineers **171**(2), 82–89 (2018)
8. Pavenergy. https://pavenergy.dec.uc.pt/. Accessed 21 Mar 2019)

Management Model Based on the Lean Thinking Method for Medium-Sized Peruvian Companies in the Apparel Sector

Luis Loayza[1](✉), Sebastián Olave[1](✉), Maribel Perez[1](✉), Jose Rojas[1](✉), and Carlos Raymundo[2](✉)

[1] Ingeniería de Gestión Empresarial, Universidad Peruana de Ciencias Aplicadas (UPC), Lima, Peru
{u201317482, u201211481, maribel.perez, jose.rojas}@upc.edu.pe

[2] Dirección de Investigación, Universidad Peruana de Ciencias Aplicadas (UPC), Lima, Peru
carlos.raymundo@upc.edu.pe

Abstract. The waste and reprocess problem in Peruvian apparel companies is greater than expected. After reviewing a history of losses and reprocesses, an innovative technical solution based on a combination of Lean Manufacturing and Agile tools is presented herein. This innovative proposal is implemented in the areas of cutting, embossing, and sewing in an apparel company. Value Stream Mapping results before and after implementing the proposed model are compared. The major achievement of this model is the significant reduction in loss percentage after two weeks of implementation.

Keywords: Lean Manufacturing · Balanced Scorecard · Takt time · Small and medium enterprises

1 Introduction

The apparel textile sector represents one of the main non-extractive activities in Perú, corresponding to 1.9% of the national GDP and slightly over 10% of the total manufacturing production [1]. This sector is one of the main sources of employment offering nearly 412 thousand jobs, representing 8.9% of the economically active population employed nationwide. Most of this employment is generated by micro, small, and medium enterprises (SMEs). These companies constitute the second most important sector within the manufacturing GDP [2].

The production process of the apparel industry covers all functions necessary for apparel manufacturing. However, based on this background, there are relevant problems that have existed in this sector for the last 6 years [3]: lack of organization and the absence of procedures, work instructions, and measurement indicators. These problems lead to inefficient productive processes that generate waste.

The need to improve and adopt new practices for achieving efficiency in many larger companies has resulted in the application of different quality management

T. Ahram et al. (Eds.): IHIET 2019, AISC 1018, pp. 896–902, 2020.
https://doi.org/10.1007/978-3-030-25629-6_140

concepts. Similarly, SMEs could also benefit from the adaptation of quality management [4]. However, the challenge for SMEs, in contrast to large companies, is limited resources, which is one of their key characteristics [5]. These resource limitations hinder the progress of SMEs in new areas, thus generating an interesting field of research. This has motivated us to research solutions to resource limitations and methods to increase efficiency in apparel production processes of SMEs in Perú.

As mentioned above, we studied the low productivity of clothing processes of SMEs in Perú due to the need to manage volatility and flexibility [6]. Accordingly, a management model based on a combination of Lean Manufacturing and Agile tools is proposed herein. Authors, such as Bruce et al. (2004), suggest a combination of these methodologies to generate efficiency in apparel processes [7].

We opted to conduct an in-depth case study to research this subject. We conducted our study at the company T23, which belongs to the apparel sector and mainly manufactures garments for ladies and gentlemen of all ages. T23 has been in the market for approximately 8 years and is currently located in the Ate district in Lima, Perú. Their long tenure in the market has allowed the company to consolidate itself as a growing SME. For example, in 2017, the company reported approximately S/. 5,507,328.00 in revenue from sales in both international and local markets. The company employs approximately 81 people in its apparel production plant.

T23N's main problem was the generation of waste and reprocessing. In economic terms, this corresponds to losses of S/. 662,329.78.

2 State of the Art

Lean Manufacturing

Lean Manufacturing is a methodology that focuses on eliminating all types of waste existing in an organization [8]. Ohno (1988) [9] was able to identify seven types of waste, which are explained in his book "Toyota Production System." Ohno further argues that these wastes are often not easy to identify at first glance. However, they can be classified as follows: Overproduction, Waiting, Transporting, Inappropriate Processing, Unnecessary Inventory, Excessive Motion, Defects.

Balanced Scorecard

The Balanced Scorecard (BSC) is a metric system used to control the performance of an organization. To this end, BSC assesses the vision, mission, and business strategies of the company and aligns them to specific objectives, metrics, and indicators. Kaplan and Norton designed BSC to represent the four different perspectives of business [10]: Customer Perspective, Internal Process Perspective, Learning and Growth Perspective, Financial Perspective.

It is true that the implementation of BSC over the years has benefited many organizations. However, the four perspectives of the initial approach should not always be followed. Each organization must be aligned to its own needs [11].

Gram (2013), in his research study on production system losses, modified the initial Kaplan and Norton BSC, and aligned it to the following perspectives: Material Perspective, Machine Perspective, Energy Perspective, Labor Perspective.

In this manner, the four perspectives were focused on the main objective, efficient production without losses.

Agile Methodologies
These methodologies arise from issues related to rigid methods and processes, not flexible enough to handle the demands of clients [12]. Given global competitive circumstances, companies must be flexible and respond to change. If this fact is seen as a possibility to handle the need for flexibility, while giving the team clear and stable objectives, the idea about Agile methodology is considered a facilitator for management of textile SMEs [13].

3 Methodology

To study the application of Lean and Agile methodologies in textile management, a qualitative and quantitative research approach is selected. To diagnose the problem, interviews were held with the production manager, area managers, and operators, using open questions in which the respondents had no answer restrictions.

After discussing the problem with their respective causes, a management model was prepared, based on the research and efforts previously developed in literature. This model's aim was not only the reduction of waste and reprocessing in the company under study but also the reduction of the lead time in the textile manufacturing process (Fig. 1).

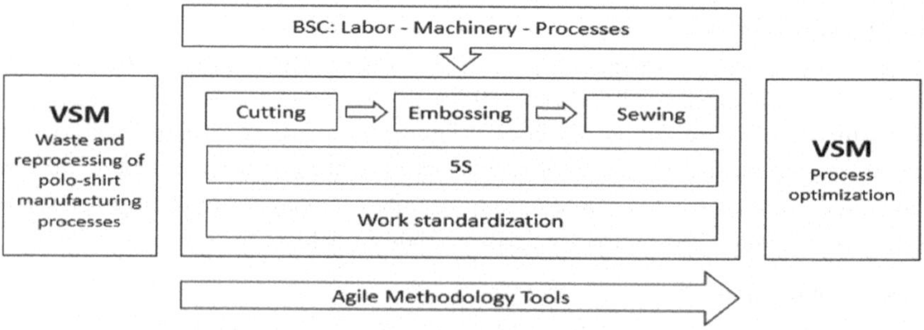

Fig. 1. Lean agility model

In addition, to validate the proposed model, data were obtained from three different sources: semi-structured interviews, observations, and group discussions. The last phase of the model comprised weekly semi-structured interviews.

4 Contribution

The proposed model works as shown in Fig. 2, wherein it starts by determining the current situation of the production process. For this, the Value Stream Mapping (VSM) tool was selected to visualize and understand the problem areas of value streams of the organization process [13]. This tool revealed the material waste, cycle time, and lead time of the production process.

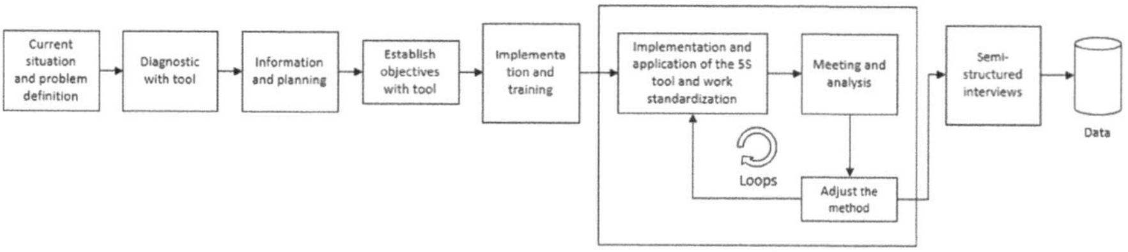

Fig. 2. Implementation of the lean agility methodology

After seeing results from the VSM, it was decided to reduce waste and reprocessing. To this end, objectives and indicators of production management and control were established, which led us to opt for the Balanced Score Card (BSC) tool. The BSC is a metric system that controls the performance of companies. This method assigned company objectives to metrics and indicators [14]. The indicators have been structured according to the perspectives set by the organization. The indicators are the following:

Waste control percentage: This indicator allows us to measure the percentage variation of waste produced during cutting processes.

Reprocessing control percentage: This indicator allows us to measure the percentage variation of reprocessing produced during sewing processes.

Productivity level: This indicator allows us to measure the productivity of trained and non-trained personnel for specific time periods.

After the objectives and indicators were defined, a 5S program was implemented to create a stability base in the process. This tool is used to maintain work areas such that they are cleaner, more organized, and more secure [15]. The program has a monitoring chart of daily cleaning audits in the production plant.

5 Validation

Validation: Cutting Area Waste

After applying the previously mentioned tools to the cutting area, as defined in our implementation model, the improvement results related to waste are currently set to an average of 9.58% (Fig. 3).

Based on the figure, it can be seen that there is a tendency to reduce the percentage of waste in the cutting area, approaching the target objective of under 9%, according to the Textile Apparel market.

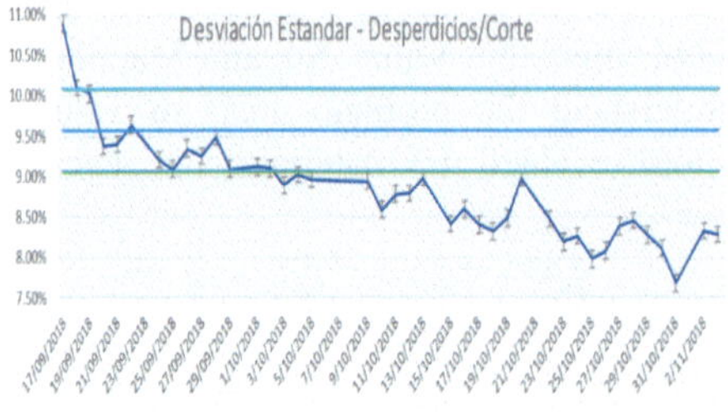

Fig. 3. Percentage variation of waste (2018)

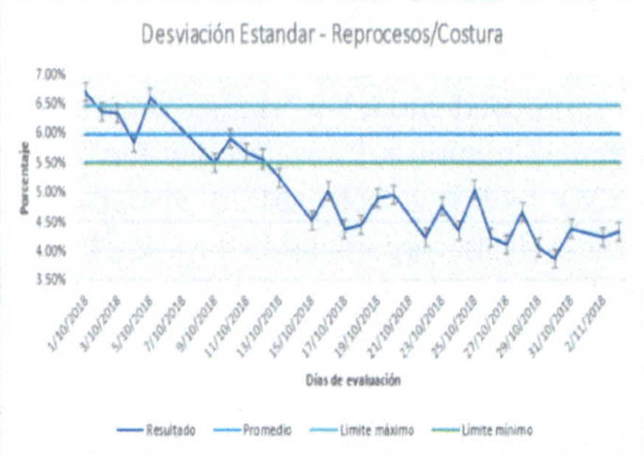

Fig. 4. Percentage variation of reprocesses/sewing (2018)

Validation: Sewing Area Reprocesses

After applying the tools proposed in our model to the sewing area, the average improvement of apparel reprocesses (here, reprocessing of polo shirts) is currently set at 5.97% (Fig. 4).

Validation: Embossing Area Reprocesses

After applying the tools proposed in our model to the embossing area, the average improvement of apparel reprocesses (polo-shirt) is currently set at 5.91% (Fig. 5).

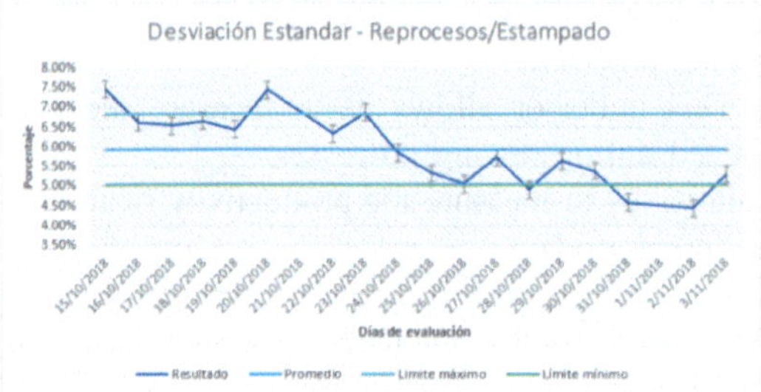

Fig. 5. Percentage variation of reprocesses/embossing (2018)

Año 2017	Año 2018
Área de Corte – Desperdicio de tela	
15.02%	9.58%
Área de Costura – Re-proceso de polos	
8.20%	6.70%
Área de Estampado – Re-proceso de polos	
8.35%	5.91%

Fig. 6. Comparative table of results

Comparative Table of Results

The Fig. 6 compares the reprocess percentages reported in 2017 to the percentages recorded in 2018 after the improvement model was implemented in the company.

6 Conclusions

Owing to the industry's own workload, there were barriers to entry during 5S implementation. Therefore, each audit had to be conducted consecutively and not in a general way. This delayed the validation of the sewing and embossing areas. However, despite these barriers to entry, the application of the 5S audits in T23N was performed efficiently as the company owners are part of the third generation. This means that the owners are open to new trends and improvement changes for the company. Furthermore, the collaboration and commitment of the workers helped implement the proposed model on the scheduled dates, collect the measurement data, and deploy production indicators. The SIPOC tools used in the development of the sequence of information flow, apart from offering methodological support to collect information, generated additional process documentation, which also added value to the project.

The model implemented at T23N, in 9 weeks of validation, shows a 5% waste reduction in the cutting area. In 2017, the company had an average waste percentage of 14.57% and currently shows an average of 9.58%, approaching the standard market target of under 9% of waste. In addition, sewing area reprocesses were reduced by 3.72%. In 2017, the company reported an average of 9.69% in reprocesses. Average reprocesses are currently at 5.97%, approaching the target reprocess indicator for the market, i.e., under 5%.

The improvements introduced by the BSC indicators and 5S audits have led to improvements indirectly focused on other perspectives, such as the production capacity of machines. Cutting capabilities increased from 60% to 70%. For sewing, they increased from 70% to 80%. Finally, for embossing, functionality increased from 70% to 75%.

References

1. Gestión: A propósito del sector textil confecciones | Blogs | Gestión. https://gestion.pe/blog/prosperoperu/2017/10/a-proposito-del-sector-textil-confecciones.html. Accessed 23 Oct 2018
2. Ministerio de la Producción: Industria Textil y Confecciones: Estudio de investigación sectorial. Lima (2015). http://ogeiee.produce.gob.pe/images/oee/docTrab_Textil.pdf
3. Gestión: Produce: Sector prendas de vestir se recuperará en el 2018 y crecería alrededor de 4% (2018). https://gestion.pe/economia/produce-sector-prendas-vestir-recuperara-2018-creceriaalrededor-4-224404. Accessed 23 Oct 2018
4. Assarlind, M., Gremyr, I.: Critical factors for quality management initiatives in small- and medium-sized enterprises. Total Qual. Manag. Bus. Excellence **25**(3–4), 397–411 (2014). https://doi.org/10.1080/14783363.2013.851330
5. Hudson, M., Bourne, M., Smart, A.: Theory and practice in SME performance measurement systems. Int. J. Oper. & Prod. Manage. **21**(8), 1096–1115 (2001)
6. Bruce, M., Daly, L., Towers, N.: Lean or agile: a solution for supply chain management in the textiles and clothing industry? Int. J. Oper. & Prod. Manage. **24**(2), 151–170 (2004)
7. Mason Jones, R., Naylor, B., Towill, D.: Engineering the leagile supply chain. Int. J. Agile Manage. Syst. **2**(1), 54–61 (2000)

8. Hodge, G.L., Goforth Ross, K., Joines, J.A., Thoney, K.: Adapting lean manufacturing principles to the textile industry. Prod. Planning Control **22**(3), 237–247 (2011). https://doi.org/10.1080/09537287.2010.498577
9. Ohno, T.: Toyota production system: beyond large-scale production. Productivity Press, New York (1988)
10. Kaplan, R.S., Robert, N.P.D.K.S., Davenport, T.H., Kaplan, R.S., Norton, D.P.: The strategy-focused organization: how balanced scorecard companies thrive in the new business environment. Harvard Business Press (2001)
11. Welge, M.K., Al-Laham, A., Eulerich, M.: Strategisches Management: Grundlagen-Prozess-Implementierung. Springer-Verlag (2017)
12. Beck, K.: Embracing change with extreme programming. Computer **32**(10), 70–77 (1999)
13. Manfredsson, P.: Textile management enabled by lean thinking: a case study of textile SMEs. Prod. Plan. Control **27**(7–8), 541–549 (2016). https://doi.org/10.1080/09537287.2016.1165299
14. Gram, M.: A systematic methodology to reduce losses in production with the balanced scorecard approach. Manuf. Sci. Technol. **2**(1), 12–22 (2013). https://doi.org/10.13189/mst.2013.010103
15. Pérez, V., Quintero, L.: Metodología dinámica para la implementación de 5' s en el área de producción de las organizaciones. Revista Ciencias Estratégicas **25**(38), 411–423 (2017)

Management Model for Pecan Production Using Process Tools in an MSE in Peru

Alejandra Muñante[1(✉)], Fabrizio Reyes[1(✉)], Fernando Sotelo[1(✉)], and Carlos Raymundo[2(✉)]

[1] Ingeniería Industrial,
Universidad Peruana de Ciencias Aplicadas (UPC), Lima, Peru
{u201211490,u201210801,fernando.sotelo}@upc.edu.pe
[2] Dirección de Investigación,
Universidad Peruana de Ciencias Aplicadas (UPC), Lima, Peru
carlos.raymundo@upc.edu.pe

Abstract. The following study proposes a production management process model based on good practices and developed with process management tools for increasing crop productivity of pecan nuts using the Ica region in the district of Pachacutec as a study area. The study covers the proposed model's diagnosis and development. The relation between these stages is the main function of improving pecan orchard productivity. The study showed that to increase pecan productivity from 1.09 (t/ha) to 2.21 (t/ha), and to determine raw material needs, tools and/or labor, a standardized process is needed for pecan production. The study's main contribution is the development of a production management process through which farmers can order and control production by means of indicators. Furthermore, the study proposes that the developed process of pecan production currently applied by farmers should be supported by a mathematical model simulation.

Keywords: Production management · Pecans · Productivity · Agricultural productivity · Process management

1 Introduction

According to the National Institute of Statistics (INEI), 94.7% of the business companies in Peru are micro and small enterprises (MSEs) [1]. Within these, most micro and small companies in Peru are involved in agricultural economic activity. Pecans are part of this sector. According to Promperu [2], international demand in European and Asian markets has led Peru to be involved in pecan production.

As compared to the 1.09 (t/ha) pecans produced in Peru, Mexico produces 2.18 (t/ha), South Africa 1.79 (t/ha), and United States 1.32 (t/ha). Therefore, we propose that the implementation of a production management model can contribute directly to an increase in productivity in the sector under study.

T. Ahram et al. (Eds.): IHIET 2019, AISC 1018, pp. 903–909, 2020.
https://doi.org/10.1007/978-3-030-25629-6_141

2 State of the Art

According to Wells [3], the nutrition provided to pecan trees is a key indicator of good quality pecans. Pecans, like other plants, require nutrients that contribute to optimum growth and fruit production. Using fertilizers is a good method of supplying nutrients to the soil and helping correct nutrient deficiencies. Malnourished plants directly affect the productivity of the pecan tree. Mokochinski [4] mentions that pecan branches form a complete system that has its source in a single yolk, lateral or terminal, and it comprises a subpopulation within the tree. Therefore, should the tree exhibit a broken branch, the regressive death of the branch may occur and, in severe cases, the tree may die [5]. One of the factors that helps increase pecan fruit productivity is the branch, which must be strengthened for growth. According to Luo [6], pecan mange, caused by the fungus Fusicladium effusum is the main disease that reduces pecan productivity and quality in southeastern United States, although several other pathogens can also cause less productivity [7]. Another factor for evaluation is the hydration of the pecan, according to Sammis [8]. Plants can suffer stress due to a lack of some nutrients, mainly water. The management of water and nitrogen is affected by lack of awareness. In addition, water shortages and an increase in the use of fertilizers have led to changes in good practices. According to Wells [9], alternance refers to the tendency of a pecan nut tree to produce poor quality nuts in one harvest year, followed by another year in which the tree has a light crop, which is an important problem affecting pecan orchards.

3 Proposal

The contribution of this research will be based on the production management model, considering good agricultural practices for the pecan production process. First, the sector's plant nutrition problem will be addressed. Consequently, the subject of irrigation will be considered, and later, the topic of pesticides. Finally, a production management model with three subprocesses will be implemented: production planning, production scheduling and production control.

3.1 Good Farming Methods

3.1.1 Fertilization

Regarding compost and fertilizers, the current situation in the Ica-Pachacutec region is that farmers compost and fertilize once a year in August. According to Walworth [10], ZnEDTA acid is a plant fertigation method, which consists of the following: it is applied in ratios of 2.2 to 4.4 kg/ha of Zn injected into the water used to irrigate trees by microaspersion. The following results were obtained: compared to untreated trees, treated trees showed that Zn treatments largely eliminated the visible symptoms of Zn deficiency and increased trunk diameter growth. The trunk growth in the third year was 1920% higher in "Wichita" trees treated with ZnEDTA compared to fertilized trees. 16N-3.5P-2.5K-4S composting was used for one year, the ZnEDTA fertigation frequency was 15 times a year, mostly in the month of January.

3.1.2 Irrigation

Ica-Pachacutec farmers irrigate by gravity. Of these, 92.3% irrigate their gardens every 90 days, the equivalent of three months. According to Wells [5], in a study conducted in the United States, trees were planted in January 2014 with a space of 3 m between them. All trees were irrigated by microsprinklers placed 0.3 m from the trunk of the tree at different speeds depending on the treatment. The plants were watered three days per week, four hours per day from April to September. If it rained, irrigation was postponed for three days so as not to flood the plants. Therefore, fungi and other diseases did not appear. Using this means of irrigation, the trunk diameter increased from 89% to 388% compared to non-irrigated trees, also reporting increases in leaf area, leaf length, leaf width, and chlorophyll index.

3.1.3 Pesticides

In the Ica-Pachacutec region, farmers do not perform controls and/or phytosanitary treatments with fungicides and insecticides. According to Sanderlin [11], the key components for the effective use of fungicides for pecan disease control are time, coverage, and concentration. The application time is based on the fact that fungicides control the disease by preventing infection. However, they must be applied before infection occurs. Infection in the stems can reduce growth and severe infection of the stems can permanently kill growth for the current season.

3.2 Production Management Model

3.2.1 Production Planning

Production planning is the initial stage of the production process. The objective of this stage is to establish the required materials and labor for the production process. These requirements are in accordance with the definitions and standards established by the quality management department and the production level of the trees.

The production planning flowchart organize the inputs and outputs of the processes in a simple image, with the production schedule as the last deliverable (Fig. 1).

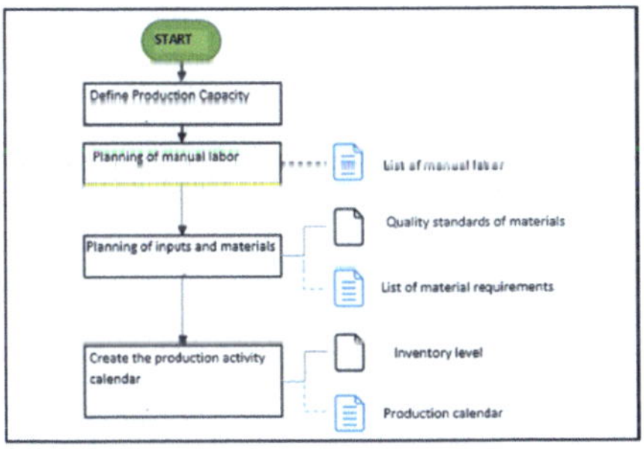

Fig. 1. Production planning flowchart

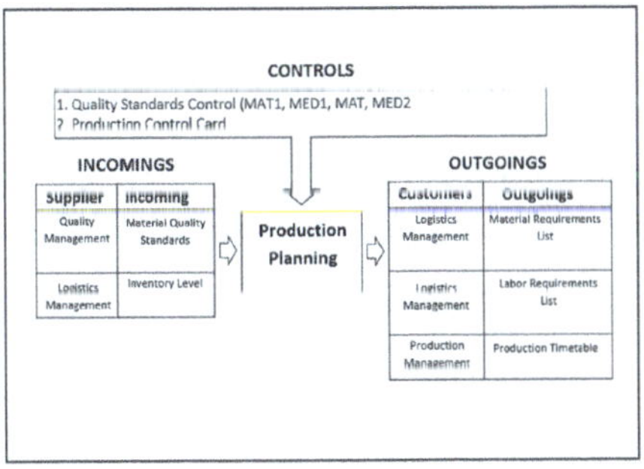

Fig. 2. SIPOC production planning

3.2.1.1 Turtle SIPOC

The SIPOC turtle diagram (Fig. 2) mainly serves to define the management system processes. In this case, the SIPOC turtle tool represents the functioning of the production planning process, from the definitions and standards established by the quality department to the delivery of a list of personnel requirements, supplies, and materials for the logistics area.

3.2.1.2 Documentation Forms

- Manual Labor List: This document outlines the activity performed by the operator, plus the quantity and date.
- Requirement List: This document indicates the activity requirements of the production process.
- Production Schedule: This is the main deliverable for the activities of the pecan production process. Every activity performed will be identified in the corresponding weeks of the month.

3.2.2 Production Scheduling

In this stage of the production process, production activities are scheduled: irrigation, nutrition (fertilizers and composting), and pesticides. The start and end dates of each production activity are defined. A greater labor force is required during the harvest stage. For this stage, the scheduling will determine the worker activities for each corresponding date, which must be performed and evidenced through the scheduling deliverables. The established activity flow will be seen in more detail through the production planning flowchart (Fig. 3).

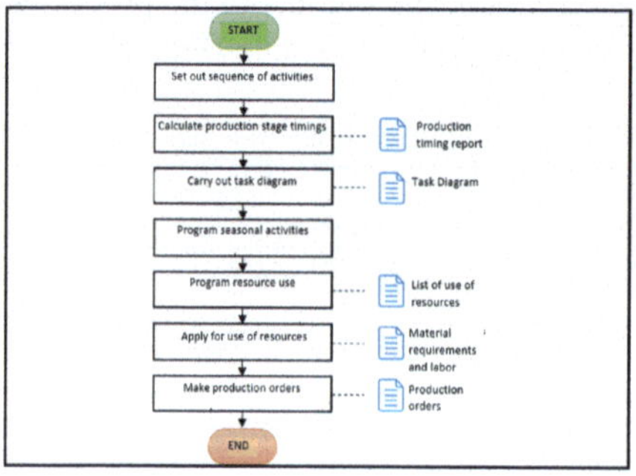

Fig. 3. Production scheduling flowchart

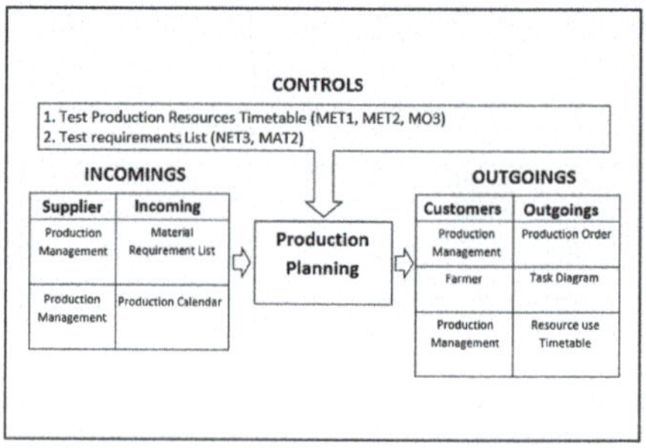

Fig. 4. SIPOC production scheduling

3.2.2.1 Turtle SIPOC

A SIPOC turtle diagram is developed for production scheduling, establishing the input and output activities of the scheduling process. At the beginning of the process, the material requirements list and the production schedule will be needed to generate the production order, the task diagram, and the resource use schedule (Fig. 4).

3.2.2.2 Documentation Forms

- Production Time: This document measures time per hectare, total time (minutes), number of hectares, and total time in days for each of the activities of the production process and for each of the project tasks.
- Task Diagram: Denotes the days of the week, the activity that the operator must perform, the number of hectares, and the corresponding month.
- Production order: This document outlines the production order, the operator's name, the activity, and number of hectares. In this production order, the operations to be performed and the quantity will be specified.

3.2.3 Production Control

Production Control is the production support process. At this stage, the aim is to guarantee the development of production process activities according to the standards and definitions established by the quality department. It uses a card-based control management model redesigned for simple use and easy access for farmers.

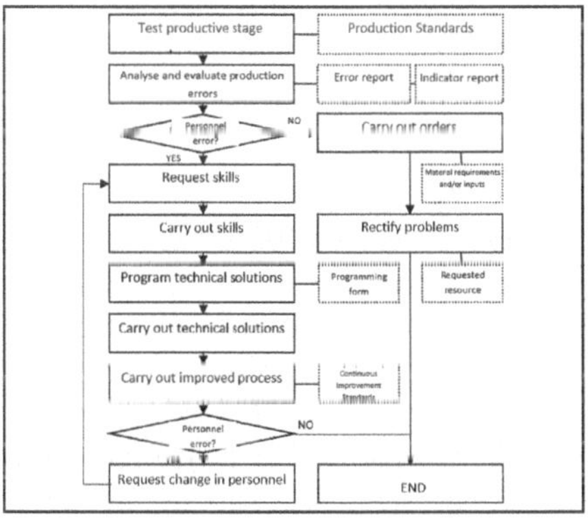

Fig. 5. Flowchart of production control.

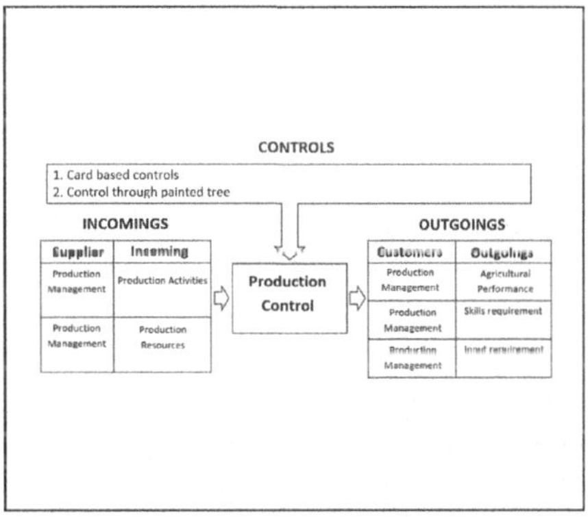

Fig. 6. SIPOC production control

With this chart (Fig. 5), possible solutions to problems according to their type are highlighted. In addition, the start of possible deficiencies within the process are indicated, which may be due to a lack of resources or personnel, or the method used (Fig. 6).

3.2.3.1 Turtle SIPOC

Similar to the previous subprocesses, a SIPOC turtle diagram is developed for production control by establishing the activities related to the entry and exit of the process.

3.2.3.2 Documentation Forms

- Agricultural Yield: Agricultural yield will be calculated by dividing the total production of pecan trees by the numbers harvested.
- Input Requirement: This document will define the input that will be required, the type of input, the input amount, and the corresponding date.

4 Results

When applying the management model of the proposed production, an implementation cost of the tools to be used within the project was generated. These tools are the following: printouts and tools, soil studies, irrigation, pruning, pesticides, nutrition for trees, warehouses, purchases, and other implementation costs (training, travel, etc.) (Fig. 7).

Pecan Sale price	18.00				
Production per normal tree (kg)	30.00	Sales	4860000.00		
Production per augmented tree (kg)	37.50	Sales (25% increase productivity)	60750.00	Difference	12150.00
Total savings	3642.00	Unit cost	2.5		

Fig. 7. Cost analysis

Orchard productivity in the surveyed Ica-Pachacutec sector is 0.9 t/ha. However, according to Wells [5], the ideal productivity of an orchard is 2.0 t/ha. The most important items affecting pecan production have been identified. Shapiro [7] indicates that there may be a loss in production between 5% and 20% due to diseases to which pecan plants are susceptible (pests, insects, fungi, grubs, among other things). Wells [5] further argues that irrigation increases production by 70% and that there may be a 30–50% loss of production due to plant malnutrition. With the help of the three integrated management processes (quality, production, and logistics), production losses will be reduced by 25%. Thus, productivity will increase by 0.5 t/ha and, in turn Ica-Pachacutec productivity will be increased to 1.4 t/ha.

Production loss savings were obtained through results from 90 trees belonging to three hectares on average. An average pecan tree produces 30 kg and the current cost of a pecan is 18 soles per kilogram, obtaining 48,600 soles in net sales. The cost of implementing the three integrated management processes (quality, production, and logistics) is 8,508 soles for an average 3-ha orchard (90 trees). With the 25% productivity increase, due to the implementation of the 3-process integrated management system, there has been a new result of 60,750 soles in sales. Sales with increased productivity, minus regular sales, yield a net profit of 12,150 soles after implementing the project. Thus, gross profits are calculated through the difference between the net profit generated after project implementation and project implementation costs. Finally, a gross profit of 3,642 soles was reported. The unit cost of the project was calculated as 2.5 soles per kilogram of pecan. This result was found by dividing the project's implementation cost of 8,508 soles by the total quantity of pecans (3 ha), which was 3,375.

References

1. Instituto Nacional de Estadística e Informática (INEI). Perú: Estructura Empresarial 2016 (2017). Recuperado de. https://www.inei.gob.pe/media/MenuRecursivo/publicaciones_digitales/Est/Lib1445/libro.pdf
2. Promperú . Desenvolvimiento del comercio agroexportador. Departamento de Agronegocios de la subdirección (2017). Recuperado de. http://media.peru.info/promperu/Desenvolvimie-ntoagro2016.pdf
3. Wells, L.: Cultural Management of Commercial Pecan Orchards. Department of Agriculture. University of Georgia (2018). Recuperado de. https://secure.caes.uga.edu/extension/publications/files/pdf/B%201304_5.PDF
4. Mokochinski, F., Watzlawick, L., Botelho, R., Moreira, V.: Randomized branch sampling to estimate fruit production in Pecan trees cv. 'Barton'. Ciência Rural, **47**(4) (2017). https://dx.doi.org/10.1590/01038478cr20151591
5. Wells, L.: Response of young pecan trees to irrigation in a humud climate. Hort Science. **52**(3), 457–462 (2017). https://doi.org/10.21273/HORTSCI11664-16
6. Luo, X., Li, Z., Sun, Z., Wan, X.: Analysis of pecan cultivars Mahan and Western in East China. Genet. Mol. Res. **15** (2016). https://doi.org/10.4238/gmr.15038732
7. Bock, C., Shapiro-Ilan, D., Wedge, D., Cantrell, C.: Identification of the antifungal compound, transcinnamic acid, produced by photorhabdus luminescens, a potential biopesticide against pecan scab. J. Pest. Sci. **87**, 155–162 (2014)
8. Sammis, T., Gutschick, V., Wang, J., Miller, D.R.: Model of water and nitrogen management in pecan trees under normal and resourcelimited conditions. Agric. Water Manag. **124**, 28–36 (2013). https://doi.org/10.1016/j.agwat.2013.03.012
9. Wells, L., Conner, P.: Pecan varieties for Georgia Orchards. Department of Agriculture. University of Georgia (2015). Recuperado de. https://secure.caes.uga.edu/extension/publications/files/pdf/C%20890_4.PDF
10. Walworth, J.L., White, S.A., Comeau, M.J., Heerema, R.J.: Soilapplied ZnEDTA: vegetative growth, nut production, and nutrient acquisition of immature pecan trees grown in an alkaline, calcareous soil. HortScience **52**(2), 301–305 (2017). https://doi.org/10.21273/HORTSCI11467-16
11. Sanderlin, R., Bollich, A.: What fungicides is best to use for control pecan scab? LSU college of agriculture (2016). Extraido de. https://www.lsuagcenter.com/portals/our_offices/research_stations/pecan/features/pecan_faqs/what-fungicide-isbest-to-use-for-control-of-pecan-scab

Implementation of a Quality Management System (QMS) Based on TQM Principles for Cocoa MSEs: A Case Study in Cusco, Perú

Edgar Wong[1(✉)], Gianpierre Pajuelo[1(✉)], Fernando Sotelo[1(✉)], and Carlos Raymundo[2(✉)]

[1] Ingeniería Industrial, Universidad Peruana de Ciencias Aplicadas (UPC), Lima, Peru
{u201423934,u201217538,Fernando.Sotelo}@upc.edu.pe
[2] Dirección de Investigación, Universidad Peruana de Ciencias Aplicadas (UPC), Lima, Peru
carlos.raymundo@upc.edu.pe

Abstract. The objective of this work is to develop a quality management system focused on the principles of TQM for cocoa micro and small enterprises (MSEs) in the province of La Convención, Cusco - Perú. The diagnosis for this investigation was made using in-depth interviews to the cocoa farmers that facilitated the identification of the current situation of cocoa MSEs. With the results obtained and based on the scientific articles studied, the critical elements in each activity related to the cocoa production process were determined, and it is focused on establishing a quality management system adaptable to the requirements of the plots studied. As a result of the analysis of the experts, the system in question is based on the following principles of TQM: documentation, customer focus, process-based approach and continuous improvement.

Keywords: Cocoa · MSEs · Productivity · Quality management system · TQM principles

1 Introduction

The micro and small enterprises (MSEs) generate around 47% of employment housing work for 127 million people in Latin America and the Caribbean. Within the Peruvian business sector, micro-enterprises represent 95%, equivalent to 1,607,305 entities, while small businesses represent only 4.3% [1]. SMEs have a different meaning according to the country, which is distinguished by the number of employees, the capital investment, the annual turnover and the amount of total assets in the company; this means that they are part of an important segment that symbolizes the growth engine in the country's economy [2].

In Peru, agriculture is one of the most important and fundamental economic activities. The agricultural sector in the 2016 period had a growth in GDP of 2%, a significant figure in the increase of national GDP that in the year 2016 was 3.9% with a growth of agricultural exports by 10% compared to the period 2015, resulting in an FOB value of 5790 million dollars; This sector growth was mainly generated by the

T. Ahram et al. (Eds.): IHIET 2019, AISC 1018, pp. 910–916, 2020.
https://doi.org/10.1007/978-3-030-25629-6_142

global economic impulse due to the increase in demand from the large developed and emerging countries [3].

In this way, this research has as its main objective the development of a quality management system (QMS) with the principles of total quality management (TQM), the challenge lies in its implementation in a less developed country, where the culture organizational has its particularities for the necessary adaptation, since the established basic parameters must be followed [4]. The internal benefits after the implementation of the quality management system are related to on-time delivery, fulfillment of orders, reduction of errors, stock rotation and cost savings [5].

2 State of the Art

In the study conducted by Fundin, Bergquist, Eriksson & Gremyr [6] emphasizes that the field of quality management (QM) has been characterized by a development driven by practice. Although QM has reached maturity as a research field based on empirical research, its professionals still struggle to adapt QM implementations to obtain its benefits.

In quality management systems, it is known that it is a process that allows continuous improvement, implementation of action plans and monitoring. Currently, total quality management (TQM) has adopted different types of approaches, in addition to receiving worldwide interest regarding its elements and its application. In general terms, TQM is used to improve quality within an organization and efficiency in all its associated projects.

Another study made by Vedant Singh [7] focus on the implementation of TQM in Indian industries and study their influence on organizational performance (OP). The study was conducted at five manufacturing companies and three service companies in northern India. The results of this study also indicate that TQM has a strong positive and significant effect on OP.

The purpose of the investigation by Mohd Faizhilmi [8] is to explore the relevant problems in the relationship between TQM and the performance of MSEs. This study also analyzes the need for mediation in the relationship between TQM and the performance of MSEs, namely the learning of the organization. The document anticipates that TQM will support the learning of the organization and the performance of SMEs.

The total quality management is a philosophy that establishes principles for management that maximize the competitiveness of a company through the continuous improvement of the quality of its products, services, personnel, processes and environment [9]; it improves the image of the company and the satisfaction of employees. In addition to the aforementioned, Daniel Jiménez [10] makes reference that the TQM system is seen as a model of operational quality improvement, capable of generating performance.

Also, some authors have described seven fundamental principles of TQM, which are focused on the client, the people, the continuous improvement and the suppliers. For this research, four principles of quality management of ISO (2015) are taken as reference in Fig. 1.

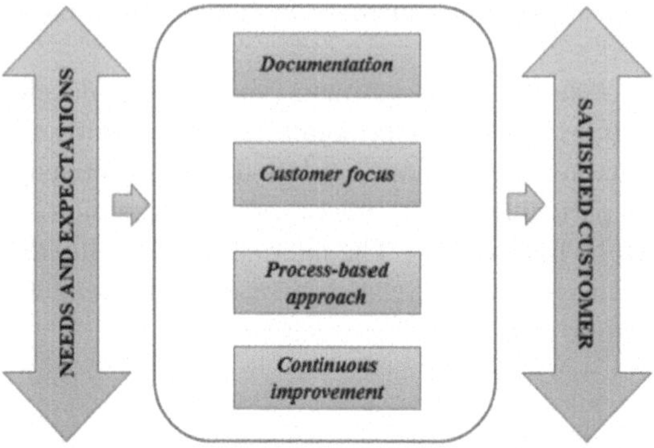

Source: Own studies based on ISO 2015.

Fig. 1. TQM principles for the QMS

2.1 Documentation

The ISO 9001: 2015 as well as the total quality management model shows that every process must manage and maintain a flow of documentation to control the procedures that they involve. Maintaining the documents updated and constantly reviewing the records contribute to a better traceability of the information within MSEs. The sub-process begins with the definition of the relevant guidelines and requirements for the quality process, after which each record or format is documented, in order to proceed to deliver the same to the interested parties.

2.2 Customer Focus

Customer satisfaction is achieved by complying with the specifications and requirements that the external customer expects, through a product with quality, punctuality and speed of delivery. This principle has a very close relationship with innovation, since innovative companies must seek new customer needs to generate new products and adapt to the dynamic market.

2.3 Process-Based Approach

This principle indicates that when activities are understood and managed as inter-related processes that function as a coherent system, the results are achieved in an effective and efficient manner. The interconnected processes generate interdependence among themselves, which favors the detection and elimination of errors.

2.4 Continuous Improvement

In accordance with this principle, every company is constantly seeking to improve its performance, so the organization should seek that workers aim to continuously improve products, processes and systems [10]. To achieve a good performance of this principle requires that the company has an organizational culture that encourages its workers to innovate, to lose the fear of being wrong and to provide them with tools.

3 Quality Management System (QMS)

The quality management system was established according to the diagnosis of the current status for the cocoa MSEs. For this, it is necessary to mention that farmers have little knowledge about the subject, because many of them have only complete secondary. In addition, they know very little about the correct records, procedures and controls for the activities they carry out regarding the cultivation of cocoa. Their knowledge is based mainly on the experience they perform on a day-to-day basis.

In this way, TQM principles were generated for the research topic, the first principal is documentation. The second principle is the customer focus, which is based on keeping the client satisfied through the trust and communication that must be provided by the provider. Likewise, we have as a third principle the process-based approach, which states that when activities are understood and managed as interrelated processes that function as a coherent system, the results are achieved in an effective and efficient manner. Finally, we have the principle of continuous improvement that is based on the study and analysis of indicators which will have to establish solutions through procedures and action plans for the standardization and improvement of the processes.

After showing the principles of the quality management system proposed for the cocoa producing SMEs, it will be explained in detail of each one of them.

3.1 Documentation

The documentation itself must add value to the activities of an organization in this case to MSEs and facilitate the execution of these. Figure 2 summarizes how this principle would be carried out.

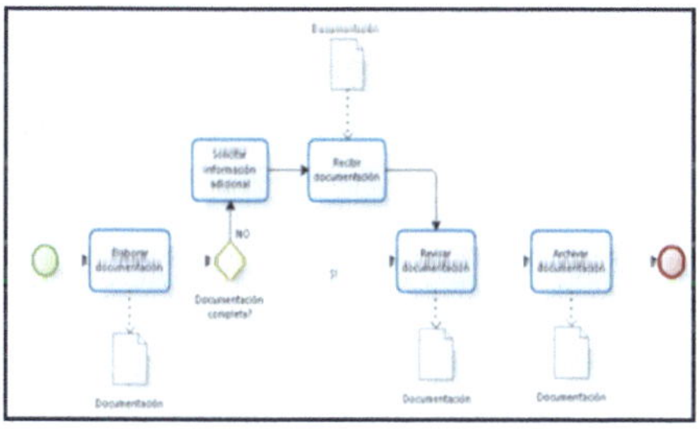

Fig. 2. Documentation principle for coca MSEs in Cusco

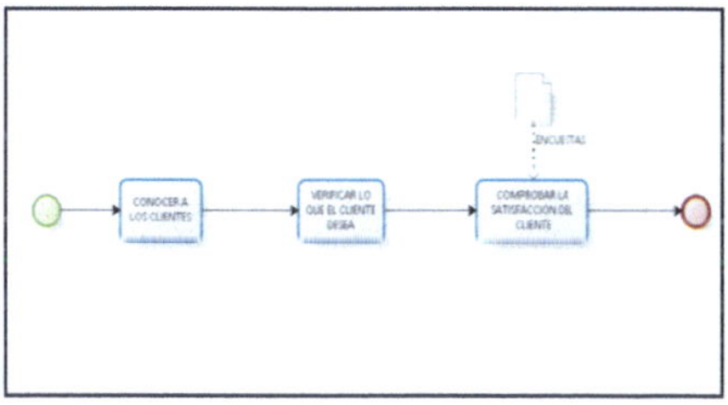

Fig. 3. Customer focus principle for coca MSEs in Cusco

3.2 Customer Focus

Figure 3 details the customer focus principle flow, which it begins by knowing what our clients are and knowing about them. Having that trustworthiness and empathy with them is key for the client to work with the provider. Finally, a brief survey will have to be carried out, which will verify if the satisfaction that had as expectation was fulfilled or not.

3.3 Process-Based Approach

Figure 4 explains the process-based approach principle flow, which begins by identifying the process that must followup the right guidelines to ensure a good practice. After the process are determined, the task is to start the implementation of every single one of them. Then the MSEs should establish a monitoring and control system that provide suitable achievement indicators. Finally, the results are analyzed and decisions are taken to help improve the flow of processes and the possibility of implementing new ones.

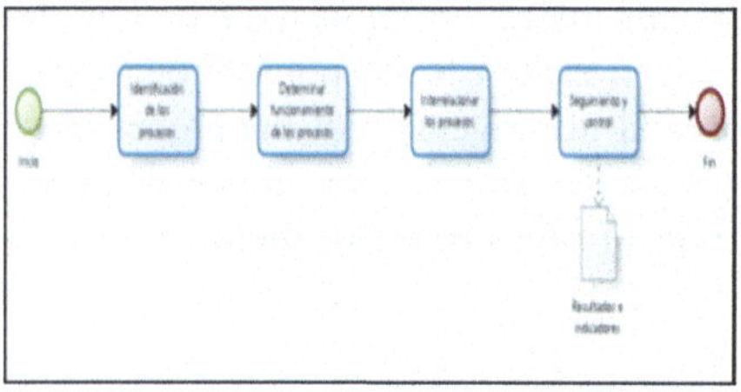

Fig. 4. Process-based approach principle for coca MSEs in Cusco

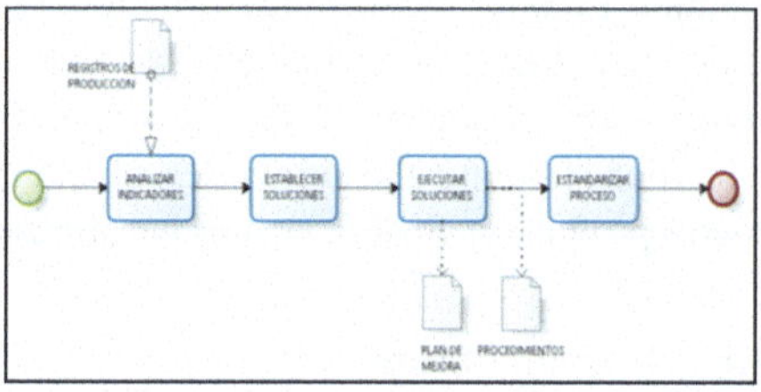

Fig. 5. Continuous improvement principle for coca MSEs in Cusco

3.4 Continuous Improvement

This process is developed based on lessons learned, therefore, the need arises to be in a constant identification of opportunities for improvement and collection of feedback from both internal and external customers. Figure 5 shows the continuous improvement principle flow.

4 Results

Cocoa farmers do not have standardized processes, all of them have different ways of carrying out each of the production processes, they use different tools, different inputs and, above all, their way of carrying out the processes is totally different. It is for this reason, that a QMS is required in order to improve their productivity in the region plots.

After carrying out the general analysis of MSEs of the agricultural cocoa sector in the Province of La Convención in Cusco, based on the findings and problems found in the in-depth interviews, quality management tools are proposed with a focus on the principles of TQM associated with the activities that need to be addressed in the investigation. It is important to mention that based on the research of articles related to the subject, the standards and good practices that should be established are established so that the existing gaps can be shortened compared to the best practices carried out in the world. For this reason, farmers must take into account the current situation in the region and the gaps identified to achieve the improvement of the productivity of MSES of the cocoa sector. Based on each identified gap, the best guidelines for quality management to be used will be determined and it is expected to increase the productivity that is the problem of the present research.

Table 1 corresponds to the definition of document procedures for cocoa MSEs in Cusco, which implies establishing the standards for each of the activities of the production process related to the final quality of the cocoa bean. Once the diagnosis was made to the MSEs of the sector under study, it could be identified that the procedures are deficient compared to the most productive countries in the world. Also, the frequency of documenting these procedures are not optimal, since there is no knowledge about how is the correct way to handle the quality management system, since they do not have any kind of previous experience. On the other hand, the use of these records is of vital importance, since monitoring and controls are carried out throughout the pecan process, from the study of soils to obtaining a quality product.

Thus, implementing the QMS with the good agricultural practices is the best way to do it because the standards would serve as a guide for farmers in the sector. After compiling all the necessary information, each of these parameters must be separated by activity, with the purpose of delivering in the appropriate formats to those responsible, both in the area of production and logistics, this information that allows them to develop their corresponding procedures successfully.

Table 1. QMS document procedures for coca MSEs in Cusco.

Code	Description
4.1/01	Control of documents
4.1/02	Control of records
4.1/03	Management review
4.1/04	Personnel training
4.1/05	Planning of product realization
4.1/06	Control of suppliers and purchasing
4.1/07	Identification and traceability
4.1/08	Control and monitoring
4.1/09	Customer satisfaction
4.1/10	Internal audit
4.1/11	Control of nonconforming product
4.1/12	Corrective and preventive action

References

1. Ministerio de la Producción (2017). Anuario Estadístico Industrial, Mipyme y Comercio Interno 2016
2. Garg, S., Agarwal, P.: Micro, small and medium enterprises in India: a review of growth and challenges in the present scenario. Int. J. Appl. Bus. Econ. Res. (2017)
3. Banco Central de Reserva del Perú. Producción Agropecuario del 2017 (2017). Consultado en. http://www.bcrp.gob.pe/publicaciones/notasemanal/cuadros-estadisticos.html
4. Aamer, A.M., Al-Awlaqi, M.A., Alkibsi, S.M.: TQM implementation in a least developed country: an exploratory study of Yemen. TQM J. **29**(3), 467–487 (2017)
5. Calvo, M.Á.C., Suárez, E.M., Mora, A.C., Cristóbal, R.P.: Sistemas de gestión de la calidad: un estudio en empresas del sur de España y norte de Marruecos, Investigaciones Europeas de Dirección y Economía de la Empresa, **22**, pp. 8–16 (2015)
6. Fundin, A., Bergquist, B., Eriksson, H., Gremyr, I.: Challenges and propositions for research in quality management. Int. J. Prod. Econ. **199**, 125–137 (2018)
7. Singh, V., Kumar, A., Singh, T.: Impact of TQM on organisational performance: the case of indian manufacturing and service industry. Oper. Res. Perspect. **5**, 199–217 (2018)
8. Mahmud, N., Hilmi, M.F.: TQM and Malaysian SMEs performance: the mediating roles of organization learning. Procedia – Soc. Behav. Sci. **130**, 216–225 (2015)
9. Espín, J.A.G., Jiménez, D.J., Costa, M.M.: La gestión de calidad: importancia de la cultura organizativa para el desarrollo de variables (2014)
10. Jiménez, D.J., Costa, M.M., Martínez, A.R., Lorente, H.A., Rabeh, D.: Total quality management performance in multinational companies: a learning perspective. TQM J. **27**(3), 328–340 (2015)

Lean Service Quality Model to Improve the Performance of Service in Automotive Dealer

Franco Valenzuela[1(✉)], Jeysev Estocalenko[1(✉)], José Rojas[1(✉)], and Carlos Raymundo[2(✉)]

[1] Ingeniería de Gestión Empresarial, Universidad Peruana de Ciencias Aplicadas (UPC), Lima, Peru
{u201411654,u201415916,jose.rojas}@upc.edu.pe
[2] Dirección de Investigación, Universidad Peruana de Ciencias Aplicadas (UPC), Lima, Peru
carlos.raymundo@upc.edu.pe

Abstract. The service sector, specifically the automotive sector, has witnessed significant growth in the economy and is constantly searching for methods to improve its quality indexes with its customers; however, errors in general repairs are ever present in this tertiary activity. This document undertakes a practical study to measure the effectiveness of the Lean Service Quality (LSQ) model, which combines the development of a multi-elemental scale to measure service quality (SERVQUAL) and a conceptual/practical Lean Service model, with the aim of reducing the number of poorly performed technical repairs at a Toyota automobile dealership. The main result of the research was defining a practical guide to replicate the LSQ model. In addition, as the model's first approach, the study demonstrated that, for the dealership under study, the rate of bad repairs was ultimately reduced by 5.17%.

Keywords: LSQ model · Lean Service · SERVQUAL · Continuous improvement · 8D model · Automotive sector · Automotive dealer

1 Introduction

The services sector has become an important driver for economies worldwide. In Europe, this activity represents 70% of the national GDP and, in the United States, this tertiary activity is even greater, with a GDP of 80% [1].

The service sector covers a broad range of markets, within which is the automotive industry. This sector involves companies that are engaged in the design, development, manufacturing, marketing, and sales of vehicles and parts. These are offered through dealers or international brand representatives who require procedures based on world-class quality standards and post-sales services [2]. The growth of the automotive sector, specifically in the Peruvian market, has had a significant increase in terms of GDP evolution by vehicle marketing, repair, and maintenance, maintaining an annual growth rate of 3% over the last seven years, and this growth trend is expected to continue [3].

T. Ahram et al. (Eds.): IHIET 2019, AISC 1018, pp. 917–923, 2020.
https://doi.org/10.1007/978-3-030-25629-6_143

Based on the foregoing, the Mitsu Canada Toyota dealership, located in Lima, was selected as our object of study. In this company, a high rate of rework was identified in technical repairs, with the following main consequences: the reuse of resources (materials, equipment, personnel, spare parts, etc), the reuse of workshop capacity and the loss of potential customers due to the dissatisfaction generated. In addition, customer dissatisfaction because of a poorly performed service has the potential to cause future negative decisions, not merely in the reduction of repurchases, but also in terms of damages to the business, loss of goodwill, and one dissatisfied customer deterring at least ten potential customers [4–6]. Given this problem, Toyota performs its repair quality measurement through the Fix-It-Right (FIR) indicator. As a starting point for research, the satisfaction indicator was around 85%, which means that 15% of customers who enter the dealership for a repair service show some level of dissatisfaction. Therefore, this research aims to reduce rework levels in the company under study by using the continuous improvement model known as Lean Service Quality (LSQ).

2 State of the Art

To consider the development of a Lean approach in the services sector, two fundamental cycles must be taken into account: conceptual and practical. The first one is focused on ensuring an adequate performance in the jump from Lean Manufacturing to Lean Service considering its inherent features to the service, definition of wastes in this sector, and role of the customer [1]. First, most research agrees that the five critical service principles are [1, 7, 8].

- Value: in the service environment, value is as a need fulfilled by a service provided to the final customer. Therefore, it must be defined by the customer.
- Value Stream: value is created mainly according to customer needs; therefore, the Value Stream is constituted by the sequence of activities that allows for their satisfaction.
- Flow: this focuses on the optimization of continuous movement through the sequence of service activities that generate value, such as those perceived by the customer.
- Pull: this means distributing customer demand throughout the value chain, delivering just what the customer really requires.
- Perfection: focusing on the customer's perspective, delivering exactly what customers want and when they want it.

Second, the role of the customer in services is different from the manufacturing category, since this is part of the production process. Finally, the eight types of wastes can be extrapolated from the manufacturing sector (duplication, waiting, unnecessary motion, poor communication, lack of standardization, underused resources, defects, and resistance to change).

In contrast, the model proposed by [9] defines service quality through the gap that exists between customer perception and the expectations of the organization's service quality performance. In other words, a comparison between the expected and desired quality (SERVQUAL). The study by [10] Roslan, Wahab, & Abdullah also maintains that many studies have identified this model as the most precise in determining the quality of the services offered [11–13]. As previously mentioned, this model is based on the analysis of customer perception under five crucial dimensions [14].

- Tangible elements: physical installations, equipment, staff members, and communications.
- Reliability: the ability to perform the promised service reliably and accurately.
- Awareness: willingness to help customers and provide prompt service.
- Security: employee knowledge and courtesy and their ability to inspire trust.
- Empathy: individualized attention that provides effective patient care.

In summary, the present investigation validates the applicability of the LSQ model to reduce high level reprocessing in a Toyota automative dealership company. This is composed of the Misztal methodology reduced into six dimensions, combining the applicability of a conceptual Lean Service model and the model focused on improving service quality SERVQUAL.

3 Methods

The main objective of this study is the definition and evaluation of the applicability of a continuous improvement model known as LSQ. With a view to achieving this objective, an automotive repair dealership, offering automotive repair and vehicle maintenance, was taken as a case study.

First, the SERVQUAL survey was structured to measure the gaps between customer perception and organization expectations with respect to the service provided by the Mitsui Canada dealership. In this sense, the survey structure comprised 22 items that assessed customer expectation (E) and 22 items that assessed customer perception in terms of superior service (P9.) Also, according to the procedures recommended by Churchill (1979), a scale of 1 to 7 was used, where the maximum value means "strongly agree" and minimum "strongly disagree"; a specific description on the rest of the scores was not placed [13]. Further, negative statements were identified with a minus sign in parentheses in the questionnaire. In this sense, the service quality measurement (Q) was defined as the degree of difference between user perceptions and user expectations.

Once the SERVQUAL survey results were analyzed and processed, the three preliminary steps of the Lean Service conceptual cycle model were conducted: (i) defining the five main Lean principles, (ii) identifying the role of the customer within the value stream of the process, and (iii) classifying the waste identified in the general repairs process. Next, a continuous improvement model was proposed to reduce the bad repair rate. This was implemented in the repairs process in the dealership under study to reduce its economic impacts and generate significant savings in terms of use of resources and potential lost customers. Finally, a comparison was made between the initial results and the results obtained after implementation of the improvement model.

4 Model

4.1 Lean Service Quality Model (LSQ)

4.1.1 Model Description

The model comprises six dimensions: initial diagnosis, problem description, analysis, action plans, evaluation of results, and preventing future problem recurrence (Fig. 1).

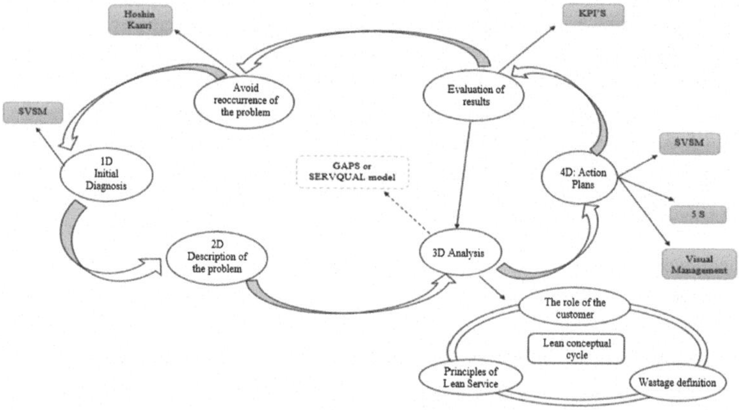

Fig. 1. Lean Service Quality (LSQ) continuous improvement model

4.1.2 Components

The LSQ continuous improvement model was implemented under the 8D methodology. However, as part of our research contribution, we decided to delimit the methodology set forth by Misztal et al [19] to six dimensions since this model proposed an initial evaluation, followed by initial action plans, a final diagnosis, and final action plans. Nevertheless, the LSQ model was reduced to six dimensions, discarding the third dimension (first analysis) and fourth dimension (intermediate action plans) from the 8D model since applying a second analysis of the problem did not guarantee its elimination.

The LSQ model began with an initial diagnosis (1D) using the SVSM tool, as this tool stated with VSM planning, which identified a process within the service that preented highly recurring problems. Next, a process map of the current situation was prepared. The second dimension (2D) entailed an accurate definition of the problem and effects that impacted the organization. The third dimension (3D) denoted an analysis of the problem's possible solutions. For this, the Lean Service conceptual model proposed by [1]. Once the ideal tools were selected for the problem, we proceeded to the fourth dimension (4D) where an implementation plan with permanent corrective actions was established to avoid any recurrence. The objective was to solve the root causes of the problem, update procedures, and train staff. Phase five (5D) of the model was very important since it closed the action plans. In this dimension, the effectiveness of the executed strategies was verified to determine if the results were positive and if the root causes of the problem under study had been eliminated. The purpose of the last phase (6D) was to prevent the problem from recurring. In fact, development possibilities were identified and a process of continuous improvement initiatives was set forth, such as modifying specifications, updating information, reviewing the value stream, and procedures to prevent the problem or similar problems from recurring in the future.

Finally, SERVQUAL model was applied because it included as part of the contributions hereof since, as previously mentioned, customers are the ones who determine what good quality service is. Consequently, this model was involved in the contribution's third dimension: analysis (3D), since this measured the service quality received by customers based on their expectations and perceptions in five dimensions (tangible elements, reliability, sensitivity, security, and empathy).

5 Results

Once the implementation of the LSQ model was complete, it could be seen that the incidence of dissatisfaction due to bad technical repairs decreased and the repair process indicators improved, as compared to the previous year. For these purposes, the results from four indicators at the end of 2017 at the Mitsui Canada dealership were used as benchmark. These data were compared with two assessments performed during the implementation of the model (September 2018) and at its completion (October 2018) as is shown in Table 1.

Table 1. Project results (kpis)

Heading level	Indicator 2017	Indicator Sep. 2018	Indicator Oct. 2018
Repair quality (FIR)	85.14%	87.50%	90.03%
Technical productivity	59.17%	60.40%	67.83%
Underused capacity	5.83%	5.77%	5.40%
Average reprocess time	2.77	2.75	2.74

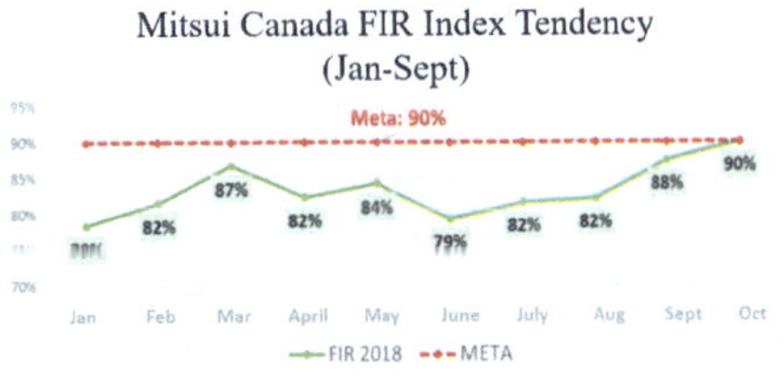

Fig. 2. Improved FIR indicator trend - Mitsui Canada 2018

An improved indicator progression can be seen during the months in which the model was implemented with one FIR indicator managing to reach over 90% in the month of October. In this regard, Fig. 2 shows an improving trend starting after the implementation of the LSQ model in the Mitsu Canada dealership, where the proposed FIR indicator target of 90% was ultimately exceeded in October 2018. The proposed model managed to reduce the number of defective repairs thus improve the FIR indicator. Therefore, after a thoroughly comprehensive review of the results the following can be said:

- Before implementation of the continuous improvement model, the dealership had a high level of repairs that were not performed correctly, generating significant economic losses due to the reuse of resources, underutilization of the workshop, and loss of customers. The reasons for this problem were mainly due to the dealership not being clear on the efficient stream value required to achieve customer satisfaction in the repair process. Also, customer perception was not considered with respect to the service provided, and therefore, the weak points within the repairs process were not known in the Mitsui Canada dealership. Consequently, the LSQ model identified the Lean tools required to solve the problem and determine weak points in the dealership based on customer perceptions and expectations with the help of the 5-dimentsion SERVQUAL survey (tangible, empathy, trust, security, and response capacity).
- The profitability study conducted denotes a total investment of S/. 30,525.45 over 12 months, estimating that the company will generate a total return of S/83,760.61 based on the reduction of the FIR index. That is, the savings generated by not reusing labor, spare parts, and workshop space. These results yield a possible Return on Investment (ROI) of 164.57% in about three months, thus rendering this automotive dealership completely profitable.

References

1. Andrés-López, E., González-Requena, I., Sanz-Lobera, A.: Lean Service: Reassessment of Lean Manufacturing for Service Activities. Procedia Eng. (2015). https://doi.org/10.1016/j.proeng.2015.12.463
2. Moisés, B.: Planeamiento estratégico del sector automotriz en el Perú (2012)
3. Asociación Automotriz del Perú (AAP), Market share en la venta e inmatriculación de vehículos (2018)
4. Hsiao, Y.H., Chen, L.F., Choy, Y.L., Su, C.T.: A novel framework for customer complaint management. Serv. Ind. J. **36**(13–14), 675–698 (2016). https://doi.org/10.1080/02642069.2016.1272592
5. Kumar, S., Dhingra, A.K., Singh, B.: Process improvement through Lean-Kaizen using value stream map: a case study in India. Int. J. Adv. Manuf. Technol. 1–12 (2018). https://doi.org/10.1007/s00170-018-1684-8
6. Liu, C.H., Tzeng, G.H., Lee, M.H., Lee, P.Y.: Improving metro–airport connection service for tourism development: using hybrid MCDM models. Tour. Manag. Perspect. **6**, 95–107 (2013)
7. Asnan, R., Nordin, N., Othman, S.R.: Managing change on lean implementation in service sector. Procedia – Soc. Behav. Sci. **211**, 313–319 (2015)
8. Parasuraman, A., Zeithaml, V.A., Berry, L.L.: SERVQUAL: a multiple-item scale for measuring consumer perceptions of service quality. J. Retail. **64**(1), 12–40 (1988). https://doi.org/10.1016/s0148-2963(99)00084-3
9. Roslan, N.A.A., Wahab, E., Abdullah, N.R.: Service quality: a case study of logistics sector in Iskandar Malaysia using SERVQUAL model. Procedia Soc. Behav. Sci. **172**, 457–462 (2015). https://doi.org/10.1016/j.sbspro.2015.01.380
10. Rauyruen, P., Miller, K.E.: Relationship quality as a predictor of B2B customer loyalty. J. Bus. Res. **60**, 21–31 (2007). Rauyruen

11. Banomyong, R., Supatn, N.: Selecting logistics providers in Thailand: a shippers'. Perspective **45**(3), 419–437 (2011)
12. Baki, B., Basfirinci, C. S., Cilingir, Z., AR Murat, I.: An application of integrating SERVQUAL and Kano's model into QFD for logistic services: a case study from Turkey, **21**(1), 106–126 (2009)
13. Kalaja, R., Myshketa, R., Scalera, F.: Service quality assessment in health care sector: the case of Durres public hospital. Procedia – Soc. Behav. Sci. **235**, 557–565 (2016). https://doi.org/10.1016/j.sbspro.2016.11.082
14. Misztal, A., Grecu, I., Belu, N.: Customer Satisfaction in the Automotive Industry. FAIMA Bus. Manage. J. **4**(1), 44–57 (2016). https://doi.org/10.1016/j.cirpj.2015.01.008

Lean Model of Services for the Improvement in the Times of Attention of the Emergency Areas of the Health Sector

Lucero Calero[1(✉)], Aracelli Maccasi[1(✉)], and Carlos Raymundo[2(✉)]

[1] Ingeniería Industrial,
Universidad Peruana de Ciencias Aplicadas (UPC), Lima, Peru
{U910802, Pcadlmac}@upc.edu.pe
[2] Dirección de Investigación,
Universidad Peruana de Ciencias Aplicadas (UPC), Lima, Peru
carlos.raymundo@upc.edu.pe

Abstract. In Peru, the health service has had certain problems in the attention of users. The emergency service of clinics has been saturated due to changes in the needs of people and demand, exposing the prestige of health entities that have this unit and generating risks for the health of users, this is reflected in the low level of satisfaction with regard to care. Based on the Lean philosophy, a model is developed using SMED, Kanban and pull tools to reduce waiting times. The application of this model of pilot in the Clinic reduces the waiting time for the first attention in 30% thereby reducing the number of fines imposed by the corresponding regulatory entity and the desertion in emergency, achieving an average time of 37 min.

Keywords: Attention time · Health sector · Lean healthcare · SMED · Pull system

1 Introduction

In Peru, 5.4% of the GDP is allocated to the health sector. This percentage is lower than the minimum percentage recommended by the World Health Organization. Patients in the emergency service of different health centers complain about the lack of quality of care in different health centers, even questioning the technical quality and effectiveness of the clinical process. Also, patients and/or users say that they encounter long waiting times. This problem happens in the emergency care service at the Limatambo clinic in San Isidro, Perú. At this site, the frequent discomfort expressed by the users can be mostly attributed to poor attention, staff shortages, and lack of better infrastructure with respect to the average volume of received patients. In addition, this site's health plan objectives for urgent care are largely aimed at improving the satisfaction of the served population and increasing the care quality and efficiency in terms of the costs and results. Therefore, Taylor and Benger conducted a systematic review to identify the three most frequent factors affecting patient care, including the interpersonal skills/staff attitude, information/explanations provided to users, and service waiting times.

T. Ahram et al. (Eds.): IHIET 2019, AISC 1018, pp. 924–930, 2020.
https://doi.org/10.1007/978-3-030-25629-6_144

2 State of the Art

The lean philosophy was conceived as a promising management approach. The first experiences in incorporating the Toyota Production System into the management of a healthcare company were observed at the Virginia Mason Medical Center in 2001. Because of its implementation, the laboratory response time was reduced by 85%, the productivity was increased by 93% in some selected areas, the inventory costs were reduced, and efficient space distribution through spatial designs could be observed.

Escude, Tanc, and Santoro [1] described the experience in a pediatric emergency (UP, for the acronym in Spanish), where different lean tools were used, in their work titled "Experiencia de Implementación de Lean en un Centro de Salud de Uruguay" (Lean Implementation Experiences at a Health Center in Uruguay). The authors methodologically conducted a patient satisfaction survey after consultation. Further, the process was mapped using the value stream mapping (VSM) tool together with the team of doctors and nurses of the emergency care unit. Next, the A3 tool was used to solve the problem of long waiting times, identifying the root causes and assessing measures for their elimination.

This research study was a successful experience in the application of lean management in the health sector, reducing the waiting times by more than four min while considering opportunities to reduce them by an additional 20% in the short term. In addition, the study concluded that significant improvements may be obtained without the requirement of capital investments.

Simón [2] described the theoretical roots for the different implementation models as well as the lean methodology applied to a hospital consortium in her study titled "Lean Implementation at a hospital: The CSG Case."

The methodological design was based on a comparative case study, exhibiting no differences in terms of methodology, tools, or culture in case of lean implementations in other sectors.

Khalifa [3] related the case of King Faisal Specialist Hospital and Research Center, wherein health analysis methods were used to identify the gap areas and suggest potential improvements to emergency room performance in "Utilizing health analytics in improving the performance of healthcare services": A case study on a tertiary care hospital." This study included data obtained from 26,948 emergency room visits during January 2015.

Further, lean healthcare tools were implemented using the following analytical techniques to suggest redesigning the process based on the results:

- Fast-tracking of less critical emergency care patients
- An internal waiting area for patients able to sit upright instead of occupying an emergency room bed.

After the implementation of the two solutions, the total emergency room waiting times were reduced from 20 h in 2014 to less than 12 h in 2016, resulting in a 40% improvement. The percentage of untreated patients remained at approximately 3.5%, whereas the percentages of patients who left the emergency room before being fully treated were significantly reduced from 13.5% in 2014 to 5.5% in 2016.

Boronat [4] explains the case of the application of the lean methodology as a continuous improvement method in a urology department at a tertiary hospital in his article. The lean healthcare methodology was implemented in a urology department in the following three stages: (1) team training and fostering feedback among professionals; (2) management by process and super specialization; and (3) improvement of indicators (continuous improvement). The lean healthcare implementation yielded high professional satisfaction levels, better quality indicators reaching a risk-adjusted complication rate of 0.59, and a risk-adjusted mortality rate of 0.24 in four years [5–7].

Lean healthcare is a relatively new patient-centered methodology. This methodology reduces the patient waiting times; staff wastes, such as time lost due to confusion and long travel distances and other such factors, which further reduce the time dedicated to direct patient care; and patient injuries and deaths due to avoidable risks, including process [8, 9].

3 Case Study

This case study involves a private health service provider. The clinic in which the model is implemented has been in operation for more than 30 years and receives approximately 45,000 patients per year in its four sites with an approximate annual revenue of S/100 million soles. This study focuses on the San Isidro site, which currently receives an average of 30,000 patients per year.

60% of the care given every year corresponds to emergency care. However, statistical reports indicate that 33% of the care provided in the emergency area ends up in complaints. The majority of these complaints can be attributed to excessive waiting times. The economic impact associated with these issues in the clinic represents 22% of the annual revenue; approximately S./14,850,000.00 soles per year are lost in the Limatambo Clinic at San Isidro because of its deficiencies.

To reach this assessment, the following VSM was performed, displaying the patient flows, the recorded times, and the problems identified (Fig. 1).

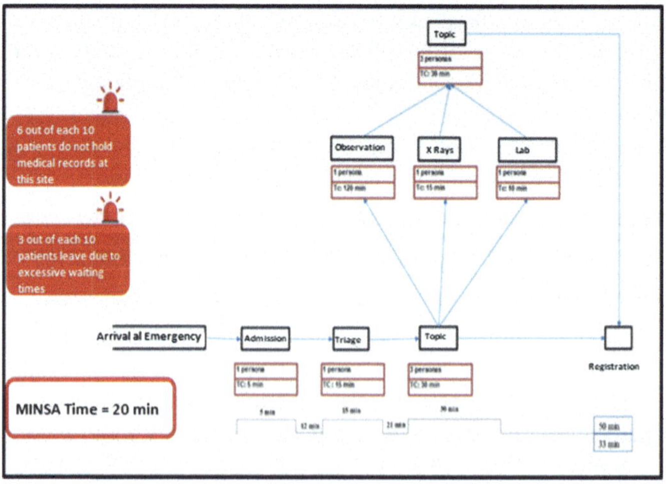

Fig. 1. VSM

After conducting the VSM analysis for the initial situation and identifying the process involved, the following diagnostic chart is obtained:

For proposal implementation purposes, a pilot program is performed to test the proposed model (Fig. 2).

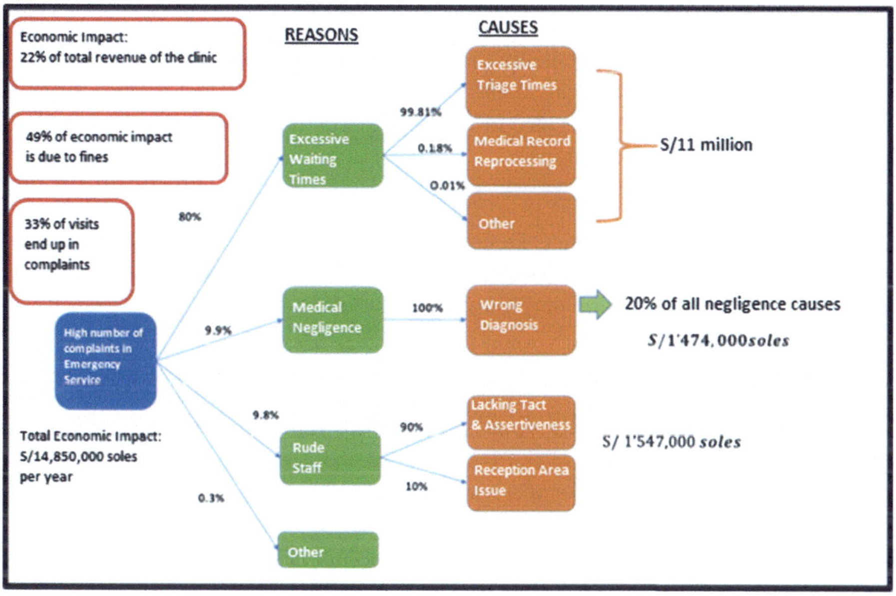

Fig. 2. Diagnostic chart

4 Proposal Implementation

4.1 Initial Audit - 5S

As a starting point for the implementation of the lean healthcare tools, an initial audit based on 5S is performed. The graph below denotes the results obtained from the initial audit questionnaire (Table 1).

Table 1. Initial audit based on 5S

5S	Results
SEIRI (Organization)	80%
SEITON (Order)	93%
SEISO (Cleaning)	95%
SEIKETSU (Standardization)	80%
SHITSUKE (Discipline)	75%

The initial audit results denote that the clinic satisfies the standards of safety, health, and process standardization required in case of health facilities. Approval levels of 75% or more allow the implementation of the selected tools without having to implement the 5S as a proposed solution tool.

4.2 Preliminary Stage

As a preliminary stage, when beginning with the implementation of the solution tools, staff members must become engaged and receive training. The initial training seeks to raise awareness about the importance of the project, continuous improvement, and the improvement tools to be developed.

TOPIC:
Lean Healthcare: Lean Healthcare Definition and Project Overview; SMED: SMED Definition and Activity Classification; Pull System: Pull System Definition; Monitoring: Indicator Monitoring Definition and Indicator Monitoring.

4.3 SMED Implementation

We propose the usage of SMED as an association between maintenance and preparation by considering patients as the backbone of the process and taking the triage process as patient preparation for receiving care.

4.3.1 Preliminary Stage: Define Activities

- Admission: Request ID from patient, Request personal data from patient, Record data in medical records, Verify insurance or social security status.
- Triage: Measure the blood pressure, Measure the temperature, Check the medical history, Initial questionnaire (visit reason, symptoms, frequency), Measure the pulse, Measure the weight and height, Assess the current patient status.

4.3.2 First Stage: Classify Internal and External Activities

- Total time in case of internal activities = 15 min
- Total time in case of external activities = 4.5 min

4.3.3 Second Stage: Convert Internal Activities to External Activities

In the second stage, we seek to convert internal activities into external activities and, if applicable, eliminate the surplus activities. For these purposes, decisions are made based on the reference data from the first stage, wherein we find many unnecessary activities and others that could be performed in parallel with other activities. The results may be observed in the table below (Fig. 3).

- Total time in internal activities = 14 min
- Total time in external activities = 5.5 min

ACTIVITIES	Type	Time (s)
Request ID from Patient	External	30
Request data from Patient / Record Medical History	External	120
Verify Social Security or Insurance	External	120
Take pressure	Internal	300
Take temperature	Internal	180
Query Medical History / Initial Questionnaire	Internal	120
Take pulse	Internal	60
Height and weight	Internal	180
Assess Patient Status	Internal	60
	Total	1170 s

Fig. 3. First stage

ACTIVITIES	Type	Time (s)
Request ID from Patient	External	30
Record Data & Verify Social Security	External	120
Medical History	External	120
Take pressure/pulse/temperature Initial Questionnaire	Internal	300
Height and weight	Internal	180
Assess Patient Status	Internal	60

Fig. 4. In Third stage

The Fig. 5 denotes the total percentage of time used as per the new classification of internal and external activities.

4.3.4 Third Stage: Streamlining and Readjustment of Internal and External Activities

In this stage, the internal activities are streamlined through simultaneous activities. After readjusting, the results are as follows (Fig. 4)

- Total time in internal activities = 9 min
- Total time in external activities = 2.5 min

The Fig. 6 denotes the total percentage of time used as per the new classification of internal and external activities, achieving a reduction in time required for internal activities.

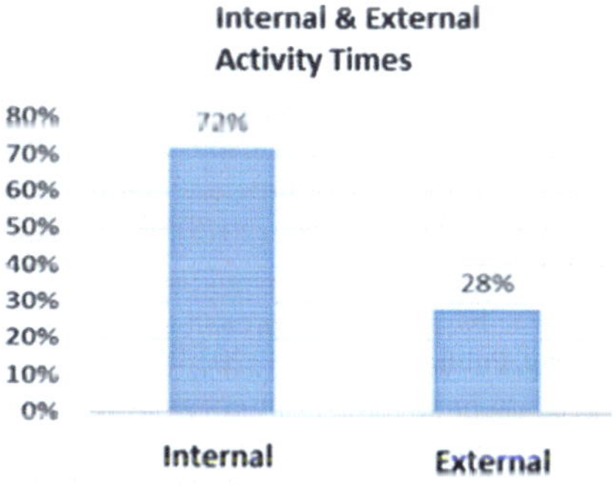

Fig. 5. Second Stage

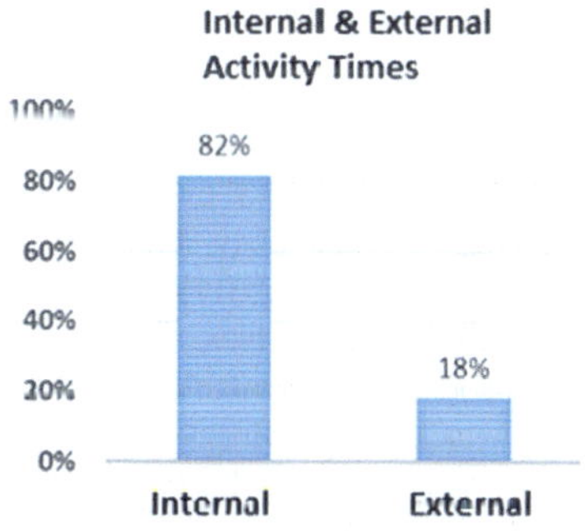

Fig. 6. In Third stage:

After completing the three SMED stages, it is theoretically observed that the preparation times may be reduced. In this case, the triage times are reduced by 40%, reaching a theoretical total time of nine min for internal activities after having reclassified some activities and performing simultaneous activities.

5 Conclusion

This study concludes that the usage of lean healthcare tools and application of SMED at the Limatambo clinic reduced the patient waiting times by 30% during the first medical examination.

In addition, the application of these tools also reduced the triage care times by 40%.

Note that these results are only attributed to the SMED and pull system implementation because the proposed layout redesign model is currently under review by the clinic's board of directors.

Therefore, this study has clearly demonstrated that the application of lean healthcare tools, which does not represent significant amounts in terms of Clinic`s revenue, largely improves the patient waiting times.

References

1. Escuder, M., Tanco, M., Santoro, A.: Experiencia de implementación de Lean en un Centro de Salud de Uruguay. Memoria Investigaciones en Ingeniería **13** (2015)
2. Simón, R., Fumadó, C.: Castellsagúes, O.C.: Implantación de lean en un hospital, Caso CSG. Revista de Contabilidad y Dirección **19**, 149–166 (2014)
3. Khalifa, M., Zabani, I.: Utilizing health analytics in improving the performance of healthcare services: a case study on a tertiary care hospital. J. Infect. Public Health **9**(6), 757–765 (2016). https://doi.org/10.1016/j.jiph.2016.08.016
4. Boronat, F., Budia, A., Broseta, E., Ruiz-Cerdá, J.L., Vivas-Consuelo, D.: Application of lean healthcare methodology in a urology department of a tertiary hospital as a tool for improving efficiency. Actas Urológicas Españolas (English Edition) **42**(1), 42–48 (2018)
5. Guillen, K., Umasi, K., Quispe, G., Raymundo, C.: LEAN model for optimizing plastic bag production in small and medium sized companies in the plastics sector. Int. J. Eng. Res. Tech. **11**(11), 1713–1734 (2018)
6. Balfour, M.E., Tanner, K., Jurica, P.J., Llewellyn, D., Williamson, R.G., Carson, C.A.: Using lean to rapidly and sustainably transform a behavioral health crisis program: impact on throughput and safety. Joint Comm. J. Qual. Patient Saf. **43**(6), 275–283 (2017). https://doi.org/10.1016/j.jcjq.2017.03.008
7. Dammand, J., Hørlyck, M., Jacobsen, T., Lueg, R., Röck, R.: Lean management in hospitals: evidence from Denmark. Administratie Si Management Public **23**, 19–35 (2014)
8. Martínez, P., Martínez, J., Nuño, J., Cavazos, J.: Process improvement in emergency units. two analysis cases. In: Proceedings of IIE Annual Conference, pp. 1–9 (2014)
9. Mazzocato, P., Holden, R.J., Brommels, M., Aronsson, H., Bäckman, U., Elg, M., Thor, J.: How does lean work in emergency care? a case study of a lean-inspired intervention at the astrid lindgren children's hospital, Stockholm, Sweden. BMC Health Serv. Res., 12–28 (2012)

Design of a Model of Marketing a Product of Detection and Identification with Technology of Positioning in Interiors Based on RFID

Amy Canepa[1](✉), Grecia Rodríguez[1](✉), Jose Rojas[1](✉), and Carlos Raymundo[2](✉)

[1] Ingeniería de Gestión Empresarial, Universidad Peruana de Ciencias Aplicadas (UPC), Lima, Peru
{u201314146,u201319865,jose.rojas}@upc.edu.pe
[2] Dirección de Investigación, Universidad Peruana de Ciencias Aplicadas (UPC), Lima, Peru
carlos.raymundo@upc.edu.pe

Abstract. Currently, one of the main problems is that "time" is becoming more important, which will cause people to perform multiple tasks every day because of a hectic lifestyle, and with it the issue of lost articles. and poorly placed also increases significantly. Although there have been initiatives by some small companies to offer solutions characterized by the use of positioning technologies, these have not achieved the desired success. That is why, in this research, a scheme for the design, evaluation and implementation and marketing of a product with RFID technology with location and alert functions in the absence of proximity to solve the aforementioned problem has been proposed. The scheme and the product were validated through focus tools, surveys and scenario analysis. Likewise, the components of the business model of the scheme allow to reach the demand.

Keywords: Indoor location · Business Model Canvas · RFID · E-Commerce · Outsourcing

1 Introduction

The loss of objects, animals, and people has become a major concern in the 21st century. We are faced with the constant need of solving this problem using technological solutions. The increasing growth of the technological trend is brought about by its association to a modern avant-garde lifestyle, creating the pressure to work more and follow this trend. As a result, the speed of life is increasing and every day one has to deal with many different types of work. This state of life creates the problem of not focusing on a particular task and, in general, this disorganization produces the quite common tendency to lose objects if you are not sufficiently organized.

Therefore, the tracking solutions field has grown rapidly because it is trying to solve problems related to the loss and misplacement of objects [1]. Some research

T. Ahram et al. (Eds.): IHIET 2019, AISC 1018, pp. 931–937, 2020.
https://doi.org/10.1007/978-3-030-25629-6_145

studies have even proposed customized positioning systems. In recent years, academic and practical proposals have emerged in the market. Nevertheless, such proposals have gone unnoticed by people or consumers. While there is an intensive demand and existence of tracking or positioning devices, they are not widely known. Many proposals fail to be considered by consumers as good options because of development difficulties such as their positioning technology, platforms, energy consumption, and costs involved.

In this study, the problem is examined for current Peruvian environments, and a revision of tracking positioning technologies is performed to select the most suitable technology for solving this issue. Two contributions are presented in this study. The first one is composed of two integrated products with radio frequency identification (RFID) indoor positioning technology for locating objects. Note that alerts are issued if the objects are not close. The second one is a scheme for the commercialization of this product. The methodology is based on Lean StartUp, proposed by Eric Ries in 2011, and is integrated to the E-Commerce methodology and tools such as the Business Model Canvas, Digital Marketing, and Outsourcing [2]. We started our research with the analysis of this problem, the revision of possible solutions and environments, the development of a prototype, and the design of the Lean StartUp scheme with the abovementioned methodologies and tools. The implementation was performed via simulations according to scheme components that included surveys, different approaches, and analysis of scenarios. The results show the product's viability and the scheme for its commercialization.

2 State of the Art

2.1 Positioning System

Depending on the destination environment, the positioning system can be classified as either indoor or external environment. External positioning systems are primarily based on global satellite navigation systems. These systems are used for monitoring and asset management, navigation and transport, network synchronization, and geodetic applications, but it does not work well near walls, buildings, trees, indoors, and in underground environments [3].

2.2 Lean StartUp

The Lean StartUp methodology applies different techniques to create viable businesses that can repetitively sell and grow [2]. The methodology involves three techniques: designing business models, customer development, and agile development. This scheme allows the creation of disruptive or classic models and simplifies the steps to generate a profitable business model supported by the value proposal [4].

2.3 E-Commerce

E-Commerce addresses the commercialization of products and services either online or on any other telecommunications network. Its purpose is to create meaningful value such as the difference between the consumer's perceived benefit for a given product or service and the cost for the company to provide such a product or service [5].

2.4 Digital Marketing

Digital marketing or digitalization is the application of marketing strategies on digital media. All techniques of the off-line world are imitated and converted into a new world, the online world [6].

2.5 Outsourcing

Outsourcing is an innovative management technique, which involves the transfer to third parties of certain supplementary processes that are not part of the main line of business. This allows for the concentration of efforts on essential activities, thus increasing competitiveness and generating tangible results [7].

In 2017, a study was carried out on "The Effect of Subcontracting Strategies on the Performance of Small and Medium-Sized Enterprises (SMEs)" in Nigeria to determine the effect of subcontracting strategies (administrative, primary, accounting, and support activities) in the performance of small and medium-sized enterprises (SMEs) [8]. The results concluded that, similar to large-scale organizations, SMEs subcontract back-office, primary, accounting, and support activities. These outsourcing activities have led to increasing profitability over the years.

3 Proposed Model

A scheme for the design and commercialization of a product is proposed. For such purposes, the methodology to be applied will be Lean Startup because its structure allows for the easy use of diverse tools such as E-Commerce, Digital Marketing, and Outsourcing. The model can be seen in Fig. 1.

3.1 Opportunity or Need Detection

To detect opportunities or requirements, a study was carried out to analyze the tendency of the increasing daily losses (Fig. 2). The research reference of the problem was used at the national level and because no information was found, surveys of 17 closed questions were conducted through online media (50%) and in person (50%) to determine the existence of the problem. The results showed that 86.8% faced the problem of losing their personal items, 100% looked for them manually, and 92.8% would like to have a device that would notify them when they forget their personal belongings.

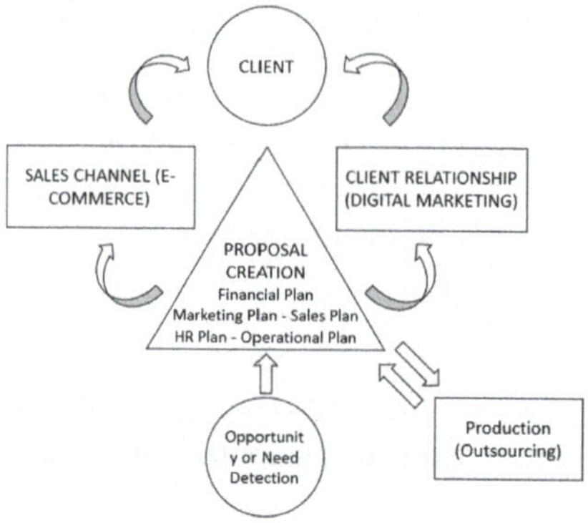

Fig. 1. Proposed design and marketing scheme

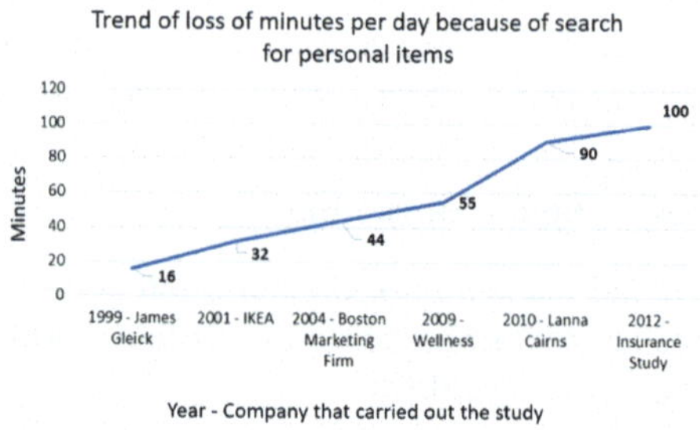

Fig. 2. Trends

3.2 Proposal Creation

The business model was developed according to the Business Model Canvas (Fig. 3).

Strategic partners	Strategic activities	Value proposal	Relationship with clients	Client segments
Watch and tag production suppliers. Watch belt supplier. Box and tag supplier. Accounting services supplier. Electronic billing services supplier. Financial entities.	Programming. Sales. Imports. Quality Supervision. Research and development. Online store handling. **Strategic resources** Employees. Prototypes. Online payment methods. Sales platform.	Sales of technological product for tracking, which will increase security to protect personal objects that are the most important ones for each client.	Social media. Web page. **Channels** Online store. Delivery.	Men and women: -With sophisticated, modern, and advanced lifestyles. -A, B, and C socioeconomic levels. -Persons who live in metropolitan Lima. -From 18 to 50 years old.
Cost structure			**Revenue flow**	
Manufacturing and imports costs Programming and delivery costs Online sales platform updates			Watch sales Tag sales Belt sales	

Fig. 3. Canvas value proposal

3.2.1 Development of the Prototype or PMV

The prototype was developed based on the design thinking methodology. In the first stage, we identified stakeholders and sought to align ourselves with the most determining factors of the target segment. In the second stage, the problem was de-fined and the reason why they lose things and find it so difficult to find them was determined, which then leads to replacements. In the third stage, the prototype was designed with the characteristics mentioned by the people. The possible options for the aforementioned solution were a watch, an application, and a key ring. In the end, the watch was selected as the best idea for the solution. In the fourth stage, the idea was prototyped by testing the technical viability via a simulation to choose Arduino programming and RFID components (watch and tag simulators). In the fifth stage, the device was tested with two focus groups and the following changes were reported. The changes were applied to the Match Watch, which is a watch that helps you to find your lost objects. It sends warning signals when you are moving away from them and it also shows the time. It works with a radar called RFID and some small tags that can be attached to the product, which help you identify and locate your personal items. It works within a radius of ~15 m and has sound alerts (Fig. 4).

3.2.2 Sales Plan

The sales plan will be focused on identified customer segments and their particular characteristics. The proposed scheme does not include vendors because the online platform is able to serve all clients (Fig. 5).

The sales process will include six activities in which commercial intelligence will be carried out. This means that it will be focused on customer acquisition regardless of those that independently visit the site. Such acquisition will be based on e-mailing and previous analysis of consumer trends, user characteristics, stock of products, and promotions.

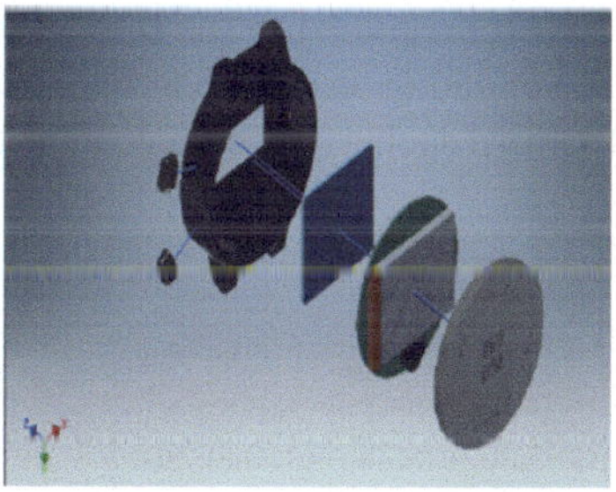

Fig. 4. Internal design of the watch - back side

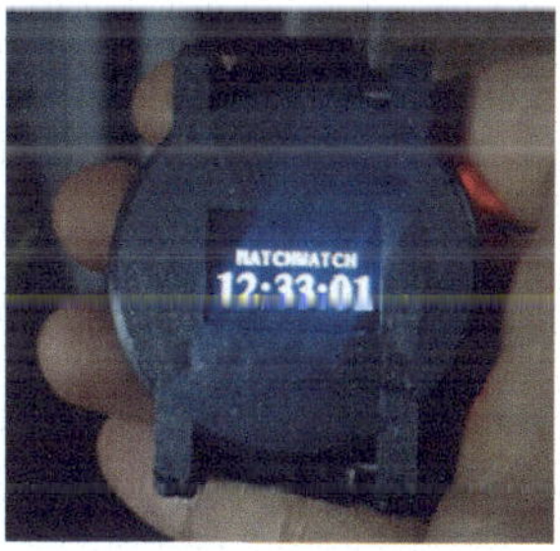

Fig. 5. Prototype

3.2.3 Marketing Plan

The marketing plan has been designed to achieve the projected sales. In this plan, digital marketing will be applied and both types of channels will be used, in addition to a blog and social networking platforms such as Facebook and Instagram. Similarly, a marketing mix will be applied.

The products include a technical sheet and manual for an in-depth understanding. The price was determined based on the survey whose results showed that 75% of users were willing to pay between 100 and 200 soles.

3.2.4 Financial Plan

The cost and revenue structure defined an optimal cash flow for the business (Fig. 6).

	Año 0	Año 1	Año 2	Año 3	Año 4	Año 5
Ingresos por Ventas		275154	302669	340503	391834	470201
Costo Directo (Ventas)		(96304)	(105934)	(119176)	(137142)	(164570)
Margen bruto		**178850**	**196735**	**221327**	**254692**	**305631**
Gastos Generales		(77914)	(80914)	(120180)	(148430)	(147780)
Gastos de Ventas		(14400)	(15120)	(15840)	(16128)	(16560)
EBITDA		**86536**	**100701**	**85307**	**90134**	**141291**
Depreciacion y Amortización		6010	6010	6010	6010	6010
EBIT		**92546**	**106711**	**91317**	**96144**	**147301**
Impuestos		(27764)	(32013)	(27395)	(28843)	(44190)
Depreciacion y Amortización		(6010)	(6010)	(6010)	(6010)	(6010)
Resultado Neto		**58772**	**68688**	**57912**	**61291**	**97101**
CAPEX	(19520)	0	0	0	0	0
Inv k de w	(19500)	(19500)	(19500)	(19500)	(19500)	(19500)
Intereses		(6000)	(6000)	(6000)	(6000)	
Gastos preoperativos	(25500)					
Valor de rescate						2500
Recuperacion k w						15600
FCF Flujo de caja libre	**(64520)**	**33272**	**43188**	**32412**	**35791**	**95701**
valor presente flujo	(64520)	26618	27640	6797	6005	12845
Recupero descontado	(64520)	(37902)	(10262)	(3464)	2540	15385
CCPP	25.00%					
VAN	**52352**					
TIR	55.51%					
Cuentas por cobrar						
Efectivo		19500	19500	19500	19500	19500
Fondo de maniobra		19500	19500	19500	19500	19500
Inversiones		(19500)	0	0	0	0

Fig. 6. Operating process

4 Validation

According to validations that were made, changes were applied to the business model to meet customer expectations, in addition to validating certain aspects that were initially planned, but whose acceptance was not known such as the extension of the age range (Fig. 7).

Componente	Acción	Estado
Propuesta de Valor	Se validó mediante Focus Group	Pivot: Cambios en la funcionabilidad, personalización y diseño
Segmento de Clientes	Se validó mediante Encuesta y Focus Group	Pivot: Cambios en la segmentación, ampliación hasta los 50 años de edad
Canales de Venta	Se validó con la Wix	Pivot: Cambios en el diseño de la página, mejoría de la interfaz y en los métodos de pago (Visa, MasterCard)
Relación con los clientes	Se validó con la página web en Facebook	Pivot: Se lanzaron publicaciones pagadas obteniendo más "likes" en la página.
Recursos estratégicos	Se validó mediante Focus Group	Pivot: Mejora del prototipo para llegar al producto final, Métodos de pago en la plataforma web en vez de contraentrega
Actividades estratégicas	Se validó mediante Focus Group	Pivot: El producto se comercializará vía web, además de la oficina y ferias tecnológicas (activaciones)
Aliados Estratégicos	Se validó el costo del reloj mediante un pedido mínimo al proveedor	Redujo los costos para cada envío considerando un pedido mínimo y de esta manera ofrecer un precio menor al cliente
Estructura de Costos	Flujos Financieros en 3 escenarios distintos	En el escenario pesimista se estaría recuperando la inversión en el año 4, en el promedio en el año 3 y en el optimista en el año 2
Flujo de Ingresos	Se validó mediante Focus Group	Pivot: Se determinó el precio de MatchWatch así como de los tags y correas

Fig. 7. Products and Prices

5 Conclusions

The Lean StartUp methodology may be used to implement an idea for a new product or business based on the customer discovery model. The number of visits to the fan page is directly proportional to the amount of money that is invested in promoting the publications or the page. Every day, Match Watch helps users minimize the loss of personal objects. Based on the validations that were carried out, we are able to conclude that there is a market and a public who accepts the value proposal and is willing to pay for a product that prevents the loss of personal items. Similarly, the structure of the Lean StartUp model supported by outsourcing, e-commerce, digital marketing, and RFID tools helps to create a flexible, dynamic, and adaptable to change business structure to sell for tracking devices with in-built triggers for alerts.

References

1. Ahmad, S., Ziaullah, M., Rauniyar, L., Su, M., Zhang, Y.: How does matter lost and misplace items issue and its technological solutions in 2015 - a review study. IOSR J. Bus. Manag. Ver. I **17**(4), 2319–7668 (2015)
2. Ries, E.: Método Lean Startup, p. 248 (2011)
3. Farid, Z., Nordin, R., Ismail, M.: Recent advances in wireless indoor localization techniques and system, J. Comput. Netw. Commun., **2013** (2013)
4. Wrigley, C., Straker, K.: Designing innovative business models with a framework that promotes experimentation. Strateg. Leadersh. **44**(1), 11–19 (2016)
5. Osterwalder, A., Pigneur, Y., Smith, A., Movement, T.: Business Model Generation (2010)
6. Torres, P.M., Lisboa, J.V., Yasin, M.M.: E-commerce strategies and corporate performance: an empirical investigation. Compet. Rev. **24**(5), 463–481 (2014)
7. Korukcu, O., Kukulu, K.: The challenges and opportunities of social media in health. Turkish Online J. Educ. Technol. **2016**, 743–745 (2016). no. DecemberSpecialIssue
8. Agburu, J.I., Anza, N.C., Iyortsuun, A.S.: Effect of outsourcing strategies on the performance of small and medium scale enterprises (SMEs). J. Glob. Entrep. Res. **7**(1), 26 (2017)

Quality Management Model for a Small Enterprise of Pecan Farmers in Ica el Valle - Peru

Angello Bolaños[1(✉)], Luis Leiva[1(✉)], Fernando Sotelo[1(✉)], and Carlos Raymundo[2(✉)]

[1] Ingeniería Industrial, Universidad Peruana de Ciencias Aplicadas (UPC), Lima, Peru
{u201415766,u201412718,fernando.sotelo}@upc.edu.pe
[2] Dirección de Investigación, Universidad Peruana de Ciencias Aplicadas (UPC), Lima, Peru
carlos.raymundo@upc.edu.pe

Abstract. In this study, we propose a basic quality management model that was designed based on good agricultural practices for micro-enterprises of pecan farmers in Ica el Valle, Peru. The research study was developed based on in-depth interviews with 18 farmers within the agricultural sector under study. The study focused on identifying and analyzing the current situation of farmers to design a basic quality management model that can be implemented. The results led to the identification of critical aspects for each of the activities related to the production of nuts. We thus designed a basic quality management model based previous scientific studies. This management system is composed of the following subprocesses: quality adjustment; documentation; parameters definition; monitoring and control; and continuous improvement and analysis of results.

Keywords: Process management · Management model · Quality management · Small agricultural business · Pecan

1 Introduction

The pecan or *Carya illinoinensis* is defined according to the Australian Nut Industry Council (2014) as a species of walnut native of the south and southeast of the United States, constituting an integral part of the multimillion-dollar tree nut industry that spans throughout the world. Note that the main nut-producing countries in the world are the United States and Mexico.

According to statistical data provided by the National Institute of Statistics and Informatics (INEI *for its name in Spanish*) (2017), the agricultural GDP shows a favorable result of 2.6% compared to the previous year, which is associated with higher harvests. From this perspective, the agricultural sector has a positive impact not only at the regional level but also worldwide because Peru is a country that exports to different countries. As regards to the aforementioned statement and considering the product discussed in this study, it is feasible to mention that Peru is extending its market

T. Ahram et al. (Eds.): IHIET 2019, AISC 1018, pp. 938–944, 2020.
https://doi.org/10.1007/978-3-030-25629-6_146

penetration by exporting large quantities of the product to countries such as China (Hong Kong), Vietnam, and Germany.

2 State of the Art

Previous studies [1–4] have indicated that, with respect to the business stratum, micro and small enterprises (MSMEs) represent the sector with greater relevance because of the high number of companies that are a part of this sector. Similarly, they concluded that the participation of these companies generates an added value for the country, as this an important trigger for the development of the economies of the analyzed countries. Furthermore, it is a great way to improve household welfare and reduce poverty through its positive effect on employment and wages because these factors contribute to the largest share of employment generation. Note that MSMEs represent 99.97% of all Peruvian companies (INEI, 2018).

Articles [5] and [6] highlight that the relationship between productivity and quality are dependent in such a way that focus on the quality of processes should effectively lead to improved productivity. Moreover, the price is defined by the quality of the product.

Other studies [7] and [8] have highlighted that quality is important for companies because a quality management system is a process that allows continuous improvement, action plan implementation, and monitoring. Moreover, total quality management (TQM) is used to improve quality within an organization and efficiency in all its associated projects. Considering the previous studies, we can propose a basic optimize a quality model that, according to the methodologies and procedures, covers the needs of the micro-agricultural enterprises of Pecan nuts in the Ica-Pachacútec valley.

Article [9] highlights that data collection using the snowball technique is most suitable for this population. This research method is based on direct contact with an involved party in the study sector and subsequently assesses a third party in the same study sector to obtain more information. Then, the method continues to contact another third party from the same sector and so on in such a way that the information that is collected has the quality and quantity necessary to carry out a study. In the case of MSMEs, this method is the most feasible one according to the aforementioned authors.

3 Rationale

Stage I: Identify the Field and Type of Study

First, the field under study was selected. For this purpose, different activities were carried out such as collecting information, delimitation of the field, and sampling to have a greater information sustenance, data, and veracity. According to the INEI, agriculture, livestock, hunting, and forestry activities are placed in the fourth position with a value of 2.6%. Similarly, it is claimed that the sector evidenced its growth because of the positive behavior of the agricultural subsector (2.6%). Moreover, SMEs form $\sim$99.4% of the company's participation. As a second step, the type of sampling to be followed is detailed and, since qualitative and quantitative data were used, a mixed study was used.

Stage II: Compilation and Analysis of Information

First, in-depth surveys were carried out because it is an adequate tool for gathering information. Eighteen farmers from the Ica-Pachacútec valley were surveyed. These in-depth interviews were conducted in a personal manner.

Second, quantitative and qualitative data were collected. The pecan production process was also identified. Note that the pecan production process takes a long time because this tree yields its first fruits around the fifth and sixth year (Fig. 1).

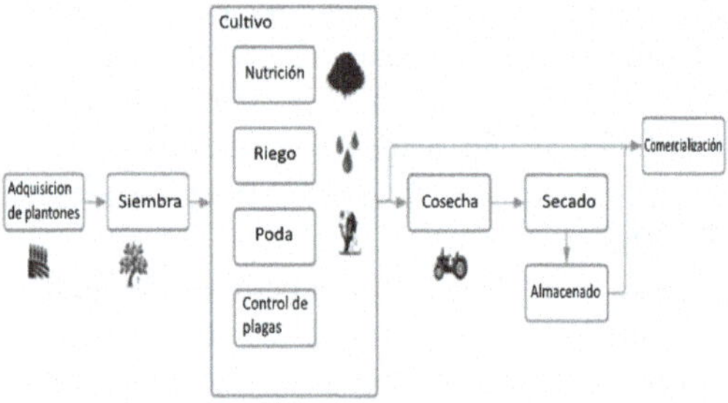

Fig. 1. Pecan nut marketing process

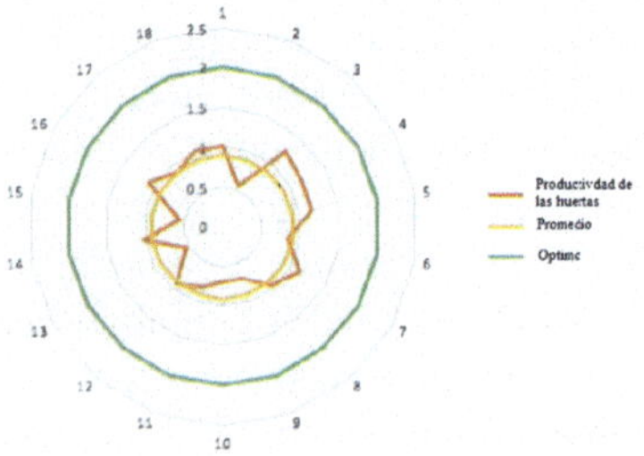

Fig. 2. Optimal productivity vs real productivity

The following are the stakeholders of the pecan nut production process:

- Suppliers: They are important participants because they provide the necessary agricultural inputs for pecan production.
- Producer: They provide labor for the proper development of the production.
- Intermediary: They provide the logistical support for the transportation and collection of pecans.
- Customers: They are the main markets, both international and domestic, that demand a quality product.

Third, evidences were obtained (filmed and photographic) to demonstrate the veracity of the collected data.

Fourth, we searched for relevant information on productivity in other countries to have a general picture of the actual production situation between Peru and the main pecan producers in the world. Within this framework, the intentional demand from European and Asian markets has made Peru one of the important suppliers in the world. Peru is now located in the fifth position with a percentage of 0.8% with respect to the total production; however, it is below countries such as Mexico (44.9%) and the United States (40.8%), which are considered powers in terms of pecan production.

Figure 2 shows the comparison between optimal productivity (following the guidelines of experts and review of literature) and actual productivity (the current). Ideal or optimum productivity would be 2.0 tons per hectare; however, the average productivity is ~0.9 tons per hectare. Finally, after having adequate data, we proceeded to analyze the information and make the assessment. In this manner, you may have the main cause for the problem, the impact it brings, and the activities involved in the whole process; therefore, a solution for the identified problem is proposed.

Stage III: Presentation of Results
The results obtained from the interviews and visits made to the 18 agricultural microenterprises reflected poor management of their activities, which leads to low productivity. The following information was obtained: 84% of the farmers did not carry out a soil survey, 77% did not perform the adequate nutritional proportion to feed the pecan trees, 77% did not use pesticides in suitable amounts to fight pests and/or diseases, 69% did not irrigate their plantations properly, and 69% did not perform proper pruning. To be able to improve these conditions, we propose a basic quality management system designed for the Pecan micro-enterprises in Ica, Peru.

Stage IV: Quality Methodology Proposed for the Sector
First, the relationship between quality and logistics and production processes is shown (Figs. 3 and 4).

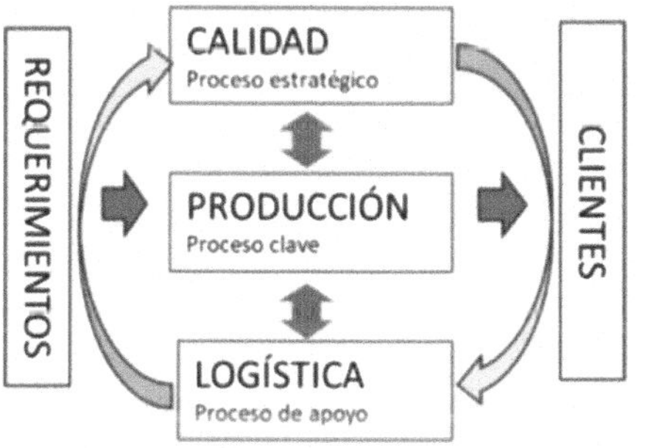

Fig. 3. Quality – production – logistics relationship

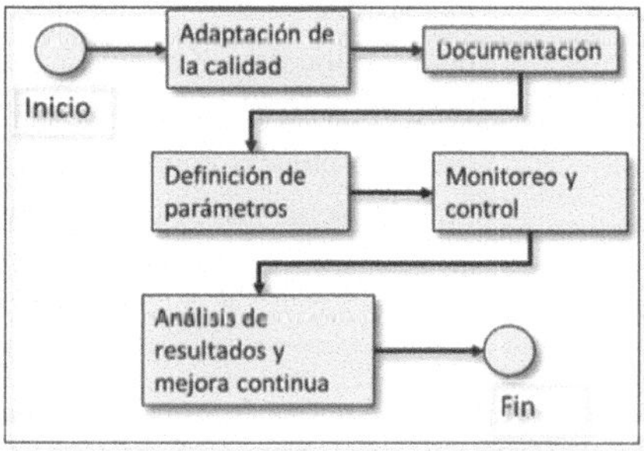

Fig. 4. Proposed model development

Considering the requirements of the market or the customers, the abovementioned processes work in synergy and provide information, activities, and corresponding procedures to achieve customer satisfaction.

The quality process defines the parameters, standards, and gathers information of good agricultural practices such that the production and logistics processes can plan, execute, and control the activities related to production.

In recent years, quality management applied to agriculture has acquired special significance. Previous studies [10, 11] have indicated the differences between the various quality leadership criteria from which the best model may be selected. Quality is defined as a set of properties or characteristics that a product or service possesses to satisfy requirements. First, ISO 9001 refers to standards that meet minimum requirements to be considered as a quality management system (QMS). These standards have an extensive and complex procedure because they are international standards. Second, the European foundation for quality management (EFQM) model is a European system of excellence, which considers total quality but not as a management system. It mainly focuses on people's functions and gathers information to improve organizational areas. Its assessment is based on people, strategies, processes of products, or services. Finally, we have the TQM model, which is based on the internal strategies that allow for process improvement via the reduction of costs, losses, and the organization of internal procedures. Moreover, it indicates the investment and constancy of stakeholders during the process. Furthermore, this model can be applied in any organization. Table 1 shows a matrix that compares the various quality management systems. Three quality methodologies have been presented: ISO 9001, EFQM model, and TQM.

Table 1. Comparative table of quality management systems

Indicator	ISO 9001	EFQM	TQM
Improvement in service or product quality	✓	✓	✓
Profitability of the enterprise	✓	✓	✓
Productivity	✓	✓	✓
Feasability for SMEs	✓	✓	✓
Increase in sales	✓	✓	✓
Improve training of staff	✓	✓	✓
Low implementation investment			✓
In-house process improvement	✓	✓	✓
Low implementation complexity			✓
Process specialized staff	✓	✓	✓

The TQM model has features that can be easily carried out such as simplicity and implementation cost. This would be beneficial for farmers because, being a microenterprise, the application of the said model would be more feasible.

Stage V: Development of the Proposed Model

The model that has been developed is aligned with TQM tools and concepts, as well as good agricultural practices, which will be implemented via a focus on the basic process management tools.

The flowchart below contains five subprocesses, with each subprocess containing a manual of procedures, record sheets, indicators, and guidelines to follow.

Below, we describe how the quality process was modeled.

- Quality adjustment: Based on planning activities, the most relevant being the development of a training schedule related to quality for micro-enterprises.
- Documentation: Focused on the definitions of the guidelines and requirements relevant to the quality process.
- Parameter Definition: Implies establishing the standards for all productive process activities related to the final quality of the nuts.
- Monitoring and control: It includes monitoring of the activities.
- Results analysis and action plans: Analysis of the results of each activity, correcting them, and proposing improvements to avoid disadvantages.

4 Conclusions

Using in-depth interviews with farmers in the sector under study, it could be analyzed that 72.2% of farmers, 15 of the 18 interviewed, are not aware of the quality management process aspects applicable to MSMEs. This evidences that when farmers do not consider the appropriate parameters for the establishment of good agricultural practices within the activities of the pecan production process, the quality of the fruit may not be optimal to compete in the international market. Therefore, the first subprocess of quality adaptation was established, which consists of carrying out previous training to farmers to ensure that they understand the structure of the process to be implemented, as well as the considerations for the designed model to obtain positive results in the corresponding indicators.

The diagnosis made in the study sector reveals that only 27.7% of the farmers interviewed, considering the 18 orchards visited, used registers such as notebooks in which they control the planting dates, fertilization dates, and the list of nutrients and pesticides that need to applied to pecan trees. In the absence of adequate documentation of the activities, i.e., when there are no simple management formats, there is a risk of committing errors for the corresponding tasks. For example, if the date to apply a certain nutrient is in June but the farmer does not know exactly in which week and on which day of the month this procedure must be carried out, the pecan trees may not grow properly, thus leading to lower fruit productivity.

Note that 100% of the farmers interviewed do not consider the standards and parameters, established by good agricultural practices within the activities they carry out in the pecan production process. Moreover, farmers and orchard owners are people who have sown the fruit for many decades; therefore, they perform tasks based on the experience they have acquired over the years, which they also transmit to the workers. Although to now considerable amounts of pecan have been sold to exporting companies, the implementation of the designed model will show an improvement in the product quality, which will also improve productivity of orchards.

References

1. Organización Internacional del Trabajo (OIT): Panorama Laboral Temático. Pequeñas empresas, grandes brechas. Empleo y condiciones de trabajo en las MYPE de América Latina y el Caribe. Recuperado de (2015). http://www.ilo.org/americas/publicaciones/WCMS_398103/lang-es/index.htm
2. Giang, L.T., Nguyen, C.V., Tran, T.Q.: Firm agglomeration and local poverty reduction: evidence from an economy in transition. Asian-Pac. Econ. Lit. **30**(1), 80–98 (2016)
3. Macías, C.J.G., Hernández, I.Z., Salgado, P.M.: Sustentabilidad organizacional en pymes familiares restauranteras de la Jonquera en Cataluña, España. Nóesis: Revista Ciencias Sociales Humanidades **24**(47), 80–97 (2015)
4. Ministerio de la Producción (PRODUCE): Anuario Estadístico Industrial, Mipyme y Comercio Interno 2015. Recuperado de (2015). http://www.produce.gob.pe/documentos/estadisticas/anuarios/anuarioestadisticomype-2015.pdf
5. Benavides-Chicón, C.G., Ortega, B.: The impact of quality management on productivity in the hospitality sector. Int. J. Hospit. Manag. **42**, 165173 (2014)

6. Choi, K., Lee, D., Olson, D.L.: Service quality and productivity in US airline industry: a service quality-adjusted DEA model. Serv. Bus. **9**(1), 137160 (2015)
7. Álvarez García, J., Fraiz Brea, J.A., Del Río Rama, M.D.L.: Análisis de las motivaciones para certificar la marca "Q de calidad turística": sector de alojamiento. Inv. Eur. Dirección Econ. Empresa (IEDEE) **18**(1), 101–121 (2012)
8. Dhounchak, D., Biban, L.K.: Total quality management and its applications. Int. J. Sci. Res. Mech. Mater. Eng. (IJSRMME) **1**(1), 15 (2017)
9. Baltar, F., Brunet, I.: Social research 2.0: virtual snowball sampling method using Facebook. Internet Res. **22**(1), 57–74 (2012)
10. Benzaquen de Las Casas, J.B.: La ISO 9001 y TQM en las empresas latinoamericanas: Perú. J. Glob. Compet. Governab./Revista de Globalización, Competitividad y Gobernabilidad/ Revista de Globalização, Competitividade e Governabilidade, **8**(1) (2014)
11. De Las Casas, J.B., Sorza, J.D.C.: El ISO 9001 y TQM en las empresas de Colombia. Globalización Competitividad Gobernabilidad Georgetown/Univ. **9**(3) (2015)

Adoption of Snowball Sampling Technique with Distance Boundaries to Assess the Productivity Issue Faced by Micro and Small Cocoa Producers in Cusco

Angie Jalca[1(✉)], Marco Lopez[1(✉)], Fernando Sotelo[1(✉)], and Carlos Raymundo[2(✉)]

[1] Escuela de Ingenieria Industrial, Universidad Peruana de Ciencias Aplicadas (UPC), Lima, Peru
{u201315761,u201313281,fernando.sotelo}@upc.edu.pe
[2] Dirección de Investigación, Universidad Peruana de Ciencias Aplicadas, Lima, Peru
Carlos.raymundo@upc.edu.pe

Abstract. The food supply chain has gained impulse over the past few years induced by the rising global demand for food; therefore, much emphasis is placed upon examining this class of supply chains. It also faces constant production, storage, and distribution challenges, wherein the key link for proper operation is the farmer, who engages in the agricultural sector, heavily impacted by low crop productivity, which interfer with economic development at a national level. Consequently, it is important to assess those farmers who belong to micro and small enterprises in the agricultural sector. Due to the characteristics of the population, a nonprobability sampling technique was used to assess micro and small cocoa producers in La Convención Province, Cusco, Peru. To such end, a snowball sampling model with distance boundaries was adopted because the population is unknown and hard to reach.

Keywords: Systems engineering · Snowball sampling · Cocoa · Food supply chain · Productivity

1 Introduction

Agriculture sector is the largest an essential sector of the Peruvian economy, employing an average of 16,897,500 people, of which 77.4% reside in rural areas. Agriculture provides job opportunities, encourages technological changes and the use of best practices, and plays a significant role in Peru's economic growth with a high share in its GDP [1]. The monthly income earned by micro and small farmers (MSE) stands at PER 448 in rural areas, against PER 1,097 in urban areas [2], where productivity is the main issue affecting MSE across the agricultural sector.

Cocoa beans, also known as "the food of the Gods," are considered one of the main commodities within the food industry with about 40–50 million people economically depending on this crop. The rise demand for cocoa is influenced by the chocolate,

T. Ahram et al. (Eds.): IHIET 2019, AISC 1018, pp. 945–951, 2020.
https://doi.org/10.1007/978-3-030-25629-6_147

pastry and cosmetics industries, by 2019, an annual growth of 3.1% is expected in the volume of the market, so the cocoa beans will have a value of USD 2.1 million in 2019. However, cocoa demand is expected to increase by 30% in 2020 [3]. Moreover, should we compare Thailand's productivity of 3,738 kg/ha—the country with the highest cocoa productivity—against Peru's productivity of 772 kg/ha, the resulting difference accounts for an improvement gap in Peruvian productivity.

Peruvian annual cocoa production totals around 4.6 million tons with an annual estimated growth of 3% over the last decade and a 2% global share. Out of the cocoa-producing regions in Peru, Cusco, the third largest cocoa-producing region at national level, has the lowest productivity level with a yield of 366 kg/ha and stands below the average Peruvian profitability of 720 kg/ha. Thus, this research aims to assess the main factors lowering cocoa productivity in Cusco, Peru.

2 State of Art

According to Ramírez and Peña [4], companies across the world direct increasing attention to supply chain because it is an enabler for achieving their strategic goals. Similarly, Avelar-Sosa, García-Alcaraz, and Cedillo-Campos [5]; and Ellram and Cooper [6] consider the importance of the supply chain in managing financial, information, and material flows to provide a quality service or product. Kusumastuti, Donk, and Teunter [7] affirm that the global demand for food has skyrocketed over the last decade, thus increasing interest in, as well as the importance of, conducting research in food supply chain management. The study by Seyed Hossein Nikou and Harihodin Selamat [8] demonstrates that farmers are the foundation of the food supply chain because they perform the production processes required to grow food.

Assessing farmers based on the Peruvian corporate structure described by the Ministry of Production, we conclude that they belong to MSEs. Aruna [9] explained that the central issue by these companies is productivity and, according to Ali's research [1], MSE development and growth is closely associated with rise productivity.

Within the agricultural sector, there are populations that are hard to reach, both socially and geographically. Moreover, Muhib [10] asserts that constructing samples, conducting assessments, and collecting data of hidden or hard-to-reach populations are challenges for many research projects. According to Heckathorn [11], "hidden populations" have two characteristics; first, the sample size is unknown; and second, individuals refuse to cooperate in the data-collection interviews. Therefore, Baltar and Brunet [12] introduce four main sampling types: targeted sampling, time-space sampling, respondent-driven sampling, and snowball sampling. Each type involves different implementation costs, access to information, geographical accessibility, and specifications and characteristics of hidden populations.

2.1 Snowball Sampling

Baltar and Brunet [12] and Browne [13] conclude that snowball sampling is among the most commonly used methods for collecting data in hidden populations, and that it is especially used in surveys that require a high level of confidence from a low number of respondents. It is also one of the main alternatives to reduce sampling bias and obtain a representative sample.

According to Baltar and Brunet [12]; and Browne [13], snowball sampling looks for appropriate subjects based on their interpersonal relations and social network; that is, the first participant recruited provides the name of another individual within the target population, who then mentions other members of the population, building a chain of referrals. Initial contact is established formally by seeking information in companies, organizations, and institutions that may offer information about certain members within a given population to build up the network. This technique is produced due to the snowball effect that occurs as the interviews conducted inspire other people to participate, feel confident, and offer detailed quality information. Browne [13] mentions that this technique, as many others, relies on the individuals' willingness to participate and, consequently, many individuals may refuse to cooperate and will be excluded from the research. Moreover, Iron-Segev, Lusweti, Kamau-Mbuthia, and Stark [14] state that snowball sampling is an easy-to-use, simple, low cost, and time-saving technique; thus, they consider it the most efficient method. Also, Salami, Babatunde, Ayinde, and Adeoti [15] argue that this technique is extremely useful when the interviewer are illiterate.

3 Sampling Method

Snowball sampling was chosen to sample cocoa farmers because this type of sampling is used in case of unknown or hard-to-access populations. It is based on developing a contact network after establishing initial contact with the population; however, before creating this network, the main basic processes of the assessment method should be followed, as shown below (Fig. 1).

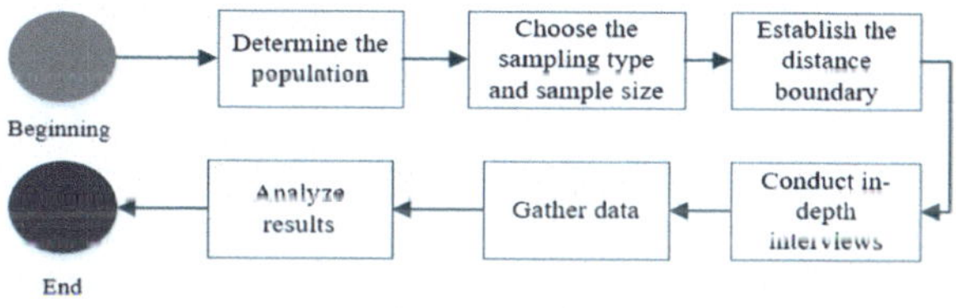

Fig. 1. Snowball sampling process

3.1 Determine the Population

The starting point of the research is to determine the population and/or sector that will be tested, and to define the country and city where the data will be collected. Access to such population should also be examined considering the geographical, social, and cultural restrictions.

3.2 Choose the Sampling Type and Sample Size

The research method should also be established as mixed, qualitative, or quantitative. This approach should be chosen based on the main assessment goals, the complexity of the research, and the expected result. The exact number of individuals representing the total population to be tested depends on the size of the universe. The sample size mainly considers the margin of error expected in the research; in other words, it refers to the confidence level that can be derived from the assessment results.

3.3 Establish the Distance Boundary

Since the geographic location and extension of the individuals are the mains characteristic of the population that hinders data collection, is why the distance between each individual needs to be restricted to certain radius to ensure cost and time effectiveness. Therefore it is important, to consider the budget and timeframe allocated for performing the assessment to reduce data collection times and costs.

3.4 Conduct In-Depth Interviews

Considering the characteristics of the population, in-depth interviewing is the most adequate tool for collecting information. It is a chat between the interviewee and the interviewer using verbal and nonverbal information tools to ensure the interviewee is comfortable and may provide correct information, to match assessment expectations. The interview questions should be designed precisely in a clear and simple language so that they are easy to understand. These questions should focus on collecting qualitative and quantitative data for the research.

3.5 Gather Data

In the sampling of snowballs, the initial contact is the first step of the network of contacts; the first in-depth interview is conducted to the individual closest to the central initial point. This subject will act as the liaison with the following more individuals who share the same characteristics. In this sense, at the end of the interview, the interviewer asks the exact location of other contacts of the interviewee. These other contacts will be chosen according to the distance restriction, starting with the closest contact and removing any contacts located beyond the distance boundaries. The qualitative and quantitative information will be compiled according to the different open and closed questions addressed to each farmer of the network of contacts. All information must be documented in writing and stored appropriately for analysis.

3.6 Analyze Results

When all the information required to assess the sector is gathered, the final qualitative and quantitative results are obtained by using percentages and a description of the status and causes of the problem. Besides, each result should be attributed to a process to identify which of them need to be analyzed in detail to recommend an improvement.

4 Case Study

Cocoa production in Peru is concentrated in five major departments: San Martín, Junín, Cusco, Ucayali, and Huánuco, which represent over 80% of total production, with varying shares. Cusco's share stands at 9%, ranking third. However, Cusco has an average productivity of 366 kg/ha and is the region with the lowest productivity, accounting for less than 50% of the Peruvian average of 772 kg/ha. Therefore, this study focuses on La Convención Province, that represents 80% of cocoa bean production in Cusco. The sample size is 68 farmers, which will be interviewed to ensure data quality.

Collecting data from cocoa farmers is very complex because La Convención Province is divided into 14 districts and has a total population of 179,845 across a surface of 30,061.82 km^2; therefore, the contact network was built based on distance boundaries. The distance boundary fixed was a radius of 20 km and the benchmark used was a first farmer that asked to provide a contact located near the current point within the 20 km radius. This distance boundary was established to reduce the time incurred in gathering data due to the extension of the area and the time available to conduct the interviews.

To initiate contact with the farmers, we visited them at their plots of land, homes, and workplaces, which are the usual places where they may be found. To acquire data, once the interview was finished, we requested the farmer to provide other contacts, starting with the closest contact and excluding any farmer outside the 20 km radius. Thus, data were collected pursuant to the previously designed in-depth interviews, for which the results are disclosed below.

5 Results

Through the results obtained from the interviews made to cocoa farmers, we identified that the low productivity of cocoa beans is related to three critical processes: planning, execution, and control; quality management, and logistics management.

Planning, Execution, and Control

- 85% of farmers do not plan and control their production.
- 37% of farmers do not fertilize plots and 63% do it only once a year.
- 76% of farmers fail to implement pest and disease control and do not receive technical assistance or undergo training.
- 82% do not have an exclusive warehouse for seeds and supplies.
- 90% of farmers do not keep production records.

Quality Management

- 85% of farmers adopt an incorrect method for drying cocoa beans and do not ferment cocoa beans.

- Only 4% receive support from cooperatives for quality assurance purposes.
- 66% do not have an exclusive storage area for cocoa beans.
- No farmer has standardized processes.

Logistics Management

- Only 7% of farmers set the price of cocoa beans and sell it collectively.
- 40% of farmers deliver the cocoa beans to cooperatives and 19% sell cocoa bean directly to end customers.
- All farmers make individual purchases.
- 94% do not carry stock of input and raw materials.

6 Conclusions and Future Research

Based on MSE characteristics and profiles within the agricultural sector, snowball sampling is the most efficient method for assessing the population, and in-depth quantitative and qualitative interviewing is the most adequate technique to rise the expected information. The distance boundaries applied to snowball sampling contributed to creating a more efficient network of contacts in terms of costs and application times.

This study demonstrated the feasibility of snowball sampling with distance boundaries to assess the main issues faced by MSE cocoa producers in Cusco, Peru, and the problems affecting productivity, which is extremely low as compared with Thailand. According to the assessment, the problems faced were related to three processes, that are key across the cocoa supply chain and could enhance cocoa productivity. Snowball sampling drives the creation of a network of contacts in an unknown population. However, the problem faced is the repetition of contacts; that is, many individuals named a contact who had already been mentioned, which obstructs network expansion and potentially reduces the number of interviewees.

For future research, we recommend conducting a study to find a solution for the productivity issue based on the problems detected. Further, the first step should be drafting a process management system for these MSE producers are at maturity level 1. Therefore, they lack standardized processes, records, controls, indicators, and others.

References

1. Ali, M.M., Rattanawiboonsom, V., Perez, C.M., Khan, A.A.: Comparative positioning of small and medium enterprises in Bangladesh, Thailand and the Philippines. Econ. Reg. **13**, 381–395 (2017). https://doi.org/10.17059/2017-2-5
2. Morales, O., Borda, A., Argandoña, A., Farach, R., Naranjo, L.G., Lazo, K.: La Alianza Cacao Perú y la cadena productiva del cacao fino de aroma. Esan Ediciones (2015). https://doi.org/10.1017/CBO9781107415324.004

3. Beg, M.S., Ahmad, S., Jan, K., Bashir, K.: Status, supply chain and processing of cocoa - a review. Trends Food Sci. Technol. **66**, 108–116 (2017). https://doi.org/10.1016/j.tifs.2017.06.007
4. Ramírez, S.A., Peña, G.E.: Analysis of chaotic behaviour in supply chain variables. J. Econ. Finan. Adm. Sci. **16**(31), 85 (2011)
5. Avelar-sosa, L., García-alcaraz, J.L., Cedillocampos, M.G.: Effects of regional infrastructure and offered services in the supply chains performance: case Ciudad Juarez. DYNA **81**(186), 208–217 (2014)
6. Ellram, L.M., Cooper, M.C.: Supply chain management: it's all about the journey, not the destination. J. Supply Chain Manag. **50**(1), 8–20 (2014). https://doi.org/10.1111/jscm.12043
7. Kusumastuti, R.D., Van Donk, D.P., Teunter, R.: Crop-related harvesting and processing planning: a review. Int. J. Prod. Econ. **174**, 76–92 (2016)
8. Nikou, S.H., Selamat, H.: Risk management capability within Malaysian food supply chains. Int. J. Agric. Econ. Dev. **1**(1), 37–54 (2013). https://www.researchgate.net/publication/312070489
9. Aruna, N.: Problems faced by micro, small and medium enterprises–a special reference to small entrepreneurs in Visakhapatnam. IOSR J. Bus. Manag. **17**(4), 2319–7668 (2015). https://doi.org/10.9790/487X-17454349. Ver. V
10. Muhib, F.B., Lin, L.S., Stueve, A., Miller, R.L., Ford, W.L., Johnson, W.D., Smith, P.J.: A venue-based method for sampling hard-to-reach populations. Public Health Rep. **116**, 216–222 (2001). https://doi.org/10.1093/phr/116.S1.216
11. Heckathorn, D.D.: Respondent-driven sampling: a new approach to the study of hidden populations. Soc. Probl. **44**(2), 174–199 (1997)
12. Baltar, F., Brunet, I.: Social research 2.0: virtual snowball sampling method using facebook. Internet Res. **22**(1), 57–74 (2012). https://doi.org/10.1108/10662241211199960
13. Browne, K.: Snowball sampling: using social networks to research non-heterosexual women. Int. J. Soc. Res. Methodol. ISSN **8**(1), 47–60 (2005). https://doi.org/10.1080/1364557032000081663
14. Iron-segev, S., Lusweti, J.N., Kamau-mbuthia, E., Stark, A.H.: Impact of community-based nutrition education on geophagic behavior and dietary knowledge and practices among rural women in Nakuru town, Kenya: a pilot study. J. Nutr. Educ. Behav. **50**, 408–414 (2017). https://doi.org/10.1016/j.jneb.2017.10.013
15. Salami, M.F., Babatunde, R.O., Ayinde, O.E., Adeoti, E.I.: Determinants of poverty among local rice processors in Kwara state, Nigeria. Trakia J. Sci. **15**(4), 386–391 (2017)

Application of Lean Manufacturing Techniques to Increase On-Time Deliveries: Case Study of a Metalworking Company with a Make-to-Order Environment in Peru

Kenny Kishimoto[1(✉)], Gabriel Medina[1(✉)], Fernando Sotelo[1(✉)], and Carlos Raymundo[2(✉)]

[1] Ingeniería Industrial, Universidad Peruana de Ciencias Aplicadas (UPC), Lima, Peru
{u201420868,u201416167,fernando.sotelo}@upc.edu.pe

[2] Dirección de Investigación, Universidad Peruana de Ciencias Aplicadas (UPC), Lima, Peru
carlos.raymundo@upc.edu.pe

Abstract. The purpose of this paper is to provide a proposal of a production management model using lean manufacturing techniques to improve on-time deliveries of a metal-mechanic company that works in a make-to-order (MTO) manufacture of industrial fans environment. The proposal of the research refers to the implementation of a production management model in a metal mechanic company in Peru and analyze the effect in on-time delivery rate of the company. In one month of operation after the implementation of the pro-posed model, the on-time delivery rate of the company increased from 35% to 80%. Likewise, the problems present in the metalworking research company may be the same in many metalworking companies in the country, so the present investigation will serve as an example for the possible solution of the problems of other companies.

Keywords: Lean manufacturing · Make-to-order · On-time deliveries · Metalworking company · Peru

1 Introduction

The metalworking industry is very important in Peru due to the great importance of this industry for mining, the production of auto parts, wood products for export, food and fishing for direct human consumption [1]. This industry has declined in the last 3 years, as it has been affected, both by the lower internal demand derived from the paralysis of mining and infrastructure projects, and by lower external demand [2]. Also, the metalworking industry is an industry that lives from mining and, as such, the mining industry is the thermometer of this sector. Therefore, when mining investments fall, this sector must look for other markets. This is how the metal mechanic sector is addressing the energy and infrastructure sector, as well as commercial ports and buildings [3]. This industry has been dominated by national companies. However, in recent years, transnational companies have entered the market.

T. Ahram et al. (Eds.): IHIET 2019, AISC 1018, pp. 952–958, 2020.
https://doi.org/10.1007/978-3-030-25629-6_148

On-time delivery is defined as the ratio of the number of orders delivered on time to the total number of orders. This indicator can determine how efficient a company is complying with the dates established in the contracts [4]. To ensure the success of the product, one key component that a company must take into consideration is their on-time delivery due to today's highly competitive markets where technological innovations and its growth occurs daily [5]. Companies in a make-to-order environments start their production after an order is made by a customer.

2 Literature Review

Lean manufacturing consists of eliminating waste and delays in each process carried out by the company, maximizing the added value of your products [6]. This technique decreases the time between the order of the product by the clients and its delivery [7].

The main objective of lean manufacturing is to transform a company to be highly competitive and responsive to customer demand by eliminating waste [8].

Lean manufacturing offers a variety of tools and techniques that help companies in the reduction of waste such as: value stream map (VSM), 5S methodology, jidoka, andon, kanban, heijunka, among others.

The value stream map (VSM) aims to develop a visual mapping of a family of products within a company, where notes adding activities like that do not add value, necessary to produce a product [9].

The 5S Methodology is a technique that is used to improve the working conditions of the company through good organization, order and cleanliness of a job [10].

Also, the simplicity of kanban systems lies in the reliability of a target inventory level. If we consider that the output inventory as a product in process, we can see the kanban system maintaining a constant level of inventory of the total WIP for each type of part [11].

The Kanban system works hand in hand with production leveling (heijunka), which is one of the lean tools used to stabilize a manufacturing system, production leveling is a kind of cyclic programming that creates uniformity of production and simplifies the coordination of activities [12].

3 Case Study

3.1 Company Airtec S.A.

Airtec S.A. is a peruvian company dedicated to engineering of air movement, specifically, to the manufacture of axial and special centrifugal fans for industrial and mining processes. They have a factory of 2000 m2 located in the constitutional province of Callao, Peru, with about 100 workers. With more than 50 years in the market, Airtec S.A. covers 80% of the market.

The production environment in which the company Airtec S.A. is Make to Order (MTO), due to the high influence of the customer on the product that will be delivered and the variety of products, the company can be considered within the production system of Workshop (Process).

The company has a wide variety of products in its catalog. Different fan lines (axial, centrifugal and mining) as well as accessories for them.

3.2 Identifying Problems

As stated above, the company Airtec S.A. covers 80% of the market. However, in recent years, the company has lost a significant number of contracts due to the bad experiences of its customers regarding the delivery times of the product offered that were not fulfilled. In summary, of the 503 orders, only 178 were delivered on time, obtaining a KPI of on-time deliveries of 35.39%.

In comparison, in the IndustryWeek Best Plants Program, which recognizes annually the leading plants that are highly competitive and enhance customer satisfaction, world-class companies (Program winner and candidates) operate with an ontime delivery rate of 97% [13].

3.3 Identifying Root Causes

To find the root causes of the low rate of on-time deliveries in Airtec S.A. a lean diagnosis was developed in order to know which of the waste mentioned in the Lean philosophy are the ones that most affect the company. For this, it was used the Value Stream Map (VSM) to represent all the flow of information and material and the process of manufacture of an industrial fan.

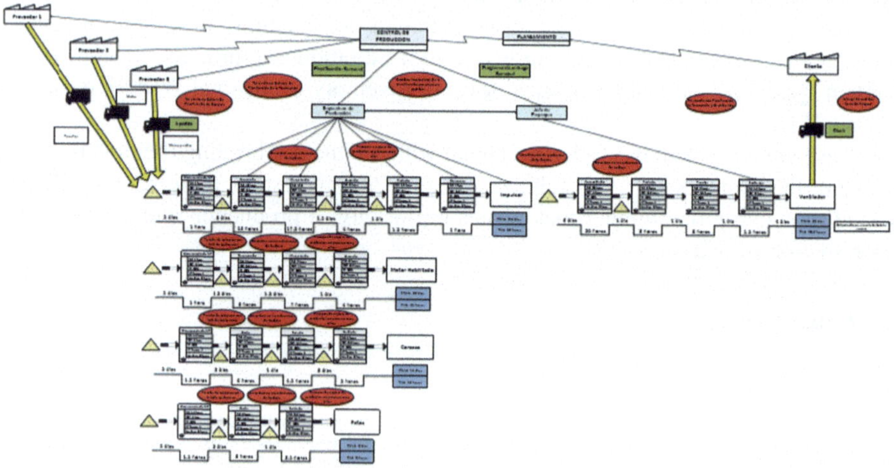

Fig. 1. Value stream map

Considering the Pareto principle, it can be identified that waste of waiting times and defects represent around 80% of the non-value-added time in the company Airtec.

For the waste of waiting time, three root causes were found: the late start of order manufacturing, the order prioritization and a poor order management to suppliers.

In the case of the waste of defects, two root causes were found, including: the disorder in work stations and the obstructed roads by in-process products or materials.

3.4 Proposed Tools

Once analyzed and obtained the root causes of the most impactful waste for the company Airtec. It was evaluated and considered that the most favorable tools for solving these causes are: the 5S Methodology, Heijunka and the Kanban-ConWIP hybrid system.

3.5 Model of the Proposal

The model began with the preparation stage as indicated in Fig. 2. In this step the conditions are organized and determine the criteria that will be considered to develop the implementation. Likewise, employees are informed and trained in Lean philosophy and principles, then the 5S methodology is implemented [14]. Before the implementation of the 5S Methodology it is important to plan the steps [15]. The first step of the 5S Methodology is to perform an audit, to know the current situation of the company in terms of cleanliness in the work stations [16]. After the audit, the methodology is disseminated through all the stations and areas of the company through training [17]. Then, the 5 phases of the methodology will be implemented, being the following: Seiri, Seiton, Seiso, Seiketsu and Shitsuke [18].

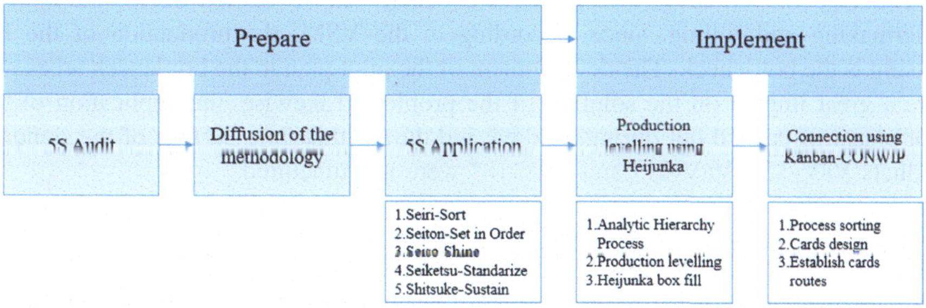

Fig. 2. Methodology deployed for the study Source: Adapted from [14]

The second stage of the model is the part of the implementation that selects the necessary tools so that the model can fulfill its objective [14]. To begin this stage, it starts implementing the leveling of production using Heijunka [19]. Analysis Hierarchy Process, which is a method to make difficult decisions based on multicriteria, is used to generate the order prioritization of manufacture [20]. After performing the hierarchical analysis and having the order of manufacture, production is leveled through the Heijunka box, since this tool harmonizes the processes by establishing periodic production sequences [19]. As a last phase, the model is the implementation of the Kanban-ConWIP system, which works together with the Heijunka box, since it is a tool for production control and inventory in process [21]. In this stage of the model, the

Kanban-ConWIP cards are designed and the flow of the cards in the production area of the company is established [22].

3.5.1 Preparation Stage

In this stage of the model, the conditions are organized, and the criteria are determined under which the company will develop the implementation. With the training and implementation of 5S, the indicators and goals to be met are generated, which are focused on the reduction of waste.

3.5.2 Implementation Stage

The Heijunka system is a tool used to level the production of the company. For this you must establish and analyze production criteria, to be able to launch the manufacturing orders. Also, the Kanban-ConWIP system is a tool used to reduce inventory in process.

4 Validation

To validate the proposed model, the pilot test was used to evaluate the operation of the proposed model. This pilot test has been made in the welding and rolling area, because as shown in the VSM (Fig. 2), the fan housing is the part of the product that take the longest time, and this part goes through the welding and rolling work stations. It is considered that the development in these work stations will have a great impact in solving the problem.

The type of validation is a pilot plan, which will be carried out in the area of boilermaking and rolling, since, according to the VSM, the production of the fan housing is the bottleneck. The development of the pilot plan in the bottleneck areas will have a great impact on the solution of the problem. Likewise, the application of the pilot plan was carried out during 20 days and during that time 22 fans of the standard products VaV-32″, VaV-21″ and VaV-18″ were manufactured.

4.1 Implementation of 5S Methodology

The implementation of the 5S methodology in the areas of boilermaking and rolling, allowed order and cleanliness of the area. The objective of the implementation was the reduction of faulty products, improving the working conditions.

4.2 Implementation of Kanban-ConWIP and Heijunka

The cards were designed and placed in the case. When a fan order leaves the assembly area, a Kanban card is generated requesting that the case that came out, be replaced. The Kanban card travels at all times with the object, in this case it is the case until the next process

- At the rolling station, the card indicates the necessary operations in order to generate the cylinder for the fan housing.

- In the area of boilermaking a card placed on Monday, which corresponds to the closing by welding the cylinder of the fan housing. Likewise, on Tuesday 2 cards were placed, one for the production of the legs and the other for the production of the accessories.
- On Wednesday at the assembly station, the card indicates the union of the cylinder, the legs and accessories and also to replace the inventory that came out at the time the order was requested.

For the measurement of results, after the implementation of a model, production was started in the work areas for the pilot test in a period of 20 days.

With the application of specialized tools, not only the non-value-added time was reduced, but also a more flexible production program for the company was achieved. It is worth noting that after the implementation of the pilot plan there were no penalties payments for deliveries out of time. This is one of the most important economic results of the proposed model.

5 Conclusions

The test of the pilot plan carried out in the welding and rolling stations, shows that on-time deliveries were increased by approximately 46%, providing great improvement for the problem.

The implementation of the 5S methodology was of great importance for the implementation of the Kanban-ConWIP and Heijunka tools, since without the initial base of the 5S's it is more difficult to implement other Lean tools.

In the implementation of the pilot plan, it is demonstrated that the Lean tools: Kanban-ConWIP and Heijunka work very well together, since it allows to prioritize orders and also allows to divide the workload equally throughout these two work stations.

References

1. Morales, C.: Sector industrial cayó 6.6% en últimos tres años, Perú 21, Lima, 29 May 2017
2. Gestión: Industria metalmecánica caería 5.6% este año, según Maximixe, Gestión, Lima, 19 August 2016
3. Saldarriaga, J.: Metalmecánica prevé tres años de vacas flacas en la minería, El Comercio (2015). https://elcomercio.pe/economia/peru/metalmecanica-preve-tres-anos-vacas-flacas-mineria195491
4. Ramachandran, G.M., Neelakrishnan, S.: An approach to improving customer on-time delivery against the original promise date. South African J. Ind. Eng. **28**, 109–119 (2017)
5. Karim, M.A., Samaranayake, P., Smith, A.J.R., Halgamuge, S.K.: An on-time delivery improvement model for manufacturing organisations. Int. J. Prod. Res. **48**(8), 2373–2394 (2010)
6. Krajewski, L., Ritzman, L., Malhotra, M.: Administración de operaciones: Procesos y Cadena de Suministro. Décima Edi., Mexico (2013)

7. Chauhan, G., Singh, T.P.: Measuring parameters of lean manufacturing realization. Meas. Bus. Excell. **16**(3), 57–71 (2012)
8. Bhamu, J., Sangwan, K.S.: Lean manufacturing: literature review and research issues. Int. J. Oper. Prod. Manag. **34**(7), 876–940 (2014)
9. Serrano, I.: Análisis de la aplicabilidad de la técnica Value Stream Mapping en el rediseño de sistemas productivos, Universitat de Girona (2007)
10. Curillo, E., Saraguro, R., Lorente, L., Ortega, E., Machado, C.: Aplicación de herramientas de manufactura esbelta en la empresa textil Anitex, Atuntaqui, Ecuador. Rev. Obs. la Econ. Latinoam., 7 (2018)
11. Askin, R.G., Goldberg, J.B.: Design and Analysis of Lean Production Systems. Wiley India Pvt. Limited, Hoboken (2007)
12. Korytkowski, P., Wisniewski, T., Rymaszewski, S.: Multivariate simulation analysis of production leveling (heijunka) - a case study. In: IFAC Proceedings Volumes (IFAC-PapersOnline) (2013)
13. IndustryWeek: The IndustryWeek Best Plants. 2016 Statistical Profile, Cleveland (2017)
14. Sarria Yépez, M.P., Fonseca Villamarín, G.A., Bocanegra, C.C.: Modelo metodológico de implementación de lean manufacturing. Rev. EAN **83**, 51–71 (2017)
15. Durana, P.: 5S - tool of eliminating waste in company processes. Int. J. Transp. Logist. **16**, 19–24 (2016)
16. Czifra, G.: Implementation process of 5S for a company in real life - problems, solutions, successes. Res. Pap. Fac. Mater. Sci. Technol. Slovak Univ. Technol. **25**(41), 79–86 (2017)
17. Gupta, S., Jain, S.K.: An application of 5S concept to organize the workplace at a scientific instruments manufacturing company. Int. J. Lean Six Sigma **6**, 73–88 (2015)
18. Manzano, M., Soler, V.G.: Lean manufacturing implantación 5S. 3C Tecnoloigia **5**, 16–26 (2016)
19. Runkler, T.A.: Controlling discrete manufacturing processes using Kanban and Heijunka approaches. In: IEEE International Conference on Industrial Informatics (INDIN) (2011)
20. Mathiyazhagan, K., Govindan, K., Noorul Haq, A.: Pressure analysis for green supply chain management implementation in Indian industries using analytic hierarchy process. Int. J. Prod. Res. **52**, 188–202 (2014)
21. Leonardo, D.G., Sereno, B., Da Silva, D.S.A., Sampaio, M., Massote, A.A., Simões, J.C.: Implementation of hybrid Kanban-CONWIP system: a case study. J. Manuf. Technol. Manag. **28**, 714–736 (2017)
22. Prakash, J., Chin, J.F.: Implementation of hybrid parallel Kanban-CONWIP system: a case study. Prod. Manuf. **1**(1), 1–15 (2014)

Comprehensive Management Model for Solid Waste Collection and Transportation in Peruvian Urban Municipalities

Renato Bernal[1(✉)], Edgar Sánchez[1(✉)], David Mauricio[2(✉)], and Carlos Raymundo[2(✉)]

[1] Escuela de Ingeniería de Gestión Empresarial, Universidad Peruana de Ciencias Aplicadas (UPC), Lima, Peru
{U201312800,U201120930}@upc.edu.pe
[2] Dirección de Investigación, Universidad Peruana de Ciencias Aplicadas (UPC), Lima, Peru
{pcsidmau,carlos.raymundo}@upc.edu.pe

Abstract. Here in, comprehensive management model of municipal solid waste collection and transportation, "MIGRU," is proposed, based on the Lean Six Sigma, VSM, and Servqual methods. This model considers and includes three important management systems for an efficient collection value chain: quality management, route management, and HR and community management. The proposed model was implemented and validated in the municipality of Lima, Peru, and the results showed that municipal costs were reduced up to 40%, solid waste was reduced in the streets, and routes and processes were updated and improved in addition to an improvement in the participation and environmental education of citizens. Thus, correct management of the proposed model's three general approaches to a very positive municipal impact at economic and environmental levels, without the investment of excessive amounts of money observed in first world countries.

Keywords: Waste management · Municipal solid waste · Waste collection · Municipal management · Municipal HR

1 Introduction

One of the biggest economic and social problems affecting Latin American countries is the poor management of municipal solid waste [1]. The main causes of this problem are a lack of fixed routes through the municipalities, little capacity of administrative personnel, and the limited revenue of municipalities. The defective management of municipal solid waste (MSW) is an economic and administrative problem that municipalities have thus far failed to solve in the short term as well as the long term. To solve this problem, currently, in cities of developed countries, successful international models have been implemented, leading to $\sim$90% reduction in the use of landfills and environmental pollution through the elimination or recycling of MSW. One such MSW main management model is the "waste to energy" (WTE) model. According to the Confederation of European Waste-to-Energy Plants (CEWEP), the WTE model

T. Ahram et al. (Eds.): IHIET 2019, AISC 1018, pp. 959–966, 2020.
https://doi.org/10.1007/978-3-030-25629-6_149

includes incinerating MSW that could not be prevented or recycled at WTE plants to generate energy [2]. However, a significant challenge to the successful implementation of a WTE plant is the initial large investment required to conduct the project in addition to the annual budget required to maintain operations in the plant. According to an Estonian construction company called Waste to Energy International, the investment required for a plant with a capacity to convert 40,000 tons of solid waste per year is 41,000,000 million dollars [2].

Hence, this research aims to optimize the MSW collection model using hard engineering tools and methodologies to reduce operating costs, maximize staff productivity, and raise awareness among the population regarding SW collection based on the service quality requirements.

2 State of the Art

Source separation programs are also available as mentioned in [3], with a total of 40% residents willing to collaborate and continue with the recycling model. Another tool is QFD, which is explained in article [4]. A survey was conducted in [4] with a population sample of 324 farmers in 16 common parks, in Moroleón, Guanajuato, to find the customer requirements and priorities for further analysis.

Finally, simulation models exist for the collection route system. In [5], the authors explain the need for an optimal solid waste collection model to improve the quality of life, economic aspects, and environmental issues in different municipalities, this is why they propose a vehicle routing model that includes multiple transfer stations, collection sites, and non-homogeneous vehicles. However, in [6], the authors discuss an optimized route plan in a static context, following which a dynamic context modeled by a multi-agent system is integrated. This study, conducted in the city of Hagiang, reduced collection costs by 11.3%. Another alternative is presented in [7], wherein the authors define a mathematical model that determines the minimum distant route between the different collection points. Then, a heuristic method is applied to determine the optimum minimum number of vehicles to be used and the optimum distance to collect waste.

3 Proposed Model

In the present research, a comprehensive model of urban MSW collection and transport management is proposed. Herein, the acronym MIGRU will be used for the proposed model. The objective of MIGRU is to support the municipal process to collect and transport domestic waste with greater efficiency and productivity, create economic value, maximize the organizational culture of the municipality, and generate an effective social culture with respect to MSW in society. The proposed model is based on Lean Six Sigma, VSM, and Servqual tools and focuses on three areas of management: service quality, route, and community culture management together with HR. Figure 1 outlines the proposed model.

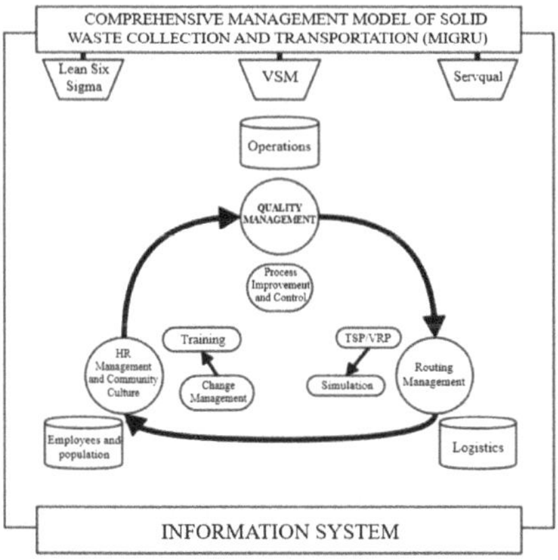

Fig. 1. Proposed model

First, MIGRU measures and analyzes the quality of service at an operational level by applying Six Sigma, VSM, and Lean Service engineering tools. Second, MIGRU considers that for route improvements, the SDVRP model must be applied by dividing the study district into quadrants. Then, the ARENA simulator is used to verify and measure different results and find the optimal economic and cultural level. Finally, MIGRU applies change management and stakeholder management methodologies to ensure an effective MSW culture.

The novelty of the proposed model is reflected in the combination and integration of the three managements tools used herein that are based on Lean Six Sigma, VSM, and Servqual methodologies.

Next, we present the summary of activities and main processes of the MIGRU model (Table 1).

Table 1. Summary of activities and main processes of the MIGRU model

Management stages/Types	Quality management	Route management	HR and community management
Definition/Redefinition	Establishing objectives of service quality Update organization and operation manual Define recruiting and personnel selection processes Implement project directory and work teams	Define objectives and indicators of route management Define the organization and operation manual (MOP) for route management Information compilation Structuring of the service's situational state Updating of policies and occupational safety and health manual Updating the district's street maps Updating heat maps and solid waste collection points Updating and improving water collection routes	Definition of objectives of HR and community culture management Definition of the organization and operation manual (MOP) of route management Definition of change needs Situational analysis and identification of important individuals and processes of the service

(*continued*)

Table 1. (*continued*)

Management stages/Types	Quality management	Route management	HR and community management
Planning	Information compilation Structuring of the service's situational state Definition of initial VSM processes and structures Valuing of municipal service processes Measurement and classification of the main problems Drawing up an improvement plan with a schedule Drawing up a financial plan Drawing up a mitigation and contingency plan Presentation and approval of plans of the first instance to authorities Formal approval and documentation sent to parties	Analysis and measurement of industrial losses based on six losses of lean manufacturing Redesigning the operations plan Redesigning and implementation of the communication plan Analysis and research of new solutions and optimal routing methods Selection of the optimal routing method Drawing up of weight and node distance matrix	Stage planning Leadership plan design Communication plan design Training plan design Motivation design plan
Execution and follow-up	Implementation of indicators Follow-up and meetings before important events or incidents Implementation of tactics and contingencies	Selection and execution of simulation software and route generators	Execute activities defined in the plan Execute training schedules Hold meetings to clarify doubts Evaluate personnel Hold meetings to follow-up on changes Evaluate the team's performance with new processes Keep the team informed on any unplanned issue
Evaluation	Controls and periodic revisions Implementation of controls and periodic revisions Self-questioning Control and evaluation of process and final services	Evaluation of different scenarios of optimal routes Verification and updation of the study field Printed or digital documents of the routing process Report and documents of incidents	Evaluation activities are undertaken Establish new objectives and goals Define reinforcement actions Create plans to replace current change leaders Gradually dismantle existing incentives

4 Validation

The validation of the proposed model is explained step by step, below:

4.1 Measure

4.1.1 Measure Quality Management

Information on the following points was gathered.

- Descriptive information on the last three months of VSM processes.
- Defects, overproduction, delays, unused talent, unnecessary transportation, unnecessary inventory, and transfers of each VSM process.

Next, we determined the sigma of the current solid waste collection management based on the losses calculated in the VSM analysis and in accordance with the Six Sigma protocols.

To measure the quality of the service offered, after formulating the questions and asking them, a quantification of the service offered by the municipality was obtained.

4.1.2 Measure Route Management

Through the collection of data and official reports, we observed that the municipality of the study has not measured or tried to improve its collection routes owing to political, economic, and other factors.

4.1.3 Measure HR Management and Community Culture

The 360-degree feedback survey was conducted for three workers in the area of solid waste management of the municipality. All three workers held different positions (assistant manager, environmental technician, and chief operator).

4.2 Improvements

4.2.1 Improve Quality Management

The Servqual survey was conducted for the third time, after the implementation of changes in the solid waste management area. Notably, the surveys were conducted for different people within the area of the case study.

4.2.2 Improve Route Management

In this study, the proposed model was validated in the area of Lima called Mangomarca. Below, you will find the important points required to collect information and validate our optimal routing (Fig. 2).

The node matrix of the different points of the segment to be studied was obtained, tests were performed using the optimal routing software. In this case, the free program TSP Solver and generator was used. The simulation software calculated 7442 m of the optimal route, but in a disorderly manner. The order of the route is based on distance and economic issues; accordingly, optimal final route was calculated (Fig. 3).

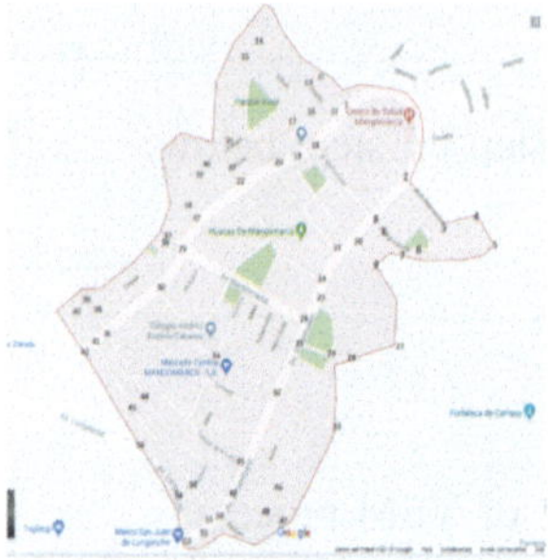

Fig. 2. Distribution of nodes

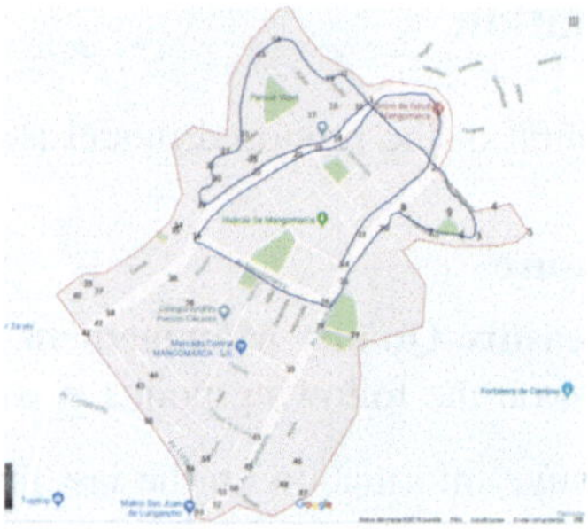

Fig. 3. Final optimal route

4.2.3 Improve HR Management and Community Culture

Management plans were formulated for both the staff and the population, as follows. Staff: Ongoing training for personnel, assign specific routes, Register and control collection trucks, draw up an incentive plan for good behavior, improve facilities for personnel (restrooms, dining rooms, relaxation centers). Population: Campaigns in schools and streets, Social media, conferences, training, flyers.

4.3 Control

Control quality management: Checks and periodic reviews, Implementation of controls, Self-questioning, Quality circles, Evaluation of the final processes and services.

Control route management: Verification and updates in the fields of study, Printed documentation, Incident report.

Control HR management and community culture.

5 Results

In the quality of service, according to Servqual, we see positive improvements in the five dimensions. Previously, three dimensions were negative and two dimensions had a very low value. The values of the gap are as follows: reliability decreases from a gap of 1.15 to 0.3; sensitivity increases from 0.1 to 0.65; security increases from −0.43 to 0.43; empathy increases from −0.45 to 0.18; and tangible elements increase from 0.1 to 0.33.

In terms of routing, before the tests, the vehicles traversed all streets, thus wasting time and consuming considerable resources. However, with the new optimal route, both time and costs can be reduced. However, this would not be useful if good change management is not applied at both the HR and operational levels (Table 2).

Table 2. Results of route management

Result 1	Quantity in meters	Result 2	Annual costs in soles
Initial route	3349	Initial and traditional route	22,000,000
Route with MIGRU	1600	Rate of reduction	47%
Rate of reduction	47%	Possible cost with MIGRU	10,340,000

Three scenarios were simulated herein and the results were positive, achieving a reduction of up to 47% in costs. As for HR management and community culture:

- 100% approval of the team was achieved regarding the need for change.
- The population understood the issue and was willing to be trained by municipal employees.
- 100% employees attended the training and motivation talks.
- The staff management plan was executed without any issues.
- The population management plan was implemented with great approval.
- No adverse incident occurred during the implementation of the change management program in the municipality.

6 Conclusion

A comprehensive management model for SW collection was designed in this work to improve the quality of service, reduce operating costs, maximize staff productivity, and raise awareness among the population regarding SW collection on the basis of service quality requirements.

- A literature review was conducted to identify existing management models of solid waste collection to create an innovative model for solid waste management.
- The quantitative and qualitative situation of the management of current MSW collection was identified and post implementation of the new model, processes, service times, and costs of solid waste collection management were determined.
- The quality level of the collection service was quantified before and after the implementation to know the client's requirements.
- A new solid waste collection route was proposed to increase collection coverage and reduce operating costs.
- The change management plan in the operational area was proposed based on the optimal routes calculated to achieve a commitment to the new solid waste management model.
- A training and conference plan was proposed to local residents to raise their awareness regarding solid waste issues

References

1. Ministerio del Ambiente: Plan nacional de gestión integral de resiudos sólidos 2016. http://sinia.minam.gob.pe/documentos/plan-nacionalgestion-integral-residuos-solidos-2016-2024
2. CEWEP, 05 October 2018. http://www.cewep.eu/what-is-waste-toenergy/
3. Sukholthaman, P., Sharp, A.: A system dynamics model to evaluate effects of source separation of municipal solid waste management: a case of Bangkok, Thailand. Waste Manage. **52**, 1–12 (2016)
4. Ocampo Jimenez, N.B., Serrato, R.: Effectiveness of QFD in a municipal administration process. Bus. Process Manag. J. **22**, 979–992 (2016)

5. Louati, A., Son, L.: Modeling municipal solid waste collection: a generalized vehicle routing model with multiple transfer stations, gather sites and inhomogeneous vehicles in time windows. Waste Manage. **52**, 34–49 (2016)
6. Nguyen-Trong, K., Nguyen-Thi-Ngoc, A., Nguyen-Ngoc, D., Dinh-Thi-Hai, V.: Optimization of municipal solid waste transportation by integrating GIS analysis, equation-based, and agent-based model. Waste Manage. **59**, 14–22 (2017)
7. Huang, S.-H., Lin, P.-C.: Vehicle routing-scheduling for municipal waste collection system under the "keep trash off the ground" policy. Omega **55**, 24–37 (2015)

Improvement of Attention Times and Efficiency of Container Movements in a Port Terminal Using a Truck Appointment System, LIFO Management and Poka Yoke

Luis Sermeño[1(✉)], Jimmy Orellana[1(✉)], Juan Eyzaguirre[1(✉)], and Carlos Raymundo[2(✉)]

[1] Ingeniería Industrial, Universidad Peruana de Ciencias Aplicadas (UPC), Lima, Peru
{u201412495,u201515940,juan.eyzaguirre}@upc.edu.pe
[2] Dirección de Investigación, Universidad Peruana de Ciencias Aplicadas (UPC), Lima, Peru
carlos.raymundo@upc.edu.pe

Abstract. In the management of port terminals, a common problem has been evidenced, high traffic of trucks and long waiting times given the variability of trucks arrival. This is a significant challenge for ports. This situation has given the opportunity to investigate in this matter and make use of a Truck Appointment System (TAS) together with other tools corresponding to industrial engineering for the optimization of truck service processes within a port terminal in Peru. To do this, a diagnosis is made of the company object of study and through a simulation of discrete systems, the technical viability of the proposal is validated. It was demonstrated that a procedure of attention based on appointments, Last in, First Out (LIFO) management for containers and development of visual management within the container yard; it is a highly viable option to shorten waiting times and unproductive movements of containers.

Keywords: Truck appointment system · LIFO · Port terminal · Simulation · Container moves

1 Introduction

A crucial element of door congestion in maritime container terminals is the fluctuation of truck arrivals, with spikes that exceed the processing capacity of terminal gates. In addition to congesting local doors, terminals and roads, the long lines of trucks are a visible source of noise and emissions in the communities of the port area.

Recognizing these problems, in the first years of the 2000s the operators of maritime container terminals in the United States, they sought to use what is now known (in the United States) as a truck dating system and internationally as a vehicle reservation system (VBS) to regulate the number of trucks arriving at their terminals throughout the day. The main and immediate objective for the use of the truck

T. Ahram et al. (Eds.): IHIET 2019, AISC 1018, pp. 967–974, 2020.
https://doi.org/10.1007/978-3-030-25629-6_150

appointment system at that time was to reduce the congestion of the door in the terminal, promoting both the efficiency and the reliability in the container hauling [1].

After reviewing the literature corresponding to the subject under study, it is possible to observe a certain variety of cases where the expected benefits are not fulfilled given that no attention was paid to any of the variables involved in the implementation of a tool such as the "Truck Appointment System" (TAS). The case under study is being carried out in an emerging country, where there is a limited capacity and certain special conditions that make the management of the terminal complex, but at the same time, it seeks to take advantage of the facilities found to simplify the use of the tool.

2 State of Art

One of the first results of previous investigations regarding the application of a TAS within a maritime terminal, agreed that such system must be adapted to the needs and conditions of the port in question [2]. Adjusting to these conditions present a concrete result regarding the implementation of a TAS in the port of San Antonio in Chile [2], where it can be observed that reserve levels, that is, the percentage of application of a TAS, it influences with greater force in the average waiting time than other variables such as yard operation capacity, segmentation of lanes or truck arrival patterns.

However, there is literature where the objectives of reducing truck waiting times or "Truck Turn Times" are not achieved [3]. In article [4] the authors do the study of a truck appointment system in a different way, with the development of the method called VDTW or Vessel dependent time windows. This takes as a basis the time it takes the transport between the date of departure and arrival of the vessel. If, according to the vessel's departure date, it will arrive at a time when the yard is full, then the departure must be postponed.

In the research carried out on the inventory management method LIFO, [5] it gives us information about the effects of the method in a queuing system. As a result of their research, they affirm that it also influences the arrival distribution of the participants and, consequently, the queuing times. This reinforces the intention to combine the application of a TAS in combination with the LIFO method to achieve greater results in the application of the research proposal [5].

In the literature reviewed [6], they find that, through simulation, models have been validated where it is discovered that the organization of the space and the previous classification improve the efficiency of the terminal in terms of reducing waiting times of the trucks.

The research [7] argues that there is no need to make use of new technologies or large investments to achieve improvements in the processes of container shipping. The search should focus on a consolidated improvement throughout the transportation process. They propose a system called "truck sharing", as the name says, it is about the decentralization of container transport processes. This system operates so that any truck associated with the terminal can move and pick up any container of a maritime agency, directly affecting the arrival, waiting and shift times of the trucks, as well as the unproductive movement number produced in the dispatch [8].

Finally, the literature described serves to evaluate the proposals made in other investigations, and in that way be able to use them in ours.

3 Description of Proposal

The TAS as a process optimization methodology will allow the arrival of trucks to be managed and regulated by the terminal, thus avoiding the long waiting times resulting from the overcoming of the attention capacity versus the existing demand. This involves that there is a current collection of reliable data at the entrance of the truck terminal so that statistical variables such as time between arrivals and time of attention in the balance are established.

The LIFO dispatch management minimizes the unproductive movements since the container that enters last to the block is the first to leave avoiding any other additional move. For this, the blocks must be segmented by deposits and that the dispatch must not be based on specific containers (Fig. 1).

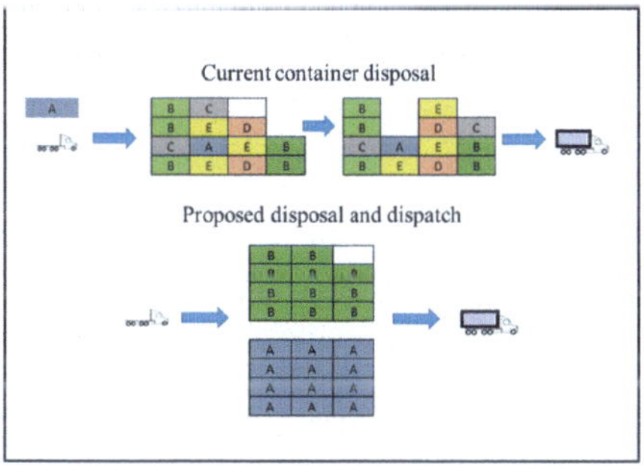

Fig. 1. One current and proposed disposal of containers

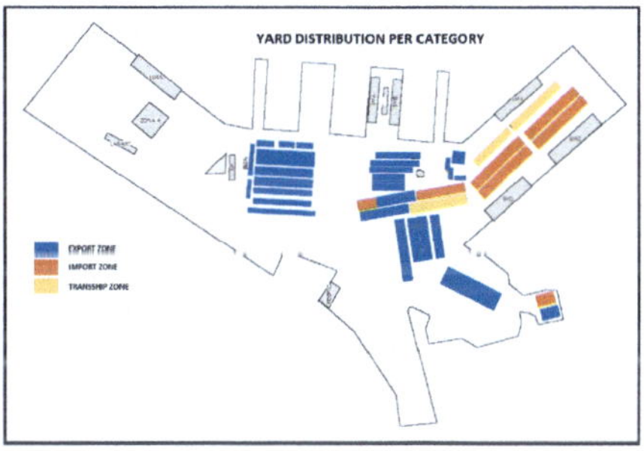

Fig. 2. Yard distribution per container category

The figure shows that the transporter comes from warehouse A and goes to the area established for the extra port deposit (represented by the different colors), to receive container A, it is necessary to move C and E containers. Currently, the driver wants a specific container; however, the policy that the LIFO methodology will support is that the last arriving container is the first to be dispatched, thus eliminating unproductive movements.

Waste of time in the transfer of the truck to the dispatch area are very frequent in a Callao port terminal, based on the complexity of the distribution (Fig. 2) that causes the carrier does not know how to get to the correct area. This can be approach by using the visual management tool (Poka Yoke) corresponding to the lean manufacturing or services. With adequate signaling and some elements that prevent errors, the driver can avoid losing time when looking for the dispatch area.

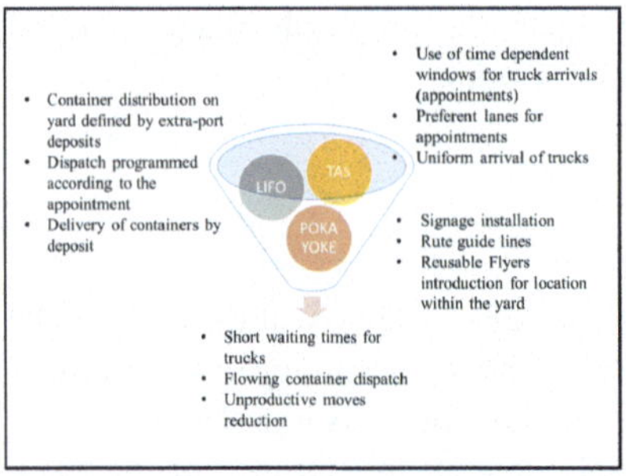

Fig. 3. Description of the proposal

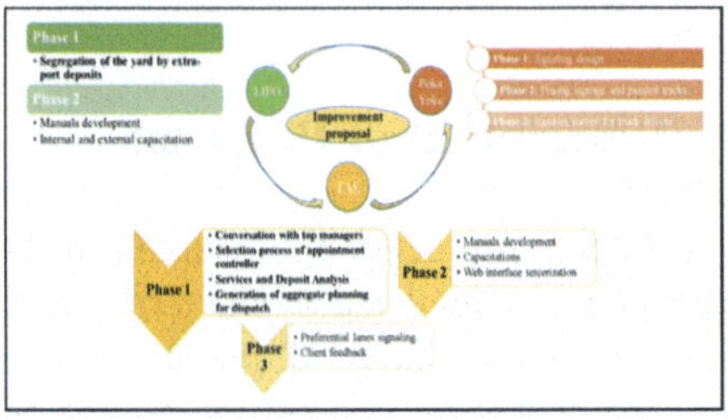

Fig. 4. "TAS+LIFO" model design

The proposed model unifies three different concepts such as the TAS, LIFO management and Poka Yoke. Each one of them can work separately as stated on the reviewed literature but, in order to obtain a higher impact on the operation of the terminal, we managed to develop a synergy among those three concepts (Fig. 3). Three phases have been defined for the application of the proposal as shown in the Fig. 4.

3.1 Phase 1

The first phase of the implementation is about introducing the concepts for the stakeholders of the project, as well as preparing the ground for the training of the next phase. The most important thing to develop at this point is the analysis of the services and the generation of aggregate planning for the dispatch of containers, both are the core of the proposal and the appointment system depends entirely on it.

3.1.1 TAS

- Conversation with top managers
- Selection process of appointment controller
- Generation of aggregate planning for dispatch.

3.1.2 LIFO

Segregation of the yard by extra-port deposits: Fundamental aspect of the LIFO methodology is that the yard planning goes hand in hand with the dispatch planning.

3.1.3 Poka Yoke

Signaling design: The signage to be used will be the same format as normally used in transit routes, whose material will be vinyl canvas since they are the ones that last longer and resist the high winds usually present in the terminal.

3.2 Phase 2

3.2.1 TAS

This phase includes the generation of manuals, training and outsourcing of the web interface for appointments. The first one is fundamental for the project since it seeks a written document that always serves as a guide for the realization of the proposal. The same, will be used in the subsequent training for all involved.

3.2.2 LIFO

There is also the need to prepare manuals for the LIFO methodology addressed to the extra-port deposits since they will manage the dispatch solicitude. Besides, external training will be programmed mainly to deposits with high volume.

3.2.3 Poka Yoke

The traffic signs with the indication of zones in which the import containers are located will be placed in 3 key points where the drivers usually got lost. It will be programmed the painting of tracks with specific colors for each area of the yard, which will serve as a nocturnal guide since they are made with phosphorescent paints.

3.3 Phase 3

3.3.1 TAS

The next important aspect in the implementation of the TAS is the evaluation and analysis of the results obtained. To do this, a customer feedback process is designed which allows the planning analyst to obtain indicators that allow finding constant improvement opportunities.

3.3.2 Poka Yoke

Similar to the 2 methodologies mentioned above, there is a focus on continuous improvement. Therefore, surveys will be carried out to the transporters in a random manner, which will allow data collection by the planning analyst in order to evaluate the improvements obtained.

4 Validation

A simulation of the process of Receiving and Dispatching containers will be modeled within the company under study. Likewise, the data will be classified, and a methodology will be applied to justify the best statistical distribution that fits them through sample sizes and goodness of fit tests. Then, opportunities for improvement will be identified where the "TAS + LIFO" methodology proposed in the research work can be applied.

4.1 Results

The results of the simulation model were analyzed. Figure 5 summarizes the results regarding the values of each variable under study, and Fig. 6 presents a Touring test where the validity of the information is confirmed by comparing it with the human knowledge of the system.

# Replica	TTT Export (min)	TTT Import (min)	T System (min)	W Time (min)	Outer port queue
1	18.05	24.01	96.21	69.01	71.54
2	17.94	23.87	95.01	68.12	70.43
3	17.83	23.95	98.17	71.27	73.64
4	17.97	24.1	98.6	71.58	74.06
5	18.24	24.11	101.27	74.03	76.46
6	18.35	24.09	102.99	75.67	78.12
7	18.31	24.06	99.4	72.13	74.64
8	18.34	24.07	98.19	70.96	73.44
9	18.33	24.05	98.99	71.75	74.27
10	18.26	24.08	96.02	68.86	71.37
11	18.32	24.06	97.03	69.81	72.3
12	18.34	24.07	97.05	69.84	72.34
13	18.37	24.08	97.22	69.99	72.48
14	18.38	24.11	96.39	69.14	71.62
15	18.34	24.1	96.33	69.11	71.59
Average	***18.22***	***24.05***	***97.93***	***70.75***	***73.22***

Fig. 5. Results of simulation model

# Replica	TTT Export (min)	TTT Import (min)	T System (min)	W Time (min)	Outer port queue
1	16.24	16.88	44.44	38.55	20.48
2	16.33	16.91	46.94	44.55	23.64
3	16.24	16.92	46.62	42.93	22.71
4	16.28	16.93	46.12	42.36	22.38
5	16.26	16.94	46.18	42.28	22.32
6	16.25	16.93	46.36	43.02	22.72
7	16.23	16.94	45.99	42.52	22.43
8	16.31	16.93	46.48	43.82	23.1
9	16.26	16.93	46.56	46.84	23.1
10	16.24	16.93	46.9	44.59	23.49
11	16.24	16.94	47.28	44.9	23.66
12	16.25	16.94	47.1	44.66	23.52
13	16.27	16.94	47.27	45.13	23.76
14	16.32	16.95	47.4	44.83	23.6
15	16.35	16.95	47.48	44.7	23.54
Average	***16.27***	***16.93***	***46.61***	***43.71***	***22.96***

Fig. 6. Results of proposed model

As can be seen, according to the experts, the results obtained through the simulation model reflect the values obtained from reality. Therefore, it can be concluded that there is no evidence to invalidate the proposed model and it can be reorganized to simulate the scenario proposed on this paper. The results of the simulation that considers the proposal put forward are shown in Fig. 7.

To evaluate	Job	Criteria	Arena
TTT Export	Planner	17-20 min	18.22 min
TTT Import		23-26 min	24.05 min
W Time	Driver	>60 min aprox	70.75 min
Outer port queue	Security Agent	60-90 trucks	73.22

Fig. 7. Touring test

	Current	Proposal	Change
TTT Export	18.22	16.27	-11%
TTT Import	24.05	16.93	-30%
T System	97.93	46.61	-52%
W Time	70.75	43.71	-38%
Outer port queue	73.22	22.96	-69%

Fig. 8. Results comparison

Figure 8 shows the decreases in the results of the variables given the changes made in the simulation. A great effect of the proposals is perceived and later their economic impact will be analyzed, as well as their viability to be implemented.

The savings will be based on the reduction of unproductive movements within the container import operations. Currently the company has a unit cost per unproductive movement of $2.18, which multiplied to the annual amount of these movements means an increase in the cost of operation of between 400,000 to 800,000 dollars. As shown in Fig. 9, made with the results of the simulation already validated, the savings generated by the proposal is calculated at $ 224,452.80 per year.

IMPORT	Current	Proposal	
Productive movements	777	777	
Unproductive movements	535	249	
Mensual average unp.	16,050.00	7,470.00	Annual savings
Annual average unp.	192,600.00	89,640.00	
Unit cost	$ 2.18		
Unproductive movements expenses	$419,868.00	$195,415.20	$ 224,452.80

Fig. 9. Annual savings calculation

5 Conclusion

Through an efficient process of assignment of appointments for trucks, management in the booths, new management of container dispatch and introduction of manuals and new visual management, it is possible to eliminate delays and transfers in the truck service process. The time of the "Truck Turn Time" is reduced by 30% for the dispatch process and by 38% the waiting times of trucks.

The new management for the dispatch of containers achieves a saving of $ 224,452.80 per year, due to the avoidance of unproductive movements that suppose operating expenses and increase in truck service times. Considering a life time of a five-year project, a net present value of $ 715,821.25 was obtained. A high impact result is demonstrated despite being a change in procedures and management policies without incurring on investments in construction, equipment or new machinery.

The implementation of the appointment system does not turn out to be a standard tool to be used for any port terminal. It is necessary to know the characteristics, restrictions and workflow of these to mold the tool in a way that is useful and has positive results as demonstrated in the research. The TAS has been focused on regulating the inflow of trucks in order to reduce waiting times in the outer harbor and the queues generated in it. The result ends up being satisfactory at the client level and allows the terminal to make use of the UEPS management and the distribution by deposits.

References

1. Ahmt, J., Skott, J., Lusby, R., Larsen, J., Ryan, D.: A new approach to the container positioning problem. Flex. Serv. Manuf. J. **28**, 617–643 (2016)
2. Gracia, M., González-Ramírez, R., Mar-Ortiz, J.: The impact of lanes segmentation and booking levels on a container terminal gate congestion. Flex. Serv. Manuf. J. **29**(3–4), 403–432 (2017)
3. Giuliano, G., O'Brian, T.: Reducing port-related truck emissions: the terminal gate appointment system at the ports of Los Angeles and Long Beach. Transp. Res. Part D Transp. Environ. **12**, 460–473 (2007)
4. Chen, G., Jiang, L.: Managing customer arrivals with time windows: a case of truck arrivals at a congested container terminal. Bus. Ann. Oper. Res. **19**, 349 (2016)
5. Breinbjerg, J., Sebald, A., Østerdal, L.: Strategic behavior and social outcomes in a bottleneck queue: experimental evidence. Rev. Econ. Des. **20**, 207–236 (2016)

6. Gharehgozli, A., Roy, D., de Koster, R.: Sea container terminals: new technologies and OR models. Marit. Econ. Logist. **18**, 103–140 (2016)
7. Islam, S., Olsen, T.: Truck-sharing challenges for hinterland trucking companies: a case of the empty container truck trips problem. Bus. Process Manag. J. **20**(2), 290–334 (2014)
8. Kua, D., Arthanaria, T.S.: Container relocation problem with time windows for container departure (CRPW). Eur. J. Oper. Res. **252**, 1031–1039 (2016)

5S Hybrid Management Model for Increasing Productivity in a Textile Company in Lima

Juanirene Neyra[1(✉)], José Muñoz[1(✉)], Juan Eyzaguirre[1(✉)], and Carlos Raymundo[2(✉)]

[1] Ingenieria Industrial, Universidad Peruana de Ciencias Aplicadas, Lima, Peru
{u201313848, u201322076, juan.eyzaguirre}@upc.edu.pe
[2] Dirección de Investigación, Universidad Peruana de Ciencias Aplicadas, Lima, Peru
carlos.raymundo@upc.edu.pe

Abstract. In general, lean strategies in the textile sector are applied in production to improve productivity, reduce production time, and reduce errors, among other aspects. However, there are also documented studies, which are not common in the literature that uses these strategies to improve storage operations. This study shows the implementation of the Lean 5S Hybrid tool in the warehouse of a textile company based in Lima. The objective of the implementation was to improve productivity in the warehouse, as there were high response times when searching for materials, which reduced production time, warehouse redistribution, better using available space, and being able to strategically locate main materials. The results revealed an increase in warehouse productivity 3.95 times the initial one, an Inventory Record Accuracy of 98.17%, a decrease in the requirement search time by 66.12% (from 25 to 8 min), and stock rotation of 6.22 times.

Keywords: Warehouses · Lean · 5s implementation · Inventory management · Textile

1 Introduction

Today, there are several factors that affect companies, such as globalization, competition, rapid market changes, a product's life cycle, productivity, and faster time-to-market. These factors have increased the impact of production logistics than it was years ago [1]. In Latin America, small- and medium-sized enterprises (SMEs) are deemed very important. According to the World Bank, SMEs generate 28% of GDP and half of all jobs in the region [2]. In Peru, SMEs are influenced by various factors that affect their growth, such as the lack of access to technology, financing, and human capital. These, in turn, affect their productivity, export capacity, and growth [3]. Therefore, studies have been carried out in the SME sector to determine the most common factors. These factors are divided into five areas: administrative, operational, strategic, external, and personal.

The management of warehouses in our country is diverse in the SME sector; 72.1% of manufacturing companies claim to make storage and can store up to 50% of used

T. Ahram et al. (Eds.): IHIET 2019, AISC 1018, pp. 975–981, 2020.
https://doi.org/10.1007/978-3-030-25629-6_151

consumables during the year. Of these, 31.6% companies claim to have concerns with the lack of space and storage conditions. In addition, 50% still perform manual tasks within their production and storage areas. This indicates that human labor is crucial within SMEs. Reports indicate that only 34.8% of workers have taken university-level education, and 19.5% of companies have conducted training or technical assistance programs for their workers in relation to management or production issues [4], which lead to problems in each of the aforementioned factors.

The purpose of this research is to successfully implement the Hybrid 5S as a quality and integration tool in a textile SME. First, successful cases of implementation are outlined. Next, a case study of a small company located in Lima, Peru, is explored in depth.

2 State of the Art

There are multifarious definitions of lean, which makes it impossible to validate a single definition as appropriate [5], but over the last 60 years [6], its main purpose has become clear—reducing waste and achieving a decrease in lead times [7]. Hence, principles of lean thinking have been widely accepted and successfully applied by different firms [8] although lean was originally associated only with production. In this line, King [9] states that understanding the complexity of the process rather than getting started with a solution is important.

In the textile sector, implementing lean principles can help improve the level of competition and market position, but more importantly, it can help increase a company's efficiency and effectiveness [10]. However, there are certain crucial barriers as well. Changing how work is done and transitioning from a traditional way to lean is time consuming, requires commitment, and involves many changes [11]. Organizational change as well as strengthening relationships with suppliers are also essential.

3 Methodology

At present, there are several methodologies to improve supply activities, among which are lean warehousing, logistics, and inventory. All come from the lean philosophy and are specialized in the relevant area. At the same time, in our literature review, we found studies indicating that lean tools go hand in hand with common engineering tools such as inventory management that gave birth to 5S Hybrid (5S + Inventory Management), 5S with value stream and Kaizen, and 5S with value stream mapping and process standardization. The objective of combining the 5S with other tools was to achieve different quality objectives where 5S plays a role, with it being the first step toward the TQM.

The Hybrid 5S technique has greater advantages than lean warehousing and 5S, owing to the fact that the Hybrid 5S not only focuses on Kaizen but also on process integration and inventory management techniques, thus always seeking to optimize the processes with the appropriate procedures. Inventory management is a critical function in any business because it involves inventory control, which, if not done correctly, can lead to delays and customer dissatisfaction. Therefore, it is important to map the current processes within the warehouse and redefine them if required, with the creation of procedures and noting who is responsible.

Thus, the 5S Hybrid technique is the best suited to resolve a textile company's current problems.

This model has four phases that will be implemented in this case study; the design of the proposed Hybrid 5S model is presented in Fig. 1 below:

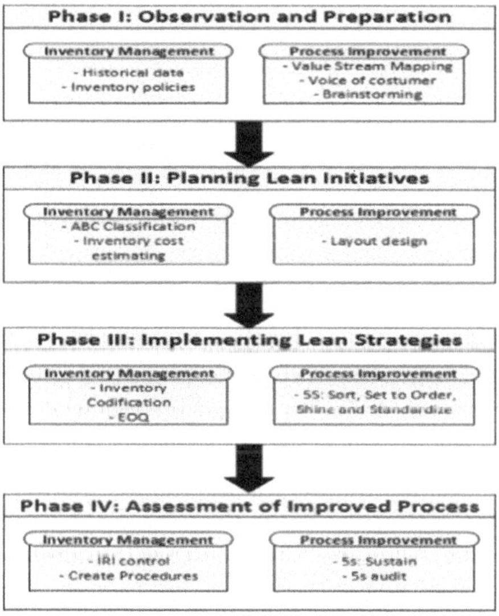

Fig. 1. Model of proposed 5S Hybrid

3.1 Specific View

3.1.1 Phase I

This phase is based on observing the process to identify problems such as inefficient procedures, delays in the area, and product loss. A value stream map should be made to identify the areas affected from the client's perspective [1]. Its advantage is that it describes the flow of materials, which makes it the most effective tool in identifying opportunities for improvement and distinguishing between the activities that add value and those that do not.

3.1.2 Phase II

In this phase, the ideas generated in Phase I are chosen, and an action plan is developed to carry out the improvements. The necessary permits are requested, and the managers are informed about the plan to be carried out and the results expected to be obtained.

3.1.3 Phase III

This phase is net implementation, including the execution of the first four Ss, sort, set-to-order, shine, and standardize. The 5S implementation manual described by Kumar should be followed. It is important to carry out the inventory coding and calculate the required levels of space and, if necessary, acquire new shelves.

3.1.4 Phase IV

In this phase, the improvements made are measured by evaluating effectiveness, efficiency, relevance, and impact. It also includes the execution of the last S, i.e., sustain. This phase is the most important and challenging because one wants to maintain the improvements made over time, for which commitment from everyone involved in the process is essential.

4 Validation

The organization carried out the following steps when adopting the 5S model.

4.1 Phase I

A company VSM of a production batch of poles was carried out to find out improvement possibilities while observing the processes involved in production and storage. It was found that it took 54.5 h to find the material in storage before leaving production, and this was because of a lack of procedures in the warehouse and a lack of knowledge by employees on the different varieties of yarn. This impacted the inventory levels, which were high, and at the same time the Kardex was not updated, which meant that the raw material in the warehouse was unknown, thereby leading to duplicate purchases and yarn that was more than 10 years old.

4.2 Phase II

Before performing the multi-criteria ABC classification, an inventory of the company's yarn was performed. The results are presented in Table 1.

Table 1. Inventory carried out

Inventory summary		
Poorly positioned products	No. of products	% of total
E Level	13	21.31%
D Level	11	17.46%
Box of Skein 8/4	6	8.57%
Box of mercerized yarn	12	17.65%
Products not identified	76	29.01%
Products not labeled	250	95.42%
Total inventoried products	262	

Deteriorated material was also found, which was attributed to the passage of time and poor storage conditions.

4.3 Phase III

4.3.1 Coding

The inventory did not have an easy recognition coding system; therefore, we proceeded to code the 31 colors that the company had.

4.3.2 First S—Sort

We proceeded to create red cards for the implementation. These were fixed in plastic boxes to enable the search for yarn throughout the company. Yarn was found in warehouse 1 and in the production area. Then, for classification, the following criteria were used:

- Uniquely colored yarn had to leave the warehouse because it would no longer be used.
- The garbage found should be put in a bag for later disposal.
- Misplaced or queried colors should be separated for locating later on.

4.3.3 Second S—Set-to-Order

In this phase, the layout elaborated in phase III for warehouse 2 was used, and then the yarns were positioned in the warehouse according to their rotation. Beige colored yarns are those with the highest rotation stored closest to the door, followed by fashionable European colors. At the same time, an analysis of shelf capacity was carried out, resulting in 64 cones per level. Taking into account good storage practices in textiles, 60 yarn cones were stored per level. To maximize the use of space, the yarns were stored with the smaller base upwards, followed by the yarn with the next smaller base.

4.3.4 Third S—Shine

Cleaning schedules were established, wherein workers rotated monthly to clean the warehouse before and after the working day. At the same time, on a weekly basis, cleaning audits were carried out to verify that the schedule provisions were being complied with.

4.3.5 Fourth S—Standardize

The company workers follow the new policies and rules. To this end, the coding in the shelves has been replaced for them to be in accordance with the new order. The Kardex has also been replaced by an improved one, and different colors for quick identification of the yarn *types* and the company's color coded display, with its respective samples and codes, has been created. This is pasted on the warehouse wall as a visual indicator.

4.4 Phase IV

4.4.1 Inventory Registration Accuracy

Stocktaking was carried out to record inventory registration accuracy during the implementation.

4.4.2 Procedures

It was necessary to create procedures for the different processes that occur within the warehouse, such as inputs of raw materials and outputs as the case may be.

4.4.3 Fifth S—Discipline

To achieve and maintain this improvement over time, the format of the 5S audit was delivered to show whether the company retains the improvements.

5 Conclusions

The results obtained by the 5S Hybrid have had a significant positive impact on activity times within the warehouse. At the same time, there has been better supply management and use of space. The implementation of 5S Hybrid, as indicated by past studies, has brought more benefits than the implementation of traditional 5S did, which only focused on ordering and cleaning the warehouse. It has been used to perform inventory management with the space available at that time by the company, thereby generating the possibility of creating procedures, labels, and ordering as per the new inventory management.

The accuracy of inventory registration, a recurring problem faced in global companies today, was a concern that caused delays in agile responses between production and warehouses, consequently increasing the total lead time, bringing losses in sales in considerable amounts to the type and size of a company. Hence, a textile company must continue carrying out the weekly inventory until it reaches 100% and then change the frequency to monthly.

Although it is true that integration has been achieved between the two areas with the greatest delays in the studied company, it is important that storage and production management aim for the same strategic and operational objectives. Thus, MRP implementation or other tools based on the JIT would increase the benefits of the 5S Hybrid implementation.

In conclusion, with regard to experiencing the implementation, it is noteworthy that the 5S is easy to understand by workers, as it only requires conventional knowledge of the discipline and high commitment. However, understanding the management of inventories takes more time, for which workers must be trained and must develop criteria to make decisions in the face of less common situations.

References

1. Dotoli, M., Epicoco, N., Falagario, M., Costantino, N., Turchiano, B.: An integrated approach for warehouse analysis and optimization: a case study. Comput. Ind. **70**, 56–59 (2015)
2. Banco Mundial: El Emprendimiento en Latino América, pp. 1–5. Banco Mundial, Washington D.C. (2014)
3. Ministerio de Producción: Las MYPES en cifras, pp. 2–6. Ministerio de Producción, Lima (2016)

4. CEMTRUM Católica: Factores que limitan el crecimiento de Micro y Pequeñas Empresas en el Perú (MYPES), pp. 70–80. Strategia, Lima (2010)
5. Ministerio de Producción: Estudio de la situación actual de las empresas peruanas, pp. 56–99. Ministerio de la Producción, Lima (2015)
6. Cannella, S., Dominguez, R., Framinan, J.M.: Inventory record inaccuracy–the impact of structural complexity and lead time variability. Omega (United Kingdom) **68**, 123–138 (2017)
7. Heese, H.S.: Inventory record inaccuracy, double marginalization, and RFID adoption. Prod. Oper. Manag. **16**(5), 542–553 (2009)
8. Sari, K.: Investigating the value of reducing errors in inventory information from a supply chain perspective. Kybernetes **44**(2), 176–185 (2015)
9. AlManei, M., Salonitis, K., Yuchun, X.: Lean implementation frameworks: lean production, six sigma quality, TQM and company culture. TQM Mag. **18**(3), 263–281 (2006)
10. Lyons, A.C., Vidamour, K., Jain, R., Sutherland, M.: Developing an understanding of lean thinking in process industries. Prod. Plan. Control **24**(6), 475–494 (2013)
11. Zhou, B.: Lean principles, practices, and impacts: a study on small and medium-sized enterprises (SMEs). Ann. Oper. Res. **241**, 457–474 (2016)

Application of a Management Model Based on DMAIC Methodology to an MSE in the Personal Beauty Sector to Increase Profitability

Katherine Mejia[1(✉)], Henry Quintanilla[1(✉)], Carlos Cespedes[1(✉)], Jose Rojas[1,2(✉)], and Carlos Raymundo[2(✉)]

[1] Ingeniería de Gestión Empresarial, Universidad Peruana de Ciencias Aplicadas (UPC), Lima, Peru
{u201217323, u201312393, pccincces, jose.rojas}@upc.edu.pe
[2] Dirección de Investigación, Universidad Peruana de Ciencias Aplicadas (UPC), Lima, Peru
carlos.raymundo@upc.edu.pe

Abstract. Micro and Small Enterprise (MSEs) are the primary employment driving force in Peru; however, their low level of management does not allow for their long-term sustainable development. This situation has led such companies to incur unnecessary costs and expenses. In this study, we deal with the case study of a microenterprise of services in the personal beauty sector, which applied a Management Model based on define, measure, analyze, improve, and control (DMAIC) method. That excellent methodology helps to improve processes through the philosophy of continuous improvement, with the aim of proposing improvements to increase profitability and growth. Moreover, the integration of various techniques and tools at each stage of the DMAIC methodology was proposed with a focus on human management processes, inventories, and operational services, which have greater impact on most companies of this type.

Keywords: MSEs · CJM · Servqual · Blueprinting · DMAIC

1 Introduction

According to a study conducted by MapCity, there are more than 8,500 formal beauty salons with 50% belonging to socio-economic sectors C and D while large beauty chains target the less saturated sectors. Furthermore, the study indicates that Peruvian women invest from 10% to 15% of their salary in hairdressing or spa services [1]. In the case of the majority of Peruvian service microenterprises, the primary obstacles they face are a lack of professionalism among operating personnel, inadequate inventory management, standardization, documentation, and process repeatability, particularly for processes related to direct client contact such as deficient customer loyalty strategies, poor monitoring of service quality, and low level of service

T. Ahram et al. (Eds.): IHIET 2019, AISC 1018, pp. 982–987, 2020.
https://doi.org/10.1007/978-3-030-25629-6_152

innovation [2]. This problem will be addressed over the following sections and applied in the context of a Peruvian microenterprise to generate a management model based on engineering tools.

The case study is focused on an MSE dedicated to integral beauty services, which is located in the district of Santiago de Surco in Lima, Peru. Its costs have increased along with income; thus, the profit margin has not increased much.

To tackle the abovementioned problem, the design of an integrated management model is suggested, which would reduce costs and expenses incurred for the execution of requirements and purchases processes as well as human management and operative processes that are vital to the development of the company. Through this model, it will be possible to have a greater profit margin without diminishing the quality of services they provide.

This study is organized as follows. In Sect. 2, we provide the literature review in which related studies are discussed. In Sect. 3, we detail the contribution and form of implementation that will help the service sector's MSEs reduce their costs. In Sect. 4, we include the validation with the case study of Natsumi Spa in which the effectiveness of the contribution is demonstrated. Finally, in Sect. 5, we outline the conclusions of the validation data as well as provide certain recommendations.

2 Prior Art

2.1 Methodologies for Process Control

First, process control is essential to improve the quality of products and services offered by companies. Therefore, the Six Sigma methodology is widely used to measure, improve, and control quality in processes through a philosophy of continuous improvement that applies DMAIC method. Similarly, it is very important to integrate certain tools for each phase to develop and improve control in the desired processes [3].

2.2 Measuring and Improving Service Quality

Service quality is considered one of the key factors of good business performance. Since the 1980s, there have been considerable changes in the business environment with quality being considered one of the key priorities for increasing competitiveness and achieving growth [4].

2.3 Control of Inventories

One of the primary problems that MSEs have is the lack of attention and importance that they give to inventory control because they do not have reliable records, policies, systems, and models [5]. This leads to different problems such as inventories being in excess or insufficient, theft of merchandise, wastage, untidiness, and ignorance of some stored inputs [6].

2.4 HR Models

Furthermore, the mismanagement of the workforce is possibly the primary reason for the failure of many service companies. Getting workers' goals to be aligned with company's goals requires a lot of research. According to Avolio, Mesones, and Roca [7], Peruvian MSEs generally do not handle the workforce correctly, which then because of a lack of proper training do not perform their work well [7]. Moreover, the low motivation that employees have influences their work performance; therefore, it is necessary to create a model of incentives for workers [8].

3 Contribution

The proposal focuses on designing a management model with the purpose of reducing costs and expenses incurred for executing requirement processes and purchases, as well as human management and operative processes that are vital in the development of the company. Similarly, we want to standardize and formalize support and key processes and have better management and control.

The proposal of the management model is shown below (Fig. 1):

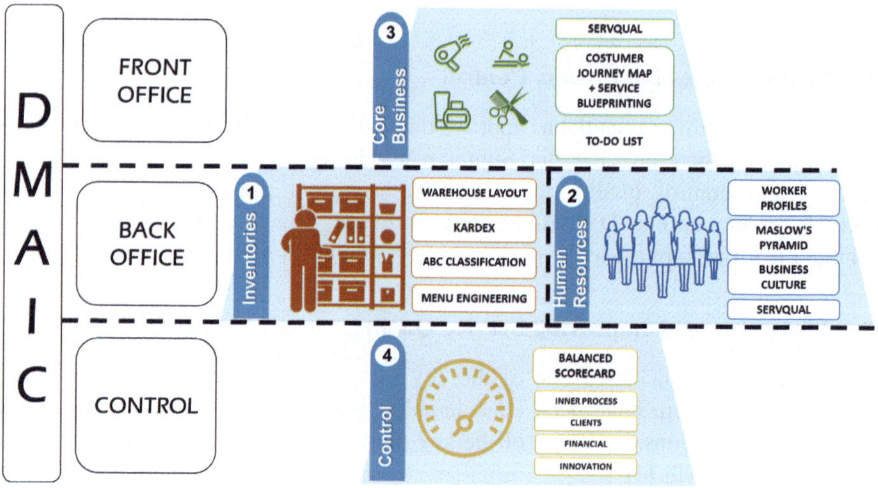

Fig. 1. Integrated management model for Natsumi Salón & Spa

The model presented has three stages on which the following sections will be detailed:

3.1 Pillar 1 – Back Office

Inventory Process: Its purpose is to reduce inventories and improve rotation.

Human Management Process: Its objective is to improve the human resources of the company through loyalty and greater productivity.

3.2 Pillar 2 – Front Office

Operating Services Process: The purpose is to carry out the processes that are related to direct client contact more efficiently. Moreover, the aim is that each action performed in the BACK OFFICE improves the cost and income structure of the company.

3.3 Pillar 3 – Control

This stage aims at establishing the following parameters that help improve the company:

Internal Processes: Establish ratios to measure profitability of the service operation to maintain high quality.

- Clients: Establish ratios focused on client management for the purpose of enhancing satisfaction and creating loyalty.
- Financial: Establish financial ratios focused on the control of expenses and costs of the company to make it more profitable over time.
- Innovation/Learning: Define ratios to understand how suitable the company is to introduce changes regarding infrastructure or services.

4 Validation

4.1 Pillar 1: Back Office – Inventory Process

4.1.1 Physical Layout

First, we counted all the inputs in the business and classified them into inputs for hair, face, nails/hands, legs/feet, and body. Moreover, the possible places where the materials used by Natsumi Salon & Spa would be stored and ordered were identified. For this purpose, a space was identified where boxes were stored, and then we proceeded to remove them and put up the shelf.

4.1.2 Kardex

Second, the Kardex was implemented for all the materials that were already identified. We proposed two tables in the Kardex. The first one is on the right and it indicates the service provided by the Spa with respect to the input in question. The one on the left shows the quantity in stock, the unit cost of the quantity of the product used, and the quantity used. The procedure is that when you provide a service that uses this input, it is deducted from the Kardex until the stock is exhausted. Because Natsumi Salon & Spa at the time of using the inputs uses percentages, the unit of measurement in this case would be milliliters. Furthermore, how much shampoo on average is used by service was calculated, and the result was 20 mL.

4.2 Pillar 1: Back Office – Human Management Process – Position Profiles

4.2.1 Maslow's Pyramid and Organizational Culture

We developed a customer care protocols and a manual of procedures for Hairdressing and Spa. So that all the organization's personnel would comply with the standards determined for each service. The owner and manager of the salon understood that the personnel are the ones who have direct contact with the client. For this reason, we continued with the next stage that was aimed at increasing the motivation of employees, strengthening their weaknesses, and giving them tools to improve the service. A human resources consultant with whom a motivational program based on Maslow's pyramid was negotiated visited Natsumi Salon & Spa.

4.2.2 Servqual

Finally, to evaluate the results of this implementation stage, an internal customer satisfaction survey based on the Servqual tool was carried out to identify improvements in the five dimensions of this type of survey: Reliability, Response Capacity, Security, Empathy, and Tangible Elements. It was determined that the survey will be carried out on a quarterly basis to follow up on the variables mentioned after the total deployment of the management model. Inventory management and human management form pillar 1 of the management model and allowed an adequate context to proceed with the improvements in direct relationship with the client (Front Office).

4.3 Pillar 2: Front Office – Operating Services Process

4.3.1 Costumer Journey Map and Service Blueprinting

The collection of data from customer satisfaction surveys began. We worked on creating the Customer Experience Map to improve the aspects that customers had rated as deficient and as an opportunity for improvement. Moreover, this technique helped make the phases that the client must go through more graphical from the moment he starts looking for the service and selects it to the moment he enters the salon, receives the service, makes the payment, and judges the results. In addition, the aforementioned technique, was complemented with service blueprinting to clarify interactions between customers and points of contact with service employees.

4.4 Pillar 3: Control

Finally, in the last pillar there is a graphic control panel so that the administration can contemplate the situation of the company more easily. For this purpose, the graph is divided into four parts: internal processes, customers, finance, and innovation. Each of these parts will have indicators that will be evaluated from 0 to 5 and will be carried out on a monthly basis by the administration.

5 Results and Conclusions

Before implementation, the percentage variation from January to May and June to September in relation to revenues in 2017 is 1.6%. The percentage variation for the aforementioned periods is 2.5%, which shows that income grows 37% less than expenses, leading to deficiencies in the control and management of microenterprise expenses. After the implementation, the income grew by 30% more than the expenses, which demonstrated and validated that it was possible to improve, control, and maintain the costs and expenses of the company, although the sales increased and, most importantly, the service quality and client satisfaction were not affected.

MSEs in Peru have a high level of informality; therefore, they do not have defined processes, duties, and management indicators, which is a challenge when generating projects that require data and information to gain awareness of their current situation.

The use of the DMAIC method allowed framing of tools and methodologies selected for the generation of an agile and sustainable model that could be communicated and applied in a short time with viable solutions and that would tackle the primary weaknesses and opportunities of the MSEs of the integral beauty sector.

Human management is vital for general development within small organizations because a sense of dissatisfaction directly affects the performance and effectiveness of the organization. MSEs suffer from high sensitivity to customer-focused actions because it is increasingly difficult to build loyalty with increased competition and demand.

References

1. La República: En el Perú, las cadenas de salones de belleza facturan más de S/8 millones al año, 30 May 2017. http://larepublica.pe/impresa/economia/880911en-el-peru-las-cadenas-de-salones-de-belleza-facturan-mas-de-s-8millones-al-ano. Accessed 24 August 2017
2. Ministerio de la Producción: Estadística de la Micro, Pequeña y Mediana Empresa (MIPYME), 10 January 2016. http://demi.produce.gob.pe/estadistica/mypime. Accessed 30 September 2017
3. Garza Ríos, R., González Sánchez, C., Rodríguez González, E., Hernández Asco, C.: Aplicación de la metodología DMAIC de Seis Sigma con simulación discreta y técnicas multicriterio. Revista de Métodos Cuantitativos para la Economía y la Empresa **22**, 19–35 (2016)
4. Martinez, L., Martinez, J.A.: Medición de la calidad del servicio. Desarrollo de escalas frente a medidas de un solo item. Decisiones de Marketing, 1–13 (2007)
5. Hatefi, M., Torabi, S.: A common weight linear optimization approach for multicriteria ABC inventory classification. Adv. Decis. Sci. **2015**, 1–11 (2015)
6. Laveriano, W.: Importancia del control de inventarios en la empresa. Actualidada Empresarial, 11–12 (2014)
7. Avolio, B., Mesones, A., Roca, E.: Factores que limitan el crecimiento de las micro y pequeñas empresas en el Perú (MYPES). Strategia **22**, 70–80 (2011)
8. Xiaolang, L., Shanshi, L., Hongli, W.: Workforce differentiation and human resource management practices: an exploratory research in China. Anthropologist **21**, 450–460 (2015)

Systematic Layout Planning: A Research on the Third Party Logistics of a Peruvian Company

Mariela Rabanal(✉), Sonia Zamami(✉), Juan Quiroze(✉), and Jose Alvarez(✉)

Ingeniería Industrial, Univerisdad Peruana de Ciencias Aplicadas, Lima, Peru
{u201515415,u201415440,pciijqui,pciijalv}@upc.edu.pe

Abstract. Logistics operators face various problems, the most common being the inadequate distribution of the operations yard. This is reflected in international logistics indexes, in which Peru ranks as one of the last countries. The company studied herein presents a problem of high reprocessing levels in the operations yard, which affects the level of service offered to customers. This study proposes the application of industrial engineering tools, such as systematic layout planning, to reduce reprocessing, increase profits. The proposed tool has been validated via simulation using the Arena software.

Keywords: Systems engineering · 3PL · Systematic layout planning · Simulation

1 Introduction

Outsourcing processes, such as packaging, distribution, storage, and inventory control, have increased the contribution of logistics operators to the supply chains of different organizations worldwide; this is because outsourcing services may reduce logistics time and cost. Logistics operators, mainly third party logistics (3PLs), play an extremely important role in the supply chain of companies or organizations [1]. Therefore, it is considered an important research topic because without operators anticipated success rates would not be achieved.

In 2015, such companies generated great benefits for the logistics of various companies worldwide by reducing inventory and fixed logistics costs by 5%, and 15%, respectively [1]. To this end, the company and the suppliers must be aligned to work with a high level of confidence that ensures order fulfillment. In addition, to better manage the supply chain, companies must automate their inventory management. Currently, only 12% companies are automated.

This study proposes the application of the systematic layout planning (SLP) tool [2] to reduce high reprocessing levels for logistics operators. The proposed improvement process comprises four stages: diagnostics, proposal preparation and design, implementation, and validation.

T. Ahram et al. (Eds.): IHIET 2019, AISC 1018, pp. 988–993, 2020.
https://doi.org/10.1007/978-3-030-25629-6_153

2 State of the Art

Several studies are available in the literature concerning the design or redesign of company areas using SLP owing to its easy application in small and medium enterprises that improves the flow of materials and labor. To apply the SLP steps, the authors identify the company's management strategy [3] and activities [4], the restrictions of the operations yard and the type of materials [5] and the time and the travel distances inside the area because the space used represents a cost for the company [6].

The distribution proposal must provide a safe work environment [7] because activities such as picking require a hard physical effort when performing the action of repeatedly placing and removing the boxes on the pallets, especially if the pallets are not find in a correct height for the operators [8].

Due to the complex activities that take place in the operations yards, it is difficult to implement the distribution proposal to evaluate the efficiency and accessibility [9] and then propose changes. Therefore, the authors propose using technology through software simulations to more accurately assess the impact of the proposal [10].

3 Methods

The method used herein comprises four steps: initial analysis, innovative technical proposal, final analysis, and results, as shown in Fig. 1.

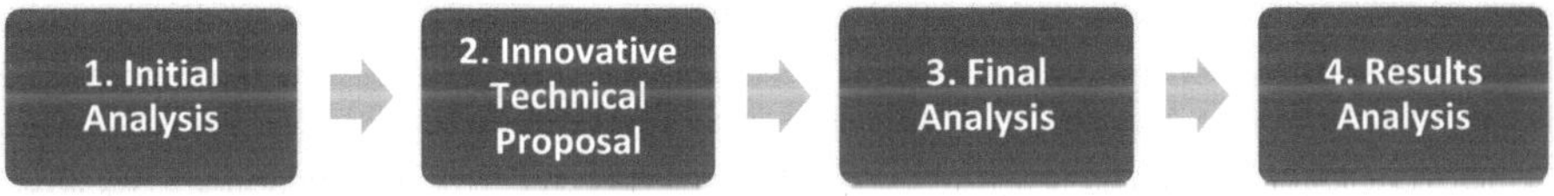

Fig. 1. Proposed method.

The above mentioned steps can be described as follows.

First, an initial analysis of the company is conducted to evaluate its current conditions. This analysis is performed through visits to the company, wherein the flow of operational processes is identified together with any potential problems. Subsequently, a prioritization matrix is created to determine the main problem in the operations area. Next, an Ishikawa Diagram is used to identify the root causes of the said problem. Post identification, tools to mitigate or eradicate these problems are proposed. In this study, the proposed tool is SLP and the research indicators are cycle time and the distance traveled.

Second, an innovative solution is proposed. This proposal begins with the collection of information relevant to the development under consideration. Then, we assess load flows and resources used for its movement inside the operations yard using a relational table and diagram to identify proximity requirements among areas located in the operations yard. In addition, the workload and income for each province is assessed using the P-Q and ABC diagram. Subsequently, different physical distribution proposals are developed for the operations yard. In all proposals, the proximity of the areas according to movements, workload, and percentage of income must be prioritized. After, the proposals are evaluated to select the proposal that provides the best flow of materials.

Third, results obtained post tool application are evaluated. In this stage, the proposed indicators are assessed via an Arena simulation, considering the improvement in employee performance and physical changes in area distribution. However, evaluating the reduction of the number of reprocesses post tool application is very important as this is the problem to be solved.

Finally, the results are analyzed using a semaphore table to compare initial results against the results obtained through the simulation.

4 Results

4.1 Initial Results

To obtain the current situation of logistics operators, continuous visits and meetings were conducted with the company's general manager and operations staff. In this manner, we were able to identify the sequence of activities and existing problems affecting the performance of the employees. Following this, current problems were listed and a prioritization matrix was created to determine the main problem. Based on the matrix, high reprocessing levels were deemed the main problem. Subsequently, causes were assessed through a problem tree, and the following reprocessing issues were identified: deliveries to the wrong destination, incomplete order deliveries, and order deliveries in poor condition. The root cause for all these reprocesses was determined to be inadequate area distribution in the operations yard.

Defining improper physical layout as one of the root causes, the following indicators were defined: the travel time and distance of an employee when mobilizing loads. To this end, the time taken and distance traveled between the areas involved in the operational processes were measured.

4.2 Innovative Technical Contribution

This study focuses on the development of the application of SLP to increase operations productivity and ensure the safety of the load and employees throughout the working day. This impacts the problem as errors may be avoided when locating loads; in addition, excessive handling of loads is reduced, which can cause physical damage to loads and errors when locating boxes in the storage area. Here in, SLP was developed in seven stages, as shown in Fig. 2.

Stage 1: In this stage, the dimensions of the area corresponding to each zone of the operations yard and the distance between them was measured. In addition, information necessary to develop the P-Q and ABC analyses. Next, we defined the three columns in the middle of the operations yard and the electrical connections that hinder the modification of office locations in this area were identified as restrictions.

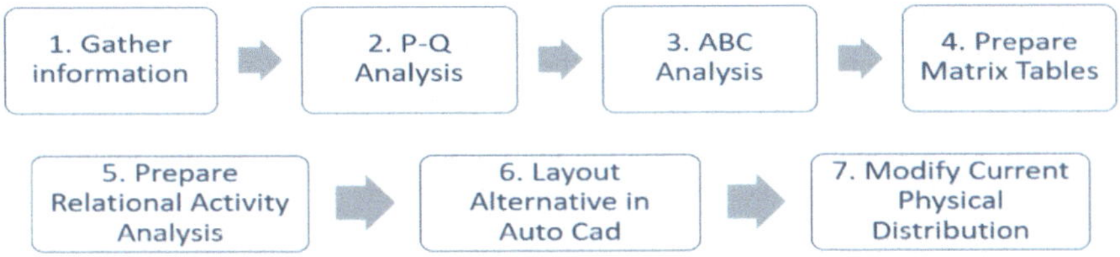

Fig. 2. Systematic layout planning stages.

Stage 2: In the second stage, destinations were evaluated according to the amount of volumetric space. This evaluation was performed through P-Q Analysis, as shown in Fig. 3.

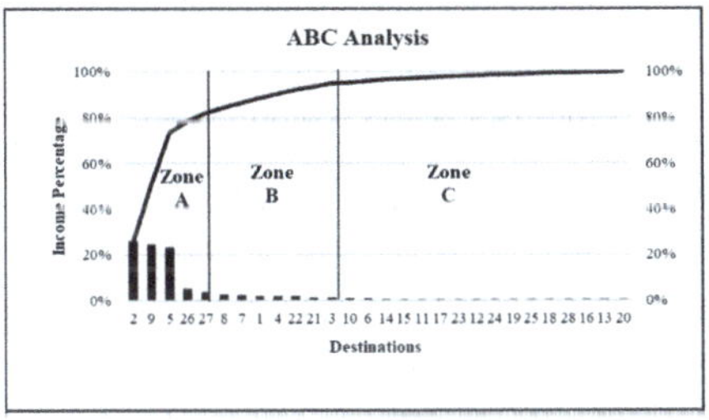

Fig. 3. P-Q analysis

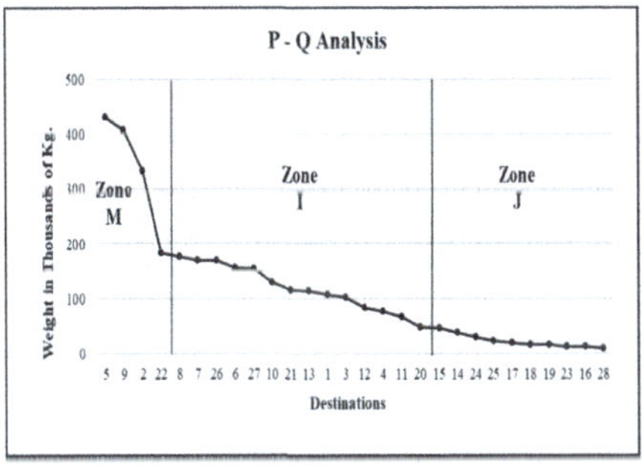

Fig. 4. ABC analysis

Stage 3: In the third stage, the destinations were evaluated via ABC analysis according to the percentage of income that they contributed to the company during the year 2017. Figure 4 shows the corresponding ABC diagram.

Based on the P-Q and ABC analysis, it is concluded that destinations 2, 5, and 9 must be prioritized when relocating the areas as they are destinations with the highest monthly load movement and represent 73.18% of the total income received by the company.

Stage 4: We evaluated current efforts and compared them against the effort that would be made when redistributing the area layout according to the analysis using matrix tables that related load weights and the distance traveled between areas. Based on this analysis, the effort being made currently is 18,266.80 kg/m. By implementing the proposed improvements, the efforts will be reduced to 14,165 kg/m.

Stage 5: In the fifth stage, relational activity analysis was conducted using the relational activities table and diagram. Based on this analysis, the direct proximity between the parking lot and the packing area and that between the pick-up and boarding area and the printing table were deemed crucial. However, the short distance between the packing area and the following areas—pick-up and boarding area, printing table, and destinations 2, 5, and 9—are also absolutely required.

Stage 6: In this new distribution, the locations of destinations 2, 5, and 9 were prioritized as they were locations storing the largest cargo to be moved to provinces. For the same reason, the storage area was increased. In contrast, certain destinations were grouped into a single area as they did not require the space they had owing to the small amount of cargo stored in them. Furthermore, the reverse logistics area was relocated outside the operations yard because it did not add value to the processes performed therein.

Stage 7: In the final stage, areas were redistributed via a simulation using the Arena software, and, in this manner, practical results were obtained for comparison against the expected theoretical results; the comparison validated the application of the SLP tool.

5 Results Analysis

After applying the SLP tool, the results were analyzed according to the proposed indicators. Figure 5 presents a semaphore table that shows the indicators of the number of reprocesses, cycle time, and distance traveled for orders addressed to significant destinations. The current value, projected value, and the value obtained from the simulation are all presented.

Indicator	Unit	Semaphore			Current Value	Expected Value	Obtained Value
		Red	Yellow	Green			
Number of reprocesses	%	> 15	15 - 6	≤ 5	9.13	5.00	7.00
Cycle times	Minutes	≥ 140	139 - 110	< 110	138.74	107.29	120.46
Distance traveled	Meters	> 100	100 - 50	≤ 50	87.50	50	39

Fig. 5. Control indicators

The main indicator of the success of this project is the amount of reprocessing as it is the main problem of the company. As observed in Fig. 5, a 5% reduction was estimated. However, the value obtained is 7% because the modifications were simulated, which generates variations in the results.

For the second indicator, at the beginning of the project, cycle times were expected to decrease to 107.29 min. However, they were reduced to 120.46 min. Furthermore, as regards the distance traveled in the operations yard, a 50-m reduction was expected, and, through the results of the simulation, distances were reduced to 39 m.

6 Conclusions

Plant distribution is a common problem in small companies and even in some large companies. However, the SLP tool may contribute to an optimal redistribution of company areas. Therefore, this study shows the changes made in the physical distribution of an operations yard for a logistics operator applying SLP, focusing on improving the operations area's performance and preventing operation errors that generate reprocessing.

Regarding the main objective of the research project, the company's reprocessing level was reduced to 7%. In addition, the simulation of the current and proposed operations yard was compared, revealing that the time was reduced to 18.28 min. Similarly, the distance traveled was reduced by 39 m.

References

1. Langley, C.J., Capgemini Consulting: 2017 Third-Party Logistics Study - The State of Logistics Outsourcing, p. 23 (2017)
2. Yang, T., Su, C., Hsu, Y.: Systematic layout planning: a study on semiconductor wafer fabrication facilities. Int. J. Oper. Prod. Manag. **20**(11), 1359–1371 (2000)
3. Kłodawski, M., Jacyna, M., Lewczuk, K., Wasiak, M.: The issues of selection warehouse process strategies. Procedia Eng. **187**, 451–457 (2017)
4. Dotoli, M., Epicoco, N., Falagario, M., Costantino, N., Turchiano, B.: An integrated approach for warehouse analysis and optimization: a case study. Comput. Ind. **70**(1), 56–69 (2015)
5. Accorsi, R., Manzini, R., Maranesi, F.: A decision-support system for the design and management of warehousing systems. Comput. Ind. **65**(1), 175–186 (2014)
6. Cakmak, E., Gunay, N.S., Aybakan, G., Tanyas, M.: Determining the size and design of flow type and U-type warehouses. Procedia - Soc. Behav. Sci. **58**, 1425–1433 (2012)
7. Moatari-Kazerouni, A., Chinniah, Y., Agard, B.: Integrating occupational health and safety in facility layout planning, part I: methodology. Int. J. Prod. Res. **53**(11), 3243–3259 (2015)
8. Calzavara, M., Hanson, R., Sgarbossa, F., Medbo, L., Johansson, M.I.: Picking from pallet and picking from boxes: a time and ergonomic study. IFAC-PapersOnLine **50**(1), 6888–6893 (2017)
9. Ali Naqvi, S.A., Fahad, M., Atir, M., Zubair, M., Shehzad, M.M.: Productivity improvement of a manufacturing facility using systematic layout planning. Cogent Eng. **3**(1), 1207296 (2016)
10. Jia, Y., Jiang, P.F.: The application of simulation technology in distribution center. Appl. Mech. Mater. **865**, 675–680 (2017)

Waste Reduction Model in a Small Clothing Company-Umbrella Model

Geraldine Cueto(✉), Yosiveth Caldas(✉), Gino Viacava(✉), Juan Quiroz(✉), and Jose Alvarez(✉)

Escuela de Ingeniería Industrial,
Universidad Peruana de Ciencias Aplicadas (UPC), Lima, Peru
{u201412059,u201410652,pcingvia,juan.quiroz,
pciijalv}@upc.edu.pe

Abstract. Excess waste problem is encountered by small and medium-sized companies in the textile and clothing sector, which has a negative impact on the profitability of these companies. Herein, a diagnosis analysis is performed in a small company using the Ishikawa diagram to identify the root causes and they are measured using indicators. Based on these results, a change management model is proposed, which supports the implementation of lean manufacturing tools and production system components during the 30-day pilot application. Then, each indicator is reassessed to verify the feasibility of the proposed umbrella model. Results show that this model reduced the amount of waste by 81.21%.

Keywords: Lean manufacturing · Clothing industry · Waste reduction · Change management · Umbrella model

1 Introduction

Production process waste must be reduced to help companies prosper in the current, highly competitive global market [1]. Therefore, improvements to the manufacturing processes should be made to reduce the waste or defects, which decrease the productivity of any production line, using a lean system [2]. Likewise, Brown et al. [3] emphasized that sustainability is achieved in manufacturing through a comprehensive vision encompassing product design, manufacturing processes, manufacturing systems, and the entire supply chain, as reflected in the value map [4].

According to Wickramasinghe et al. [5], production waste is defined as waste that does not add value to the product or service from the customer's standpoint. Lean manufacturing tools contribute significantly in the reduction of different types of waste [6]. In addition, lean practices exhibit positive effects in terms of the operations area [7]. Therefore, lean manufacturing is considered the best system to help improve textile management performance at an operational level [8]. Further, Saleeshya et al. [9] claimed that lean manufacturing is a waste disposal philosophy through the application of continuous improvement.

There Adikorley et al. [10] have focused their efforts on studying small and medium-scale enterprises in the textile and clothing sector. Currently, there is little

T. Ahram et al. (Eds.): IHIET 2019, AISC 1018, pp. 994–1000, 2020.
https://doi.org/10.1007/978-3-030-25629-6_154

research in the textile-clothing sector for small businesses, since these companies usually lack the resources required for the acquisition of new quality concepts [8].

Sarkar et al. [11] stated that mudas or wastes, are best reflected in idle times, which significantly reduce productivity. Ismail et al. [6] added that waste increases the operating costs, which in turn reduces the gross profit margin, whereas Zhou [12] mentioned that waste generates loss of competitiveness in the market. Therefore, it can be concluded that production process waste has a direct negative impact on the company's profit margin. Also, Joshi et al. [13] state that the manufacturing process requires great value-added potential to obtain a competitive advantage in the market.

In Herein, an inadequate level of waste in the clothing manufacturing process has been identified as a problem. It must be noted that out of the eight lean manufacturing wastes, the company under study exhibits six. Therefore, a solution must be found to reduce waste percentages. Therefore, in this case study, the implementation of nine solutions has been proposed for the root causes identified in the problem tree. These proposals are (a) standardization, (b) line balancing, (c) cellular manufacturing, (d) Change Management, (e) Push–Pull system, (f) job design, (g) 5 Ss, (h) operations meetings, and (i) JIDOKA (humanized automation). The proposed model may help improve the efficiency of the manufacturing process through combinations of tools, methods, and systems.

This study presents different cases focusing on the same business sector and problem. Additionally, the model proposed for the reduction of waste levels in a garment workshop will be explained in detail. Finally, the contributions of this study will be listed and the effectiveness of the proposed model will be discussed.

2 Method

A diagnosis analysis was conducted in the manufacturing area using the Ishikawa diagram and quantifying each root cause based on the assessment of 7 indicators, which were calculated with information, timekeeping, and daily on-site evaluations in the company. Then, an innovative technical proposal was developed based on the change management methodology [14], which is used as support throughout the lean manufacturing tools and production system component pilot implementation. Finally, the "umbrella model" was tested in a 30-day pilot, as evidenced in the pre- and post-pilot results.

3 Results

3.1 Pre-intervention Results

Data were collected from 2016 to 2017, wherein the company's income decreased by 15.2%, which is a profitability loss percentage. In addition, a decrease in the productivity and efficiency was reported, obtaining only an average efficiency of 64.4%. Then, the value stream was mapped, identifying 8 critical points:

- Absence of production planning, since there is 44.02% excess scheduling.
- Absence of operations meetings.

- High manufacturing times, since they exceed the Takt time by 31.64%.
- The lead time exceeds three days and consequently, the cycle efficiency only reaches 5.01%.
- Absence of process standardization—currently standing at 5.01%, it must be at least 10.00% according to Baeza [15].
- Lack of quality control: reprocessing is reported at 24%.
- Absence of layout design, with 69% of long distance routes between levels.
- Lack of inventory in process.

An Ishikawa analysis was performed (Fig. 1), where the main problem is identified as an "inadequate level of waste in the clothing area of Y4RD1" based on 6 wastes: (a) unnecessary movements, (b) transportation, (c) overproduction, (d) long waiting times, (e) overprocessing, and (f) unused human talent. For each waste, a "5 whys" analysis was performed to identify the root cause of each waste. In the first instance, the problem is evident because there is a 19% overtime impacting an additional cost of 1258.10 dollars per week (13.3%).

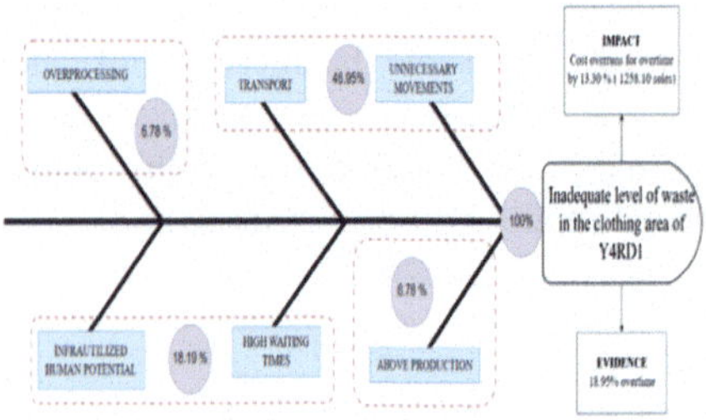

Fig. 1. Ishikawa diagram showing the dumb

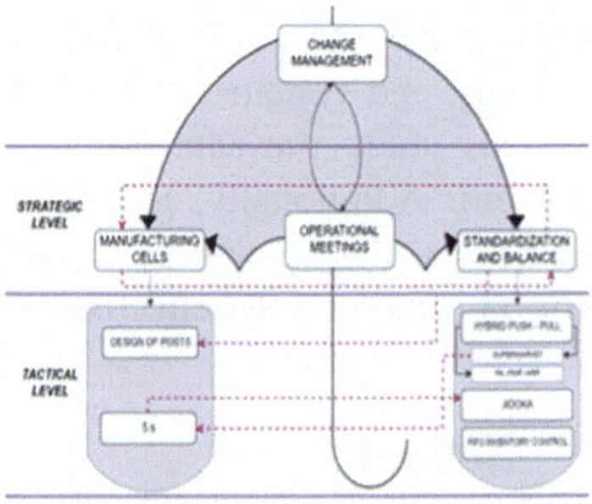

Fig. 2. Umbrella model

In Fig. 1, 7 root causes are identified (green links) with their corresponding impact percentage, which were found through the assessment of the 7 following indicators:

- Percentage of Long Distances Between Levels:
  (Distance traveled between Levels)/(Total Distance traveled) = 69%
- Process Cycle Efficiency
  (Value Added Time)/(Total Cycle Time) = 5.01%
- Percentage of Excess Cycle Time over Takt Time
  (Cycle Time - Takt Time)/(Takt Time) = −31.68%
- Average Overproduction
  (Units Produced - Units Sold)/(Units Sold) = 44.02%
- Reprocessing Index
  (# Reprocessing Operations)/(# Total Operations) = 24.00%
- Percentage of Underutilized Work
  (Time dedicated to Non-Manufacturing Activities)/(Total Work Time) = 17.96%
- Percentage of Non-Compliance with Principles of Motion Economy
  (Number of Principles Breached)/(Total Number of Principles) = 56.52%

Finally, in Ishikawa's analysis, the impact percentage of each muda or waste was calculated for the problem. It is observed that waste from transportation and unnecessary movements has an impact of 46.95%, while overproduction impacts in a 28.09%. Therefore, there are 7 indicators: 5 indicators that are considered out of control and critical (red) and 2 that are out of control but are not critical. For this reason, in the innovative proposal, a model will be proposed that manages to bring these indicators back into control (green).

3.2 Innovative Technical Proposal

The innovative technical proposal comprises a model known as "umbrella model" (Fig. 2). This model is based on the change management methodology, which supports the implementation of the whole model [13]. Based on this methodology, lean manufacturing tools and other production system components will be implemented following the innovative of the umbrella model. The umbrella is divided into two subgroups: (a) Strategic, the central and basic tools of the model and (b) tactical, the secondary tools used after the first sector.

On one hand, the strategic area contains the following lean tools, such as cellular manufacturing, operations meetings, standardization, and line balancing. These three links focus on attacking the immediate causes identified in the Ishikawa, which are transportation and long waiting times. First, operations meetings help monitor the current state of the company as well as to augment the change management approach. Second, the standardization and line balancing will be performed to reduce times by grouping activities. Finally, manufacturing processes will be based on line balancing and grouping different types of machines used by an operator, which will help reduce the transportation time between each machine.

On the other hand, the tactical area is based on applying post design, the 5Ss, the push–pull hybrid system, the JIDOKA quality inspection, and the PEPS inventory control to help reduce the impact of the main problem. These links are located in the second level because it focuses more on the operations issues, thus engaging all workers.

3.3 Pilot Results

To validate our proposal, a 30-day pilot was performed, implementing all the umbrella components. Second, waste from unnecessary movements based on compliance with the principles of motion economics was reduced to non-compliance of 26.1%. This change is critical because it is associated with workplace culture. Still, waste from overproduction, overprocessing, and unnecessary movements was only reduced by 5.4%.

Therefore, the model focuses on the strategic side. The manufacturing process will be streamlined with support from all the workers in the company. Further, the tactical sector will help reinforce the reduction of the impact of the main problem of the company, which is shown in Fig. 2 because workers still do not adapt to the new process standardization.

In addition, waste from underutilized human talent was reduced by 12.69%, i.e., the workers no longer have idle time due to the fact that the line was correctly balanced.

Likewise, regarding waste from long waiting time, takt time was greater than the cycle time. Then, the process cycle efficiency increased to 13.33%. Finally, the proposed model was able to reduce the main problem by 81.2% overall. This is due to the fact that the overtime was reduced from 19.0% to 3.6%, and therefore, the cost overrun percentage was reduced to 2.7%.

It must be noted that the remaining 18.8% problem was retained owing to two reasons: (1) 100% of the cellular manufacturing was not implemented and (2) changing the culture of the workers requires more time and effort.

4 Results Analysis

The objective of the umbrella model was for indicators to be in control without being critical. However, owing to human factors, the goal was not reached at 100%. With this model, no indicators were completely out of control, with 3 indicators being fully controlled and 4 being controlled but critical, as evidenced in Table 1.

Table 1. Comparative of the before vs. After the performance indicators of each cause root

Indicator	Before	Expected	Pilot	% Dif.
% long routes between levels	69.00% (red)	25.00% (green)	21.03% (green)	47.97%
Efficiency of the process cycle	5.01% (yellow)	15.00% (green)	13.33% (green)	8.32%
% in excess of cycle time over Takt time	131.64% (yellow)	95.00% (green)	94.97% (green)	36.37%
% overproduction	44.02% (red)	10.00% (green)	11.53% (yellow)	32.49%
Reprocessing index	24.00% (red)	7.00% (green)	18.67% (yellow)	5.33%
% of underutilized work	17.96% (red)	5.00% (green)	5.43% (yellow)	12.53%
% non-compliance with the principles of economy of movements	56.52% (red)	15.00% (green)	26.09% (yellow)	30.43%

The reason for obtaining controlled but critical indicators is because the human factor still needs to adapt to the changes implemented, especially in terms of the operating system, which includes process standardization, JIDOKA quality inspection and the principles of motion economics.

5 Conclusions

- This paper proposes a model, based on change management methodology, which, when implemented through a 30-day pilot, managed to reduce overtime and cost overrun percentages. Therefore, the problem was reduced by 81.2%.
- The model was implemented through a pilot based on the change management methodology, since all the stakeholders were engaged in pilot development and application.
- Waste from transportation and overproduction was reduced to the expected levels since human factors did not directly intervene.
- 5 indicators were identified as out of control and critical, whereas 2 were identified as out of control but not critical. After pilot implementation, no indicators remained out of control and critical, with 3 being fully controlled and 4 controlled but critical.

References

1. Behnam, D., Ayough, A., Mirghaderi, S.H.: Value stream mapping approach and analytical network process to identify and prioritize production system's Mudas (case study: natural fibre clothing manufacturing company). J. Tex. Inst. **109**(1), 64–72 (2017). https://doi.org/10.1080/00405000.2017.1322737
2. Obeidat, M.S., Al-Aomar, R., Pei, Z.J.: Lean manufacturing implementation in the sewing industry. J. Enterp. Transform. **4**(2), 151–171 (2014). https://doi.org/10.1080/19488289.2014.890980
3. Kasemset, C., Chernsupornchai, J., Pala-Ud, W.: Application of MFCA in waste reduction: case study on a small textile factory in Thailand. J. Clean. Prod. **108**(Part B), 1342–1351 (2015). https://doi.org/10.1016/j.jclepro.2014.09.071
4. Brown, A., Amundson, J., Badurdeen, F.: Sustainable value stream mapping (Sus-VSM) in different manufacturing system configurations: application case studies. J. Clean. Prod. **85**, 164–179 (2014). https://doi.org/10.1016/j.jclepro.2014.05.101
5. Wickramasinghe, G., Wickramasinghe, V.: Implementation of lean production practices and manufacturing performance: the role of lean duration. J. Manuf. Technol. Manag. **28**(4), 531–550 (2017). https://doi.org/10.1108/JMTM-08-2016-0112
6. Ismail, A., Ghani, J.A., Ab Rahman, M.N., Md Deros, B., Che Haron, C.H.: Application of lean six sigma tools for cycle time reduction in manufacturing: case study in biopharmaceutical industry. Arab. J. Sci. Eng. **39**(2), 1449–1463 (2014). https://doi.org/10.1007/s13369-013-0678-y
7. Khanchanapong, T., Prajogo, D., Sohal, A.S., Cooper, B.K., Yeung, A.C.L., Cheng, T.C.E.: The unique and complementary effects of manufacturing technologies and lean practices on manufacturing operational performance. Int. J. Prod. Econ. **153**, 191–203 (2014). https://doi.org/10.1016/j.ijpe.2014.02.021
8. Manfredsson, P.: Textile management enabled by lean thinking: a case study of textile SMEs textile management enabled by lean thinking: a case study of textile SMEs. Prod. Plan. Control **27**(7–8), 541–549 (2016). https://doi.org/10.1080/09537287.2016.1165299
9. Saleeshya, P.G., Raghuram, P., Vamsi, N.: Lean manufacturing practices in textile industries–a case study. Int. J. Collab. Enterp. **3**(1), 18–37 (2012). https://doi.org/10.1504/IJCENT.2012.052367

10. Adikorley, R.D., Rothenberg, L., Guillory, A.: Lean six sigma applications in the textile industry: a case study. Int. J. Lean Six Sigma **8**(2), 210–224 (2017). https://doi.org/10.1108/IJLSS-03-2016-0014
11. Sarkar, A., Mukhopadhyay, A.R., Ghosh, S.K.: Productivity improvement by reduction of idle time through application of queuing theory. Opsearch **52**(2), 195–211 (2015). https://doi.org/10.1007/s12597-014-0177-2
12. Zhou, B.: Lean principles, practices, and impacts: a study on small and medium-sized enterprises (SMEs). Ann. Oper. Res. **241**(1–2), 457–474 (2016). https://doi.org/10.1007/s10479-012-1177-3
13. Joshi, R.N., Singh, S.P.: Technical efficiency and its determinants in the Indian garment industry. J. Text. Inst. **103**(3), 231–243 (2012). https://doi.org/10.1080/00405000.2011.564797
14. Bamford, D.: A case-study into change influences within a large British multinational. J. Change Manag. **6**(2), 181–191 (2006). https://doi.org/10.1080/14697010600719841
15. Baeza Serrato, R.: REDUTEX: a hybrid push – pull production system approach for reliable delivery time in knitting SMEs. Prod. Plan. Control **27**(4), 263–279 (2016). https://doi.org/10.1080/09537287.2015.1120362

Strategic Planning Model to Improve Competitiveness for Service Industry SMEs Using the Balanced Scorecard

Miguel Casas(✉), Maribel Perez(✉), Jose Rojas(✉), and Jose Alvarez(✉)

Escuela de Ingeniería de Gestión Empresarial, Universidad Peruana de Ciencias Aplicadas (UPC), Lima, Peru
{u201220230,maribel.perez,jose.rojas, pciijalv}@upc.edu.pe

Abstract. Today the implementation of strategic planning in small- and medium-sized enterprises (SMEs) is a variant that helps organizations to acquire and build knowledge, as it generates that the company manages to understand and manage the main processes in a given context and facilitates decision making for the acquisition of concrete results. This research is focused on the development of a strategic planning model based on the balanced scorecard (BSC) to help SMEs generate and execute strategies while considering their level of development as regards processes and needs, and though this help them to be more competitive and profitable. The expected results are the increase in profitability, the improvement in the quality of the service, the increase in sales volume, and reduction of the cost overruns found before the implementation of the proposed model.

Keywords: Pymes · Strategic planning · Competitiveness · Organizational development · Balanced scorecard

1 Introduction

Nowadays, the global economy is undergoing major changes, and in this environment, small- and medium-sized enterprises (SMEs) are under intense pressure because national markets are constantly facing competition from across the world. The information technology revolution and the constant communication innovation of the 1990s along with the rapid proliferation of the Internet greatly provided equal opportunities to all competitors through free information flow, regardless of boundaries, and it opened up new opportunities [1]. SMEs are among the key forms of economic self-reliance in many countries and they mainly contribute to generating employment, innovation, alleviating poverty, social stability, and economic well-being [2].

In the context of microenterprise growth, the number of microenterprises has constantly increased; according to the National Institute of Statistics and Informatics (INEI, Instituto Nacional de Estadística e Informática), in 2017 alone, approximately 284,000 new microenterprises were created, and compared with 2016, this is a growth of 7%.

T. Ahram et al. (Eds.): IHIET 2019, AISC 1018, pp. 1001–1006, 2020.
https://doi.org/10.1007/978-3-030-25629-6_155

On the other hand, the number of SMEs that closed down has increased, with approximately 150,000 closed companies in 2017, which has generated unemployment and social issues. According to a study published by the Pontifical Catholic University, the main factors that limit SME growth are human resource management, accounting and financial issues, administrative management, and operational issues [4].

These factors are closely related because SMEs arise from the need for self-employment and along with a growth in their sales and customer volumes comes deficiencies, mainly in process planning and execution.

To meet the growth and development needs of SMEs in Peru, this article approaches a planning model based on the balanced scorecard (BSC) methodology, as the traditional models were designed for other contexts rather than the country's current circumstances.

According to Cepteranu [5], SME competitiveness can be approached in four different ways. Chaudhry [6] states that the training of SME employees and managers forms a framework in which SME competitiveness tends to grow.

To solve this problem, Recarti and Caturida [7] propose the implementation of a theoretical model. This along with marketing strategies and proper accounting management would directly increase SME competitiveness and improve financial results and organizational innovation.

Kumar [8] argues that to successfully face global competition, SMEs must break the isolation of their suppliers and other entities in the supply chain. As organizations seek to develop more effective partnerships and IT relationships with their business partners, internal processes become intertwined and span the traditional enterprise boundaries. In Peru, the situation is no different, since by 2017, 96.5% of the total number of operating companies was SMEs, and these companies generate approximately 22% of the country's GDP [3].

2 Proposed Model

The proposed model is mostly based on the BSC planning methodology. This technique is mainly tailored to organizations that count on formally established processes, as well as clear growth objectives, which allows the company that applies this method to have a view of the four perspectives at the same time and thus be able to make effective decisions.

However, SMEs do not have such components, thus the BSC model must be modified to be implemented and used by these companies.

Next, the proposed model is presented graphically to achieve an increase in the company's gross profit.

The model is divided into four phases:

- Phase 0: We analyze the internal and external environment through the EFE, EFI, and SWOT matrices; then we define the organizational orientation, i.e., the organization's mission, vision, and values. From this, the general strategic orientation will emerge. As a final step, we define the strategies applied in order to reach the goal by means of a matrix of indicators.

- Phase 1: In phase 1, we focus on the first BSC perspective, which is employee training and development to provide and ensure the company's main process, i.e., food preparation and customer service. The procedures will be standardized and a training plan will be completed with the main goal being maintaining a high level of customer satisfaction. The training also aims to improve the level of job satisfaction that will be measured using the core self-evaluations (CSE).
- Phase 2: Phase 2 consists of the implementation of the formal processes where the main problems were found at the time of diagnosis, namely the human resources, purchasing, and commercial processes.
- In the human resources process, different measures will be conducted to reduce the employee turnover rate. Thus, the selection process will be modified by adding the personnel applicant assessment filter using the CSE. This test will help select the most suitable personnel for the organization because the higher the applicant's assessment result, the less likely the personnel applicant's intention is to leave the role. For the constant evaluation of the work environment, the same method will be used among recruited personnel.
- Second, in terms of the purchasing process, the standardization of product cost variability is proposed to reduce cost overruns due to purchasing costs. Through this standardization, we aim for greater control over the quality of products purchased so as not to affect the final product.
- Finally, in phase 2, the commercial management plan will be implemented in the sales area. The aim is to increase B2B sales through an online campaign and email marketing to attract sales and new operations and boost B2C sales for dealers through cross-selling.
- Phase 3: The third and final phase of the model focuses on the evaluation of the proposed indicators to analyze each company process and find solutions across the organization.

3 Results

Strategic Environmental Analysis—Porter's Five Forces Analysis (Table 1).

We found that the company in our case study is located in a market with high barriers to entry due to the implementation costs, but substitute services such as food delivery services have also emerged. Service quality and food quality are among the most important competitive factors, as well as cost management focused on maintaining a competitive price.

– Strategic Environmental Analysis - SWOT Analysis.

After the Porter's five forces analysis, we performed a SWOT analysis to obtain preliminary strategies that can be proposed based on this analysis.

– Financial analysis of the case study and problem identification.

As can be seen in Table 2, in the January–June 2018 period, the company had a profit of approximately 30% of its sales, which allows it to meet its obligations such as salaries and purchasing raw materials; however, it is below the gross profit margin estimated for the industry (i.e., 40%).

Table 1. Porter's five forces analysis

Porter's five forces analysis	
Threat of new entrants	Low due to the high cost of implementation of a dining room, i.e., approximately S/.80000
Rivalry among existing competitors	We identified six main points that determine the success among companies in this area, namely: - Service quality - Food quality - Market experience - Price - Menu variety - Nutritional services
Threat of substitute products and services	There is growth of competing services mainly in delivery services
Bargaining power of buyers	Low, since the bidding framework is provided by means of bases to which competitors must adjust
Bargaining power of suppliers	Medium, owing to the large number of supplier options

Table 2. Financial information of the case study

Year 2018	Sales	Gross profit	Average industry gross profit	Gap
January	$8,314	$2,494	$3,326	$831
February	$8,465	$2,539	$3,386	$846
March	$8,615	$2,585	$3,446	$862
April	$8,400	$2,520	$3,360	$840
May	$8,098	$2,430	$3,239	$810
June	$8,325	$2,497	$3,330	$832
Total period	$50,217	$15,065	$20,087	$5,022

This gap is because although the company generates continuous sales volumes, it has some deficient processes that incur cost overruns. This impedes it from reaching the industry gross profit level.

Next, we show the results of the process analysis and their respective impact:

- Human Resources Process: In the January to June 2018 period, there were five voluntary resignations and dismissals from a total team of eight employees. This represents 63% of the staff turnover rate, when according to the INEI the industry turnover rate should be 10% at maximum. This high turnover rate generates an additional process cost that has a direct impact on the company's profit.
- Purchasing Process: During the analysis period, the costs of raw materials purchased represented 45% of the sales volume generated, but approximately 5% of these costs are for unplanned purchases and must be executed at higher prices than initially planned.

- Operations: The operations area includes two main processes: the cooking process and the customer service process. These two processes are considered the organization's main processes, since customer satisfaction with the service and food quality is determined by customers continuing with the provided service.
- Commercial Management: As an area, commercial management is not implemented in the case study, as it has not carried out actions that could generate an increase in its sales volume. This volume is exclusively generated by the sale of lunches. This opportunity is not taken advantage of since the business model presented, which is that of the food concessionaire, has direct access to the public.

4 Result Analysis

Next, we present the indicator table, which shows the results obtained by the model compared to its goal (Table 3).

Table 3. Results table

	Indicator	Goal	Initial result	Achieved result	Gap	Status
Phase 1	Food quality	Maintain the level	95%	97%	2%	Achieved
	Service quality	Increase the level by 10%	80%	95%	15%	Achieved
	Training	Reach 90%	NA	100%		Achieved
	Increased employee committment	Increase the level by 10%	65%	75%	10%	Achieved
Phase 2	Time to fill	Reduce at 3 days	5 days	3 days	2 days	Achieved
	Turnover rate	Reduce at 10%	32%	13%	19%	Near target
	Number of servings sold	Increase to 5%	2700	2881	6%	Achieved
	Number of new sales	Achieve 25% of the lunch clientele	25%	35%	10%	Achieved
	Reduction of purchasing costs for the approved products	10% reduction	$2,432	2,168	11%	Achieved

We analyzed the indicators of both model phases; the results are as follows.

In phase 1, all the proposed goals were reached, generating a greater impact on customer satisfaction (95%). Furthermore, a training control indicator was added to check if the training was conducted as scheduled.

In phase 2, the selection process time could be reduced by two days and become more dynamic due to the job exchange tool. The only indicator not achieved was the expected reduction of the turnover rate to 10%. However, it improved, reaching 13%. As a countermeasure, various retention techniques should be made available and enhanced for key personnel positions such as chefs.

5 Conclusions

These are the preliminary conclusions of the model:

- The model ensured the main operations of the case study, which is the basis for the other strategies.
- Employee commitment was achieved through training, with the effect of reducing the turnover rate and improving service quality.
- The proposed tools are low cost, which would help their replication in other SMEs from different industries.

Finally, the model fulfilled most of the indicators proposed, and our proposal for change consists of adding other strategies for personnel retention and reducing the turnover rate to the expected 10%.

References

1. Hoque, R., Mohammad, S., Mustafa, A.: Adoption of information and communication technology for development: a case study of small and medium enterprises in Bangladesh. Inf. Dev. **32**, 1–15 (2015). https://doi.org/10.1177/0266666915578202
2. Peru Retail: Las Pymes son el 96.5% de las empresas que hay en Perú. APEC Perú Retail (2017). https://www.peru-retail.com/pymes-empresas-peru/
3. Avolio, B., Mesones, A., Roca, E.: Factores que limitan el crecimiento de las PYMES. – Revistas PUCP (2017)
4. Alva, E.: La desaparición de las microempresas en el Perú. Una aproximación a los factores que predisponen a su mortalidad. Cso del Cercado de Lima. Economía y Desarrollo **158**, 76–90 (2017)
5. Ceptureanu, S.: Competitiveness of SMES. Bus. Excel. Manag. **5**(2), 55–67 (2015)
6. Chaudhry, A.: Knowledge management practices and organizational performance of SMEs in Pakistan. Bus. Econ. **9**(3), 173–183 (2017). https://doi.org/10.22547/BER/9.3.7
7. Rekarti, E., Meiwanto, C.: Improving business performance: a proposed model for SMEs. Eur. Res. Stud. J. **20**(3A), 613–623 (2017)
8. Kumar, R., Singh, R., Shankar, R.: Strategy development by Indian SMEs for improving coordination in supply chain an empirical study. Competitiveness Rev. **24**(5), 414–432 (2014). https://doi.org/10.1108/cr-06-2012-0016

6TOC Model for Small Wood Furniture Companies to Increase Machining Productivity in Villa El Salvador Industrial Cluster

Leonel Gutierrez[1(✉)], Jesus Laredo[1(✉)], Fernando Sotelo[1(✉)], and Carlos Raymundo[2(✉)]

[1] Ingeniería Industrial, Universidad Peruana de Ciencias Aplicadas (UPC), Lima, Peru
{u201120439,u201319383,fernando.sotelo}@upc.edu.pe

[2] Dirección de Investigación, Universidad Peruana de Ciencias Aplicadas (UPC), Lima, Peru
carlos.raymundo@upc.edu.pe

Abstract. This research article focuses on the application of the main engineering tools in the wood furniture manufacturing sector. It uses as an information source furniture companies of the industrial park of Villa El Salvador. Its objective is to implement 6TOC methodology based on LEAN philosophy, Six Sigma and restrictions theory, focusing on improvements to the bottleneck. Defines the product design as an ideal input for the planning and development of activities. Start to know the work environment: stations and functions, machines and tools, plant layout and ergonomics in order to increase productivity. Application of tools level operations for planning, control and execution of production. Resulted in the GDP in the year 2017 increased by 2.2%. However, the manufacturing sector of goods decreased by 5.5%, that is, it impairs GDP growth, since the wood and furniture industry, which had an aggregate gross manufacturing value of −19.9%.

Keywords: Wood · Furniture production · TOC · LEAN · 6SIGMA

1 Introduction

Although microenterprises represent 96% of the sector, they generate only 29% of sales. In 2015, this industry was invoicing 57% of domestic sales. The problem of this company lies in the stagnation of productivity, since the installed capacity is not efficiently used. Also, not the poor control of equipment and lack of maintenance.

In Peru, a small business must have between 1 and 100 employees and generate annual income between 150 UIT up to 1700 UIT and a median has up to 250 employees and invoices between 1700 UIT up to 2300 UIT per year (SUNAT, 2017). The MYPES plays a fundamental role in the Peruvian economy, since it contributes to the creation of employment, poverty decreases, increase the Gross Domestic Product, participate in the development of innovation and can constitute as a support important to the large company solving some bottlenecks in production [1]. More than half of the MYPES are informal, 58.4%. Another characteristic of the sector is that 96.4% of

T. Ahram et al. (Eds.): IHIET 2019, AISC 1018, pp. 1007–1013, 2020.
https://doi.org/10.1007/978-3-030-25629-6_156

companies are micro companies, who produce on a small scale, use half their capacity installed, do not have equipment or efficient machinery and do not have quality standards in the products that they offer to the market.

The strategy of operations must be defined by the volume of production, the product design and the process with which it is counted. In the case of the manufacture of furniture this is by type workshop and work by production lots. We work to satisfy the order. The work station study is used to evaluate the performance and develop proposals for the realization of the process. The work station is a floor space where the operator and the machine or tool interact. Each work station performs different tasks that as a whole deliver a result with added value.

The objective of 6TOC is to go through productive processes to apply tools to solve specific problems of each activity in the process. Based on the strategy of reducing costs, improve quality and customer service. In addition, propose improvements achievable for small wood furniture manufacturing companies in the industrial park of Villa El Salvador in order that they obtain advantages over their competitors and learn to better manage resources.

The research seeks to improve productivity in companies compared to the same sector in Colombia. Focus effort on bottleneck process.

2 Literature Review

Lean

Lean Manufacturing allows improving the organization of the company where it is implemented, as well as how it manages the relationship with its customers, the supply chain, the development and the manufacture of the products, seeking to generate greater outlets with fewer resources [2].

5s is a tool that is also classified in the Lean Manufacturing methodology. The concurrent use of 5S (Classify, Organize, Clean, Maintain and Discipline, translated into Spanish) has become indispensable in the stage of improvement of production [3]. These steps must give order and process the discipline, help maintain any progress and promote continuous improvement as a work style [4]. This tool can be applied at the beginning of the Lean implementation together with strategic decisions that include the evaluation of performance throughout the application stage [5].

Six Sigma

Six sigma is another tool that helps companies, even SMEs in continuous improvement. It proposes to reduce costs, eliminate errors, increase quality and customer satisfaction through manufacturing processes. The objective of this technique is to reduce the appearance of defects while performing operations [6]. Six sigma aim to optimize the production process within improvement quality. The company has a poor management system quality, lack of formality, lack of procedures and quality records;

focused on the production processes, where the speed was calculated of production flow, process cycle efficiency and average time.

Theory of Constrains

The theory of constrain or TOC is a technique also used to improve processes. This focuses on the bottleneck that causes the main inventory of the system and generates time delays in production [7].

Theory of restrictions (TOC) defines the bottleneck: weak area, which is an obstacle to improve the quality and efficiency of the company and increase profits. Then, the Lean tools manage this area. And the next phase includes Six Sigma, which allows it to receive a significant increase in the efficiency and effectiveness of production and profits [4]. To be able to improve the times of the restriction generated by the bottleneck, a time study has to be carried out within the activity [8].

6TOC

6TOC is a technique that seeks to optimize the production system and is a combination of constraint theory techniques, Lean Manufacturing philosophy and Six Sigma. TOC, starting from its main objective, which is to improve the operational level of the company through its general perspective of continuous improvement through its own resources and its special focus on the restriction of the production system [9] is able to manage the operations in such a way that it delimits the production problem in a process that is not running at the pace of the other processes. As a second phase, defined by 6TOC, the Lean Manufacturing methodology is adapted to this system, providing new tools to improve the effectiveness of resource optimization such as the 5S technique, which is capable of ordering the production chain to have a better vision of the critical process defined by TOC and analyze an adequate solution to the problem. As final stage of the 6TOC and with the objective of providing sustainability to the production system, the Six Sigma methodology is implemented, which will be the actuator in charge of controlling, monitoring and validating the improvement of the production system through the use of KPIs indicators, control charts and the standardization of processes, which provide continuous information on the level of defective and/or obsolete products.

3 6TOC Model

A population of 17 companies was used, of which 13 were selected to take information on their productive processes. It was agreed that a large part of these companies had the same processes. To start with the methodology, you have to concentrate on the bottleneck. For this, a time was taken for the elaboration of the bedroom bed product where it was found that the station that takes the longest time is the cutting station. This station defines the rhythm of production. That is to say, every time we see that this station carries out a cycle, a unit is being manufactured (Figs. 1 and 2).

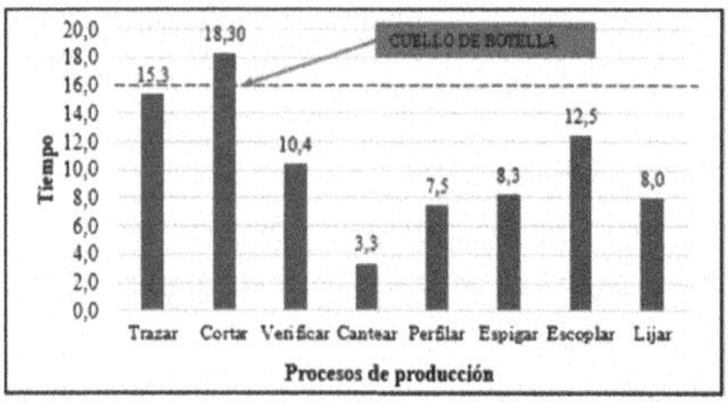

Fig. 1. Bottle neck, production rate

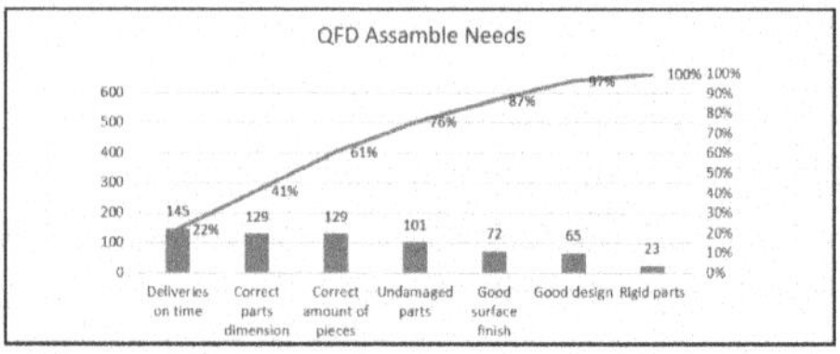

Fig. 2. Solutions to meet the needs of the assembly station

The calculated cycle time is 18.30 min/unit.

To visualize the information and identify the production flow, the VSM should be used in order to show the added value of the processes and indicators of the System.

The 5s methodology in order to classify the elements that are located around the cutting process, organize the tools and equipment required by the process through shelves that allow to locate them easily, clean the sources of dirt and keep the area always clean, standardize procedures through formats and flow diagrams that are around the cutting station so that the operator knows what to do before, during and after carrying out their activities and, finally, to discipline work habits through training. The purpose of applying this methodology in this group of companies is to determine the basic conditions, mentioned, that they must have, so that it is possible to make more sophisticated tools that require a stable work environment in order to improve the quality and productivity of these companies. Also, as the model proposed by the project shows, the bottleneck was identified, which was the cutting process and to which this methodology will be applied.

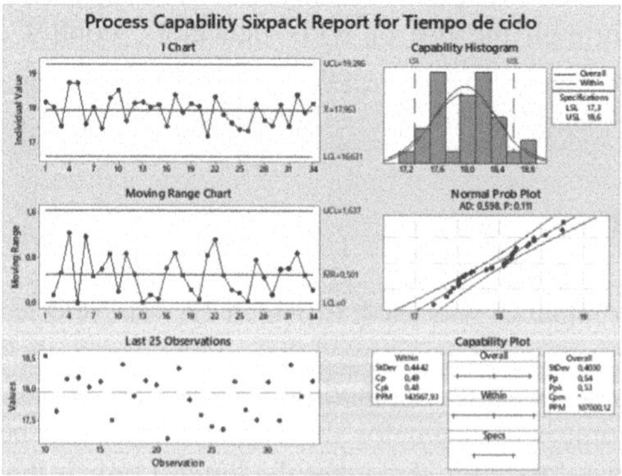

Fig. 3. Process capability sixpack report for Tiempo de cilclo

It was identified that the needs that represent 80% of the consequences of variability in the internal customer satisfaction are "Deliveries on time", "Parts with correct dimension", "Adequate quantity of pieces" and "Damaged parts or components".

Basically, the needs of the assembly station are related to problems of time and product quality. These aspects have to be foreseen by the machining process.

Among the most important solutions are creating records, using product design plans, creating procedures for quality inspection of input and output within the machining sub-processes, executing a results control plan where the frequency of occurrence is investigated and the cause that causes a certain problem within the bottleneck station, analyze the behavior of the process based on the variability of the time inside the bottleneck. Almost all of these solutions mentioned above have been developed in the previous components, which is why a greater emphasis is placed on the fact that what has been stated above can improve the working conditions of the bottleneck station.

The behavior of the bottleneck process cut, as explained earlier, this process marks the production rate. Figure 3 shows the behavior of the cycle time in the production of 35 product units. These data types are unique, which is why the individual data chart and the mobile range are used. It is observed that the process is stable according to the individual chart (Chart I). It can be observed that atypical data are not presented in the development of the activities, but the satisfaction of the assembly client must be improved, since the first part of the productive process is not complying with the specifications requested by the client. The Cpk is less than 1, which denotes poor performance and indicates that the process is not able to meet the requirements of its internal client assemble; Ideally, it is between 1 and 1.33 according to the theory of statistical quality control (Fig. 4).

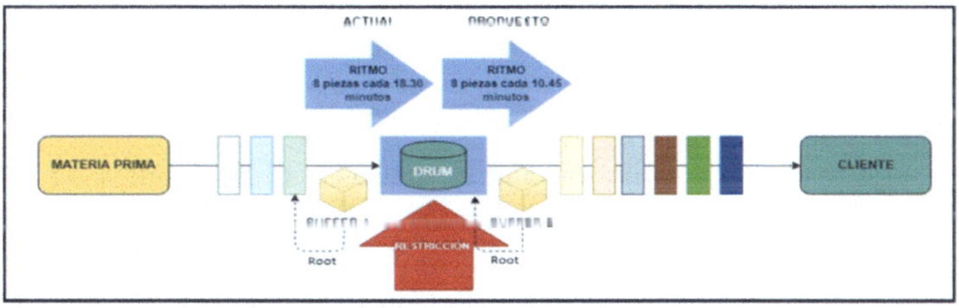

Fig. 4. Buffer

Due to the uncertainty existing from the arrival of material to the workshop to the possible origins of atypical problems in the stations before cutting, it is necessary, in order to maintain the continuous flow, to implement a buffer before the bottleneck process, to ensure its continuity to the long of the time.

Making use of the VSM performed previously, we obtain the productivity data of the Cutting and Layout station, activity preceding the bottleneck. Then, the productivities difference is made to obtain the desynchronization margin between both operations. Finally, with the value of the daily work it is calculated that the buffer should be 0.5 beds, which is translated into an equivalent of 4 components to be cut.

4 Conclusions

Despite the fact that the Peruvian state offers opportunities for training and growth through its national wood institute CITEMADERA, the research identified that companies in this sector are poorly articulated so that there is great informality in the sector. Likewise, the vast majority of personnel have a low educational level, especially those who work in the plant. Additionally, they are companies with a low level of maturity, since they do not have control of their processes and act reactive to the market, which generates a high possibility of the appearance of defects. This prevents companies from meeting the main objective identified, which is on-time delivery and reduction in resource consumption.

The project model required at least SMEs, which have a defined sequence of production and a number of stable operators. For this reason, a sample was made, and it was identified that there are 45 small companies that are in charge of the manufacture of wooden goods, of which 38% make bedroom furniture, 29% living and dining room furniture, 18% kitchen furniture and 16% office furniture. The chosen product is among the family of bedroom furniture is bed.

Quantitative information was collected from 13 SMEs of wooden furniture to calculate their productivity and then compare it with a similar country. Then the productivity calculated with Colombia was compared. A sector with conditions similar to the Peruvian wood sector, but with greater productivity. Where was obtained as a result that the productivity of Peru is 22% below the productivity of Colombia.

Due to the complexity and variability of activities throughout the transformation process, the research project was divided into five macroprocesses, Enabled, Machined, Assembled, Veneered and Finished, of which the scope of the project for the first two macroprocesses was defined.

The research made it possible to identify that 54% of companies do not comply with product delivery times due to variations during production and the lack of alignment between each process with respect to production capacity. This implies that in order to meet the objectives, an extra cost must be incurred in order to reach a specific goal, which impacts the productivity per unit produced. 46% have disorganization in the workshop, this is a critical factor for the efficiency of the development of activities and the efficient use of resources.

When comparing the reviewed academic literature, approximately 100 articles, with the diagnoses raised of the 13 PYMES companies of wooden furniture, it was defined that the most adequate methodology to solve these problems is 6TOC, which is the combination of the Lean, TOC and Six Sigma Additionally, the effectiveness of this methodology was validated with the investigation of successful cases where good results of its application were found in both large and medium-sized companies.

The implementation of this methodology, in relation to the pilot test developed in the company Huarcaya, which had greater availability and access to information, allowed estimating that the productivity gap of 22% between Peru and Colombia would be reduced to 18% which in terms of cost would allow reducing the production cost overruns of these Peruvian SMEs from S/.610,893 to S/.545,800, generating greater profits and making them more profitable in the market.

References

1. Cabello, S.Y.T.: Importancia de la micro, pequeñas y medianas empresas en el desarrollo del país. LEX **12**(14), 199–218 (2014)
2. Felizzola Jiménez, H., Amaya, C.L.: Lean six sigma en pequeñas y medianas empresas: un enfoque metodológico. Ingeniare **22**(2), 263–277 (2014)
3. Suhardi, B., Puspita, A., Widyo, P.: Implementation of standardization work to improve productivity in indonesian furniture industry. Medwell J. **11**, 12 (2016)
4. Demchuk, L., Baitsar, R.: Combined usage of theory of constraints, lean and six sigma in quality assurance of manufacturing processes. Key Eng. Mater. **637**, 21–26 (2015)
5. Hu, Q., Mason, R., Williams, S.J., Found, P.: Lean implementation within SMEs: a literature review. J. Manuf. Technol. Manage. **26**(7), 980–1012 (2015)
6. Bailey, A.Y.A., Motwani, J., Smedley, E.M.: When lean and six sigma converge: a case study of a successful implementation of lean six sigma at an aerospace company. Int. J. Technol. Manage. **57**(1/2/3), 18 (2012). https://doi.org/10.1504/IJTM.2012.043949
7. Velumani, S., Tang, H.: Operations status and bottleneck analysis and improvement of a batch process manufacturing line using discrete event simulation. Procedia Manuf. **10**, 100–111 (2017)
8. Sims, T., da Wan, H.: Constraint identification techniques for lean manufacturing systems. Robot. Comput. Integr. Manuf. **43**, 50–58 (2017). https://doi.org/10.1016/j.rcim.2015.12.005
9. De Jesus Pacheco, D.A.: TOC, lean and six sigma: the missing link to increase productivity? Afr. J. Bus. Manage. **9**(12), 513 (2015)

Author Index

T. Ahram et al. (Eds.): IHIET 2019, AISC 1018, pp. 1015–1020, 2020.
https://doi.org/10.1007/978-3-030-25629-6

The manufacturer's authorised representative in the EU is Springer Nature Customer Service Centre GmbH, Europaplatz 3, 69115 Heidelberg, Germany. If you have any concerns regarding our products, please contact ProductSafety@springernature.com

Printed and bound by CPI Group (UK) Ltd, Croydon, CR0 4YY
05/10/2026
02228148-0003